Lippincott's

Textbook for Long-Term Care
NURSING ASSISTANTS

A HUMANISTIC APPROACH TO CAREGIVING

Pamela J.

Program Coo—
School of Hea
Davis Applied
Kaysville, Uta

Wanda M

Director of C
EMA
Faculty Memb
Eldersburg, M

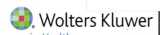 Wolters Kluwer | Lippincott Williams & Wilkins
Health
Philadelphia · Baltimore · New York · London
Buenos Aires · Hong Kong · Sydney · Tokyo

Executive Acquisitions Editor: Elizabeth Nieginski
Senior Development Editor: Melanie Cann
Product Manager: Betsy Gentzler
Director of Nursing Production: Helen Ewan
Art Director, Design: Holly Reid McLaughlin
Art Director, Illustration: Brett MacNaughton
Manufacturing Coordinator: Karin Duffield
Production Services: Aptara, Inc.

9 8 7 6 5 4 3 2 1

Printed in China

Library of Congress Cataloging-in-Publication Data

Carter, Pamela J.
   Lippincott's textbook for long-term care nursing assistants : a humanistic approach to caregiving / Pamela J. Carter, Wanda M. Goldschmidt.
         p. ; cm.
   Includes index.
   Adaptation of: Lippincott's essentials for nursing assistants / Pamela J. Carter. 2nd ed. c2010.
   ISBN 978-0-7817-8068-1
   1. Nurses' aides—Textbooks.   2. Long-term care facilities—Textbooks. I. Goldschmidt, Wanda M.   II. Carter, Pamela J. Lippincott's essential's for nursing assistants.   III. Title.   IV. Title: Textbook for long-term care nursing assistants.
   [DNLM: 1. Nurses' Aides. 2. Humanism. 3. Long-Term Care—methods. 4. Nursing Care—methods. WY 193 C3238L 2010]
   RT84.C374 2010
   610.7306'98—dc22
                                                                2009027155

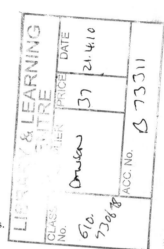

LWW.COM

CONTENTS

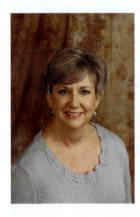

Pamela Carter is a registered nurse and an award-winning teacher. After receiving her bachelor's degree in nursing from the University of Alabama in Huntsville, Pamela immediately began a career as a perioperative nurse. Over the course of her nursing career, she also worked in a physician's office and as a staff nurse in an intensive care unit.

Pamela started teaching informally while serving as an officer in the United States Air Force Nurse Corps. She formally entered the field of health care education by accepting a position at the Athens Area Technical Institute in Athens, Georgia, where she taught surgical technology. After obtaining a master's degree in adult vocational education from the University of Georgia, Pamela moved to Florida and took a position teaching nursing assisting students. She continued teaching nursing assisting after accepting a position at Davis Applied Technology College in Kaysville, Utah. During her first year at Davis Applied Technology College, Pamela piloted a new "open-entry/open-exit" method of curriculum delivery for the nursing assistant program at the college and was awarded the Superintendent's Award for Outstanding Faculty for her work. She then opened a surgical technology program at the college and has obtained national accreditation from the Commission on Accreditation of Allied Health Education Programs (CAAHEP) for delivery of this program using the "open-entry/open-exit" method. In 2002, Pamela received a National Merit Award for having her program rank in the top 10% in the nation for students passing their national certification exam.

In addition to authoring this textbook, Pamela has also authored *Lippincott's Textbook for Nursing Assistants*, *Lippincott's Essentials for Nursing Assistants*, and *Lippincott's Advanced Skills for Nursing Assistants*. Pamela's writing style reflects her love of teaching and of nursing. She is grateful for the opportunity teaching and writing have afforded her to share her experience and knowledge with those just entering the health care profession, and to help those who are new to the profession to see how they can have a profound effect on the lives of others.

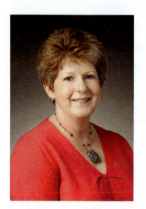

Wanda M. Goldschmidt began her career in health care working as a nursing assistant in a nursing home. During this time, Wanda found great fulfillment in working with her older residents. After becoming a licensed practical nurse and then obtaining a bachelor's degree in nursing from Towson University in Towson, Maryland, Wanda worked as a nurse and taught in a hospital-based practical nursing program. After that program closed, Wanda returned to her first love—long-term care nursing—where she has remained for nearly 30 years.

In the long-term care setting, Wanda has held both clinical and administrative positions. As a Director of Nursing, Wanda was the founder and first president of the Maryland chapter of the National Association Directors of Nursing/Long-Term Care (NADONA/LTC). She was also inducted into the national nursing honor society in recognition of her work promoting a positive image for long-term care. Wanda has worked many years as a nursing consultant for assisted living and nursing home facilities. She is currently the Director of Clinical Education for EMA in Carroll County, Maryland, where she is responsible for the ongoing education of the nurses and nursing assistants throughout the company's four communities. Wanda also coordinates educational experiences for nursing students from several area schools, and is a member of the Nursing Assistant Advisory Committee for the Maryland Board of Nursing.

Wanda has held certification in gerontological nursing since 1987. She also earned a master's degree in the Studies in Aging program at the College of Notre Dame of Maryland in Baltimore, Maryland, where she received the Academic Achievement Award and was inducted into Sigma Phi Omega, the National Academic and Professional Society in Gerontology. Wanda delivers a number of professional presentations related to long-term care, both locally and nationally.

This textbook is dedicated to all those nursing assistants who have chosen to provide care for people in a long-term care setting. Your compassion and respect for our aging and disabled population enriches the lives of those you care for every day. You are appreciated more than you will ever know by your residents, and their families.

—*Pam*

In memory of my dear friend and colleague, Pat McNulty, who always told me I would write a book one day. To my friend and mentor, Connie Mucha, who has taught me so much about compassionate care. To Les, my loving husband, and my girls, Brooke and Sara, for their patience and support. To Carmel Roques, who recommended me for this project, and to the Lord above who has sustained me with strength and perseverance so that I could complete it!

—*Wanda*

PREFACE

The United States is in the midst of a health care crisis—profound demographic changes have led to an ever-widening gap between the number of people who need care and the number of people who are qualified to provide that care. This is particularly true as the population of the United States ages. Each year, the number of people living in the United States who are 65 years and older increases. It is estimated that one third to one half of all people 65 years and older will be admitted to a nursing home for care at some time. Long-term care facilities are facing a critical need for nursing assistants who are well prepared to take care of a mostly older, vulnerable, and dependent population. As educators, we are charged with providing the community with competent, dedicated, compassionate caregivers who have the skills and knowledge that they need to meet the special needs of long-term care residents and their families.

In the past, the focus of nursing assistant education was on skill competency. However, that focus is shifting now toward graduating nursing assistants who not only possess the technical skills they need to provide competent care, but also the compassion and the communication and critical thinking skills they need to function effectively in the health care setting. It is no longer enough for nursing assistants to be competent at changing bed linens and measuring vital signs. Today's nursing assistants must also be able to recognize and understand that each resident they are responsible for providing care for is unique and special, with individual needs that are very different from those of the resident in the next bed. This textbook, *Lippincott's Textbook for Long-Term Care Nursing Assistants,* has been written not only to help students develop the skills they need to become nursing assistants in the long-term care setting, but also to introduce them to a very humanistic approach to caregiving.

THEMES AND FEATURES

Three key beliefs informed the writing of this textbook:

1. Students need a textbook that captures their interest and increases their desire to learn.
2. Graduates of nursing assistant training programs must be able to provide competent, skilled care in a compassionate way.
3. The nursing assistant is a vital member of the health care team.

These beliefs form the basis for the textbook you hold in your hands.

LIPPINCOTT'S TEXTBOOK FOR LONG-TERM CARE NURSING ASSISTANTS IS WRITTEN WITH THE STUDENT IN MIND

One of the primary goals in writing this textbook was to make the information it contains interesting and accessible to the student. Great care has been taken to present the student with a textbook that is easy and enjoyable to read, with a well-developed art program and proven learning aids.

A Student-Focused Writing Style

Educators know that a student can easily understand complex information if it is explained in a way that the student can understand. *Lippincott's Textbook for Long-Term Care Nursing Assistants* uses a conversational, yet professional, writing style that respects the student's intelligence. Concepts are presented in a straightforward, accessible way. Recognizing that many students entering nursing assistant training programs speak English as a second language or are resource students, each chapter has been thoroughly reviewed by a special needs consultant to ensure an appropriate reading level.

An Art Program Developed Alongside the Text

The purpose of an art program is to reinforce and expand on concepts discussed in the text. To do this effectively, the art must be planned and developed alongside the manuscript. Numerous photographs, both alone and in combination with line art that has been created specifically for this textbook, help students to visualize and remember important concepts.

Proven Learning Aids in Every Chapter

Learning and remembering new information is challenging for many students. To help them meet the challenge of mastering the information in the textbook, we have developed features to assist students with studying and internalizing information:

- **What Will You Learn?** Each chapter begins with a *What Will You Learn?* section, which previews the chapter and helps to focus the student's reading. Each *What Will You Learn?* section begins with a paragraph that introduces the topic of the chapter to the student and explains why the topic is important. This introductory paragraph is then followed by a list of learning objectives and vocabulary words.
- **Summary.** Each chapter ends with a summary in a unique narrative outline format. This summary helps students to review the key, "take home," concepts of the chapter.
- **What Did You Learn?** Multiple-choice and matching exercises at the end of each chapter provide students with the opportunity to evaluate their understanding of the material they have just studied. Answers to these exercises are given in Appendix A.
- **Highlighted figure, table, and box callouts.** The references to figures, tables, and boxes are highlighted with color in the narrative, helping students to quickly find their place in the text after stopping to look at a figure, table, or box.

LIPPINCOTT'S TEXTBOOK FOR LONG-TERM CARE NURSING ASSISTANTS IS DESIGNED TO PREPARE STUDENTS FOR CLINICAL PRACTICE

It is the authors' desire to help prepare students to enter the health care profession with the knowledge, skills, and confidence that education and training can provide. Several of the textbook's features were designed specifically to help prepare the student for clinical practice in the long-term care setting:

- **Procedures.** Certainly, a major objective of any nursing assistant training course is to ensure that graduates are able to provide care in a safe and correct manner. Seventy-eight core procedures are presented in this text. The procedures for each chapter are grouped at the end of the chapter, to avoid breaking up the text with lengthy boxes. Each procedure box begins with a "Why You Do It" statement, to help students understand the "why behind the what," an understanding that is the foundation for the development of critical thinking skills. The concepts of privacy, safety, infection control, comfort, and communication are emphasized consistently in every procedure. *"Getting Ready"* and *"Finishing Up"* steps are included in every procedure box to help students remember these very important pre- and post-procedure actions. The steps of the procedure are given using clear and concise language, and illustrated with photographs or line art as necessary. An icon identifies procedures that are demonstrated on *Lippincott's Video Series for Nursing Assistants.*
- **Guidelines Boxes.** These boxes summarize general guidelines for various aspects of the nursing assistant's job. The unique "What You Do/Why You Do It" format helps students to understand why things are done a certain way. Rather than just presenting students with an endless list of guidelines to memorize, these boxes help them to remember why these guidelines are important to follow.
- **Tell the Nurse! Notes.** A recurrent theme throughout the book is the important role the nursing assistant plays in making observations about a resident's condition and reporting these observations to the nurse. The *Tell the Nurse!* notes highlight and summarize signs and symptoms that a nursing assistant may observe that should be reported to the nurse immediately.
- **Stop and Think! Scenarios.** Each chapter concludes with one or more *Stop and Think!* scenarios. These scenarios, which are excellent tools for initiating classroom discussion, encourage students to think critically to

solve problems, and help them to see that many situations they will encounter in the workplace do not have cut-and-dry answers.

- **Helping Hands and a Caring Heart: Focus on Humanistic Health Care Boxes.** These boxes, found throughout the text, encourage students to empathize with those in their care, and emphasize the importance of meeting residents' emotional, social, and spiritual needs, as well as their physical needs.
- **Caring for Those With Dementia.** Dementia is a leading cause for admission to a long-term care facility. This feature helps students understand the unique challenges a resident with dementia may face, and provides suggestions for helping to meet these challenges.
- **OBRA Highlights.** Nursing assistants who work in nursing homes work in a highly regulated environment. An icon highlights government standards for the quality of services provided by nursing homes, as established by the Omnibus Budget Reconciliation Act (OBRA).
- **Be Smart About Surveys!** These boxes, found throughout the text, raise the student's awareness of what the surveyors are looking for during a survey and help students identify specifically what they need to do as nursing assistants to help prevent potential survey problems.

LIPPINCOTT'S TEXTBOOK FOR LONG-TERM CARE NURSING ASSISTANTS SEEKS TO INSTILL IN STUDENTS PRIDE IN THEMSELVES AND THEIR CHOSEN PROFESSION

It is important to impress upon students entering the health care profession that no one is "just" a nursing assistant. In long-term care, nursing assistants are the members of the health care team with the most day-to-day contact with residents. As such, they bear a large part of the responsibility for the well-being of those in their care. To highlight the contributions that nursing assistants make, each unit in the textbook concludes with a resident's or family member's first-person account of how a nursing assistant had a positive impact on their lives or the lives of their loved ones. The goal of these *Nursing Assistants Make a Difference!* stories is to help students to see that nursing assistants

are vital members of the health care team. Nursing assistants who feel that they can and do make a difference in the lives of others will go the "extra mile" to ensure that the care they provide is humanistic.

AN OVERVIEW OF LIPPINCOTT'S TEXTBOOK FOR LONG-TERM CARE NURSING ASSISTANTS

This textbook consists of nine units. The following is a brief survey of these units and the information they contain.

UNIT 1: INTRODUCTION TO HEALTH CARE AND THE LONG-TERM CARE SETTING

The six chapters that make up Unit 1 provide the student with basic background knowledge. Chapter 1 provides an overview of the many different types of health care facilities, and introduces the idea of holistic, humanistic health care and the "health care team." Chapter 2 introduces the student to the long-term care setting in particular, including a discussion about the past, present, and future of long-term care. Chapter 3 focuses on the nursing assistant's roles and responsibilities as a member of the health care team, and on the concept of delegation. Professionalism and qualities that characterize a sound work ethic are also discussed in Chapter 3, introducing students to the idea that a professional attitude is critical for success in the workplace. Legal and ethical issues—including resident rights, the Health Insurance Portability and Accountability Act (HIPAA), and abuse detection and prevention—are covered in Chapter 4. Communication, one of the most essential responsibilities of the nursing assistant, is discussed in Chapter 5. This unit concludes with Chapter 6, which introduces the student to the survey process.

UNIT 2: THOSE WE CARE FOR

The four chapters in Unit 2 introduce students to some of the special needs that are common to many residents of long-term care facilities. Chapter 7 introduces the concept of human needs and explains how a resident of a long-term care setting has many needs other than those specifically associated with illness or disability. Chapter 8 helps students understand the factors that can lead to admission to a long-term care facility, and the special needs that residents of long-term care facilities, and their families, may have. In Chapter 9, the student is provided with information about dementia, a condition that affects many long-term care residents. Chapter 10 describes the nursing assistant's responsibilities with regard to rehabilitation and restorative care.

UNIT 3: INDIVIDUALIZING CARE

Providing quality, individualized care and excellent customer service is the focus of Unit 3. Chapter 11 reviews the processes for admitting, transferring, and discharging residents. Chapter 12 describes the nursing assistant's role in the assessment and care planning process, and explains how this process supports individualized care. Chapter 13 introduces the student to the concept of customer service, and discusses the importance of serving customers in a way that goes beyond meeting basic needs and expectations.

UNIT 4: MAINTAINING A SAFE AND COMFORTABLE ENVIRONMENT

The six chapters that make up Unit 4 are concerned with the measures taken to ensure a safe and comfortable environment. Chapter 14 seeks to familiarize the student with equipment used in the health care setting, and OBRA standards related to maintaining a safe and comfortable environment for residents. Chapters 15 and 16 cover communicable disease and how the spread of communicable disease is prevented in the long-term care setting. Chapter 17 deals with workplace safety, and includes an extensive discussion about the importance of using proper body mechanics to prevent work-related injuries. Also in Chapter 17, the student is introduced to the "Getting Ready" and "Finishing Up" steps that are taken before and after each procedure. Chapter 18 explores some of the conditions that put residents at risk for injury, followed by a discussion about methods used to prevent accidents from occurring. This unit concludes with Chapter 19, which contains information related to recognizing emergencies and responding to them.

UNIT 5: BASIC RESIDENT CARE

The eight chapters in Unit 5 focus on the skills and equipment used to provide basic daily care to residents. In Chapter 20, the techniques used to safely assist residents with repositioning and transferring are covered. Chapter 21 covers bedmaking. Chapter 22 covers vital signs, with an emphasis on exactly what function of the body is being measured and situations that may alter these measurements. Also included are practical tips to take the mystery out of taking vital sign measurements, procedures that many students find intimidating and difficult to master at first. Chapters 23 and 24 cover hygiene and grooming, with a focus on empathizing with the person receiving the care. Chapter 25 contains basic information about nutrition and the nursing assistant's role in assisting residents with meeting their nutrition and fluid needs. Chapter 26 reviews assisting with elimination. Again, much emphasis is placed on empathizing with the resident who requires assistance with this most intimate of activities. We conclude Unit 5 with Chapter 27, which describes the nursing assistant's role in recognizing and responding to pain and promoting comfort, rest, and sleep.

UNIT 6: DEATH AND DYING

Unit 6 includes two separate chapters on the subject of death and dying to emphasize that a person may cope with approaching the end of life for a long period of time before the actual physical process of dying takes place. Chapter 28 discusses concepts related to preparing for the end of life, including the stages of grief, legal considerations, and the role of hospice and palliative care. Chapter 29 focuses on the care a nursing assistant provides to the dying person and his or her family members in the hours immediately leading up to, and following, death.

UNIT 7: STRUCTURE AND FUNCTION OF THE HUMAN BODY

Having a basic understanding of how each of the body's organ systems functions in health is essential to understanding how failure of an organ system to work properly leads to disease and disability. Unit 7 begins with Chapter 30, which provides an overview of the body's organization. The next 10 chapters (Chapters 31 through 40) each cover one of the organ systems. A basic explanation of the normal structure and function of the organ system is given. Next, the normal effects of aging are discussed and differentiated from the effects of disease and disability. Key disorders specific to that particular body system are then discussed. Throughout these chapters, the nursing assistant's role in recognizing problems and providing care is emphasized.

UNIT 8: SPECIAL CARE CONCERNS

Unit 8, which consists of four chapters, introduces the student to the special needs of residents who have developmental disabilities, mental illness, cancer, or HIV/AIDS. In Chapter 41, some of the major types of developmental disabilities are reviewed, and challenges faced by these residents and their families if admission to a long-term care facility becomes necessary are discussed. Chapter 42 is dedicated to a discussion about mental illness, including the importance of recognizing depression in elderly residents. Chapter 43 discusses the diagnosis and treatment of cancer, as well as the special needs of people with cancer. The final chapter in this unit, Chapter 44, discusses the special needs of the resident who is HIV-positive or has AIDS.

UNIT 9: ENTERING THE WORKFORCE

Unit 9 seeks to assist the student with moving forward in his or her career. Chapter 45, the final chapter of this text, reviews strategies for conducting a targeted job search, interviewing, accepting a job, and resigning from a job.

APPENDICES AND GLOSSARY

The textbook concludes with three appendices and a comprehensive glossary. Appendix A contains the answers to the *What Did You Learn?* exercises that appear at the end of each chapter. Appendix B introduces the student to the language of health care. We chose to include this discussion about medical terminology as an appendix so that it could be introduced at any point during the training course, and referred to frequently. The tables containing common roots, prefixes, suffixes, and abbreviations are in close physical proximity to the glossary for easy and quick reference. Appendix C contains the Minimum Data Set (MDS) for the student's reference.

The glossary is the most comprehensive found in any nursing assistant textbook. A precise definition of each vocabulary word is given. The number in parentheses at the end of each entry indicates the chapter where the term is introduced as a vocabulary word. Extensive cross-references remind students of synonyms and antonyms, and help them to differentiate related words. All of the terms in the glossary are included on the audio glossary found on the CD included with the book, enabling students to hear the words pronounced, defined, and used in a sentence.

A COMPREHENSIVE PACKAGE FOR TEACHING AND LEARNING

To further facilitate teaching and learning, a carefully designed ancillary package is available. In addition to the usual print resources, we are pleased to present multimedia tools that have been developed in conjunction with the text.

RESOURCES FOR STUDENTS

- **Student Resource CD-ROM and thePoint.** Interactive learning resources are provided on the CD packaged with the textbook at no additional charge. Students can also access these resources on thePoint at http://thePoint.lww.com/CarterLTC using the codes printed in the front of their textbooks. Features include:
  - *Watch and Learn!* —A series of video clips that support information given in the text
  - *Listen and Learn!* —An interactive glossary that enables students to hear the vocabulary words pronounced and defined, and then to quiz themselves using the flashcard feature
  - *Nursing Assistants Make a Difference!*—A feature that allows the student to listen to first-person accounts of how nursing assistants have made a difference in the lives of residents and their family members
- **Workbook for *Lippincott's Textbook for Long-Term Care Nursing Assistants.*** This workbook provides the student with a fun and engaging way of reviewing important concepts and vocabulary. Multiple-choice questions, matching exercises, true-false exercises, word finds,

crossword puzzles, coloring and labeling exercises, and other types of active-learning tools are provided to appeal to many different learning styles. The workbook also contains procedure checklists for each procedure in the textbook.

- *Lippincott's Video Series for Nursing Assistants: Student Edition DVD.* This DVD provides step-by-step demonstrations of 41 key nursing assistant skills.

RESOURCES FOR INSTRUCTORS

Tools to assist you with teaching your course are available upon adoption of this text on thePoint. at http://thePoint.lww.com and on the Instructor's Resource DVD:

- The **Test Generator** lets you put together exclusive new tests from a bank containing hundreds of questions to help you in assessing your students' understanding of the material.
- An extensive collection of materials is provided for each book chapter:
  - **Pre-Lecture Quizzes** (and answers) are quick, knowledge-based assessments that allow you to check students' reading.
  - **PowerPoint Presentations** provide an easy way for you to integrate the textbook with your students' classroom experience, via either slide shows or handouts.
  - **Guided Lecture Notes** walk you through the chapters, objective by objective, and provide you with corresponding PowerPoint slide numbers.
  - **Discussion Topics** (and suggested answers) can be used as conversation starters or in online discussion boards.
  - **Assignments** (and suggested answers) include group, written, clinical, and web assignments.
- An **Image Bank** lets you use the photographs and illustrations from this textbook in your PowerPoint slides or as you see fit in your course.
- **Discussion Points for the Stop and Think Scenarios** in the book are provided to guide discussion.
- **Answers to the exercises in *Workbook for Lippincott's Textbook for Long-Term Care Nursing Assistants*** are provided.
- Information about classroom management, including a **sample syllabus,** is available.

- An **introduction to cognitive learning styles** includes a quiz that can be used to determine a student's learning style, as well as tips for appealing to each type of learner and for making information accessible to resource and special needs students.
- Two **100-question multiple-choice exams** can be printed out and given as practice exams to students at the conclusion of the course.

ADDITIONAL RESOURCES

- *Lippincott's Video Series for Nursing Assistants.* Eleven procedure-based modules provide step-by-step demonstrations of the core skills that form the basis of the daily care the nursing assistant provides. *Getting Ready* and *Finishing Up* actions are reviewed on every procedure-based module, and the concepts of privacy, safety, infection control, comfort, and communication are emphasized throughout. Four non-procedure– based modules, on the topics of preparing for entry into the workforce, caring for people with dementia, death and dying, communication, and patient and resident rights, are also available.
- **Copper Ridge *Dementia Care Modules.*** Developed by the esteemed Copper Ridge Institute in affiliation with Johns Hopkins University School of Medicine, this two-CD set consists of nine interactive modules designed to teach students how to care for people with dementia. The causes and types of dementia are reviewed, along with dementia-related behaviors and the best way to manage them. Communication and compassion are emphasized throughout. Learning is enhanced through video clips, interactive exercises, and short multiple-choice quizzes at the conclusion of each module.

It is with great pleasure that we introduce these resources—the textbook, the ancillary package, the videos, and the Copper Ridge modules—to you. One of our primary goals in creating these resources has been to share with those just entering the health care field our sense of excitement about the health care profession, and our commitment to the idea that being a nursing assistant involves much more than just "bedpans and blood pressures." We hope we have succeeded in that goal, and we welcome your feedback.

Pamela J. Carter
Wanda M. Goldschmidt

To The Student

Welcome! By enrolling in this nursing assistant training course, you have taken a big first step. You may be taking this course for any number of different reasons. For example, you may be taking this course to "test the waters"—to see if working in health care is something you really want to do. Or, you may already know that you want to work in health care, and you are taking this course because it is the first step toward reaching your goal.

Health care is an exciting, yet demanding, field. During your training course, you will be expected to learn and apply a lot of new information. You will even have to learn a new language, the language of health care! My name is Pam Carter, and I am the author of the book you hold in your hands. It is my pleasure and my honor to assist you on your journey toward becoming a health care professional.

HOW TO USE THE BOOK TO PREPARE FOR CLASS AND STUDY

Learning is an active process. You need to read, make notes, and ask questions about anything you are having trouble understanding. Most students who are successful learners take a three-step approach to learning:

PREVIEW

During the *preview* stage of learning, you focus on preparing yourself for class. Most likely, your instructor will give you reading assignments that must be completed before each class. The course *syllabus* that you will receive at the beginning of the course will tell you when each reading assignment must be completed. The reading assignments give you the chance to get a general idea of what is going to be discussed in the next class.

To prepare for class, just read the assignment as if you were reading a novel or a newspaper for enjoyment. As you read the chapter, look for the *Watch and Learn!* banner too. This symbol lets you know that you can use the CD in the front of your book to watch a video clip that supports the information you are reading about. During the preview, you do not need to take notes or try to memorize facts—just read through the material to get the "big picture" of the information you are about to learn. Some people find it helpful to read the chapter out loud to themselves (or into a tape recorder, so that they can listen to the chapter again later). Others like to highlight parts of the chapter using a highlighting pen, or make notes in the margin. Learning becomes much easier when you discover what methods work best for you.

To assist you with previewing, each chapter in the book begins with a *What Will You Learn?* section. This section contains a list of specific goals for the chapter, called *learning objectives*. Learning objectives tell you what you will be expected to know or be able to do to demonstrate complete understanding of the material in the chapter. During the preview stage, the learning objectives are useful for giving you an overview of the key goals of the chapter.

The *What Will You Learn?* section also contains a list of the new vocabulary words you will need to learn. The vocabulary words, which appear in **bold type** throughout the chapter, are listed in the order that they appear. The *Listen and Learn!* banner lets you know that you can use the CD in the front of your book to hear the words in the vocabulary list pronounced and defined. This is an effective and fun way to preview vocabulary words! Or, you can look each word up in the glossary at the back of the book to find a complete definition. Familiarizing yourself with the chapter's vocabulary words before class puts you one step ahead, because when you hear those words in class, they will not sound strange to you, and you may already know what they mean.

VIEW

The *viewing* stage is when you get down to business and really work to understand the material. During the classroom lecture or discussion, highlight important points and take notes as you need to. Ask questions about any of the material that you do not fully understand. Remember, there are no "stupid" questions! If you do not fully understand something, you need to speak up so that the instructor can help you. This is your instructor's job.

REVIEW

After class, go back over the notes you took in class, and re-read the chapter in your book. Some students like to read the entire chapter over again. Others just skim the chapter, paying close attention to the topics they still have questions about. Read the chapter summary, which reviews the key concepts of the chapter. If you are using the student workbook in your class, complete the exercises by looking the answers up in the textbook chapter. Looking for the answers is another way of reviewing the information in the chapter, and many students find that the act of writing the answers down helps them to remember the information.

When you feel comfortable with your understanding of the material, test yourself! Go back to the learning objectives in the *What Will You Learn?* section at the beginning of the chapter and pretend they are questions. Try to answer them. If you have trouble answering them, then you know that you need to review certain parts of the chapter again. You can also test yourself using the *What Did You Learn?* section, at the end of each chapter. The answers to the questions in the *What Did You Learn?* section are in Appendix A in the back of the book so that you can see how well you understood the material you just studied. Again, if you have trouble answering these questions, then you will know that your studying is not quite finished! You may need to read certain parts of the chapter again, or ask your instructor for help.

Try to set aside short periods of time for studying each day. For example, you might study for 30 to 45 minutes, take a break to attend to other activities or chores, and then come back and study for another 30 to 45 minutes. After 30 to 45 minutes of studying, most people become tired and lose their ability to concentrate. Studying in short bursts will help keep you focused on the material you are trying to learn.

HOW TO PREPARE FOR TESTS

Did you learn the material or not? This is what instructors want to know when they give tests, quizzes, and exams. Not doing well on a test does not mean that you are a failure. It just means that you need to figure out what went wrong, and make an effort to improve the next time. Perhaps you did not study as well as you could have for the test. Or maybe you got so nervous, you forgot everything you learned when it came time to take the test!

The course syllabus will tell you when a test is scheduled to be given, and what material it will cover. Mark these dates on your calendar, so you are not surprised! Preparing for a test should not be a major event. If you use the preview–view–review approach and study each day, when it comes time to prepare for the test, you will be very well prepared. In the days leading up to the test, all you will need to do is review the material that will be covered on the test one more time, by skimming the chapters in the book and reviewing the notes you took in class.

When it comes time to actually take the test, remember the following tips:

- Relax! You have prepared for this test, and you know the answers to these questions!
- Take a deep breath and make sure you read the directions carefully. The directions will tell you whether there is only one correct answer for each question, or whether it is possible for a question to have more than one correct answer.
- Read each question completely and carefully. Many students answer questions incorrectly simply because they are in a hurry and miss important words, like "except" or "not."
- If the question is a multiple-choice question, try to state the answer in your head before looking at the answer choices. Then read each answer choice before choosing the one that best matches the answer you have in your head. This will increase your confidence that the answer you have selected is the correct one.
- After selecting an answer, avoid second-guessing yourself. Research has shown that your first choice is most likely to be correct, if you studied the material well. Sometimes, however, you will come across a question later in the test that makes you realize that you answered an earlier question incorrectly.

In this case, when you are sure that you have made a mistake, it is all right to go back and change your answer. But if you do not have a clear idea of what the correct answer is, doubting your first choice will most likely result in changing a correct answer to an incorrect one!

- If you cannot answer a question, go on to the next. Often, another question on the test will jog your memory and help you to remember the answer to the question you skipped earlier. Just remember to go back over your answer sheet before you hand in your test to make sure you have answered all of the questions.

Many people think that the goal of studying is to pass a test. It is true that as you work through your training course, you will have to pass many tests. Most states require people who want to be nursing assistants to pass a certification exam at the end of the training course, but passing the test is a short-term goal. It is more important for you to be able to remember and use the information that you learned during your training course long after you complete the course and pass the certification exam. The people you will be caring for are depending on you to be knowledgeable and good at what you do. They are trusting you with their health and well-being. Study hard, ask questions, and remember that each and every person you care for throughout your career deserves the same type of competent, compassionate care that you would expect to be given to your own mother, father, spouse, sibling, or child. As a nursing assistant, you will have the chance to have a positive effect on the lives of many people.

Caring for those in need is very important work. Let me be among the first to thank you for your interest in pursuing a career in health care, and to wish you luck on your journey.

Sincerely,

Pam

REVIEWERS

Many thanks to the nursing assistant instructors who read the manuscript during its various stages of development and provided us with valuable suggestions for improving it:

LANA ANDERSON
Ivy Tech Community College
Indianapolis, Indiana

CAROLYN BALLINGER
Kentucky Community and Technical
  College System
Edgewood, Kentucky

CARRIE BECKER-LANDON
Lower Columbia College
Longview, Washington

DEBORAH BRABHAM
Florida Community College
Jacksonville, Florida

TONYA BRAGG-UNDERWOOD
Bowling Green Technical College
Glasgow, Kentucky

ROBIN BREVARD
Tidewater Community College
Virginia Beach, Virginia

ELIZABETH BULLOCK
Kentucky Tech System Office
Frankfort, Kentucky

JUDY BURCHETT
New Market Skills Center
Tumwater, Washington

LESLIE COLLINS
Mountain View Care Center
Scranton, Pennsylvania

CINDA DODGE
GST BOCES
Elmira, New York

TRACI GENTRY
Bowling Green Technical College
Glasgow, Kentucky

LINDA HARRES
Highline Community College
Des Moines, Washington

GAIL JOSEPH
Madison Area Technical College
Prairie du Sac, Wisconsin

CHERRY KARL
Anne Arundel Community College
Arnold, Maryland

DENA KOMMER
West Kentucky Community and Technical
  College
Paducah, Kentucky

RITA KRUMMEN
Columbus State Community College
Columbus, Ohio

CAREY LAKE
Central Kentucky Technical College
Lexington, Kentucky

DIANE MILLER
Indiana County Technology Center
Indiana, Pennsylvania

ACKNOWLEDGMENTS

Giving an existing textbook a new focus is a challenge that requires new ideas and expertise. I would like to extend many thanks to Wanda Goldschmidt, who worked diligently to ensure that this new book would meet the very specific needs of nursing assistants being trained to work in long-term care. I would also like to thank Melanie Cann, Senior Development Editor, and Elizabeth Nieginski, Executive Acquisitions Editor. Melanie's editorial genius again transformed our words into a work of art. Elizabeth provided steadfast support and wise counsel, as always.

—Pam

I would like to extend a special thanks to Pam Carter, for all of her hard work on *Lippincott's Textbook for Nursing Assistants*, which served as such a great foundation for this long-term care text. I would also like to thank the members of the Lippincott staff who were so instrumental in conceiving this project and seeing it through to the end. Special thanks to Elizabeth Nieginski, Executive Acquisitions Editor, for welcoming me to the project so warmly, and for her support. A special thanks also goes to Melanie Cann, Senior Development Editor, not only for her astute editorial skill, but also for her extraordinary patience and support when professional and life demands did not run on the same schedule as deadlines. The guidance and encouragement she gave me when times got tough were genuinely appreciated. I would also like to thank Gary Attman, President and CEO of FutureCare Health and Management Corporation, for committing the resources to help with our photo shoot, and the staff and residents of FutureCare Cherrywood for their most willing and efficient assistance—especially Donna Leister, Marla Bosley, Hattie McClintock, and Regina Muhammad. I sincerely thank all my friends and colleagues at EMA for their supportive words and actions that have helped me so much. I would also like to acknowledge the EMA nursing staff at the Buckingham's Choice, Copper Ridge, Fairhaven, and William Hill communities. They have given me so much inspiration, and have helped me to become a better teacher.

—Wanda

CONTENTS

CHAPTER 16
BLOODBORNE AND AIRBORNE PATHOGENS   249

CHAPTER 17
WORKPLACE SAFETY   259

CHAPTER 18
RESIDENT SAFETY   281

CHAPTER 19
BASIC FIRST AID AND EMERGENCY CARE   308

UNIT 5

BASIC RESIDENT CARE   327

CHAPTER 20
POSITIONING, LIFTING, AND TRANSFERRING RESIDENTS   329

CHAPTER 21
BEDMAKING 364

CHAPTER 22
VITAL SIGNS, HEIGHT, AND WEIGHT 380

CHAPTER 23
CLEANLINESS AND HYGIENE 415

INTRODUCTION TO HEALTH CARE AND THE LONG-TERM CARE SETTING

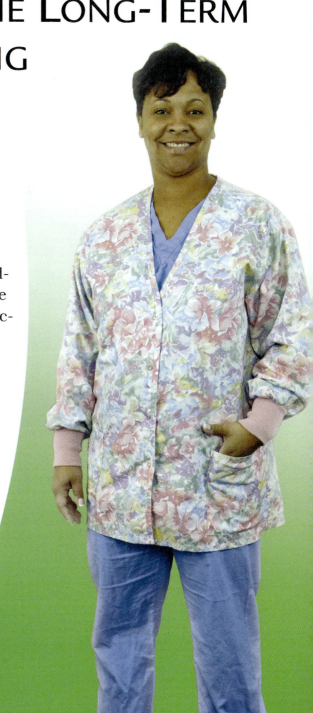

Welcome to the health care field! If you are holding this book in your hands, it is likely that you are preparing to work as a nursing assistant in a particular type of health care setting, the long-term care setting. Unit 1 introduces you to the health care field in general and the long-term care setting in particular. Basic concepts and skills that you will use every day in your work as a nursing assistant are also reviewed in Unit 1.

Photo: Welcome to the health care field! Nursing assistants are key members of the health care team.

1

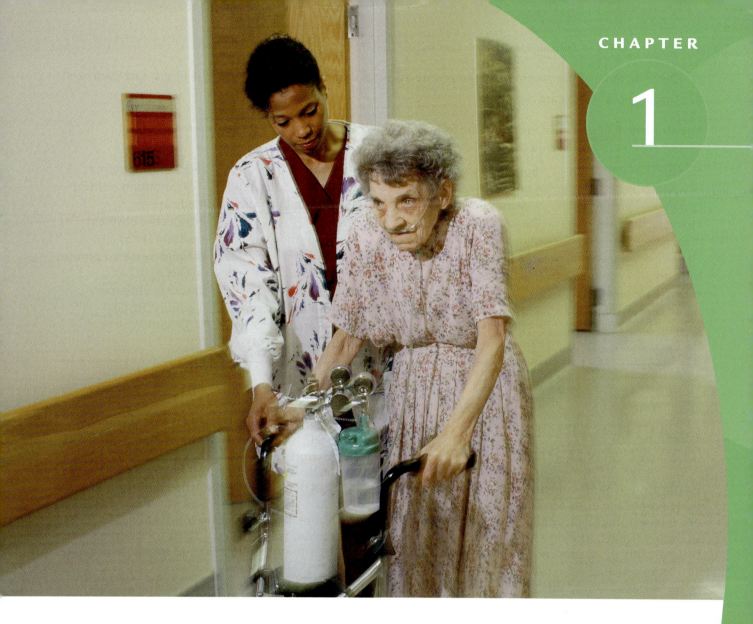

The Health Care System

WHAT WILL YOU LEARN?

As a nursing assistant working in a long-term care facility, you will be working within the structure of a larger health care system. In this chapter, you will learn about the many different types of organizations that make up this health care system, and how these organizations are typically structured. We will also discuss some of the government and private agencies that monitor health care facilities to make sure that they are providing quality care, and some of the ways that health care is paid for in the United States. When you are finished with this chapter, you will be able to:

1. Identify changes that have occurred in how health care is delivered.
2. Describe the different types of health care organizations.
3. Briefly explain the structure of a health care organization.

Photo: Health care is a people-oriented business.

4. Describe some of the government and private agencies that provide oversight of the health care system.

5. Discuss how health care is paid for.

Vocabulary Use the CD in the front of your book to hear these terms pronounced and defined:

Holistic
Hospital
Long-term care facility
Home health care agency
Hospice organization
Mission
Health care team
Acute care setting
Patient
Post-acute care setting

Sub-acute care setting
Long-term care setting
Resident
Assisted-living facility
Nursing home
United States Department of Health and Human Services (DHHS)
The Joint Commission

Accreditation
Occupational Safety and Health Administration (OSHA)
Group insurance
Precertification (preapproval) process
Managed care system
Preferred provider organization (PPO)

Health maintenance organization (HMO)
Medicare
Prospective payment system (PPS)
Diagnosis-related groups (DRGs)
Resource utilization groups (RUGs)
Medicaid

HEALTH CARE DELIVERY, PAST AND PRESENT

In the United States during the 18th, 19th, and early part of the 20th centuries, health care delivery focused mainly around the home and family. In many cases, the health care provider was trained, but as a generalist, rather than a specialist. He would deliver the babies, attend to wounds and broken bones, and provide comfort to both the dying person and the family (Fig. 1-1).

Until the early 1800s, the quality of health care in the United States was variable. Charlatans, people with no training or knowledge of medicine, traveled from town to town, offering worthless ("snake oil") cures in an effort to make

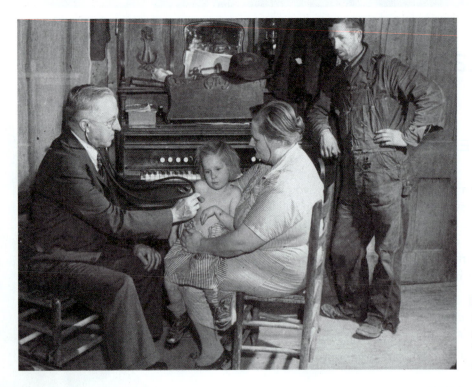

Figure 1-1
In the past, health care was delivered in the home, usually by a "family doctor." (*Hafton/Archive by Getty Images.*)

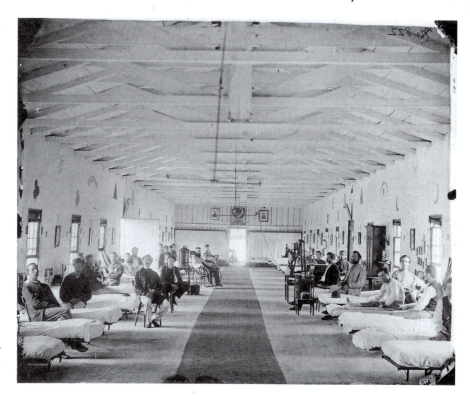

Figure 1-2
Modern ideas about hospital cleanliness and patient care did not exist in the 1800s.

a quick dollar. Hospitals typically caused more illness than they helped (Fig. 1-2). Patients were at the mercy of the "family doctor," and there was little they could do if the care they received was poor.

Present-day delivery of health care has changed dramatically. More intensive educational preparation for health care providers has become the standard and, in the United States, is required for those who want to care for those in need. Large facilities dedicated to providing on-site patient care have been established, replacing the home as the primary site for patient care. Due to advances in technology, a family doctor would no longer be able to carry the tools of his trade in the familiar black medical bag. A variety of medications and other treatments allow us to treat and cure many diseases that in the past would have been fatal, increasing the average person's life span by decades. The family doctor who attended a person from birth to death is now called a "general practitioner" or "family physician," and in many cases, he or she is supported by a team of specialists.

Although in the recent past, the trend was to *replace* the family doctor with a team of specialists, today we are seeing a return to a more holistic approach to health care. A **holistic** approach focuses on the care of the whole person, physically and emotionally. The best aspect of the care

Helping Hands and a Caring Heart

FOCUS ON HUMANISTIC HEALTH CARE

A "humanistic" approach to health care is one that focuses on the person receiving the care. When we take a humanistic approach to health care, we:
- Consider the qualities that make the person unique, and use that knowledge to guide the care that we provide
- Imagine how it would feel to be in the person's situation, and act with empathy and compassion
- Consider the person's emotional, social, and spiritual needs, as well as his or her physical ones

A humanistic approach to health care is the basis for providing quality care. There are many things you can do as a nursing assistant to take a humanistic approach to health care. Spend time with your residents and get to know them as individuals. Using that knowledge, think about things you can do that will help them feel more comfortable, both physically and emotionally. Act with compassion. Everyone will benefit! You will have the satisfaction of knowing that you are providing the best care possible, and your residents will feel well cared for and valued as individuals. That is what a humanistic approach to health care is all about.

provided by the old-fashioned "family doctor"—the doctor's familiarity with the person as an individual—is combined with modern-day availability of specialized care when needed.

HEALTH CARE ORGANIZATIONS

As the health care system has developed and changed over the years, we have seen more and more variety in the organizations that provide health care to people in need. Major types of health care organizations include the following.

- A **hospital** provides short-term medical and surgical care for people with acute conditions (that is, conditions with a rapid onset and a relatively short recovery time). People who receive care in hospitals usually have a condition that requires close monitoring by the health care team.
- A **long-term care facility** provides ongoing nursing care and personal assistance for people who can no longer live independently as a result of illness or disability.
- A **home health care agency** provides professional health care in a person's home. Home health care services are available for people of all ages with any number of different medical needs. For example, a new mother and her baby may need home care, especially if the baby was born too early. A person recovering from an accident, a stroke, or surgery may also need home care.
- A **hospice organization** provides care for people who are dying and their families. People are able to receive the services of a hospice organization when they know that they have only 3 to 6 months to live. The focus of hospice care is on relieving pain and other physical symptoms, and providing emotional and spiritual support for both the dying person and the family. Hospice care can be provided in the home, hospital, or long-term care facility, or in a facility devoted exclusively to providing care for the dying.

All health care organizations have a purpose, or **mission.** Some health care organizations, such as university hospitals, are associated directly with schools. The primary mission of a university hospital may be to train people in the field of health care. Other health care organizations are associated with a religious group. Although some health care organizations have very specific missions, others combine many of the following:

- To prevent disease by providing immunizations, teaching people how to control chronic health problems, and identifying factors that could place a person at risk for a disease
- To detect and treat disease
- To promote health by teaching people about ways to achieve and maintain both physical and mental fitness
- To offer rehabilitation (restorative care) services in order to help people return to their highest possible level of physical or emotional function
- To educate health care professionals by providing work-based training for medical students, student nurses, and other types of students training for a career in the health care field

Most health care organizations are governed by a board of trustees (also called a board of directors) and most have divisions (groups in charge of certain aspects of the organization's function). An administrator or chief executive officer (CEO) usually manages the organization and is the link between the board and the organization.

The board is made up of community members. The board sets policies to ensure that the care offered by the organization is safe and of good quality. The board also makes sure that the organization meets the needs of the community. For example, think about a rural community where there is only one hospital. This hospital does not provide obstetric services, which means that pregnant women must travel out of the area to deliver their babies. The hospital's board surveys the people in the town and determines that the hospital needs to offer obstetric services in order to meet the community's need. The board then develops a plan to get funding to build a maternity ward, and to find qualified people to staff it.

Each division within a health care organization is responsible for one key aspect of the organization's function. Each division is managed by a division director or division manager. For example:

- The medical services division is led by a medical director, who is responsible for the doctors on staff.
- The nursing services division is led by a director of nursing (DON) or chief nursing officer (CNO), who is responsible for all aspects of the organization that have to do with patient or resident care.
- The business services division is led by a business director, who oversees functions such as admissions, billing, and payroll.

- The ancillary services division is led by a director of ancillary services, who is responsible for overseeing the departments that provide additional support to patients or residents, such as social services and dietary services.
- The facility services division is led by a director of facility services, who is responsible for overseeing functions that have to do with keeping the facility and grounds clean, attractive, well maintained, safe, and secure.

Within each health care organization, care of patients or residents is provided by a **health care team,** made up of many people with different types of knowledge and skill levels (Fig. 1-3). The patient or resident is always the focus of the health care team's efforts. The goal of the health care team is to provide holistic care (care of the whole person, physically and emotionally). Each member of the health care team's job is as important as any other member's job. Think of the members of the health care team as links in the chain of care provided for the patient or resident. Because a chain is only as strong as its weakest link, each member of the health care team must provide care to the best of his or her ability. For example, the maintenance staff keeps the facility running smoothly by keeping equipment in good working order. The housekeeping staff keeps the facility clean. The people who work in the lab must be precise when performing laboratory studies and writing reports. In short, everyone must provide competent care in order for the health care team to function properly.

HEALTH CARE SETTINGS

Health care is provided in many different types of settings. In your career as a nursing assistant, you will no doubt hear about, or have experience with, many of these health care settings.

ACUTE CARE SETTINGS

A person who has a severe illness or whose condition is unstable and who requires a great deal of care and close monitoring is usually treated in a hospital, which is a type of **acute care setting**

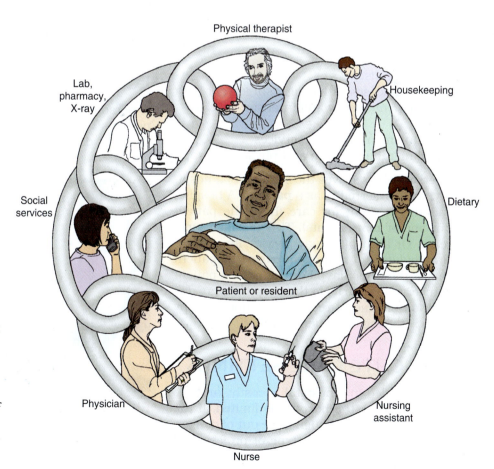

Figure 1-3
Care is provided by the health care team. The patient or resident is the primary focus of the health care team's efforts. Because a chain is only as strong as its weakest link, each member of the health care team must provide care to the best of his or her ability.

Physical therapist

Lab, pharmacy, X-ray

Housekeeping

Social services

Dietary

Patient or resident

Physician

Nursing assistant

Nurse

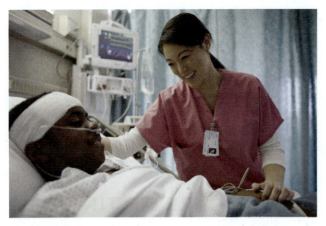

Figure 1-4
People being cared for in acute care settings usually have a serious illness, or their condition is unstable. Often, they also have chronic conditions that complicate the acute problem. As a result, they require close monitoring and a high level of care.

(Fig. 1-4). The services provided by a hospital differ according to the hospital's mission and location. Some hospitals, such as children's hospitals, women's centers, cancer centers, or orthopedic hospitals, have very specific missions, either in terms of the type of people they serve or the services that they offer. Other hospitals, sometimes called "general hospitals," provide a variety of services such as:

- Delivering babies
- Diagnosing diseases
- Treating diseases with drugs, surgery, or both
- Providing emergency and intensive care services
- Providing mental health services
- Providing rehabilitation and physical therapy

A person who receives the services of a hospital is typically referred to as a **patient.** A hospital may admit a patient for care (have the patient stay for one or more nights). This is called *inpatient* care. Or a hospital may provide its services on an *ambulatory* or *outpatient* basis (the patient goes home the same day). For example, a patient with cancer who returns to the hospital every day for a period of time to receive radiation therapy would be receiving outpatient care.

POST-ACUTE CARE SETTINGS

The care provided in a hospital is costly, and the number of beds in the hospital is limited. If the patient has recovered enough to be out of danger, but is still in need of some type of professional health care, the patient may be moved to a **post-acute care setting.** Post-acute care settings provide care for people who do not require hospitalization, but still require more care and monitoring than can be provided in the person's home by unskilled caregivers. Post-acute care can be provided in a number of different settings, depending on the type of care needed. Examples of these settings include sub-acute care settings, nursing homes, and even the person's own home with visits by caregivers from a home health care agency.

A **sub-acute care setting** is a type of post-acute care setting. Patients in sub-acute care settings require more care and closer monitoring by licensed health professionals than is usually provided in a typical nursing home setting, but less care and monitoring than is usually provided in a hospital. For example, patients in sub-acute care settings may require intravenous medications, respiratory care or ventilator services, wound management, or intensive rehabilitation services, such as physical therapy (Fig. 1-5). Sub-acute care is a short-term measure that provides a transition from a higher level of care to a lower level of care (or no care at all). The length of time a person spends in a sub-acute care setting is usually 30 days or less. After receiving sub-acute care, many people recover fully. Others may need to move to a long-term care facility or arrange for continued care from a home health agency after returning home.

LONG-TERM CARE SETTINGS

A person who requires ongoing assistance with personal care, medical care, or both for longer than 30 days may be cared for in a **long-term**

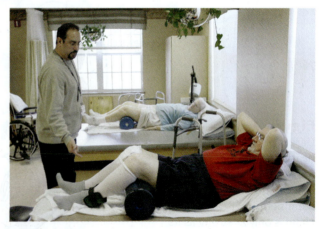

Figure 1-5
These patients are receiving rehabilitation therapy in a sub-acute care setting. (*AP Photo/Matt Rourke*)

requires limited assistance with tasks such as personal care, medication administration, transportation, meals, and housekeeping, but is otherwise fairly independent. In contrast, a resident of a **nursing home** usually requires around-the-clock nursing care and supervision.

OVERSIGHT OF THE HEALTH CARE SYSTEM

Today in the United States, many agencies exist to protect both the recipients and the providers of health care.

ENSURING QUALITY HEALTH CARE

Agencies involved with making sure that the health care provided in the United States is safe and of high quality may be associated with the government, or they may be independent non-profit organizations. These agencies may have one or more of the following objectives:

- To ensure that providers of health care are properly trained and competent
- To ensure that health care facilities meet standards of cleanliness and quality
- To ensure that all products used in the delivery of health care are safe
- To ensure that quality health care is available to everyone

The **United States Department of Health and Human Services (DHHS)** is the primary government agency responsible for protecting this nation's health. Under the umbrella of the DHHS, there are multiple agencies involved in overseeing many different aspects of the health care system in the United States (Fig. 1-7). Some of these agencies are involved with inspecting health care organizations regularly to make sure that the standards set by the government are being followed. Any problem is addressed, and if the problem is serious, the organization faces being fined or closed, or the loss of government funding.

Several independent, non-profit organizations also exist to help ensure that facilities provide quality health care. The largest and best known of these independent organizations is **The Joint Commission,** known in the past as The Joint Commission on Accreditation of Healthcare Organizations (JCAHO, pronounced "jay-co"). The

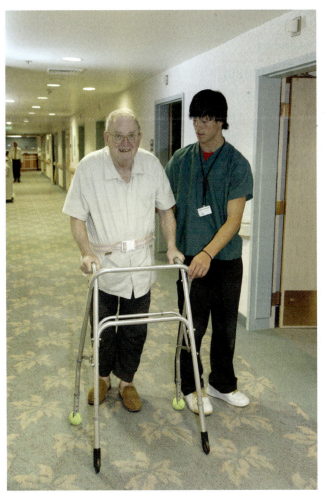

Figure 1-6

Long-term care facilities provide ongoing assistance with personal care, medical care, or both to those who can no longer live independently due to illness or disability, but who do not need to be hospitalized. Care is focused on helping residents to achieve and maintain their highest level of function. Here, a nursing assistant helps a resident to go for a walk.

care setting (Fig. 1-6). People receiving care in a long-term care setting are usually elderly, with one or more chronic illnesses. However, younger adults and children with conditions resulting from accidents or birth defects may also need long-term care. Because the long-term care facility becomes the person's home, either temporarily or permanently, a person being cared for in a long-term care facility is referred to as a **resident,** rather than a patient.

Long-term care settings include assisted-living facilities and nursing homes. Both of these types of facilities provide long-term care, but there is a difference in the level of care that is provided. A resident of an **assisted-living facility**

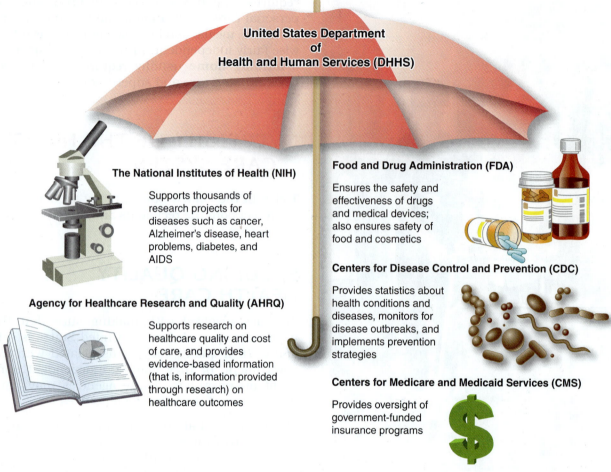

United States Department of Health and Human Services (DHHS)

The National Institutes of Health (NIH)

Supports thousands of research projects for diseases such as cancer, Alzheimer's disease, heart problems, diabetes, and AIDS

Agency for Healthcare Research and Quality (AHRQ)

Supports research on healthcare quality and cost of care, and provides evidence-based information (that is, information provided through research) on healthcare outcomes

Food and Drug Administration (FDA)

Ensures the safety and effectiveness of drugs and medical devices; also ensures safety of food and cosmetics

Centers for Disease Control and Prevention (CDC)

Provides statistics about health conditions and diseases, monitors for disease outbreaks, and implements prevention strategies

Centers for Medicare and Medicaid Services (CMS)

Provides oversight of government-funded insurance programs

Figure 1-7

The United States Department of Health and Human Services (DHHS) oversees many different agencies that are responsible for protecting the health of the people in this country. Some of the key agencies that you may hear about are shown here.

Joint Commission, established in 1951, sets national standards for all types of health care organizations and officially recognizes (accredits) organizations that meet these standards. The standards establish expectations for how the organization carries out certain activities, especially activities that affect patient and resident safety and the quality of patient and resident care. For example, The Joint Commission has established standards for safe medication administration, infection control, the use of abbreviations in documentation, staffing levels and staff education, and responding to emergencies.

Like the government agencies, The Joint Commission also inspects health care facilities regularly to make sure that its standards are being followed. However, unlike the government inspections, inspections by The Joint Commission are voluntary. Health care organizations request and pay for these inspections to be done

in order to receive **accreditation** (official recognition that the organization meets certain standards of quality). Organizations that have been accredited by The Joint Commission are permitted to display the Joint Commission's Gold Seal of Approval, which is recognized nationwide as a symbol of quality (Fig. 1-8). After receiving accreditation status, a health care organization must continue to provide proof that it meets the standards of quality. The organization must also demonstrate a commitment to continuously improving its performance.

PROTECTING HEALTH CARE WORKERS

The **Occupational Safety and Health Administration (OSHA)** is a government agency that is responsible for protecting the health and safety of

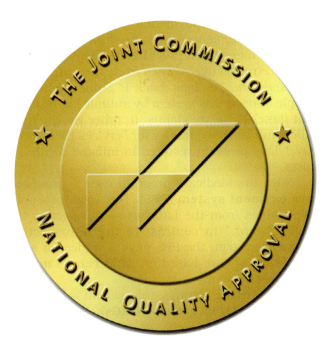

Figure 1-8
Health care facilities that comply with the standards set by The Joint Commission are allowed to display the Joint Commission's Gold Seal of Approval.

American workers by enforcing standards and providing education to improve conditions in the workplace. OSHA, which is part of the United States Department of Labor, seeks to protect workers across all industries, not just the health care industry. OSHA was formed after a key piece of legislation (the Occupational Safety and Health Act of 1970) was passed in response to public concern over increasing numbers of on-the-job injuries and deaths. You will see OSHA standards referenced frequently throughout this text. These standards protect you while you care for others.

PAYING FOR HEALTH CARE

If you have ever received a bill for health care in the United States, you know that health care can be expensive. Insurance can help to lessen these costs to the individual. As a nursing assistant, you should know a little bit about how health care is paid for in the United States.

PRIVATE AND GROUP INSURANCE

Although people can pay for health insurance privately, using their own funds, most people are covered by **group insurance** (insurance that is purchased at group rates by an employer or corporation). The employee may be covered in full as a benefit of employment, or he may pay a certain percentage of his coverage. The insurance company then pays for health care according to the individual policy.

Due to the increasing costs of medical care, the insurance industry has taken measures to control costs. Some insurance companies have a **precertification (preapproval) process.** This means that in order to be paid, the health care provider must prove that a person's medical condition meets certain criteria and obtain the insurance company's go-ahead for the proposed treatment before starting treatment.

Other insurance companies use a **managed care system.** Managed care systems assist in delivering health care to people who need it by arranging contracts with various health care providers (for example, doctors' offices, hospitals, ambulance services, pharmacies). In addition, they help to reduce unnecessary costs associated with medical and surgical procedures by authorizing treatments before they are carried out. One form of managed care system is the **preferred provider organization (PPO).** In a PPO, health care providers contract with an insurance company to accept a standard payment as total payment for services rendered. In return for seeking care only from health care providers who are part of the PPO network, the insured person usually receives that care at a reduced cost. A **health maintenance organization (HMO)** is another type of managed care system. Like PPOs, HMOs contract with health care providers to provide health care services for a prepaid fee, and people seeking care agree to see only health care providers who are part of the HMO network. An underlying principle of HMOs is that it costs less to keep a person healthy than it does to treat an illness. Therefore, these organizations typically promote regular physical examinations and screening to detect and prevent illnesses.

MEDICARE

Medicare is a type of insurance plan that is federally funded by Social Security, under the administration of the Centers for Medicare and Medicaid Services (CMS). People who are 65 years or older are eligible for Medicare, regardless of their financial situation. Some younger people who are disabled also qualify for Medicare. A person who is eligible for Medicare will have a card like the one shown in Fig. 1-9.

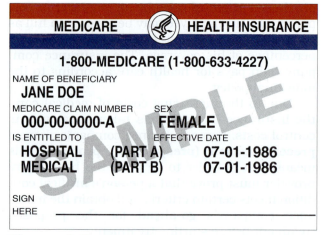

Figure 1-9

Medicare is government-funded health insurance for those 65 years of age and older, regardless of their financial situation. Some people younger than 65 who are disabled may also qualify. Those participating in the Medicare program will have a card like this.

To receive Medicare funding, a long-term care facility must be certified by Medicare to deliver skilled care. Health care facilities that are eligible to receive Medicare funding must follow strict rules and guidelines to receive payment. Not all long-term care facilities choose to participate in the Medicare plan.

Like insurance companies that insure the general public, the Medicare program is faced with the problem of controlling ever-increasing health care costs. In general, older people have greater health care needs than younger people. Therefore, a very large percentage of the money spent on health care in this country is spent on the elderly, and this money mostly comes from the Medicare program. In addition, the number of people 65 years and older living in the United States is increasing every year. These factors have put a huge strain on the government's ability to cover Medicare costs.

In an effort to control costs, there have been some changes in recent years in the way the Medicare program is administered. In the past, the Medicare program reimbursed (paid money back to) an individual or health care facility for dollars spent on health care services received or delivered. For example, if a health care facility provided services that qualified for Medicare money, the facility would bill the government for the services it provided and the government would send the facility a check to reimburse their

costs. This type of payment system is called a *retrospective payment system* because payment is based on money that has already been spent (the word "retrospective" comes from the Latin word *retrospectare*, "to look back"). Some dishonest people abused this system by submitting fraudulent (fake) Medicare claims. In other words, they billed and collected money for services they never gave! This problem resulted in inflated Medicare costs.

Now, the Medicare program uses a **prospective payment system (PPS).** The word "prospective" comes from the Latin word *prospectus*, "to look forward." In contrast to the retrospective payment system, the PPS pays a set fee for specific levels of care based on what care is anticipated or expected.

In acute care settings, this system is based on **diagnosis-related groups (DRGs).** Payment for hospitalization, surgery, or other treatment is specified according to the person's diagnosis. Lengths of hospital stays are also determined by the diagnosis and are typically short. For example, if a patient is admitted to the hospital for treatment of a broken hip, Medicare will pay the hospital a standard fee based on the estimated cost of caring for someone with a broken hip. The hospital must deliver the care efficiently (that is, for the same or less money than what Medicare allows) to keep its budget in check. If the cost of caring for the patient exceeds what Medicare allows, the hospital must absorb the additional costs. Because of the DRG system, hospitals are under pressure to discharge patients in a timely manner. This change has increased the need for, and the use of, the post-acute care settings that we discussed earlier.

The Medicare payment system for long-term care works in a similar way. However, the system is based on **resource utilization groups (RUGs).** Payment for care provided by the long-term care facility is based on the estimated amount of resources that a resident is expected to use. The amount of resources the resident is expected to use is determined by specific codes recorded on a document called the Minimum Data Set (MDS). The codes reflect the resident's mental status, the resident's ability to care for himself, the medical conditions that the resident has, and the treatment that is required for those conditions. A RUGs score is calculated based on the MDS coding. There are multiple levels of RUG categories, and generally, the higher the category, the higher the level of payment. MDS coding must be accurate to ensure that the facility bills for the right

RUG category. You will learn more about the MDS in Chapter 12.

MEDICAID

Medicaid is a federally funded and state-regulated plan designed to help people with low incomes to pay for health care. Elderly people, as well as those who are disabled, may also be eligible, especially if they have limited incomes. To receive Medicaid reimbursement, a facility must be approved by the state agency. Not all facilities or health care providers choose to participate in the Medicaid plan.

SUMMARY

- Society has always sought to care for the sick and injured.
  - In the United States during the 1700s, 1800s, and early part of the 1900s, most people who needed health care received it in their homes. Most care was provided by family members and a "family doctor."
  - Today, health care is delivered by many different types of health care organizations in many different types of health care settings.
  - People being cared for in an acute care setting usually have a serious illness, or their condition is unstable. As a result, they require close monitoring and a high level of care.
  - People being cared for in post-acute care settings are not so ill that they need the intense care and monitoring provided in an acute care setting, but they still require complex care from a trained caregiver. The sub-acute care setting is a type of post-acute care setting.
  - People being cared for in long-term care facilities require ongoing assistance with personal care, medical care, or both.
- Most health care organizations are structured in a similar way. Most have a board of trustees (board of directors), and most have divisions (groups in charge of certain aspects of the organization's function).
- Today, we take a holistic approach to health care. That is, we take into consideration the person's emotional, as well as his or her physical, needs.
  - Health care is provided by a team of people, each with different areas of expertise and job responsibilities.
  - As a nursing assistant, you are a critical part of the health care team.
- There are numerous agencies that monitor health care organizations to protect both the recipients of health care and the providers of health care.
  - The United States Department of Health and Human Services (DHHS) is the primary government agency responsible for protecting this nation's health. The DHHS oversees government agencies such as the Centers for Disease Control (CDC), the National Institutes of Health (NIH), and the Centers for Medicare and Medicaid Services (CMS).
  - The Joint Commission is a private, non-profit agency that sets national standards for all types of health care organizations and officially recognizes (accredits) organizations that meet these standards.
  - The Occupational Safety and Health Administration (OSHA) is a government agency that is responsible for protecting the health and safety of American workers by enforcing standards and providing education to improve conditions in the workplace. OSHA standards are in place to help protect you, the health care worker.
- As the health care system has become more complex, the cost of health care has increased, and the way health care is paid for has changed.
  - Private and group insurance policies are one way that individuals pay for health care.
  - Medicare is insurance that is funded by the United States government. Medicare payment for hospital care is based on the patient's diagnosis. Medicare payment for long-term care is based on estimated resources that will be used to care for a resident.
  - Medicaid is also funded by the United States government, and is designed to help people with low incomes pay for health care.

WHAT DID YOU LEARN?

Matching

Match each numbered item with its appropriate lettered description.

_____ **1.** Sub-acute care setting

_____ **2.** Acute care setting

_____ **3.** Long-term care setting

_____ **4.** Hospice organization

_____ **5.** Health maintenance organization (HMO)

_____ **6.** Home health care agency

_____ **7.** Preferred provider organization (PPO)

_____ **8.** Diagnosis-related groups (DRGs)

_____ **9.** Resource utilization groups (RUGs)

a. Used as a basis for Medicare payments in hospitals

b. Type of insurance that requires the insured person to seek care only from providers who are part of the network

c. Where care is provided on an ongoing basis for people who can no longer live on their own, due to illness or disability

d. Provides professional health care in a person's home

e. Type of insurance that promotes regular screening to prevent illnesses

f. Where care is provided for acutely ill people who require a high level of care and monitoring

g. Used as a basis for Medicare payments in long-term care settings

h. Provides care devoted exclusively to the dying

i. Where a high level of care is provided for people who are making the transition from hospital care to a lower level of care or home care

Match each agency with its description.

_____ **10.** The Joint Commission

_____ **11.** The Occupational Safety and Health Administration (OSHA)

_____ **12.** The United States Department of Health and Human Services (DHHS)

_____ **13.** The Food and Drug Administration (FDA)

_____ **14.** The Centers for Medicare and Medicaid Services (CMS)

j. Provides voluntary accreditation for health facilities meeting quality standards

k. Oversees government-funded insurance programs

l. Ensures the safety and effectiveness of drugs and medical devices, as well as food and cosmetics

m. Primary agency responsible for protecting the health of the American people

n. Sets and enforces standards to keep American workers safe in the workplace

STOP and Think!

- Think about what health care was like in the United States 100 years ago. How has health care delivery changed in the United States since the early 1900s? What aspects of the "old-fashioned" way of delivering health care were good? Not so good? What aspects of modern health care delivery are good? Not so good?

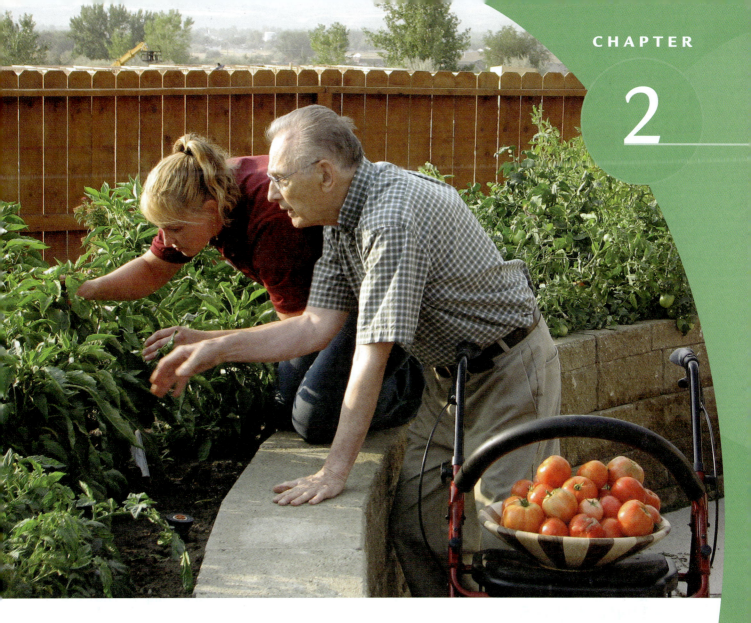

Overview of Long-Term Care

WHAT WILL YOU LEARN?

In this chapter, we will take a closer look at the long-term care setting. We will review the different types of long-term care settings that exist in the United States today. In addition, we will discuss the history of long-term care in the United States, as well as its future. You will learn more about the regulatory and accreditation organizations that help to ensure the quality of long-term care provided in the United States today. Finally, we will discuss how long-term care is paid for. When you are finished with this chapter, you will be able to:

1. Identify the various types of long-term care settings and discuss how they are different from one another.
2. Discuss the past, present, and future of long-term care.

Photo: A resident of a Green House® home enjoys gardening. The Green House® project is an example of how long-term care is changing. (Photo courtesy of THE GREEN HOUSE® Project.)

3. Describe some of the government and private agencies that provide oversight of long-term care.
4. Discuss how long-term care is paid for.

Vocabulary Use the CD in the front of your book to hear these terms pronounced and defined:

Continuing care retirement community (CCRC)	Chain facility	Pioneer Network	Continuing Care Accreditation Commission (CCAC)
	Poorhouses	Pioneer Models for Culture Change	
	Social Security Act		
Continuum of care	Pension	Culture change	Benefit period
For-profit facility	Omnibus Budget Reconciliation Act (OBRA)	Centers for Medicare and Medicaid Services (CMS)	Private pay
Non-profit (not-for-profit) facility			Long-term care insurance
Free-standing facility	Balanced Budget Act		

TYPES OF LONG-TERM CARE SETTINGS

As you remember from Chapter 1, a long-term care setting is a place where health care is provided for people who require ongoing nursing care, personal assistance, or both as a result of illness or disability. The three major types of long-term care settings are nursing homes, assisted-living facilities, and continuing care retirement communities (CCRCs). Some people also consider adult day care and home health services part of long-term care.

NURSING HOMES

Nursing homes provide residents with around-the-clock nursing care and supervision. Typically, residents live in private or semi-private rooms grouped along a common hallway (Fig. 2-1). All rooms have access to a toilet (either private or shared between two rooms). Often, a communal bathing area (with bathtubs, showers, or both) is located down the hall. Some rooms may have private bath and toilet facilities that are used only by the resident occupying the room. Usually, there are also common areas where residents gather to socialize (such as dining rooms and activity rooms), a small chapel where religious services can be held, and patios and gardens that allow the residents access to outdoor activities.

ASSISTED-LIVING FACILITIES

Assisted-living facilities provide residents with limited assistance with tasks such as personal care, medication administration, transportation, meals, and housekeeping. Residents of assisted-living facilities often live in small apartments that have a kitchen or kitchenette, a bathroom, a living area, and a bedroom (Fig. 2-2). Most assisted-living facilities also have common areas where residents can go to socialize and eat.

CONTINUING CARE RETIREMENT COMMUNITIES (CCRCS)

Continuing care retirement communities (CCRCs) provide many different levels of care and multiple services on the same campus. The CCRC

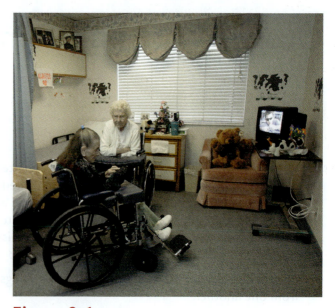

Figure 2-1
Residents of nursing homes often live in private or semi-private rooms.

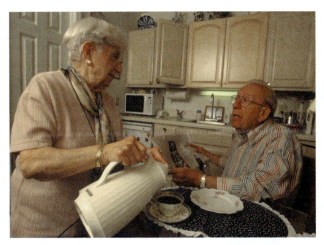

Figure 2-2
Residents of assisted-living facilities often have a small apartment with areas for eating, living, and sleeping. (*Catrina Genovese/Index Stock Imagery, Inc.*)

campus provides a **continuum of care** by including facilities for independent living, assisted living, and nursing home care (Fig. 2-3). As age, health problems, or both cause a resident of a CCRC to become less independent, he is able to stay within the CCRC to obtain the care he needs. In addition, the CCRC campus may include restaurants or dining facilities, recreational and social facilities, facilities for worship, a small market where food and other items can be pur-

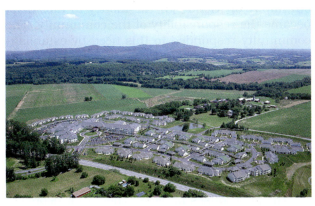

Figure 2-3
A continuing care retirement community (CCRC) has facilities for independent living, assisted-living, and nursing home care, all on the same campus. As residents' needs change, they can obtain the care they need without moving away from the campus. Other buildings on campus might include restaurants, recreational facilities, facilities for worship, stores, and a health center where residents can go for medical care.

chased, and a health center where residents can go for medical care.

OWNERSHIP AND OPERATION OF LONG-TERM CARE FACILITIES

Long-term care facilities differ from one another in terms of the types of services they provide. They also differ from one another in terms of how they are owned and operated.

FOR-PROFIT FACILITIES VERSUS NON-PROFIT (NOT-FOR-PROFIT) FACILITIES

A facility may be "for-profit" or "non-profit" (not-for-profit). A **for-profit facility** is one that is owned by a company or organization that is operating the facility as a business, with the intention of making money (a profit). In contrast, a **non-profit (not-for-profit) facility** is owned and operated by a service organization, like a church or charitable group. Its primary goal is to provide a service to fulfill a need in the community. Although a non-profit facility still has to make money to stay in business, money-making for the purpose of financial gain is not the primary intent. The profits are often put back into the services provided by the organization.

FREE-STANDING FACILITIES VERSUS CHAIN FACILITIES

Long-term care facilities may be free-standing or part of a chain. A **free-standing facility** is independently owned and operated. A **chain facility**, on the other hand, is owned and operated by a corporation that owns multiple facilities. Facilities that are part of a chain tend to be very similar to each other because they are run by the same corporation. If you have ever visited a McDonald's or a Wal-Mart in another city, you are already familiar with this concept. By the name, you basically know what to expect when you go inside the restaurant or store. The same is true of long-term care facilities that are part of a chain. Each facility in the chain follows the same corporate policies and procedures, so the services offered and the care provided is similar from facility to facility within the chain. Chain facilities are often for-profit facilities,

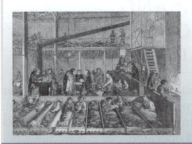

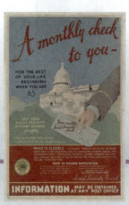

More private dwellings begin to open up to provide board and care for older people, decreasing the number of poorhouses from 135,000 to 72,000.

1935–1950

Mid-1800s

Poorhouses provide shelter for older people who are no longer able to work to pay for housing, and who have no families to take care of them. The poorhouses are often crowded and dirty.
Photo by Mansell/Time & Life Pictures/Getty Images

1900–1930s

Shelters dedicated solely to housing the elderly begin to appear and are called "homes for the aged," "convalescent homes," or "rest homes."

1935
President Franklin D. Roosevelt signs the Social Security Act into law, providing monthly pensions for older people.

1965

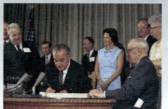

President Lyndon B. Johnson signs the Medicare/Medicaid programs into law, making it possible for more people to afford long-term care.
LBJ Library, photo by Unknown

although some non-profit organizations may also run multiple facilities.

LONG-TERM CARE: PAST, PRESENT, AND FUTURE

In past years, public opinion of long-term care, most specifically nursing homes, was very low. Throughout history, there have been many problems with long-term care in the United States, so it is understandable how such an opinion developed. However, it is important to recognize that today's long-term care facilities provide a significantly improved quality of care and quality of life for residents. Only by understanding our past can we can truly understand the present, and appreciate the future, of long-term care (Box 2-1).

THE JOURNEY FROM THE PAST TO THE PRESENT

As long as there have been older, chronically ill, and disabled people, society has been challenged to care for them. Throughout history, family members or friends of those in need often took on the responsibility of caring for them. Those without family or friends (or the money to hire help) became the responsibility of the community. The community responded to this need by establishing **poorhouses** (community-supported facilities that provided shelter for those without the means of supporting themselves, also known as *almshouses* or *poor farms*). From the mid-1800s, up until the Social Security Act was passed in 1935, many older, chronically ill, or disabled people lived in poorhouses. Conditions in the poorhouses varied quite a bit, but overcrowding, filth, and disease were common.

The poorhouses provided shelter for people of all ages. By the early 1900s, shelters dedicated solely to housing the elderly were beginning to appear. These shelters had various names, including "homes for the aged," "rest homes," and "convalescent homes." These shelters offered a place for the elderly to live, and possibly some assistance with basic tasks. Charitable groups, known for running some of the better poorhouses, established many of these facilities and

Nursing homes are recognized as a new kind of business. There is an increase in the number of for-profit and chain facilities. Many facilities are poorly managed and provide poor care, and public concern grows.

1965–1970s

1980s
The Institute of Medicine (IOM) studies nursing home care and reports unsatisfactory care and poor quality of life.

The Omnibus Budget Reconciliation Act (OBRA) of 1987 establishes standards that improve the quality of care and quality of life for residents of nursing homes. The culture change movement begins.

1987–1990

1990s
Health care costs are increasing at a rapid rate. To control costs, hospitals begin to discharge patients "sooner and sicker." Sub-acute care facilities that specialize in immediate post-acute care start to emerge.

President Bill Clinton signs the Balanced Budget Act (BBA) of 1997, resulting in the most significant cut to the Medicare budget in the program's history and establishing the prospective payment system (PPS). Alternatives to nursing homes, such as assisted-living facilities, start to emerge. A small group of long-term care professionals meet to share ideas about the future of long-term care.

1997

2003

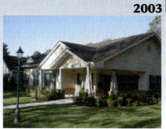

The first nursing homes are built following The Green House® Project model in Tupelo, Mississippi.
THE GREEN HOUSE® Project

some still exist today. While the names of these facilities may reflect an earlier time in history, the care they provide meets today's standards.

In 1935, President Franklin D. Roosevelt signed the **Social Security Act** into law. As a result of the Social Security Act, older people who were retired or unemployed were entitled to receive a **pension** (regular cash payments) from the government. Now, older people who could no longer work had a source of money to pay for their keep. Many elderly people could now afford to move to "boarding homes," places that provided housing, meals, and possibly other services for a fee. Rather than lose paying tenants as they became older and more frail, some boarding homes started to hire nurses to care for their tenants. This was the beginning of the "nursing home" that we know today.

In 1965, President Lyndon B. Johnson signed the Medicare and Medicaid programs into law. As you recall from Chapter 1, these new programs were federally funded insurance programs. As a result of the Medicare and Medicaid programs, more people could afford long-term care. There was also more of an opportunity to make money

by providing long-term care. During the late 1960s and early 1970s, many new for-profit nursing homes were built. In addition, many of the smaller independent facilities were bought by larger companies, leading to the development of chain facilities. An "industry" was born.

During the 1960s and 1970s, the quality of care provided in many nursing homes was poor. Many of the facilities were run by people who were more interested in making money than in caring for the elderly and disabled. The "aides" who provided care were not required to receive any formal health care training. Neglect and abuse of residents were common. In addition, some dishonest facility owners were submitting fraudulent Medicare claims, causing Medicare costs to go up. Nursing home scandals frequently were headline stories in the newspapers.

In the 1980s, the Institute of Medicine (IOM) was given the task of studying nursing home care. The result of their report was the **Omnibus Budget Reconciliation Act (OBRA)** of 1987, which was put into effect in 1990. The strict OBRA legislation improved the quality of life for residents of nursing homes, by making sure that

BOX 2-2　The Omnibus Budget Reconciliation Act (OBRA)

An understanding of OBRA standards is an absolute must for nursing assistants who work in nursing homes. As you read this book, look for the OBRA icon ◻, which highlights key information related to this law. OBRA legislation is reviewed and passed by Congress each year. If you work in a nursing home, your employer may provide informational sessions to update the staff on new requirements. It is important for you to attend these sessions so that you can stay current on the most up-to-date information regarding your role in resident care.

---

they received a certain standard of care. This care was required to take into account the residents' physical, emotional, spiritual, and social needs. In addition, OBRA set standards for the physical environment in the nursing home, as well as for the training and evaluation of the nursing assistants who worked in nursing homes (Box 2-2).

OBRA legislation improved the quality of care in the nation's nursing homes. However, the expanded services that nursing homes were required to provide in order to meet OBRA's standards increased their costs at a time when they were already facing financial pressures. The hospitals were also experiencing financial pressures. In an effort to keep their budgets in check, hospitals began to discharge patients "sooner and sicker." Many of these patients were still too ill to be cared for at home, and the government started to offer money to nursing homes to accept these patients as residents. (For the government, paying the nursing homes a higher rate to care for these patients was still less costly than paying for another day at the hospital!) Nursing homes, anxious to survive in a tight financial market, sought certification to provide skilled care so that they could accept the patients who were discharged from the hospital. During this time, sub-acute care facilities that specialized in immediate post-acute care began to emerge.

By the late 1990s, health care costs were rapidly increasing. In response, in 1997, President Bill Clinton signed the **Balanced Budget Act** into law. This legislation called for a $116.4 billion cut in funding for the Medicare program over 5 years' time, the largest cut ever in Medicare's history. The prospective payment system (PPS) for Medicare reimbursement (see Chapter 1) was also put into action as part of this legislation. These legislative changes created huge financial difficulties for many nursing homes. Many, including several large nursing home chains, had no choice but to file for bankruptcy.

Also in the late 1990s, less costly alternatives to the traditional nursing home began to emerge.

One of these alternatives was the assisted-living facility. Because assisted-living facilities provided care for people who needed support, but not skilled nursing care, their services were not as costly. Currently, we are also seeing a trend toward providing more care in a person's home, thus reducing costs even further.

THE FUTURE

In 1997, a small group of professionals working in long-term care met to share ideas and create a new vision for the future of long-term care. In a sense, these people could be considered *pioneers*, people who lead the way and prepare others to follow. This group of long-term care professionals, which officially became known as the **Pioneer Network** in 2000, developed several models for long-term care. These models are known as **Pioneer Models for Culture Change** (Box 2-3). **Culture change** is an ongoing process that focuses on changing attitudes, goals, and practices in order to improve the long-term care environment and the way care is delivered.

The Green House® project is representative of culture change in long-term care. It was founded by Dr. Bill Thomas, the creator of The Eden Alternative®, to be a place of warmth and growth for residents and staff. The design of a Green House home is much like that of a private home. Only 7 to 10 residents live in each Green House home. Each resident has a private bedroom and bathroom. Because only 7 to 10 residents live in each Green House®, there are no long hallways, so many residents are able to get around without using wheelchairs. Other features of the house include a large common living area called "The Hearth" (which contains a fireplace, an open kitchen, and a dining area), a laundry area, and an open patio and outdoor garden (Fig. 2-4). Residents are encouraged to help in the preparation of meals, which are served at a large common table where residents and staff can eat together in a family-style arrangement. Daily routines are based on

BOX 2-3 Pioneer Models for Culture Change

Individualized Care. In this model, each resident's personal history is used as the basis for an individualized plan of care. The plan of care is based on an understanding of what has been important to the person throughout her life, and how the person wants to live life. Staff members are permanently assigned to residents to foster this individualized knowledge and understanding.

Regenerative Community. This model fosters a sense of community within a facility among residents, staff, families, and volunteers. It moves away from the traditional medical model, which focuses on tasks. Instead, the regenerative community model focuses on understanding and meeting needs. Focusing on each resident's strengths and abilities, regardless of his physical or mental status, is emphasized.

Resident-Directed Care. This model focuses on the idea of creating a "neighborhood." Neighborhoods are made up of small groups of residents who live in a home-like environment that has a kitchen, laundry facility, and family gathering room. Residents are encouraged to contribute to daily routines related to daily life and the care of the facility (for example, gardening, helping to prepare meals, light housekeeping). This helps to provide a sense of meaning and purpose in their lives. Resident care is based on individual choice, rather than facility routine and schedules. This allows the resident more independence (for example, in bedtime, mealtime, and leisure activities).

The Eden Alternative®. This model also focuses on creating a sense of community. The surroundings are designed in a way to support life and eliminate loneliness, helplessness, and boredom. Plants and companion animals (such as birds, dogs, cats, and fish) are part of the facility environment. Day care centers for children may be located on the same site. These features provide the residents with opportunities to participate in the care of the facility pets and environment and to enjoy the companionship of children. Staff members work together to ensure that the services provided meet each individual resident's needs and desires.

---

individual choice, just as if the person was in his own home. This helps to foster a greater sense of independence and individuality for residents.

The first Green House® project, built in Tupelo, Mississippi, has been very successful. Some of the problems that residents frequently experience in more traditional long-term care settings, such as urinary incontinence (an inability to control urination), unexplained weight loss, depression, and a decline in abilities, are seen less frequently among residents of The Green House® homes. The Green House® model has other benefits as well. In The Green House® model, nursing assistants receive additional education that enables them to make decisions and plan care. In this model, nursing assistants are called *Shahbazim* and their role is to protect and nurture the residents and each other. Staff turnover rates have been maintained well below the national average, and there have been fewer work-related injuries.

These successes have been noticed. The Robert Wood Johnson Foundation, a major funding organization that is devoted to supporting education and research projects to improve health care, has provided a $10 million grant to help develop other Green House® homes. The goal is to develop 50 Green House® homes across the United States, and eventually, to move The Green House® concept into the mainstream of long-term care services.

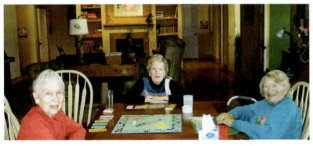

Figure 2-4
Residents of a Green House® home enjoy a board game together in the large common living area called "The Hearth." (*Photo courtesy of THE GREEN HOUSE® Project.*)

OVERSIGHT OF LONG-TERM CARE

Many different agencies—including the federal, state, and local government, as well as independent non-profit organizations—are responsible for making sure that the care provided in long-term care facilities in the United States is safe and of high quality.

OVERSIGHT BY THE FEDERAL GOVERNMENT

All types of long-term care facilities must follow the requirements of agencies such as the Occupational Safety and Health Administration (OSHA), the Food and Drug Administration (FDA), and the Centers for Disease Control and Prevention (CDC). The functions of these agencies were reviewed in Chapter 1.

In addition, federal (OBRA) laws apply to every nursing home in the United States. (These laws apply only to nursing homes, not to assisted-living facilities.) Each nursing home is subject to routine inspection by the government. These inspections are called *surveys*. The purpose of the survey is to make sure the facility is following OBRA regulations and meeting the government's standards. The **Centers for Medicare & Medicaid Services (CMS)** is the government agency responsible for monitoring nursing homes to make sure that they are following OBRA regulations and meeting the government's standards. Government payment for services depends on whether or not the facility is meeting the required standards. If, through the survey process, a facility is found to not meet the required standards, government payment for services becomes jeopardized.

Under the federal OBRA laws, nursing homes must make their most recent survey results readily available to residents, families, and anyone else who wants to review them. In addition, the CMS posts survey results on the Internet. Because survey results are easily available to anyone who is interested, the facility has additional incentive to provide quality services, beyond just avoiding regulatory problems. Survey results that indicate a high quality of care can make the facility more attractive to potential customers (that is, residents and their families). As a nursing assistant, you will play a very important role in ensuring that your facility meets or exceeds survey requirements by doing your job well and always following facility policy. You will learn more about the survey process in Chapter 6 and in the *Be Smart About Surveys!* boxes found throughout this book.

OVERSIGHT BY STATE GOVERNMENTS

Assisted-living facilities are regulated by the state. Because no federal laws apply to assisted-living facilities, assisted-living services can vary greatly from state to state. Nursing homes must comply with state laws, in addition to federal laws. Many state laws that apply to nursing homes follow OBRA, but some states have additional requirements that OBRA does not include.

All long-term care facilities must have a license to operate. The license is issued by the state. To maintain *licensure*, long-term care facilities must undergo an inspection. The state officials who perform this inspection are responsible for checking to make sure the facility is meeting the state's requirements. In addition, they may be responsible for making sure that the facility is following any federal regulations that may apply.

Nursing homes that wish to participate in the Medicare and Medicaid programs must be certified. In order to achieve and maintain *certification*, the facility must undergo inspections. These inspections are usually carried out by state officials who are contracted by the federal government (that is, the CMS). These officials check to make sure that the facility is meeting federal regulations, as well as state regulations.

OVERSIGHT BY LOCAL GOVERNMENTS

Local agencies (such as city or county health departments) are responsible for ensuring that the facility is in compliance with any regulations that the local government has established for long-term care facilities. Local officials may also have a role in checking to make sure that the facility is providing care according to state or federal standards.

INDEPENDENT NON-PROFIT ORGANIZATIONS

In Chapter 1, you learned about The Joint Commission, an organization that sets national standards for all types of health care organizations and officially recognizes (accredits) organizations that meet these standards. Many long-term care facilities seek accreditation from The Joint Commission.

A similar organization, the **Continuing Care Accreditation Commission (CCAC),** grants accreditation to CCRCs, as well as to some other types of organizations that provide long-term care services (such as adult day care centers). The CCAC is the only accrediting organization specifically for CCRCs. A CCRC (or other health care organization) seeking accreditation by the CCAC requests and pays for routine inspections.

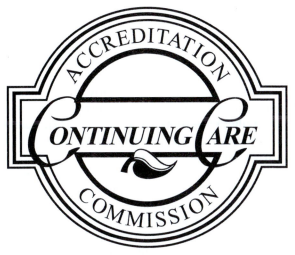

Figure 2-5
This symbol, displayed by a continuing care retirement community (CCRC), is a sign that the CCRC has met quality standards set by the Continuing Care Accreditation Commission (CCAC).

Organizations that have been accredited by the CCAC are permitted to display the CCAC's accreditation seal, which is recognized nation-wide as a symbol of quality (Fig. 2-5).

PAYING FOR LONG-TERM CARE

Long-term care is very expensive and not easily paid for by individuals or by the government (Fig. 2-6).

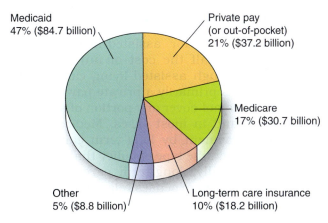

Medicaid
47% ($84.7 billion)

Private pay
(or out-of-pocket)
21% ($37.2 billion)

Medicare
17% ($30.7 billion)

Long-term care insurance
10% ($18.2 billion)

Other
5% ($8.8 billion)

Figure 2-6
Long-term care is expensive! This graph shows the billions of dollars that are spent each year on long-term care in the United States, as well as where that money is coming from.

PAYING FOR NURSING HOME CARE

In the United States, the average cost for nursing home care is more than $6,000.00 per month. By *average,* we mean that in some areas it may cost less, but in other areas it may cost more. Many Americans underestimate the cost of nursing home care. As a result, many do not have the savings to pay for nursing home care if it is needed.

Medicare

Many people assume that Medicare will pay for nursing home care. In reality, what Medicare pays for is extremely limited. For Medicare to pay, several requirements must be met:

- The person must meet strict criteria for skilled health care services. Skilled health care services are those provided by nurses or other licensed health care professionals.
- Care must follow a hospital stay.
- Care must be provided in a nursing facility licensed to provide skilled care.

A **benefit period** begins when the person is hospitalized and ends when the person has not received any skilled health care services, either in the hospital or nursing home, for 60 days. The Medicare program uses benefit periods as a way of tracking how many days of skilled health care services a person uses, and how many are still available. A person can have up to 100 days of skilled care in one benefit period. Once the person uses those 100 days, the current benefit period ends. A new benefit period cannot begin until the 60 days without skilled services is completed. During a benefit period, only the first 20 days are fully covered by Medicare. The remaining days (days 21 to 100) require a co-pay of approximately $100 per day. Medicare can end a person's coverage when the person no longer meets the strict criteria for coverage, even if the 100-day period is not over.

Medicaid

So, what happens to those who need nursing home care but do not have Medicare coverage? Many are admitted to a nursing facility as "**private pay,**" meaning that they pay for care using their own money (Fig. 2-7). With care in a nursing home costing an average of more than $6,000 per month, you can see that it may not take very long to go through a lifetime of savings.

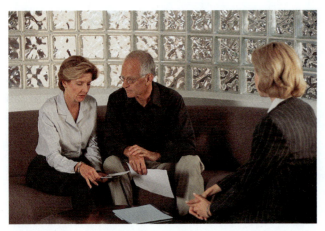

Figure 2-7
Most people are not prepared to pay for nursing home care for an extended period of time. Here, a member of the nursing home admissions staff reviews options for paying for care with the family of a resident.

Many people do exhaust all of their savings, and then must rely on Medicaid to pay for their care. Approximately 70% of those currently living in nursing homes are relying on Medicaid to pay for their care.

Although Medicaid eases the financial burden for the person receiving care, the financial burden is transferred to the nursing facility, and to the state that is distributing the Medicaid payments. For facilities, Medicaid causes a financial strain because Medicaid payments have not been able to keep up with the rising costs of care. As a result, it often costs the facility more to provide the services than the facility receives as payment in return. For states, Medicaid causes a financial strain as well. The state must accommodate Medicaid costs within its budget. This is becoming hard to do because Medicaid costs are consuming a greater percentage of state budgets every year.

Long-Term Care Insurance

Long-term care insurance is a private insurance policy that can be purchased by an individual to help pay for long-term care in the future, should it be needed. The benefit of long-term care insurance is that it can help to pay for long-term care services, which helps to protect the person's savings and assets. The disadvantages are that long-term care insurance is very expensive and somewhat risky.

Most financial planners advise people who are interested in long-term care insurance to obtain a policy when they are in their 40s or 50s. If a person waits until he is older to buy the insurance, the *premiums* (that is, the regular payments made on the policy) are more expensive, and the person may not qualify for coverage if he already has existing chronic medical conditions. However, the insurance only remains in effect as long as the person keeps paying for the policy. If the person's financial situation changes, or if the premiums increase, the person may be forced to drop the policy. In this case, the person loses all of the money paid into the policy. Even if the person continues to pay for the policy, he may never use it. In that case, the person will receive no benefits, despite all of the money paid into the policy over the years. A person could pay for the insurance for 40 years without knowing whether or not he will ever use it! There is also the risk that the insurance company will no longer be in business by the time the person needs the benefits of the policy.

Long-term care insurance, like Medicare, does not pay for all costs associated with nursing home care. Even if the insurance pays for the nursing home stay, it may not cover additional expenses related to medications, supplies, or other special services and therapies. These additional expenses can add up very quickly. Many policies also require the person to pay a *deductible* (i.e., a sum of money paid "out-of-pocket" before actual insurance benefits are paid).

PAYING FOR ASSISTED-LIVING CARE

The average cost for assisted-living care is approximately half the cost of nursing home care. Even though assisted-living care is less expensive, it is primarily a private pay expense. Medicare does not cover any portion of assisted-living care, and in most cases, Medicaid does not either. Payment by long-term care insurance depends on the type of policy that was purchased. Generally, long-term care insurance only covers certain expenses related to assisted-living.

SUMMARY

- The three major types of long-term care settings are nursing homes, assisted-living facilities, and continuing care retirement communities (CCRCs). Some people also consider adult day care and home health care services to be part of long-term care.
  - Nursing homes provide residents with around-the-clock nursing care and supervision.
  - Assisted-living facilities provide residents with limited assistance with certain tasks, such as meals and housekeeping.
  - Continuing care retirement communities (CCRCs) provide residents with multiple levels of services, ranging from independent living to nursing home care, all on the same campus.
- A long-term care facility can be "for profit" (operated with the intent of making money) or "non-profit" (operated with the intent of meeting a need in the community). A long-term care facility can be free-standing (independently owned and operated) or part of a chain (owned and operated by a corporation that owns and operates other similar facilities as well).
- Only by understanding the past can we understand the present, and future, of long-term care.
  - In the past, long-term care in the United States had many problems. As a result, many people today still hold poor opinions of long-term care facilities (especially nursing homes).
  - Legislation, such as the Omnibus Budget Reconciliation Act (OBRA) of 1987, has greatly improved the quality of care provided in nursing homes.
  - Today, leaders in long-term care continue to seek ways to improve the long-term care environment and the way care is delivered.

- Government agencies, as well as independent non-profit organizations, provide over sight of the long-term care industry.
  - Nursing homes in the United States must follow federal and state regulations, and local regulations as well. Currently there are no federal laws that govern assisted-living facilities. Each state has its own regulations for this type of care.
  - Independent non-profit organizations, such as The Joint Commission and the Continuing Care Accreditation Commission (CCAC), set standards for health care organizations and grant accreditation to organizations that meet the standards. Participation in these programs is voluntary.
- Long-term care is very costly and is not easily paid for by either the individual or the government.
  - Most people do not adequately plan for long-term care expenses. At an average cost of more than $6,000 per month for nursing home care, a lifetime of savings may not last very long.
  - Medicare coverage for nursing home care is minimal. Those qualifying must meet very strict criteria for skilled health care, and even then the coverage is limited. Medicare provides no payment for assisted-living care.
  - Medicaid pays for most nursing home care in this country. This is causing financial strain for both the facilities and the government, as the cost of care continues to rise. Medicaid usually does not pay for assisted-living care.
  - Long-term care insurance is private insurance that can help pay for long-term care. Premiums are expensive, benefits may be limited, and there is the possibility that the policy-holder may never actually benefit from the policy.

WHAT DID YOU LEARN?

Multiple Choice

Select the single best answer for each of the following questions.

1. What is the name of the law that called for the biggest cut in the Medicare budget in history?
   a. Balanced Budget Act of 1997
   b. Deficit Reduction Act of 2005
   c. Omnibus Budget Reconciliation Act (OBRA) of 1987
   d. Social Security Act of 1935

2. Which one of the following is an insurance policy for long-term care that can be purchased by an individual?
   a. Long-term care insurance
   b. Medicaid
   c. Medicare
   d. Pension

3. How is most assisted-living care paid for?
   a. Medicaid
   b. Medicare
   c. Private pay
   d. Long-term care insurance

4. What did the members of the Pioneer Network do?
   a. They started a movement to get older people out of poorhouses in the late 1800s
   b. They met to share ideas and create a new vision for the future of long-term care
   c. They investigated nursing home care and wrote the report that led to the Omnibus Budget Reconciliation Act (OBRA) in 1987
   d. They developed the Social Security program in the 1930s

5. What is a benefit period?
   a. The period of time when a person receives nursing home care after using up all private funds
   b. The period of time when long-term care insurance benefits are paid out to a person who has purchased a policy
   c. The period of time when a person is eligible for Medicare benefits
   d. The period of time that Medicaid pays for a person's nursing home care

Matching

Match each numbered item with its appropriate lettered description.

_____ **1.** Pension

_____ **2.** For-profit facility

_____ **3.** Continuing care retirement community (CCRC)

_____ **4.** Poorhouse

_____ **5.** Centers for Medicare and Medicaid Services (CMS)

_____ **6.** Omnibus Budget Reconciliation Act (OBRA)

_____ **7.** Continuing Care Accreditation Commission (CCAC)

_____ **8.** Culture change

_____ **9.** Chain facility

_____ **10.** Continuum of care

a. A long-term care facility that provides multiple levels of care and multiple services on one campus

b. A facility that is operated with the intent of making money for the business owners

c. Community-supported facilities that provided shelter for those without the means of supporting themselves from the mid-1800s until the 1930s in the United States

d. The delivery of health care over time as a person moves from being independent to needing assistance with personal care, medical care, or both

e. A facility owned by a corporation that owns other similar facilities

f. An ongoing process that focuses on changing attitudes, goals, and practices in order to improve the long-term care environment and the way care is delivered

g. Tough regulations put into action to improve the quality of care and quality of life for residents of nursing homes

h. The government agency that provides oversight to ensure nursing home compliance with OBRA regulations

i. Monthly income provided to older Americans as a result of the Social Security Act of 1935

j. An organization that provides voluntary oversight of continuing care retirement communities (CCRCs) and offers accreditation to those meeting their quality standards

STOP and Think!

- How would your life change if you had to take in an elderly, dependent family member because there were no other options available to provide care? What difficulties would you encounter? What would be the benefits?

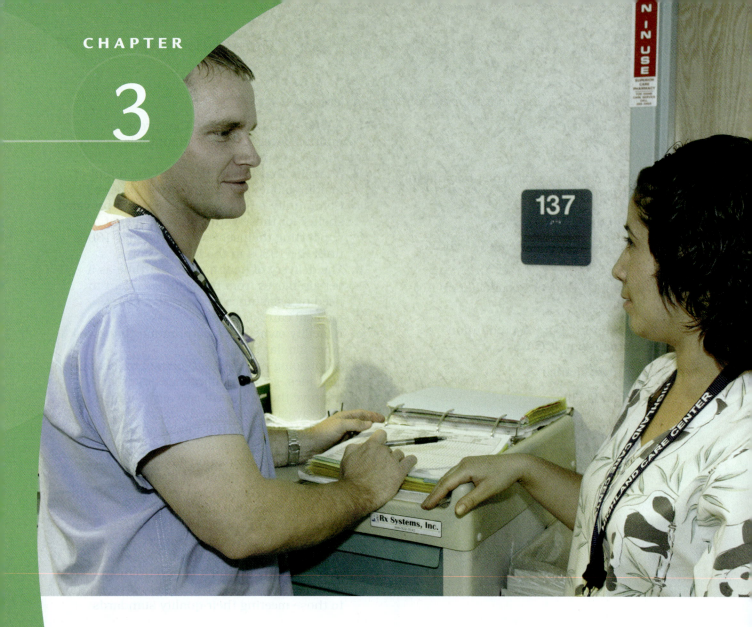

The Nursing Assistant and the Nursing Team

WHAT WILL YOU LEARN?

The nursing team is responsible for providing care to residents. As a nursing assistant, you will be an important member of both the nursing team and the health care team. What education is needed to become a nursing assistant, and what contributions will you make to resident care? What personal qualities are important for a nursing assistant to have? In this chapter, we will answer those questions, as well as describe the various ways in which nursing care can be delivered. We will also discuss how the nursing assistant, the nurse, and the other members of the nursing department work together to

Photo: Nurses and nursing assistants work together to provide resident care.

achieve the goal of safe, efficient resident care. When you are finished with this chapter, you will be able to:

1. Discuss the responsibilities of the nursing assistant.
2. Discuss the Omnibus Budget Reconciliation Act (OBRA) requirements for nursing assistant training.
3. Describe the contents of the registry.
4. Define the terms *professionalism* and *work ethic* and describe how good work habits promote professionalism.
5. Understand the importance of personal health and hygiene for the health care worker.
6. List the members of the nursing team, and describe the role of each team member.
7. List the steps of the nursing process, and describe how nurses in all care settings use the nursing process to plan care.
8. Discuss the delegation process as it relates to the nursing assistant.
9. List the five rights of delegation.

Vocabulary Use the CD in the front of your book to hear these terms pronounced and defined:

Competency evaluation	Empathy	Unit manager	Nursing process
Registry	Hygiene	Shift supervisor	Delegate
Reciprocity	Licensed practical nurse	Director of nursing	Nurse practice acts
Professional	(LPN) or licensed	(DON)	Five rights of
Professionalism	vocational nurse (LVN)	Certified nurse	delegation
Attitude	Registered nurse (RN)	practitioner (CRNP)	Scope of practice
Work ethic	Charge nurse	Care plan	

NURSING, PAST AND PRESENT

Very simply stated, the field of nursing involves caring for others. People who enter the field of nursing, such as nurses and nursing assistants, provide physical and emotional care for people who are sick, disabled, or injured. Many nurses also work to keep people healthy, by teaching them about ways to maintain health and prevent illness.

Perhaps you have heard of Florence Nightingale. Florence Nightingale (1820–1910) was a British nurse who is credited with making nursing into the profession that it is today (Fig. 3-1). Ms. Nightingale started training programs for nurses and set up practices for hospital cleanliness and patient care that are followed to this day. By establishing educational standards for nursing professionals, Ms. Nightingale improved conditions for both the people receiving health care and those providing it. For the first time, those in the nursing field were regarded as professionals in their own right, with specialized knowledge, skills, and responsibilities.

The knowledge, skills, and responsibilities of the nursing assistant have grown over the years too. Early nursing assistants, often referred to as "aides" or "orderlies," were employed in nursing homes and hospitals to help the nurses care for residents and patients. These aides usually did not have training in the health care field, which led to poor care in many cases. Today's nursing assistants, however, are well-trained members of the health care team with many important responsibilities.

RESPONSIBILITIES AND EDUCATION OF THE NURSING ASSISTANT

RESPONSIBILITIES OF THE NURSING ASSISTANT

The duties of the nursing assistant vary according to the setting, but all nursing assistants assist nurses in giving care to patients or residents by

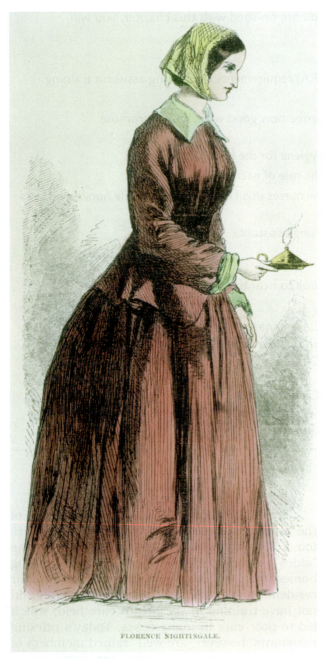

Figure 3-1

Florence Nightingale was a British nurse who established educational standards for nursing professionals.
(© *National Library of Medicine/Photo Researchers, Inc.*)

port, and helping your residents to feel valued and cared for as individuals). Demonstrating kindness and a willingness to listen, and paying attention to each resident's interests and activities, lets your residents know that they are important to you and that you care for them as individuals. Making the effort to really listen to what residents or family members are telling you will help you to better know and understand them. It will help you to individualize care for your residents, which will greatly contribute to their sense of well-being and enhance their quality of life.

Finally, you will play an important role as "observer and communicator." As the member of the health care team with the most opportunity to interact with the residents, you will be in a unique position to observe changes in the resident's physical, mental, or emotional status, and report these observations to the nurse. You will also play an important role in communicating with family members of residents, who will want to hear from you how their loved one is doing while they are not around.

EDUCATION OF THE NURSING ASSISTANT

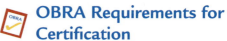

OBRA Requirements for Certification

As you learned in Chapter 2, a major goal of OBRA was to improve the quality of care given to residents of nursing homes. To ensure that nursing assistants have the necessary knowledge and skills to give care, OBRA requires nursing assistants who want to be employed in nursing homes to complete a training program and pass a test that evaluates both their knowledge *and* skills.

Training can be offered in vocational schools, community colleges, and private training academies. In addition, many long-term care facilities have their own nursing assistant training programs. All programs must submit proof that they meet federal standards, as well as any state- specific standards, in order to be approved by the state's authorizing agency.

OBRA mandates a *minimum* of 75 hours of training. States must meet the OBRA minimum of 75 hours of training, but many require more hours. This training must include classroom lectures and hands-on practice of skills, as well as supervised experience in an actual health care setting.

As you complete your nursing assistant training program, you will study communication skills,

performing basic nursing functions. As a nursing assistant in a long-term care facility, most of your responsibilities will relate to meeting the basic physical needs of residents, which include hygiene, safety, comfort, nutrition, exercise, and elimination (Fig. 3-2).

In addition to taking care of residents' physical needs, you will play an important role in meeting residents' social and emotional needs (for example, by providing companionship and emotional sup-

HIGHLAND CARE CENTER
JOB DESCRIPTION

CERTIFIED NURSING ASSISTANT
(CNA)

SUPERVISOR : CHARGE NURSE/DIRECTOR OF NURSING

GENERAL QUALIFICATIONS

I.   SKILL LEVEL AND EXPERIENCE:

A. Must be a Certified Nursing Assistant as required by state and federal law.
B. If applicant is an Aide in Training, certification must be obtained within 4 months of hire.
C. Must complete orientation required by company policy.
D. Must complete health screening and TB test (if required) within 2 weeks of employment.
E. Must complete a mandatory drug test within 90 days of hire.
F. Must be free of criminal activity proven by a criminal background check.
G. Must become familiar with and comply to all local, state, and federal regulations relating to the job.
H. Must obtain a current Food Handler's Permit within 14 days of hire.
I. Must show within 3 days of hire satisfactory evidence of identity and eligibility for employment.
J. Previous experience as a CNA and experience in working with geriatric residents is preferred and may be required.

II. COMMUNICATION AND DECISION-MAKING SKILLS:

A. Must possess the ability to work well and communicate effectively with other employees, residents, family members, visitors, government agencies, the general public, etc.
B. Must be able to read, write, speak, and understand English sufficiently to perform required duties.
C. Must be perceptive, with good judgment and decision-making/problem-solving skills.
D. Must be able to understand and implement the plan of care and assess resident needs.
E. Must be able to follow verbal and written instructions.

III. PERSONAL CHARACTERISTICS:

A. Must show courtesy and respect to other employees, residents, family members, visitors, government agencies, the general public, etc.
B. Must maintain good personal hygiene and dress and groom appropriately.
C. Must not be a habitual abuser of drugs (prescription or non-prescription) or alcohol.

IV. WORKING CONDITIONS & ENVIRONMENTAL PARAMETERS:

A. Must be very flexible and willing to cover shifts for other employees who are on vacation, sick, etc. Shift work will be required.
B. Must be willing to work holidays and weekends.
C. Must possess the ability to work in a wet or humid environment.
D. Must be able and willing to work with body fluids, excretions, extreme odors, etc., while using universal precautions.
E. Is subject to exposure to infectious waste, diseases, conditions, etc., including the AIDS and Hepatitis B viruses.
F. Must be able to relate to and work with the ill, disabled, elderly, emotionally upset, and, at times, hostile people within the facility.

V. PHYSICAL ABILITIES:

A. Must be able to sit, walk, run, lift and carry in excess of 75 pounds, bend, climb, kneel, squat, stoop, push, pull, grasp, reach arms above head, and have hand and finger dexterity.
B. Must be able to rapidly assist in the evacuation of all residents from the building in case of emergency.
C. Must be able to cope with the mental and emotional stress of working daily with geriatric residents and dealing with emergency situations.

Figure 3-2
It is always a good idea to be very familiar with your formal job description at each facility where you work. Here is an example of a typical job description for a nursing assistant.
(*Courtesy of Highland Care Center, Salt Lake City, Utah.*)

    D.   Must be able to see, hear, and smell sufficiently to ensure the personal comfort, dignity, health, and safety of the residents, and to assure that the requirements of this position can be fully met.

    E.   Must be in good general heath and be emotionally stable.

    F.   Must be able to perform the essential job functions without posing a direct threat to residents, self, or others.

VI.   EQUIPMENT TO BE USED:

Must be able to operate the following equipment: fire extinguisher, blood pressure cuff, stethoscope, weight chair, mechanical lift, thermometer, restraints, whirlpool bath, gait belt, hair dryer, rollers, curling iron, and other equipment as required to do the job.

ESSENTIAL JOB FUNCTIONS

I.   POLICIES:

    A.   Report on time as scheduled and follow all company policies and procedures.

    B.   Attend staff meetings and in-service sessions and complete 12 hours per year continuing education.

    C.   Become thoroughly familiar with emergency procedures and all applicable nursing procedures currently in use.

    D.   Must be able to perform duties in a timely fashion, and within the prescribed sequences and schedules.

    E.   Must be able to perform assigned tasks with a minimum of supervision and develop an awareness for and a willingness to perform other tasks, as needed, without constant supervision.

    F.   Must possess the ability to seek out new methods and principles and be willing to incorporate them into existing practices.

    G.   Must respect all resident rights, including the confidentiality of resident care information.

    H.   Follow all established safety precautions when operating equipment, and report hazardous and defective equipment or conditions to your supervisor.

    I.   Must be cooperative with other departments and be courteous and respectful in dealing with them at all times.

    J.   Report immediately to the Charge Nurse, to the Administrator, and to the proper legal authorities if you have reason to believe a resident has been physically, emotionally, or sexually abused, or been a victim of theft of their personal property.

    K.   Participate in and respond professionally to surveys (inspections) conducted by government agencies.

    L.   Create and maintain an atmosphere of warmth, cheerfulness, enthusiasm, and love, giving the resident the quality of service you would want to receive personally.

II.   PATIENT CARE:

    A.   The primary purpose of your position is to provide your assigned residents with routine daily nursing care in accordance with current regulations, established nursing care procedures, and as may be directed by your supervisors, and to provide quality patient care on a consistent basis.

    B.   Assume the authority, responsibility, and accountability necessary to carry out the assigned duties.

    C.   Assist residents as needed with activities of daily living. This includes bathing, hair care, nail care, oral care, shaving, dressing, eating, pericare, restraining (if ordered), assisting to and from bed, toileting, turning, transferring, lifting, changing when needed, etc.

    D.   Bathe each resident according to schedule. Change bed linens completely on bath days, more often as needed. Clean showers and tub rooms thoroughly before and after each use.

    E.   Make rounds regularly on each shift and assist each resident as needed, making sure they are safe, clean, and comfortable.

    F.   Always respect resident privacy and confidentiality including all details of resident care. Refer all questions regarding patient's status to the Charge Nurse and all questions regarding operation of care center to the Administrator.

    G.   Safeguard and use appropriately all resident belongings and appliances: hearing aids, eyeglasses, dentures, clothing, personal property, etc.

    H.   Escort residents to scheduled activities (recreational, religious, etc.) according to care plan.

    I.   Bring residents to the dining area, serve trays, feed residents as needed, and provide assistance to those not totally independent. Pick up trays and replace in kitchen cart for depository. Document meal intake percentage.

    J.   Fill resident water pitchers with ice water at least once a shift.

    K.   Perform restorative and rehabilitative nursing tasks as ordered. This includes turning and massaging bedfast residents every 2 hours, giving exercises as ordered, ambulating, checking and releasing restraints every 2 hours for 15 minutes, toileting every 2 hours or as ordered or as needed.

    L.   Inform the Charge Nurse of any observed change in resident's condition. This includes decrease in level of response, alteration in bowel function, skin lesions, changes in skin color or temperature, bruises, rashes, falls or other accidents, altered behavior, etc.

    M.   Accurately document all duties performed on the appropriate records. This includes flow sheets, charts, notes, accident reports, intake and output records, record of restraints, etc.

Figure 3-2 (*Continued*)

III.   LAUNDRY & CLEANING

    A.   Make sure all resident clothing is properly marked and returned to the owner after being laundered.

    B.   Take or send soiled linen and clothing to the laundry in properly secured laundry bags as soon as the bag is full and at the end of each shift, whether the bag is full or not. Linens soiled with feces, vomitus, blood, or any other bodily waste products must be thoroughly rinsed in the hopper room before being sent to the laundry.

    C.   Keep resident rooms clean and orderly. (This includes nightstands, dressers, over-bed tables and closets.) Mop up spills and clean messes made by residents as needed.

    D.   Help maintain cleanliness of work areas, break areas, and linen closets. Make sure that equipment and supplies are properly stored before leaving for breaks and at the end of each shift.

    E.   If a resident has been discharged, have the cleaning staff completely clean and disinfect the area and get resident room ready for reoccupancy.

OTHER DUTIES

Perform other duties as may be assigned by the Charge Nurse or the Director of Nursing within the scope of CNA certification.

Check one

_____   I have read the above job description and can perform all duties as outlined.

_____   I have read the above job description and cannot perform the duties listed below and would like to discuss reasonable accommodation:

_____

_____

_____

_____   _____
Signature   Date

Figure 3-2 (*Continued*)

infection control, safety and emergency procedures, residents' rights, basic nursing skills, personal care skills, feeding techniques, and skin care. You will also learn how to help residents move from place to place, change positions, dress, and perform range-of-motion exercises. In addition, you will learn the signs and symptoms of common diseases, and how to care for people who have problems with thinking and memory. During the practical experience portion of the course, you will have the opportunity to practice what you have learned by caring for patients or residents in a health care facility (Fig. 3-3).

The training ends with a **competency evaluation,** which involves a written test (consisting of approximately 75 multiple-choice questions) and a skills test (during which you will be asked to perform selected nursing skills learned in the training program). The actual number of test questions that you must answer and skills that you must demonstrate is determined by the state. You will have three opportunities to complete the evaluation successfully. This is mandated by OBRA. The pass rate (or score that you must attain in order to pass the evaluation) varies from state to state.

Some states allow a person who has on-the-job experience as a health care worker or one who has been trained in a related field to take the competency evaluation without completing the training course. However, the person must pass both the written and skills portions of the competency evaluation on the first try. If he does not, then he must complete the course before taking the competency evaluation again.

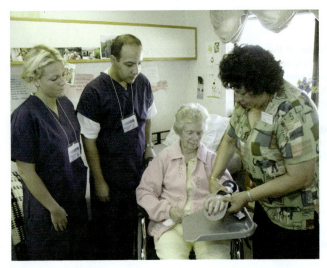

Figure 3-3
Part of a nursing assistant's training involves working with residents in an actual health care setting.

When you complete your training program and pass the competency evaluation, you will be certified to work as a nursing assistant in the state where you completed your training and passed your competency evaluation. To remain certified, you must work as a nursing assistant providing direct care for residents or patients for a minimum number of hours (determined by the state) to keep your knowledge and skills current. You may also need to provide proof of your employment status to renew your certificate. OBRA requires nursing assistants who have not met the minimum requirement for 2 years in a row to undergo retraining and pass a competency evaluation. It is your professional responsibility to maintain your certification and to renew when you are required.

 ### Registry

OBRA requires every state to maintain a **registry,** an official record of the people who have successfully completed the nursing assistant training program. The registry contains the following information about each nursing assistant:

- Full name, including maiden name and any married names
- Last known home address
- Social Security number
- Date of birth
- Date the competency evaluation was passed
- Reported incidents of resident abuse or neglect, or theft of resident property

Long-term care facility employers check this registry to verify certifications as part of the hiring process. Information about performance concerns, such as resident abuse, must remain in the registry for at least 5 years. It is important that you notify the nurse aide registry in the state that issued your most recent certification of any changes in the information contained in your registry record, especially address changes. Notification that it is time to renew your certification will be sent to the address that the registry has on file for you. If you do not receive this notification and as a result fail to renew your certification, your certification could lapse, making you ineligible to work as a nursing assistant.

Reciprocity

Some states practice the principle of **reciprocity.** This means that in many cases, your certification will be valid in states other than where you originally trained. However, before working in another state, you must go through the official process of getting your certification approved by that state. Usually this involves contacting the state's nurse aide registry and completing an application. In addition to submitting the application, you may also be required to demonstrate competency in the new state. If you want to work in a state that requires more hours of training than you have, additional training can be obtained.

Continuing Education

Regular in-service education and performance reviews are also mandated by OBRA. Once you are certified, you must complete a *minimum* of 12 hours of continuing education per year (some states require more). Most nursing homes provide for this requirement through their in-service training programs. During in-service training, new knowledge and skills may be taught or existing ones reviewed, depending on the needs of the facility. Although it is the facility's responsibility to provide in-service training, it is your responsibility to attend the training to complete the required hours.

WORKING AS A PROFESSIONAL

The health care industry gives the title of **professional** to those who have credentials, obtained through education and training, that enable them to become licensed or certified to practice a certain profession. This industry certainly relies on all types of professionals, such as doctors, nurses, and nursing assistants, to provide quality care to residents. However, many people who are considered professionals do not need a license or a certificate to perform their jobs, and they may not even need a specific educational background. Being a professional also means having a professional attitude, or exhibiting **professionalism.**

An **attitude** is the side of ourselves that we display to the world, communicating outwardly how we feel about things. A person's attitude is apparent from things he says (and the way he says them), the way he behaves, and the way he looks. You may have heard it said about a person that he or she "has an attitude," meaning that the person's outward behavior is unpleasant. Well, an attitude is something we all possess and it can be positive instead of negative.

Possessing a positive attitude in the workplace means that you are caring and compassionate toward your residents, and that you demonstrate a commitment to doing your job to the best of your ability at all times. This commitment to doing your best is the attitude that defines professionalism, the attitude of being a professional. While your job as a nursing assistant will allow you to earn a paycheck, a true professional views her work as a reflection of the role she plays in society. Income is important, but so is the sense of pride you will feel as a result of setting high standards for your performance and obtaining satisfaction from the work you do, and in knowing that you are helping others. Regardless of the level of education, certification, or experience a health care professional has, professionalism is all about exhibiting the right attitude to co-workers, residents, and visitors. Professionalism is a choice you make and requires effort. What attitude will you choose to show?

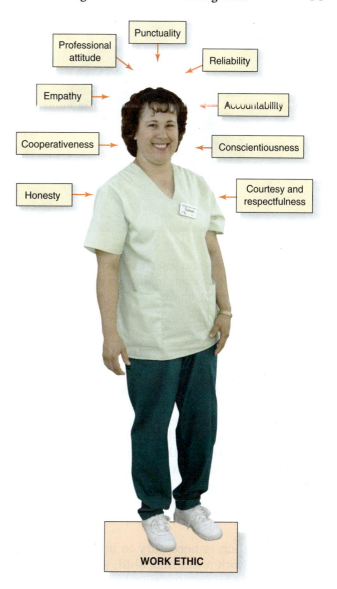

Figure 3-4
Professionalism and a strong work ethic go hand-in-hand. Many qualities contribute to a strong work ethic.

HAVING A STRONG WORK ETHIC

A **work ethic** can be described in many ways and measured by any number of standards, but simply put, it relates specifically to your attitude toward your work. Professionalism and a strong work ethic go hand-in-hand (Fig. 3-4).

A strong work ethic is what separates an average employee from a great employee. Two nursing assistants can have solid skills and be very good at getting their work done on time, but the nursing assistant with the strongest work ethic will be the one who enjoys the greatest professional success. A good work ethic not only allows a person to grow in her career (because her employer will be satis-

fied with the quality of her work), but it also allows her to experience the emotional rewards of knowing that she has made her best effort.

There are many qualities that are associated with a strong work ethic such as cheerfulness and enthusiasm, a willingness to volunteer for new assignments, and a desire to learn new skills. A nursing assistant with a strong work ethic is someone you can depend on and trust, and someone who treats others with kindness, respect, and compassion. People with strong work ethics know how to do their jobs well, they like their jobs, and they continue to learn and improve. Let's discuss some specific qualities that define a good work ethic.

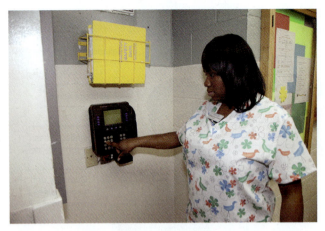

Figure 3-5

Being punctual means that you are on time or a little early. It is important to come to work on time because many people are relying on you.

Punctuality

Being punctual means that you are on time, or a little bit early (Fig. 3-5). Arriving to work on time prepared to start your duties is vital in the health care industry. Many people are relying on you! The staff working the shift before yours is anxious for you to relieve them so that they can go home to their families and other responsibilities. If you work a morning shift, residents will need your assistance in getting out of bed, preparing for breakfast, and getting ready for the activities of the day.

Organization is necessary to achieve punctuality. If you work a morning shift, plan ahead the evening before by packing your lunch and making sure your uniform is clean and pressed. If you have children, pack their lunches, lay out their clothes for the next day, and make sure any papers they need for school are completed. Setting the alarm 15 minutes earlier will not significantly affect the amount of sleep you get, but it will allow you that extra time you need to have breakfast before work, or tend to any small last-minute crises.

Reliability

Reliability is an essential characteristic for a nursing assistant. Reliability means that others can count on you to do your job conscientiously and well, with minimal supervision. Your supervisor should not feel the need to look over your shoulder or "check up" on you to make sure your work has been finished.

Reliability also means that others can count on you to come to work every day, as scheduled, and to remain there during your entire shift (in other words, that your attendance is consistent). Everyone certainly has to miss a day of work occasionally for sickness or emergencies, but frequent absences are a very poor reflection on your work ethic. Have alternative plans for transportation and childcare in place before the need arises, and try to keep yourself healthy to decrease your need to take sick days. Poor attendance and chronic lateness are primary reasons employers take corrective action against nursing assistants.

If you do not come to work as scheduled, your manager will need to spend time trying to find someone to cover your shift. One of your co-workers will have to come in on a scheduled day off, or stay extra hours. If no one can be found to cover your shift, then your co-workers who are scheduled for that shift will have to do their own assignments, in addition to yours. This significantly increases their workload, which jeopardizes safety and overall quality of care. You can certainly see why reliability is an important quality for any nursing assistant to have!

Accountability

Accountability is also an essential characteristic for a nursing assistant. An accountable person accepts responsibility for his or her actions and the results of those actions. Being accountable means that you can accept criticism that is intended to help you improve, admit a mistake, and work to correct the situation. Although it can be difficult to admit that you have made a mistake, trying to conceal a mistake or blame it on someone else will only make matters worse. By acknowledging a mistake and taking measures to correct it, you are not only acting in the best interest of your resident, you are letting your supervisors and co-workers know that you can be trusted to do your job to the best of your ability at all times, and that you are interested in learning how to prevent similar mistakes from happening in the future.

Conscientiousness

Conscientious nursing assistants take their assignments seriously and make sure they follow directions carefully. They demonstrate responsibility by asking for additional explanation or clarification when necessary, seeking help with difficult tasks, and admitting that they may not know how to perform a particular task. If you have not been shown how to do a procedure that you have been asked to do, show that you are interested in learning how. A conscientious nursing assistant attends to details and goes the extra mile to complete a task with care. When you act conscientiously, you leave your residents feeling like they are special and have received the "royal treatment."

Courtesy and Respectfulness

Always treat your residents, their families, and your co-workers with respect. The phrases *please, thank you,* and *excuse me* can improve the quality of almost any interaction. Avoid using "baby talk" or "talking down" to residents. Address people as they prefer to be addressed. If in doubt, err on the side of formality ("Dr. Smith," "Mrs. Jones," "Mr. Davis," "Miss Thomson"). In some parts of the United States, such as the Deep South, elderly people prefer to be addressed by their first names, preceded by "Miss" or "Mr." ("Miss Katharine"), and "ma'am" and "sir" are always used. Being polite and having good manners is correct in any situation. Considering another person's feelings and beliefs shows that you truly care about the person.

Show respect for your co-workers and supervisors by not saying anything negative about them to your residents, or other co-workers. Do not speak poorly about your place of employment to others, even if there are things that you are not happy with. People who hear you say negative things about your place of employment will begin to wonder about you and why you continue to work there if the situation is so bad. If the person you are speaking to is a resident or a family member, he or she may begin to question the quality of care that is being given. Imagine how you would feel if the person taking care of you complained about the place where you lived, or about other people who you relied on for care!

Honesty

Honesty is a critical quality for health care workers to have. You are expected to accurately record vital signs and other information about the condition of the people you care for. You will be trusted with information of a very private nature regarding your residents' medical conditions, and the care they are receiving. You will have access to your residents' valuables. Residents and families will come to trust you and confide in you. If you act in a way that gives your residents or their family members reason to lose confidence in their ability to trust you, it will be very difficult to reestablish your relationship.

Cooperativeness

Being able to cooperate, or work as part of a team, is essential in the health care field. Professionals with many different levels of education and areas of training work together to benefit the people they care for. Remember how important your part of the chain of care is and what an essential role you play in providing for the care and comfort of your residents, and use this as a driving force. Making an effort to get along with your co-workers will make your work easier and will ease the burden on your co-workers, as well. A good nursing assistant does not wait for a co-worker to ask for help; he or she sees a need and offers a helping hand. You will undoubtedly have to work with people you may not especially like, but a professional is able to put his or her personal feelings aside for the benefit of the resident.

Empathy

Empathy means that you are able to try and imagine what it would feel like to be in another person's situation. There are times when co-workers, residents, or family members will really try your patience, but if you think of how you would feel if you were in a similar situation, you may find that you are able to understand the offending behavior better. Empathy gives us another perspective and helps us to be kinder and more tolerant. Treating people with kindness is a better reflection of professionalism than, for example, displaying superior intellect.

A Desire to Learn

Although you may have completed your training as a nursing assistant, you will never stop needing to learn new things. The field of health care is constantly changing, and new techniques and treatments are developed daily. To provide the best possible care to your residents, you must continue to learn new ways of caring for them. It is not the responsibility of your supervisor or your place of employment to keep you up to date on new health care issues. It is your responsibility. There are many professional journals, some specifically for nursing assistants, that cover new information that is important for you to know. Learn about the illnesses or conditions that the people you are caring for have. Ask questions about new techniques or treatments you see being used. This way, you become more involved as a member of the health care team because you have a better understanding of the care being given.

MAINTAINING A PROFESSIONAL APPEARANCE

Personal **hygiene,** or cleanliness, addresses several issues. First, it promotes a professional image. If you care enough about yourself to keep yourself clean and neat, the people you care for will feel that you will do the same for them. Would you want to be cared for by someone with bad breath, body odors, or dirty hair? Second, good personal hygiene helps to prevent the spread of infection, both to your residents and to you and your family. In a health care setting, the potential to come into contact with all types of "germs" is increased, and practicing good personal hygiene is necessary. To practice good personal hygiene:

- Bathe daily and use a deodorant.
- Shampoo your hair regularly and treat dandruff or other scalp conditions.
- Keep your nails short and clean.
- Brush and floss your teeth and use mouthwash. Visit a dentist regularly. Poor dental health can cause breath odors and gum infections.
- Men should shave daily, or keep facial hair neatly groomed and trimmed.
- Wear a clean, pressed uniform each day.
- Wash your hands often.

When you picture a health care professional, what does she look like? Is she wearing a wrinkled, stained uniform? Is her hair unkempt? Are her shoes dirty? Of course not! The health care worker you picture in your mind is clean and neat, with an unwrinkled uniform and clean shoes (Fig. 3-6). Her hair is neatly styled and held back off the face. She wears few accessories. A watch with a second hand is an essential part of a nursing assistant's uniform, but bracelets, necklaces, rings, and dangling earrings are not. In the health care field, many of the traits we have come to associate with a professional image are related to maintaining safety and health. Guidelines for a professional appearance are given in Guidelines Box 3-1.

STAYING HEALTHY

To care for your residents to the best of your ability, you must first care for yourself. By taking proper care of yourself, you demonstrate that you are a professional who takes her responsibilities seriously.

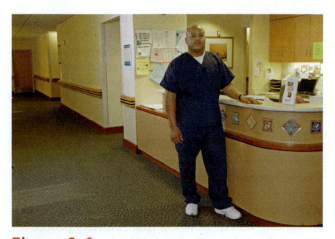

Figure 3-6

In the health care field, many of the traits we have come to associate with a professional image are related to maintaining safety and health.

Maintaining Your Physical Health

The duties of a nursing assistant require much physical effort. You will be constantly lifting, bending, walking, and reaching as you perform your daily tasks at work. As you will learn in later chapters, there are many risks to your health and physical condition in the health care profession. Your employer, your co-workers, your family, and especially your residents rely on you to be able to do your duties. In addition to giving you more energy, staying physically fit keeps your body strong and allows you to avoid many types of job-related injuries (Fig. 3-7). To keep your body in good physical condition:

- **Get enough sleep.** Most people need an average of 6 to 8 hours of sleep to function properly. Not only does rest relax the muscles, but also it relaxes the mind and allows you to think clearly. Too little rest can weaken your immune system, making you more likely to get infections, such as cold and flu viruses.
- **Eat well-balanced meals.** A working body needs good nutrition, a subject you will learn more about in Chapter 25. You need fuel for your muscles and for your brain. Avoid fad diets because they often are responsible for the loss of muscle mass and strength.
- **Exercise regularly.** Regular physical exercise gives you more strength and energy and keeps your heart and lungs healthy. In addition, regular exercise helps reduce the

Guidelines Box 3-1   Guidelines for a Professional Appearance

WHAT YOU DO	WHY YOU DO IT
Style your hair neatly and away from your face.	Securing your hair away from your face keeps it away from equipment, out of your eyes, and out of your work. If your hair is not secured back, when you move your hair out of your eyes, any dirt on your hands will be transferred to your hair and face.
Keep your nails short and clean, with smoothly filed edges.	Germs can hide under the tips of long nails. Long nails can also scratch a person's skin. Frequent handwashing can cause acrylic and false nails to lift, allowing water to become trapped underneath and leading to a fungal infection in the nailbed. Most facilities have policies that prohibit artificial nails.
Leave bracelets, necklaces, rings, and dangling earrings at home.	A child or confused person might pull dangling earrings through your earlobes. Necklaces and bracelets get in the way and can get caught in equipment and broken. If you wear rings, germs can become trapped underneath them, which makes handwashing less effective. Rings can also scratch a person's skin when you are providing care.
If you wear makeup, apply it lightly and tastefully.	Wearing too much makeup, or makeup that is too bright or too dark, does not contribute to a professional appearance.
If you wear cologne or perfume, it should be of a light fragrance and lightly applied.	Many people are sensitive to fragrances and may find perfume or cologne that is of a strong scent or heavily applied offensive.
Wear a clean, pressed uniform each day. Make sure that your shoes are polished.	Attention to details, such as making sure that your uniform is wrinkle-free and your shoes are polished, says to others that you care about your appearance. A clean uniform is also essential for limiting the spread of infection.
If you have a tattoo or body piercing, try to select a uniform style that will conceal it. If you are thinking about getting a tattoo or body piercing, consider its location carefully.	Many people feel that tattoos and body piercings make a person look less professional. Many facilities have dress codes that prohibit visible tattoos or body piercings.
Practice good personal hygiene and grooming daily.	Good personal hygiene helps to prevent breath and body odors and limits the spread of infection. In addition, if you care enough about yourself to keep yourself clean and neat, the people in your care will feel that you will do the same for them.

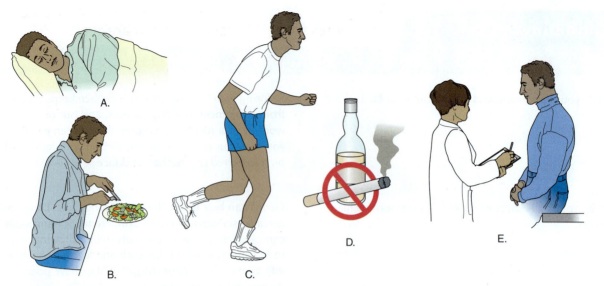

Figure 3-7

There are many things you can do to keep your body in good physical condition. **(A)** Get enough sleep. **(B)** Eat well-balanced meals. **(C)** Exercise regularly. **(D)** Avoid smoking, excessive alcohol consumption, and the use of recreational drugs. **(E)** Get routine physical examinations to detect health problems early.

mental stress that sometimes goes along with intensely emotional jobs, such as those in the health care field.

- **Do not smoke.** Smoking causes the blood vessels in the body to narrow, reducing the flow of oxygen-carrying blood to the body's cells. It is well known that smoking is associated with lung cancer, emphysema, and heart disease. Infertility, impotence, and an increased risk of miscarriage are other negative effects of smoking. In addition to being a health risk, smoking makes your clothes and breathe smell bad.
- **Do not take recreational drugs and limit your alcohol intake.** Recreational drugs are associated with many health problems. Many employers now perform drug screening of potential employees. Although many people feel that there is nothing wrong with occasionally having a drink if this is something you enjoy, drinking too much or too frequently can negatively impact your health and leave you unable to perform your job to the best of your ability. The health care profession needs workers who are clear-headed and able to make good decisions on behalf of others. Do not report to work while under the influence of recreational drugs or alcohol, or use these substances while on duty—doing so is dangerous for you, as well as for your residents and coworkers.

- **Have a routine physical examination.** Many chronic illnesses, such as high blood pressure and diabetes, go undetected until they have caused permanent damage to your body. Many types of cancers can be cured if detected early enough. Uncorrected vision and hearing problems can lead to errors when taking vital signs or reading product labels. Routine physical examinations can help you to detect problems early so that actions can be taken to correct them.

Maintaining Your Emotional Health

Caring for others is an emotionally demanding job, as well as a physically demanding one, for many reasons:

- Due to the shortage of health care workers, as well as a need to cut costs, many facilities are understaffed, which means that employees are often overworked.
- Not all residents are happy or grateful for the care they are receiving. Many people in need of care do not feel well and, as a result, may be difficult or hard to manage. Sometimes a person who is ill or worried will become angry or very critical and he or she will take these feelings out on you, even though you have done nothing wrong.
- As a health care worker, you will have to face the death of some of your residents. This can be difficult, especially in situations where

you have had a chance to develop a relationship with the resident and his or her family members.

Fortunately, there are actions you can take to help keep your emotions in check while you are on the job, and prevent emotional "burn-out":

- Maintain your physical health. It is proven that physical activity relieves mental and emotional stress.
- Be sure to schedule time for yourself. Most of us are not just caregivers in the workplace; we are caregivers at home as well. It is important to make time for yourself, to do what you like to do, in order to avoid feeling overwhelmed by your responsibilities at home and at work.
- Take advantage of counseling services offered by your employer, or confide in a clergy member. Talking to a professional can help you to manage work-related stress and define your feelings and beliefs about difficult subjects, such as death and dying (Fig. 3-8).
- When a situation becomes particularly "heated" at work, take a physical and emotional break. Have someone relieve you and take a walk outside to calm down.
- Ask to be assigned to different work areas, or to different residents, occasionally.

WORKING AS A MEMBER OF THE NURSING TEAM

MEMBERS OF THE NURSING DEPARTMENT

The nursing department is responsible for all aspects of the nursing care provided to residents. In a nursing home, the nursing department is made up of licensed nurses in a variety of different roles, as well as nursing assistants (Table 3-1). The two types of licensed nurses you will work with most frequently are **licensed practical nurses,** or **LPNs** (referred to in some states as **licensed vocational nurses,** or **LVNs**), and **registered nurses (RNs).** The difference between an LPN and an RN is in the level of education and training. The RN completes a longer training program that includes a broader scope of knowledge. Because of this training, RNs are able to perform some skills that LPNs may not be allowed to do.

You will work with nurses who have specific job titles and duties to perform within the nursing department (Fig. 3-9).

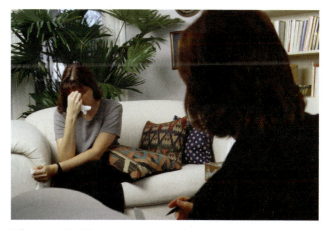

Figure 3-8
Talking with a counselor can help you to manage work-related stress.

- **Charge Nurse.** The **charge nurse** is a licensed nurse (an RN or LPN) who supervises the nursing assistants and may supervise another nurse for a particular shift.
- **Unit Manager.** The **unit manager** (sometimes called a *nurse manager* or *head nurse*) is usually an RN who is in charge of a particular floor or section of the facility. The unit manager supervises the charge nurse and has 24-hour-a-day responsibility for the operation of the floor or section.
- **Shift Supervisor.** The **shift supervisor** may have some of the same responsibilities as the unit manager, but these duties are generally limited to an assigned shift, instead of 24-hour-a-day responsibility.
- **Director of Nursing (DON).** All long-term care facilities have a **director of nursing (DON),** an RN who directs all of the nursing care within the facility. The DON is responsible for the overall operation of the entire nursing department. The DON hires and manages the nursing staff and is responsible for ensuring that the nursing care provided to residents meets quality and regulatory standards.
- **Coordinator (or Director) of In-Service Education (or Staff Development).** Most nursing homes have a nurse who is in charge of continuing education and staff development. The person in this role is responsible for developing and delivering in-service education sessions and other required training (such as first aid training). This person is also responsible for maintaining records of the educational activities that were offered and the attendance at those activities.
- **Quality Assurance (QA) Nurse** or **Quality Improvement (QI) Nurse.** The nurse in this

Table 3-1   Nurses and Nursing Assistants in Long-Term Care

TITLE	REQUIREMENTS TO PRACTICE	RESPONSIBILITIES
Registered nurse (RN)	A baccalaureate degree from a college or university (4 years) OR An associate degree from a junior or community college (2 years) PLUS A license obtained by passing a state board examination	Performs assessments, develops care plans, and coordinates activities of the health care team to ensure that the resident's needs are met Participates in resident care Delegates selected aspects of resident care to other team members, and supervises these team members as they carry out the delegated tasks Monitors the resident's response to the care plan and makes changes as needed
Licensed practical nurse (LPN) OR Licensed vocational nurse (LVN)	A certificate from a 12- to 18-month training program offered by a vocational school, community college, or hospital PLUS A license obtained by passing a state board examination	Under the supervision of a registered nurse (RN), provides nursing care to residents Delegates selected aspects of resident care to other team members, and supervises these team members as they carry out the delegated tasks
Certified nursing assistant (CNA) OR Geriatric certified nursing assistant (GCNA or GNA)	A certificate from a 75- to 200-hour training program offered by a vocational school, community college, or health care facility, obtained by completing the training and passing a state-administered competency evaluation	Assists the RN or LPN with providing nursing care to residents; responsibilities include basic nursing tasks related to meeting hygiene, safety, comfort, nutrition, exercise, and elimination needs, as well as helping to meet the resident's emotional needs

position is responsible for tracking data that reflects quality-of-care issues such as the number of residents with infections, pressure ulcers, or weight loss; the number of falls that resulted in injuries, and the like.

This information is then used to identify care practices that may need to be improved.

- **Registered Nurse Assessment Coordinator (RNAC).** Federal law requires an RN to be in

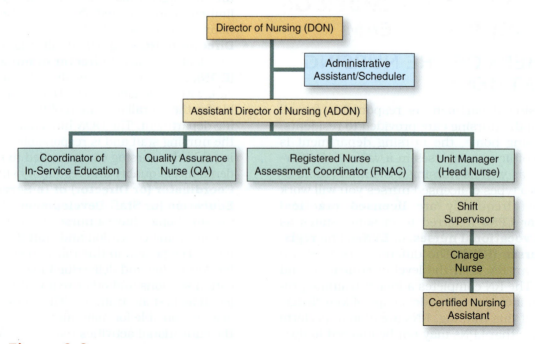

Figure 3-9

The typical organization of the nursing department in a long-term care facility. Here, only one unit manager is shown, but in actual practice, there would be more than one unit manager in the organization.

charge of the assessment process that is used to complete the Minimum Data Set (MDS). (The MDS is a document that is used to determine and record the degree of assistance or skilled care that each resident of a nursing home needs. You will learn more about the MDS in Chapter 12.) Other nurses and members of the health care team may contribute to the assessment process, but the RNAC is responsible for ensuring the accuracy of nursing assessment documentation. He or she is also responsible for making sure that the entire MDS is completed, per the requirements of the law. In some facilities, these responsibilities are handled by the charge nurse or a head nurse, instead of by an RNAC.

- **Certified nurse practitioner (CRNP).** A **certified nurse practitioner (CRNP)** is an RN who has completed additional training for licensure in advanced practice. These highly trained nurses are able to do some tasks that usually only doctors are allowed to do, such as perform advanced health assessments, interpret laboratory results, and manage and treat selected medical conditions. The CRNP may also be allowed to write orders for diagnostic tests or medications. The CRNP is able to provide more immediate evaluation and treatment when the doctor is not available. The CRNP, although part of the nursing department, does not have any management responsibilities.

THE NURSING PROCESS

The doctor is responsible for diagnosing a person's medical problems and ordering medication or other therapies to correct those problems. The nursing team is responsible for carrying out the doctor's orders and providing holistic care to the resident. To achieve the nursing team's goals, the nursing team develops a **care plan** for each resident with the help of other health care team members.

The **nursing process** is used to create the care plan. The nursing process allows members of the nursing team to communicate with each other regarding the resident's specific nursing care needs, what steps will be taken to meet those needs, and whether or not the steps were effective in meeting the person's needs. The five steps of the nursing process are described in Box 3-1. As a nursing assistant, you will be involved in the implementation step of the nursing process. You will also help the nurse with the assessment and evaluation steps of the nursing process by observing how your residents are doing and reporting this information to the nurse.

BOX 3-1   The Nursing Process

1. **Assessment.** During this step, the nurse gathers information about the resident. As part of the assessment process, the nurse examines the resident and asks questions about his abilities, habits, and needs.

2. **Diagnosis.** Using the information gathered during the assessment step, the nurse then develops a *nursing diagnosis*, or a statement that describes a problem the resident is having, as well as the cause of the problem. Unlike a medical diagnosis, which identifies a medical problem that must be managed by a doctor, a nursing diagnosis identifies a problem that the nursing staff can manage independently.

3. **Planning.** The next step in the nursing process involves making a plan for the person's nursing care. Using information obtained from the nursing diagnosis, the nurse develops *interventions* (actions that will be taken by the nursing team to help the resident) and *goals* (descriptions of what the interventions are meant to achieve). The interventions and goals that have been set for the resident are written down in a formal way. This document is the care plan.

4. **Implementation.** During the implementation step, the interventions that were detailed in the care plan are carried out. The care plan specifies the nursing team members who are responsible for each intervention.

5. **Evaluation.** During the evaluation step, the nursing team checks the effectiveness of the care plan and revises it as necessary. Is the care plan working? What needs to be improved or changed to meet the goals? Has the resident's status changed? Is the existing care plan still appropriate for the resident? If certain interventions are not working or if the goals have been met, the care plan will change.

DELEGATION

As a nursing assistant, you will be a very important member of the nursing team. The nursing team, a subset of the health care team, is responsible for providing care to the residents. At minimum, the nursing team consists of a licensed nurse and a nursing assistant. The way in which the members of the nursing team work together to care for residents varies, depending on the size of the facility and the available resources.

In order to ensure that the necessary care is given and the nursing team functions efficiently, a nurse has the authority to delegate selected tasks to a nursing assistant. To **delegate** a task means to give another person permission to perform that task on your behalf. State **nurse practice acts** (state laws that govern nursing practice and education) give RNs and LPNs the responsibility for performing nursing tasks and the authority necessary to fulfill this responsibility. Although a nurse may delegate a task to a nursing assistant, the nurse remains ultimately responsible for the quality of care.

Typically, the nurse will delegate nursing tasks related to routine care (hygiene, comfort, exercise) to nursing assistants. The nurse can also delegate certain nursing tasks, such as data collection and documentation, to a nursing assistant. However, nursing tasks that require professional judgment, such as assessment, planning, or evaluating, cannot be delegated to a nursing assistant. For example, a nursing assistant can take a person's vital signs and record this information on the person's chart, but the assistant is not qualified to interpret the data.

Understanding how a nurse decides which tasks to delegate will help you to understand why you may be asked to do certain tasks but not others. When delegating a task, the nurse must know the abilities and qualifications of the nursing assistant, and she or another licensed nurse must be available to provide supervision. In addition, she must consider the resident's individual needs. In order to enable nurses to make good decisions about which tasks to delegate and to whom, the National Council of State Boards of Nursing (NCSBN) has developed guidelines called the **five rights of delegation** (Table 3-2).

You and the nurse share the responsibility for making sure that delegated tasks are carried out,

without causing harm to the resident. The nurse is responsible for making good decisions about which tasks to delegate and for providing adequate supervision. You are responsible for recognizing which delegated tasks are within your **scope of practice** (the range of tasks a nursing assistant is legally permitted to do) and range of abilities, and using this knowledge as the basis for either accepting or refusing the assignment. Just as a nurse uses the five rights of delegation to decide which tasks to delegate and to whom, you can use the five rights of delegation to help you decide whether to accept or decline a delegated task (see Table 3-2). When you agree to perform a task, you accept responsibility for your actions. You must ask for help when you have questions or are unsure about how to proceed, and you must communicate with the nurse by reporting what you have done and what you observed.

You should never refuse an assignment simply because you do not want to do it. You must have a good reason for refusing to carry out an assignment, or you could lose your job. Valid reasons for refusing an assignment include the following:

- The task is not in your job description. Box 3-2 summarizes tasks that are generally outside of the scope of practice of a nursing assistant.
- Carrying out the task could result in harm to the resident.
- The task is illegal or unethical.
- The nurse is not available to supervise your efforts.
- You do not have the proper equipment.
- The directions are not clear.

Table 3-2	Five Rights of Delegation	
	QUESTIONS THE NURSE MUST CONSIDER	**QUESTIONS THE NURSING ASSISTANT MUST CONSIDER**
The right task	Is this a task that can be delegated? Does the nurse practice act allow me to delegate the task? Is the task in the job description for the nursing assistant?	Does the state allow me to perform this task? Have I been trained to do this task? Do I have experience performing this task? Is this task in my job description?
The right circumstance	What is the patient's or resident's condition? Is he or she stable? What are the needs of the patient or resident at this time?	Can I perform this task safely, given the patient's or resident's condition?
The right person	Does the nursing assistant have the right training and experience to safely complete the task?	Am I confident that I can perform this task safely? Do I have any reservations about performing this task, and if so, what are they?
The right direction	Am I able to give the nursing assistant clear direction regarding how to perform this task? Am I able to explain to the nursing assistant what is expected?	Did the nurse give me clear instructions? Do I understand what the nurse expects?
The right supervision	Will I be available to supervise and answer questions?	Will the nurse be available to supervise and answer questions?

BOX 3-2	Tasks That Are Generally Beyond the Nursing Assistant's Scope of Practice

Administering medications (including oxygen).
Some states allow nursing assistants to administer medications to residents in assisted-living facilities, if the nursing assistant has undergone specialized training to do so. Generally, only a licensed nurse (RN or LPN) or doctor is allowed to give medications. Nursing assistants may assist patients in taking medication by bringing water or assisting them into a proper position to receive medications.

Receiving verbal orders (in person or over the telephone) from doctors. Licensed nurses (RNs or LPNs) are the only personnel authorized to receive doctors' orders.

Diagnosing illness and prescribing medications.
Only doctors can diagnose illness and prescribe medical or surgical treatment.

Supervising other nursing assistants. Licensed nurses (RNs or LPNs) are responsible for supervising nursing assistants.

Performing procedures that require sterile technique. Nursing assistants are permitted to assist a nurse in performing a sterile procedure, but they are not trained to do these procedures themselves.

Inserting or removing tubes from a person's body (bladder, esophagus, trachea, nose, ears).
Nursing assistants generally are not trained in procedures that involve inserting or removing tubes from a person's body. Exceptions may be made if state law allows nursing assistants to perform advanced skills after receiving additional training and with the proper supervision.

- You are not able to perform the task safely.
- You have not been adequately trained to perform the task or use the necessary equipment.

If you do make the decision to decline a task that you have been assigned to do, it is your responsibility to state clearly that you are not going to do the task and your reason why. Failure to communicate your refusal to complete a task to the person requesting your help can jeopardize the care or safety of the resident. The person requesting your help assumes that you are doing the task, unless he or she hears otherwise. Declining a task

is a discussion that you should have privately with the person requesting the task of you. Do not discuss the issue in front of the resident or visitors.

General guidelines for accepting or declining an assignment are given in Guidelines Box 3-2. A good general rule to keep in mind is that you should not perform any task that is not listed in your job description. Because a nursing assistant's duties can vary from state to state, and also from facility to facility, you must be familiar with your formal job description. Ask your supervisor about anything you do not understand. This is important to protect yourself, as well as your residents.

Guidelines Box 3-2	Guidelines for Accepting or Declining an Assignment
WHAT YOU DO	**WHY YOU DO IT**
Always ask the nurse for clarification if there is something you do not understand.	It is your responsibility to make sure you know what is to be done and how it is to be done before going to the resident.
Never perform a task that you have not been taught to do, or that you feel uncomfortable doing, unless you are supervised by a nurse.	The nurse is ultimately responsible for ensuring the resident's safety. This means that it is the nurse's responsibility to ensure that whoever is performing the task on her behalf is qualified to do so, and capable. It is irresponsible for you to misrepresent your abilities, or to proceed unsupervised with a task that you are not fully capable of doing well.
Never ignore an assignment because you do not know how to perform the task or the task is beyond your scope of practice.	The resident's needs must be attended to, either by you or by someone else. If you feel that you cannot perform the task that you are being asked to do, explain your concerns to the nurse so that she can either help you with the task or reassign it.

SUMMARY

- Nursing assistants are health care professionals who assist the nurse by performing basic nursing functions such as those related to hygiene, safety, comfort, nutrition, exercise, and elimination.
  - Nursing assistants undergo training that authorizes them to perform certain tasks.
  - Nursing assistants present themselves as professionals when they have a positive attitude; a clean, neat appearance; and a solid work ethic.
    - Qualities that contribute to a solid work ethic include punctuality, reliability, accountability, conscientiousness, courtesy and respectfulness, honesty, cooperativeness, empathy, and a desire to learn.
    - Practicing good personal hygiene and taking steps to protect your physical and emotional health demonstrates that you take your professional responsibilities seriously.
- Nursing assistants are an integral part of the nursing team, a subset of the health care team.

- The nursing process is an organized approach used by the nursing team to determine a resident's specific nursing care needs, what steps will be taken to meet those needs, and whether or not the steps were effective in meeting the resident's needs. The nursing assistant plays a role in the nursing process by carrying out interventions and communicating observations to the nurse.
- In order to ensure that the nursing team operates smoothly and efficiently, a "chain of command" exists. This means that licensed nurses (RNs or LPNs) are able to assign (delegate) certain tasks to nursing assistants.
  - The delegation of tasks cannot be taken lightly by either the delegator (the licensed nurse) or the delegatee (the nursing assistant). Both share the responsibility of ensuring that the procedure is carried out without harm to the resident.
  - The nursing assistant must know which tasks are within his or her scope of practice and which tasks are not.

WHAT DID YOU LEARN?

Multiple Choice

Select the single best answer for each of the following questions.

1. Nursing assistants who work in a long-term care facility must complete a course of training and undergo a competency evaluation. These requirements are set by the:
   a. Centers for Disease Control (CDC)
   b. Food and Drug Administration (FDA)
   c. Omnibus Budget Reconciliation Act (OBRA)
   d. Occupational Safety and Health Administration (OSHA)

2. As a nursing assistant, it is your responsibility to:
   a. Plan the resident's care
   b. Perform the tasks your supervisor assigns to you
   c. Do the best you can without asking for help

   d. Compare assignments with your co-workers

3. If you do not know how to do an assigned task, you should:
   a. Call another nursing assistant for help
   b. Ask the resident how he prefers to have it done
   c. Call the charge nurse and ask for help
   d. Follow the instructions in the procedure manual

4. Nursing assistants work under the supervision of:
   a. A doctor
   b. A registered nurse (RN) or licensed practical nurse (LPN)
   c. Other nursing assistants
   d. The long-term care facility administrator

5. To "delegate" means to:
   a. Do what you are told to do
   b. Give another person permission to perform a task on your behalf
   c. Transfer your duties to another assistant
   d. Have the charge nurse take your assignment

6. What information is included in the registry?
   a. The nursing assistant's full name
   b. The nursing assistant's Social Security Number
   c. Any reported incidents of abuse or theft
   d. All of the above

7. A person with much experience and great skill in a specified role is referred to as a(n):
   a. Apprentice
   b. Professional
   c. Graduate
   d. Novice

8. A nursing assistant can promote his or her own physical health by doing all of the following except:
   a. Eating well-balanced meals
   b. Getting plenty of rest
   c. Smoking and drinking occasionally
   d. Attending aerobics classes

9. A nursing assistant's personal cleanliness is referred to as:
   a. Grooming
   b. Neatness
   c. Hygiene
   d. Fashion

10. Qualities that characterize a good work ethic include all of the following except:
    a. Reliability
    b. Punctuality
    c. Honesty
    d. Tardiness

11. What type of nursing assistant accepts responsibility for his or her actions?
    a. An accountable nursing assistant
    b. A respectful nursing assistant
    c. A courteous nursing assistant
    d. A punctual nursing assistant

12. What type of a nursing assistant is able to imagine what it would feel like to be in another person's situation?
    a. A creative nursing assistant
    b. An empathetic nursing assistant
    c. An experienced nursing assistant
    d. An honest nursing assistant

13. What type of nursing assistant can be counted on to come to work every day?
    a. A punctual nursing assistant
    b. A nursing assistant with access to public transportation
    c. A reliable nursing assistant
    d. An ethical nursing assistant

14. Which step of the nursing process involves gathering information about a resident?
    a. Implementation
    b. Assessment
    c. Planning
    d. Evaluation

STOP and Think!

- One of your co-workers, Jennifer, is talking to you about an assignment the nurse has given her. The nurse has asked Jennifer to obtain Mrs. Chatham's vital signs so that she can call the doctor with this information. Unfortunately, Mrs. Chatham has been resisting care and she yells, kicks, and hits whenever anyone tries to touch her. Jennifer says to you, "Every time I try to go near Mrs. Chatham to take her vital signs, she hits me! I'm ready to make up some vital signs to give to the nurse because I'm tired of getting hit, and I'm afraid I'll get in trouble with the nurse if I don't get her those vital signs soon." How would you respond to Jennifer? What are the potential consequences to the resident if Jennifer follows through with her plan to make up the vital signs? To the nurse?

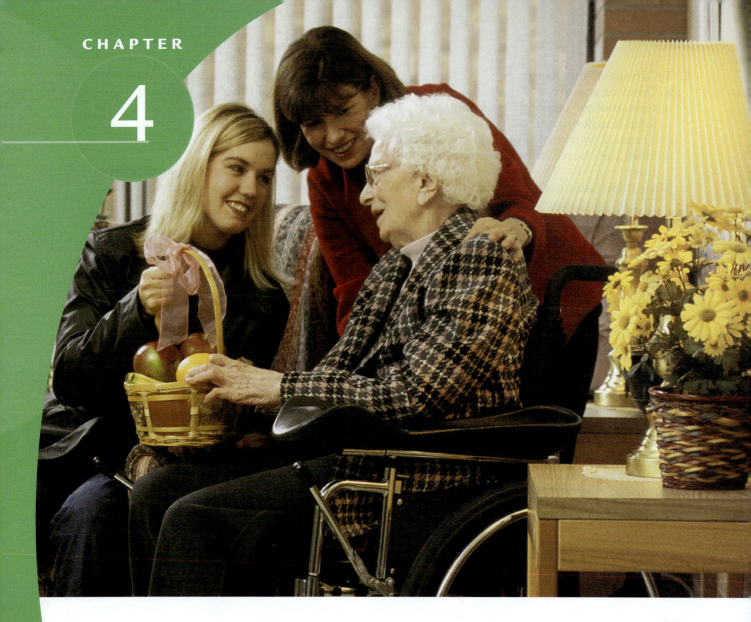

Legal and Ethical Issues

WHAT WILL YOU LEARN?

As members of society, we make decisions every day about how to behave. Some of these decisions are dictated by society's laws, or rules established by the governing authority, and we act a certain way because we know that failing to obey these rules can result in punishment. Other decisions are dictated by our own personal ethical code, or moral sense of what is right and wrong. Many factors influence an individual's ethical code, including spiritual beliefs and values instilled by the person's family. Generally, when we act according to our ethical code, we act a certain way because we believe it is the right way to act, not because we risk punishment if we do not behave in that way. Obeying society's laws and upholding our own personal ethical

Photo: Residents and their families expect and deserve quality care. Laws exist to protect residents and their families and ensure that they receive quality care.

standards allow us to function as members of society. Just as laws and ethics guide our behavior in society, laws and ethics guide our behavior in the workplace as health care providers. This chapter explores some of the legal issues that can affect you, as a nursing assistant, and describes general ethical principles that should guide your behavior in the workplace When you are finished with this chapter, you will be able to:

1. List and discuss residents' rights, as set forth by the Omnibus Budget Reconciliation Act (OBRA).
2. Describe two major types of advance directives and explain why advance directives play an important role in long-term care.
3. List common legal violations that are related to the provision of health care.
4. Define the types of abuse and describe signs that indicate abuse.
5. Discuss the health care worker's obligations in the reporting of suspected abuse.
6. Explain the difference between legal and ethical issues.
7. Describe the ethical standards that govern the nursing profession, in particular, and the health care profession, in general.
8. Discuss awareness that health care workers must have in order to avoid legal and ethical dilemmas.

Vocabulary Use the CD in the front of your book to hear these terms pronounced and defined:

Advocacy	Litigation	Fraud	Psychological
Ombudsman	Liability	False imprisonment	(emotional) abuse
Decision-making	Tort	Invasion of privacy	Sexual abuse
capacity	Unintentional tort	Confidentiality	Financial abuse
Advance directive	Negligent	Health Insurance	Elder abuse
Durable power of	Malpractice	Portability and	Ethics
attorney for health	Intentional tort	Accountability Act	Beneficence
care	Defamation	(HIPAA)	Nonmaleficence
Health care agent	Slander	Larceny	Justice
Living will	Libel	Abuse	Fidelity
Laws	Assault	Physical abuse	Autonomy
Civil laws	Battery	Neglect	Value
Criminal laws	Informed consent	Abandonment	Ethics committee

  # RESIDENTS' RIGHTS

Guidelines concerning the rights of residents of long-term care facilities are ordered by the federal government and must be followed if a facility receives any federal payments from Medicare. These guidelines are called the *Resident Rights* and are included as part of the Omnibus Budget Reconciliation Act (OBRA). The *Resident Rights* portion of OBRA was written to guide the way residents, health care providers, and the administrators of health care organizations interact with one another. In respecting the rights of residents, health care workers behave according to legal standards; they also behave according to ethical standards. The major points of the *Resident Rights* portion of OBRA are as follows:

1. The resident has the right to know what rights and responsibilities he has, in language that he can understand.
2. The resident has the right to exercise his rights, as a resident of the facility, and as a citizen of the United States. This includes the freedom to make choices about how to live his life (subject to the facility's rules), the freedom to vote, and freedom from discrimination.
3. The resident has the right to a dignified existence.
4. The resident has the right to make decisions regarding his care, including choosing his own doctor, participating in planning and implementing his own care, and having his individual needs and preferences accommodated. The resident has the right to refuse

treatment and to refuse to participate in experimental research.

5. The resident has the right to privacy, including privacy while receiving treatments and nursing care, making and receiving telephone calls, sending and receiving mail, and receiving visitors. The resident has the right to confidentiality of personal and medical records.

6. The resident has the right to be free from physical or psychological abuse, including the improper use of restraints.

7. The resident has the right to receive visitors and to share a room with a spouse if both partners are residents in the same facility.

8. The resident has the right to communicate with and have access to people and services both inside and outside of the facility, including advocacy groups. The resident has the right to organize and participate in groups organized by other residents, or the families of residents. For example, residents or their families may organize groups dedicated to improving life for residents, by suggesting changes that could be made at the facility or by planning group outings and activities. The resident also has the right to participate in social, religious, and community activities of his choosing.

9. The resident has the right to keep and use personal possessions (as space and safety permit).

10. The resident has the right to control his own finances (or, if he wishes, have the facility manage personal funds).

11. The resident has the right to information about eligibility for Medicare or Medicaid funds, and to be protected from Medicaid discrimination.

12. The resident has the right to information about the facility's compliance with regulations, planned changes in living arrangements, and available services (and the fees for those services).

13. The resident has the right to remain in the facility unless transfer or discharge is required by a change in the resident's health, the resident is unable to pay for the services he is receiving, or the facility is closed. The resident has the right to refuse transfer from a distinct unit (for example, the certified skilled unit) of the facility.

14. The resident has the right to choose to work at the facility, either as a volunteer or a paid employee. Working or helping others gives many people a sense of purpose. However, under no circumstances is a resident obligated to work (for example, in exchange for services).

15. The resident has the right to self-administer medications, if the health care team determines that the resident can do so safely.

16. The resident has the right to voice grievances, and to have the facility respond to those grievances.

ADVOCACY PROGRAMS

Advocacy is the process of making a plea or providing support on another's behalf. Because many of the residents of long-term care facilities are vulnerable, federal laws provide advocacy programs for their benefit. An example of a federally funded advocacy program is the Long-Term Care Ombudsman Program. An **ombudsman** is a person from a state or local Office on Aging who regularly visits residents of long-term care facilities to check on their welfare and overall satisfaction with their care. Ombudsmen gather information from residents and work on their behalf to negotiate solutions to their concerns (Fig. 4-1). These concerns could be related to care issues, misunderstandings between residents and staff, violations of resident rights, or suspected abuse and neglect. While an ombudsman does not have the authority to force a facility to take action, the ombudsman can work with the appropriate people and agencies to ensure that resident issues are addressed.

OBRA requires nursing homes to post information notifying residents of their right to file complaints, and listing the contact information for agencies that can assist them (e.g., the state agencies that handle licensure of long-term care facilities, Medicare and Medicaid

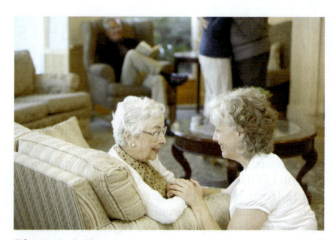

Figure 4-1

An ombudsman talks with residents about their concerns, and works with the necessary people and agencies to resolve them. *Ombudsman* is a Swedish word that means "one who speaks on behalf of another."

idents who need end-of-life care. The Patient Self-Determination Act of 1990 requires long-term care facilities to educate residents about advance directives, and to offer them the opportunity to establish a living will, a durable power of attorney for health care, or both.

CIVIL AND CRIMINAL LAWS: A WAY OF PRESERVING CITIZENS' RIGHTS

All people are entitled to certain basic human rights, and the government, which is put in place by the people, plays a role in making sure that these rights are honored.

One way the government works to preserve its citizens' basic human rights is by making and enforcing laws. **Laws** are rules that are made by a controlling authority, such as the state or federal government. By formally establishing principles to guide behavior, laws give society a way of settling disputes in a civilized, orderly way. Laws enacted by the federal and state governments serve to protect basic human rights for all people, regardless of race, religion, gender, or income.

There are two types of laws that preserve a person's rights: civil laws and criminal laws. **Civil laws** are concerned with relationships between individuals. **Criminal laws** are concerned with the relationship between the individual and society as a whole. People found guilty of violating civil laws usually must pay a fine or make a financial settlement to the party that was wronged. Those who violate criminal laws are often sentenced to prison. **Litigation** is the law-suit, or legal action, taken against a person who is accused of breaking a law. The responsibility of an individual to act within the confines of the law is called **liability**. Each individual is considered responsible, and held accountable, for her own actions in accordance with the law.

VIOLATIONS OF CIVIL LAW

When a person is admitted to a health care facility, he signs a form giving the facility permission to provide medical care. Likewise, a health care worker employed by that facility likewise agrees to provide that care. This arrangement is a contractual agreement. Contracts, such as the contract that exists between a nursing assistant and the person she cares for, fall under the jurisdiction of civil law. When this civil law is violated, a **tort**, or wrong, is committed. An **unintentional tort**

certification, and reports of Medicare or Medicaid fraud). In addition, the contact information for the ombudsman program must also be posted for resident use. As a nursing assistant, you should know where this information is posted in your facility and be able to assist a resident or visitor who asks you how to contact one of these agencies. If a resident or visitor does ask you for this information, you should report the person's request to the nurse. The person's request may indicate that he or she is unhappy about something that has happened in the facility. By alerting the nurse to the person's request, the nurse may be able to talk with the person about the issue, and perhaps resolve it without involving the state agency.

ADVANCE DIRECTIVES

Many residents of long-term care facilities are not able to make their preferences for health care known, or they will become unable to make their preferences known in the future. For example, residents with dementia (a medical condition that results in the permanent and progressive loss of the ability to think and remember) lose their decision-making capacity. **Decision-making capacity** is the ability to make a thoughtful decision based on an understanding of the potential risks and benefits of taking a certain course of action. Medical conditions that result in the loss of consciousness also result in a loss of decision-making capacity.

For these situations, state laws make provisions for advance directives. An **advance directive** is a document that allows a person to make her wishes regarding health care known to family members and health care workers, in case the time comes when she is no longer able to make those wishes known herself. One type of advance directive, a **durable power of attorney for health care**, transfers the responsibility for making medical decisions on the person's behalf to a family member, friend, or other trusted individual, in the event that the person is no longer able to make these decisions on her own behalf. The person who is responsible for making decisions on the person's behalf is called the person's **health care agent** (or, sometimes, the person's durable power of attorney for health care). Another type of advance directive, a **living will,** allows the person to give instructions about what medical treatments he would or would not want done in an effort to save his life. Advance directives play a particularly important role in long-term care, because of the number of residents who have dementia, as well as the number of res-

occurs when someone causes harm or injury to another person or that person's property without the intent to cause harm. A person who commits an unintentional tort is considered **negligent** for failing to do what a "careful and reasonable" person would do (Fig. 4-2). For example, in each of the following scenarios, the nursing assistant would be considered negligent:

- A nursing assistant becomes distracted by another resident's needs and forgets to lock the wheels on the wheelchair she has just placed by the resident's bed. As the resident moves from the bed to the wheelchair, the wheelchair rolls, causing the resident to fall.
- While changing a resident's bed, a nursing assistant forgets to check the linens for personal objects. As a result, the resident's dentures are sent to the laundry with the soiled linens, and the dentures are damaged when they go through the washing machine.
- A nursing assistant who is caring for a resident with a reputation for complaining fails to report the resident's complaints of pain to the nurse. It turns out that this time the resident's complaints were valid.

Negligence committed by people who hold licenses to practice their profession, such as doctors, nurses, lawyers, dentists, and pharmacists, is considered **malpractice**. Nursing assistants (who receive certification, but not licensure) are not charged with malpractice. However, acts of negligence by a nursing assistant can be reported to the state agency that is responsible for nursing assistant certification, and disciplinary action may be taken against the nursing assistant.

A violation of civil law committed by a person with the intent to do harm is considered an **intentional tort**. Intentional torts that nursing assistants are particularly at risk for committing in the workplace include defamation, assault,

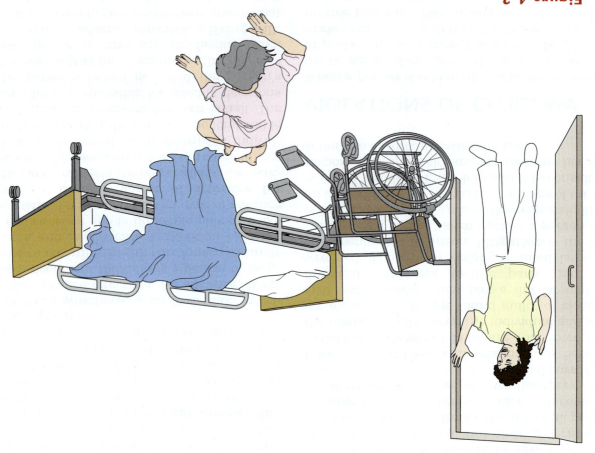

Figure 4-2
The nursing assistant who was responsible for this resident has committed an unintentional tort and would be considered negligent for failing to lock the wheels on the wheelchair, an action that could have prevented the resident from falling.

battery, fraud, false imprisonment, invasion of privacy, and larceny.

Defamation

Defamation is making untrue statements that hurt another person's reputation. Statements in spoken form are called **slander**, while statements in written form are called **libel**. It is best to avoid saying negative things or spreading rumors about a co-worker, supervisor, doctor, resident, or resident's family member (Fig. 4-3). Although it is easy to become hurt, angry, or defensive when you feel that someone has treated you unfairly, making untrue remarks about that person is not the professional way to handle these feelings.

Assault

Assault is threatening or attempting to touch a person without his consent, causing that person to fear bodily harm (Fig. 4-4). A person can be found guilty of committing assault on the basis of an angry statement ("If you get up out of that wheelchair once more without calling for help, I'll tie you down!") or an angry gesture (shaking a fist in someone's face or acting as if you are going to slap her). Even very patient people can become frustrated occasionally. To avoid doing something you will regret later, notify your supervisor of your need to "take a break" (physically and emotionally) when you feel your emotions get on edge.

Battery

Battery is touching a person without his or her consent. For example, a health care worker could

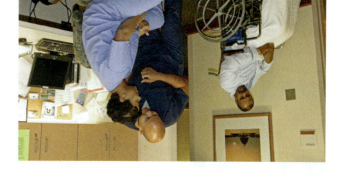

Figure 4-3
Never say negative things or spread rumors about co-workers, residents, or residents' family members. Doing so is unprofessional, and it could get you in trouble with the law!

be accused of battery for physically restraining a person who is trying to leave the room, or for performing a procedure that the person or the person's health care agent has not consented to.

When a person requires a medical treatment or procedure (such as surgery or a diagnostic test), the health care provider must obtain **informed consent** (formal, written permission to go ahead with a treatment or procedure). Obtaining informed consent involves providing a full explanation of the treatment or procedure to be done, including the risks and benefits, as well as information about alternatives to the proposed treatment or procedure (including the risks and benefits of those options). This allows the person to make an intelligent, or "informed," decision that is consistent with his or her personal feelings and beliefs. The person then provides written consent for the treatment or procedure to be done. Even if a person initially consents to a treatment or procedure, he is able to withdraw that consent and refuse the treatment or procedure at any time.

Although as a nursing assistant, you will not be responsible for obtaining written informed consent from residents, you must still obtain the resident's verbal permission before providing care. Always explain to the resident what you are there to do, and ask if it is all right for you to proceed. If a resident tells you "no," you may need to ask in a different way in order to gain the resident's cooperation, approach the resident again at a later time, or ask the nurse for help. Also, remember that even if a resident initially gives you permission to go ahead with providing care, the resident is able to withdraw that permission and refuse care at any time.

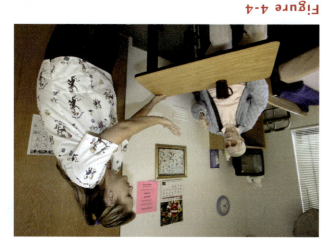

Figure 4-4
Try to avoid letting your emotions get out of check. Making angry gestures toward another is considered assault.

Invasion of Privacy

Invasion of privacy is violating another person's right to keep certain information and aspects of himself away from the examination of others. Failure to maintain a person's physical privacy (for example, by leaving a door or curtain open during a procedure, or exposing a person's entire body when it is only necessary to expose a certain part) is considered an invasion of privacy. So is entering a resident's room without knocking first. Discussing a resident's physical condition, diagnosis, prognosis, or behavior with anyone who is not involved with that resident's care is also considered an invasion of privacy. This type of privacy violation is considered a violation of the person's right to confidentiality. **Confidentiality** means keeping personal information that you have knowledge of to yourself. A breach of confidentiality can happen if you talk about a resident in a public area of the facility (such as an elevator, hallway, or cafeteria) [Fig. 4-5], or outside of the facility (for example, in a discussion with friends or neighbors). The only time it is acceptable to discuss a resident is when it is necessary to exchange information about that person's care with someone else who is directly involved in caring for that person. Even then, you must be careful about where that conversation takes place and who else is around.

Confidentiality applies not only to spoken and observed information, but also to written information. Always make sure that medical records (charts) and assignment sheets are not left where others can read them. The screens of computers that are used to enter and house information about residents should be shielded from public view, and documents containing information about residents should be closed when not in use. Be aware that a resident's medical record is only to be read by members of the health care team who are directly involved in the care of that resident and need access to the information in the record in order to provide that care. Therefore, it would be inappropriate for a nursing assistant to read the medical record of a resident who she is not assigned to care for. It would also be inappropriate for a member of the health care team who is not involved in providing direct resident care (such as a custodial worker) to read a resident's medical record.

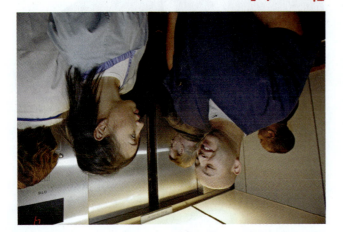

Figure 4-5
It is fine to chat with co-workers in public areas about topics that are not related to work, but never discuss your residents, or their care, in a place where you could be overheard by others.

False Imprisonment

False imprisonment is confining another person against his or her will. In the health care setting, it is sometimes necessary to confine a person to a chair, a bed, or a room to maintain that person's safety (or the safety of others). However, the use of restraints can be considered false imprisonment if the restraints are not justified for the safety of the resident (or others) and if less restrictive restraint alternatives were not tried first. (The use of restraints, and alternatives to restraint use, are discussed in more detail in Chapter 18.)

Fraud

Fraud is deception that could cause harm to another person. A health care worker who misrepresents her professional qualifications (for example, by telling a resident that she is a nurse when she is not, or lying about previous training or employment on a job application) is committing fraud. Similarly, a health care worker who documents care for a resident that was not actually provided is also committing fraud.

Caring For Those With Dementia

Residents with dementia may not be able to understand enough about the situation to make appropriate decisions about their care. However, this does not mean that you can provide care without the resident's permission and cooperation. Even people with dementia know when they do not want to be touched!

The **Health Insurance Portability and Accountability Act (HIPAA)** originated in 1996. HIPAA is a federal privacy regulation that helps to keep personal information about patients and residents private. HIPAA:

- Regulates who has the right to view a person's medical records, data, or other private information
- Sets standards on how a person's medical information is to be stored and transmitted from one place to another
- Requires that health care organizations set policies that allow a patient or resident to have access to his or her medical records

Larceny

Larceny is stealing. In a long-term care setting, health care workers have access to residents' personal belongings. It is never acceptable to take something belonging to another person, even if the item is not of great monetary value or if the person does not seem to "need" it. People who are elderly or ill are particularly vulnerable to theft, and not just at the hands of health care workers—other employees of the facility, family members, friends, or even other residents may also commit larceny. As a nursing assistant, it is important for you to report any suspicions you might have about loss of property according to your facility's policy.

VIOLATIONS OF CRIMINAL LAW—ABUSE

Abuse, the deliberate infliction of pain or injury on another person, is a criminal act and is punishable by a court of law. A person can commit abuse by *actively doing something to* another person (for example, hitting or verbally abusing the person), or by *failing to do something for* another person (for example, failing to provide adequate care or attention). The injury that results from the abuse may be physical or emotional.

Forms of Abuse

Abuse takes many forms (Table 4-1).

- **Physical abuse** is the use of force to cause pain or injury to the abused person's body.
- **Neglect** is the failure to provide for a dependent person's basic physical needs. **Abandonment,** which is the act of withdrawing support or help from another person in spite of duty or responsibility, falls under the category of neglect. A health care worker who

walks off the job or leaves the unit without telling anyone (even for a short time) has committed abandonment.

- **Psychological (emotional) abuse** is the use of words or actions to cause emotional pain or injury. Psychological abuse can be inflicted in many ways. Making another person fearful by threatening him with physical harm or abandonment is one form of psychological abuse, as is teasing a person in a cruel way or treating a person in an undignified manner. Isolating a person by preventing him from interacting with others (an act called *involuntary seclusion*) is another form of psychological abuse. Keeping a person in a room alone with the door closed can be considered a form of involuntary seclusion.
- **Sexual abuse** involves subjecting a person to unwanted attention of a sexual nature, forcing a person to engage in unwanted sexual activity, or sexually exploiting a person (for example, by taking nude photographs of the person).
- **Financial abuse** involves misusing or stealing another person's money or property. Dishonest people may trick older people into giving them money for services that are not provided or charities that do not exist. A common way of doing this is over the telephone. There have also been incidents where health care workers have convinced residents to give them money to help them out of difficult personal situations (for example, to pay for child care, rent, or medication). Discussing personal problems with residents is not professional behavior and should never be done! Even if a resident offers money or property to a health care worker by his or her own free will, it should never be accepted. Most employers have policies against accepting gifts or money from residents.

Perpetrators of Abuse

There are many reasons why a person may become abusive toward another. Sometimes, abuse is rooted in the desire of one person to overpower and dominate another. Many abusers were victims of abuse themselves, and believe that abusive behavior is "normal." Other times, in a situation where a person requires a great deal of care, the primary caregiver may become overly tired, frustrated, and overwhelmed by the responsibility of providing care (as well as other life demands in addition to caregiving), leading to abuse and neglect. This is often the case with an adult child who finds herself in the situation of

Table 4-1	Types of Abuse	
TYPE OF ABUSE	**EXAMPLES**	**SIGNS THAT ABUSE MAY BE OCCURRING**
Physical abuse: Causing pain or injury to the person's body through the use of force	• Hitting and slapping • Pushing and shoving • Pinching and kicking • Shaking • Burning • Force feeding • The inappropriate use of medications • The inappropriate use of physical restraints	• Red marks, welts, or bruises, particularly on the face or torso • Broken bones • Broken or bent eyeglasses • Patches of missing hair • Laboratory work that indicates under- or overdosing of medications • Resident displays fearful or anxious behavior, especially in the presence of the abuser • Resident reports physical abuse
Neglect: Failing or refusing to provide for the person's basic human needs	• Failing to provide food, water, clothing, shelter, or ordered medications • Failing to help the person meet hygiene and toileting needs • Withdrawing support or help from another person, in spite of duty or responsibility (abandonment)	• Unusual weight loss • Dehydration • Pressure ulcers • Poor personal hygiene, unkempt appearance • Incontinence, dried feces on the skin, or skin irritation • Inadequate or inappropriate clothing for environment • Pain • Contractures • Uncontrolled medical conditions (possibly the result of a lack of prescribed medication or treatment) • Resident reports improper care
Psychological (emotional) abuse: Causing emotional pain or injury through the use of words or actions	• Insulting or threatening a person • Bullying, humiliating, or harassing a person • Treating a person in an undignified or child-like way • Giving a person the silent treatment • Isolating the person from others (involuntary seclusion)	• Resident appears emotionally upset (for example, the resident cries frequently) • Resident appears withdrawn or apathetic (does not seem to care about anything), or resident stops responding • Changes in the resident's behavior, or unusual behavior (such as rocking or biting) • Resident reports psychological abuse
Sexual abuse: Subjecting the person to unwanted attention of a sexual nature, forcing the person to engage in unwanted sexual activity, or sexually exploiting the person (for example, by taking nude photographs of the person)	• Touching personal body parts in an inappropriate way • Making inappropriate, sexually suggestive comments or gestures • Committing sexual assault or battery (for example, forced nudity, inappropriate photography, rape)	• Bruising on breasts or in genital area • Torn or stained underwear • Unexplained bleeding from the vagina or rectum • Resident reports sexual abuse or harassment
Financial abuse: Misusing or stealing another person's money or property	• Stealing money or belongings • Withholding a person's Social Security checks or other sources of income • Making withdrawals from a person's bank account or cashing checks without the person's permission • Forging the person's signature on checks or legal documents • Tricking or blackmailing a person into giving away money or property • Tricking or blackmailing a person into signing a legal document or making changes to an existing legal document	• Unexplained disappearance of money or belongings • Sudden change in bank account activity, such as unauthorized withdrawals from the person's account • Unexplained money or property transfers, or changes to the person's will • The inclusion of additional names on the person's bank account • The discovery of forged documents • Resident reports mishandling or loss of money or property

caring for an ill and demanding elderly parent, without the proper training or support system.

Even people who are trained to administer care may become overwhelmed by their responsibilities or a particular situation. A health care worker is particularly at risk for becoming abusive when a resident is "difficult" or hard to manage, and the relationship is long-term, rather than short-term. In long-term care, most relationships with residents last for months, if not years! Any situation can be hard to cope with if you can see no end to the difficulties. As described in Chapter 3, many facilities have counseling services to help employees deal with the emotional stress that caring for others can create. It is a healthy step, not a sign of weakness, to take advantage of these services. Teamwork among co-workers is also essential for helping to reduce work-related stress.

Regardless of the reason abuse occurs, abuse is never an acceptable form of behavior! Be very careful not to place yourself in the position of potentially abusing a resident. Being found guilty of abuse could destroy your potential for future employment in the health care field.

Elder Abuse

Anyone can become the victim of abuse, but those who depend on others for their care (the very young, the disabled, and the elderly) are particularly at risk. **Elder abuse** is the abuse of an older person. Elder abuse can take any of the forms described in Table 4-1.

Most cases of elder abuse occur in private homes, but elder abuse can and does occur in long-term care settings as well. Some reports have indicated that episodes of elder abuse have occurred in 30% of our nation's nursing homes. At least 10% of our nation's nursing homes have been charged with abuse as the result of incidents that involved physical harm to a resident. The perpetrators of the abuse may be staff members, other residents, visitors, or family members.

Many factors can place an older person at risk for abuse:

- **Multiple health conditions.** Older people often have multiple health conditions, which increase their need to depend on others. The older person may require a great deal of care, and the caregiver may become overwhelmed by the demands the person places on her time and energy.
- **An inability to defend oneself.** Physical disabilities, mental disabilities, or both can make an older person vulnerable to abuse, and unable to defend herself if abuse occurs.

- **"Difficult" behavior.** An older person in need of care may become "difficult," either as a result of his medical condition (for example, dementia), or because he is having trouble adjusting emotionally to his current situation. For example, the person may fear that his needs will not be met if he is left alone, so he may make constant demands on the caregiver in an effort to keep her close. Or, the person needing care may become resentful or angry about the situation and take these feelings out on the caregiver. This is a common reaction among people who up until this point were always very independent.
- **The caregiver's perception of the person needing care.** Sometimes, the caregiver does not fully realize the extent of disability caused by the person's health problem. If the caregiver views the person as being purposefully difficult, this can cause the caregiver to have feelings of anger and resentment toward the person needing care.
- **Social isolation.** Many older people are isolated away from the rest of society, whether they are living in their own homes, or living in a long-term care facility. Their daily contact with others is generally limited to a small number of people. This makes it more difficult for the older person to report abuse, and it makes it more difficult for others to detect signs of abuse.
- **A reluctance to report abuse.** Older people are often reluctant to report those who mistreat them. Imagine that you are dependent on someone else to meet your needs, and that person mistreats you. If you report the mistreatment, you will get the caregiver in trouble. Now the caregiver is angry with you. Maybe the other caregivers in the facility (or other members of the family) will turn against you as well, because you got their friend or relative in trouble. But you are still dependent on these people for care. How would you feel in that situation?

Role of the Nursing Assistant in Reporting Abuse

As a nursing assistant, you may find yourself in a situation where you suspect that one of your residents is being abused. (Signs that abuse may be occurring are listed in Table 4-1). You are obligated to protect the residents in your care. Laws require any health care worker who suspects the abuse of an elderly person or child to report her suspicions to the proper authorities. Your facility will have specific policies regarding the chain of reporting. Some organizations will require that you report to your supervisor, while others require reporting to an administrator. It is not your responsibility to investigate whether or not abuse has actually occurred, or who has caused it. The person in your facility who is responsible for handling reports of abuse will follow up on your report. Your responsibility is simply to report your suspicions (Box 4-1).

Sometimes nursing assistants are hesitant to report suspected, or even witnessed, abuse. They may be fearful of getting a co-worker in trouble. However, if you say nothing, you are allowing the abuse, and the harm to the resident, to continue. If it becomes known that you were aware of an abusive situation and did not report it, you could find yourself in legal trouble, and your certification may be jeopardized.

BOX 4-1   Reporting Abuse

- Report the incident immediately (for example, do not wait until your next scheduled shift to make your report).
- Set the scene—report what was happening just before the incident.
- Report exactly what you saw or heard.
- Give the names of those involved. If you do not know a person's name, provide a good physical description. If the incident was heard but not seen, describe sounds, including the person's voice, if possible.
- Report the date and time of the incident. If the exact time of the incident is not known, indicate the approximate time by relating it to the routine of the shift (for example, "It occurred after I passed fresh water, just before dinner.").
- Use exact quotes when reporting what the resident (or someone else) said to you.
- Describe suspicious evidence in detail (for example, if you are describing the appearance of a new injury, such as a bruise, include a description of the location and size of the bruise).
- Keep a written record of what you reported, when you reported it, and to whom.

Examples

- "I am concerned about Mrs. Brewster. I am afraid that something may be occurring between her and her daughter, Ella Franks. I have noticed a change in Mrs. Brewster's behavior, especially when her daughter comes to visit. She doesn't say anything, but she looks at me with pleading eyes whenever her daughter is around, and she often grabs hold of my hand. Mrs. Brewster seems frightened for at least an hour after her daughter leaves. When she hears someone approaching in the hall, she jumps, and jerks her head to look at the door with wide eyes and a fearful expression. Sometimes she whimpers. She never used to do that before. Today at about 2:30 PM, just after Mrs. Franks left her mother, I noticed a red mark on Mrs. Brewster's left cheek. I know it wasn't there earlier when I helped her to the bathroom. When I asked Mrs. Brewster what happened, she covered her cheek and just kept shaking her head. She wouldn't say anything."
- "When I did my first rounds after reporting for duty tonight, Mr. Jeffries told me that he had observed someone in his room going through his nightstand on the previous shift and now his money is missing. He wasn't sure what time it was, but the room was dark, and he had been asleep for a little while. Mr. Jeffries said that he asked the person what he was doing in there, and the person responded, "None of your business. Shut up and go back to sleep." The person then quickly shut the drawer. Mr. Jeffries said he saw him put something in his pocket. He described the person as tall, with dark hair. His voice was deep. He could not see the person's face, and he did not recognize him as someone he had seen before. He looked like he might have been wearing a blue uniform. Mr. Jeffries reports he had about $10.00 in bills that his daughter had given him, and probably about $3.00 in quarters from his Bingo winnings. He says that he knows it isn't much, but it was all he had and it gave him a little something to spend at the canteen. Mr. Jeffries is very upset."

Be Smart About Surveys!

Surveyors are very conscientious about monitoring compliance with resident rights during their survey visits, particularly the right of residents to be protected from abuse. It is common for a surveyor to question nursing home staff about their knowledge of the facility's policies and procedures for reporting of abuse and neglect. To help your facility remain without survey problems in this area:

● Know the forms that abuse can take, and signs that may indicate abuse is occurring (see Table 4-1)

● Know your responsibilities in reporting suspected abuse

● Know the name and title of the person in your facility who you are supposed to report suspected abuse to

● Know what type of information to include in your report (see Box 4-1)

ETHICS: GUIDELINES FOR BEHAVIOR

As you have learned, laws serve to preserve basic human rights. As such, laws generally deal with issues that are either "black" or "white"—an action is either within the law, or outside of it. But what about situations that are not so easily defined? The dramatic changes in health care that have been brought about by advances in technology and research have greatly impacted legal and ethical issues surrounding the medical profession, and have created some unique moral dilemmas. Consider the following questions:

- In every situation, should a person be resuscitated if his heart stops working and he stops breathing?
- Should a person be kept alive by artificial means (such as by tube feeding or mechanical ventilation), regardless of the person's circumstances?
- Should a doctor be allowed to end a terminally ill person's life if the person requests that this action be taken because she does not want to suffer anymore?

Clearly, these are difficult questions to answer because the answers to these questions depend on the individual's values and beliefs. When definitive answers to questions are not available, we rely on ethical standards to decide what to do. **Ethics** are moral principles or stan-

dards that govern conduct. The word "ethics" comes from the Greek word *ethos*, which means "beliefs that guide life." Ethical standards, which are less rigid than laws, help us to determine the difference between right and wrong in areas where the law fears to tread.

PROFESSIONAL ETHICS

Each profession has a code of ethics, or guidelines pertaining to standards of conduct and practice, for that profession. The code of ethics for nursing assistants falls within the American Nurses Association (ANA) code of ethics for nursing (Box 4-2). In addition, there are some general ethical principles that guide all health care workers:

- **Beneficence.** Do good for those in your care by preventing harm and promoting the health and welfare of the person above all else.
- **Nonmaleficence.** Avoid harming those in your care. Use kindness and gentleness when administering care.
- **Justice.** Treat people fairly and equally, regardless of race, religion, culture, disability, or ability to pay.
- **Fidelity.** Act with integrity to earn others' trust.
- **Autonomy.** Respect a person's rights and personal preferences.
- **Confidentiality.** Maintain a person's privacy by allowing the person to discuss sensitive issues with the knowledge that the information will be kept secret.

PERSONAL ETHICS

Many factors influence a person's ethics, which are derived from a person's values. A **value** is a cherished belief or principle. Factors that influence a person's values include his or her religious

BOX 4-2 Code of Ethics for Nursing Assistants

● Treat residents with respect for their individual needs and values.

● Respect the resident's right to choice in regard to the individual's right to control his or her own care.

● Hold confidential all information about residents learned in the health care setting.

● Be guided by consideration for the dignity of residents.

● Fulfill the obligation to provide competent care to residents.

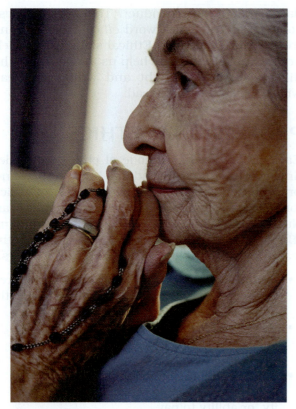

Figure 4-6
Values, which are derived from religious and spiritual beliefs, culture and heritage, and a person's family, are the basis of ethics. Not everyone has the same values. It is important to recognize and respect your residents' values, even if they are not the same as yours.

or spiritual beliefs, level and type of education, culture and heritage, and life experiences. Each person's value system is unique, and as a nursing assistant, you need to think about how you feel about certain moral and ethical issues. Only then will you be able to understand that although another person's values may differ from yours, that person's values are as important to her as yours are to you. Respect for the individual is one of the principles that forms the basis of the code of ethics for nursing (Fig. 4-6).

ETHICAL DILEMMAS

Ethical dilemmas arise when we attempt to judge other people by our own ethical standards. Satisfactory resolutions to ethical dilemmas in the health care field can be difficult to achieve. With so many health care workers being involved in resident care, there is always the potential for a clash of viewpoints based on differing values. In the best-case scenario, the resident can speak for himself with regard to care decisions, either by

stating his preferences at the time a decision must be made, or through an advance directive. However, instructions in an advance directive can create an ethical dilemma if they are not clear, or if they do not really apply to the resident's clinical situation. Problems can also occur if the resident no longer has the capacity for making decisions, and did not prepare an advance directive.

Many states have surrogacy laws, which allow for family members to make health care decisions on behalf of a loved one when the loved one is no longer able to do so. Often, grown children are the ones responsible for making a decision on behalf of their parent. This situation can lead to an ethical dilemma if the children do not all agree about what decision should be made. Legally, all of the person's children have an equal say in this situation. These types of disagreements can be very difficult to resolve, and if not handled with care, can lead to family disputes and broken family ties.

An **ethics committee** can help to resolve difficult ethical dilemmas (Fig. 4-7). The ethics committee is made up of people representing many different areas of expertise such as clergy members, social workers, health care professionals (such as doctors, nurses, or pharmacists), facility board members or administrators, family and resident council members, and members of the community at large. The committee members meet, and the case is presented. They are given information about the resident's medical history and current situation, the resident's beliefs and values, and the nature of the dilemma facing the staff. The committee members listen to the facts that are presented, and ask questions to clarify or obtain additional information. When the committee members have an understanding of all of the facts related to the

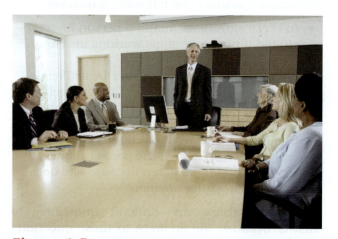

Figure 4-7
An ethics committee can help to resolve difficult ethical dilemmas.

ethical dilemma, they then discuss the various viewpoints held by the people directly involved in the case. The committee members try to reach an agreement about the course of action to take that would reflect the best interests of the resident. Care decisions based on the recommendations of an ethics committee are usually protected by the law.

PROTECTING YOURSELF FROM LEGAL AND ETHICAL DIFFICULTIES

During your career, you will find yourself in a variety of situations where the "right" thing to do may not be absolutely clear. Always bear in mind the legal and ethical responsibilities and obligations that you have as a caregiver. Make sure that you are familiar with your employer's policies, and with your duties and obligations as listed in your job description. Be aware of the scope of practice for nursing assistants in your state. Do not make decisions or perform duties that are not within your scope of practice, as defined by facility policy, your job description, and your state's regulations. Keeping yourself informed is critical to ensure that the care you give is within the legal limits of your job (Fig. 4-8). Finally, if you find yourself in a situ-

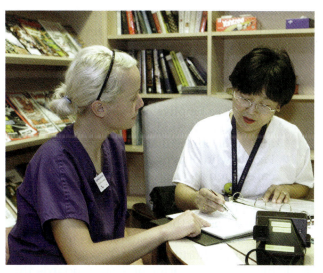

Figure 4-8

In order to stay within the legal limits of your job, know your scope of practice (as defined by the state and your job description), familiarize yourself with your employer's "policies and procedures" manual, and always seek clarification from your supervisor if there is something you do not understand.

ation that may pose legal liability issues for you or your employer, or you are facing an ethical dilemma that you are not sure how to resolve, be sure to share your concerns with your supervisor.

SUMMARY

- A professional acts in a way that is legally and ethically appropriate.
- The *Resident Rights* portion of the Omnibus Budget Reconciliation Act (OBRA) protects the people who receive our care and creates an atmosphere of open communication among everyone involved in that care.
  - An ombudsman is a person who advocates for residents, and helps to ensure that their rights are upheld.
  - Advance directives are legal documents that help to protect residents' rights by giving the resident the opportunity to make her preferences known, in the event that she is unable to state these preferences herself.
- Laws are rules that are made by a controlling authority, such as the state or federal government, that serve to protect basic human rights.

- Civil laws are concerned with relationships between individuals. Criminal laws are concerned with the relationship between an individual and society as a whole.
- An unintentional tort occurs when someone causes harm or injury to another person or that person's property without the intent to cause harm. A person who commits an unintentional tort is considered negligent for failing to do what a careful and reasonable person would do.
- A violation of civil law committed by a person with the intent to do harm is called an intentional tort. Examples of intentional torts that may be committed by nursing assistants in the workplace are defamation, assault, battery, fraud, false imprisonment, invasion of privacy, and larceny.

- Abuse, the deliberate infliction of injury on another person, is a criminal act and is punishable by a court of law.
  - Abuse can be committed by either actively doing something *to* another person, or by failing to do something *for* another person.
  - Abuse can be physical, psychological (emotional), sexual, or financial. Neglect is a form of physical abuse.
  - People who depend on others for their care, such as the disabled and the elderly, are particularly at risk for abuse.
  - Laws require that any health care worker who suspects the abuse of a vulnerable person to report his suspicions to the proper authorities.
- Ethics are moral principles or standards that govern conduct.

- The nursing assistant, as a member of the health care team, should follow a professional code of ethics.
- Respecting the values of the people you care for is essential in following a code of ethics.
- Some situations in health care result in ethical dilemmas. Ethical dilemmas can be resolved by allowing residents to be informed and active participants in their own care, and by respecting residents' individual values and choices.
- In situations where a resident's choice is not known or unclear, or where there is disagreement among those responsible for making care decisions, facilities can turn to an ethics committee for guidance in making difficult ethical decisions.

WHAT DID YOU LEARN?

Multiple choice

Select the single best answer for each of the following questions.

1. All of the following are legal terms that relate to making false statements that injure another person's reputation except:
   a. Defamation
   b. Battery
   c. Slander
   d. Libel

2. Mrs. Chapman's care plan specifies that a mechanical lift should be used when moving Mrs. Chapman from the bed to the chair and vice versa. The nursing assistant caring for her is in a rush. She sees that the mechanical lift on the unit is being used for someone else. Instead of waiting, she decides to go ahead and get Mrs. Chapman out of bed herself. Mrs. Chapman is very heavy, and in the middle of the transfer, the nursing assistant loses her grip and Mrs. Chapman falls to the floor. Mrs. Chapman suffers a broken leg. The nursing assistant has committed:
   a. Malpractice
   b. Negligence
   c. An intentional tort
   d. Assault

3. *Resident Rights* are a part of which legislation?
   a. American Medical Association (AMA)
   b. Omnibus Budget Reconciliation Act (OBRA)

   c. Older Americans Act
   d. Social Security Act

4. Which ethical principle relates to the concepts of informed consent and a person's right to refuse treatment?
   a. Beneficence
   b. Autonomy
   c. Fidelity
   d. Justice

5. Confidentiality means:
   a. Only sharing information with those directly involved in a resident's care
   b. Respecting a resident's right to privacy
   c. Never sharing information with anyone
   d. Both "a" and "b"

6. All residents have basic rights. Which of the following is a basic right of residents?
   a. Right to choice
   b. Right to privacy and confidentiality
   c. Right to be free from verbal abuse, or any other abuse
   d. All of the above

7. Mr. Bennett is the husband of one of your residents. Every time he visits, he requests that his wife's door be closed so that they may have a private visit. You notice that after her husband's visits, Mrs. Bennett seems frightened when you enter the room, and cries when you ask her what is wrong. Today, you notice that she also seemed frightened when you announce that Mr. Bennett is on his way. Mr. Bennett seems like a very nice man, but you are starting to suspect that Mrs. Bennett is being abused in some way by her husband. What should you do first?

a. Call the police

b. Keep your suspicions to yourself, but continue to observe the situation

c. Immediately report your suspicions to your supervisor

d. Ask another nursing assistant what she thinks about Mr. Bennett

8. One of your fellow nursing assistants has been having a very hard time with one of her residents. The resident is confused and, as a result, is being uncooperative. In a moment of complete frustration, your co-worker says to the resident, "If you don't shut up and behave yourself right now, I'm going to slap you!" What kind of an intentional tort has this nursing assistant committed?

a. Assault

b. Battery

c. Negligence

d. Malpractice

9. A nursing assistant answers the telephone at the nurses' station. The doctor who is calling wants to give a verbal order, and the nursing assistant tells the doctor that she is a nurse and can take the order. What intentional tort has the nursing assistant committed?

a. Slander

b. Fraud

c. Libel

d. Informed consent

10. What does the Health Insurance Portability and Accountability Act (HIPAA) protect?

a. The resident's right to privacy

b. The resident's right to sue negligent health care workers

c. The resident's right to be free from abuse

d. The resident's right to choose who will provide his or her care

11. Mr. Murphy recently suffered a massive stroke. Since that time, he has been unresponsive. The doctors state that there is little hope that Mr. Murphy will ever regain consciousness. Mr. Murphy never prepared an advance directive. His three children are recognized as legal surrogate decision makers. The two older children feel that their father no longer has a good quality of life, and that he should be allowed to die peacefully. The youngest child disagrees, saying that her father would want all possible measures taken to keep him alive. What should the facility do to ensure legal and ethical care?

a. Follow the instructions of the two oldest children

b. Follow the instructions of the youngest child because she seems to know what her father would want

c. Rely on the doctor to make the best decision based on his medical judgment

d. Call a meeting of an ethics committee to discuss Mr. Murphy's situation

12. An ombudsman is a person who:

a. advocates to protect residents living in long-term care

b. prosecutes long-term care staff guilty of abuse

c. lives in a long-term care facility

d. is authorized to force a facility to take action to address resident issues when residents have concerns about their care

Matching

Match each numbered item with its appropriate lettered description.

_____ **1.** Civil laws

_____ **2.** Liability

_____ **3.** Fraud

_____ **4.** Ethics

_____ **5.** Beneficence

a. The responsibility of an individual to act within the confines of the law

b. A system of moral principles or standards used to govern conduct

c. Protecting a resident from harm

d. Deception that could cause harm to another person

e. Laws that deal with relationships between individuals

STOP and Think!

- A licensed practical nurse (LPN) who works with you in a long-term care facility stops in Mrs. Taylor's room to give Mrs. Taylor her daily medications. Mrs. Taylor is in the bathroom and you are changing the linens on her bed. The nurse hands you the medication cup, which contains three pills, and asks you to have Mrs. Taylor take the pills as soon as she comes out of the bathroom. You are aware that in your state, nursing assistants who work in long-term care facilities are not allowed to give medications. When you mention your concern about giving Mrs. Taylor her medication to the nurse, she says, "It's okay, the other nursing assistants do this for me all of the time." What should you do?

- Mrs. Fields has dementia and is sometimes very difficult to care for. The family comes to visit as you are finishing up her bath. During their stay, they have watched you assist Mrs. Fields to the toilet, coax her to eat more of her lunch, and bring her some hot tea, which Mrs. Fields really seems to enjoy. Before she leaves, Mrs. Fields' daughter pulls you aside and gives you a $20 bill, thanking you for taking such good care of her mother. How should you respond to Mrs. Fields' daughter?

- Mrs. Walters has been a resident in Room 205B of your facility for 3 years. Last week, Mrs. Sumner moved in as her roommate in Room 205A. Mrs. Sumner has a favorite television show that she enjoys watching at 8:30 PM. Because Mrs. Sumner is hard of hearing, she turns the volume up loud so she can hear her program. Mrs. Walters has always enjoyed quiet time in the evening. She likes to read her Bible and say her prayers just before going to bed around 9 PM. Mrs. Walters tells you that the television is making it hard for her to concentrate on her Bible study and nightly prayer, and requests that the television be turned off. However, you know that Mrs. Sumner has a right to enjoy her usual evening routine too. Whose rights do you think should be honored in this situation? Is there a way that this disagreement could be resolved?

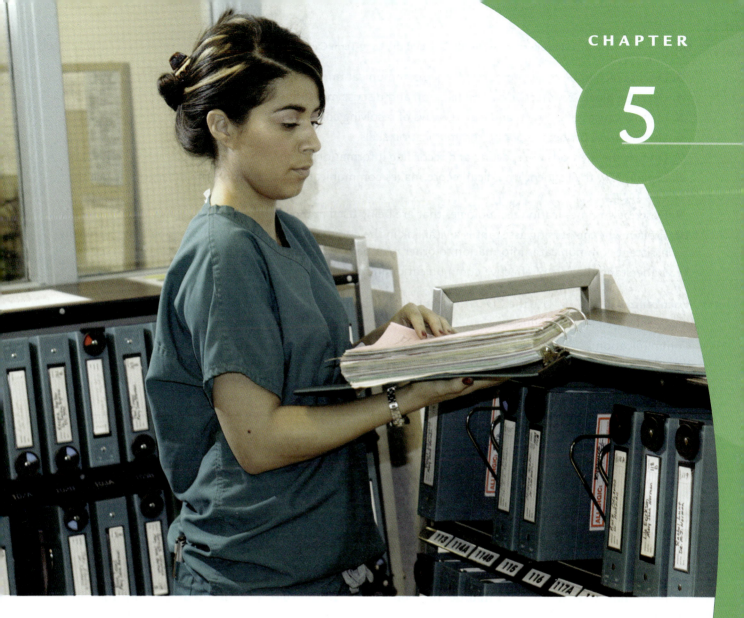

Communication Skills

WHAT WILL YOU LEARN?

Being able to effectively communicate, or participate in the exchange of information, is a critical skill for all people in the health care field to possess. Every day, you will need to communicate with your residents, and with other members of the health care team. If just one link in the chain of communication is broken, the quality of care given to the resident can suffer. In this chapter, we will describe techniques for, as well as obstacles to, effective communication. In addition, we will review some of the tools that are commonly used by members of the health care team to ensure that information is readily available to all who are involved with the care of a resident. When you are finished with this chapter, you will be able to:

1. Define communication.
2. Describe the two major forms of communication, and give examples of each.

Photo: A nursing assistant checks a resident's medical record. The medical record is one way members of the health care team share information with each other.

65

3. Discuss techniques that promote effective communication.

4. Describe blocks to effective communication and discuss methods used to avoid them.

5. Identify causes of conflict, and discuss ways of resolving conflicts.

6. Demonstrate proper telephone communication skills.

7. Discuss the methods of reporting and recording information in a health care setting.

8. Explain how the resident's medical record makes communication easier among members of the health care team.

9. Describe communication technologies that are being used in the health care field today.

10. Explain why the nursing assistant is a vital link in the communication chain, and describe how the nursing assistant communicates information to other members of the health care team.

11. Understand the role of effective communication in the provision of quality health care.

Vocabulary Use the CD in the front of your book to hear these terms pronounced and defined:

Communication	Conflict	Signs	Reporting
Verbal communication	Observation	Subjective	Recording
Nonverbal	Objective	data	Medical record
communication	data	Symptoms	Kardex

WHAT IS COMMUNICATION?

Communication is the exchange of information. The key to understanding what communication truly is lies within the word "exchange." If you exchange gifts with another person, you give that person a gift, and in return, you receive one back. In the exchange of information that defines communication, there is a constant back-and-forth flow of information. Communicating is not just about telling someone something (giving information). It is also about listening and observing (receiving information).

For effective communication to occur, all of the people who are involved must actively participate in the exchange of information. Communication involves at least two people, a *sender* and a *receiver*. The sender is the person with information to share, and the receiver is the person for whom the information is intended. The sender delivers the information in the form of a *message*, which the receiver may or may not understand. Through *feedback*, or a return message, the receiver lets the sender know whether the message was received and understood (Fig. 5-1). Note that as information is transmitted back and forth, the sender and the receiver switch roles.

There are two major forms of communication, verbal and nonverbal. **Verbal communication** involves the use of language, either spoken or written. Sign language, a system of hand gestures used to make letters of the alphabet and words, is also considered a form of verbal communication. Verbal communication tends to be deliberate—when we use language to express a thought, it is usually with the intent of giving specific information to another person.

Nonverbal communication, on the other hand, tends to be more subtle. In nonverbal communication, a person gives information through the use of facial expressions, gestures, body language, and tone of voice. For example, consider a resident with disabling arthritis. Not wanting to seem a "burden" to the health care staff, the resident may tell you that she feels fine when you ask. However, you note that she makes a face when she tries to get out of her chair and her voice seems strained. These observations suggest that the resident is not being entirely truthful with you about how she is feeling. Of the two forms of communication, nonverbal communication is perhaps the most reliable method of "reading" another person, especially in the health care field. For various reasons, such as embarrassment, shyness, or a fear of being perceived as foolish, people may not say what they really mean. Being observant and aware of others' nonverbal cues will give you a greater understanding of what your residents are feeling and thinking.

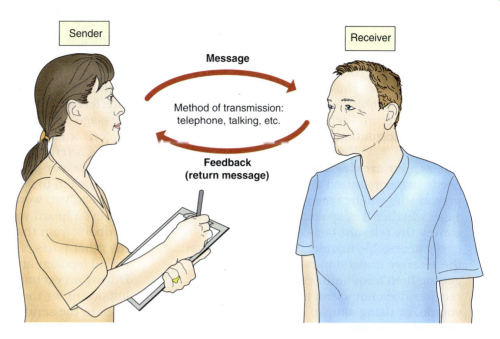

Figure 5-1
Communication involves the back-and-forth flow of information between a sender and a receiver.

COMMUNICATING EFFECTIVELY

As a nursing assistant, you must be a successful communicator, both as a sender and as a receiver of information, with both those you care for and your co-workers. For example, you will use communication skills to comfort, reassure, and teach your residents. Because the nursing assistant is the member of the health care team who typically spends the most time with a resident, the nursing assistant is one of the strongest links between the resident and the other health care team members. As you form relationships with your residents, they will talk to you, confide in you, listen to you, and trust you. In addition, by carefully watching your residents for nonverbal communication cues, you may be the first member of the health care team to notice that Mr. Jones' color is not quite right, or that Mrs. Smith is having abdominal pain after eating, even though she is not complaining verbally.

In addition to communicating well with residents, communicating well with your co-workers is also essential. Supervisors will delegate tasks to you, and you must be sure that you understand what they are asking you to do and how you are to go about doing it. Additionally, you will be the "eyes and ears" of the nurses, physical therapists, dietitians, social workers, and other members of the health care team. Relaying vital information about your resident's condition to the nurse is an essential part of your duties. As a nursing assistant, you are not trained to diagnose and treat medical problems. However, your knowledge of your resident will allow you to gather important information that, when communicated to the nurse, will alert the health care team members to changes in that person's condition and influence the care he or she receives. Your responsibility as a communication link between the resident and the rest of the health care team is very important (Fig. 5-2)!

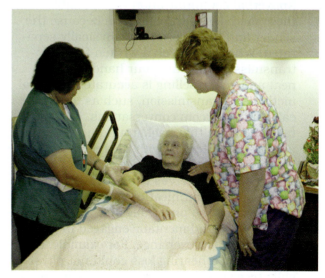

Figure 5-2
As a nursing assistant, you are an important link between the resident and the other members of the health care team.

Clearly, it is important for a nursing assistant to learn good communication skills. There are many ways that communication can fail. Remember that good communication is a "two-way street" and involves the *exchange* of information. To see where problems in communication can occur, let's look at each part of the process of exchanging information:

1. **The sender creates a message.** Information needs to be organized and relevant to the person who will be receiving it. Your message, whether it is spoken or written, should convey the relevant facts, organized in an easily accessible manner. Use language that the receiver understands—this could mean getting help from an interpreter if the receiver does not speak the same language you do, or using simple, common words in place of more complex, medical words. Speak clearly and loudly enough for the receiver to hear you without straining. Written messages should be legible and organized so that the information is complete and concise.

2. **The sender delivers the message.** Information can be transmitted from one person to another in many different ways. Speaking directly to another person, or "face-to-face," permits nonverbal communication to take place. Other methods of transmission, such as letters, memos, e-mails, telephone calls, and intercom conversations, are primarily methods of verbal communication. Nonverbal communication is impossible with these methods of transmission because the sender and the receiver are physically separated. When relying on a written form of transmission, be sure your handwriting is neat and your spelling is accurate. With oral methods of transmission, such as telephone calls and intercom conversations, it is important to ensure that background noise or static does not interfere with the receiver's ability to hear your message.

3. **The receiver receives the message.** For successful communication to occur, the receiver must be physically able to receive the message and mentally engaged in the communication exchange. For example, a person with a hearing loss could not physically receive a spoken message. A person who cannot read would not be able to understand a message sent in written form. A person who has had a stroke may be able to hear your words perfectly, but may not be able to understand their meaning. Sign language or communicating through nonverbal means (for example, nodding your head "yes" to a person's question) would not be effective if the person is blind. These are all examples of physical problems that can interfere with a person's ability to receive a message. Communication can also fail when a receiver is mentally distracted, or not really paying attention to the sender.

4. **The receiver provides feedback.** Have you ever spoken to someone and had him ignore you? Did you wonder whether or not the person even heard you? You did not receive feedback from that person. Feedback, like the other parts of communication, can be verbal (spoken or written) or nonverbal. During an exchange of information, it is important for the receiver to provide feedback to the sender, and it is important for the sender to listen and watch for this feedback. If the receiver does not provide feedback, the sender should make an effort to get a response of some sort. When feedback does not occur, or indicates that the message the sender sent was not interpreted correctly, other methods of enhancing communication may be necessary.

TACTICS THAT ENHANCE COMMUNICATION

Good communication skills will serve you well, both in your professional life and your personal life. There are many ways you can enhance communication with others.

When You Are the Receiver, Be a Good Listener

Listening is perhaps the most useful communication skill, especially in the health care setting. Active listening requires focusing your attention on the speaker. Sit down or assume a relaxed posture so you do not appear rushed or in a hurry to move on, and make eye contact with the person (Fig. 5-3). Do not interrupt or try to finish the person's sentence for her. Interrupting a person may make her forget what she was trying to tell you in the first place. Let the person finish what she was saying before you ask another question or make a comment, and focus on the person and the information she is trying to give you—try not to think about what *you* intend to do or say next. After the person has finished speaking, you should ask questions to help clarify any information that you

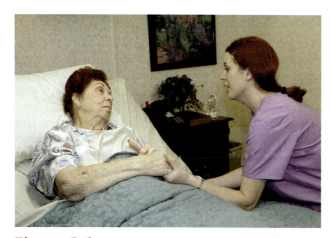

Figure 5-3
Being a good listener is essential to being a good communicator.

do not understand. Your comments and questions will let the speaker know whether you understood her message, or whether she needs to provide additional information.

When You Are the Sender, Make Sure Your Message Is Clear

Speak clearly and use words that the person you are speaking to understands. A nurse or another nursing assistant will understand medical terminology, and using medical terminology is appropriate when you are communicating with one of your co-workers. However, a resident or family member may not be familiar with medical terminology. To make sure the resident or family member understands your message, try to use common words instead of technical words whenever it is

appropriate to do so. For example, you could say, "Miss Lewis, we're going to go for a walk down the hall now, to get you up and moving" instead of "Miss Lewis, I'm going to ambulate you now."

Sometimes, it is necessary to communicate with someone who does not speak the same language as you do, or who has a physical problem that makes certain forms of communication less effective than others. For residents who speak languages other than English, health care facilities are required by law to provide interpreters. A hearing-impaired person may need a sign language interpreter to assist with communication, or you could try writing out important questions for the person to read and respond to. A picture board, a tool that allows a person to point to a picture of what he or she is trying to say, is often useful when trying to communicate on a basic level with someone who speaks a different language or is hearing impaired (Fig. 5-4). More information about communicating with residents with special needs can be found in Chapters 35 and 36.

If a resident seems to have difficulty understanding you when you are talking to him, make sure that there is not too much background noise. If the person usually wears glasses or a hearing aid, check to make sure that these aids are in place and the hearing aid is turned on.

Learn Techniques for Encouraging People to Talk

When you need to get information from someone, try asking the person an open-ended question. Questions that can be answered with a simple "yes" or "no" usually get just that response, and the conversation ends. In contrast, open-ended

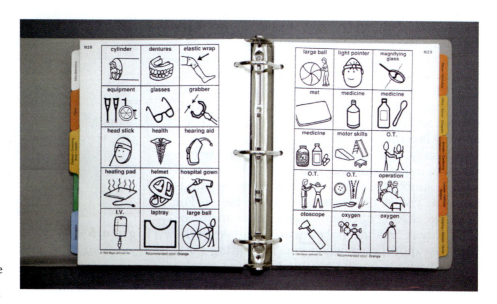

Figure 5-4
A picture board can be used to communicate when illustrations are more effective than words.

questions encourage the person to talk. Another question that can cause a conversation to end is "Why?" If a resident complains that he does not like his dinner or choice of snack, instead of asking "Why?" (which can be intimidating), you could ask the resident to tell you what his favorite food or snack is. For example, consider the following two conversations:

Conversation 1
Nursing assistant: "Good morning, Mr. Hopkins. Did you have breakfast this morning?"

Mr. Hopkins: "No."

Nursing assistant: "Why not?"

Mr. Hopkins: "I don't know . . . I just wasn't hungry, I guess."

Conversation 2
Nursing assistant: "Good morning, Mr. Hopkins. What did you have for breakfast this morning?"

Mr. Hopkins: "Not much. They sent up scrambled eggs. I don't care for scrambled eggs, so I just had some buttered toast and coffee."

Nursing assistant: "I didn't know you didn't like scrambled eggs! Let me see what I can do about that. Do you dislike eggs in general, or just scrambled eggs? In the meantime, are you hungry?"

In the second conversation, the nursing assistant achieved two key goals: She engaged Mr. Hopkins in the conversation, and in the process, she made him feel as though she really cared about him as an individual.

Rephrasing what someone says to you is another way to encourage someone to talk. For example, if one of your residents tells you that she feels sad and lonely, instead of asking "Why?" try repeating the person's statement back to her as a question: "You are feeling sad and lonely?" By rephrasing and asking an open-ended question, you will invite the person to say more. In addition, encouraging the person to talk more about what she is feeling shows the person that you are actively listening to what she is saying to you.

Usually, asking open-ended questions is better than asking questions that can be answered with a simple "yes" or "no." But in some situations, a "yes or no" question may be better. For example, asking questions that can be answered with a short "yes" or "no" (or a nod or shake of the head) is appropriate when you are caring for a resident who is having trouble breathing or who finds it very difficult to speak.

Provide and Seek Feedback

Providing and seeking feedback is a critical communication skill that will come into play with both your co-workers and your residents. Consider two conversations, one between you and the nurse, and the other between you and one of your residents. In the first, you are the "receiver"—the nurse is asking you to do a task. After the nurse has finished speaking, you could say, "Let me make sure I understand this correctly," and repeat the information back to her. What awesome feedback! The nurse now knows that you were listening, and that you understand what is being asked of you (Fig. 5-5). The *exchange* of information has occurred. You are communicating effectively.

In the second conversation, you are the "sender" and one of your residents is the "receiver"—you are trying to give instructions to the resident about how to use the call light control system in the room, and you want to make sure that he understands how the system works. You might say, "Now repeat that information back to me so I can make sure you've got it," but asking for feedback in this way could be intimidating to the resident. A more gracious way of finding out whether the resident understood your message would be to say, "Now, if you could just repeat these instructions back to me so I can make sure I didn't leave anything out. . . . " This approach makes the resident feel that he is helping you by repeating the information, and in the process, you are able to tell whether or not he understands your instructions clearly.

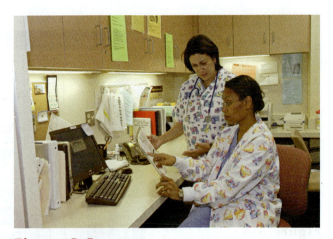

Figure 5-5

By indicating to the nurse that she understands what she is being asked to do, this nursing assistant is providing good feedback.

Be Mindful of Your Body Language and Tone of Voice

Use appropriate body language when listening or talking to other people. Negative body language, such as crossing your arms across your chest, tapping your feet or fingers, rolling your eyes, or constantly looking at your watch or toward the door sends the very clear message that you are bored or uninterested (Fig. 5-6). In contrast, displaying positive body language, such as facing the person, nodding as he speaks, smiling or looking serious as appropriate, and making occasional vocal sounds such as "uh huh" or "hmm," indicates to the person that you are interested in what he is saying. Positioning your body so that you are at eye level with the person you are communicating with also shows interest and respect (Fig. 5 -7). This is especially important when you are communicating with a person who is in a wheelchair. Towering over a person in a wheelchair can make the person feel threatened, intimidated, and defenseless.

Tone of voice is important too. A sharp or hurried tone of voice suggests to the person that

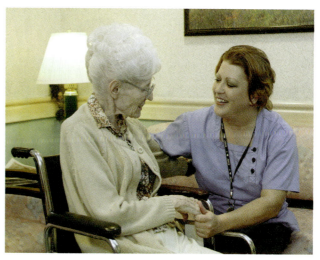

Figure 5-7
Putting yourself at eye level with a resident indicates to the person that you are interested in what he or she has to say, and that you have time to listen.

you are impatient or angry. In contrast, speaking slowly in a soothing tone of voice suggests that you are calm, competent, and kind. This relaxes the other person and is a useful technique for calming a person who is frightened or upset.

Remember the Value of Silence and a Comforting Touch

There will be many times throughout your career as a nursing assistant when words will not be enough to communicate your care and concern to a resident or to a resident's family members. Silence and a comforting touch will say more than words can (Fig. 5-8). Touch is perhaps the most universal of all languages, but remember to be sensitive to the person's comfort level. Many residents appreciate affection and will enjoy a hug or sitting and holding your hands as you talk. Other people may not be as comfortable with affection, and will be satisfied with a light pat on the shoulder or top of the hand as you greet them or say good-bye.

In addition to allowing us to communicate when words are not enough, touch is comforting and establishes a bond. So much has been written about the "healing powers of touch"—for example, consider the role of therapeutic massage in the treatment of physical ailments. Research has also shown that babies, even when given adequate food and physical care, fail to grow and thrive without human touch and attention.

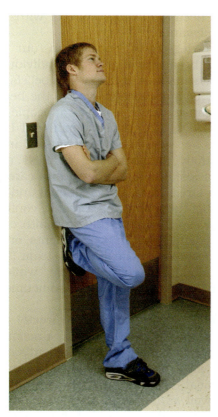

Figure 5-6
If you were a resident, what message would this nursing assistant be sending to you?

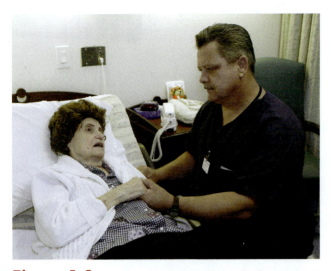

Figure 5-8
Of the many techniques for enhancing communication, nothing says "I care about you and I want to help you" more effectively than a simple touch on a person's hand or shoulder.

BLOCKS TO EFFECTIVE COMMUNICATION

Some behaviors and attitudes can block effective communication. Perhaps the most common obstacle to effective communication is not listening carefully to what another person is saying. You must be especially careful not to "tune out" your residents, despite the fact that you will be busy, and many of the people you will care for could be easily labeled "complainers." Imagine the consequences if you ignore a resident's complaint, and it turns out to be valid.

Being judgmental of others will also block communication. If a person feels that you do not believe or respect what he is trying to tell you, he will most likely stop talking and will probably refuse to answer any questions you may ask later. A judgmental attitude, indicating that you do not really care to hear what the person is trying to tell you, can be revealed through negative body language or comments you may make.

Communication blocks can occur when you assume that someone else knows what you are thinking. Your resident should know that she should not adjust the flow rate on her oxygen equipment, shouldn't she? Your co-workers should know without bothering you that Mrs. Jones has already been up to the bathroom, shouldn't they? Your husband should know why you are mad at him, shouldn't he? The assumption that other people know what you know, think the way you think,

and feel the way you feel presents a major block to effective communication and can lead to conflict and confusion. To avoid this communication pitfall, be proactive in your interactions with others, and keep them informed. For example, give instructions and gentle reminders to residents, tell your co-workers what has already been accomplished and what still needs to be done before you go on break, and ask your husband to take out the trash instead of getting angry because he did not think of it himself!

CONFLICT RESOLUTION

Conflict, or discord resulting from differences between people, can occur when one person is unable to understand or accept another's ideas or beliefs. Conflict can also arise when one person's expectations for another differ from that person's expectations for himself. Other times, conflict arises because one person misunderstands another person's words or intentions. How many times have you been angry with a friend because you thought she said or meant one thing, only to find out after talking with her that what you thought she said or meant is not what she said or meant at all? Conflict can occur when another person's needs or wants conflict with our own needs and wants.

Some degree of conflict in our lives is inevitable because we are each individuals with unique personalities, feelings, and beliefs. Conflict is a fairly common occurrence in the health care field, because health care is a people-oriented business. It is also a very emotional business. Residents are sick, hurting, confused, and frightened. Family members feel helpless and sad. Nursing assistants and other health care workers are often stressed by the emotional and physical demands of their work. As a result, conflicts may arise between a member of the health care team and a resident, between two residents, or between two members of the health care team (Fig. 5-9). Getting along with other people, while a very important part of your job, can sometimes be the hardest part of your job.

Conflict makes the people directly involved, as well as those around them, uncomfortable. This discomfort can affect a resident's quality of life or a staff member's quality of work. Good communication is essential to preventing conflict, as well as helping to resolve it. If you find yourself involved in a conflict, remember what it means to be a professional, and take the time to talk calmly with the person you are upset with. It is important to address areas of conflict early,

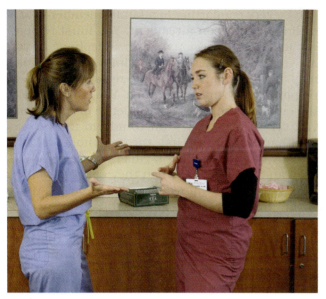

Figure 5-9
Conflict can occur between two members of the health care team or between a member of the health care team and a resident or visitor. Poor communication is one of the most common reasons conflict occurs!

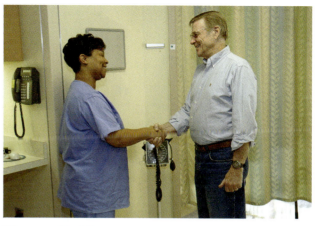

Figure 5-10
Sometimes, the best solution to a conflict is to simply "agree to disagree." Instead of focusing on your differences, focus on your similarities. In the professional setting, for example, even if you and a resident's family member cannot agree about what is "best" for the resident, you can certainly respect the fact that both of you care deeply about the resident and want to do what is best for him.

before they have time to get worse and involve more people. Approaches for resolving conflict include the following.

- Ask to speak privately with the person you have a conflict with. Because the two of you may be able to resolve your disagreement on your own, try this approach before asking a supervisor to mediate, if at all possible. Remain polite and professional and thank the person for her time.
- During your conversation, focus on the specific area of conflict. Do not focus on how you feel about the other person, or how you think she should have acted under the circumstances.
- Be specific about what you understand the problem to be, and express why you are upset in terms of "I," rather than the more accusatory "you." For example, instead of saying, "You really hurt my feelings by what you said the other day," say, "I am bothered by what you said the other day." In this manner, you take responsibility for the emotion and allow the other person to explain her side of the story.
- Be prepared to hear how the other person may feel toward you or the problem, even if it is not pleasant. Perhaps you were the one who was initially misunderstood.

- Be gracious enough to apologize for misunderstanding the other person, or for being the one who was misunderstood.
- Ask the other person for insight into solutions for resolving the conflict. Her suggestions may surprise you!
- Sometimes it is necessary to "agree to disagree." People with differing opinions and beliefs can focus on the things they have in common, such as caring about the resident's well-being, and still disagree on certain issues (Fig. 5-10). Learning to respect others' beliefs is an important part of being professional.
- If you are unable to resolve a conflict with a co-worker, a resident, or a resident's family member on your own, seek the advice of your supervisor. A conflict that affects the quality of the care you provide must not be allowed to continue!

TELEPHONE COMMUNICATION

The telephone is a primary tool of communication in the health care field. Other departments will call to verify an order or request, doctors will call to ask about a resident or to give orders, and family

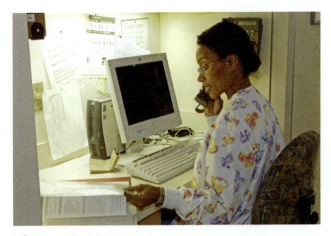

Figure 5-11
Developing a good phone manner is important, because you will find yourself using the telephone to communicate frequently!

members will call to get an update on the condition of a loved one. The telephone at the nurses' station is in use constantly—it is almost as if a teenager lives there! As a nursing assistant, you will usually be required to answer the telephone, either at the nurse's station or in a resident's room (Fig. 5-11). Proper telephone etiquette is reviewed in Box 5-1.

When you answer the telephone, make sure your voice is pleasant and unhurried. Believe it or not, a caller can "hear a smile" in your voice. This can be very comforting to a family member who is calling to check on a resident. You must remember to be as professional on the telephone as you are in person. There will be times when a caller may be impatient or angry; resist the urge to respond in a similar manner. You do not know the cause of the caller's impatience or anger, and you certainly do not want to add to it. The way you handle yourself on the telephone reflects directly on your facility. If callers perceive you as kind and professional when they speak to you on the phone, they will feel that the people you are caring for are receiving the same kind, professional care.

Confidentiality is of concern when the telephone is used as a means of communication. When you are discussing a person's care over the telephone, be sure that other residents and visitors cannot overhear your conversation. The Health Insurance Portability and Accountability Act (HIPAA), discussed in Chapter 4, specifically regulates who may be given information about a person in a health care facility. Know your facility's policy regarding what information can be provided over the telephone and to whom. For example, an interested neighbor or church member might call to ask about how a resident is doing. Although a request of this nature seems innocent enough, if you gave out *any* information about that resident, you have violated the resident's privacy rights. To give out such information

---

BOX 5-1   Telephone Etiquette

- Answer the telephone promptly, within the first three rings.
- Answer with a pleasant greeting, such as "Good morning" or "Good afternoon."
- Identify yourself by name and title and by your unit or floor according to facility policy: "3 West; Mary Smith, CNA, speaking."
- Because the caller obviously needs something (otherwise, he would not be calling), ask "How may I help you?"
- Know how to perform basic functions using your facility's telephone system, such as how to transfer a call or place a caller on hold.
- If you must place a caller on hold, ask her permission first ("May I put you on hold for a minute?"). Be aware of the length of time a caller has been on hold; if the time becomes excessive (more than 5 minutes), ask the caller if she wants to continue to hold, leave a message, or call back later.

- If the person the caller wants to speak to is unavailable, offer to take a message. When taking a telephone message, be sure to write down the date and time of the call, the name of the caller, a telephone number where the caller can be reached, and your name. Write clearly, and ask the caller to spell his or her name if you are not sure how to spell it. Be sure to deliver the message to the person for whom it was intended.
- A nursing assistant is not to take doctor's orders, receive or give results of diagnostic tests, or release resident information to anyone, even family members. Calls of this nature should be handled by a nurse.
- Do not use the telephone at the nurse's station to make or receive personal calls. Personal calls should be made from a pay phone or your own cellular phone, while you are on break or at lunch. Never tie up a telephone used for health care communication by using it for personal business.

could result in litigation against the facility, and ultimately cost you your job. It is best to refer inquiries about residents to the nurse.

COMMUNICATION AMONG MEMBERS OF THE HEALTH CARE TEAM

As you have already learned, the nursing assistant plays a very important role in gathering and sharing information about residents with other members of the health care team. As you interact with your residents, you will have the opportunity to make **observations.** An observation is something that you notice about the resident, typically related to a change in the resident's physical or mental condition. The amount of time you will spend with your residents, combined with the type of duties you are responsible for performing daily (for example, bathing, feeding, ambulating, toileting), will give you a chance to observe things that other health care team members may overlook.

Observations can be based on either objective data or subjective data. **Objective data** are information that you obtain directly, through measurements or by using one of your five senses. In the professional setting, the senses you will use most often are sight, hearing, touch, and smell. For example, certain indicators of a person's health, called vital signs, can be objectively measured. (The vital signs are temperature, pulse, respiratory rate, and blood pressure.) You can see the color of a person's skin and feel that it is cool and clammy (Fig. 5-12). You can see the color of a person's urine, smell any foul odor, and measure the amount. You can hear wheezing or gurgling as a person breathes. You can see bruises, swelling, or rashes on the skin when you help a person bathe. You can see how much breakfast the person ate and measure how much juice she drank. These are all objective observations. Objective observations, such as an elevated temperature, a rash, or a low urine output, are called **signs.**

Subjective data, on the other hand, are information that cannot be objectively measured or assessed. The basis for a subjective observation is usually a person's complaint, or **symptom.** For example, a resident may tell you that he has a headache or stomachache. You cannot see, feel, measure, or hear his pain, but he can describe it to you (Fig. 5-13). When you are communicating subjective observations to the other

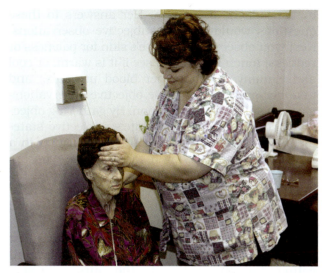

Figure 5-12
Objective data are obtained using one of your five senses. Here, the nursing assistant is feeling the resident's forehead to assess whether or not the skin is hot and dry or cool and clammy.

health care team members, it is useful to quote the person directly, whether you are relaying the complaint verbally (reporting) or writing the information in the person's medical record (recording).

It is useful to support subjective observations with objective ones. For instance, Mrs. White tells you that she feels dizzy when she stands up (a subjective observation). To gather more information, you ask Mrs. White if she has gotten dizzy before, and whether or not her dizziness is accompanied

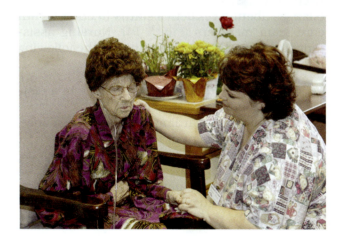

Figure 5-13
Subjective data are information that is derived "secondhand." This nursing assistant knows that her resident is experiencing stomach pain because the resident is describing it to her, not because she detected the resident's pain using one of her five senses.

by a headache or nausea. Her answers to these questions would also be subjective observations. Next, you observe Mrs. White's skin for paleness or redness; touch her skin to see if it is warm, or cool and clammy; measure her blood pressure; and take her pulse. All of these objective observations give you still more information. By gathering objective facts to add to Mrs. White's subjective statements, and then organizing this information in a logical way and relaying it to the nurse, you are truly communicating! Not only have you told the nurse about Mrs. White's symptoms, but you have also given her objective data that may help her find out what is causing those symptoms.

Once you have made an observation, you must decide on the most effective method of communicating that observation to the nurse. Nursing assistants use two methods of communicating observations about their residents and documenting the care provided so that other health care team members are kept "in-the-know." These methods are reporting and recording. Some observations need to be reported to the nurse immediately, such as a resident's complaint of pain or a change in her vital signs. Other observations only need to be recorded in the resident's medical record. Throughout this text, observations that need to be reported to the nurse immediately are highlighted as "Tell the Nurse!" notes.

REPORTING

Reporting is the spoken exchange of information between health care team members. Reporting is used throughout the shift to communicate changes about a resident's status to other health care team members (Fig. 5-14). Nursing assistants use reporting to communicate the following information to the nurse:

- Observations that suggest a change in a resident's condition
- Observations regarding a resident's response to a new treatment or therapy
- Accidents (such as a fall) or injuries (such as a bruise or skin tear)
- A resident's complaints of pain or discomfort
- A resident's refusal of treatment
- A resident's request for clergy

When reporting information, follow the guidelines that help promote effective communication. Make sure the information that you are reporting is accurate—refer to the resident by name and room number, and if you are reporting measurements, such as vital signs, write the numbers

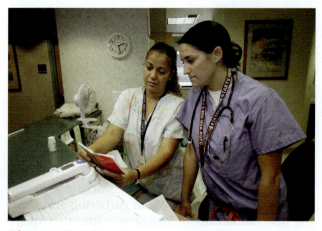

Figure 5-14

This nursing assistant is reporting a change in one of her resident's vital signs to the nurse.

down so that you do not forget them or report them incorrectly. Report your observations in an orderly, concise manner. Avoid adding information that is not relevant to what you are trying to communicate. Use correct terminology when reporting, and make sure the person you are reporting to gives you feedback so that you know he received the information and will act on it.

Reporting is also routinely used when shifts change to keep the staff members who are coming to work aware of all the information that is necessary to ensure a smooth continuation of care for the resident. For example, the end-of-shift report is when oncoming staff members would be informed of new residents and their care requirements, changes in the care plan for established residents (such as new orders or treatments), and changes in a resident's status (such as rest or appetite changes).

RECORDING

Recording, sometimes referred to as "charting," is communicating information about a resident to other health care team members in written form.

Medical Record (Chart)

A person's **medical record (chart)** is a legal document where information about the resident's current condition, the measures that have been taken by the medical and nursing staff to diagnose and treat the condition, and the resident's response to the treatment and care provided is recorded. Because the medical record, a legal document, is a formal accounting of the care the resident received from the health care facility, it can be retrieved at any time and used in a court of law as evidence in a litigation claim.

The medical record is usually organized in sections with specific forms contained in each section. Some of these forms provide general information about the resident. Others are specific to a particular health care department. The forms used may vary, but typically, a medical record contains the sections and forms shown in Table 5-1. To keep residents safe and reduce the risk for errors that could occur if orders meant for one resident were accidentally placed in another resident's medical record, each form in the medical record is stamped or printed with the resident's identification information.

The information recorded on the various forms in the medical record allow the members of the health care team to communicate with each other efficiently. For example, consider the following scenario:

Five days ago, Mrs. Wilson complained to the nursing assistant of abdominal pain and frequent urination. When the nursing assistant reported Mrs. Wilson's complaints to the nurse, the nurse asked the nursing assistant to check Mrs. Wilson's vital signs. On reviewing Mrs. Wilson's vital signs, the nurse saw that Mrs. Wilson had a fever. The nurse assessed Mrs. Wilson, placed a phone call to the doctor to request that the doctor review Mrs. Wilson's new signs and symptoms, and then documented her assessment findings and her phone call to the doctor in the nurses' progress notes (Fig. 5-15). The doctor gave an order to the nurse to start an antibiotic. The nurse

		Wilson, Ethel J.
		Room 302
		Resident #1801
		Dr. Nicholas Smith

Nurses' Progress Notes

Date	Time	Notes
2/20/08	6:25am	The nursing assistant reported that the resident is complaining of
		frequent urination and abdominal pain. She has been to the
		bathroom x4 since 5am and each time voided only a small amount.
		Her urine appears cloudy and has a foul ordor. Abdominal pain
		assessed in her lower abdomen. She denies burning upon urination.
		Skin is warm and appears slightly flushed. T = 100.8, P = 73,
		R = 18, B/P = 118/74. Call placed to Dr. Smith. Tylenol given for
		fever. See new orders. N. Nevins, RN
2/20/08	12:30pm	Resident continues to complain of frequent urination and
		abdominal pain. Appetite 50% for breakfast and lunch. Fluids
		encouraged and accepted. Antibiotic rec'd from pharmacy and first
		dose was received at 12n. T = 99.8, P = 70, R = 16, and B/P =
		113/70. Will continue to monitor. P. Smithson, LPN
2/20/08	9:55pm	Resident rec'd second dose of antibiotic at 6pm. No adverse
		effects noted. Still complaining of some urinary frequency and
		abdominal pain. Appetite 75% for dinner. Fluids encouraged. Denies
		any other complaints. Assisted to the bathroom x3. Small, soft
		BM x1. T = 99.2, P = 72, R = 19, B/P = 122/74. Resting comfortably
		at this time. L. Goode, LPN

Figure 5-15

A resident's new symptoms, care provided by the nursing staff, and continued monitoring of the resident's response to treatment are all documented in the nurses' progress notes.

Table 5-1   The Medical Record

SECTION	FORMS AND DOCUMENTS CONTAINED IN THE SECTION
Admissions	● The admission (face) sheet, which includes the resident's name, address, date of birth and age, gender, Social Security number, insurance information, emergency contacts, and sometimes funeral home information
Advance Directives	● Legal documents identifying the resident's health care agent, wishes for end-of-life care, or both ● Power-of-attorney papers for business affairs
History and Physical	● Discharge summaries from hospitalizations, which tell why the resident was admitted to the hospital, what happened during the hospital stay, the resident's condition on discharge, and the follow-up care and treatment needed ● History and physical forms, completed by the doctor on admission, and annually thereafter
Physician Progress Notes	● Forms used by the doctor to record his or her observations about the person's medical condition and response to treatment
Physician Orders	● Forms used by the doctor to order treatments (such as medications) and consultations, specify dietary orders and activity restrictions or special allowances, order diagnostic tests or laboratory work, and communicate other measures that should be taken for the resident
Nurses' Progress Notes or Interdisciplinary Progress Notes	● Form used by the nursing staff to document the resident's progress and problems, and the actions taken by the nursing staff in response to the problems* or ● Form used by members of the health care team from many different areas (such as the doctor, nurse, dietician, social worker, and activities director) to document the resident's progress and problems, and the actions taken by the health care team in response to these problems
Therapy	● Assessments, progress notes, and treatment records for rehabilitation services such as physical therapy, occupational therapy, and speech language pathology
Dietary	● Nutritional assessments and progress notes written by the dietitian
Social Work	● The social history, which details personal information about the resident, including birthplace, family relationships, education and employment history, marriage and family, and significant life events ● Progress notes relating to the resident's adjustment to the long-term care setting, assistance with Medicare or Medicaid documents, discharge planning, special family situations, and end-of-life care
Activities (Recreational Therapy)	● Documents detailing the resident's hobbies and other leisure time activities, personal interests, and religious beliefs and practices ● Notes about the resident's participation in activities while in the facility
Flow (Graphic) Sheets	● Forms used to record information that is collected routinely such as the resident's vital signs, weight, food and fluid intake, bowel habits, performance of activities of daily living (ADLs), and restorative care
Medication/Treatment Administration Record	● Form listing the medications or treatments ordered for the resident, along with the dosage and time at which the medications or treatments are to be administered and specific administration instructions; also used to record when medications or treatments are given and by whom
Consultations	● Assessments and notes from specialist doctors (such as the eye doctor or foot doctor) or other members of the health care team (such as the clinical pharmacist, a pharmacist responsible for reviewing medication therapy)
Laboratory Work and Diagnostic Studies	● Results from tests ordered for the resident such as blood work, specimen studies (such as urine or stool), and x-rays
Assessments and Care Plans**	● Minimum Data Set (MDS) assessments ● Other assessments such as those used to evaluate the resident's skin condition, fall risk, or mood status

*Some facilities allow nursing assistants to make notations in the nurses' notes, and some do not.

**Some facilities keep MDS assessments and care plans in a separate binder.

recorded the order on the physician's order sheet and also transcribed it to the medication administration record (MAR). The ward clerk faxed the order to the pharmacy so that the order for the antibiotic could be filled. When the antibiotic was delivered by the pharmacy, the nurse administered the antibiotic to Mrs. Wilson, and recorded that the antibiotic was given on the MAR. The nursing assistants who were caring for Mrs. Wilson measured and recorded Mrs. Wilson's temperature at regular intervals on the flow (graphic) sheet. When the doctor made her rounds a few days later, she was able to see that the antibiotic had been given as ordered. She could also tell by the nurse's documentation in the nurses' progress notes (which described improvement in Mrs. Wilson's symptoms) and the temperature recordings on the flow (graphic) sheet that Mrs. Wilson was responding to the medication.

By using the medical chart properly, the health care team members were able to communicate with each other in an organized, efficient way. The doctor did not need to find the nurse or nursing assistant to ask whether Mrs. Wilson was receiving the antibiotic, or to find out whether her fever had gone away.

Each facility has specific policies about whether or not a nursing assistant is allowed to record information in the medical record. In some facilities, you may be able to record information on the flow (graphic) sheet (Fig. 5-16), but not on the nurses' progress notes. In others, you will be required to make entries in the nurses' progress notes as documentation of the care you provide and the observations you make. Whenever you enter information on a person's medical record, date and time your entry correctly. Facilities may

Flow Sheet/Vital Signs						Kensington, Eleanor Room 213A Dr. Ross Ryan			
Date	**Time**	**Temp.**	**Pulse**	**Resp.**	**BP**	**Intake**	**Output**	**Weight**	**Initials**
5/1/08	8:00am	98.4	76	20	136/78	–	–	128.5#	WG
5/1/08	2:15pm	–	–	–	–	925	850	–	WG
5/1/08	3:45pm	98.2	72	16	132/70	–	–	–	TM
5/1/08	10:10pm	–	–	–	–	775	800	–	TM
5/2/08	**12:05am**	**97.5**	**68**	**16**	**130/68**	–	–	–	**MC**
5/2/08	**6:30am**	–	–	–	–	**250**	**175**	–	**MC**
5/2/08	7:55am	98.2	74	18	140/74	–	–	–	WG
5/2/08	2:50pm	–	–	–	–	875	900	–	WG
5/2/08	3:30pm	99.1	80	20	138/72	–	–	–	DH
5/2/08	10:30pm	99.0	78	18	138/68	725	800	–	DH
5/2/08	**11:55pm**	**98.8**	**78**	**22**	**138/70**	–	–	–	**MC**
5/3/08	**6:35am**	**98.6**	**76**	**16**	**134/72**	**150**	**200**	–	**MC**
5/4/08	7:35am	98.8	80	18	134/68	–	–	128.0#	WG
5/4/08	2:20pm	–	–	–	–	850	775	–	WG

Figure 5-16
This flow (graphic) sheet is used to record routine measurements such as vital signs, intake and output, and weight. This format helps the nurse to follow changes and see patterns over time.

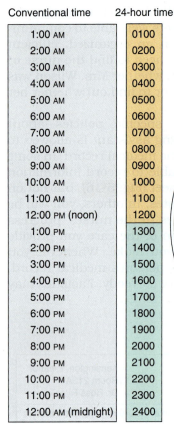

Conventional time	24-hour time
1:00 AM	0100
2:00 AM	0200
3:00 AM	0300
4:00 AM	0400
5:00 AM	0500
6:00 AM	0600
7:00 AM	0700
8:00 AM	0800
9:00 AM	0900
10:00 AM	1000
11:00 AM	1100
12:00 PM (noon)	1200
1:00 PM	1300
2:00 PM	1400
3:00 PM	1500
4:00 PM	1600
5:00 PM	1700
6:00 PM	1800
7:00 PM	1900
8:00 PM	2000
9:00 PM	2100
10:00 PM	2200
11:00 PM	2300
12:00 AM (midnight)	2400

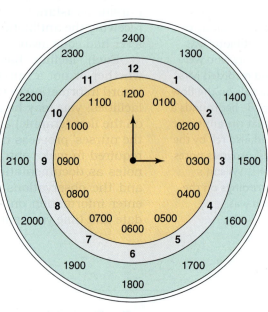

Figure 5-17
Facilities may use the 24-hour time clock, also referred to as "military time," for recording the time in a resident's medical record. The 24-hour time clock eliminates the need to differentiate between morning (AM) and night (PM), thus reducing errors in recording. On the 24-hour time clock, the morning hours are the same as on the conventional clock. To indicate a time in the afternoon, add "12" to the time on the conventional clock. When time is stated according to the 24-hour time clock, the first two numbers indicate the hour and the last two numbers indicate the minute (e.g., 8:24 PM conventional time = 2024 military time). Conventional time = *gray*; morning hours = *yellow*; afternoon hours = *green*.

use the 24-hour time clock, also called "military time," for recording the time in a resident's medical record (Fig. 5-17). Guidelines for recording are given in Guidelines Box 5-1.

As the use of computers becomes more widespread, computerized charting is replacing paper charting in some facilities (Fig. 5-18). In computerized charting, the person's medical record is maintained by entering data into a computer in response to the computer's prompts, rather than by filling in a paper form. Data is usually typed into the computer, but in the future, we may see an increase in voice-activated systems, which make it possible to chart by responding to the computer's prompts verbally! Medical records that are maintained using a computer tend to be more accurate and legible because they are typed rather than handwritten.

Using a computer to access and maintain a resident's medical record does not require advanced computer training. If your facility uses computerized charting, your employer will provide training in the use of the computer as part of your new employee orientation. During this training, you will learn how to enter data about your residents, as well as how to quickly retrieve information that you need about a resident in order to provide care.

Remember from Chapter 4 that the information contained in a person's medical record is considered confidential. Special measures to protect confidentiality are taken when using a computer to chart. For example, each user of the computer is assigned a password, which permits the user to have access to certain residents'

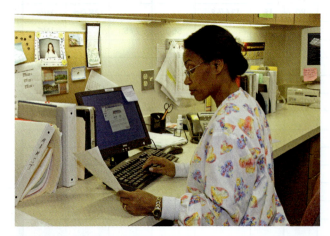

Figure 5-18
Computerized charting is becoming more widespread.

Guidelines Box 5-1   Guidelines for Recording

WHAT YOU DO	WHY YOU DO IT
Write legibly, using blue or black ink. Your facility may have specific policies regarding the color of ink used.	It is important to write legibly to avoid miscommunication. A pen is used instead of a pencil because pencil can be erased, enabling someone to change the person's medical record. Blue and black ink reproduce best when a document is photocopied.
Always sign or initial your entry, according to facility policy.	By signing or initialing your entry, you indicate that you are the person who needs to be consulted if further clarification of the information you have entered is necessary. Additionally, signing or initialing your entry indicates that you accept legal responsibility for what you have written.
Only record observations that you have made, or care that you have given. Do not make entries for another person.	By making an entry in a medical record, you accept legal responsibility for that entry. Therefore, it is best to record only information that you, personally, can vouch for.
Date and time your entries correctly (see Fig. 5-17).	The date and time that actions occurred or observations were made are extremely important elements of the medical record, which is a legal account of care provided.
Check the resident's name on the medical record and on the form where you are recording.	By verifying the resident's identification information, you will ensure that you are recording the person's information in the correct medical record.
Use appropriate medical terminology and facility-approved abbreviations when recording.	Using correct terminology and abbreviations will prevent others from having to second-guess your meaning.
Do not record care as given or procedures as performed before you have provided the care or performed the procedure. Only document after the fact.	You may become distracted or involved in another situation that prevents you from carrying out the duties you have already charted. If you record duties as "completed" in the medical record, but then do not actually complete these duties, you will have committed fraud.
Record information in a timely manner. If you must wait to record something, keep notes about your observations and care so that the information you record in the medical record will be accurate.	If you wait until the end of your shift to record, you may forget important information.
If you make an error, do not erase, use correction fluid to cover, or scribble through the mistaken entry. Simply draw a line through the mistake and initial it according to facility policy.	Striking through an error is the only legal way to indicate a change in the medical record. Erasing or using correction fluid to correct an error could be seen as an attempt to hide or change existing information.
Remember that in a liability situation, care not recorded was care not provided.	Proper and conscientious recording of resident information protects the resident, your employer, and you.

ADVANCED DIRECTIVES		Behavior QOL program _n/a_			Self-Performance	Support (# of Persons)

ADVANCED DIRECTIVES

_X_ Living will   ___ Autopsy request
___ Do not resuscitate   ___ Feeding restrictions
___ Do not hospitalize   ___ Medication restrictions
_X_ Organ donation   ___ Other treatment restrictions
___   ___ NONE OF THE ABOVE

Allergies: **Sulfa**
(Write in red or highlight)

Nutritional/Oral

Diet _Regular_
Supplements: _n/a_
Meal Location: Breakfast _Dining room_
                Lunch _Dining room_
                Dinner _Dining room_

___ Swallowing Difficulty   ___ Thicken Liquids
___ Tube Feeding   ___ NPO
___ I-O   ___ Fluid Restriction
___ TPN

Elimination   QOL program(s) _n/a_
Bladder:
_X_ Continent ___ Incontinent ___ Catheter
Bowel:
_X_ Continent ___ Incontinent ___ Ostomy

Cognition
___ Short term memory problem
___ Decision-making difficulty
___ Difficulty expressing self

Oriented to:
_X_ Person   _X_ Place
_X_ Time   _X_ Situation

Behavior   QOL program _n/a_
___ Verbally Abusive
___ Physically Abusive
___ Socially Inappropriate
___ Resistant to Care
___ Wandering/Exit Seeking   QOL program _n/a_

Communication
 Primary Language:
_X_ English ___ Other: ___
___ Alternative methods used:
___ Communication board   ___ Writing
___ Sign language   ___ Gestures
___ Other ___

Appliances
___ Hearing Aide ___ R ___ L
_X_ Glasses ___ Contacts
_X_ Dentures ___ Upper ___ Lower _X_ Partial
___ Anti-embolism hose
_X_ Prosthesis/Splint/Brace (description) _Cast-Rt_
    Forearm

Respiratory
                           ___ Pulse Oximetry
___ Tracheostomy   ___ Oxygen
___ Ventilator   ___ Suctioning
Skin Management   QOL program ___
___ Turn & Position   ___ Other ___
___ Mattress

Additional Quality of Life Program(s) or Medical Specialty Treatment Program(s)
Physical Therapy rt. arm

ADL's Self-Performance / Support (# of Persons)

ADL's	Self-Performance	Support (# of Persons)
Bathing ___	I S (L) E T	(1) 2
Dressing ___	I S (L) E T	(1) 2
Toileting ___	(I) S L E T	1 2
Eating ___	I S (L) E T	(1) 2
Transferring ___	(I) S L E T	1 2
Walking ___	I S (L) E T	(1) 2

I - Independent   E - Extensive
S - Supervised   T - Total
L - Limited

Mobility: Weight bearing status _good_

___ Mechanical lift   ___ W/chair
___ ROM   ___ Walker
_X_ AROM   _X_ Cane
___ PROM   ___ Other: ___
___ Bedfast/chairbound
Weight schedule _X_ mo ___ why ___ other
          QOL program ___
Restraint: Type: ___   When: ___
          QOL Program

Resident Preferences:	Bathing type:	Bathing Day/time:
Name: _miss (Ethel)_	___ Shower _X_ Tub	M (T) W (Th)
Time to arise _7 am_	___ Other: ___	F (Sa) Su
Time to rest: _1 pm_		
Time to retire _10 pm_	___	AM (PM)
Likes/dislikes: ___		

Special Precautions:
Please assist at mealtime by opening milk and cutting food into small pieces

Diagnoses:
 Primary: ___
 Secondary: _FX Rt. radius & ulna_

RESIDENT NAME	ADMISSION DATE	PHYSICIAN	DOB	AGE	Medical Record Number
Ethel Hayes	12/01/06	Sanders	03/06/1929	77	1301

Figure 5-19
The Kardex card, kept in a Kardex file, summarizes the most up-to-date information about a resident's condition and care needs.

medical records. Never give anyone else your password or leave the computer active after you have used it. If you fail to log off after using the computer, the information on the screen may be visible or accessible to people who are not authorized to have access to it. Additionally, if you fail to log off when you are finished with the computer, someone else could enter information under your password, and it will appear that you have entered it. Computer monitors should be positioned so that the screen is not visible to the public when you are working. Your facility will have specific policies (mandated by HIPAA) regarding computer use and confidentiality. Make sure you are familiar with these policies, and follow them carefully.

Kardex

The **Kardex** is a card file, containing condensed versions of each resident's medical record. The Kardex card contains a one-page summary of the person's current diagnosis, any special care needs (such as treatments ordered by the doctor or specific care measures specified in the care plan), and information about routine care measures such as the resident's diet, level of ambulation, and bathing schedule (Fig. 5-19). The Kardex card is updated as the resident's condition or doctor's orders change. Some long-term care facilities use the Kardex card system so that health care team members do not have to search through the entire record every time they need information about the resident's status and care plan.

SUMMARY

- Communication is the exchange of information.
    - For good communication to occur, a sender must send a clear message directly to a receiver who can understand the message. The receiver must provide feedback that lets the sender know that the message was heard "loud and clear."
    - Effective communication among health care team members is essential to ensure that residents receive top-quality, safe care. It is important for nursing assistants to have good communication skills because the exchange of information with residents and co-workers is a key part of the nursing assistant's job.
    - Nursing assistants are an important link between the resident and other members of the health care team. The nursing assistant is often the first member of the health care team to become aware of a change in a resident's condition that could be a sign of something serious.
- There are many ways to improve communication with others.

- Listening is one of the most important communication skills, especially in the health care field.
    - Speaking clearly, asking open-ended questions, and using appropriate body language when talking with other people are other ways to improve communication.
- Reporting and recording are two methods of communication used by the health care team to make sure that everyone involved in the care of a resident has current, reliable information about that person. Observations about a resident's condition are reported, recorded, or both. Observations may be subjective or objective.
    - Reporting is the spoken exchange of information between members of the health care team. Observations about a change in a resident's condition must be reported to the nurse immediately.
    - Recording is the written exchange of information between members of the health care team. Recording is done in the person's medical record or chart.

WHAT DID YOU LEARN?

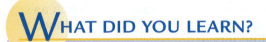

Multiple Choice

Select the single best answer for each of the following questions.

1. Which one of the following is an open-ended question?
   a. "Are you Mrs. Brown?"
   b. "Mr. Jones, when you were growing up, what was your favorite meal?"
   c. "Are you feeling okay, Mrs. Smith?"
   d. "It's beautiful outside today, Mrs. Murphy! Do you want to go for a walk?"
2. Which one of the following is an example of positive body language?
   a. Nodding encouragingly as someone speaks
   b. Crossing your arms across your chest
   c. Tapping your feet or fingers
   d. Rolling your eyes

3. An example of an action that blocks effective communication is:
   a. Interrupting
   b. Not listening carefully
   c. Being judgmental
   d. All of the above
4. Which one of the following is an observation based on objective data?
   a. "Mr. Wohl says that his back hurts when he coughs."
   b. "Ms. O'Connell's urine is cloudy, and has a strong odor."
   c. "Mr. McAndrews is complaining of a headache."
   d. "The resident in room 201B is complaining of a stomachache."

5. Which one of the following is an example of nonverbal communication?
   a. Using sign language to communicate with a deaf person
   b. Recording vital sign measurements in a resident's chart
   c. Gently touching a resident on the shoulder to reassure her
   d. Making a telephone call

6. What usually forms the basis for a subjective observation?
   a. A symptom, or resident's complaint
   b. A measurement
   c. A doctor's order
   d. All of the above

7. With regard to telephone communication, nursing assistants are responsible for all of the following except:
   a. Writing down the caller's name and telephone number if the person the caller wants to speak to is not available, and delivering this message to the intended recipient
   b. Answering the telephone promptly, with a pleasant greeting
   c. Taking down doctor's orders if the nurse is not available and a doctor calls
   d. Identifying themselves to the caller by name and title, per facility policy

8. When recording information in a person's medical chart, what should you remember to do?
   a. Use pencil so that errors can be corrected neatly
   b. Sign or initial and date and time your entry, per facility policy
   c. Update all of your residents' charts at one time at the end of each shift
   d. All of the above

9. What is it called when people have differences and they are unable to come to an agreement?
   a. Communication
   b. Conflict
   c. Culture
   d. Personality difference

Matching

Match each numbered item with its appropriate lettered description.

_____ 1. Admission (face) sheet

_____ 2. Nurses' progress notes

_____ 3. Medication administration record (MAR)

_____ 4. Flow (graphic) sheet

a. Form used by the nursing staff to document the resident's progress and problems, and the actions taken by the nursing staff in response to the problems
b. Form used to record routine data such as vital signs, weight, bowel habits, and food and fluid intake
c. Form used to list the medications ordered for the resident, and to record when the medications are given and by whom
d. Document that contains essential information about the resident, including his or her name and address, birth date, insurance information, and emergency contact information

STOP and Think!

- You are caring for Mr. Thompson today and notice that he seems distracted and is having difficulty speaking clearly. You know that you should report this to the nurse immediately.

What other subjective and objective data should you gather to report to the nurse? How can you make sure that the nurse receives the information from you?

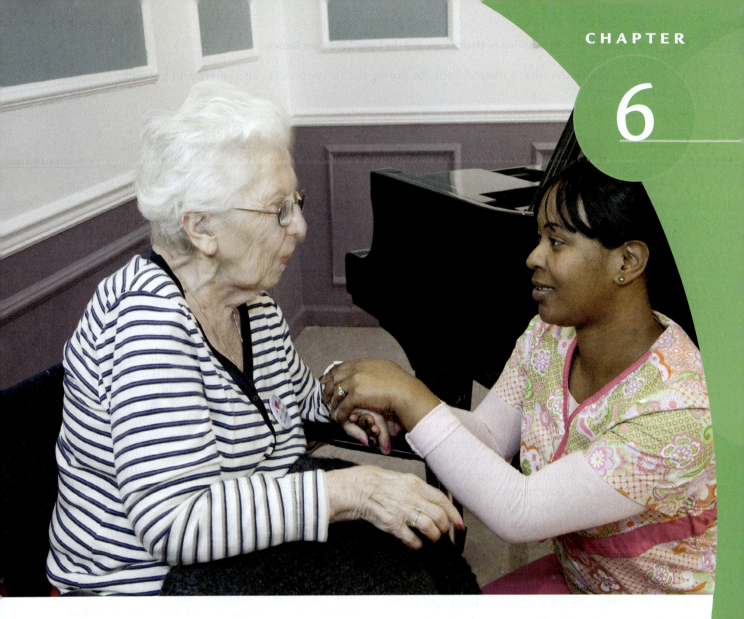

The Survey Process

WHAT WILL YOU LEARN?

The government performs routine inspections of nursing homes, called surveys, to ensure that the nursing homes are following Omnibus Budget Reconciliation Act (OBRA) regulations and meeting the government's standards. In this chapter, you will learn more about the survey process and the very important role you will play in helping your facility to achieve a positive survey outcome. When you are finished with this chapter, you will be able to:

1. Discuss the purpose of the survey.
2. Identify who performs the survey.

Photo: The survey team will want to see that you are attentive to your residents' needs. Here, a nursing assistant pauses to visit with a resident.

3. Identify and discuss what surveyors look for during the survey process and where and how they find that information.

4. Describe the nursing assistant's role in the survey process.

Vocabulary Use the CD in the front of your book to hear these terms pronounced and defined:

Compliance	Sanitarian	F-Tags	Quality Indicator Profile
Survey	Surveyor	Plan of	report
Survey team	Deficiency	correction	Sentinel events
Dietitian	citations	Off-site preparation	

AN OVERVIEW OF THE SURVEY PROCESS

As you learned in Chapter 2, the Omnibus Budget Reconciliation Act (OBRA) established government standards for the quality of services provided by nursing homes. Regulations are put in place to enforce these standards. The government must have a way of making sure that nursing homes are following OBRA regulations and meeting the government's standards. The survey process is how the government checks for **compliance** (the state of meeting established regulations, standards, or requirements).

A **survey** is an inspection of a nursing home done to ensure that care is being provided according to standards and regulations. The **survey team** (the group of government officials who perform the survey) must include at least one registered nurse (RN), but often there are several. The team usually also includes a **dietitian** (a person who has a degree in nutrition) and a **sanitarian** (a person who evaluates the safety and cleanliness of the building). The **surveyors** (individual members of the survey team) work together to complete the required survey tasks.

The surveyors may be from local, state, or federal agencies. Most of the surveyors who come to your facility will be from the state. State or local surveyors are often hired by the federal government to perform the survey on the federal government's behalf. Federal surveyors may accompany the state or local surveyors. They will be there to evaluate the facility, as well as to monitor the performance of the state or local surveyors. Sometimes the federal surveyors will come to the facility by themselves.

During the survey, the surveyors directly observe the care and services provided in the facility. They look at the overall appearance and condition of the building. They review resident services such as the laundry, housekeeping, food service, and activities programming departments. And, of course, they review the nursing care that is provided to residents.

The survey is unannounced. While surveys most often occur during standard business hours (that is, between the hours of 9 AM and 5 PM, Monday through Friday), they can occur at any time, on any day of the week. Usually, the survey takes place over several days, but it may take longer depending on the size of the facility, the number of surveyors on the team, and the number and types of problems that the surveyors find.

At the end of the survey, the survey team presents a written report of their findings. If the facility is found to be out of compliance, the report will include **deficiency citations** (statements that identify the standards that were not met, as well as the survey team's findings that indicate how the facility failed to meet the standards). Deficiency citations are noted under **F-Tags**, numerical headings that categorize the various standards included in the nursing home regulations in OBRA. For example, problems related to quality of care would be listed under F-309, Quality of Care, and concerns about falls and injuries would be listed under F-323, Accidents.

The facility must respond to the deficiency citations by submitting and carrying out a **plan of correction.** The plan of correction outlines specific actions that the facility will take to fix the problems and achieve compliance. For each deficiency citation, the plan of correction must outline how the problem will be fixed, as well as how the facility will identify other residents at risk for the same problem (in order to make sure that those residents are included in the corrective action). The plan of correction also must include the measures the facility will take to prevent the same problem from happening in the future.

Depending on the seriousness of the deficiency, the survey team may return to the facility at a future date to make sure that the plan of correction has worked and the facility is back in compliance. A facility that does not regain compliance status may face serious penalties, such as:

- Substantial fines
- An inability to qualify for Medicare or Medicaid payments
- An admission ban (the facility is not allowed to admit new residents)
- Closure

Nursing homes are being trusted to care for those who are unable to care for themselves, which is very serious business!

ensure that your residents are receiving top-quality care. As a nursing assistant, you strive to provide top-quality care to your residents every day. You may still be nervous when the survey team is in your facility. We all get nervous when we are being watched, or judged. But rest assured, if you are caring for your residents the way you have been taught, and you are properly following your facility's policies and procedures, you will be doing your part to ensure that your facility comes through the survey with flying colors. Guidelines for excelling at your job and helping your facility do well on the survey are given in Guidelines Box 6-1.

STAFF REACTIONS TO THE SURVEY

As you begin your health care career in the nursing home environment, you will hear a lot about "the survey." Staff members often react to these words with dread and anxiety. Sometimes, staff members deliberately try to stay out of sight of the surveyors because they are anxious about making a mistake in the surveyors' presence. This is one of the *worst* things that can happen. If surveyors do not see or cannot easily find staff members, they will wonder how the staff can possibly be meeting the residents' needs!

It is normal to feel some anxiety about the survey process, because the survey process is very important and there is a great deal at stake. However, you can keep things in perspective by remembering that the purpose of the survey is to

OFF-SITE PREPARATION FOR THE SURVEY

When the survey team arrives at the facility, they have a relatively short period of time to complete a lot of work. To maximize the time that the survey team has on-site, the survey team begins the survey process before they actually come to the facility. This advance work, called **off-site preparation,** allows the survey team to identify potential areas of concern, which in turn provides a focus for their attention during the actual visit to the facility. During off-site preparation, the survey team reviews information from various sources (Table 6-1).

After completing their off-site preparation, the survey team knows what care issues they will want to examine when they arrive at the facility. In addition, they will have identified specific residents in

Table 6-1	Information Used for Off-Site Preparation
DOCUMENT	**INFORMATION PROVIDED**
Past survey reports	● Specific survey findings from past surveys conducted at the facility
Online Survey, Certification, and Reporting (OSCAR) reports	● Deficiencies that the facility was cited for in the past ● Information about the characteristics of the facility and its residents
Ombudsman reports	● Complaints from residents or family members that were reported to and investigated by the ombudsman's office ● Input from the ombudsman based on his or her experiences during visits to the facility (or during other interactions with the facility)
Complaint investigation reports	● Problems reported to and investigated by the state
Waivers and variances reports	● State-approved variations in the facility's manner of meeting a required standard
Quality Indicator Profile report	● Markers of quality in specific care areas ● How the facility compares with other facilities in the state in each of the specific care areas ● Care concerns for specific residents, based on assessment data pulled from the Minimum Data Set (MDS)

Guidelines Box	6-1	Guidelines for Excelling at Your Job and Helping Your Facility Do Well During a Survey

WHAT YOU DO	WHY YOU DO IT
Always act within your scope of practice, as defined by facility policy, your job description, and your state's regulations.	This is the best way to ensure that the care you are providing is within the legal limits of your job.
Always behave like the professional that you are. Be courteous and respectful toward others. Offer your assistance to residents and co-workers readily. Have a positive attitude.	Having a professional attitude and displaying a solid work ethic indicates to others that you take pride in your job and are interested in doing it to the best of your ability.
Make sure that your conversations with co-workers are appropriate for the workplace. Be aware of the volume of your voice.	You would not want anyone to overhear anything that would reflect poorly on you or your work ethic. Gossiping about others or going into great detail about your personal life is inappropriate in the workplace. Speaking in a loud voice adds to the noise level on the unit.
When discussing a resident's care with a co-worker, be mindful of where the discussion is taking place and the volume of your voice.	Discussions that involve a resident's care need to be held in private areas to protect the resident's right to confidentiality.
Do your part to maintain a neat and clean environment. Put items away after you use them. Dispose of trash properly. If you notice a spill or other mess, clean it up promptly.	A cluttered, messy environment is unpleasant for everyone, residents and staff alike. It may even present safety issues. It is difficult to work efficiently if you cannot locate something you need because it was not put away properly after the last person used it. If everyone on the unit does his or her part to keep the unit neat and clean, it is easier to maintain order on the unit.
Always put your residents' needs first. Strive to provide humanistic, holistic care.	When you are at work, your first priority must be helping your residents to meet their physical, emotional, social, and spiritual needs. A humanistic, holistic approach to health care is the basis for providing quality care.
Answer questions honestly and to the best of your ability. If you do not know the answer to a question, simply say that you do not know, and offer your help in getting the person the answer he needs.	Most people are quick to recognize bluffing. Admitting that you do not know the answer to a question conveys to the other person that you are honest. Offering to find out the answer for the person, or directing the person to someone who is better able to answer the person's question, indicates that you are helpful and conscientious.

those targeted areas who are at risk. For example, if the facility has had deficiency citations in the past related to falls resulting in injuries, surveyors will be particularly interested in looking at safety issues within the facility during this survey. They will be on the alert for safety hazards such as wet floors, clutter, or poor lighting. They will also be interested in care issues, such as whether or not the nursing team responds promptly to call lights, and whether residents have easy access to necessary assistive devices for walking, such as walkers or canes. They will be interested to know what the ombudsman has observed during visits to the facility, and whether there have been any complaints related to factors that have contributed to a fall. They will also want to know which residents are at risk for falls and what measures the facility is taking to prevent those residents from falling.

One report that the survey team will pay close attention to during off-site preparation is the **Quality Indicator Profile report.** The Quality Indicator Profile report identifies markers of quality in specific care areas. One part of the report compares the facility's performance in each area to the performance of other facilities in the state in the same area (Fig. 6-1). Another part of the Quality Indicator Profile report focuses on care concerns related to specific residents, based on assessment data pulled from the Minimum Data Set (MDS) (Fig. 6-2). (The MDS is used to assess and document the degree of assistance or skilled care that each resident of a nursing home needs. You will learn more about the MDS in Chapter 12.)

Some markers of quality on the Quality Indicator Profile report are identified as sentinel events. **Sentinel events** are problems that should rarely, if ever, be seen in a resident of a nursing home. The three sentinel events are:

- Fecal impaction (a condition that occurs when constipation is not relieved)
- Dehydration (too little fluid in the tissues of the body)
- A pressure ulcer (a difficult-to-heal and potentially fatal sore) in a resident who is at low risk for developing pressure ulcers

You will learn more about these conditions in later chapters. For now, just remember that these are serious concerns. Surveyors have a very low tolerance for these types of events. It only takes *one* case of a sentinel event on a Quality Indicator Profile report to get a surveyor's attention!

The facility's management team has access to the same Quality Indicator Profile reports that the surveyors use. This gives the facility's management team an opportunity to identify potential care issues in the facility and correct them prior to the survey. You may hear your facility management team talk about these reports and what actions the facility is taking to address any identified issues.

THE SURVEY WALK-THROUGH

When the survey team arrives at the facility, they begin to gather information that allows them to either confirm or disregard any concerns they identified during their off-site preparation for the survey. The survey team does this by making direct observations, interviewing residents and staff, and reviewing residents' medical records.

First, the survey team holds a meeting, called an *entrance conference*, with members of the facility's management team. During the entrance conference, the facility's management team gives the survey team access to documents such as meal and medication schedules, staff schedules, menus, and activity calendars. The survey team will expect what they see happening in the facility to be consistent with the information in these documents.

Next, the surveyors go on a tour, or *walk-through*, of the facility. During the walk-through, they are making general observations about the building, the residents, and the staff. These observations help the survey team to determine whether or not their initial concerns were valid. They may also pick up new information that they will want to explore further. Even though the survey team had a focus for their attention when they arrived at the facility, that focus can change at any time if they find other areas of concern. Suppose the survey team arrives with a particular concern about the number of residents who have experienced falls (as we used in our earlier example). However, after the surveyors spend a little time in the facility, they notice that many residents appear to be under-weight. In addition, they see that a lot of food is left uneaten at meal time. In light of this new information, the survey team may decide to expand their focus to include nutritional concerns and food service, or they may decide to change their focus altogether if they do not find any significant problems related to resident falls.

The information that the survey team gathers during the facility tour is critical to the success or failure of the survey. In the sections that follow, we will provide an overview of some of the things

Facility-Level Quality Indicator Profile					

Domain/Quality Indicator	# in Num	# in Denom	Facility Percent	Comparison Group Percent	Percentile Rank
Accidents					
1. Incidence of new fractures	3	102	2.9	1.7	93 🚩
2. Prevalence of falls	17	105	16.2	19.8	34
Behavior/Emotional Patterns					
3. Prevalence of behavioral symptoms affecting others	17	104	16.3	20.7	42
High risk	13	66	19.7	26.6	34
Low risk	4	38	10.5	8.0	74
4. Prevalence of symptoms of depression	10	104	9.6	13.8	41
5. Prevalence of symptoms of depression without antidepressant therapy	7	104	6.7	7.4	56
Clinical Management					
6. Use of 9 or more different medications	46	105	43.8	40.2	63
Cognitive Patterns					
7. Incidence of cognitive impairment	4	41	9.8	12.5	44
Elimination/Incontinence					
8. Prevalence of bladder or bowel incontinence	47	97	48.5	51.9	39
High risk	15	16	93.8	90.9	50
Low risk	32	81	39.5	40.0	48
9. Prevalence of occasional or frequent bladder or bowel incontinence without a toileting plan	1	30	3.3	43.3	0
10. Prevalence of indwelling catheter	8	105	7.6	6.6	67
11. Prevalence of fecal impaction	1	105	1.0	1.0	68 🚩
Infection Control					
12. Prevalence of urinary tract infections	10	105	9.5	9.2	57
Nutrition/Eating					
13. Prevalence of weight loss	15	105	14.3	12.4	67
14. Prevalence of tube feeding	7	105	6.7	4.9	75
15. Prevalence of dehydration	3	105	2.9	1.6	83 🚩

Figure 6-1

This is a sample of the portion of the Quality Indicator Profile report that compares how the facility's performance compares to that of other facilities in the state. The *Domain/Quality Indicator column*, on the left, lists potential areas of concern. The *Percentile Rank column*, on the right, indicates the percentage of facilities in the area that have performed better in that area than the facility that is the subject of the report. A *flag* next to the percentile ranking indicates a potential care problem. Percentile rankings of 90% or higher get a flag. So does *any* occurrence of a sentinel event. This report shows flags next to the percentile rankings for *incidence of new fractures* because the percentile ranking for this category is 93%. In addition, there are flags next to *prevalence of fecal impaction* and *prevalence of dehydration* because these are sentinel events.

Resident-Level Quality Indicator Summary

Resident Name	Most recent date	Accidents New frac	Falls	Behavioral Problem behavior Hi	Lo	Deprs	Deprs No Tx	Clin 9+ Meds	Cogn Cog Impair	Elimination/Incontinence Bwl/Blad Incont Hi	Lo	Incont no TP	Indw Cath	Fecal Impact	Infect UTIs	Nutrition Wt Loss	Food Tube	Dehyd
Doe, Jane	5/28/2007			√						√								
Resident, Herman	6/3/2007							√							√			
Smith, John	6/3/2007	√									√							
Eldercare, Nancy	6/9/2007										√							
Jones, Doris	6/10/2007	√									√							
Cann, Melanie	6/14/2007							√			√							

Figure 6-2

This is a sample of the portion of the Quality Indicator Profile report that focuses on care concerns related to specific residents. The residents' names are listed in the column on the left. The quality indicators are identified at the tops of the columns arranged across the page. The check marks in the columns indicate which quality indicators have been flagged for that resident based on the resident's assessment information. So, if the survey team is interested in looking more closely at the issue of falls in the facility, they would look in the column labeled "Falls" and select a sampling of residents with check marks in that area. They would then review those residents' medical charts to make sure the facility is taking the necessary measures for each of those residents to decrease the resident's risk of falling.

that surveyors evaluate during the walk-through. You will see that if you always strive to provide humanistic, compassionate care to your residents, and if you perform your duties the way you have been taught—in a professional manner and according to your facility's policies and procedures—then you will really have nothing to worry about during a survey.

THE ENVIRONMENT

When unexpected company arrives at our home, our first impulse is often to straighten things up. It is only natural to want to be seen at our best. We get that same feeling in the workplace when surveyors arrive. However, it is important to remember that you have visitors to your facility every day. More importantly, the residents are living in that environment every day. The impression that you want to make on the surveyors should be no different than the impression that you would want to make on anyone else!

When you arrive for duty on your unit, be objective and use your senses. Surveyors are going to do that very same thing.

- **What do you see?** Are there papers and supplies scattered about? Are waste containers full to overflowing? If the first thing the surveyors see is clutter and disorganization, their impression will be that resident care is also provided in an unsafe and disorganized way. We do not want to give that impression to *anyone*, especially not a surveyor!
- **What do you hear?** Is the unit very noisy? Excessive noise on the unit can also hint at disorganization and chaos.
- **What do you smell?** Unpleasant odors raise concerns about the quality of care the residents are receiving.

It is very important that things are neat, clean, and orderly in the work area (Fig. 6-3). If you notice that things are out of place, take a minute to "straighten up." Be sure that trash is thrown away and that waste containers are properly emptied.

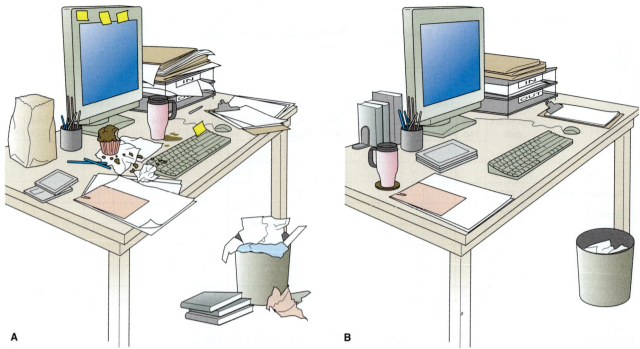

A   B

Figure 6-3

(A) A messy, cluttered work area may be interpreted by surveyors as a sign that resident care is also chaotic and disorganized. **(B)** A neat, clean, and orderly work area is more pleasant and efficient for everyone. Do your part every day to keep work areas orderly.

Make sure that tables and other work surfaces are clean. Be on the alert for sources of odors and make sure that they are properly addressed. You will notice that when your work area is clean and well-organized, the day is more pleasant for everyone!

STAFF-TO-STAFF INTERACTIONS

People often get so comfortable in their workplace that they forget that other people are around, watching and listening. This is especially true in health care, where your work takes you into the personal space of those you care for. Surveyors, visitors, and residents can learn a lot about how care is given by watching and listening to the staff.

Surveyors will be sensitive to the content of conversations between staff members, and where these conversations take place. Are staff members openly discussing facility problems? Are they talking about other co-workers or residents? Are they discussing personal problems or other topics unrelated to work? When staff members

are discussing resident care, are they making an effort to protect the resident's rights to privacy and confidentiality by having these conversations in appropriate places?

Surveyors will also be evaluating how staff members communicate with each other. Do staff members show respect for each other, or are they rude and short-tempered? Do they offer each other help and act as a team? Failing to act as a team affects the staff's ability to meet the needs of the residents. Surveyors will be very sensitive to this. Remember everything you learned about professionalism in Chapter 3. A professional attitude and an ability to work well with others are so important in the health care setting.

STAFF-TO-RESIDENT INTERACTIONS

While they are walking through the facility, surveyors are going to be paying particular attention to where the residents are, what they are doing, and how staff members respond to them. This is important because it gives the surveyors an indication of how well the staff members are supporting resident rights, quality of life, and quality of care, all of which are specifically addressed in the regulations.

Surveyors will pay attention to those residents seated in various areas around the nursing unit. Are these residents doing anything, or are they just sitting there? Are staff members interacting with them, or just walking past them without saying anything to acknowledge their presence? Do these residents have a way of alerting the nursing team when they have a need? If a resident calls out for help, how does the nursing team respond? Do staff members stop and listen, or do they just walk by on their way to do something else?

Surveyors will also observe the residents who stay in their rooms. Are these residents occupied in an activity, or are they just sitting alone? Are the blinds or drapes over the window open, or is the resident sitting in the dark? Are staff members knocking and asking permission before entering residents' rooms? Are staff members respectful of a resident's wish for privacy by keeping doors or privacy curtains closed as the resident desires?

To avoid potential problems in this area, always be aware of, and responsive to, the resident's needs and wants. Residents must have a way of communicating with you when they want or need something. Be sure that the call light control is always within reach of the resident. If the resident is seated in a common area where a call light control is not available, ensure that there is some other method for the resident to get your attention (for example, provide a hand bell). If hand bells are not available, make sure the resident is seated in an area where she is always in sight of someone who can see her and respond to her.

Be prompt in answering call lights or verbal requests for help (Fig. 6-4). If the resident is not able to ask for help, be alert to behavior that might indicate an unmet need. For example, you may notice that a resident who needs to use the bathroom will start to fidget in her seat with a worried look on her face. Offer assistance with routine activities (such as using the bathroom or getting a drink of water) frequently. Some residents will find it easier to accept an offer of assistance than to ask for help.

Residents need to engage in activities and interact socially with others (Fig. 6-5). When residents are outside of their rooms, are they seated where they can talk or interact with others? Do they have access to materials needed for hobbies or interests, such as books, games, and craft

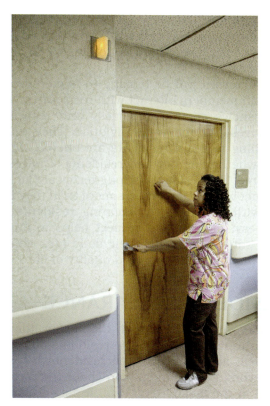

Figure 6-4
Responding promptly to call lights and requests for help is important every day, not just during a survey.

supplies? Surveyors will check that scheduled activities are actually occurring as planned. They will check the designated area at the scheduled time to see what activity is taking place, how many residents attend, and whether or not the residents are participating. The surveyors will note the level of assistance provided by the nursing team in

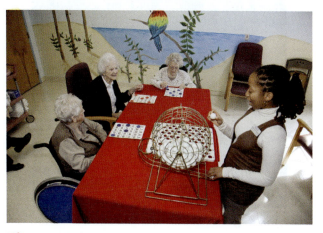

Figure 6-5
The nursing staff supports the facility's activity staff in helping residents to enjoy the activity program.

getting residents ready for, and transported to, the activities of their choice. A resident's day can be very long when there is nothing to do or look forward to.

Surveyors will be looking to make sure that all staff members interact with residents in a way that shows common courtesy and respect for each resident as an individual. They will be watching to see if residents are offered choices, and whether or not the residents' choices are honored. The residents of long-term care facilities interact with staff members more than they interact with anyone else. Treating residents with courtesy, dignity, and respect helps to improve their satisfaction with their daily life, which in turn results in an improved quality of life.

RESIDENT APPEARANCE

As surveyors walk through the facility, they will pay attention to how the residents look. The physical appearance of the residents helps the surveyors to form an opinion about the care provided in the facility (Fig. 6-6). It also gives them

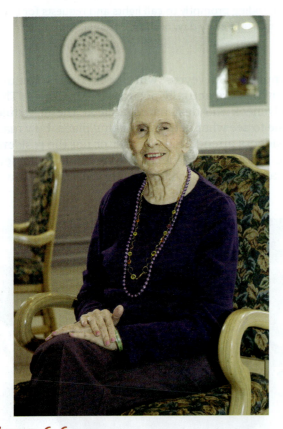

Figure 6-6
A resident's physical appearance says a lot about the care provided at the facility.

an indication of the amount of attention the staff pays to maintaining the respect and dignity of those in their care.

The surveyors will look at the residents' overall cleanliness, grooming, and hygiene. Uncombed hair, dirty clothes, and odors will certainly give the surveyors cause for concern. The surveyors will also check to make sure that residents are dressed appropriately for the season or the activity in which they are engaged.

Surveyors also pay special attention to mouth care. Are the resident's teeth clean and the gums healthy? If the resident wears dentures, are the dentures clean and in the person's mouth (especially at meal time)? Does the resident's breath smell fresh, or does it have a foul odor? Are the tongue and mucous membranes of the mouth moist and healthy, or do they appear dry? A dry mouth could indicate that the resident is not taking in enough fluid to maintain his health. Insufficient fluid intake can lead to very serious health problems. If surveyors become concerned about the number of residents with dry mouths, they may start to investigate medical records for evidence of dehydration. Remember, dehydration is a sentinel event. If dehydration becomes a concern, surveyors will be particularly observant of the nursing team's efforts to provide residents with fluids throughout the day.

Surveyors will also be attentive to positioning of residents. Improper positioning can lead to pressure ulcers and other injuries. It can also lead to muscle strain that can cause pain and discomfort. Surveyors want to be confident that the nursing team is paying attention to this very basic need. They will check to make sure that residents who need help changing position are being turned and repositioned at least every 2 hours. They will also look to make sure residents are properly supported and in good body alignment. Are pillows or other supports being used properly? Do residents in wheelchairs have their feet properly supported, or are their feet dragging on the ground?

Surveyors will also be looking at residents for evidence of injury. If many residents are noted to have bruises, abrasions, or dressings, the surveyors will begin to focus attention on the facility's efforts to prevent accidents. Resident safety is always a primary concern!

MEAL SERVICE

Meal time is a very important time in a nursing home (Fig. 6-7). Good nutrition is essential for health. In addition, meal time is a very social

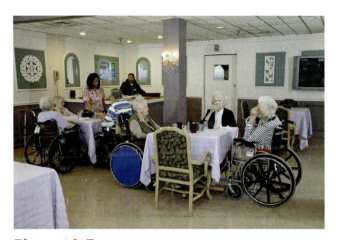

Figure 6-7
Surveyors pay close attention during meal time. Timely meal service; a clean, pleasant environment; and attentiveness to the residents' needs are key things that they are looking for.

time in the resident's day. Surveyors will monitor meal service in the facility to make sure that meal time is as pleasant as possible for the residents.

Their observations will start with the environment. Do the residents have a pleasant setting for their meals? Are the floors and tables clean? What attention is given to the overall atmosphere? Is there music playing in the background? Are tablecloths used? Think about how you would want to experience a meal at a restaurant. Would you want to eat there if there were unpleasant odors or trash on the floor? How would you feel if the hostess seated you at a dirty table? You want to do everything you can to make the dining experience as pleasant as possible for your residents. A pleasant setting can help to increase your residents' interest in eating, which in turn helps to ensure that they receive adequate nutrition.

Surveyors will watch that meals are delivered on time to residents. They will compare the time of tray delivery to the meal schedule that was given to them at the entrance conference. They will also note the length of time between when the trays are delivered and when they are served. The nursing team must organize their work so that they are ready to start serving meals when they are delivered. Delays can lead to problems with food temperatures. Hot food should be served hot, and cold foods should be served cold! A surveyor may request a "test tray." The surveyor will test the temperature of

the foods on that tray when the last tray is served to a resident. This is done to ensure that even the last resident served receives food of the proper temperature.

Surveyors will evaluate the nursing team's attention to getting the residents ready for the meal. Have the residents had the opportunity to use the bathroom before the meal? If residents need to be excused from the meal to use the bathroom, this may indicate that they have not been assisted in meeting their toileting needs before the meal. Have the residents been assisted with basic hygiene? Are they properly dressed and groomed for meal time? Are the residents positioned properly for eating? It is very difficult to eat if you are slumped over in a chair!

Surveyors will be attentive to the way meals are served. Are all of the residents seated at the same table served at the same time? It can be cited as a dignity issue if everyone has been served except for one resident who has to sit and watch the others eat while waiting for his meal. Surveyors will also watch how attentive staff members are to residents during the meal. Do they notice when someone is not eating well or is having difficulty? Do they offer encouragement and assistance when necessary? If a resident is not eating, has she been offered something else to eat that might be more appealing to her?

When a resident needs assistance with eating, does the staff member focus on the resident he is assisting? Does the staff member sit down while assisting the resident to eat, or stand over the resident? Does he talk with the resident, or engage in personal conversations with co-workers? Sitting with the resident and being attentive to that resident are very important not only for dignity, but also for safety.

Some residents can be very messy when they eat. It is important to take measures to preserve the resident's dignity. Are efforts being made to keep the resident's face and clothes clean (for example, by assisting the resident with a napkin or providing a clothing protector)? Have any modifications been made that will allow the resident to manage foods more easily? For example, has the resident been provided with eating utensils that may be easier for her to manage? Difficulty in feeding oneself can lead to feelings of incompetence and embarrassment. It is important that we are just as sensitive to those emotional issues as we are to the physical need for nutrition.

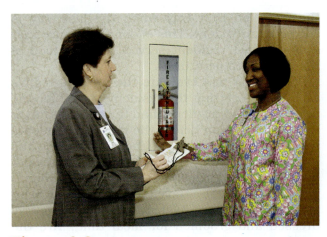

Figure 6-8
During the survey, a surveyor may ask you questions to check your knowledge of the facility's emergency procedures. Review your facility's policies and procedures for responding to emergencies as often as you need to so that this information is always fresh in your mind!

EMERGENCY PREPAREDNESS

As part of the survey process, a surveyor may ask you questions about the facility's fire and disaster procedures to make sure you know them (Fig. 6-8). Examples of questions the surveyor may ask include:

- "What is your facility's code for fire/disaster?"
- "What would you do if you heard those codes?"
- "When is the last time you participated in an emergency drill?"

When you start a new job at a nursing home, you will be given information about the facility's policies and procedures in the event of an emergency. Be sure to refresh your memory by reviewing these policies and procedures as often as you need to. Know the location of emergency exits and equipment used to respond to emergencies, and how to use this equipment. You are caring for

people who need help. In an emergency situation, their safety depends on you!

THE FUTURE OF THE SURVEY

As this book is being produced, a new survey process is being introduced. The new survey process, called the Quality Indicator Survey (QIS), has been developed to improve and standardize the collection of data about quality of care and quality of life. There are two phases to the new survey. During Phase I, the survey team will interview a large number of residents, using a specific set of questions. These questions focus on gathering feedback from the residents about personal choices in care (such as bed time, wake time, and other care routine schedules) and satisfaction with quality of life issues related to food, privacy, activities, staff treatment, and the like. During Phase I, the survey team may also interview staff and family members. In addition, the survey team will review MDS data, and observe residents and staff members. The surveyors will record the responses to interview questions and their observations in a portable computer device that analyzes the data. Phase II of the survey focuses specifically on further review of any issues identified during Phase I.

The QIS process is being phased into use as survey teams are trained in the new method. During this training period, some facilities will still go through the traditional survey process, while other facilities will go through the new QIS process. Although the survey process is changing, the purpose of the survey (to ensure that quality care is being provided according to standards and regulations) remains the same. As a nursing assistant, the things that you will do every day to ensure quality care and a successful survey outcome remain the same, regardless of whether or not your facility is surveyed using the old or new process.

SUMMARY

- The survey is an inspection of a nursing home done to ensure that care is being provided according to standards and regulations. The survey is performed by government officials referred to as the survey team or surveyors.
  - The survey team begins the survey process off-site by reviewing available

information to identify care concerns. This off-site preparation provides an initial focus for the survey team's attention during the actual survey visit.
- After arriving at the facility, the survey team makes direct observations; interviews staff, residents, and visitors; and

reviews residents' medical charts to determine whether or not a facility is in compliance with regulations.

- If you always strive to give care the way that you have been taught and in accordance with your facility's policies and procedures, and if you always treat others with courtesy and respect, you will have nothing to worry about when the survey team comes to your facility.
  - Behave like the professional that you are when you are at work.

- Always be alert and responsive to your residents' physical, emotional, and social needs.
- If the survey team finds the facility to be out of compliance, the facility will have to respond with a plan of correction that includes the actions that will be taken to fix the problems and prevent them from happening again. The consequences of failing to achieve compliance are very serious.

WHAT DID YOU LEARN?

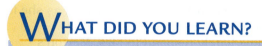

Multiple Choice

Select the single best answer for each of the following questions.

1. You recently started working at the Golden Village Retirement and Nursing Center. You hear that the facility is due for its annual survey. You know that the purpose of a survey is to:
   a. Get feedback from residents and families about the care and services provided at the facility
   b. Ensure compliance with government regulations to protect the residents receiving care
   c. Produce reports about what the facility is doing wrong
   d. Make sure that state surveyors are correctly doing their jobs

2. You know that before the survey team arrives at the facility, they will be reviewing information about the facility from various sources. They do this because:
   a. It helps them to focus on potential areas of concern.
   b. They have never been to the facility before.
   c. They will not have to come to the facility to perform the survey if their off-site preparation indicates that there are no problems.
   d. It allows them to identify staff members who are not good employees.

3. All of the following people are part of the survey team except:
   a. A facility administrator
   b. A dietitian
   c. A registered nurse (RN)
   d. A sanitarian

4. Members of a survey team are:
   a. Government officials
   b. Employed by a private, non-profit agency
   c. Ombudsman
   d. Employed by the long-term care facility

5. Shortly after you arrive for your shift, you learn from your charge nurse that the survey team has just arrived for the annual survey. You immediately:
   a. Check your work area to make sure that everything is neat and orderly and that your residents are comfortable and positioned properly with easy access to their call light controls
   b. Complain that someone should have told you that they would be coming today so that you would have felt more prepared
   c. Do your best to stay out of sight to make sure a surveyor does not notice you
   d. Loudly instruct your co-workers about what they need to do to keep the facility from getting into trouble

6. You see the survey team is in the resident dining room observing meal service. You notice that Mrs. Merton is spilling her food all over her dress. You are not assigned to Mrs. Merton today. You should:
   a. Call to her assigned nursing assistant who is standing across the room to help Mrs. Merton before you all get into trouble
   b. Begin to feed Mrs. Merton, because she cannot do it properly herself
   c. Take Mrs. Merton back to her room and change her clothes
   d. Assist Mrs. Merton by wiping her clothing, providing her with a clothing protector, and making sure she is properly positioned to reach her food

7. During lunch, you notice that Mr. Humphrey has not eaten very much. One of your co-workers asks Mr. Humphrey if he is finished eating, and then starts to pick up his tray and put it back on the cart. You are aware that the surveyor is watching. In order to show the surveyor how you normally provide proper care, you should promptly:
   a. Get a thermometer and take Mr. Humphrey's temperature to make sure he is not sick
   b. Engage Mr. Humphrey in a conversation about the meal, and offer to get him something else to eat that he might enjoy more

   c. Tell your co-worker to give Mr. Humphrey his tray back, and remind Mr. Humphrey that he needs to eat because it will be a long time until dinner and you don't want him to be hungry
   d. Approach the surveyor and assure her that Mr. Humphrey usually eats well every day and that today he is just not hungry

8. After assisting Mr. Humphrey back to bed for a nap, you see that Mrs. Merton has put on her call light. You just saw her assigned nursing assistant enter Mr. Smith's room to answer his call light. What action will show the surveyor that you are responding appropriately to resident needs?
   a. Go to Mr. Smith's room and let Mrs. Merton's nursing assistant know that she should go to Mrs. Merton as soon as she is done with Mr. Smith
   b. Immediately respond to Mrs. Merton's light and tell her that her nursing assistant will be with her shortly so that Mrs. Merton will not become impatient
   c. Wait for Mrs. Merton's nursing assistant to answer the call light because Mrs. Merton's nursing assistant knows best what Mrs. Merton needs
   d. Promptly answer Mrs. Merton's light to find out what you can do to help her while her nursing assistant is busy with Mr. Smith

Matching

Match each numbered item with its appropriate lettered description.

_____ 1. Sanitarian

_____ 2. Compliance

_____ 3. Deficiency citation

_____ 4. Sentinel event

_____ 5. Plan of correction

_____ 6. Survey

_____ 7. Off-site preparation

a. A problem that should occur very rarely, if at all
b. The state of meeting established guidelines, standards, or requirements
c. A person who examines the safety and cleanliness of a building
d. Statements that identify standards the facility did not meet
e. The work the survey team does in advance to prepare for the survey, before arriving at the facility
f. An inspection to observe and review care and services provided by a facility
g. A document that outlines the specific actions a facility will take to fix problems and achieve compliance

STOP and Think!

- When you enter Mrs. Dell's room this morning, she tells you that today is the monthly birthday party and she is really looking forward to going. She tells you she would like a shower and her hair washed this morning so that she looks nice for the party. Today is not her scheduled day for a shower. You are already feeling stressed because you know there are surveyors in the building. You do not want to fall behind in your work. What should you do?

- One of the surveyors approaches you and asks you questions about Mr. Smithfield's care. You have never been assigned to care for Mr. Smithfield and you really do not know much about his care. You want to make the best impression possible to show that your facility really does give good care. How should you respond to the surveyor's questions?

Nursing Assistants Make a Difference!

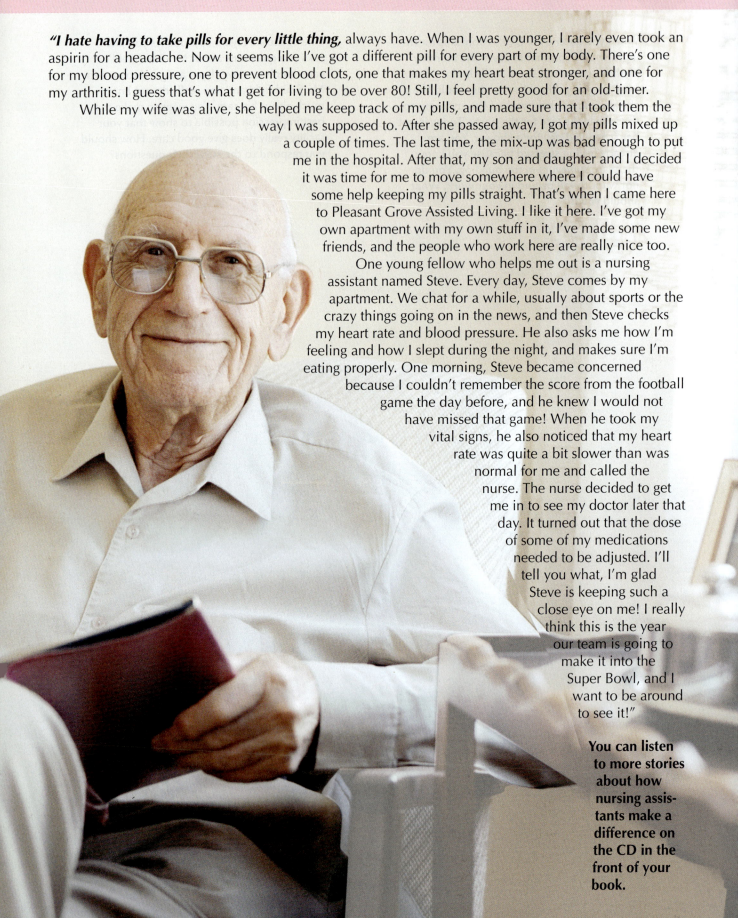

"I hate having to take pills for every little thing, always have. When I was younger, I rarely even took an aspirin for a headache. Now it seems like I've got a different pill for every part of my body. There's one for my blood pressure, one to prevent blood clots, one that makes my heart beat stronger, and one for my arthritis. I guess that's what I get for living to be over 80! Still, I feel pretty good for an old-timer. While my wife was alive, she helped me keep track of my pills, and made sure that I took them the way I was supposed to. After she passed away, I got my pills mixed up a couple of times. The last time, the mix-up was bad enough to put me in the hospital. After that, my son and daughter and I decided it was time for me to move somewhere where I could have some help keeping my pills straight. That's when I came here to Pleasant Grove Assisted Living. I like it here. I've got my own apartment with my own stuff in it, I've made some new friends, and the people who work here are really nice too. One young fellow who helps me out is a nursing assistant named Steve. Every day, Steve comes by my apartment. We chat for a while, usually about sports or the crazy things going on in the news, and then Steve checks my heart rate and blood pressure. He also asks me how I'm feeling and how I slept during the night, and makes sure I'm eating properly. One morning, Steve became concerned because I couldn't remember the score from the football game the day before, and he knew I would not have missed that game! When he took my vital signs, he also noticed that my heart rate was quite a bit slower than was normal for me and called the nurse. The nurse decided to get me in to see my doctor later that day. It turned out that the dose of some of my medications needed to be adjusted. I'll tell you what, I'm glad Steve is keeping such a close eye on me! I really think this is the year our team is going to make it into the Super Bowl, and I want to be around to see it!"

You can listen to more stories about how nursing assistants make a difference on the CD in the front of your book.

THOSE WE CARE FOR

As a nursing assistant, one of your primary goals is to provide holistic, humanistic care. In order to do this, you must get to know each of your residents on an individual basis. In Unit 2, we will look at some of the qualities that all human beings share, as well as the ones that make us unique individuals. We will also look in more detail at some of the special needs that are common to many residents. The resident is the focus of Unit 2.

Photo: Each resident is a unique individual.

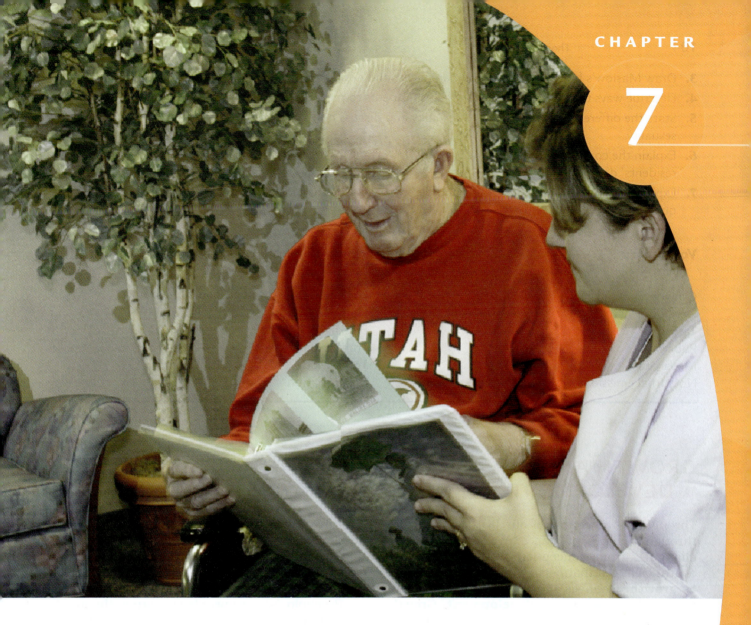

Understanding Human Needs

WHAT WILL YOU LEARN?

You are probably beginning to realize that there is much more to being a nursing assistant than blood pressures and bedpans. A health care worker can go to the most well-known schools, receive the most intense training, and graduate at the top of his class, but if he is not able to connect on a human level with those he cares for, he will fail. In this chapter, we will take a closer look at some of the things that all humans have in common, as well as some of the things that make us different. When you are finished with this chapter, you will be able to:

1. List and briefly describe the stages of human growth and development.
2. Understand that developmental changes are common throughout the life span of a person.

Photo: Nursing assistants play an important role in helping residents to meet their physical, social, emotional, and spiritual needs. Here, a nursing assistant helps a resident to meet his emotional need for love and belonging.

3. Draw Maslow's hierarchy of basic human needs, and explain each level.

4. Describe ways that a nursing assistant helps residents to meet their needs.

5. State the difference between sex and sexuality and discuss how age and illness can affect a person's sexuality.

6. Explain the concept of diversity, and why it is important for health care workers to recognize their residents' diversity.

7. Explain the concept of quality of life, and describe ways that nursing assistants help to support residents' quality of life.

Vocabulary Use the CD in the front of your book to hear these terms pronounced and defined:

Growth	Menopause	Heterosexual	Culture
Development	Need	Homosexual	Race
Tasks	Sexuality	Bisexual	Religion
Puberty	Intimacy	Transsexual	Quality of life
Menarche	Sex	Transvestite	Activity
Nocturnal emissions	Coitus	Masturbation	

GROWTH AND DEVELOPMENT

Throughout the course of our lives, we all pass through a series of stages. We are constantly changing, from conception until the time of death. Changes that occur physically are known as **growth.** Changes that occur psychologically or socially are known as **development.** Growth is demonstrated by changes in height and weight and by physical maturation of the body's organ systems. Development is evidenced by changes in a person's behavior and way of thinking. Both growth and development occur in an orderly fashion and progress from the simple to the complex. Physically, a baby must develop the muscle strength and coordination that will enable him to sit, then stand, and finally to walk. Developmentally, that baby will smile at his mother, then coo, say his first word, and soon speak in complete sentences.

The process of growth and development is divided into stages of normal progression (Fig. 7-1). A person cannot progress to the next stage without successfully completing the **tasks,** or growth and development milestones, associated with the stage she is currently in. Although all people progress through the stages of growth and development in a series of expected steps, they do not progress through the stages at the same pace. Personal experiences, as well as social

and historical events, can influence the way a person passes through the stages of growth and development. For example, people who lived through an event like World War II experienced circumstances that may have forced them to develop more emotional maturity at an earlier age than would normally be expected. The basic principles of growth and development are highlighted in Box 7-1.

Psychologists are people who study the mind and behavior. Many psychologists have developed

---

BOX 7-1	Principles of Growth and Development

- Growth and development occurs continuously throughout a person's life span, from conception until death.
- Growth and development occurs step by step and in an orderly progression. Each stage has specific characteristics and tasks that must be accomplished before the person can progress to the next stage.
- Growth and development tasks progress from the simple to the complex.
- Growth and development tasks progress from head to toe, and from the center of the body outward.
- Growth and development occurs at variable rates for each individual, and may occur unevenly or in spurts.

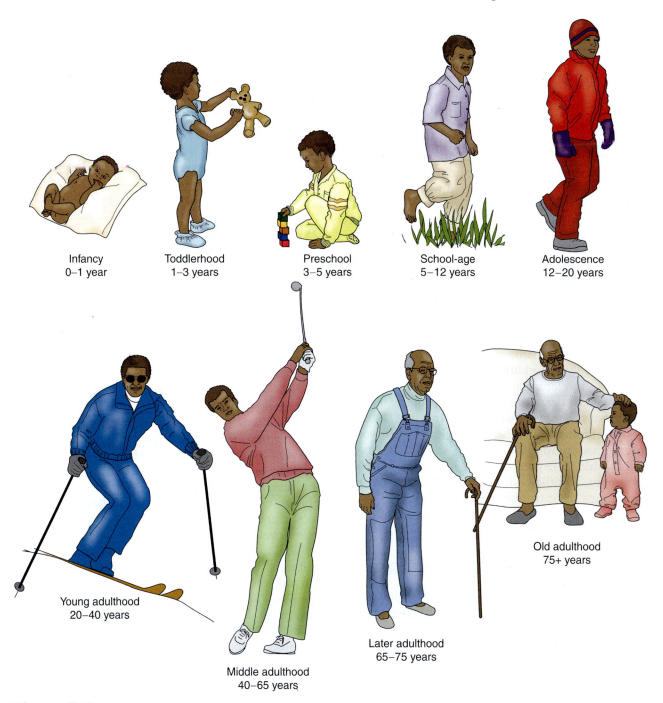

Infancy
0–1 year

Toddlerhood
1–3 years

Preschool
3–5 years

School-age
5–12 years

Adolescence
12–20 years

Young adulthood
20–40 years

Middle adulthood
40–65 years

Later adulthood
65–75 years

Old adulthood
75+ years

Figure 7-1
Everyone passes through the same stages of growth and development.

theories about human development throughout the life span. Depending on which psychologist's work you study, you may find that the growth and development stages are defined slightly differently, in terms of age ranges and tasks. Additionally, the age at which a person begins or ends a certain stage of development varies slightly according to the individual. Figure 7-1 and the descriptions of the various stages in the sections that follow are generalizations, obtained from the large amount of research that has been done on the subject of human growth and development.

As a person grows and ages, the physical and psychological changes that occur affect the type of care the person needs, and the way in which we communicate with him or her. Becoming familiar with the stages of growth and development and the tasks commonly associated with these stages will help you to become a more able caregiver.

INFANCY (BIRTH TO 1 YEAR)

Infancy is the stage during which physical and psychological changes occur most rapidly. By his first birthday, an infant will typically weigh three times what he did when he was born, and he will have progressed from a totally helpless newborn to a child learning how to walk and feed himself. During the first year, the infant begins to smile and laugh, recognize parents and siblings, and say simple words.

TODDLERHOOD (1 TO 3 YEARS)

Physical growth slows down during toddlerhood, but development of the muscular and nervous systems allows the toddler to become quite active. The toddler can walk, run, climb, jump, and peddle a tricycle easily. In addition to permitting increased mobility, development of the muscular and nervous systems permits greater control of the bladder and bowels, so this is when toilet training begins.

Developmentally, the toddler learns the words to express emotions, such as "sad" or "scared," and is able to express herself in short, complete sentences. Toddlers are quite self-centered and sometimes have trouble following rules of behavior. Being separated from a parent or familiar caregiver can be very frightening for a toddler.

PRESCHOOL (3 TO 5 YEARS)

The preschooler's physical coordination improves a great deal, and he learns to dress himself and tie his own shoes. Toileting becomes more independent. Preschoolers become involved in playing with other children and will use their active imaginations to create detailed play stories and scenes. They ask questions all the time and love to have stories told or read to them. During this stage, children become aware of gender differences and roles and are very curious about the differences between boys and girls. As the preschooler begins to know the difference between right and wrong behavior, he begins to develop a conscience and is able to more easily follow rules.

SCHOOL-AGE (5 TO 12 YEARS)

The school-aged child experiences several major physical growth spurts, which lead to increases in both height and weight. As her fine motor skills

develop, the child's ability to write and draw improves. Play usually involves groups of same-sex friends. With school attendance comes an increased ability to follow society's rules. Children in this age group actively seek approval from authority figures and peers. School-aged children may feel very strongly about issues being either right or wrong, with no gray area. Spirituality and religious beliefs, as well as a concern for other living things, also take root during this developmental stage.

ADOLESCENCE (12 TO 20 YEARS)

Adolescence begins at the onset of **puberty,** when the secondary sex characteristics appear and the reproductive organs begin to function. In girls, the onset of puberty usually occurs between the ages of 10 and 14 years, and in boys, it occurs between the ages of 12 and 16 years.

Physical growth and development during adolescence is considerable. In girls, the development of breasts and the growth of hair in the pubic and armpit (axillary) regions occur before the onset of menstruation, or **menarche.** Throughout adolescence, a girl's breasts continue to develop and her hips broaden, leading to the curves that characterize the female shape. In boys, the genitals increase in size. Pubic, axillary, and facial hair develops, and the voice deepens. Ejaculation, or the release of semen, signals the onset of puberty; adolescent boys often experience **nocturnal emissions** (commonly known as "wet dreams") while sleeping. A growth spurt occurs, and the adolescent boy may gain more than a foot in height over the course of a few months. His shoulders broaden and his muscles become more developed.

Adolescents may be self-conscious about their changing bodies and increased awareness of their own sexuality. They are torn between wanting to be treated as grown-ups and being afraid to make their own decisions. Adolescents experiment with new styles of dress and hair, and follow very closely with their friends. They begin to date and to question the moral teachings of authority figures and parents. As a result, experimentation with alcohol, drugs, and sex may occur during this stage. As a reflection of their increasing emotional maturity, adolescents take jobs to make extra cash, learn to drive, and begin to make plans for their future education or the beginning of a career.

YOUNG ADULTHOOD (20 TO 40 YEARS)

Young adults typically enjoy stable, supporting friendships and good health. The primary tasks of this stage include completing one's education, starting a career, and, possibly, finding a partner and marrying. The young adult learns to be successful on his or her own, and may need to adjust to living with a partner. Many young adults choose to start families. For many women, the most significant physical change that will occur during young adulthood is pregnancy. Otherwise, the physical changes that occur in young adults are generally minor. The adult height is achieved during adolescence.

MIDDLE ADULTHOOD (40 TO 65 YEARS)

Middle adulthood frequently finds people at the height of their careers and productivity. Many middle adults find themselves in the role of caretaker to their children as well as to their aging parents. As their children grow up and become less reliant, many middle adults find that they have more time to travel or participate in leisure activities. During middle adulthood, many people become grandpar-

ents. Physically, the middle adult begins to show signs of aging, such as wrinkles or a few gray hairs. Women typically experience **menopause** (cessation of menstruation and fertility) in their early 50s. Although good health is usually still enjoyed, some chronic illnesses, such as hypertension and diabetes, become apparent during this stage.

LATER ADULTHOOD (65 TO 75 YEARS)

During this stage, normal physical changes that occur as a result of aging (Table 7-1) and the development of chronic illnesses become more prevalent. Retirement may place the older adult on a fixed income, but those who have planned wisely are able to travel and pursue hobbies that they did not have time for when they were employed. During this stage, many people must cope with the loss of friends or a spouse due to death.

OLDER ADULTHOOD (75 YEARS AND BEYOND)

During this stage, a primary task is looking back on one's life and preparing for one's own death. Some older adults continue to be relatively healthy

Table 7-1	Normal Physical Changes of Aging
ORGAN SYSTEM	**AGE-RELATED CHANGES**
Integumentary system (skin, hair, nails)	● Wrinkles, gray hair, "age spots" appear ● Skin becomes fragile, dry, and thin ● Nails become thicker
Musculoskeletal system	● Muscle mass decreases, leading to decreased strength ● Increased stiffness in joints ● Bones become more brittle
Respiratory system	● Lung capacity decreases, making it more difficult to move air in and out of the lungs
Cardiovascular system	● Heart pumps less efficiently, which means it has to work harder to meet the body's demands
Nervous system	● Slower reaction times ● Some difficulties with short-term memory
Sensory system	● Decreased sharpness of vision and some colors may appear to be distorted as the lens of the eye yellows ● Decreased hearing ● Decreased sense of taste ● May have slight loss of smell ● Skin loses some sensitivity to touch
Digestive system	● Food moves more slowly through the digestive tract, which may lead to constipation and other problems
Urinary system	● Bladder capacity decreases, leading to increased urination ● Decreased muscle tone may lead to difficulty with fully emptying the bladder

and independent, but many must adjust to failing health and a growing dependency on others. Many older adults enjoy sharing their life's experiences and the wisdom they gained along the way with younger people. Reminiscing (remembering and retelling events and experiences) helps older adults find meaning and purpose in their lives.

Helping Hands and a Caring Heart

FOCUS ON HUMANISTIC HEALTH CARE

Many people associate old age with poor physical health, disability, and a loss of mental function. But many things affect how we age—our genes, our outlook on life, and our overall health, for example. You may care for a 60-year-old who seems much older than he or she really is, while the 80-year-old down the hall may get around better than you do! Two people of the same age may be very different in terms of their health and abilities. Be sure to notice the real differences in all of the people you care for.

BASIC HUMAN NEEDS

A **need** is something that is essential for a person's physical and mental health. Even though most of your residents will be in the later stages of growth and development, each resident's needs will be unique. The primary mission of health care is to tend to the physical and emotional needs of those we care for.

Abraham Maslow (1908–1970), a famous American psychologist, defined what he thought to be the basic human needs, and then arranged them in a pyramid to show that certain needs are more basic than other needs (Fig. 7-2). Maslow's pyramid, called *Maslow's hierarchy of human needs,* reflects Maslow's belief that the more basic, lower-level needs must be met, at least to some degree, before the higher-level needs can be met. Many people can meet their needs with little or no outside help. But people who are ill, injured, or disabled must rely on the help of the health care team to make sure that their needs are met.

The needs of the people you care for will change as their conditions improve or decline. By helping people to meet their most essential needs first, you will enable them to meet their higher-level needs. For example, it is difficult to work on a person's self-esteem if he is struggling to breathe! Recognizing needs that people have difficulty meeting on their own, and helping them to meet

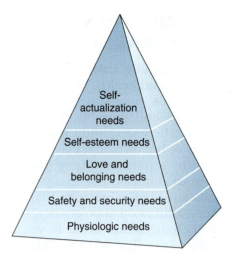

Figure 7-2
Maslow's hierarchy of human needs. A "hierarchy" shows the relationship of one idea to another. By arranging the basic human needs in a pyramid shape, Maslow created a visual representation of the idea that basic needs must be fulfilled before more complex ones.

these needs, is one of the most valuable contributions you will make as a nursing assistant.

PHYSIOLOGIC NEEDS

The most basic level in Maslow's hierarchy of needs is the physiologic (physical) needs, such as oxygen, water, food, shelter, elimination, rest and sleep, physical activity, and sexuality. Meeting the physiologic needs is essential for survival. Therefore, meeting these needs is of the highest priority. A person must have enough oxygen or he will die within minutes. Water and food are essential for life, as is the ability of the body to eliminate waste products such as carbon dioxide, urine, and feces. Shelter protects a person from the elements and extremes in temperature. Rest and sleep are essential for preventing physical exhaustion, which can lead to disability and illness. Physical activity keeps the nervous, skeletal, and muscular systems functioning and prevents wasting. Sexuality involves both the individual's need to have a sexual identity, as well as the need to engage in sexual activity, which allows for a species to reproduce and avoid extinction. Nursing assistants perform many duties that assist residents in meeting their physiologic needs: Assisting with meals, toileting, and ambulating and providing a relaxing environment in which to sleep are just some of the many ways you will help people to meet their most basic needs (Fig. 7-3).

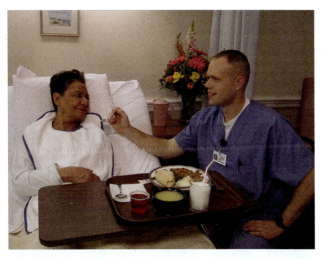

Figure 7-3
The nursing assistant shown here is helping his resident to meet her need for nutrition, one of the most basic human needs.

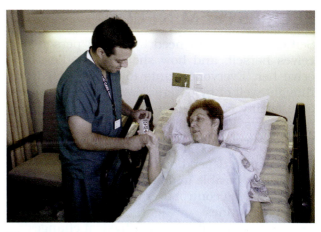

Figure 7-4
Understanding how the bed-positioning controls work can make a nervous resident feel more secure in her unfamiliar environment.

SAFETY AND SECURITY NEEDS

Safety and security needs are both physical and emotional. Not only must we *be* safe, but we must also *feel* safe. Nursing assistants follow policies and procedures that are designed to ensure the physical safety of their residents. For example, to prevent the spread of infection, a nursing assistant follows the procedure for hand washing. To protect a resident who is at risk for falling, the nursing assistant always makes sure that the resident has his walker close at hand. Throughout this text, you will learn about many ways in which nursing assistants work to ensure the safety of the people they care for.

The emotional part of safety and security involves trusting others and being free of fear of harm. A nursing assistant can help a resident feel safe by remembering that becoming a resident of a long-term care facility can be a very frightening experience. By introducing yourself and others, explaining routines and procedures, anticipating the resident's needs, and answering questions promptly, you can help to relieve much of the anxiety a resident may be feeling (Fig. 7-4).

LOVE AND BELONGING NEEDS

All people need to feel loved, accepted, and appreciated by others. People meet this need for one another by showing affection and forming close (intimate) relationships. Family life helps us to meet our love and belonging needs. We need to feel that we are part of an accepting group. When this need is unmet, feelings of loneliness and isolation develop. Babies and children fail to grow, and older people can actually "die of loneliness." Being a resident in a long-term care facility can cause a person to feel isolated, unlovable, and unappreciated. Residents often feel that they have become a medical condition, instead of a person. By taking an interest in the resident and showing respect for the resident's specific likes and dislikes, you can help to meet that resident's need to feel loved, accepted, and appreciated by others. A smile, a kind word, or a gentle touch can go a long way toward making someone feel loved, appreciated, and like she "belongs" (Fig. 7-5).

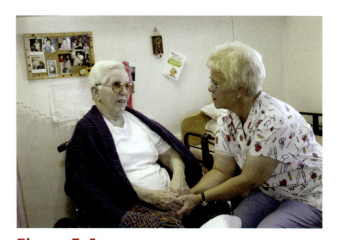

Figure 7-5
All human beings need to feel that they are loved and needed by others.

SELF-ESTEEM NEEDS

Self-esteem is influenced by how a person perceives herself, and how she thinks others perceive her. Everyone wants to be respected and thought well of by others. Moving to a long-term care facility can affect a person's self-esteem in many ways. For example, a resident's self-esteem may be affected by:

- Having to depend on others for something he used to be able to do for himself
- Not having control over his environment and daily routines
- Medical conditions and physical changes that alter his body image and sense of self
- Having to adjust to a new role and feeling as if he is no longer a productive member of society

Nursing assistants help to preserve their residents' self-esteem by:

- Providing for privacy when it is necessary to expose a resident's body
- Allowing residents to wear their own clothing (as opposed to a hospital gown), whenever possible
- Assisting residents with basic grooming to ensure that they look and feel their best (Fig. 7-6)
- Encouraging residents to do as much as they can independently or with minimal assistance
- Asking residents about their feelings and opinions

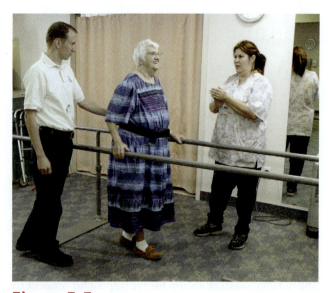

Figure 7-7
Helping residents to set small, realistic goals helps them to meet their need for self-actualization.

SELF-ACTUALIZATION NEEDS

The highest level on the hierarchy of needs is self-actualization. To achieve self-actualization, a person must reach his or her fullest potential. Most of us try throughout life to meet this need, because we are constantly setting new goals for ourselves. As a health care worker, you will have the unique opportunity to help the people you care for achieve self-actualization, by helping them to set small, realistic goals for a positive outcome (Fig. 7-7). Examples of goals that residents may have include taking one step (for a person who has had a stroke), being able to attend a social activity (for someone who has been confined to bed for a long time), or returning home (for a person who has broken a hip).

HUMAN SEXUALITY AND INTIMACY

All human beings are sexual beings. **Sexuality** is an integral part of our personalities; it is how a person perceives his or her maleness or femaleness. Sexuality differs from **intimacy**, which is a feeling of emotional closeness to another, and **sex**, which is the physical activity one engages in to obtain sexual pleasure and reproduce. Although sex is a part of some intimate relationships, it is not necessarily a part of all. Sometimes illness or physical disabilities make **coitus** (sexual intercourse)

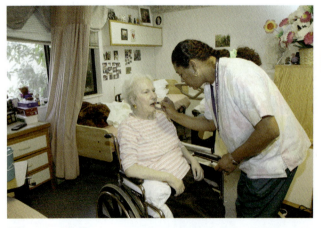

Figure 7-6
By helping this resident to look her best, this nursing assistant is helping to foster the resident's self-esteem.

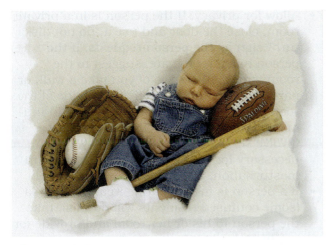

Figure 7-8
Society influences our ideas about our sexuality from an early age.

difficult or impossible, but there are other ways in which two people can share intimacy.

A person's sexuality can be influenced by many factors, including the person's culture and religious beliefs. From birth, we are surrounded by symbols of our sexuality—little boys receive baseball mitts and miniature toolboxes "just like Dad's"; little girls receive dolls and tea sets (Fig. 7-8). We grow up being taught by our parents and peers what is appropriate behavior for a "little girl" or for a "big boy."

As we progress through the developmental stages of life, we develop personal ideas and beliefs about our own sexuality. Many women like to express their sexuality by dressing in a feminine manner and wearing make-up, while others may prefer a more casual, natural look. Men also have preferences in their dress. For example, some feel most masculine in suits and ties, others in jeans and boots. People also develop preferences for the types of people they are sexually attracted to. For example, **heterosexuals** are attracted to members of the opposite sex, while **homosexuals** are attracted to members of the same sex. **Bisexuals** are attracted to members of both sexes.

Sometimes, a person's feelings about his or her sexuality do not correspond with the person's physical body. These people, called **transsexuals,** believe that they should be members of the opposite sex. Some transsexuals have a surgical procedure (a "sex change operation") to physically become a member of the opposite sex, after receiving psychiatric counseling to ensure that they are good candidates for the surgery. In other cases, the way a person chooses to express his or

her sexuality does not match what society has defined as typically "male" or "female." For example, a **transvestite** is a person who becomes sexually excited by dressing as a member of the opposite sex. Most transvestites are men who prefer to dress like women. A person with transvestite tendencies is not necessarily a transsexual or a homosexual—in fact, most transvestites are heterosexual men.

As a nursing assistant, you will meet people whose feelings about their sexuality, and the ways in which they express these feelings, might be very different from your feelings about your sexuality and the way you express those feelings. You must avoid being judgmental or critical of how another person chooses to express his or her sexuality. Acceptance of another person's views does not mean that you approve of that person's beliefs and practices. It only means that you respect that person's right to make his or her own decisions.

Because society so often associates youth and beauty with sexuality, we often do not consider the sexual needs of aging people. Sexuality (or the need to think of oneself as a sexual being) and intimacy (the need to share emotional closeness with another) are basic human needs, common to all people, young and old (Fig. 7-9). Many residents have lost their sexual partners as a result of illness or death. However, the loss of one's partner does not necessarily mean that the need to express sexuality and experience intimacy is lost too.

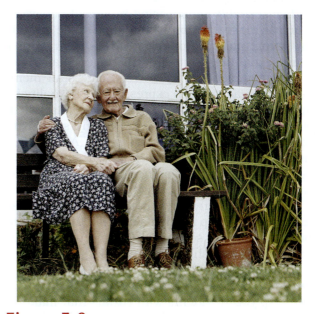

Figure 7-9
Sexuality and intimacy are basic human needs for everyone, young and old.

Residents of long-term care facilities may have difficulty meeting their needs related to sexuality and intimacy. First, let's consider for a moment the atmosphere of a typical long-term care facility. Take a look at the floor plan and furnishings. Are there lots of areas furnished with comfortable and cozy seating where a couple can enjoy private time together? Do the beds look like they would easily accommodate two people? What about privacy? Would you feel comfortable engaging in a sexual act with so many other people around and no lock on your door?

Next, let's consider the people who may be available for a resident to meet and develop an intimate relationship with. Generally, the only people the resident has the opportunity to meet and interact with on a regular basis are the other residents of the facility, visitors, and the facility staff. While it is possible for a resident to find a partner among the other residents in the facility, many residents have physical or mental disabilities (or both) that eliminate them as suitable choices. Also, there are many more female residents than male residents. If you are a male resident, this may be a good thing, but the opportunities for female residents are limited! Visitors are more likely to spend their time at the facility interacting with their own family members or friends. The only other people that residents see and interact with on a regular basis are staff members.

Some residents will have partners. Even if no partner is available, the resident may still have the need to express his or her sexuality, and to form intimate relationships. A resident may express his or her sexuality by engaging in sexual behaviors (such as **masturbation,** stimulation of the genitals for sexual pleasure or release by a means other than sexual intercourse) or making sexually suggestive comments or gestures. Some staff members may react to such expressions of sexuality by laughing at the person. Others may be disgusted. Neither of these reactions shows any sensitivity to, or respect for, the person's needs. A resident's need to express his or her sexuality should be recognized as a basic human need, just like any other human need a resident may have.

There are many ways that, as a nursing assistant, you can help residents to fulfill their need to be thought of as sexual beings and to engage in intimate relationships with others:

- Avoid being judgmental.
- Help your residents with rituals that make them feel either feminine or masculine, such as dressing and applying make-up, perfume, or aftershave lotion.

- Allow for privacy. If the person is in a private room, close the door and use a "do not disturb" sign as the person requests. If the person has a roommate, suggest to the roommate that the two of you take a walk or participate in another activity, outside of the room. Privacy is necessary for people in intimate relationships, whether or not they involve sexual intercourse. Privacy is also necessary for people who want to engage in masturbation.
- If a person is masturbating in a public area (some confused residents will do this), take the person to his or her room and provide for safety and privacy.
- Always knock before entering a person's room. If you do interrupt a sexual encounter, excuse yourself quietly and say you will return later.

As a nursing assistant, you may find yourself receiving unwanted attention of a sexual nature from a resident. A resident may make sexually suggestive comments to you, or touch you inappropriately (for example, pinching your behind). This may embarrass and anger you. But before you become angry with the person, stop and think about a few things. Think about what that person sees when he or she looks at you. You may be young and very attractive. You may remind the resident of his or her spouse, when that person was young. The resident may have poor eyesight and mistake you for someone else, or he or she may be confused or disoriented as a result of a disease process. Remember that even though the behavior may be offensive and unwelcome, it is still an expression of a need the resident has. Although it is totally inappropriate for you to attend to the sexual needs of your residents, it is important to avoid being unkind or hateful in your response. Depending on the situation, tell the resident kindly, yet firmly, that you are not going to do what he or she is asking you to do, or that he or she must not touch you in that manner. Avoid giggling or teasing the resident in a flirtatious manner. This will only serve to reinforce the inappropriate behavior. You should discuss the behavior with the nurse so that it can be appropriately assessed and addressed in the resident's care plan.

It is important for you to be able to recognize situations that could be considered sexual abuse or assault. As you know, anyone can be a perpetrator of sexual abuse, even a resident. A resident may attempt to engage in sexual activity with another resident who is not a willing participant.

Residents with disorders such as dementia can easily become victims of sexual abuse because they may not be aware of what is happening, and they may not be able to provide appropriate consent to participate in sexual activity. Although people with dementia still have the right to express their sexual needs, it is important to ensure that they are not unwillingly being exploited or abused. Other residents may not be physically able to defend themselves. As a nursing assistant, you must be especially observant for signs of sexual abuse. Any observations you make or suspicions that you have should be reported to the nurse immediately.

CULTURE AND RELIGION

You can see that there are many things that, as human beings, we all have in common. For example, everyone has the same basic needs, although some needs may be more pressing than others at any given time for any one individual. Similarly, we all pass through the same stages of growth and development, although not at the same time or at the same rate. Culture, the subject of this section, is another thing that makes human beings human. All people have a culture, although everyone's culture is not the same. **Culture** is made up of the beliefs (including religious or spiritual beliefs), values, and traditions that are customary to a group of people. It is a view of the world that is handed down from generation to generation. A culture can be shared by people of the same race or ethnicity, by people who live within the same geographic area or speak the same language, or by a combination of these two (Fig. 7-10). While racial identity is often mixed with a person's culture, **race** is a general characterization that describes skin color, body stature, facial features, and hair texture.

One of the most unique things about the United States is the diversity of cultures that are represented here. Diversity has enriched this country, yet problems can arise when people are not sensitive to, or respectful of, the cultural uniqueness of each individual. As a health care worker, it is important for you to learn as much as possible about the characteristics of other cultural or ethnic groups of people, because your residents will have cultural differences that may affect their preferences regarding health care. Additionally, a primary goal of the nursing team is to provide for the comfort of those we care for. A person who feels that his culture is not under-

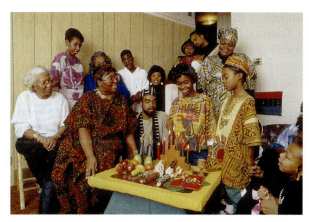

Figure 7-10
This African American family is celebrating Kwanzaa, a holiday celebrated by Africans and people of African descent throughout the world. Kwanzaa, a celebration of African history and culture, with a special emphasis on family life, occurs from December 26 through January 1. Kwanzaa is a cultural holiday, not a religious one. Celebrants are united by their African heritage, not their religion. (© *Lawrence Migdale.*)

stood or respected by the people who are caring for him will feel uncomfortable.

There are many ways in which a health care worker can accidentally be disrespectful of a resident's culture, which can lead to conflict. Sometimes, misunderstandings occur simply because a health care worker is not aware of how a certain person's culture influences her behavior. Although it is difficult to make generalizations about culture—not everyone from the same geographic region, or with the same skin tone, necessarily has the same beliefs or value system—being aware of what a resident is telling you can help you to know when cultural differences need to be taken into account. Areas where culture and health care often intersect include beliefs and practices associated with food and meals; religious beliefs and practices; and attitudes toward health, sickness, and death.

Liking certain types of food, or food prepared a specific way, is very cultural. For example, a person from the southern United States may prefer "grits" (cornmeal) to oatmeal. Sometimes, a resident may request or refuse a certain food or combination of foods in order to follow religious beliefs or practices. For example, a person of the Catholic faith may not want to eat meat on Fridays during Lent, and a person of the Jewish faith may follow the practice of not drinking milk with a meal that contains meat. In some cultures, it is believed that certain combinations of foods can aid or inhibit healing. For example, according to Taoism (a philosophy that originated in Asia), illness occurs when the body is out of balance. To restore balance, certain foods may be chosen over others. If one of your residents requests or denies a certain food or combination of foods for religious or other reasons, be sure to tell the nurse. The nurse will work with the dietary department to meet the person's request.

A person's spiritual beliefs, or **religion,** are often very closely linked with his or her culture. Members of some cultural groups have certain rituals that they feel will bring them good luck or aid in healing. For example, you may encounter a person from Turkey who believes hanging an "evil eye" talisman will ward off bad spirits, or a person from Panama who believes that wearing strings on the wrist will relieve pain. A person might want to light candles while praying to a specific saint. Many people are very spiritual and find comfort and solace in reading scriptures or spiritual books, singing, and praying. If a resident asks to see a spiritual leader or clergy member, communicate the request promptly and according to your facility's policy, and allow for privacy during the visit. A resident's religious beliefs may be very different from yours, but you can be certain that the resident's beliefs are as important to him as yours are to you (Fig. 7-11). You do not have to share a person's religious beliefs to help the person obtain comfort from them. For example, even if you do not share a resident's religious beliefs, you can read his scriptures to him if he is not able to read them himself.

There are other examples of cultural practices that we must be respectful of, even if we think they are wrong. Remember, your culture gave you your value system, and your resident's culture gave her hers. Respecting another person's values does not mean that you have to agree with that person, or her values. For example, some cultures do not allow women certain freedoms that we take for granted in this country. Imagine that you are a male nursing assistant, caring for a Middle Eastern woman. In some Middle Eastern cultures, a woman is not allowed to be questioned or examined by a male health care provider unless her husband is present. Your resident's husband has not yet arrived at the facility, and you need to perform care for this resident. Although it would be tempting to go ahead with your duties without the husband present, you know that your resident would not be comfortable if you were to put her in a difficult situation. You would be devaluing her belief system by trying to overrule it.

Throughout your career, you may be lucky enough to care for people from many different cultural and religious backgrounds. You will most likely encounter situations, practices, and beliefs that no book could have prepared you for! Take time to listen to your residents, and to learn from them. Exposure to cultures other than your own is enriching, both professionally and personally.

QUALITY OF LIFE

Quality of life has to do with getting satisfaction and comfort from the way we are living. As you recall, the Omnibus Budget Reconciliation Act (OBRA) was put into place to protect residents' quality of life. Many factors contribute to quality of life, including:

- The ability to be free from physical and emotional discomfort
- The ability to make decisions for oneself, based on one's own personal values and sense of what is best for oneself
- The ability to engage in activities that one finds enjoyable

A humanistic approach to health care, as you have learned, takes into account a person's emotional, social, and spiritual needs as well as his or her physical ones. When you take a humanistic approach to health care, you help to ensure that your residents enjoy a good quality of life. Respecting residents' rights, as outlined in the *Residents' Rights* portion of OBRA, also helps to protect your residents' quality of life.

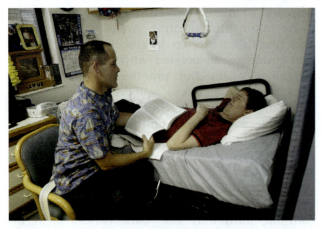

Figure 7-11
A nursing assistant can help residents obtain comfort from their religious beliefs, even if the nursing assistant does not share those same beliefs.

PERSONAL CHOICE

The idea of what quality of life means differs for each person and may vary as a person's situation changes. As a health care worker, you are trained to care for a person's physical needs. Treating illness and promoting good health are two primary goals of all health care workers. However, sometimes we are so focused on treating a resident's problems, we forget to consider the desires of the individual.

As a nursing assistant, you will learn that a person who has diabetes must control her diet carefully. You will learn that a person with heart disease should eat fewer foods high in cholesterol and stop smoking. But, what if your resident does not comply with the recommendations of the health care team? Is the woman with diabetes a bad person if she truly loves sweets and does not want to give them up? Is the man with heart disease a bad person if he cannot bear to give up his cigarettes? What if a person refuses a treatment or surgery that may prolong his or her life? Should the health care worker simply write that person off and focus only on those willing to follow medical advice?

If a health care worker gives a person the proper information about his illness or condition, and educates him about the steps that can be taken to treat or resolve the condition, then the health care worker has provided the person with the information he needs to make a conscientious decision concerning his own health. The person must make these decisions according to his own personal values and sense of what is best for himself, as an individual.

During your career as a health care worker, you will care for people who want every treatment available to help them fight for life, even if the procedures are dangerous or painful, or believed by others to be of no real benefit. You will also care for people who decline treatments because they feel that their ability to enjoy life and derive pleasure from living will be too compromised. Each of your residents must be allowed to make decisions concerning his or her quality of life. In order to provide humanistic, holistic care for your residents, you must respect, and support, their decisions related to maintaining their quality of life.

ACTIVITIES

In order to enjoy a good quality of life, we must get pleasure from life. One of the ways that we get pleasure from life is by engaging in hobbies or activities that interest us. An **activity** is a hobby or pursuit (pastime) that engages the mind, body, or both. Participating in activities that we enjoy provides an outlet for our creativity, prevents boredom, reduces stress, improves sleep, and allows us to feel a sense of purpose and accomplishment. Many activities also give us the opportunity to interact with people who share similar interests, so they help us to meet our need to socialize with others.

Participating in activities benefits us physically, as well as mentally. Because participation in activities has so many benefits and is so important for maintaining quality of life, OBRA specifies that nursing homes must provide for meaningful activity for residents (Fig. 7-12). The activity program must include a variety of activities that allow residents to socialize with others and pursue personal interests (Box 7-2).

The activity program is developed and managed by the Activities (or Therapeutic Recreation) Department. However, all staff members play an important role in making sure that each resident has the opportunity to participate in activities that provide pleasure and increase the resident's satisfaction with the quality of his or her life. As a nursing assistant, you will support the facility's activity staff by ensuring that residents are ready on time for scheduled activities (for example, by helping residents to select and put on appropriate outfits and assisting residents with toileting before the activity is scheduled to begin), and by helping to transport residents to the area where the activity is taking place.

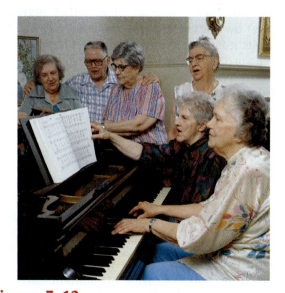

Figure 7-12

Activities provide entertainment and an opportunity to socialize with others.

BOX 7-2   Examples of Activities

Social Activities
- Parties for special occasions
- Tea parties
- Happy hour
- Sing-a-longs
- Family events

Physical Activities
- Exercise programs
- Dancing
- Walking
- Ball toss
- Gardening

Intellectual Activities
- Current events
- "Name that Tune"
- Trivia
- Guest speakers
- Book clubs

Sensory Stimulation Activities
- Touching surface textures
- Smelling scents (aromatherapy)
- Viewing pictures or nature slides
- Listening to music or nature sounds

Spiritual Activities
- Worship services
- Bible study
- Eucharistic visits
- Prayer groups

Creative Activities
- Crafts
- Painting
- Flower arranging
- Cooking
- Ceramics

Productive Activities
- Folding clothes
- Sweeping floors
- Watering plants
- Wiping tables

Not all activities must be coordinated through the Activities Department. As a nursing assistant, you can also help residents to enjoy activities throughout the day. Some activities, such as reading to the resident from a favorite book or playing a game of cards together, will require you to set aside some special time. Other activities can just be worked into your normal routine. For example, it is easy to sing along with a resident or play a word game during a bath.

Many residents will express the need to feel useful, rather than just sitting around watching other people work. While it is not acceptable to force a resident to perform work in a facility, it is acceptable to allow a resident to help wipe tables, water plants, and perform other simple chores on the unit, if that is what the resident wants to do. Productive activities like this often do a great deal to help boost a resident's self-esteem and sense of worth. The resident's desire to assist with chores on the unit should be documented appropriately in the resident's care plan, so that it is clear that the resident's participation in these sorts of activities is voluntary.

SUMMARY

- The people you will care for are individuals, with unique feelings, memories, needs, goals, and personalities. Recognizing and respecting the differences in the people you care for will allow you to provide humanistic care. When you provide humanistic care, you make a difference in the lives of your residents and their family members.

- The process of growth and development is divided into stages of normal progression: infancy, toddlerhood, preschool, school age, adolescence, young adulthood, middle adulthood, later adulthood, and older adulthood.
  - As a person moves through life, the growth and development changes that occur affect the type of care the person

needs and the way we communicate with the person. Becoming familiar with the various stages of growth and development will help you to become a better caregiver.

- Everyone passes through the same stages of growth and development, but not necessarily at the same rate.
- People in health care settings have many different physical and emotional needs. The primary mission of health care is to tend to the human needs of those we care for.
    - Basic needs must be met before higher-level needs can be met.
    - Maslow's hierarchy of human needs includes physiologic needs, safety and security needs, love and belonging needs, self-esteem needs, and self-actualization needs.
    - Residents who are not able to meet their needs on their own rely on the health care team to recognize and help meet these needs for them.
- Sexuality and intimacy are basic human needs. Sexuality is how a person perceives his or her maleness or femaleness. Sexuality differs from intimacy (the need to feel emotionally close to another person) and from

sex (a physical act engaged in for pleasure and reproduction).
- The need to express sexuality and experience intimacy continues into older adulthood. Older people, especially those who are residents of long-term care facilities, may have more difficulty meeting these needs.
- Assisting with grooming routines and providing for privacy are two ways that nursing assistants help residents to fulfill the sexuality and intimacy needs.
- Culture is made up of the beliefs, values, and traditions that are customary to a group of people. Problems can arise when a person is not sensitive to, or respectful of, another person's culture.
- We are responsible for helping our residents to maintain a good quality of life. Quality of life has to do with getting satisfaction and comfort from the way one is living.
    - Allowing residents to make decisions related to their quality of life is an important part of providing holistic care.
    - Participating in enjoyable activities benefits residents physically, emotionally, and socially, and contributes to their overall quality of life.

WHAT DID YOU LEARN?

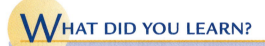

Multiple Choice

Select the single best answer for each of the following questions.

1. Sally is caring for Mrs. Norville, who lives in a long-term care facility. Sally encourages Mrs. Norville to make her own decisions about what to do each day. She helps her with dressing and grooming, but lets her do as much as she can for herself. These activities help fulfill Mrs. Norville's need for:
   a. Security
   b. Shelter
   c. Spirituality
   d. Self-esteem
2. When caring for people from different cultures, you should try to:
   a. Understand and respect their special needs
   b. Encourage them to change their beliefs while in your facility

   c. Pretend that the cultural differences do not exist
   d. Avoid talking to them
3. A resident's religion forbids him from eating pork. Pork chops are being served for dinner. What should you do?
   a. Tell the resident that religious restrictions on diet do not count in times of illness
   b. Ask the nurse to call the dietary department
   c. Insist that the resident eat the pork because it contains protein, an essential nutrient
   d. Reassure the resident by telling him that the doctor ordered this diet

4. A resident in a long-term care facility may show her sexuality by doing all of the following except:
   a. Desiring sexual intercourse
   b. Engaging in public fondling
   c. Giving her granddaughter a doll for her birthday
   d. Applying make-up and scented powder before receiving a male visitor

5. Which one of the following is not a basic human need?
   a. Fear
   b. Self-actualization
   c. Self-esteem
   d. Water

6. Which one of the following is a basic social need?
   a. Food
   b. Water
   c. Air
   d. Love

7. What is a person who becomes sexually excited by dressing as a member of the opposite sex called?
   a. A transsexual
   b. A transvestite
   c. A bisexual
   d. A homosexual

8. A development task for an older person is to:
   a. Have grandchildren
   b. Express individual rights
   c. Reflect on the meaning of her life
   d. Talk about her children

Matching

Match each numbered item with its appropriate lettered description.

_____ **1.** Infancy

_____ **2.** Toddlerhood

_____ **3.** Preschool

_____ **4.** School-age

_____ **5.** Adolescence

_____ **6.** Middle adulthood

_____ **7.** Older adulthood

a. A 16-year-old girl going to the junior prom
b. A 42-year-old executive running his own company
c. A 2-year-old boy starting toilet training
d. A 6-month-old girl learning to sit up
e. A 92-year-old great-grandmother moving to a long-term care facility
f. A 4-year-old boy learning to tie his shoes
g. An 11-year-old Boy Scout participating in his troop's annual canned food drive

STOP and Think!

- You are caring for Mr. Spencer, who was admitted to your long-term care facility yesterday. Yesterday, he was quiet and polite. Today, however, he is hostile and mean. He refused to go to the dining room for lunch and knocked the tray you brought him to the floor. He keeps yelling at you, saying, "This feels like a prison!" Why do you think Mr. Spencer is acting this way? What could you do to help him?

- You are assigned to Mr. Jones and must help him with his bath. While you are giving him care, he tells you how pretty you are, and how much you look like his wife did in her younger years. When you are all finished with Mr. Jones, he grabs your hand, squeezes it, and tells you that he loves you and asks for a little kiss. Is Mr. Jones being inappropriate? How will you respond to Mr. Jones?

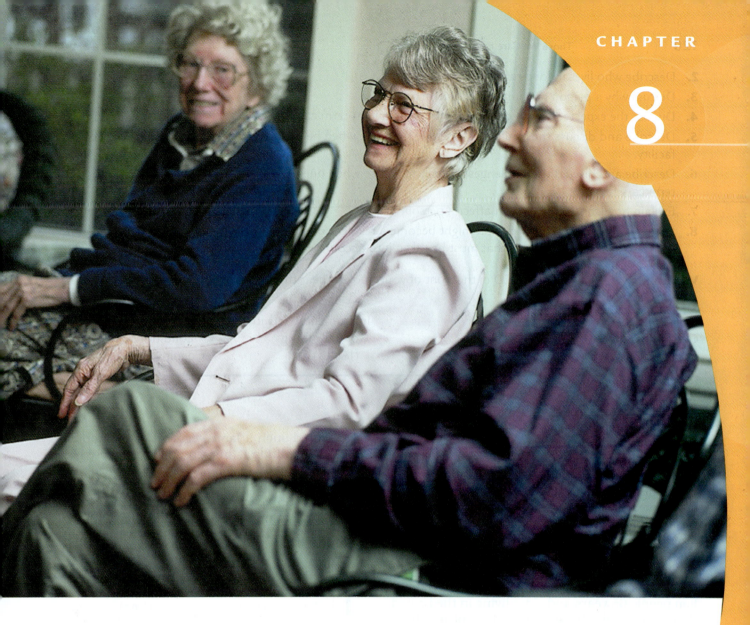

The Long-Term Care Resident

WHAT WILL YOU LEARN?

In Chapter 7, you learned about human growth and development and meeting human needs. In this chapter, you will build on this knowledge by learning more specifically about the residents and the families that you will care for in the long-term care setting. As you begin your nursing assistant career in long-term care, it is important that you have knowledge about the people in this setting as well as their circumstances. Who are they? Why are they here? What do they need? When you can answer these questions, you will be better able to meet their needs. When you are finished with this chapter, you will be able to:

1. Discuss why the number of people 65 years and older living in the United States is increasing every year, and describe what effect this could have on the long-term care industry.

Photo: Most residents of long-term care facilities are older with multiple care needs. Here, a group of residents enjoy an activity together. (Photo courtesy of Copper Ridge.)

2. Describe who lives in long-term care facilities.

3. Discuss why a person might need long-term care.

4. Discuss the expected length of stay for someone in long-term care.

5. Describe and discuss the challenges a person may face when he or she comes to live in a long-term care facility.

6. Describe and discuss the challenges a family may face when one of its members comes to live in a long-term care facility.

7. Explain how chronic illness can affect a person.

8. List reasons why a younger person might become a resident of a long-term care facility, and explain some of the special considerations that must be taken into account with younger residents.

Vocabulary *Listen & Learn* Use the CD in the front of your book to hear these terms pronounced and defined:

Acute illness
Chronic condition
Degenerative condition

Activities of
  daily living
  (ADLs)

Instrumental activities
  of daily living
  (IADLs)

Co-existent medical
  conditions
Cognitive impairment

OUR AGING POPULATION

Although people of all ages are cared for in nursing homes, most of the residents of nursing homes are 65 years and older (Fig. 8-1). Each year, the number of people living in the United States who are 65 years and older increases. As a society, we need to be prepared to care for this growing segment of the population.

In 2006, there were a little more than 37 million people 65 years and older living in the United States. This number is about 12% of our total population. That means that approximately one of every eight people in the United States is an older citizen! Never before in our nation's history have people in this age group (65 years and older)

represented such a large segment of the population. In addition, this trend is expected to continue. By the year 2030, the government expects that there will be nearly 72 million people older than 65 years of age living in the United States, or that one in every five people will be an older citizen (Fig. 8-2). It is estimated that one-third

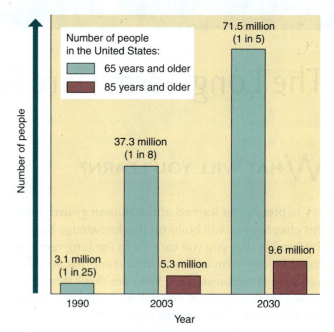

Figure 8-2

America's population is growing older. Never before in our nation's history have people 65 years and older represented such a large segment of the population.

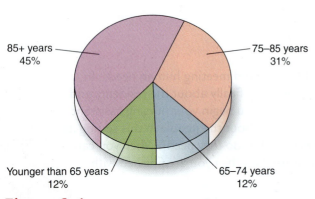

Figure 8-1

Most of the people living in nursing homes are 65 years of age and older, with the highest number of people being 85 years and older.

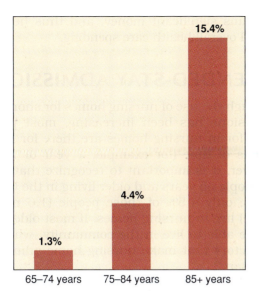

Figure 8-3

The oldest old, those 85 years and older, are most likely to require care in a nursing home. Only 1.3% of people between the ages of 65 and 74 years live in nursing homes. But 15.4% of people older than 85 years live in nursing homes.

to one-half of all people 65 years and older will be admitted to a nursing home for care at some time.

The oldest old, those 85 years and older, are the people most likely to require care in a nursing home (Fig. 8-3). The number of people in the United States 85 years and older is also steadily increasing each year (see Fig. 8-2).

So, why is the number of older people in the United States steadily increasing each year? One major reason is advances in health care. These advances have made it possible for people to recover from (or continue to live with) conditions that at one time would have caused them to die. For example:

- In the past, many people died from acute illnesses for which there were no treatments. An **acute illness** is an illness with a rapid onset and a relatively short recovery time, usually unexpected. For example, many people with acute heart conditions who have open-heart surgery today would not have survived in the past because that treatment was not available. Similarly, in the early 1900s, the major cause of death in the United States was infectious disease, such as tuberculosis, influenza, and pneumonia. Because of advances in public health and medical care, we have been able to significantly reduce the risk of death from these

diseases. Public sanitation and hygiene are better now, reducing the spread of infection. Antibiotics, which were not generally available before the 1940s, made treatment of infection possible, thus reducing the risk of death. Once the risk of death from infection was reduced, more people had a chance of living longer.

- In the past, conditions that are now considered chronic or degenerative might have caused a person to die sooner. A **chronic condition** is a condition that is ongoing and often needs to be controlled through continuous medication or treatment (for example, diabetes, heart failure, or hypertension). A **degenerative condition** is a condition that gets progressively worse over time (for example, dementia). Today, we have medications and treatments that help people to live with chronic or degenerative conditions, while in the past we did not.

These changes in cause of death are reflected in our current population. We have large numbers of people who are living longer and longer lives, but with chronic conditions. According to government figures, 80% of all people 65 years and older have at least one chronic condition and 50% have at least two. Keep in mind that these figures describe the general population, not just the segment of the population living in nursing homes. As more and more people live longer lives, many with one or more chronic conditions, the need for long-term care services will increase.

FACTORS LEADING TO LONG-TERM CARE ADMISSIONS

There are several reasons why a person might be admitted to a nursing home:

- A person may be admitted to a nursing home to recover from the lingering effects of an acute illness (such as a stroke) or injury (such as a broken hip).
- A person may be admitted to a nursing home because she needs continuous monitoring and treatment as a result of one or more chronic conditions.
- A person may be admitted to a nursing home because he needs help meeting his physical needs as a result of a degenerative condition.

- A person may be admitted to a nursing home because it is no longer safe for the person to live on her own, due to physical or mental impairment (or both).

SHORT-STAY ADMISSIONS

The use of nursing homes for short-stay admissions (3 months or less) has been steadily increasing. This increase in short stays is primarily due to changes in how health care is paid for, as we discussed in Chapter 1. As a result of these changes, hospitals are discharging patients "quicker and sicker." Many of these patients are admitted to long-term care facilities to receive the care they need until they are well enough to return home. Providing this care in a nursing home instead of in a hospital saves the government insurance

programs significant money, and thus helps to control overall health care spending.

EXTENDED-STAY ADMISSIONS

Although the use of nursing homes for short-stay admissions has been increasing, most people cared for in nursing homes are there for longer periods of time (for example, 1 year or more). However, it is important to recognize that of all the people 65 years and older living in the United States, only 4.5% of those people (1.6 million people) live in nursing homes. If most older people are able to live in the community, what are the factors that make nursing home admission necessary?

People come to live in nursing homes because they have physical or mental disabilities that

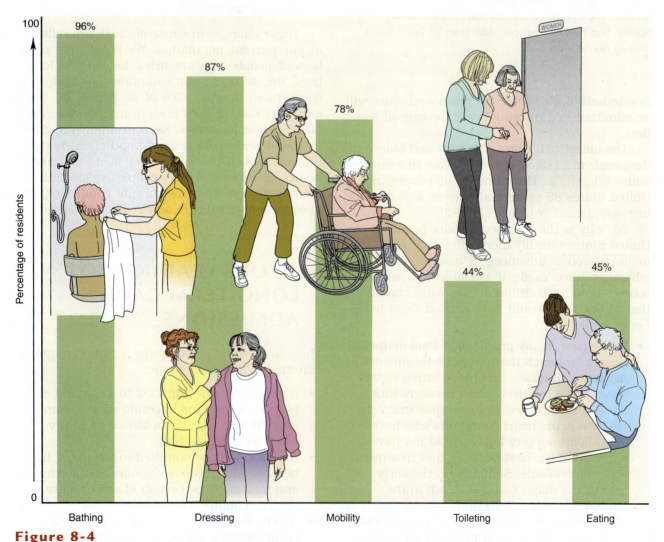

Figure 8-4

Most residents need help with their activities of daily living (ADLs) such as bathing, dressing, moving, toileting, and eating.

make it impossible for them to care for themselves properly. Many times, the level of care they require is beyond what family members are able to provide, or there simply are no family members to provide care.

Most residents of nursing homes need help with routine tasks of daily life, called **activities of daily living (ADLs).** These tasks include bathing, dressing, eating, moving, and toileting (Fig. 8-4). At least 75% of nursing home residents need help with three or more of their ADLs. **Instrumental activities of daily living (IADLs)** are more complex tasks that a person must be able to do in order to continue to live independently, such as using the telephone, handling money, and obtaining groceries and preparing meals. About 75% of nursing home residents need help with at least some IADLs, and more than 50% need help with all of them. Several factors can cause a person to need help with his or her ADLs and IADLs:

- Medical conditions or the effects of aging can affect the person's strength, endurance, or coordination.
- Medical conditions that affect a person's ability to think and remember (such as dementia) can cause the person to forget how to do these routine tasks.
- Sensory deficits, such as impaired vision or hearing, can make it harder for the person to function independently.

It is very common for a resident to have **co-existent medical conditions** (more than one medical condition at the same time). For example, the person might have both an acute and a chronic condition. Or, the person could have more than one chronic condition. Nearly all residents of nursing homes have more than one medical condition at the time of admission. More than half of them have three or more.

The most common medical conditions among nursing home residents are cardiovascular disease, respiratory disease, stroke, dementia, depression, diabetes, and arthritis. These are all examples of chronic conditions that require continuous medical monitoring and care. These conditions may also significantly impact a resident's ability to perform ADLs and IADLs.

Cognitive impairment (problems processing, learning, or remembering information), especially when it is accompanied by physical problems, is the reason why many people come to live in nursing homes. Seventy percent of the residents in nursing homes have either short-term or long-term memory loss, or both. Almost half of the residents have some form of dementia (the permanent and progressive loss of mental functions caused by damage to the brain tissue).

In summary, most residents of nursing homes need a great deal of support. Without your help, their lives would be significantly compromised in comfort and quality.

MAKING THE ADJUSTMENT TO LONG-TERM CARE

The move to a nursing home is often preceded by some crisis, such as an unexpected accident or illness. For example, an elderly widow living alone may have a stroke. Suddenly, she is taken from her home to the hospital for intensive medical care. She needs extensive rehabilitation that the hospital cannot provide, so she is transferred to a nursing home for that care. Despite months of therapy, she is unable to regain enough self-care skills to live independently anymore. Living with her son or daughter is not an option because their homes are not set up for someone with a disability and besides, no one is at home during the day. Without much time for emotional preparation, this woman must adjust to the loss of her independence and the loss of her home. Her son and daughter must also adjust to the changes brought on by their mother's stroke.

Consider a different situation. Perhaps an elderly man is living with family members because he has dementia and diabetes. He is no longer able to take care of any of his own needs. As the dementia progresses, he becomes more and more difficult to care for. The family struggles to get him to take his medication. He is no longer able to find the bathroom and has begun to urinate in inappropriate places throughout the house. His odd behaviors are scaring the grandchildren. He requires supervision 24 hours a day. He has wandered away from home several times, once in the middle of the night. The last time the police had to be called to help find him. The family is exhausted and family relationships are suffering. The family can no longer continue to provide the care that the man needs so the decision is made to admit him to a nursing home. Even though this situation is not as sudden as the situation described in the first example, there is still a crisis (in this case, calling the police for assistance) that spurs action toward nursing home placement.

Can you imagine what it would be like if you suffered an unexpected injury or medical crisis that made it impossible for you to return home to

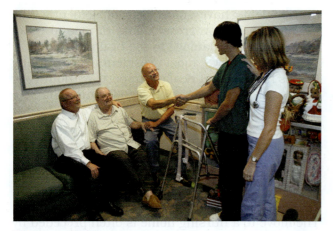

Figure 8-5
Being admitted to a nursing home is often stressful for the resident, as well as his or her family members. As a nursing assistant, it is important for you to take steps to make the transition easier for everyone. The first step is understanding what the resident and family may be feeling.

BOX 8-1	Helping Residents and Family Members Adjust

- Be knowledgeable about the resident's condition.
- Be knowledgeable about the circumstances that necessitated the move to the long-term care facility.
- Know your resident. Learn about his or her likes, dislikes, relationships, and interests.
- Allow the resident to make choices about his or her care.
- Be sensitive to both resident and family needs.
- Be flexible!
- Welcome family members and include them in the resident's care when appropriate.
- Be sensitive to the resident's environment. Accommodate needs for privacy.

live? Perhaps someone else made the decision about where you would live, and you did not even get a say in the matter. This happens frequently—most nursing home residents are "placed" in the long-term care facility; they do not choose to come live there. How would you feel? How would you react?

Similarly, how would you feel if you were the one who had to make the decision to admit your mother, father, sibling, husband, wife, or child to a nursing home? Would it be a hard decision to make? Would you feel a sense of loss, or possibly guilt?

When a person comes to live in a nursing home, it is often a difficult adjustment for both the person and his or her family members (Fig. 8-5). As a nursing assistant, there are many things that you can do to help ease the transition to long-term care for both the resident and the family (Box 8-1). Let's take a closer look at the impact admission to a nursing home can have on both the resident and the family.

THE RESIDENT

Most people do not *plan* to come live in a nursing home, and to be honest, it is not something most people *want* to do. People do not choose illness or infirmity. All of us, given the choice, would prefer to remain healthy and in our own homes.

Many of your residents are coping with multiple losses and life changes. For example, in the case of the elderly widow who suffered a stroke, she must not only cope with the loss of her home,

but with the fact that her body no longer functions as it used to. She has to re-learn many tasks that she took for granted when her body worked normally. The man with dementia from the second example is thoroughly confused in his new environment. He is unable to understand the reason for the change, and he does not recognize anything or anybody. How upsetting and frightening this must be!

Residents of nursing homes often have many fears and anxieties. They may worry about how their medical problems will affect their health and independence in the future. Because long-term care is expensive, they may have concerns about finances. They worry about how the move to the nursing home will affect their family members, and they may be sad to be separated from them.

The nursing home environment itself can be frightening and uncomfortable, full of strange noises and smells and unfamiliar people. The resident must learn to develop trusting relationships with many new people under very difficult circumstances. Imagine what it would be like to have staff members you do not know well asking personal questions about your life, poking and prodding your body with strange equipment, or seeing and touching private parts of your body during care. Staff, and sometimes even other residents, come into your room and handle your personal belongings. People may be coming in and out of your room at all hours of the day and night. You might find it disheartening to be surrounded by so many other people in various stages of sickness and disability.

Moving to a nursing home means having to give up your home. Think about your own home. What does it mean to you? What makes it home? What are your favorite belongings? What is your favorite thing to do at home? Now, imagine having to give that up. Your new home will be a room that you may have to share with someone who you do not know. Since space is limited, you will have to leave most of your belongings behind. What would you bring with you? Do you think that will make your new room feel like home? What would you miss the most?

Moving to a nursing home also means having to adjust to the loss of a certain amount of independence. It means not being able to do whatever you want to do, whenever you want to do it. You may have to adapt your usual routines to your new situation. How difficult will it be for you to do the things that you are used to doing in a different place, with different people, and perhaps on a different schedule?

People who become residents of a nursing home often feel that they are at the mercy of the health care industry. While some are cheerful, compliant, and grateful, others may be depressed, angry, anxious, or unpleasant. You must understand that residents will not always see you as an "angel of mercy" who is there to provide help. To some residents, you may be an unwelcome reminder of all the things that the resident can no longer do! When you must care for a resident who makes you wish you had never chosen to be a nursing assistant (and you can be certain you *will* encounter residents like this), stop and think for a moment about the reasons that person may be acting out of sorts. When you look beyond the illness or condition, past the technical duties and procedures, and into that person's eyes, you will find your reason for choosing to be a nursing assistant . . . a *person* who needs you very much.

THE FAMILY

Admitting a family member to a nursing home is often a traumatic event for the family as well as for the person who is actually being admitted. Like the resident, the family may have a hard time adjusting to the fact that admission to a nursing home is necessary. They may be struggling to accept the change in the resident's condition that made admission to the nursing home necessary in the first place. It may be difficult for them to accept that their loved one is in declining health or is no longer able to be independent. Finally, family members do not always get along with each other. When this is the case, it may be hard for the family members to agree on a course of action, especially when they are under stress, and this can lead to conflict within the family. Also, keep in mind that some family members may take out their stress on the person being admitted to the nursing home, leading to abuse. Family members struggle with many things when a loved one is admitted to a nursing home, including changing roles within the family, giving up the responsibility of "primary caregiver," and losing a life partner.

Adjusting to Changing Roles Within the Family

Within a family, each family member has familiar and expected roles. For example, imagine that your mother has had a stroke. As a result, she can no longer talk. Your mother has always been the person that you could tell your troubles to. She has always had words of wisdom for you and sound advice about what to do. Now that she is unable to talk, who do you turn to for needed advice in difficult times? How will what has happened change your relationship with your mother?

A decline in health or function for any one member of the family often disrupts expected roles and relationships for all of the family. Many adult children experience "role reversal" as their parents become more dependent. The child becomes the parent and the parent becomes the child. We are used to our parents caring for *us*. It is physically and emotionally difficult to assume basic care for a parent. Sometimes the change in roles causes problems among other members of the family. If there are several children in a family with elderly parents, it often happens that one child assumes primary responsibility for the parent's care. This can lead to resentment and jealousy among siblings. If you are the child who takes on the primary responsibility for caring for a parent, perhaps you are angry that your brothers and sisters are not doing their fair share and that you have such a heavy burden. If you are not the child who takes on primary caregiving responsibility, perhaps you feel jealous of the close relationship that the caregiving sibling seems to have with your parent. Caregiving responsibilities take a lot of time, and sometimes even financial resources, away from other family members. This can also create tension, conflict, and stress within the family.

Family members may look to you for direction and support. (Unfortunately, some will also look to you as a target for their stress and frustration.) Admission of a family member to a nursing home affects the whole family. As a nursing assistant, it is your responsibility to care for the resident as well as the family.

Giving up the Role of "Primary Caregiver"

You might think that admitting a loved one to a nursing home is a relief to family members because it relieves them of their caregiving responsibilities. In reality, it is not a relief, just a change. Family members must learn to trust other people—usually people they do not know—with providing care for their loved one. This is not always easy, no matter how competent and caring the staff may be! To further complicate matters, because many admissions to nursing homes are brought on by a crisis like a medical emergency, often the choice of facility is made rapidly. In this situation, the family may not feel like they had time to make the best decision.

Family members often feel guilty about not being able to provide care themselves. They may feel like they have let their loved one down. Because they are no longer in control of the care being provided, some family members may assume the role of "watchdog" to monitor the quality of care being given. Family members who provided care to their loved one before the person was admitted to the nursing home usually have a great deal of knowledge about how to care for the person. Adjusting to a new role (that of "visitor" instead of "primary caregiver") may be particularly difficult for these family members. When the family member tries to share knowledge about the resident's care with a staff member, the staff member may feel that the family member is interfering or lacks confidence in his or her abilities. This may create tension and conflict between the family and the staff.

Families want to see that staff members are interested in their loved one as a human being. They expect staff members to ask questions about their loved one's preferences and dislikes. They want to feel as if their input provides the staff with knowledge that is welcomed and valued. As a nursing assistant, you can help family members adjust by helping them to feel included and involved in the ongoing care of their loved one (Fig. 8-6).

Losing a Life Partner

For couples, admission of one partner to a long-term care facility can be particularly difficult, for both the partner who is left behind and for the partner who is moving to the long-term care

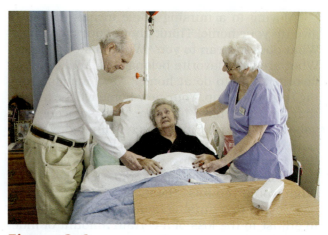

Figure 8-6
As a nursing assistant, you can help family members adjust by helping them to feel included and involved in the ongoing care of their loved one.

facility. No longer being able to live together can trigger a tremendous sense of loss for both partners. The need to share intimate moments with a life partner, whether sexual or not, is important throughout one's entire life. As a nursing assistant, you can help to make the transition easier by ensuring that couples have privacy during their visit.

LIVING WITH A CHRONIC CONDITION

As you have just learned, most residents have one or more chronic conditions. A chronic condition affects our self-image (how we see or feel about ourselves). Many people with chronic conditions find it difficult to accept that their bodies no longer function as they should. Some people have a "Why me?" attitude. Others are thankful for what they can still do or experience.

A chronic condition often affects how others act toward the person with the condition. Some people become overprotective. This may cause problems with roles and relationships, particularly if the person does not want to be treated any differently. The opposite can also happen. The person with the chronic condition may let others do everything for him, when in reality he is capable of doing many things independently. This can also cause problems with relationships, as those around the person with the chronic condition become frustrated and impatient.

Medications for a chronic condition are usually taken over a very long period of time. The person may have to learn to live with side effects that are unpleasant. Some people have a hard time accepting the fact that they must take medication every day, sometimes multiple times a day, in order to prevent acute symptoms. In addition, many medications are very expensive, particularly for people who are living on a fixed income. Worrying about how to pay for medication can be a source of stress.

Living with a chronic condition often necessitates making lifestyle changes that are not always welcome. For example, a person with diabetes must change the way she eats. The person may have to begin to exercise, an activity she might not enjoy. A person with a cardiovascular or respiratory disease should stop smoking, but he may not want to or be able to. Making changes to the way we live can be difficult even when we want to make these changes. Imagine how it must feel to be told that you *must* make these changes, or risk further health problems.

It is common for those with chronic conditions to experience problems with mental health. Some see the disease as taking over their lives and become angry, frustrated, or depressed. Some will just continue to deny that they have the disease. Some chronic conditions, such as arthritis, are painful. The battle for pain relief may become the primary focus of every single day! This is a true test of endurance. Living with pain can disrupt a person's life. Constant pain or discomfort reduces a person's physical abilities and limits the person's ability to interact socially with others, and is therefore often associated with depression.

For a person with a chronic condition, there will be good days when the person feels well and there will be bad days when symptoms make it hard to function. This can become very tiresome for the person. The person may have to be hospitalized repeatedly for acute flare-ups. The person may worry about the outcome of these flare-ups. For example, the person may wonder if she will be able to regain the same level of function that she had before, or whether she will have to adjust to a reduced level of health or function.

As a nursing assistant, it is important to understand the roller-coaster ride of living with a chronic condition. Most of your residents have co-existent medical conditions, not just one condition. You cannot expect your residents to perform at the same level every day. You must adapt to their good days and bad days by being flexible with your approach and the amount of assistance that you provide. Knowledge of each resident's *conditions* will help you to understand that resident's

struggles and limitations. Knowledge of each *resident* will help you to understand the resident's strengths and triumphs. Your encouragement and support can help your residents maintain their sense of self and their dignity, despite any limitations caused by disease.

THE YOUNG RESIDENT

Although most people living in nursing homes are 65 years of age or older, younger people receive care in nursing homes as well (see Fig. 8-1). You may care for residents who are in their 20s, 30s, or 40s (Fig. 8-7). (Children and adolescents who are severely disabled may also require long-term care, but usually they are cared for in long-term care facilities that specialize in the care of children and adolescents, rather than in regular nursing homes.) Traumatic injuries (such as severe brain and spinal cord injuries), degenerative neurological conditions (such as multiple sclerosis), and developmental disabilities (such as cerebral palsy or Down syndrome) are reasons why a younger person might be cared for in a nursing home.

For many younger residents, the disease or injury that results in the need for nursing home care is an unexpected life event. As you learned in Chapter 7, people in their 20s to 40s are busy completing their educations, starting or advancing in their careers, and possibly finding life partners and starting families. Can you imagine what it would be like to have your normal life shattered by disease or injury, and to find yourself living in a facility where most of the other residents are significantly older than you are?

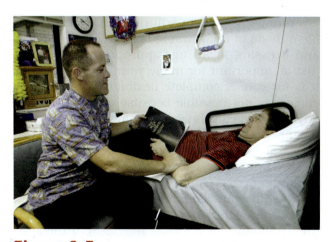

Figure 8-7
Not all residents are elderly.

Understandably, many younger residents experience anger, frustration, and depression. It may take a younger person a lot longer to adjust to placement in a long-term care facility. Younger residents may feel like they have lost all control over their lives. As a result, younger residents may "act out" (for example, by breaking rules, using foul language, or making unrealistic demands) in an effort to gain some kind of control over their situation. When caring for a younger resident, you will need to have empathy and patience. Be flexible, and give the person opportunities to exercise personal choice whenever possible. Ask the younger resident how he or she would like to plan the day, and try to accommodate these wishes. For example, a younger resident may want to stay up later at night and sleep later in the morning, or have more flexibility in visiting hours. Having the opportunity to make decisions about everyday matters helps the resident maintain a sense of control and personal identity and is important for maintaining the resident's self-esteem.

Because younger residents are living in an environment that is not reflective of their age group or interests, special accommodations will need to be made. For example, food choices often differ according to age. A younger person living in a nursing home might want pizza, subs, or ethnic foods, while an older person might prefer more traditional foods. Preferences relating to activities will also differ significantly. Younger residents may prefer video games over Bingo, and popular music over Frank Sinatra. They may enjoy action and thriller movies more than classic movies. Scheduling a movie and pizza night for a younger resident, or providing ear phones so the resident can listen to his own choice of music are examples of ways the unique needs of a younger resident can be met.

Younger residents still need to connect with life outside of the nursing home. Looking stylish and dressing in an age-appropriate manner is just as important for many younger residents as it is for you. If complete flexibility with clothing choices is not possible because of the resident's physical or medical needs, jazzing up sweat suits, pajamas, or hospital gowns with modern accessories or jewelry may help younger residents to feel a connection with their peers. Phone and computer access can help younger residents keep up with the outside world, and a pleasant area where younger residents can "hang out" with friends should be available (Fig. 8-8). If the resident is able, it may even be possible for the resident to participate in some activities outside of

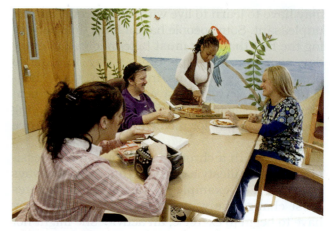

Figure 8-8

Providing opportunities for younger residents to enjoy the same things that others their age enjoy can greatly improve the younger resident's quality of life.

the facility, such as attending club meetings or taking a class. Helping a younger resident find ways to enjoy and participate in life and interests outside of the facility greatly enhances the resident's quality of life and provides a sense of hope for the future.

Being involved in life outside of the long-term care facility also includes being involved in family life. Being separated is hard on all members of the family. Family members' roles usually have to change when one member of the family is absent from the home. For example, when one parent is admitted to a long-term care facility, the children may need to assume more responsibility in the home to help the other parent keep things running smoothly. Family relationships can be strained by these changes. Family members at home may even feel "abandoned" by the family member who was admitted to the nursing home. Finding ways to help the resident continue to participate in family life is very important. Providing for phone and e-mail access, ensuring that a private space is available for family visits, and encouraging the family to participate in events held at the facility are all measures you can take to help maintain connections among family members.

As you learned in Chapter 7, sexuality and intimacy are basic human needs for everyone, young and old. Younger residents face many of the same challenges older residents face in meeting these needs. For young residents who are married or in a committed relationship, admission to a nursing home disrupts the normal intimate relationship between the two partners. Other young residents will not be married or in committed relationships, but will still have the need to establish and maintain intimate relationships with others. In a nursing home environment, it can be especially difficult for a younger resident to find someone to develop an intimate relationship with, and privacy can be an issue. As a nursing assistant, you will need to recognize the importance of sexual expression as part of the human experience and take measures to help your younger residents meet their needs related to sexuality and intimacy.

Caring for a younger resident can pose some unique challenges for a nursing assistant. Sometimes a younger resident may take out his or her anger on you, because you are the same age, but you still have a normal life. You may find it emotionally difficult to take care of someone who is close to your own age. The feeling that "this could be me" can be very frightening. You may also find it difficult to maintain professional boundaries. Younger residents often interact more with staff members than with the other older residents, or even with their friends outside of the nursing home. As a result, a younger resident may interpret your professional interest and caring as a sign of personal friendship, and become interested in developing a personal, or even a sexual, relationship with you. Although it is important for you to have a friendly and warm attitude toward all of your residents, you must make sure that you keep your relationships with your residents professional at all times.

SUMMARY

- The population of the United States is aging.
  - People in the United States are living longer because of improvements in public health and advances in medical care and technology. Because of this, the number of people 65 years and older living in the United States is increasing each year.
  - One third to one half of all people age 65 years and older will need long-term care sometime before they die. People 85 years and older are the most likely to require long-term care.
- Medical need, triggered by acute, chronic, or degenerative illness, often makes long-term care necessary. Most residents have three or more co-existent medical conditions.
- Most people who live in nursing homes need help with activities of daily living (ADLs) and instrumental activities of daily living (IADLs), because of physical disability, mental disability, or both.
  - At least 75% of residents need help with three or more ADLs such as bathing, dressing, moving, eating, and toileting.
  - At least 75% of residents need help with at least some IADLs, such as using the telephone or paying bills.
- Adjusting to admission to a nursing home is difficult for both the person being admitted and his or her family members. It involves coping with many changes, accepting losses, and adapting to new roles and relationships.
  - Adjustment is complicated by the fact that admission to a nursing home is often necessitated by a crisis, such as an unexpected illness or injury.
  - The resident must adjust to changes in his health at the same time that he is learning to adjust to a new home.
  - The loss of privacy and independence is very difficult.
  - The resident must learn to trust new people in new surroundings.
  - Not everyone learns to adapt to these changes in a positive way.
- Admission is often just as traumatic for the family as it is for the resident.
  - Family members must adjust to the changed health status of their loved one and adapt to the new surroundings.
  - Family roles and relationships change when a loved one moves to a long-term care facility.
  - Family members may have a hard time learning how to be "visitors." Their tendency to monitor the quality of care delivered and their attempts to share information may be negatively perceived by staff, leading to conflict and tension.
  - Families need to be welcomed and included to the best extent possible.
  - Families expect nursing home staff to show interest in their family member as a person.

- Provision of privacy for family visits is essential, particularly for couples.
- Most residents of nursing homes are living with one or more chronic health conditions. Chronic conditions become part of who we are and can significantly affect our day-to-day life.
  - Chronic conditions affect how we feel about ourselves, as well as how other people feel about us.
  - The strain of living with a chronic condition can affect mental health.
  - Physical health and functioning can be variable and unpredictable. When caring for people with chronic conditions, nursing assistants must adapt care approaches as necessary to accommodate the person's "good days" and "bad days."
  - Knowledge of both the disease as well as the person is necessary to help the person with a chronic condition maintain her sense of self and dignity.
- Although people 65 years and older make up most of the population in nursing homes, younger people may also live in long-term care facilities. Special accommodations need to be made to give the younger resident the opportunity to socialize with peers, engage in age-appropriate activities, and connect with the world outside of the nursing home.

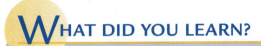

WHAT DID YOU LEARN?

Multiple choice

Select the single best answer for each of the following questions.

1. Which of the following is a reason why people are living longer than they ever have before?
   a. Advances in public health and medical care
   b. Antibiotics
   c. Improvements in public sanitation and hygiene
   d. All of the above

2. As more people live into old age, you would expect:
   a. All of them to need long-term care
   b. An increase in long-term care use
   c. A decrease in long-term care use
   d. No change in long-term care use

3. Most residents of nursing homes fall into what age group?
   a. Younger than 65 years
   b. 65 to 74 years
   c. 75 to 84 years
   d. 85 years and older

4. Mrs. Merkle was admitted to the Golden Harvest Nursing Center following a fall that resulted in a broken hip. She had been living alone in her own home, where she had lived for more than 50 years. She could not return home because she experienced complications from her broken hip and was unable to regain her ability to walk. She cried a lot when she was first admitted to the nursing facility, and often was impatient with the staff. What could be the cause of these behaviors?
   a. Mrs. Merkle's nursing home admission occurred with little warning or preparation
   b. Mrs. Merkle had to cope with multiple changes and losses at one time
   c. Mrs. Merkle had to get used to being cared for by people she did not know
   d. All of the above

5. Mrs. Merkle has been a resident at the Golden Harvest Nursing Center for almost 2 years. You know that this length of stay is:
   a. Typical for most nursing home residents
   b. Unusual (most people stay for 3 months or less)
   c. Longer than most stays (the average stay is 6 months to 1 year)
   d. Shorter than most stays (the average stay is 2.5 years or more)

6. Which of the following are reasons that someone might need long-term care?
   a. The family can no longer provide for care at home

b. The person needs to recover from the lingering effects of an acute accident or illness

c. The person is no longer able to care for himself

d. All of the above

7. Which of the following statements about family members' reactions to a loved one's nursing home admission is NOT true?

a. Family members are relieved, knowing that they no longer have to worry about the person

b. Families members must adjust to changes in roles and relationships

c. Family members often feel guilty about admitting a loved one to a nursing home

d. Family members may not trust staff members to provide adequate or proper care

8. Which of the following is true about the challenges a person must face when living with a chronic condition?

a. The chronic condition changes how the person feels about herself, and how others feel about her

b. The person must adapt to repeated episodes of illness

c. The person may have to make lifestyle changes to control the chronic condition

d. All of the above

9. A younger resident may live in a nursing home because of:

a. A spinal cord injury from a diving accident

b. A developmental disability

c. Progressive multiple sclerosis

d. All of the above

10. Most of the residents at Seaside Village Nursing Home are "typical," in that they are older people. However, today Mr. Leroy, a 35-year-old married father of two with progressive multiple sclerosis, was admitted to Seaside Village. To meet Mr. Leroy's needs, staff members at Seaside Village should:

a. Help Mr. Leroy to stay connected with his family and friends outside of the facility

b. Make a special effort to plan activities of interest to someone Mr. Leroy's age

c. Recognize that Mr. Leroy may have difficulty coping emotionally as a result of his admission to Seaside Village

d. All of the above

Matching

Match each numbered item with its appropriate lettered description.

_____ **1.** Acute illness

_____ **2.** Chronic condition

_____ **3.** Degenerative condition

_____ **4.** Activities of daily living (ADLs)

_____ **5.** Instrumental activities of daily living (IADLs)

_____ **6.** Co-existent medical conditions

_____ **7.** Cognitive impairment

a. Problems processing, learning, or remembering information

b. A condition that gets progressively worse over time

c. Examples include dressing, eating, bathing, toileting, and moving

d. More than one illness at the same time in the same person

e. A condition that is ongoing

f. Examples include using the telephone and balancing a checkbook

g. An unexpected illness with a rapid onset and a relatively short recovery time

STOP and Think!

- You are working the day shift on a very busy day. One of your co-workers went home sick so everyone had to pick up the care for additional residents. You are behind in your work, and the charge nurse has just told you that Mrs. Wilkins, a new resident, is arriving any minute and you have been assigned to Mrs. Wilkins' care. You wish the charge nurse would have told you this earlier. There is only an hour left on your shift, and you have to leave on time because you have a doctor's appointment after work. You still need to answer Mr. Jones' call light, and now you see Mrs. Wilkins arriving on a stretcher. How are you feeling about this new admission? What mood will you be in when you enter Mrs. Wilkins' room to greet her? If you are not careful, what impression could you give Mrs. Wilkins and her family members? What impression do you want to give Mrs. Wilkins and her family members?

- After helping Mr. Jones, you enter Mrs. Wilkins' room and greet her. She is very quiet. You ask Mrs. Wilkins a few questions to get to know her, and she replies, "What do you want to know for?" As you begin to put Mrs. Wilkins' belongings away, she questions you about what you are doing and then says, "Leave those alone! Those are mine!" You explain how the call light control works and ask Mrs. Wilkins to use it when she needs help to go to the bathroom. You notice that Mr. Jones' call light is on again, so you go across the hall to help him. When you return to Mrs. Wilkins' room, you find Mrs. Wilkins alone in the bathroom, barefoot, and without her walker. There is urine on the floor. You ask Mrs. Wilkins why she didn't put her call light on, and she tells you that she did not know about the call light. How are you feeling about Mrs. Wilkins? What might be some reasons that she is acting this way? What could you do to make Mrs. Wilkins' adjustment to her new environment easier?

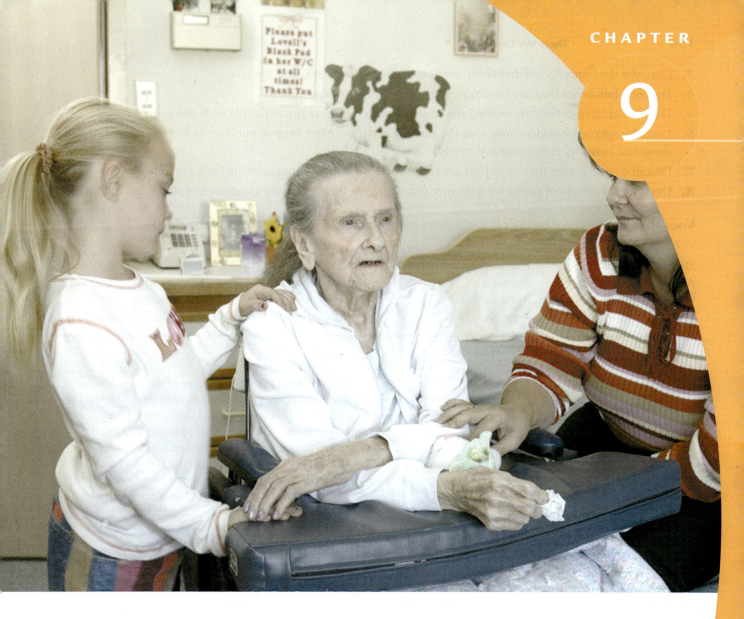

The Resident With Dementia

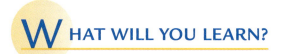HAT WILL YOU LEARN?

Dementia, which is caused by changes in the brain tissue, affects a person's ability to remember, think, and communicate. A person with dementia becomes increasingly dependent on others for care. Because dementia is a leading cause for admission to a long-term care facility, many of the residents in your care will have dementia. In this chapter, you will learn about the more common types of dementia, and about the special care needs of people with this illness. When you are finished with this chapter, you will be able to:

1. Describe the three major stages of dementia.
2. Describe four major causes of dementia.

Photo: Many of your residents will have dementia. The emotional pain suffered by a person with dementia, as well as his or her family members, is immeasurable.

3. Describe the "four As" of dementia: amnesia, aphasia, agnosia, and apraxia.
4. Describe behaviors that are common in people with dementia.
5. Describe strategies for determining the cause of difficult behaviors in people with dementia.
6. Describe special considerations that the nursing assistant must keep in mind while helping a person with dementia meet his or her physical needs.
7. Describe special care measures that are taken to help maintain quality of life for a person with dementia.
8. Describe the effects of caring for a person with dementia on the nursing assistant and strategies for coping.

Vocabulary Use the CD in the front of your book to hear these terms pronounced and defined:

Dementia	Frontotemporal dementia	Apraxia	Delusion
Alzheimer's disease	Amnesia	Validation therapy	Catastrophic reaction
Vascular dementia	Aphasia	Perseveration	Sundowning
Lewy body dementia	Agnosia	Hallucination	Reminiscence therapy

WHAT IS DEMENTIA?

Dementia is the permanent and progressive loss of mental functions (such as thinking, reasoning, and remembering), caused by damage to the brain tissue. A person with dementia experiences:

- Problems with memory, especially short-term memory
- Difficulty communicating
- Problems with judgment (the person is not able to make good decisions)
- Disorientation (the person is not oriented to person, place, or time)
- An inability to manage activities of daily living (ADLs)

Dementia has a very gradual onset, with symptoms appearing over a period of several months or a few years. On average, a person with dementia will live 8 to 10 years after the first symptoms appear. During this time, the person will pass through three major stages (Box 9-1). Although medications are available that may help to slow the progression of dementia, there is currently no cure for dementia.

Helping Hands and a Caring Heart

FOCUS ON HUMANISTIC HEALTH CARE

For family members, having a loved one with dementia can be particularly hard. Because dementia lasts for many years, dementia is sometimes referred to as "the long good-bye." Throughout the course of the person's illness, family members will constantly have to deal with loss, as the person they knew and loved slowly slips away. Imagine how hard it would be if someone you loved no longer remembered or recognized you.

As a nursing assistant, you can support the family members of a resident with dementia by helping the family members make the most of their time with their loved one. Encouraging family members to bring in photos or other mementos to share with the resident benefits the resident and also benefits the family members, by allowing them to remember and talk about experiences they shared together as a family. Sometimes, simple things, such as just sitting together as a family in the sunshine and listening to the birds, can form the basis for special memories in the future. Helping family members to create special memories during this difficult time can help them deal with the feelings of loss they will experience as the person's disease progresses, and after the person dies.

CAUSES OF DEMENTIA

Many different disorders can cause dementia. Some neurologic disorders, such as Parkinson's disease and Huntington's disease, are associated with the development of dementia. Dementia may also be a part of some infectious disorders such as HIV/AIDS, syphilis, and "mad cow disease." However, four of the most common causes of dementia are Alzheimer's disease, vascular dementia, Lewy body dementia, and frontotemporal dementia (Fig. 9-1).

BOX 9-1 Stages of Dementia

Early Stage
- The person begins to experience memory loss. Because the person is aware of these memory changes, she may become fearful, anxious, or depressed. The person may become angry at other people.

Middle Stage
- The person begins to have difficulty communicating. She may have difficulty using words, understanding words, or both.
- The person begins to have difficulty recognizing familiar people and things.
- The person begins to have difficulty remembering the steps that are necessary to complete familiar tasks, such as getting dressed.

- The person's personality may change, and she may begin to behave differently, often in challenging ways.
- The person begins to experience incontinence.

Late Stage
- The person loses the ability to walk and sit independently, and eventually becomes bedridden.
- The person is no longer able to speak, swallow, or smile.
- The person becomes totally incontinent of urine and feces.
- The person dies.

ALZHEIMER'S DISEASE

Alzheimer's disease is the most common cause of dementia, accounting for more than 50% of all cases. In the United States today, Alzheimer's disease is a leading cause of death. More than 5 million people in the United States have Alzheimer's disease. If no cure is found, it is estimated that 11 to 16 million people will have the disease by the year 2050.

Alzheimer's disease usually occurs in people older than 65 years of age; however, people as young as 40 years of age may also get the disease. Because the risk for developing Alzheimer's disease increases with age, people 85 years of age and older are at the highest risk for developing Alzheimer's disease.

Alzheimer's disease is named after Alois Alzheimer (1864–1915), a German doctor who discovered the disease in 1906. One of Dr. Alzheimer's patients, a 51-year-old woman, died after showing unusual mental changes and behaviors. To learn why these changes occurred, Dr. Alzheimer performed an autopsy on her brain. He found that certain areas of her brain seemed soft and shrunken. In addition, he saw abnormal deposits of protein, especially in the parts of the brain that function in memory. He called these abnormal deposits *plaques* and *tangles* (Fig. 9-2). We now know that these plaques and tangles affect the ability of the nerve cells in the brain to communicate with each other. The nerve cells start to die. As a result, the brain shrinks in size, and brain activity decreases (Fig. 9-3).

Although we do not know exactly what causes Alzheimer's disease, researchers have identified a number of risk factors. The most significant risk factor for developing Alzheimer's disease is age. Another known risk factor is family history. Those who have a parent, child, or sibling with Alzheimer's disease are more likely to get the disease themselves. If more than one family member has the disease, the risk increases. Researchers have also found that those who have had serious head trauma are at increased risk for developing Alzheimer's disease. Finally, risk

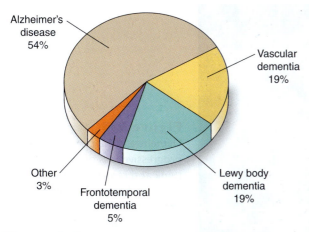

Figure 9-1
Many disorders can cause dementia. Alzheimer's disease is the most common cause of dementia, accounting for more than 50% of cases. Other causes of dementia include vascular dementia, Lewy body dementia, and frontotemporal dementia.

Normal

Alzheimer's disease

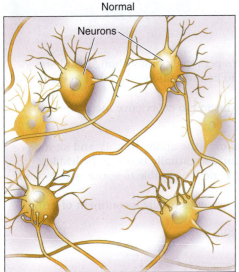

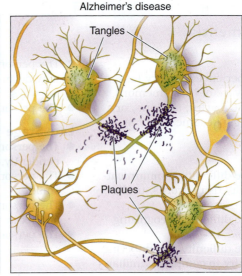

Neurons

Tangles

Plaques

Figure 9-2
Protein deposits, called plaques and tangles, are found in the brains of people with Alzheimer's disease.

factors for heart disease (such as high blood pressure, high blood cholesterol levels, and diabetes) have also been linked to the development of Alzheimer's disease.

VASCULAR DEMENTIA

Vascular dementia is thought to be the cause of dementia in approximately 20% to 25% of people with dementia. Vascular dementia most often affects people between the ages of 55 and 75 years, and is most common in people who are 70 years or older. Damage to the blood vessels that supply the brain can affect the delivery of oxygen and nutrients to the brain tissue and may contribute to the onset of vascular dementia. In **vascular dementia,** mental functions are lost because areas of brain tissue die due to lack of adequate oxygen and nutrients. Conditions that put a person at risk for developing vascular dementia include:

- A history of myocardial infarction ("heart attack"), stroke, or transient ischemic attacks (TIAs or "mini-strokes")
- Peripheral vascular disease ("hardening" of the arteries that supply the legs)
- High blood pressure

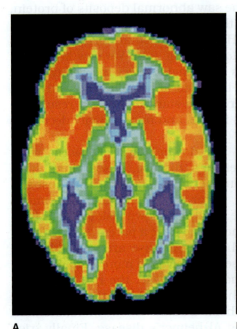

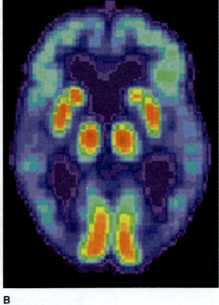

A

B

Figure 9-3
Dementia is the permanent and progressive loss of the ability to think and remember. **(A)** Brain scan of a healthy person. **(B)** Brain scan of a person with Alzheimer's disease, the most common cause of dementia. The blue areas indicate areas where brain activity is lost. (*Alzheimer's Disease Education Referral Center, a service of the National Institute on Aging.*)

- High blood cholesterol levels
- Diabetes mellitus
- Obesity
- Smoking

Symptoms of vascular dementia may appear suddenly (for example, following a stroke that causes an area of the brain tissue to die), or they may appear over time. Symptoms of vascular dementia vary from person to person, depending on which areas of the brain are affected. Like Alzheimer's disease, vascular dementia is irreversible and incurable. However, keeping the person's blood pressure, blood glucose, and blood cholesterol levels within normal limits can help to slow the progression of the dementia and decrease the severity of the symptoms.

LEWY BODY DEMENTIA

Lewy body dementia accounts for approximately 20% of all cases of dementia. **Lewy body dementia** is caused by the build-up of abnormal protein deposits (called *Lewy bodies*) in areas of the brain that are responsible for thinking and movement. In addition to a decline in mental abilities, people with Lewy body dementia develop problems controlling body movement (for example, muscle rigidity, a shuffling gait, slow movements, and tremors), similar to those seen in people with Parkinson's disease. People with Lewy body dementia also tend to experience visual hallucinations (that is, they see things that do not really exist) and distinct changes in mental alertness. For example, one day a resident with Lewy body dementia will be alert and capable of participating in his own care, but the next day he will be very confused and need more assistance to complete his ADLs.

FRONTOTEMPORAL DEMENTIA

Frontotemporal dementia is caused by damage to the frontal and temporal lobes of the brain. The frontal lobe is the area of the brain that is responsible for personality and behavior. The temporal lobe is the area of the brain responsible for language. As a result, a person with frontotemporal dementia may show extreme changes in personality and behavior, have difficulties with language, or both. Caring for a person with frontotemporal dementia can be particularly challenging, because the disease may cause the person to say or do things that are socially inappropriate. For example, the person may undress in a public area, or make comments that are insulting or rude. Other people with frontotemporal dementia become bored and listless. They no longer seem to care about anything, and they lack motivation and energy. These behavioral difficulties are a common reason why a person with frontotemporal dementia may require long-term care.

Frontotemporal dementia accounts for about 5% of all cases of dementia. Symptoms of frontotemporal dementia generally appear at a younger age than in other types of dementia, often between the ages of 40 and 65 years. Also, unlike other forms of dementia, memory is often spared until later in the disease process.

THE "4 As" OF DEMENTIA

No matter what the underlying cause of the dementia is, all people with dementia experience changes in the brain that lead to the "4 As" of dementia: **amnesia** (difficulty remembering), **aphasia** (difficulty using language), **agnosia** (difficulty recognizing information obtained using the five senses), and **apraxia** (difficulty coordinating the steps needed to complete a task). The "4 As" of dementia are summarized in Table 9-1 and described in more detail in the sections that follow. Understanding these "4 As" will allow you to provide better care for your residents with dementia, because you will be better able to understand what they are experiencing, thinking, and feeling.

AMNESIA

Amnesia is memory loss. During the early stage of dementia, memory loss generally only affects short-term (recent) memory, and long-term memory remains intact. So, although the person may not remember who he had lunch with last Thursday, he will still be able to tell you the name of his high school girlfriend. As time passes and more and more of the brain becomes diseased, long-term memory is also lost, robbing the person of all memory.

Short-Term Memory Loss

The loss of short-term memory can cause a person with dementia to behave in puzzling ways. For example, the person may:

- Accuse others of stealing a personal belonging (because he cannot remember where he put it)

Table 9-1   The "4 As" of Dementia

"A"	THE PERSON MAY:	THE NURSING ASSISTANT SHOULD:
Amnesia (difficulty remembering)	<li> Ask the same questions over and over <li> Forget where belongings are (and accuse others of stealing) <li> Forget he has eaten <li> Live in the past <li> Forget that loved ones have passed away	<li> Be patient <li> Maintain a structured routine <li> Repeat information as necessary using simple language <li> Label everything <li> Use validation therapy techniques to acknowledge the person's reality
Aphasia (difficulty using language) <li> *Expressive* – difficulty making self understood <li> *Receptive* – difficulty understanding others	<li> Use the wrong word, make up words, or talk in "word salad" (the words are real, but the way they are put together does not make any sense) <li> Appear to be uncooperative, but in reality, is not understanding what was said	<li> Use simple words <li> Allow plenty of time for communication <li> Repeat information as necessary <li> Eliminate distractions when communicating with the person <li> Make eye contact with the person when communicating <li> Observe the person's body language <li> Use non-verbal communication to convey information to the person
Agnosia (difficulty recognizing information obtained using the five senses)	<li> Use common objects in very strange ways <li> Fail to recognize where he is <li> Fail to recognize family members or familiar caregivers <li> Fail to recognize self in the mirror	<li> Introduce himself or herself, and others, to the person as necessary <li> Take measures to limit the person's access to objects, supplies, or equipment that could cause the person harm if they are misused or swallowed
Apraxia (difficulty coordinating the steps needed to complete a task)	<li> Lose the ability to complete tasks, such as getting dressed, independently	<li> Observe what steps the person can do independently, and then offer assistance, as needed

- Ask for a meal after he has already eaten (because he cannot remember eating)
- Stop in the middle of a task (because he cannot remember what he was doing)
- Ask the same question over and over again (because he cannot remember asking the question, and he cannot remember the answer you gave him)

Because of the short-term memory loss a person with dementia experiences, you will need to provide lots of reminders and redirection. Be sure to introduce yourself each time you see the person, and explain what you will be doing. Do not expect the person to remember you, even if she just saw you 5 minutes ago! It is also important to maintain a structured routine. Because of amnesia, people with dementia have a limited ability to think through changes to their routine, and to remember what they are supposed to be doing. As a result, a change in the normal routine causes a person with dementia a great deal of stress. Find out about the person's usual routine, and try to adapt your care approaches to that routine, as much as possible. This helps the person to feel more comfortable by minimizing stress caused by change.

Long-Term Memory Loss

As the dementia progresses, the person's long-term memory will begin to be affected as well. The person can lose years of memory, causing her to forget about entire periods of her life. Sometimes time periods blend together. For example, a married resident with several children may believe that she is 16 years old and still living at home with her parents. She may not recognize her married name, and she may tell you she has no children (yet another time, she may tell you that she is waiting for her husband). Because this resident is literally living in the past, she will not be able to understand references to her current situation. Trying to orient the resident to her current reality can embarrass or upset her. If you insist that what the resident believes to be true is not real, she may lose trust in you. Instead, it is better to use a technique called validation therapy.

Validation therapy stresses the importance of acknowledging the person's reality. Rather than correcting the person, you respond to the person within her own reality. For example, let's say you are trying to get one of your residents, Mrs. Pyne, to go to the dining room for lunch, but she tells you that she does not want to go because her father is coming to the facility to pick her up. You know that Mrs. Pyne's father died 20 years ago, but in Mrs. Pyne's mind, he is still very much alive. Instead of telling Mrs. Pyne the truth, which is likely to cause her significant emotional distress, you could respond by suggesting that she have a little snack in the dining room while she waits, because her father is going to be late. You can also acknowledge Mrs. Pyne's reality by asking her questions about her father, such as "What does your father look like?" or "What kind of work does your father do?" This supports Mrs. Pyne's current reality, and gives her the opportunity to connect with fond thoughts about her father. Validation therapy protects the feelings and beliefs of the person with dementia, and helps the person to retain a sense of self-worth and dignity. Validation therapy also helps the caregiver to understand what the person with dementia is experiencing.

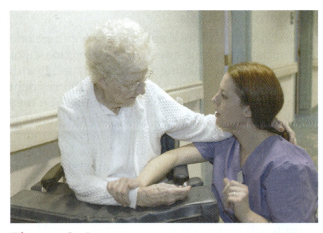

Figure 9-4

When communicating with a person with dementia, place yourself at eye level with the person, and maintain eye contact. Many people with dementia also respond well to touch.

APHASIA

Aphasia is difficulty communicating. During the middle stage of dementia, the person begins to experience aphasia. The person may have *expressive* aphasia (difficulty using words), *receptive* aphasia (difficulty understanding words), or both. The inability to make oneself understood, or to understand others, can be a great source of stress and frustration for the person with dementia. For example, Mr. Smith, a resident with dementia, really needs to use the bathroom, but because of his aphasia, he cannot explain his need to anyone. In addition, no one is recognizing his need. You are asking Mr. Smith to join the others in the activity room, but Mr. Smith's need to use the bathroom has not been taken care of. As Mr. Smith's need to use the bathroom becomes more urgent, he becomes increasingly uncomfortable and stressed, and he may strike out. Behaviors are often the resident's way of telling us that there is an unmet need. It is up to us to be observant of our resident's behavior and body language, and to use this information to figure out what the resident is trying to tell us.

Allow extra time when communicating with your residents who have dementia. Because of aphasia, it will take a person with dementia longer to process what you are telling her, and to find the words to say what she wants to say. Eliminate distractions when possible, to help the person focus on the conversation. Maintaining eye contact during communication is also important (Fig. 9-4). If the person is not looking at you,

she may forget that you are there! Remember what you learned about good communication in Chapter 5. Even if a person with dementia does not understand your words, she does understand your tone of voice and body language. If the resident detects that you are impatient, irritated, or angry, the resident is going to respond in a similar manner. A calm, soothing tone of voice and a helpful attitude will help you to be more successful when working with residents with dementia.

Expressive Aphasia

A person with expressive aphasia may have difficulty finding the right word. Sometimes a word will come out that is related to what the person is trying to say, but it is not the right word. For example, a person with expressive aphasia may refer to her husband as her brother. "Brother" is a word for a male family member, but it is not the right word for the relationship the person is describing. The person may group words together that do not make sense (for example, "My twig had a cap and the nose was had indeed!"), or utter nonsense sounds in a tone and pattern that mimics normal conversation. Do not laugh at the person, or tell him that he is talking nonsense. Instead, when you cannot understand the words or sounds, respond to the mood or feeling that the person is conveying through his body language and tone of voice. For example, if the person is smiling and pleasant, respond in a lighthearted, pleasant manner. If the person seems worried or distressed, respond with concern and caring.

Receptive Aphasia

A person with receptive aphasia may not respond appropriately to your questions or directions. For example, you are asking the resident to go with you to the dining room, but instead the resident opens his closet to show you something. You may think that the resident is being difficult, but it is more likely that the resident just does not understand what you are asking him to do. Using gestures may help the resident to understand your message. For example, you could point toward the door, and mimic picking up a fork and eating so that the resident gets the idea. If you need the resident to sit, you could point to the chair and bend at the knees to demonstrate the sitting motion.

AGNOSIA

Agnosia is difficulty recognizing sensory input (that is, information received through the eyes, ears, nose, taste buds, or sense of touch). For example, when a person with agnosia looks at a pencil, his eye sees the pencil, but the part of the brain that tells the person what he is seeing is not working. By the size and shape of the pencil, the person may think that the pencil is a straw, put it in a cup, and try to drink through it.

Difficulty Recognizing Objects

We rely on our senses to protect us from harm. People with dementia who have agnosia will not be able to recognize potential danger and could easily harm themselves. For example, because of agnosia, a person with dementia may not be able to tell the difference between shampoo and lemonade, and as a result, he may try to drink the shampoo. When caring for residents with dementia, you must be very careful to keep cleaning solutions, personal care items, medications, equipment, and other potentially dangerous items in a secure place.

Difficulty Recognizing People

Because of agnosia, a person with dementia may not recognize people she knows (such as family members, friends, and caregivers). Not being able to recognize others can be very frightening and frustrating for a person with dementia. Imagine how not being able to recognize people can affect a person with dementia who lives in a long-term care facility. Each change of shift brings many new "strangers" onto the unit! You can help to minimize some of the stress your resident may feel by taking the time to introduce yourself and others at each interaction.

In addition to not recognizing others, a person who has agnosia may not even recognize herself in a mirror. She may think her reflection in the mirror is a stranger spying through the window. Putting a towel over the mirror to "close the curtain" can help to reassure and calm the person.

APRAXIA

Apraxia is difficulty coordinating the steps needed to complete a task. Simple, everyday activities become very difficult for a person with dementia. For example, the person may have difficulty getting dressed because he might put clothes on in the wrong order. Or, he may not be able to feed himself, because he cannot remember how to use the knife and fork. The frustration the person experiences because of the inability to perform these tasks can contribute to a behavioral outburst. It is important to observe the person to determine what he is capable of doing, and what he needs help to accomplish. Although it may be easier and faster to just do the task for the person, it is important to allow the person to do as much as he can for himself for as long as he can.

When you are coaching a resident through daily care, break the task down into individual steps. For example, if you are helping the resident to brush his teeth, you could break that task down into the following individual steps: Take the cap off the toothpaste. . . . Pick up your toothbrush. . . . Put toothpaste on the toothbrush . . . Turn on the water . . . and so on. You will need to remind the person at each step what he needs to do next. If you give the person too many instructions at once, he will not remember what you said (because of amnesia) and he will not be able to complete the task.

Hand-over-hand cueing is another technique that may help a resident to complete his care routines (Fig. 9-5). For example, you could use hand-over-hand cueing to help a resident remember how to eat. First, you would put the fork in the resident's hand. Then you would place your hand over the resident's hand, and together you would move the fork to the plate to pick up a bite of food. Finally, you would guide the fork to the resident's mouth. Sometimes, the familiar feel of the movement will come back to the resident and the resident will be able to continue with the task by himself, with occasional reminders.

Never rush a person who has dementia. Plan your care to allow the extra time the person needs to think about how to coordinate and complete her care routines. Rushing a person with dementia

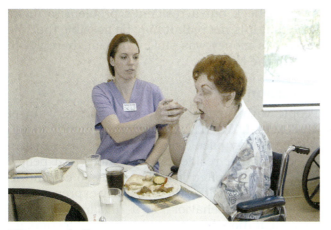

Figure 9-5
Hand-over-hand cueing is a technique that can be used to help a person with dementia remember how to eat.

increases the person's confusion and frustration, and will most likely result in a behavioral outburst.

BEHAVIORS ASSOCIATED WITH DEMENTIA

Some behaviors are very common in people with dementia. When you are caring for a person with dementia, you will come to know the behaviors that are normal for that person. A change in a person's normal behavior is a cause for concern and should be reported to the nurse.

COMMON BEHAVIORS

Common behaviors in people with dementia include the following.

Wandering

Some residents with dementia will walk around the facility almost constantly. They may be looking for some place in particular, or they may just need to move around. Some may try to leave the facility. This may be because they want to find the home that they remember, or because they feel like they must leave to fulfill an obligation, such as going to work or checking on the children. Sometimes, they may just be exploring the building and accidentally find an exit door. Whatever the reason, if a resident with dementia gets out of the building without an escort, it is a very dangerous situation. The person might get lost, walk into the path of an oncoming car, or

drown in a body of water, such as a lake or river. Depending on the weather and climate, the person may not be dressed appropriately to be outside. For example, if it is raining or cold, the person may not have a coat.

Because this tendency to wander cannot be stopped, many long-term care facilities have developed ways to allow residents to wander safely. Many facilities have outdoor areas enclosed by walls or fences so that the resident can wander outside but still remain within the safe environment of the facility (Fig. 9-6). A resident who tends to wander may also wear a bracelet or an anklet that will set off an alarm if the resident tries to leave the facility through a doorway that leads to an unsafe area. When the alarm sounds, staff members are alerted to guide the person back to safety.

Pacing

A person with dementia may pace back and forth. Often, the person is pacing because he has a physical need that is not being met. For example, the person may be hungry or need to use the bathroom. A person might also pace in response to a noisy, overstimulating environment, or because he is feeling scared or lost. If one of your residents is pacing, try to figure out what is causing the behavior, and take steps to relieve the cause of the behavior. Sometimes there is nothing to do but to let the person pace. In this case, you might take the person to a safe place (for example, a fenced-in garden) and walk alongside him until the behavior has run its course.

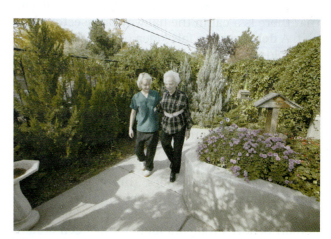

Figure 9-6
Wandering and pacing are two very common behaviors in people with dementia. Many long-term care facilities have enclosed areas outdoors where people can wander and pace safely.

Repetition

A person with dementia may do the same thing over and over again. This is called **perseveration.** For example, the person might repeat the same phrase or question constantly. Or, she might constantly move a piece of cloth around on a coffee table, as if dusting. Although these behaviors are usually not physically harmful to the person, they can be a sign that the person is bored. These behaviors can also be annoying to caregivers and other residents. Distracting the person by offering to take her for a walk, or by getting her involved in an activity such as looking through a magazine, may help to break the cycle.

Rummaging

A person with dementia may go through drawers or closets, searching for an item that he is never able to find. If you notice that a resident is rummaging, ask the person what he is trying to find, and offer help in finding it. If the person tends to rummage through other residents' belongings or every single drawer in his own dresser, it may be necessary to make certain areas "off-limits" by locking them. You can then show the person a special drawer or a box filled with small personal items that he can rummage through. Sometimes placing pictures or labels identifying the contents of the drawer on the front of the drawer can help the person to find items without having to go through everything.

Hallucinations and Delusions

A **hallucination** is seeing, hearing, tasting, or smelling something that is not really there. For example, a person with dementia may tell you that there is a cat in the hallway or insects on the bed. A **delusion** is a false idea or belief that a person holds to be true and that cannot be changed. For example, the person may believe that you are someone you are not. It does not help to tell the person that what he believes is not true. In fact, it can make the situation worse.

You must respond to the person with hallucinations or delusions according to what he is experiencing, not according to what you know to be real or true. Remember, this is the person's reality. Usually, offering to help the person with his situation is comforting. For example, if the person believes that his money has been stolen, assure him that you will report the loss and offer assistance to help him to find it. Or, if the person tells you she sees bugs on the bed, go through the motion of sweeping them off, and gently redirect the person's attention. Of course, you should always check out a resident's problem to make sure that it is *not* real. It may be possible that the resident's money was stolen, or that there was a bug on the bed!

Agitation

People with dementia often become very upset and excited. When a person with dementia is agitated, he may pace, shout, or strike out at caregivers or other residents. Remember that people with dementia often lose the ability to communicate effectively with others, so they express themselves through behavior (Fig. 9-7). Many things can cause agitation, including pain or an infection, an unmet physical need (for example, hunger, a full bladder, or lack of sleep), or a noisy environment. When reporting agitation, be sure to describe exactly what you saw or heard that made you believe that the resident was agitated. For example, reporting that "Mrs. Jones will not sit still and keeps yelling to go home" is more meaningful than reporting that "Mrs. Jones is very agitated today." Knowing Mrs. Jones' exact behavior makes it easier for the health care team to identify the cause of the behavior so that the proper action can be taken to address Mrs. Jones' need.

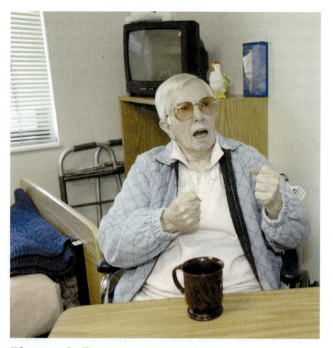

Figure 9-7

People with dementia often lose the ability to communicate effectively with others, so they express themselves through behavior. Agitation is often a sign that a physical or emotional need is not being met. Reporting to the nurse exactly what behaviors you see helps the nurse determine the cause of the person's agitation.

Catastrophic Reactions

A person with dementia may over-react to something that would cause a healthy person minimal or no stress. This is called a **catastrophic reaction.** For example, a person with dementia may begin to scream or sob loudly when you try to give him a bath. Catastrophic reactions often occur when the person feels threatened. For example, the person may feel that his privacy is being threatened when you attempt to give him a bath. Feeling overwhelmed can also cause a person to have a catastrophic reaction. For example, a ringing telephone in a room where the television is on and people are talking might be too much for a person with dementia to handle.

Sundowning

Sundowning is the worsening of a person's behavioral symptoms in the late afternoon and evening, as the sun goes down. For example, the person may become more restless and confused in the evening hours and may have trouble getting to sleep.

No one knows for sure exactly why sundowning behavior occurs. One factor that may contribute to sundowning behavior is fatigue, especially if the person frequently wanders or paces throughout the day. An inability to see as well in the evening hours, when natural light is decreased, may also contribute to sundowning behavior. Finally, it is possible that sundowning behavior may occur because the person begins to feel frightened and alone during the evening hours, when activity on the unit begins to quiet down, and there are fewer people around.

Helping to ensure periods of quiet and rest during the day might help to reduce fatigue, in turn reducing sundowning behavior. Turning on lights earlier, providing some activity, and checking on the person frequently to reassure him of your presence may help as well.

Inappropriate Sexual Behaviors

There are many different reasons why a person with dementia may show inappropriate sexual behaviors. A resident with dementia may climb in bed with another resident who is not her spouse because after being married for 50 years or more, it may feel more normal to sleep next to another person. Or, a resident with dementia may make a sexual advance toward someone she believes is her spouse, because of a similarity in appearance or mannerisms. Behaviors that staff members may view as "sexual" may not be sexual in nature at all. Rather, they may just be a demonstration of the resident's need to feel love and affection from another person.

Sometimes a person with dementia may masturbate or undress in a public area, such as the dining room. There are several reasons why a person with dementia might do this. Changes in the brain may make the person unable to tell the difference between behavior that is socially acceptable and behavior that is not. Or, changes in the brain may interfere with the person's ability to control his or her impulses. You must take measures to protect the person's dignity. Give the person privacy by gently, but firmly, leading the person back to his or her room, or redirect the person's attention by introducing another activity.

Although OBRA specifically says that a resident of a long-term care facility must be allowed to fulfill his or her sexual needs, it is important to make sure that if another resident is involved, that resident is able to give consent. A resident with dementia may not be able to understand what he or she is consenting to, and therefore will be unable to fully provide consent. If another resident is involved and has not provided consent, you must take measures to protect that resident.

WHAT DO THESE BEHAVIORS MEAN?

It is important to try and determine the cause of the person's behavior, rather than just accepting it as a normal part of the person's disease process. In many cases, finding the underlying cause of the behavior and addressing it causes the behavior to stop, providing relief to the person, and to you. In addition, a change in the person's normal behavior could be a sign that the person's illness is progressing, or that the person is experiencing some other medical condition that needs to be evaluated. Remember that a person with dementia may not be able to tell you about symptoms he is experiencing.

To identify the underlying cause of the behavior, first describe the behavior in as much detail as possible, using only facts, not personal opinions:

- What did you see happen?
- What did you hear?
- Where did the behavior occur?
- What time did it occur?
- Who was the resident with?
- What were the circumstances? What was going on at the time the behavior occurred?

Compare your answers to these questions each time the resident demonstrates the behavior, to see if there is a pattern. Then, consider the following points:

- The inability to remember (amnesia), communicate (aphasia), recognize (agnosia), or perform tasks (apraxia) may be contributing to the person's behavior.
- The person may have a physical problem (for example, discomfort or hunger).
- The person may have a medical problem (for example, an infection or low blood sugar).
- The person may have a psychiatric symptom (for example, hallucinations or delusions) that alters his environment and causes distress.
- The person's personal history may provide clues to the behavior. (For example, a retired military officer may believe that he is still in charge of others. As a result, he may become agitated when he issues an order to another resident that is not obeyed.)
- The person may be responding to the way he was approached. (For example, the resident may become agitated if he senses that the nursing assistant who is helping him is rushed or impatient.)

Once you have a few ideas about what could be causing the behavior, you can try doing different things to eliminate or reduce the behavior. For example, if you suspect that the person is acting a certain way because she is hungry or needs to use the bathroom, you can try offering a snack or taking the person to the restroom. If you observe that the room is noisy and there is a lot of activity, you might try taking the person to a quieter place. If you suspect that the person is behaving in a certain way because he has a medical problem or is in pain, report your suspicions to the nurse so that the nurse can investigate further.

CARING FOR A PERSON WITH DEMENTIA

As a person's dementia progresses, he will need more and more help with all activities of daily living (ADLs). In addition to physical needs, the person will have emotional and social needs that must be met as well. General guidelines for caring for a person with dementia are given in Guidelines Box 9-1.

ASSISTING WITH ACTIVITIES OF DAILY LIVING (ADLs)

For a person with dementia, accomplishing everyday tasks such as bathing, dressing, eating, and using the bathroom can be difficult. The inability to remember how to do these things can be very frustrating for the person. Sometimes the person will resist doing what you need her to do. This can be challenging for the nursing assistant who has been assigned to provide care! Several factors can cause a person to resist care:

- The person may not remember where she is, or who you are (amnesia)
- The person may not recognize you (agnosia)
- The person might not be able to understand what you are asking her to do (receptive aphasia)
- The person might feel threatened or rushed
- The person may feel as if she has no choice in the matter

When you are helping a resident with dementia with her ADLs, there are several general things you can do to gain the resident's cooperation and help the task go more smoothly:

- Take the time to help the person to feel comfortable with you before beginning the task. For example, introduce yourself as necessary, and talk with the person a little bit before turning your attention to accomplishing the necessary task.
- Speak clearly, in a calm tone of voice. Try not to appear rushed, busy, or impatient.
- Remind the person at each step what she needs to do next.
- Use hand gestures in addition to spoken instructions.
- Plan for the procedure in advance. Being prepared and having everything you need before you begin a procedure will allow you to accomplish the task efficiently, which can help to reduce the amount of stress the person feels.
- Keep to a regular schedule. Following an established routine also helps to reduce the amount of stress the person feels.

Throughout this book, you will see *Caring For Those With Dementia* boxes. These boxes highlight special considerations you should keep in mind, and approaches you can take when assisting your residents with dementia with specific tasks.

Guidelines Box 9-1 Guidelines for Caring for a Person With Dementia

WHAT YOU DO	WHY YOU DO IT
Maintain a calm, structured environment.	A person with dementia can become overwhelmed very easily. When the person becomes overwhelmed, difficult or dangerous behaviors, such as wandering, agitation, or a catastrophic reaction, are likely to increase.
Approach the person with dementia slowly, announcing yourself before touching him.	Many people with dementia also have hearing problems, vision problems, or both. If you approach quickly without warning, you may startle the person, triggering a catastrophic reaction.
Avoid arguing or disagreeing with the person.	A person with dementia exists in a different reality from the rest of the world. Trying to force the person with dementia to understand or acknowledge anything other than her own reality will increase the person's agitation.
When asking a person with dementia to do something, use short words and short sentences. Avoid negatively worded instructions (such as, "Don't put that there!"). Avoid instructions that require the person to remember more than one action at a time.	Because a person with dementia has problems with short-term memory, he will not be able to remember or process long words and sentences. A positively worded command ("Please put that here") is easier to understand than a negative one. Failing at a task increases the person's frustration. When you give the person instructions in a way that she can understand, you increase the person's chances of successfully completing the task.
Give a person with dementia enough time to respond to questions and directions.	It may take the person a while to think of the word or words he needs to answer your question, or the actions he must take to follow your directions. Feeling rushed can cause the person to become agitated or upset.
"Listen" to the person by paying attention to body language. Make good use of your observation skills.	As a person's dementia gets worse, she loses the ability to communicate effectively. Often, body language and behaviors become the person's main way of expressing herself.
When managing difficult behaviors, be aware that solutions that work today may not work tomorrow. Be creative, and do not give up.	Dementia is a progressive disease. Therefore, the person's abilities, disabilities, and needs change over time, and your approaches to managing difficult behaviors may also need to change.
Help the person with dementia to feel secure and loved by showing affection (kind words, a gentle touch) and smiling.	Like all people, people with dementia have emotional needs that must be met.

(continued)

Guidelines Box 9-1   Guidelines for Caring for a Person With Dementia (continued)

WHAT YOU DO	WHY YOU DO IT
Allow the person with dementia to do as much as he can for himself, for as long as possible.	This is important for maintaining the person's dignity and self-esteem. No one likes to feel helpless or useless.
Help the person to maintain independence for as long as possible by using visual cues to orient the person to place and time. For example, place a large-faced clock in the person's room, decorate for the holidays, and post names and other reminder signs in prominent, meaningful places. (For example, if a person keeps trying to walk out the front door, apply a big, red and white "stop" sign to the inside of the door.)	Using visual cues can help the person to maintain his independence longer, which is important for the person's self-esteem.
Help the person to exercise her mind by getting the person involved in activities that relate to the person's interests and experiences.	Participating in activities helps to prevent boredom and increases the person's sense of purpose and accomplishment.
Protect the person from physical injury.	People with dementia lose the ability to make good decisions related to their well-being. For example, a person with dementia might walk in front of an oncoming car, leave the house without a coat in the middle of a snowstorm, or drink the contents of a bottle found under the sink.
Maintain the person's hygiene and good grooming habits.	This is important for the person's health as well as for her self-esteem.
Be as tolerant as possible of the person.	The person's behaviors are a result of his dementia, and are beyond the person's control. The person is not purposely trying to frustrate or annoy you.
When you become tired and frustrated, take time out, be good to yourself, and share your feelings with the nurse. Know that these emotions and thoughts are normal.	Caring for a person with dementia is emotionally draining and physically difficult. If you do not take measures to protect your own mental health, you run the risk of "burn-out." In addition, you place the resident at risk for abuse, should you lose your temper.

MEETING THE PERSON'S EMOTIONAL AND SOCIAL NEEDS

Helping a person with dementia to meet her emotional and social needs is just as important as helping the person to meet her physical needs.

Just like everyone else, a person with dementia needs to feel loved and needed, and to gain enjoyment from life. Meeting these needs is essential for maintaining the person's quality of life.

Activities give the person with dementia something enjoyable to look forward to, and help the person experience a sense of fulfillment and satisfaction with life (Fig. 9-8). Even though a person with dementia is confused, he still can become bored and depressed. In fact, boredom may be an underlying cause of some difficult behaviors, such as wandering or rummaging. Engaging in activities helps the person to feel useful and gives him a sense of purpose and accomplishment. There are many different types of activities that a person with dementia can enjoy and benefit from (Table 9-2).

OBRA requires that everyone, not just activity staff, be supportive of meeting the residents' social and emotional needs. As a nursing assistant, you will be responsible for helping residents to get ready for scheduled activities, and for helping them get to where the activity is being held. You will also have the opportunity to engage residents in activities on a "one-on-one" basis throughout the day. For example, you can

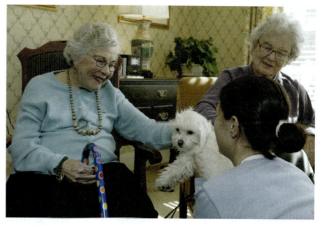

Figure 9-8

Activities, such as visiting with animals as part of a visiting pet program, can improve the quality of life for many residents with dementia. (*Photo courtesy of Jeremy Gilbert/ Caring Canines Visiting Therapy Dogs, Inc.*)

Table 9-2	Activities That Benefit People With Dementia	
TYPE OF ACTIVITY	**EXAMPLES**	**BENEFITS**
Social	• Cocktail hour (with non-alcoholic drinks) • Birthday parties • Cookouts • Pet therapy (visits with companion animals, such as dogs or cats)	• Promotes interaction with others • Provides opportunities for friendships • Meets the person's need to feel like part of a group • Allows the person to receive and give love and affection
Physical	• Taking a walk • Participating in an exercise class • Dancing • Gardening	• Helps maintain strength and muscle tone • Helps improve circulation • Increases the person's sense of well-being
Intellectual	• Discussing current events • Reading • Doing a puzzle • Identifying pictures in a book or magazine • Playing "Name that Tune"	• Provides mental stimulation • Promotes interaction with others
Sensory stimulation	• Listening to music • Participating in sing-a-longs • Touching surface textures • Smelling scents (aromatherapy) • Viewing pictures or nature slides	• Lowers heart rate and blood pressure • Provides mental stimulation and promotes reminiscing • Holiday music may help resident identify the time of year
Spiritual	• Attending a religious service • Studying the scriptures • Participating in communion or other religious practices • Celebrating religious holidays	• Maintains the person's religious identity • Familiar rituals are comforting
Creative	• Flower arranging • Baking • Painting • Doing craft projects	• Allows the person to gain enjoyment from the creative process • Provides mental stimulation • Gives the person a sense of accomplishment and productivity; increases self-esteem
Productive	• Sweeping the floor • Wiping tables • Watering plants	• Allows the person to feel that he is making a contribution and that he is useful to others • Gives the person a sense of accomplishment and productivity; increases self-esteem

sit with the resident and look at a photo album or magazine together, or help the resident find and place a few pieces of a jigsaw puzzle. You can also set the resident up with an activity that is based on some aspect of the resident's past. For example, if Mrs. Jones used to be a secretary, she may welcome having a collection of file folders, papers to file, and access to an old typewriter or telephone.

When planning an activity, take care to choose one that relates to the interests and abilities of the person or people who will be participating in it. When planning group activities, it is important that all of the residents in the group have similar interests, abilities, and social skills. In addition, it is also important to consider the attention span of each resident who will be participating in the activity. For example, if Mrs. Ward's attention span is only about 30 minutes, including her in an activity that lasts 1 hour may not be appropriate (unless it would not be disruptive to the other residents for Mrs. Ward to leave in the middle of the activity). Assign tasks according to each resident's abilities and interests. For example:

> Debra is responsible for planning one special activity a week for a group of residents. This week, she decides that she, Mr. Pitt, Mrs. Winger, and Mrs. Kemp will make fruit smoothies and then share them with some of the other residents. Debra knows that both Mrs. Winger and Mrs. Kemp used to enjoy baking for their families, so she asks Mrs. Winger to peel the bananas and Mrs. Kemp to measure the orange juice. Mr. Pitt worked for years as a bartender, so once all of the ingredients are in the blender, Debra asks Mr. Pitt to turn the blender on, and then to help her pour the drinks into cups to serve to the other residents.

Debra's activity will be successful because she considered the special interests and talents of each of the residents who would be participating in it. Planning the activity in advance, gathering all necessary supplies, and having a back-up plan "just in case" are other things that you can do to help ensure success when planning an activity for residents.

Activities that appeal to the person's senses in different ways (for example, looking at photographs, drawings, or objects; listening to music; tasting a favorite food; petting a dog or a cat; smelling a familiar scent) can help the person to recall and share memories. Activities that encourage the person to recall and share memories are a form of **reminiscence therapy** (Fig. 9-9).

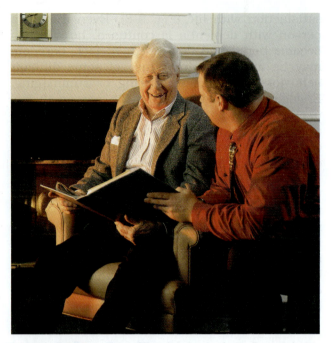

Figure 9-9
Reminiscence therapy increases a person's self-esteem and happiness by encouraging him to remember the past. (*Courtesy of Copper Ridge.*)

Reminiscence therapy can be used in a "one-on-one" setting, or in a group setting. Reminiscence therapy provides mental stimulation and, when done in a group setting, gives the person a chance to socialize with other residents.

CARING FOR THE PERSON WITH LATE-STAGE DEMENTIA

In the final stage of dementia, the person loses the ability to walk and sit independently. Immobility puts the person at risk for problems such as pressure ulcers, contractures, and pneumonia. You will learn more about these conditions, and how to prevent them, as you continue in your training.

The person also loses the ability to swallow, affecting the person's ability to eat. When the person can no longer eat on his own, it usually signals the final phase of the disease process before death occurs. The person may have an advance directive that specifies whether or not a feeding tube should be inserted to provide nourishment. If no advance directive is in place, the person's health care agent will need to decide whether or not nutrition will be artificially supported with a feeding tube. This is not an easy decision to make. There is no research that suggests that tube feeding really benefits a person at this stage in the disease process, and it often leads to complications, such as aspiration pneumonia. Although family members may understand the reasons for not placing a feeding tube, it is still emotionally difficult to watch a loved one go without nourishment. Families need a tremendous amount of support at this time.

Because a person with dementia will eventually die from the disease, care efforts during the final phase of the disease process are directed toward ensuring that the person is as comfortable as possible until death occurs. For example, oxygen therapy might be provided to make breathing easier. The doctor will often discontinue orders for medications and laboratory work that is no longer beneficial. Routine measuring of the person's weight is also usually discontinued at this time, because weight loss is expected. Your responsibilities during this time will be the same as they are when caring for any resident who is dying (see Chapter 29).

EFFECTS OF CARING FOR THE PERSON WITH DEMENTIA ON THE NURSING ASSISTANT

Caring for people with dementia is very important work. The difference you make in the life of the person with dementia, as well as those of her family members, is significant. However, caring for a person with dementia can take its toll on you, physically and emotionally.

- A person with dementia is prone to outbursts of anger and can become agitated very easily. Therefore, it is likely that on any given day, you may be cursed at, spit on, slapped, hit, scratched, or pinched. Because you will most likely develop a fondness for the residents in your care, it can be very difficult when a resident has a "bad day" and that affection is not returned!

- Many of the behaviors of people with dementia can be very annoying, because they are repetitious. It is not always easy to figure out what you can do to make the behavior stop, and until a solution is found, the behavior can really try your patience.

- Caring for a person with dementia is hard physical work. As the dementia progresses, the person becomes completely dependent. Exhaustion and fatigue can put you on edge, making it difficult for you to keep your emotions in check.

If you feel yourself becoming overwhelmed by your responsibilities or a particular situation, take a deep breath and remind yourself that a person with dementia cannot be held responsible for her actions. If you still feel angry, make sure that the person is safe and walk away. Ask a co-worker or the nurse for help with the person. Sometimes you may need to ask to be assigned to another resident for a while. If your frustration or anger moves you to the point of actually causing a resident physical harm, you will lose your job (as well as all chances of future employment in the health care field). You may even be punished by a court of law for abuse. Remember, a member of the health care team is particularly at risk for becoming abusive when the resident is "difficult" or hard to manage and the relationship is a long-term relationship. When you become tired and frustrated, take time out, be good to yourself, and share your feelings with the nurse. To provide the best care to your residents, you need to care for yourself.

SUMMARY

- Dementia, which is caused by changes in the brain tissue, affects a person's ability to remember, think, and communicate.
  - There are many different causes of dementia. The most common causes of dementia are Alzheimer's disease, vascular dementia, Lewy body dementia, and frontotemporal dementia.
  - Most types of dementia follow a similar course and ultimately lead to death. Currently, there is no cure for dementia.

- All people with dementia experience changes in the brain that lead to the "4 As" of dementia: amnesia (difficulty remembering), aphasia (difficulty using language), agnosia (difficulty recognizing information obtained using the five senses), and apraxia (difficulty coordinating the steps needed to complete a task).

- Some behaviors are common in people with dementia. These behaviors often result from changes in the person's ability to understand and respond to his environment.

- A change in a person's behavior is often a sign that the person has a physical or emotional need that is not being met.
- Nursing assistants use their observation skills and a systematic approach to try and figure out the underlying cause of the person's behavior.

- A person with dementia has physical, emotional, and social needs that must be met.

- As the person's dementia gets worse, he will need more and more help with activities such as eating, bathing, dressing, and toileting.
- Activities help to meet the person's emotional and social needs.

- Dementia is a terrible disease that is devastating both to the person who has it, as well as his family members.

- Caring for a person with dementia is very demanding, yet very important, work.

WHAT DID YOU LEARN?

Multiple choice

Select the single best answer for each of the following questions.

1. Which one of the following is experienced by a person with dementia?
   a. Problems with memory, especially short-term memory
   b. Confusion and disorientation
   c. An inability to manage activities of daily living (ADLs)
   d. All of the above

2. When caring for a resident with dementia, it is helpful to:
   a. Be understanding and see the resident's behaviors as part of the disease
   b. Take the same approach with every resident
   c. Correct the resident to bring him or her back to the "here and now"
   d. Avoid acknowledging your own feelings

3. When communicating with a person with dementia, what is the best approach to take?
   a. Speak loudly and quickly to get the person's attention
   b. Speak clearly, in a calm tone of voice
   c. Avoid touching the person or using hand gestures
   d. Avoid talking about the past

4. Which statement about validation therapy is true?
   a. Validation therapy stresses the importance of bringing the person with dementia back to the "here and now."
   b. Validation therapy is based on the belief that people with dementia are able to return to the present, if given enough information to do so.

   c. Validation therapy stresses the importance of acknowledging the person's reality.
   d. Validation therapy encourages the caregiver to correct the person, to help the person to stay on track.

5. A person with dementia may show which of the following behaviors?
   a. Pacing and wandering
   b. Hallucinations
   c. Agitation expressed by restlessness and yelling
   d. All of the above

6. Mrs. Franklin, a resident who has dementia, comes to the dining room inappropriately dressed. She has her slip on over her dress and her coat on. She has on one slipper, and one black shoe. You should recognize that:
   a. You will need to dress Mrs. Franklin from now on since she cannot make the right choices.
   b. Mrs. Franklin is most likely experiencing apraxia, and will need assistance in performing the task of getting dressed.
   c. Mrs. Franklin is most likely experiencing aphasia, and cannot ask for help.
   d. Mrs. Franklin needs to be told to go back to her room and change her clothes.

7. What is sundowning?
   a. Increased confusion, restlessness, and insecurity that occurs late in the day, as it becomes darker outside
   b. Aimless wandering after dark
   c. Worry and increased suspicion
   d. Crying inconsolably for a long time

8. Mr. Greene, one of the residents in your care, has Alzheimer's disease. For the last hour, Mr. Greene has been folding and unfolding a piece of paper, and he is showing no signs of stopping. What should you do?
   a. Let him keep doing it; perseveration is a normal behavior in a person with dementia.
   b. Try to distract Mr. Greene by starting a new activity with him, such as reading the newspaper together or going for a walk.
   c. Tell the nurse; she will be able to give Mr. Greene a sedative to make the behavior stop.
   d. Tell Mr. Greene firmly that the behavior is unacceptable and it must stop immediately.

9. What is a catastrophic reaction?
   a. A response to a situation that is more extreme than would normally be expected
   b. An abnormal protein deposit that is found in the brains of people with Alzheimer's disease
   c. The belief that you are someone you are not (for example, the President of the United States)
   d. The reaction family members have on learning that a loved one has Alzheimer's disease

10. When helping a person with dementia with her activities of daily living (ADLs), such as bathing, eating, and dressing, what should you remember?
    a. Keep to an established routine as much as possible

    b. Prepare for the procedure ahead of time
    c. Many ADLs are very frightening or frustrating for the person with dementia
    d. All of the above

11. When you come on duty at 3:00 PM, Mr. Antonio asks you what time dinner will be served. You tell him that dinner is served at 5:30 PM, and show him where "5:30" is on the clock. When you return to his room at 3:30 PM, he asks you again what time dinner will be served. You give him the same response as you did before. He leaves the room, and heads towards the dining room. You hear him ask another staff member what time dinner will be served. You understand this behavior is most likely a symptom of:
    a. Amnesia
    b. Aphasia
    c. Apraxia
    d. Agnosia

12. You are listening to report and hear that a new resident was admitted today. His diagnosis includes frontotemporal dementia. You know that this resident:
    a. May demonstrate socially inappropriate behaviors
    b. Will be older than your usual resident with dementia
    c. Will demonstrate Parkinson-like movements
    d. Will not be able to participate in reminiscence therapy

STOP and Think!

- You work in the dementia unit of a long-term care facility. Mrs. Darden, one of the residents you are responsible for, needs a great deal of help with all of her activities of daily living (ADLs). Lately, Mrs. Darden has started having a catastrophic reaction every time you help her to bathe. What are some things you could do to make bathing easier and less frightening for Mrs. Darden?

- Mrs. Rowan has Alzheimer's disease. You have cared for Mrs. Rowan for a long time and know pretty much what to expect from her in terms of behavior. Although she does tend to pace and to rummage quite frequently, she is usually calm and pleasant. Today in the dining room, however, when you are trying to help Mrs. Rowan eat lunch, she becomes angry and strikes out at you. What might be the explanation for this behavior?

- You have just finished helping Mrs. Stonefield to get dressed, and are now helping her to fix her hair. She is facing the mirror as you are brushing her hair, and suddenly she seems very frightened, and starts yelling, "Get away! Get away from here. I don't know why you keep bothering me!" You ask her if you are upsetting her, and if you should leave. She responds, "I am not talking to you. That other lady is there again. She keeps spying on me!" Who do you think she is talking about, and what should you do?

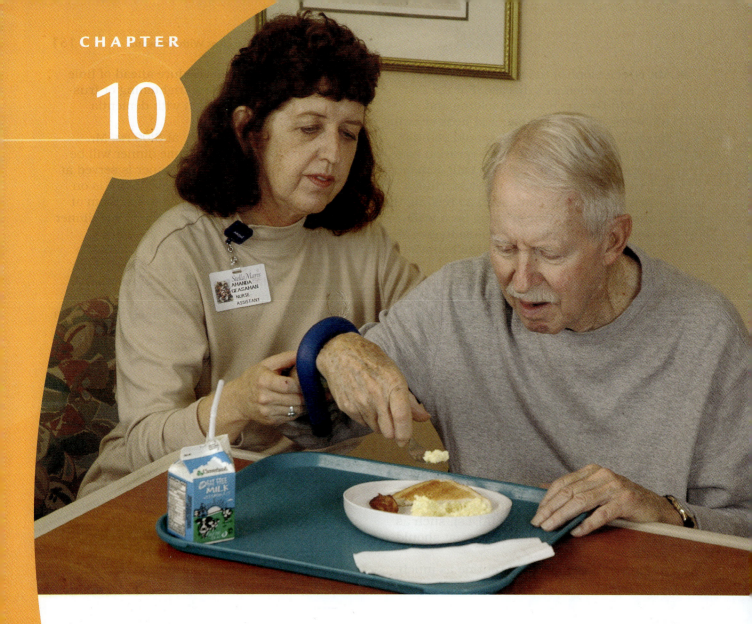

The Resident in Need of Rehabilitation and Restorative Care

WHAT WILL YOU LEARN?

The word "rehabilitation" comes from the Latin word *habilitas*, "to make able." As you have learned, most residents have some degree of **disability,** or impaired function. As members of the health care team, we are responsible for helping each of our residents reach or maintain their highest level of function. The ability to function is essential for maintaining or regaining independence, and for ensuring the best quality of life. Rehabilitation

Photo: Rehabilitation and restorative care can help residents to be as independent as possible, for as long as possible. Here, a resident uses an assistive device that enables him to eat independently.

services and restorative care are often needed to help residents achieve their goal of reaching or maintaining their highest level of function. When you are finished with this chapter, you will be able to:

1. Define the terms *rehabilitation* and *restorative care*.
2. Describe reasons why a resident may require rehabilitation services, restorative care, or both.
3. Relate the importance of rehabilitation and restorative care to OBRA compliance.
4. Identify rehabilitation services that are generally available in long-term care.
5. Identify the OBRA requirements for a restorative care program.
6. Describe different types of restorative care programs that may be of benefit to the long-term care resident.
7. Discuss the nursing assistant's role in rehabilitation and restorative care.

Vocabulary Use the CD in front of your book to hear these terms pronounced and defined:

Disability	Physical therapy	Speech–language	Dysphagia
Rehabilitation	Contracture	pathology	Trapeze bar
Restorative care	Occupational therapy		

Rehabilitation is the process of helping a person with a disability to return to his highest level of physical, mental, or emotional function. Rehabilitation involves treatment, education, and the prevention of further disability. **Restorative care** is the care provided by all of the members of the health care team that supports the rehabilitation effort and helps the resident reach the goal of achieving or maintaining his highest level of function. In the nursing home setting, the term "rehabilitation" usually refers to services provided by licensed therapists who specialize in various aspects of rehabilitation (such as physical therapists, occupational therapists, and speech–language pathologists), and the term "restorative care" usually refers to the actions taken by the nursing team to support the rehabilitation effort.

Many of your residents will require rehabilitation and restorative care. As you learned in Chapter 8, many of your older residents will be frail (physically weak and fragile), either as a result of age, chronic conditions, or both. These factors, especially when combined, can lead to disability. Rehabilitation and restorative care can help these residents to maintain the skills and abilities that they have, and prevent the further loss of function and independence. Many residents also come to live at a long-term care facility after experiencing an acute illness or injury such as a stroke, broken hip, or spinal cord injury. Rehabilitation and restorative care can help these residents regain the strength and skills they need to return to their highest level of functioning.

The rehabilitation effort focuses on the individual needs and capabilities of the resident. Like any other type of health care, rehabilitation and restorative care are achieved through a team effort. Members of the team include the resident, the resident's family members, the nurse, the nursing assistant, the social worker, members of the activities staff (or a recreational therapist), licensed rehabilitation therapists, and doctors. Some facilities have a chaplain, who also plays a very important role in supporting the goals of the health care team related to rehabilitation and restorative care.

The Omnibus Budget Reconciliation Act (OBRA) requires nursing homes to provide each resident with the services the resident needs to reach and maintain her highest possible level of well-being and function. There are many specific OBRA requirements related to helping residents maintain or achieve their highest level of function (Box 10-1). To be in compliance with OBRA, staff members must take steps to improve or maintain existing function, and to prevent the loss of function. If a decrease in function occurs, the facility must be able to prove that the appropriate steps were taken to try to prevent the decrease in function from occurring. The reasons for the decrease in function must be properly assessed and an appropriate care plan must be developed with the goal of either helping the resident regain her usual level of function, or preventing further decline.

It is important to recognize that not all residents may be candidates for rehabilitation or

BOX 10-1	OBRA Requirements Related To Helping Residents Maintain or Achieve Their Highest Level of Function

- A resident's ability to perform activities of daily living (ADLs) does not decrease unless a change in the resident's clinical condition makes the decrease in ability unavoidable.
- A resident who enters the facility without pressure ulcers does not develop pressure ulcers unless they are unavoidable due to the resident's clinical condition. A resident who has pressure ulcers receives the necessary care and treatment to promote healing, prevent infection, and prevent new pressure ulcers from developing.
- A resident who has urinary incontinence receives the necessary care and treatment to prevent urinary tract infections and to restore as much normal bladder function as possible.

- A resident who enters the facility without a limited range of motion does not experience decreased range of motion unless it is unavoidable due to the resident's clinical condition. A resident with limited range of motion receives the necessary care and treatment to increase range of motion, and prevent further decrease.
- A resident who displays mental or psychosocial difficulty receives the necessary care and treatment to correct the problem.
- A resident who did not previously have mental or psychosocial difficulty does not display a pattern of decreased social interaction, anger, or depression unless these changes are unavoidable due to the resident's clinical condition.

restorative care. Some residents may have mental impairments that limit their ability to benefit from rehabilitation services or restorative care. For example, a person with advancing dementia may not be able to remember new skills learned in rehabilitation or respond to instructions given as part of a restorative care program. Some residents may be too ill to participate in a rehabilitation program. For example, a person with advanced respiratory disease may become too short of breath to perform exercises as part of a physical rehabilitation program. Some residents may not have the desire or motivation to participate in a rehabilitation or restorative care program. Although the cause for the resident's refusal should always be investigated (to rule out a treatable condition such as depression), the resident does have the right to refuse. For example, consider a 92-year-old resident who has become increasingly weak. It is no longer safe for her to walk alone, and she has started to use a wheelchair to get around. When evaluated for physical therapy to restore her strength, she refuses. She explains to the physical therapist that she has been walking around for more than 90 years. She is tired now and is content to be in a wheelchair for whatever time she has left.

It is to be expected that at some point, advanced age or disease will contribute to a resident's decline in condition. As long as there is the potential for improving or maintaining function, we must make every effort to support a resident's independence (with the resident's consent). The reasons for not pursuing a program of rehabilitation or restorative care must be carefully documented in the resident's record.

REHABILITATION SERVICES

As noted earlier, in the nursing home setting, the term "rehabilitation services" usually refers to those services provided by licensed therapists who specialize in various aspects of rehabilitation such as physical therapists, occupational therapists, and speech–language pathologists. A doctor's order is required for these services. These services are usually provided in a special area within the facility. The people providing these services may be employees of the facility, or they may be employees of an outside company that specializes in providing rehabilitation services. In this case, rehabilitation therapists come to the facility to provide rehabilitation services for the residents.

OBRA requires nursing homes to provide rehabilitation services that meet the specific needs of the residents who live in the facility. The type of rehabilitation services a resident receives depends on the resident's disability and individual needs. Many residents will require more than one type of rehabilitation (Table 10-1). Three of the most common types of rehabilitation that you will see in the long-term care setting are physical therapy, occupational therapy, and speech–language pathology.

PHYSICAL THERAPY

Physical therapy is a health care specialty that focuses on helping the person regain or maintain strength, endurance, coordination, balance,

Table 10-1   Common Conditions and Rehabilitation Measures

CONDITION	COMMON PROBLEMS	REHABILITATION
NEUROLOGICAL CONDITIONS		
Stroke	Paralysis or weakness on one side Immobility Impaired fine motor skills Impaired speech and swallowing	Physical therapy to improve strength and mobility (strength training, balance, transfers, walking with or without assistive devices) Occupational therapy to improve ability to perform personal care and other activities (using supportive and assistive devices, assistance with seating and positioning) Speech–language pathology to improve speech and swallowing
Parkinson's disease	Difficulty controlling movements/walking Posture and balance problems Swallowing problems Inability to project voice (speak audibly)	Physical therapy to improve ability to walk and balance (gait training, balance) Speech–language pathology to improve speech and swallowing
MUSCULOSKELETAL CONDITIONS		
Fractures	Immobilized limb after surgery or casting Decreased muscle tone and strength	Physical therapy to improve strength and mobility of affected limb Occupational therapy if ability to perform daily activities or routines is affected
Deconditioning (generalized weakness after a period of illness or immobility)	Weakness	Physical therapy to improve strength, endurance, and mobility
Frequent falls	Balance problems Weakness Movement disorders	Physical therapy to evaluate the cause of the falls and to improve strength and mobility
Inability to maintain seated posture	Leaning to one side Falling forward	Occupational therapy for evaluation and recommendations regarding chair type and seating supports
Pain	Decreased movement and activity Depression Decline in overall well-being	Physical therapy for exercise and pain treatments

posture, and flexibility. Physical therapy is provided by, or under the supervision of, a licensed physical therapist. The primary goals of physical therapy are to improve or maintain a person's ability to move, and to prevent complications that can result from the loss of function. These goals are achieved through a program of exercise (Fig. 10-1), often combined with the use of supportive devices, assistive devices, prosthetic devices, or all three (Fig. 10-2):

- **Supportive devices,** such as splints and braces, help to stabilize a weak joint or limb.
- **Assistive devices** make certain tasks, such as transferring or walking, easier.
- **Prosthetic devices** are artificial replacements for legs, feet, arms, or other body parts.

Complications that can result from the loss of function include loss of strength and contractures. When a person does not use a part of the body for a long time, he loses muscle mass in that part. As the muscle mass is lost, so is the person's strength. For example, have you ever had a cast put on an arm or a leg for a long period of time? When the cast finally came off, your arm or leg probably looked skinny and felt weak. That was because during the time your arm or leg was in the cast, you were not able to move it, and your muscle mass decreased. When a person cannot use an arm or a leg, exercising the arm or leg helps to keep it working properly. In Chapter 32, you will learn how to help a resident exercise a limb when the resident is not able to do it himself. Another complication that physical rehabilitation can help to prevent is contractures. A **contracture**

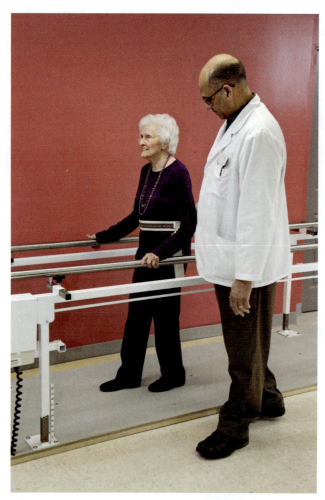

Figure 10-1

Physical therapy helps a person regain function through a program of exercise to improve strength, endurance, coordination, balance, posture, and flexibility. Here, a physical therapist assists a resident with gait training and balance.

occurs when a joint is held in the same position for too long. The tendons shorten and become stiff, leading to loss of motion of the joint that is often permanent (Fig. 10-3).

Physical therapy may also be used as part of a pain management program, when the person has pain caused by a musculoskeletal condition. You will learn more about how physical therapy can be used to assist in pain management in Chapter 27.

OCCUPATIONAL THERAPY

Occupational therapy is a health care specialty that focuses on helping the person regain or maintain the skills needed for everyday life, including those related to activities of daily living

(ADLs, such as bathing and dressing), instrumental activities of daily living (IADLs, such as doing laundry and preparing food), and activities the person engages in for personal enjoyment (such as a craft or hobby). Occupational therapy is provided by, or under the supervision of, a licensed occupational therapist. The primary goal of occupational therapy is to improve or maintain the person's independence, productivity, and ability to gain satisfaction from life.

While physical therapy focuses on maintaining or improving the skills that involve bigger muscles and bigger movements, occupational therapy focuses more on maintaining or improving the skills that involve smaller muscles and smaller movements (Fig. 10-4). Like physical therapy, occupational therapy uses exercise combined with supportive devices, assistive devices, prosthetic devices, or all three to help the person regain function. Examples of assistive devices used to help promote independence in tasks such as eating and grooming are shown in Figure 10-2.

SPEECH–LANGUAGE PATHOLOGY

Speech–language pathology is a health care specialty that focuses on helping the person regain or maintain the ability to communicate with others, chew, and swallow. (Difficulty swallowing is called **dysphagia**.) Difficulty forming words, speaking, chewing, and swallowing can occur as a result of many different conditions, including disorders that affect the function of the muscles of the mouth and throat (such as stroke), disorders that affect the brain (such as brain injury or dementia), and developmental disorders (such as cerebral palsy). A licensed speech–language pathologist (sometimes called a *speech therapist*) works with the person to improve the person's ability to speak, chew, or swallow.

The speech–language pathologist assesses problems with speech, chewing, or swallowing and provides recommendations for improving function in these areas. For example, the speech–language pathologist may recommend use of a picture board for a resident who has trouble communicating, or a modified diet for a resident who has trouble chewing and swallowing. In addition, the speech–language pathologist works with the resident to practice exercises and positioning techniques that can improve function. Exercises for the muscles of the lips, tongue, and jaw help the person develop the skills needed for forming words and for controlling food in the mouth. Positioning

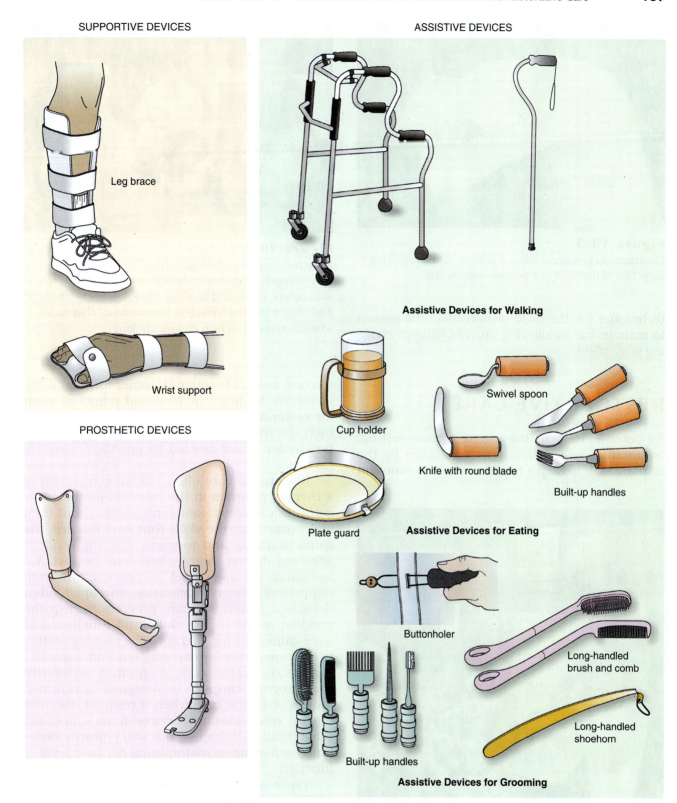

SUPPORTIVE DEVICES

Leg brace

Wrist support

PROSTHETIC DEVICES

ASSISTIVE DEVICES

Assistive Devices for Walking

Cup holder

Plate guard

Swivel spoon

Knife with round blade

Built-up handles

Assistive Devices for Eating

Buttonholer

Built-up handles

Long-handled brush and comb

Long-handled shoehorn

Assistive Devices for Grooming

Figure 10-2

Supportive devices, assistive devices, prosthetic devices, or all three can help a person do certain tasks independently.

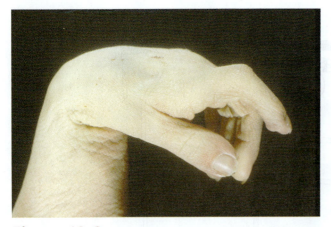

Figure 10-3
Contractures can occur when a joint is not exercised regularly. Use of the joint can be permanently lost.

techniques for the head or neck help the person to manage the swallowing process without choking (Fig. 10-5).

RESTORATIVE CARE

As noted earlier, in the nursing home setting, "restorative care" refers to actions taken by the nursing staff to help a resident reach or maintain

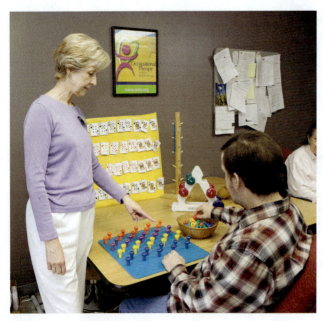

Figure 10-4
Occupational therapy helps a person regain skills needed for everyday life. Here, a resident performs an activity that helps him to improve his fine motor skills. Fine motor skills are needed for everyday activities such as using eating utensils, using a toothbrush, and writing.

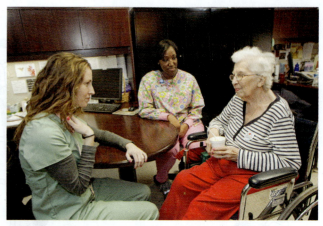

Figure 10-5
Speech–language pathology focuses on helping the person regain or maintain the ability to communicate with others, chew, and swallow. Here, a speech–language pathologist teaches a resident how to do a "chin tuck" when swallowing to help prevent choking.

his best level of function. In order for the facility to receive Medicare or Medicaid reimbursement for restorative care services, the services must meet the requirements listed in Box 10-2. A doctor's order is not needed to provide restorative care.

Restorative care often follows completion of a therapy program in the rehabilitation department. If a resident completes therapy, but then stops practicing the skills that were learned, the gains in ability and function that the resident achieved during therapy will soon be lost. We lose what we don't use! To prevent this from happening, the rehabilitation therapist often designs a restorative care program to help the resident maintain the skills and function that were gained during therapy. The nursing staff is then responsible for carrying out and supervising the restorative care program. A restorative care program can also be designed by a nurse. This is often the case when a resident does not receive rehabilitation services from a licensed rehabilitation therapist, but still requires assistance achieving or maintaining her best level of function.

Types of restorative care programs that are eligible for reimbursement in nursing homes include the following.

- **Passive range of motion (PROM).** Range-of-motion exercises are movements that put a joint through the complete extent of movement that the joint is normally capable of without causing pain. In a passive range-of-

Medicare or Medicaid Requirements for Reimbursement for Restorative Care

- Measurable objectives (goals) are documented in the resident's medical record, and are included in the care plan.
- Periodic evaluations of the resident by a registered nurse are documented in the clinical record.
- Nursing assistants must be trained in the specific techniques that promote the resident's involvement in the restorative care activity.

- The restorative care activities must be carried out by the nursing staff and supervised by a nurse.
- Restorative activity groups cannot include more than four residents per assigned caregiver.
- The restorative care activity must be carried out for at least 15 minutes within a 24-hour period. The 15 minutes may be broken up into smaller time periods throughout the day (for example, a 5-minute activity 3 times per day = 15 minutes per 24 hours.)

motion (PROM) program, a caregiver moves the resident's joints through the exercises, without active involvement on the part of the resident. This is done to maintain flexibility of the joints and help to prevent muscle loss. You will learn how to assist a resident with passive range-of-motion exercises in Chapter 32.

- **Active range of motion (AROM).** This program serves the same purpose as a PROM program, except that the resident performs the movements independently, with supervision and verbal guidance from the caregiver.
- **Splint or brace assistance.** In this program, a caregiver may provide the verbal guidance and help that the resident needs to correctly apply, remove, and care for a splint or brace. Or, the caregiver may apply and remove the splint or brace according to a regular schedule, ensure correct positioning of the device and the limb, and monitor for problems caused by the device (such as poor circulation or skin breakdown).
- **Bed mobility.** The purpose of this program is to improve or maintain the resident's ability to change positions in bed (for example, sit up, lie down, and turn from side to side). Often, equipment is used to promote independence in this area. For example, a resident may learn how to turn from side to side using the side rail to help pull herself over. Some residents will use a **trapeze bar** (a triangular device that hangs from an overhead frame attached to the bed) to pull themselves up in bed, or to move to or from a lying position.
- **Transfer.** This program is used to help a resident to maintain as much independence as

possible when moving between surfaces (for example, from the bed to a chair, or from a wheelchair to the toilet). The resident may have been taught during rehabilitation how to use an assistive device for transferring, such as a transfer board or a swivel cushion. Equipment such as grab bars and raised toilet seats can help a resident to be independent when transferring to the toilet.

- **Walking (ambulation).** This program is designed to help a resident maintain walking skills, either with or without assistive devices. Walking programs often include goals based on distances (Fig. 10-6). For example, when beginning a program, a reasonable goal may be for the resident to walk to the bathroom with assistance. The next

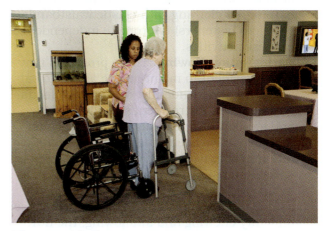

Figure 10-6
Goals for walking programs are often based on measurable distances. Here, a nursing assistant is encouraging a resident to walk from the entrance of the dining room to her place at the table using a walker.

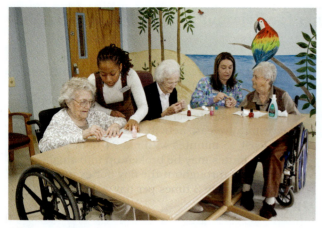

Figure 10-7
Group activities can be part of a restorative care program. Here, residents are practicing providing their own nail care.

goal may be for the resident to walk to the bathroom independently with a walker. The next goal may be for the resident to walk 10 feet in the hallway, then 20 feet, then 30 feet, and so on. The final goal may be for the resident to walk to the dining room or the activity room.

- **Dressing or grooming.** These types of programs help to improve or maintain the resident's ability to perform self-care activities such as dressing and undressing, bathing, mouth care, and nail care (Fig. 10-7). The resident may have been taught during rehabilitation how to use assistive devices (such as combs and brushes with built-up handles or long handles, long-handled sponges for bathing, or clothing with elastic waistbands or Velcro fasteners) to promote independence in these activities.

- **Eating or swallowing.** These programs may help a resident to maintain the ability to eat and drink independently, or they may focus on improving the resident's ability to chew and swallow effectively and safely. The resident may have been taught during rehabilitation how to use assistive devices (such as special utensils, a plate with a raised rim, or a cup holder) to promote independence in eating and drinking. For a resident who has difficulty chewing and swallowing, the nursing staff provides supervision and coaching to reinforce what the person was taught by the speech–language pathologist. For example, you may need to remind the person to

keep food on one side of the mouth, to perform a "chin tuck" when swallowing to prevent choking, or to take frequent small sips of liquid to keep the food moist and make it easier to swallow.

- **Amputation/prosthesis care.** This program helps a person to gain or maintain independence in putting on and taking off a prosthesis and in caring for the site where the prosthesis is attached.

- **Communication.** A communication restorative care program helps to improve or maintain a resident's ability to speak and communicate with others. The resident may use a device such as a picture board to make communication easier. When helping a resident in a communication restorative care program, it is important to allow extra time in your schedule. For example, a resident who is relearning speech skills following a stroke will need more time to form his words. If you seem hurried or rush the resident, the resident may give up in frustration and lose any abilities that were gained in therapy. It is important to provide encouragement and to allow sufficient time for the resident to practice these newly learned skills.

Other restorative care programs, such as a bowel and bladder training program, may also be eligible for reimbursement, if they meet all of the requirements listed in Box 10-2. For example, assisting the resident to use the toilet every 2 hours as part of routine care does not count as a restorative care program for bowel and bladder training. Specific goals for the resident must be set and documented, and the program must be designed to meet the resident's individual needs.

THE NURSING ASSISTANT'S ROLE IN REHABILITATION AND RESTORATIVE CARE

Nursing assistants play a key role in supporting the rehabilitation effort and providing restorative care. As a nursing assistant, you will be responsible for encouraging your residents to practice the skills and techniques they are learning in rehabilitation. You will also be responsible for carrying out many of the actions specified in the

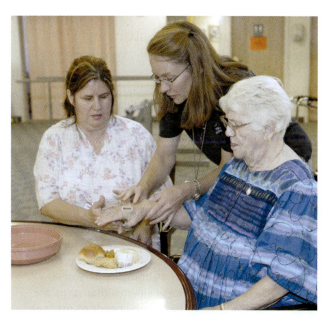

Figure 10-8
Ask the nurse or rehabilitation therapist to show you how to use assistive devices. This will allow you to help your resident use the assistive device more effectively. Here, an occupational therapist is showing a nursing assistant how to assist a resident to use a wrist supporter with a spoon attached.

person's care plan related to restorative care. Ask questions about rehabilitation or restorative care measures that have been planned for a resident. Have the nurse or rehabilitation therapist explain how to use any special equipment and show you how to help your resident to use it (Fig. 10-8). Also, make an effort to learn about any specific techniques that the resident should be practicing. Guidelines for assisting with rehabilitation and restorative care are given in Guidelines Box 10-1.

Because of the unique relationship that develops between nursing assistants and the residents they care for, you will become the "eyes and ears" of the rehabilitation team. You will be able to observe the resident for any changes, positive or negative, that are related to rehabilitation or restorative care. Make sure you report your observations. If a rehabilitation or restorative care measure does not seem to be working for the person, perhaps a change is necessary. Your input can help initiate that change. Your daily care routines will also allow you to observe problems related to rehabilitation and restorative care measures (such as chafing or redness of the skin caused by a new splint or supportive device) that should be reported.

Helping Hands and a Caring Heart

FOCUS ON HUMANISTIC HEALTH CARE

A person who is experiencing disability will have to face many losses. The loss of function, independence, and self-esteem can make the rehabilitation and restorative care effort seem futile. The person will need to grieve for these losses. Think for a moment how a disability might affect you. How would it feel to have to rely on someone else for help performing tasks you used to be able to do for yourself? To be embarrassed by your appearance? People who become disabled in some way often feel inadequate, helpless, or resentful of other "normal" people, especially at first. The rehabilitation and restorative care effort requires the person to work very hard, and the outcome of all of that hard work is uncertain. The person is likely to have good days and bad days. Be patient and empathetic. Focus on the person's abilities, rather than his disabilities. Make an effort to learn what motivates the person—what are his goals and dreams? Offer realistic encouragement and reassurance, and celebrate every success, no matter how small. A holistic approach—considering the person's emotional needs, as well as his physical ones—is essential for the rehabilitation and restorative care effort to be successful.

When a resident is receiving rehabilitation and restorative care, providing emotional and spiritual care is just as important as providing physical care. There are many things you can do to help meet the person's emotional needs. Focus on the resident's abilities. Encourage and reassure the resident, but remember to be realistic in your encouragement. For example, avoid saying things like, "Keep on working and you'll be back to normal in no time!" if it is unlikely that the resident will ever return to the level of function he had before. Instead, say something like, "I am so impressed by your progress. You've gone so much further this week than you did last week!" Allow the resident to hope for new treatments or advances in medical technology that can improve his quality of life. Finally, monitor the person's emotional status. Working to regain or maintain function, or learning to adjust to a loss of function, can be a long, difficult, and painful process. If you sense that your resident is becoming depressed, angry, or frustrated, report this to the nurse. The nurse and the other members of the health care team will make sure that the person receives the help he needs to work through these feelings.

Guidelines Box 10-1 — Assisting With Rehabilitation and Restorative Care

WHAT YOU DO	WHY YOU DO IT
Ask questions about new rehabilitation measures that have been planned for a resident. Have the nurse or therapist explain to you how to use new equipment and show you how to help your resident to use it.	Knowing about the special techniques that are being used with the person will allow you to help the person to practice these techniques. Knowing how to use any special equipment will allow you to help the person to use the equipment properly.
Monitor the person's emotional status.	Working to regain or maintain function, or learning to adjust to a loss of function, can be a long, difficult, and painful process. It is very easy for residents to become frustrated and discouraged. Reporting your observations about the person's emotional status to the nurse ensures that steps are taken to get the person the help he needs to manage these feelings.
Focus on the person's abilities, and celebrate all successes, no matter how small.	Achieving small goals gives the person an emotional boost and encourages him or her to keep working.
Encourage and reassure the person, but be realistic in your encouragement and be careful not to compare the person with someone else.	Each person will have individual responses to rehabilitation. Not all goals will be reached.
Give the person the time he or she needs to complete a task independently. Offer assistance only as needed and only if the person seems overly frustrated.	Although it may be faster or easier to just complete the task for the person, it is important for the person's self-esteem to let the person do as much for himself or herself as possible.
Be empathetic, but do not pity the person.	When you pity someone, it means that you recognize his or her loss. When you empathize with someone, it means that you can imagine how the person feels about the loss. Empathy will help you deal more effectively with the person's anger and frustration.
If you find yourself feeling frustrated with a resident who is struggling with rehabilitation, talk to the nurse.	If you let the person's frustration and anger affect you, you may not be able to provide the person with the best care possible. You may need a break or a short reassignment from that person to continue to provide the best care possible.

TELL THE NURSE ❗

When you are caring for a resident who is receiving rehabilitative therapy or restorative care, be sure to report the following observations to the nurse immediately:

- A supportive device or assistive device is broken or not working properly

- The person has a change in vital signs during or after the rehabilitation or restorative care activity

- The person has pain, swelling, redness, or signs of inflammation around supportive devices or prosthetic devices

- The person is showing signs of depression or excessive frustration, such as crying, withdrawal, anger, or talk of suicide

- The person is having excessive difficulty with a new rehabilitation technique or treatment

Because it is necessary to help each resident achieve and maintain the highest possible level of function, your observations of residents who are not receiving rehabilitation or restorative care are also important. You may be the first to notice that a resident is showing increased weakness, or a decline in abilities. Reporting your observations to the nurse promptly will allow her to investigate possible causes for the resident's decline. Reporting your observations will also allow the nurse to initiate a rehabilitation referral (so that the resident can be evaluated by licensed rehabilitation therapists), a restorative care program, or both. If you do not promptly report a resident's decline in abilities, the resident's condition may decline even more, to the point that a return to the resident's usual level of performance becomes impossible. If this occurs, the resident has been harmed, and the facility may be found to be out of compliance with OBRA requirements.

SUMMARY

- A person generally experiences loss of strength, endurance, and flexibility as part of the aging process. These changes, especially when combined with the effects of illness or injury, may lead to disability.
  - Disability is impaired function and can be physical, mental, or emotional.
  - Some disabilities are short-term, some last a long time, and others may be permanent.
- A primary goal of the health care team in long-term care is to help residents remain as independent as possible. Rehabilitation and restorative care can help residents achieve that goal.
  - In the nursing home setting, the term "rehabilitation" usually refers to services provided by licensed therapists who specialize in various aspects of rehabilitation, such as physical therapists, occupational therapists, and speech–language pathologists.
    - Physical therapy focuses on helping the person regain or maintain strength, endurance, coordination, balance, posture, and flexibility.
    - Occupational therapy focuses on helping the person regain or maintain the

skills needed for everyday life, such as those related to self-care.
  - Speech–language pathology focuses on helping the person regain or maintain the ability to communicate with others, chew, and swallow.
  - In the nursing home setting, the term "restorative care" refers to care provided by the nursing team that supports the rehabilitation effort and helps the resident to become more independent. Examples of restorative care programs include passive and active range of motion, splint or brace assistance, bed mobility, transfers, walking, dressing or grooming, eating or swallowing, amputation/prosthesis care, and communication programs.
- The nursing assistant plays a very important role in the rehabilitation and restorative care effort.
  - The nursing assistant is often the first person to notice a decline or an improvement in a resident's abilities. Keeping the nurse informed of these changes is important.
  - The nursing assistant is responsible for carrying out many of the actions specified in the person's care plan related to restorative care.

WHAT DID YOU LEARN?

Multiple Choice

Select the single best answer for each of the following questions.

1. The process that helps a person with a disability to return to her highest level of physical function and emotional well-being is called:
   a. Homeostasis
   b. Metabolism
   c. Prosthetics
   d. Rehabilitation

2. Which one of the following is a nursing assistant's responsibility that is related to the rehabilitation and restorative care effort?
   a. Encouraging the resident to use a trapeze to reposition herself in bed, if this is part of the resident's care plan
   b. Taking the resident to the toilet every 2 hours as part of normal care
   c. Teaching the resident techniques used for swallowing, such as the "chin tuck"
   d. All of the above

3. The definition of dysphagia is:
   a. Difficulty walking
   b. Difficulty breathing
   c. Difficulty swallowing
   d. Difficulty thinking

4. A person who is having difficulty with balance when walking can benefit from which of the following?
   a. Emotional rehabilitation
   b. Occupational rehabilitation
   c. Physical rehabilitation
   d. Speech–language pathology

5. Mr. Dirkens has a history of a stroke. He sometimes has difficulty keeping food in his mouth when chewing because he cannot close his lips all the way on the right side of his face. Which of the following might be of benefit to Mr. Dirkens?
   a. A visit to the dentist
   b. Speech–language pathology
   c. Occupational therapy
   d. Physical therapy

6. Mrs. Jenkins always liked to play cards. She is frustrated now because she is having difficulty holding her hand of cards. Which of the following statements is true?
   a. Occupational therapy could help Mrs. Jenkins regain her ability to play cards.
   b. Physical therapy could help Mrs. Jenkins regain fine motor control in her fingers.
   c. A restorative care program should be initiated to improve Mrs. Jenkins' card game.
   d. Mrs. Jenkins will need to find another pastime to enjoy, because playing cards will not be possible for her anymore.

7. To meet the requirements of Medicare, a restorative care program must be carried out by the _____, and supervised by the _____.
   a. Resident, physical therapist
   b. Rehabilitation department, nurse
   c. Nursing staff, nurse
   d. Nurse, rehabilitation department

8. Which of the following statements is not true?
   a. All residents in long-term care must receive rehabilitation to stay in compliance with OBRA.
   b. A resident has the right to refuse rehabilitation, even if it means that she will have a decline in function.
   c. Sometimes rehabilitation causes residents to become depressed because they find it hard, and very frustrating.
   d. Some residents may receive more than one kind of rehabilitation therapy at a time.

9. To meet reimbursement requirements for restorative care, how much restorative care must be provided?
   a. 15 minutes every 8 hours
   b. 15 minutes over a 24-hour period
   c. 30 minutes over a 24-hour period
   d. There is no time requirement for reimbursement

10. You routinely take care of Mrs. Futura. She is usually able to transfer from the bed to the chair, only needing you to guide her to sit in the right spot. Lately, you have noticed that she is leaning on you more and more, to the point where you are almost supporting her weight during the transfer. As a nursing assistant, you should:

a. Call Mrs. Futura's daughter and advise her to request a physical therapy evaluation

b. Report this change in Mrs. Futura's ability to the nurse right away so that Mrs. Futura can be evaluated for possible rehabilitation or restorative care

c. Report this change in Mrs. Futura's ability to the physical therapist right away and request an evaluation

d. Investigate the cause for Mrs. Futura's increased weakness

STOP and Think!

- Jacob has been assigned to care for Mr. Huff, who has recently had his right leg amputated (removed) above the knee. Jacob is to assist Mr. Huff in his transfers until he is able to do them himself. Mr. Huff is to do all of his own activities of daily living (ADLs), such as bathing, feeding, and dressing himself, with minimal help from Jacob. This morning when Jacob enters the room, he finds Mr. Huff on the floor between the bed and the wheelchair. Mr. Huff is struggling to climb into his wheelchair. When Jacob approaches him to help, Mr. Huff says angrily, "Leave me alone; I can do this. I'm OK, just leave me alone." What should Jacob do first? How might Jacob be able to help Mr. Huff maintain his independence and still be safe?

- Amanda is assigned to care for Mrs. Webb, who recently had a stroke. When the stroke occurred, Mrs. Webb had been preparing dinner at the stove. As a result, when she fell, she also suffered severe burns on her arms. Now, Mrs. Webb is receiving rehabilitation therapy for her left-sided weakness, in addition to recovering from the skin grafts used to treat the burns on her arms. Mrs. Webb is a widow and her children live out of state. She cries frequently because she says there is "no one to help her and she will probably end up staying in the nursing home for the rest of her life." Every time Amanda tries to get Mrs. Webb to participate in bathing and feeding herself, Mrs. Webb shakes her head and says she "just doesn't feel up to the effort today." Mrs. Webb's grafts are healing well and she is doing great in therapy. Is there anything Amanda can do to help Mrs. Webb not feel so helpless?

Nursing Assistants Make a Difference!

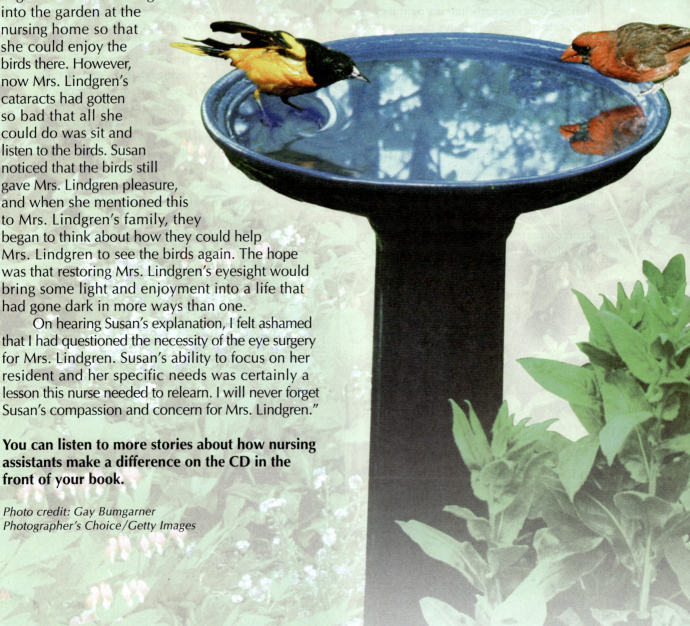

"I am an operating room nurse, and I care for many elderly patients who are having cataract surgery. Many of my elderly patients are very healthy, and excited about having surgery to restore their vision.

Not too long ago, we were scheduled to perform cataract surgery on a resident from a local nursing home, Mrs. Lindgren. I was somewhat surprised to meet my patient! Mrs. Lindgren had Alzheimer's disease and was quite confused. Susan, a nursing assistant who had cared for Mrs. Jones regularly for about 3 years, came with her to the surgery. Needless to say, I pondered the wisdom of putting Mrs. Lindgren through surgery, which would most certainly be a frightening experience for her. What was the surgeon thinking?

When I expressed my concerns to Susan, she told me a little bit about Mrs. Lindgren. Susan told me that before Mrs. Lindgren's Alzheimer's disease had progressed to the point where she was no longer able to care for herself, she had loved to sit in her garden and watch the birds gather around the many bird baths that she kept filled. Knowing this, Susan began to take Mrs. Lindgren into the garden at the nursing home so that she could enjoy the birds there. However, now Mrs. Lindgren's cataracts had gotten so bad that all she could do was sit and listen to the birds. Susan noticed that the birds still gave Mrs. Lindgren pleasure, and when she mentioned this to Mrs. Lindgren's family, they began to think about how they could help Mrs. Lindgren to see the birds again. The hope was that restoring Mrs. Lindgren's eyesight would bring some light and enjoyment into a life that had gone dark in more ways than one.

On hearing Susan's explanation, I felt ashamed that I had questioned the necessity of the eye surgery for Mrs. Lindgren. Susan's ability to focus on her resident and her specific needs was certainly a lesson this nurse needed to relearn. I will never forget Susan's compassion and concern for Mrs. Lindgren."

You can listen to more stories about how nursing assistants make a difference on the CD in the front of your book.

Photo credit: Gay Bumgarner
Photographer's Choice/Getty Images

INDIVIDUALIZING CARE

Every resident has the right to quality care that supports his or her quality of life. As you know from Unit 2, each resident is a unique individual, with unique physical, social, emotional, and spiritual needs. To provide the highest quality of care, we must provide individualized care (that is, care that is specific to each individual resident). Providing quality, individualized care and excellent customer service is the focus of Unit 3.

Photo: Residents, and their families, are our primary customers.

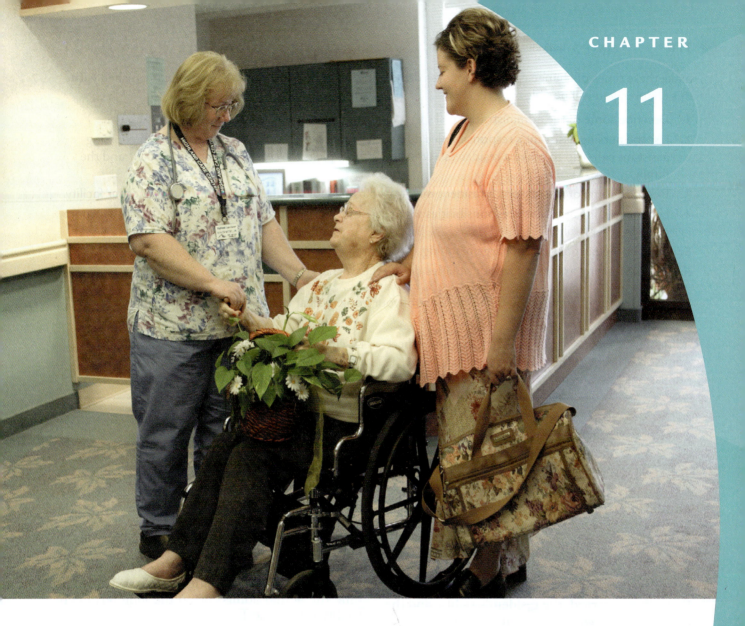

Assisting With Admissions, Transfers, and Discharges

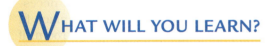HAT WILL YOU LEARN?

In the long-term care setting, people are admitted ("checked in"), discharged ("checked out"), or transferred (moved from one room in the facility to another, or moved to another facility altogether) every day. These events cause a major change to the person's daily routine and normal lifestyle, and can be very upsetting. In this chapter, you will learn how admissions, transfers, and discharges are carried out. You will also learn about things you can do to help

Photo: A new resident arrives at a long-term care facility.

make these times of change easier for your residents and their family members. When you are finished with this chapter, you will be able to:

1. Describe some of the administrative tasks that are completed during the admission period.

2. List the nursing assistant's responsibilities during the admission period, and discuss how the nursing assistant can help to make a resident's admission a more pleasant experience for the resident and the family.

3. Describe some of the reasons a resident might need to be moved to another room, or to another facility.

4. List the nursing assistant's responsibilities when assisting with the transfer of a resident to another room, or to another facility.

5. Discuss the purpose of discharge planning.

6. List the nursing assistant's responsibilities during the discharge process.

Vocabulary Use the CD in the front of your book to hear these terms pronounced and defined:

Admission	Resident inventory sheet	Discharge	Discharge planning
Admission sheet	Transfer	Against medical advice	
Admissions assessment	Bed hold	(AMA)	

ADMISSIONS

Admission is the official entry of a person into a health care setting. Admission is a time of orientation, for both the new resident and the health care team. During the admission period, the resident (or the resident's health care agent) learns about the services that will be provided, the fees that will be charged, the resident's rights, and the facility's policies. The resident and the members of the health care team who will be caring for the resident are introduced to each other. The process of gathering the information that the health care team needs to care for the resident properly begins.

As you learned in Chapter 8, most people do not choose to be admitted to a long-term care facility. Many admissions, especially those to nursing homes, are preceded by some sort of a crisis, such as an unexpected accident or illness. In many cases, the accident or illness results in the person being hospitalized. It is common for the person and the family to learn during this time that because of the person's condition, the person will need ongoing care following discharge from the hospital. The person and family must now decide, in a very short period of time, how and where that ongoing care will be provided.

In many cases, admission to a long-term care facility is the best option for the person. The family may need to visit several facilities before making a decision. They will also need to gather paperwork needed for a long-term care admission, such as financial records and insurance information. The family may need to complete applications for Medicaid if the person does not have enough money to meet long-term care costs. You can understand why the person and his family members may be feeling very stressed by the time the actual admission to the long-term care facility takes place!

ADMINISTRATIVE TASKS THAT TAKE PLACE DURING THE ADMISSION PERIOD

During the admission period, the new resident (or the resident's health care agent) meets with the admissions coordinator to complete some necessary paperwork. This meeting may take place in the admissions office or in the resident's room, if the resident is too tired, frail, or ill to tolerate sitting in an office. During this meeting:

- The admissions coordinator reviews the services that will be provided, the fees that will be charged, the resident's rights, and the facility's policies (Fig. 11-1). The resident (or the resident's health care agent) must sign documents acknowledging that this information has been received and accepted.

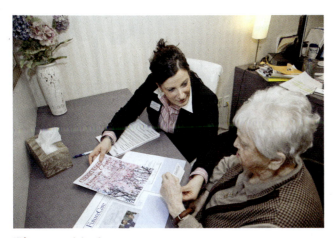

Figure 11-1
The admissions coordinator reviews important paperwork with the new resident (or the resident's health care agent) as part of the admissions process.

- The admissions coordinator reviews the resident's **admission sheet** with the resident (or the resident's health care agent) to ensure that the information it contains is correct and complete. The admission sheet, which is usually prepared before the resident arrives at the facility, includes standard information about the resident such as the resident's name, address, date of birth, age, social security number, gender, insurance information, emergency notification information, and health care agent information (if needed).
- The admissions coordinator obtains copies of any legal documents the resident may have related to advance directives.
- The admissions coordinator provides a way of identifying the resident (Fig. 11-2).

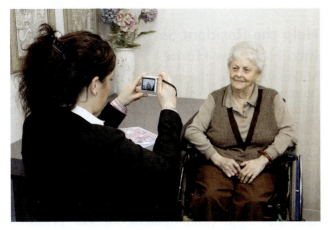

Figure 11-2
A photograph of the resident is usually taken for identification purposes.

Usually, a photograph of the resident is taken to keep with the resident's medical record. The facility may also provide the resident with an identification bracelet to wear, although this is becoming less common in the long-term care setting.

Also during the admission period, a nurse will complete an **admissions assessment** of the resident. The admissions assessment provides baseline information about the resident's condition at the time of admission. You may be asked to assist with the admissions assessment by obtaining the resident's vital signs, height, and weight for the nurse. In addition to these measurements, the admissions assessment also includes a review of the major organ systems and a review of the resident's self-care abilities and preferences for care. For example, as part of the admissions assessment, the nurse will usually listen to the resident's heart and lungs, ask about bowel and bladder habits, check for edema (swelling) or skin conditions, and identify what assistance the resident needs for activities of daily living (ADLs). Information that is obtained during later assessments can then be compared to the admissions assessment information to monitor changes in the resident's condition.

In addition to completing the admissions assessment, the nurse is responsible for obtaining orders for the resident's care from the doctor and contacting all of the various services that will be needed to carry out the doctor's orders. The doctor's orders typically include instructions for diet, activity, and any special therapies that are needed. So, for example, the nurse may have to fax medication orders to the pharmacy, work with people in the rehabilitation department to make arrangements for rehabilitation services and for any special equipment that the resident may need, and notify the food service department of the resident's arrival and the type of diet that has been ordered. There are many people involved in coordinating all of the care and services that the new resident will need, and good communication is necessary to ensure that things run smoothly.

HELPING THE NEW RESIDENT TO FEEL WELCOME

The members of the health care team may regard the process of admitting a person to the facility as routine. However, for the person being admitted (and for the person's family members), this "routine" event can be very stressful. Remember what you learned in Chapter 8 about the challenges a new resident (and the resident's family members) must face when admission to a long-term care facility becomes necessary. As a nursing assistant, you will play an important role in helping to make the admissions process as pleasant as possible for the resident and the resident's family members.

When a new resident is being admitted, the admissions staff will usually notify the nursing staff of the resident's estimated time of arrival, if it is known. The unit is also called as soon as the person arrives at the facility. This gives the nursing staff time to prepare for the resident's arrival. As a member of the nursing staff, you will play a very important role in making sure that the resident feels expected and welcomed when he arrives at the facility. A good first impression can go a long way toward easing anxiety, especially if one of the things the resident and her family members are worried about is the quality of care that the resident will be receiving. As a nursing assistant, there are several things you can do to make sure that the admission goes as smoothly as possible.

Prepare the Resident's Room in Advance

Ask the nurse about any special requirements that your new resident may have. Does the person use a walker or some other ambulation device, or will he be arriving in a wheelchair or on a stretcher? If so, you will want to check the placement of the furniture in the room and move it as necessary to ensure easy entry into the room. If necessary, adjust the lighting and temperature of the room. Open the blinds or drapes and prepare the bed, if needed, by turning the sheets back, lowering the bed to the lowest position, and making sure the wheels are locked (see Chapter 21). If the resident is arriving by stretcher, you will need to prepare the bed in a slightly different manner (also described in Chapter 21).

Gather the equipment you will need for taking and recording the person's vital signs (see Chapter 22). Make sure any other equipment needed by the incoming resident (such as oxygen equipment, an intravenous [IV] pole, or a bedside commode) is in the room before the resident arrives. If your facility provides them, obtain an admissions pack for the resident. A typical admissions pack contains a basin, a water pitcher, a drinking cup, a package of tissues, and assorted personal care items (such as toothpaste, soap, and shampoo). Preparing the room in a thoughtful manner indicates to the new resident that her arrival was anticipated and planned for (Fig. 11-3).

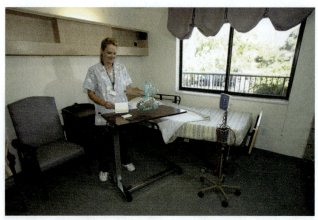

Figure 11-3

Turning the bed sheets down and opening the blinds or drapes to let the sunshine in says to a new resident, "Welcome! We were expecting you!" Making sure the room is stocked with the necessary equipment and supplies, including personal toiletry items, also indicates to the new resident that his arrival was planned for and expected.

Greet the Resident Warmly and Introduce Yourself

When you meet the resident and family members for the first time, be sure to introduce yourself. Give your title and explain how you will be involved in the resident's care. A warm, courteous, and professional greeting helps to put the resident and family at ease and gives them confidence that they will be well taken care of by the health care team. Now is also a good time to ask the resident how she prefers to be addressed. Addressing the resident as she prefers to be addressed is courteous, and it helps maintain the resident's sense of identity and individuality.

Help the Resident Settle Into Her New Home

Make sure that the resident is comfortable by helping her into bed or a chair. Next, take the time to give a new resident a "tour" of the room (Fig. 11-4). Point out the location of the bathroom. Show the resident how to use the call light control, how to adjust the bed, how to adjust the lights, and how to operate any other appliances or pieces of equipment in the room.

You should also help the resident to unpack and find appropriate places for her personal belongings (Fig. 11-5). In most long-term care facilities, you will need to complete a resident inventory sheet as part of the unpacking process.

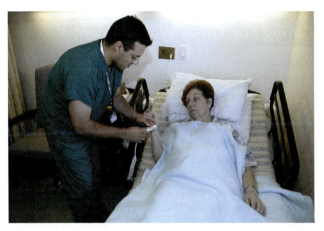

Figure 11-4
A new resident must be taught how to operate the equipment in the room. Here, a nursing assistant shows a new resident how to use the call light control.

The **resident inventory sheet** is a document that lists and briefly describes all of the resident's personal belongings (Fig. 11-6). When completing the resident inventory sheet, make sure that you describe each item objectively. For example, when describing a resident's ring, you would write, "yellow metal ring with two blue stones" instead of "gold ring with two sapphires" because you do not know for sure that the ring is gold or the stones are sapphires. The resident inventory sheet is used to help make sure that a resident leaves the facility with all of her belongings, in the event of a transfer or discharge. It is also used to assist with tracking if belongings are misplaced or borrowed. Most long-term care facilities require

Inventory of Personal Effects

Resident _____   Room   No. _____

Description :	
Bathrobe	Cane
Bed Jackets	Comb Brush
Belts	Crutches
Blouses	Dentures-Full Upper ( ) Lower ( )
Bras	Partial Upper ( ) Lower ( )
Coat	Furniture
Dresses	Glasses-Rimmed ( ) Rimless ( )
Girdles	Luggage
Hat	Other
Hose	Prosthesis
Nightgowns	Purse
Pajamas	Radio
Panties	Razors - Electric ( ) Safety ( )
Shirts	Rings
Shoes	Toothbrush
Skirts	Walker
Slips	Watch
Slippers	Wheelchair
Sweaters	
Ties	
Trousers	
Undershirts	
Undershorts	
Wallet	

I certify that the above is a correct list of my personal belongings.
I take full responsibility for retaining in my possession the articles listed above and any others brought to me while a resident in this facility.
_____

ALL ITEMS BROUGHT FOR THE PERSONAL USE OF THE RESIDENT MUST BE PROPERLY MARKED AND LISTED AS ARE THE ABOVE. Please bring additional items to the Nurses' Station for proper handling.
_____

Resident's washable clothing to be: _____ taken home for laundering
_____ laundered here at the center.
_____

I understand the Management will not be responsible for any valuables, money, or clothing left in the possession of the resident._____ Date_____

Signature of Resident (or Relative) _____ Date _____
Signature of Nurse _____ Date _____

Disposition on Discharge   *Upon Discharge, all personal items are sent with resident or picked up by responsible party. Upon transfer, all personal items are to be boxed and placed in designated storage area for safekeeping.
Signature of Nurse _____   Signature of Resident/Relative _____
Date _____   Date _____

Figure 11-6
A resident inventory sheet is completed when a person is admitted to a long-term care facility. This document is used to keep track of each resident's belongings.

each resident to write her name inside of each article of clothing to help with laundry sorting. You may need to help the resident do this if it has not been done already.

If the resident has brought personal items to decorate with, let the resident know that you will be willing to assist in any way that you can. For example, the resident may need your help with hanging a favorite picture on the wall, or obtaining a bulletin board to display treasured cards and pieces of art.

After the new resident has had a chance to rest, be sure to orient her to the rest of the unit. Show her other rooms that she will be using, such as the dining room and the activity room. Let her know the usual meal schedules and how to obtain snacks or beverages in between meals if she desires them. Show the resident the activity calendar so that she can see the variety of events that are planned, and perhaps even identify some that she would like to participate in. Take some time to introduce the new resident to some

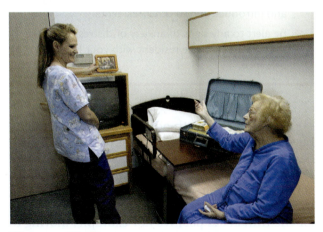

Figure 11-5
Helping the person to unpack and find suitable spots for personal items can make a new environment feel more "home-like" instantly.

of the other residents so that she will start to feel more comfortable in her new environment.

Practice Good Communication Skills

While you are helping the new resident to get settled, talk to her! Involving the resident in conversation will indicate to the resident that you are interested in her personally, and it will let you get to know her a little bit better. It is also a good time to ask questions that will help you to plan the resident's care. Remember that the long-term care facility is now the person's home. The care that you provide for the new resident should be arranged around her preferences, not your routine. For example, rather than telling the resident when you will help her with her shower, you might ask her when and how she likes to bathe. Find out about the resident's usual routine and habits. For example, maybe the resident likes to take a nap between lunch and dinner. This will be important for you to know. Ask the resident whether she would prefer to take meals in the dining room or in her room. Be sure to listen to what the resident is saying to you, both on her own and in response to your questions. Is the resident asking questions or expressing feelings that suggest that she is scared, worried, or upset? Answer questions about your specific responsibilities to the best of your ability. Questions the resident may have about her medical care should be directed to the nurse. Also, report any concerns that you may have about the resident's ability to adjust to the new environment to the nurse.

TRANSFERS

A **transfer** occurs whenever a resident is moved within or between health care settings. A transfer can be:

- From one room to another (for example, from a semi-private to a private room)
- From one unit to another (for example, from a standard care floor to a dementia care unit)
- From one health care facility to another (for example, from a long-term care facility to a hospital for the treatment of an acute illness, or from one long-term care facility to another)

Transfers can occur when a person's medical condition improves, or when it worsens. Transfers can also occur when a preferred room becomes available for a person on a waiting list, or when it is necessary to move residents to resolve conflicts between roommates.

Caring For Those With Dementia

Admission to a long-term care facility can be difficult for anyone, but for a person with dementia it is particularly challenging. A person with dementia functions much better with a consistent routine, but leaving home and moving to a long-term care facility is extremely disruptive to the person's normal routine. The surroundings are unfamiliar, the daily tasks and routines may not be done the way that the person is used to, and the caregivers are strangers. Because the dementia prevents the person from understanding what is going on, the person may become very frightened, embarrassed, or even humiliated when unfamiliar people touch his body or handle his belongings. To help admission go more smoothly for your residents with dementia:

- Approach the resident with a friendly smile and good eye contact.
- Introduce yourself each time you are with the resident. The resident may not remember you, even if he just saw you 5 minutes ago.
- Ask the family about the resident's likes, dislikes, interests, and life before coming to live at the facility. This information can help you to talk with the resident and develop a relationship.
- Before you start performing a care task, take the time to talk and socialize with the resident.
- Show the resident around the new environment. You may have to do this many times before the resident starts to get used to his surroundings.
- Consider the use of labels or pictures to help the resident find his belongings and key areas in the room (such as the closet or the bathroom).
- Take the resident to activities that he would enjoy and introduce him to other residents.
- Be alert to any signs of anxiety or distress and take the time to calm the resident with your familiar presence.

As is the case with admissions, transfers can be stressful for the resident, as well as the resident's family members. The reason for the transfer may cause anxiety, especially if the person's condition has worsened and the person is being transferred to a hospital. Even when the reason for the transfer is positive (for example, moving to a better room), the resident may still experience some stress as a result of the change.

The physical transfer can be carried out in a number of ways. The resident may simply walk, or he may be transported in a wheelchair or on a stretcher. Sometimes, the resident does not even need to get out of bed. The bed (with the resident in it) is simply moved to another room or unit. An ambulance may be used when a person is being moved from one health care facility to another. Some people are transferred from one facility to another by their regular means of transportation, such as a car or taxi. When this is the case, a family member usually accompanies the resident in the car or taxi.

TRANSFERS WITHIN THE FACILITY

If the transfer is occurring within the facility, you will be responsible for helping to physically prepare the resident for the transfer, for packing the resident's belongings, and possibly for transporting the resident to the new room or unit. The nurse will report information about the resident's medical condition and medications or other treatments to the nurse on the resident's new unit. Because you are the caregiver who is most likely to know the most about your resident's personal preferences, you may be asked to report information about the resident's preferences and habits to the nursing assistant on the resident's new unit. For example, you would know that Mr. Vasquez does not like overcooked vegetables, that he requires minimal assistance in the bathroom, and that he likes to read the paper after breakfast. By providing the new nursing assistant with this information, you are helping to ensure that the transition from one caregiver to another is as seamless as possible for your resident (Fig. 11-7).

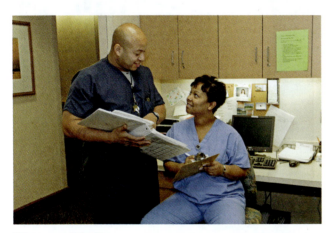

Figure 11-7
Two nursing assistants meet to discuss the personal care needs of a resident who is being transferred from one part of the facility to another.

TEMPORARY TRANSFERS

A resident may be temporarily transferred to another health care facility (such as a hospital) for acute care or a diagnostic test or procedure. In this case, you may be asked to assist by obtaining the resident's vital signs and physically preparing the resident for the transfer. The nurse gathers relevant information from the resident's medical record for photocopying (such as information about advance directives), and completes a transfer summary. The transfer summary explains why the resident is being sent to the hospital and includes the nurse's assessment of the resident's condition at the long-term care facility. This information is given to the ambulance crew in a sealed envelope to take to the hospital with the resident.

It will not be necessary to pack up all of a resident's belongings when the transfer is only temporary. Valuables may be placed in a safe or other locked area in the long-term care facility. Non-valuables typically remain in the resident's room. Many residents (or their families) choose to pay for a **bed hold** for the time the resident is in the hospital. The bed hold reserves the resident's bed at the nursing home and ensures that it will still be available when the resident returns from the hospital. If a bed hold is not in place, the resident is considered officially discharged from the long-term care facility, and the resident's bed becomes available for a new admission. If a new resident is admitted, there may no longer be a place for the hospitalized resident when he is discharged from the hospital.

DISCHARGES

A **discharge** is the official release of a person from a health care facility. For example, a long-term care resident may be discharged to her home, to a family member's home, or to another health care facility. The doctor orders a resident's discharge. Occasionally, a person will insist on leaving a health care setting without a doctor's order, or **against medical advice (AMA).** A person who is mentally competent may choose to leave a facility if she wants to. However, that person must sign certain documents first. By signing these documents, the person states that she understands that leaving the facility without a doctor's order releases the doctor and the health care facility from any legal responsibility regarding her health status because she has refused to follow the recommendations for her care. If a person tells you that she is leaving the facility, you must report this to the nurse immediately. The nurse will follow the facility's policy for ensuring that a person who is leaving AMA is aware of the consequences of her actions.

Although some residents initiate their own departure from the facility, most residents wait to be officially discharged. Many times, the official discharge is a happy event, but sometimes, residents have mixed emotions about leaving. If the resident is going home, the resident and the family members may worry about how they will get along without the support of the long-term care staff. Many residents develop close relationships with their caregivers, and separation from them may be very difficult. The resident may also have developed friendships in the facility that she will miss. If the resident is going to another facility, she may be worried about having to get used to new caregivers and making new friends.

To help ease the transition, preparations for discharge begin as soon as it is anticipated that the resident may leave the facility. Preparations for discharge may begin as soon as the resident is admitted to the facility, if it is known that the stay will be temporary. These preparations may also occur later in the resident's stay if the resident's situation changes and a discharge becomes necessary. **Discharge planning** is the process used by the members of the health care team to help prepare a resident to leave the facility. Discharge planning helps to make sure that the person continues to receive quality care after discharge, either at another facility or at home with support from a home health care agency or from family members. The purpose of discharge planning is to identify the needs that the person will have after her discharge and to make arrangements for meeting these needs. For example:

- Mrs. Luking is being discharged from one long-term care facility so that she can move to another one in a different state. Discharge planning will help to ensure that the facility Mrs. Luking is moving to has the equipment Mrs. Luking needs (such as oxygen equipment or ostomy supplies) so that there is no interruption in her care.
- Mr. Ziegfried has recovered from his broken hip and is being discharged from the long-term care facility to his daughter's home. As part of discharge planning, a member of the health care team may assess the daughter's home and recommend changes that will help promote Mr. Ziegfried's safety and independence (such as installing grab bars in the bathroom, removing throw rugs that pose a

tripping hazard, and installing additional lighting to make it easier for Mr. Ziegfried to see).
- Mrs. Pyne has diabetes and is being discharged to her home. As part of discharge planning, Mrs. Pyne and her family members will learn about how to manage the diabetes and prevent complications.
- Mr. Burns has completed his rehabilitation following a stroke and is being discharged to his home. He still requires a fair amount of help with his activities of daily living (ADLs). As part of discharge planning, the health care team will help Mr. Burns and his family obtain the services of a home health care agency.

The ultimate goal of discharge planning is to help the person achieve the best health status possible after he leaves the health care facility.

Many members of the health care team take part in discharge planning. The social worker is often involved in coordinating the transfer of information from one facility to another.

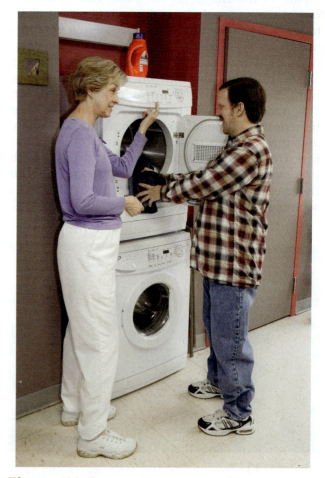

Figure 11-8
A resident practices skills he will use at home in preparation for discharge from the long-term care facility.

Rehabilitation services may be involved in helping the resident develop skills the person will need for his own self-care following discharge. For example, the person may need to learn how to use assistive devices, or re-learn skills that are used in the home (Fig. 11-8). The nurse is responsible for making sure the resident (and family, if necessary) has been taught what they need to know about the person's condition and how to monitor and care for it. For example, the nurse will provide information about medications and other treatments, and work with the person and family to ensure that they are able to administer the medications or perform the recommended treatments at home.

As a nursing assistant, your responsibilities when a resident is discharged include helping the resident to gather and pack his belongings and say goodbye to friends and caregivers. Ask the nurse or the resident about the estimated time of discharge so that you can have the resident ready to leave on time, taking into account the time the resident needs to pack and say his good-byes. You may also need to assist the resident out of the facility or help to carry his belongings.

TELL THE NURSE ❗

The changes that accompany discharges, transfers, and admissions to health care facilities can be very stressful for a resident and for his family members. Often, a lot of information is communicated in a very short period of time, and the resident (as well as his family members) may have trouble absorbing and understanding everything. Make sure you observe and listen carefully to the resident and family members during these transitions. Report any of the following to the nurse immediately:

- Any questions that have to do with a resident's medical condition or transfer

- Any comments that would indicate that the resident or a family member does not fully understand what she has been told by a doctor or nurse

- Any signs of anxiety such as crying, confusion, agitation, or other unexplained behavior

- Any changes in the resident's vital signs or mental status

- Any mention of leaving the facility against medical advice (AMA)

SUMMARY

- Admission to a long-term care facility is a time of orientation. The resident must learn to accept his new environment and his new status as a "resident," and the members of the health care team must learn about the new resident.
    - During the admission period, necessary paperwork is completed, a means of identifying the resident is provided, and an admissions assessment is done.
    - A smooth admissions process helps to reduce a person's anxiety about entering the long-term care facility. Many of the nursing assistant's duties revolve around making the admissions process easier for the resident and family members.
        - Nursing assistants are responsible for preparing the resident's room, taking the resident's vital signs and measuring his height and weight, helping the resident to unpack, teaching the resident how to use the equipment in the room, and orienting the resident to other areas on the unit.
        - By actively listening to the comments made by the resident and family mem-

  bers during the admissions process, the nursing assistant can notify the nurse of any specific concerns that may need to be addressed.

- Transfers occur when a resident is moved, either within a health care setting or between health care settings. When a resident is transferred within the long-term care facility, the nursing assistant is responsible for passing vital information about the resident's care to the receiving nursing assistant.

- Although many residents look forward to being discharged from a long-term care facility, some might wonder whether they will be able to manage on their own, or with only the help of family members.
    - Discharge planning, which begins as soon as the potential for discharge is identified, helps to ensure that the resident continues to receive quality health care even after being released from the long-term care facility.
    - Discharge planning is the responsibility of the entire health care team.

WHAT DID YOU LEARN?

Multiple choice

Select the single best answer for each of the following questions.

1. One of your residents, Mr. Janofsky, is being transferred to the dementia care unit in your facility. As a nursing assistant, you will be assisting with Mr. Janofsky's transfer by doing all of the following except:
   a. Packing all of his personal belongings
   b. Escorting Mr. Janofsky to his new room
   c. Telling the nursing assistant on the dementia care unit about Mr. Janofsky and his care routines
   d. Telling the nurse on the dementia care unit about Mr. Janofsky's medications and treatments.

2. One of your residents, Mrs. Sarandis, tells you that she is leaving the long-term care facility to go live with her son. He is coming to pick her up at 11:00 AM. Before Mrs. Sarandis can be discharged, there must be:
   a. A nurse's order for discharge
   b. A doctor's order for discharge
   c. An admissions sheet on record
   d. A bed hold

3. As a nursing assistant, one of your tasks during the admission process is to:
   a. Take and record the new resident's vital signs and weight
   b. Obtain a photograph of the resident for identification purposes
   c. Hurry the new resident through the admissions process to keep things running smoothly
   d. Complete the admissions assessment

4. Who gives the orders on admission for a resident's diet, medications, level of activity, and any special treatments or therapies?
   a. The admissions coordinator
   b. The resident or one of his or her family members
   c. The Director of Nursing
   d. The doctor

5. Discharge planning begins:
   a. A couple of days before the resident is scheduled to be discharged
   b. As soon as discharge potential is identified

   c. The day the resident is scheduled to be discharged
   d. Before the resident is admitted to the health care facility

6. The ultimate goal of discharge planning is to:
   a. Make sure that the room is clean and ready for the next resident
   b. Close out the care plan
   c. Help the resident who is being discharged achieve or maintain his best level of health
   d. Make sure that all of the resident's belongings are accounted for

7. Who is responsible for discharge planning?
   a. The doctor
   b. The social worker
   c. The health care team
   d. The nursing assistant

8. Mr. Singer, one of your residents, tells you that he hates the facility and feels that being here is actually doing him more harm than good. He says that he has called a friend to come take him home. As far as you know, Mr. Singer's discharge has not been ordered. What should you do?
   a. Apply a restraint
   b. Help Mr. Singer pack; it is his right to leave if he wants to
   c. Tell the nurse immediately
   d. Remind Mr. Singer's roommate that the door to the room must be kept shut and locked at all times

9. Why should a newly admitted resident be given a warm welcome?
   a. Because he represents more revenue for the facility
   b. Because he will be a good roommate for another resident
   c. Because he may be feeling scared and uncomfortable about entering the long-term care facility
   d. He should not be given a warm welcome; after all, admissions happen every day and a "business as usual" attitude is best to avoid upsetting the resident

STOP and Think!

- Mr. Gardner has been a resident in your facility for several months, and he has reached his maximum potential in therapy. Medicare will no longer pay for his care. Mr. Gardner's son is transferring him to an assisted-living facility for monetary reasons. Mr. Gardner tells you that he is uncomfortable and scared about the new facility since he does not know anyone there. How can you help Mr. Gardner?

- Mrs. Becker is being admitted as a new resident to the long-term care facility where you work. Mrs. Becker's daughter, Rhonda, has accompanied her mother to her room. Rhonda mentions to you that she is feeling "like a bad daughter" because she is unable to care for her mother in her own home. She goes on to explain that both she and her husband travel extensively for work, and there would be periods when no one would be around to help care for Mom. Describe some things that you could do to help both Mrs. Becker and Rhonda feel more comfortable about Mrs. Becker coming to live at the long-term care facility.

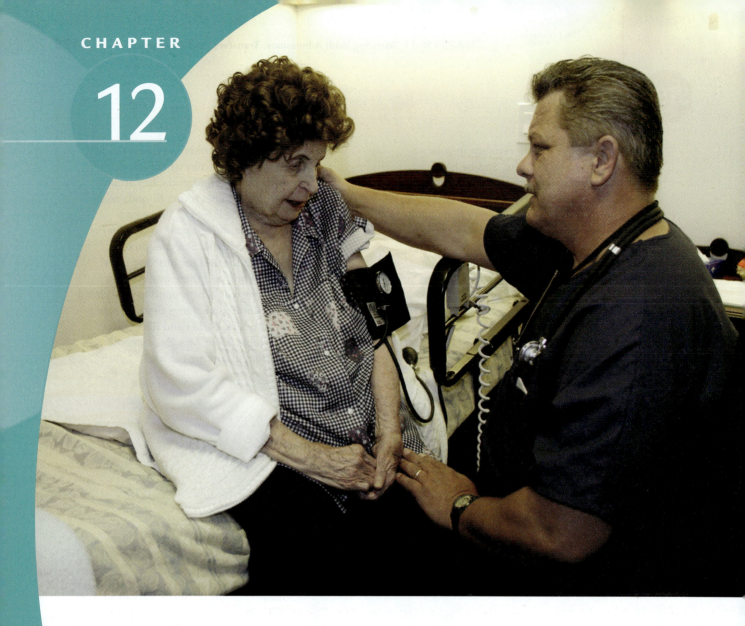

Assisting With Assessments and Care Planning

As you know, the health care team is responsible for helping residents to meet their physical, social, emotional, and spiritual needs, and for helping residents to attain and maintain their highest level of physical, mental, and social function. But how do we know what each resident's needs are, and whether or not they are being met? How do we know how well a resident is functioning? In this chapter, you will learn about how the health care team identifies each resident's needs, and then works out a plan for helping the resident meet

Photo: Assessment and care planning are necessary to ensure that the care provided meets the resident's needs. Here, a nursing assistant participates in the assessment process by gathering information to report to the nurse.

those needs. You will also learn about your role in supporting this effort. When you are finished with this chapter, you will be able to:

1. List the two parts of the Resident Assessment Instrument (RAI), and describe how this tool is used in the nursing home setting to assess the resident's needs and develop the resident's interdisciplinary care plan.

2. Identify four ways that information from the Minimum Data Set (MDS) is used, and explain the nursing assistant's role in supporting accurate completion of the MDS.

3. Describe the Omnibus Budget Reconciliation Act (OBRA) regulations relating to the assessment process in nursing homes.

4. Describe the basic format of an interdisciplinary care plan.

5. Describe the OBRA regulations relating to the care planning process in nursing homes.

6. Explain how the nursing assistant contributes to, and supports, assessment and care planning.

7. Describe how the nursing assistant's knowledge of the interdisciplinary care plan promotes good resident care.

Vocabulary Use the CD in the front of your book to hear these terms pronounced and defined:

Assessment
Interdisciplinary care plan
Resident Assessment
 Instrument (RAI)

Minimum Data Set
 (MDS)
Resident Assessment
 Protocols (RAPs)

Problem statement
Goal statement
 (expected outcome)

Interventions
Evaluation statement

Assessment is the act of gathering information about a resident's condition and then interpreting what that information means. Because interpreting information about a resident's condition is outside of the nursing assistant's scope of practice, nurses are responsible for assessment. However, as a nursing assistant, you are responsible for gathering and reporting information about your residents to the nurse. In this way, you play a very important role in supporting the assessment process.

Assessment allows the health care team to identify the resident's needs, abilities, and disabilities. The next step, then, is to make a plan for meeting those needs and helping the resident to attain or maintain his highest level of functioning. To achieve its goals, the health care team develops and then follows a specific care plan, called the **interdisciplinary care plan,** for the resident. (*Interdisciplinary* means "involving many different areas of knowledge and expertise.") The process of developing the interdisciplinary care plan is called care planning.

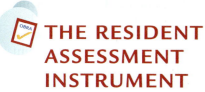

THE RESIDENT ASSESSMENT INSTRUMENT

The **Resident Assessment Instrument (RAI)** is an assessment tool that all nursing homes in the United States are required by OBRA to use. The

RAI is the tool that is used to create and update the resident's interdisciplinary care plan. The RAI must be completed at regularly scheduled intervals for each resident. The RAI is comprehensive, which means that it requires the health care team to assess multiple areas, including the resident's physical function, as well as his or her medical, nutritional, social, emotional, and activity needs. The RAI has two parts: the Minimum Data Set (MDS) and the Resident Assessment Protocols (RAPs). It is necessary to complete both parts of the RAI to understand and appropriately plan for the resident's care needs.

THE MINIMUM DATA SET

The **Minimum Data Set (MDS)** is the first part of the RAI. The MDS is shown in Appendix C. The MDS is used to identify and document the resident's problem areas and the degree of assistance or skilled care that the resident needs. The data collected on the MDS form is used in four important ways (Box 12-1).

The MDS is completed on a computer. Each item on the MDS is answered by selecting the appropriate code from the options described. Although the nurse is usually responsible for completing most of the sections, other health care team members who specialize in specific areas may be responsible for completing some of the

BOX 12-1   How Minimum Data Set (MDS) Data Is Used

The Minimum Data Set (MDS) is an extremely important document for those who work in nursing homes. MDS data is used in many different ways, so it is very important for the MDS to be completed accurately and on time.

- MDS data provides the foundation for developing the interdisciplinary care plan. Accurate completion of the MDS helps to ensure that the resident's needs are correctly identified, so that they can be addressed in the interdisciplinary care plan.
- MDS data is used to determine reimbursement rates for care provided through government insurance programs (Medicare and Medicaid; see Chapter 1). To determine reimbursement rates for care provided through Medicare and Medicaid, it is important that the MDS coding accurately reflects the resident's functional abilities and the care that he or she has received. If MDS coding reflects less care than a resident is actually receiving, the money paid to the facility will not cover all of the care that was delivered. If MDS coding reflects more care than a resident is actually receiving, the facility will be overpaid. The government performs audits regularly to make sure that payments are accurate. If audit findings

are questionable, the facility may be investigated for fraud. Financial responsibility helps to protect your residents and you. It helps to ensure that there are resources to provide the care and services that residents need, and it also provides for your employee benefits and paycheck!

- MDS data feeds into the Quality Indicator Profile report, the document used by surveyors to identify care problems that may be present in the facility, as well as residents who are experiencing those problems (see Chapter 6). During a survey, problems can result if the Quality Indicator Profile report does not match the resident care and conditions that the surveyor observes.
- MDS data is used to calculate Quality Measures of Care outcomes that are made available to the public on the Centers for Medicare and Medicaid Services (CMS) web site. The Quality Measures of Care outcomes are a valuable resource for people who are in the process of choosing a nursing home for a loved one, or who are interested in reviewing the quality of care provided in a nursing home where a loved one already lives. If the information reported on the MDS is not accurate, the public could get the wrong impression about the quality of care provided in the facility.

---

sections. For example, the dietitian may be responsible for completing the nutrition section, the social worker may be responsible for completing the mood and behavior section, and the activities director may be responsible for completing the activity section (Fig. 12-1).

To complete the MDS accurately, the other members of the health care team will rely on you to provide them with information about the resident's abilities and the amount of assistance the resident needs (Fig. 12-2). The codes used on the MDS for describing the resident's ability to perform his activities of daily living (ADLs), as well as the amount of help he needs from the staff to complete these activities, are shown in Box 12-2. Using these descriptions when reporting to the other members of the health care team about a resident's ability to complete his ADLs helps to ensure that they have the information they need to complete the MDS accurately.

OBRA requires a registered nurse to be responsible for ensuring the accuracy of the sections completed by the nursing staff, and for making sure that the entire MDS is completed on time and per the requirements of the law. In some facilities, these responsibilities are handled by a

registered nurse with the job title *Registered Nurse Assessment Coordinator (RNAC)*. In other facilities, these responsibilities are handled by the charge nurse or a head nurse.

RESIDENT ASSESSMENT PROTOCOLS

The second part of the RAI is the **Resident Assessment Protocols (RAPs).** The RAPs help the health care team to develop an interdisciplinary care plan that is tailored exactly to the resident's needs. After the MDS is complete, the coded responses are analyzed by a computer program that identifies problem areas (or potential problem areas) for the resident. These problems (actual and potential) are indicated on the last page of the MDS, called the *Resident Assessment Protocol Summary* (see Appendix C). At this point in the assessment process, completion of the MDS has only identified problem areas for the resident. For example, we may see that Mr. Taylor has a problem with incontinence, but we may not know *why* Mr. Taylor has that problem. For a better understanding of *why* a resident has a problem

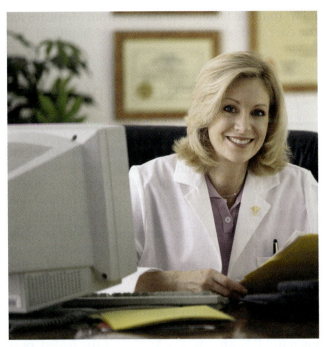

Figure 12-1
Different members of the health care team are responsible for completing different sections of the Minimum Data Set (MDS). Here, the dietitian is reviewing a resident's intake as recorded by the nursing assistant so that she can complete the nutrition section of the MDS.

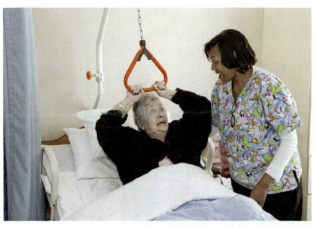

Figure 12-2
Because you will be assisting your residents with daily care, you will have first-hand knowledge of what the resident is capable of doing, and what kind of assistance she needs. Being specific when reporting helps the nurse and the other members of the health care team to complete the Minimum Data Set (MDS) accurately.

(or is at risk for a problem), the RAPs must be used in addition to the MDS.

The RAPs are a series of questions to answer or points to consider for each problem area. Completing the RAPs provides more in-depth assessment of each of the resident's problem areas, and helps to identify the specific reasons the resident has a particular problem, or is at risk for a problem. For example, by responding to each of the items in the RAP for incontinence, the nurse is able to identify the specific conditions or problems that contribute to Mr. Taylor's incontinence. It might turn out that Mr. Taylor is incontinent because of physical changes in the urinary system, while another resident, Mr. Jones, is incontinent because of dementia. Mr. Taylor and

---

| BOX 12-2 | Minimum Data Set (MDS) Codes and Descriptions For Describing Resident Performance of Activities of Daily Living (ADLs) and Staff Support Provided | OBRA |

Resident Performance

0 **Independent:** The resident can perform the activity independently without any supervision, guidance, or physical help from you.

1 **Supervision:** The resident can perform the activity independently as long as you provide verbal cues to remind the resident what to do, or provide the resident with the necessary supplies or equipment to perform the activity.

2 **Limited assistance:** The resident needs hands-on assistance from you to complete the task, but you do not support any of the resident's weight.

3 **Extensive assistance:** The resident needs hands-on assistance from you to complete the task, and you have to physically support all or part of the resident's weight.

4 **Total assistance:** The resident is unable to perform any aspect of the task. You do everything for the resident and totally support the resident's weight.

Staff Support

0 No physical help or set-up help provided
1 Only set-up help provided
2 One staff member required to provide physical help
3 Two or more staff members required to provide physical help*

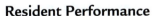

*Specify the number of staff members when reporting.

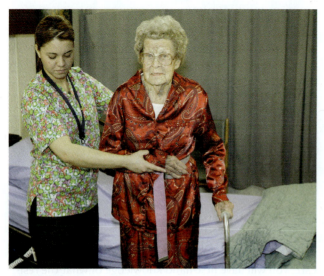

Figure 12-3
The Resident Assessment Protocols (RAPs) help the health care team identify the specific cause of a resident's problem. Knowing detailed information about a resident's problem is necessary in order to plan appropriate interventions to address it. Here, a nursing assistant assists a confused resident with incontinence to the bathroom at regularly scheduled times to help prevent incontinence accidents from occurring.

Mr. Jones are both incontinent, but because of the differences in the cause of incontinence, the care that would be planned for them would be very different (Fig. 12-3).

SCHEDULE FOR ASSESSING RESIDENTS

Per OBRA regulations, the full RAI (that is, both the MDS and the RAPs) must be completed for all residents (except those whose care is being paid for by Medicare) within 14 days of admission and once a year thereafter. The full RAI must also be completed whenever there is a significant change in a resident's condition. In addition to the full assessments that must take place annually (or whenever there is a significant change in a resident's condition), a shorter version of the MDS must be completed on a quarterly basis (that is, every 3 months) to check the resident's status between full assessments. Your state regulations may also require scheduled assessments using specific MDS items.

Residents whose care is being paid for by Medicare are assessed on a different schedule. They require more frequent MDS assessments during the first 3 months of their coverage, because the MDS data is used to determine the rate of pay-

ment that the facility will receive from Medicare for the care and services provided (see Chapter 2).

THE INTERDISCIPLINARY CARE PLAN

The health care team develops the interdisciplinary care plan to address the resident's care needs that were identified through the assessment process. (The *care plan*, which you learned about in Chapter 3, is a sub-set of the interdisciplinary care plan. The care plan describes only the nursing team's roles and responsibilities in providing care to the resident, while the interdisciplinary care plan describes the entire health care team's roles and responsibilities.)

OBRA requires an interdisciplinary care plan to be written or reviewed within 7 days of completing a full RAI (that is, the MDS and the RAPs), or a quarterly MDS. The interdisciplinary care plan identifies the resident's problems, sets goals, and specifies actions that will be taken by the health care team to help the resident meet those goals. The interdisciplinary care plan must be reviewed at least every 3 months, but may be reviewed more frequently depending on the nature of the problem and the condition of the resident.

The format used for the interdisciplinary care plan may vary from facility to facility. In general, however, interdisciplinary care plans have at least four parts (Fig. 12-4):

- The **problem statement** identifies exactly what problem is being addressed. The problem may be an actual problem (for example, the resident has a pressure ulcer) or a potential problem (for example, the resident is at risk for developing a pressure ulcer due to immobility and incontinence).

- The **goal statement** or **expected outcome** is a statement of what the health care team expects the resident to be able to achieve within a specific time frame. For example, for the resident with a pressure ulcer, the goal may be that within the next 90 days, the resident's ulcer will heal, and the resident will have no further skin breakdown. For the resident who is at risk for developing a pressure ulcer, the goal may be that he will remain without pressure ulcers for the specified period of time.

- The **interventions** are the specific actions that the members of the health care team will take to help the resident achieve the

Interdisciplinary Care Plan

Resident Name: _____Betty Samuels_____   Room #: _423A_

Problem Statement	Goal Statement (or Expected Outcome)	Interventions
9/15/08 At risk for weight loss r/t pattern of deceased intake over the last 2 weeks.	Resident's weight will remain stable within range of 134 lb–145 lb x 30 days.	~~Oral assessment for sign of sore mouth or dental problems (Nurse; dentist)~~ d/c 10/16 10/16 – Monitor healing from tooth extraction and continually observe for sign of oral or dental discomfort. (Nurse, CNA) ~~Monitor mood; assess for possible depression. (CNA, Activities, Nurses, Social Work, Psychiatrist)~~ d/c 10/16/08 Make sure resident prepared for meal: toileted, properly dressed and positioned. (CNA) Diet as ordered. (Dietary, Nursing) Monitor intake; offer alternative if resident does not like or is not eating meal provided. (CNA) Provide snacks throughout the day; likes puddings, fruit, and graham crackers. (CNA, Activites, Dietary) Encourage resident to eat meals in dining room. (Nursing, Social Work, Activites, Dietary) Report to nurse right away if resident does not eat at least 50% of her meal. (CNA, Activites Aide) Ask daughter to bring in resident's favorite dishes from family recipes. (Nurse, Social Worker, Dietitian)

Evaluation Statement

10/16/08 – Goal met. Resident's intake has varied between 50% and 75%. Weight has remained stable at 134.2#. Resident evaluated by psychiatrist—no evidence of depression. Seen by dentist on 9/28/08. One tooth was pulled due to decay and deterioration. Area healing well. Accepting snacks in the afternoon and at bed time. Daughter is usually able to bring special treat of resident's choosing on Sundays when she visits.

Figure 12-4

The interdisciplinary care plan is a specific plan of care for each resident that is based on the resident's assessed needs. For each problem noted, the interdisciplinary care plan includes a problem statement, a goal statement or expected outcome, a list of the interventions (care measures) that are necessary to help the resident meet the goal, and an evaluation statement that reviews the effectiveness of the interventions in helping the resident to meet the goal.

stated goal. For example, if a resident is at risk for a pressure ulcer because of incontinence and immobility, appropriate interventions would include assisting the resident with elimination at regularly scheduled times, providing good skin care, using pressure-reducing devices, and changing the resident's position at least every 2 hours. These interventions lower the resident's risk for developing a pressure ulcer, supporting the goal of preventing the resident from developing a pressure ulcer.

- The **evaluation statement** reviews the effectiveness of the interventions in helping the resident to meet the goal.

The interdisciplinary care plan is a work in progress. It is continuously updated to reflect changes in the resident's overall condition. Each resident is assessed in a formal manner at least every 3 months, so at minimum, the interdisciplinary care plan will be updated every 3 months. If the resident has not met a goal, perhaps the goal needs to be changed to be more realistic. Perhaps the goal is still appropriate, but the interventions that were tried were not successful, so other interventions need to be identified. If the resident has met the goal, the goal may be replaced with a new goal or eliminated from the interdisciplinary care plan.

Interdisciplinary care plan conferences are held so that all of the members of the health care team can meet to discuss the resident's assessed needs and develop an appropriate care plan (or revise an existing care plan) (Fig. 12-5). OBRA

mandates that the resident (or the resident's health care agent) must be offered the opportunity to participate in the interdisciplinary care plan conference. Other family members may be included as well, if the resident desires. Resident and family input helps to ensure that the interdisciplinary care plan addresses the issues that are of importance to the resident. This helps to ensure that the interdisciplinary care plan supports quality of care for the resident, as well as quality of life.

THE NURSING ASSISTANT'S ROLE

Nursing assistants play a very important role in supporting assessment and in supporting the interdisciplinary care plan.

SUPPORTING ASSESSMENT

As a nursing assistant, you are the one who spends the most time with your residents on a day-to-day basis. From your daily contact with your residents, you will often be the first one to notice when a resident is developing a new problem. You will notice changes in a resident's condition, or a resident may report a new complaint to you as you are giving care. You may also be the first one to see that a resident is making progress toward meeting his care plan goals. All of this information is absolutely essential to report! By reporting your observations to the nurse, you support the assessment process and help to ensure that the care plan continues to address the resident's needs.

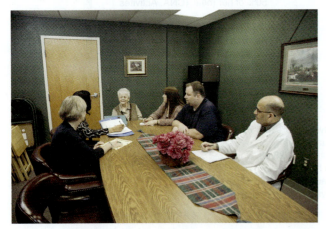

Figure 12-5
Interdisciplinary care plan conferences are held so that the whole health care team can meet together to develop or review the resident's interdisciplinary care plan. Resident and family input helps to ensure that the interdisciplinary care plan addresses the issues that are of importance to the resident.

TELL THE NURSE

As a nursing assistant, you may be the best one to know how a resident behaves or performs in the areas listed below. Your observations are important to share with the nurse. Be sure to report the following observations:

- The resident has become more confused, or there is a change in the resident's level of alertness
- The resident is having increased memory problems
- The resident's ability to express himself or understand others has changed
- The resident's ability to see has changed
- The resident is showing mood or behavioral changes

- The resident is having difficulty sleeping
- The resident is having difficulty getting along with others
- The resident is having difficulty eating and drinking
- The resident is having problems with his teeth or mouth
- The resident reports pain or other physical symptoms
- There is a change in the resident's ability to complete activities of daily living (ADLs)
- There is a change in the resident's ability to control the bowel, bladder, or both
- There is a change in the resident's skin condition
- There is a change in the resident's attitude toward, or participation in, activities
- The resident's responses to planned interventions

Any decline in a resident's ability to complete his ADLs needs to be reported promptly so that the change can be appropriately assessed and addressed in the interdisciplinary care plan. With prompt action, the lost function may be restored, or at least further decline may be prevented.

SUPPORTING THE INTERDISCIPLINARY CARE PLAN

As part of the health care team, your actions must be consistent with those of everyone else on the team. Consider for a moment a football team. Before a game, the coach gives the team members a game plan. Each team member knows what his role is on the playing field, as well as the roles of the other team members. All of the team members have the goal of winning the game. They also know that in order to win, they have to coordinate their actions. They have to know how to move the ball down the field toward the goal line. They have planned who to throw the ball to, and who is to block who on the other team. When the team members are successful, they score a touchdown. Think about what would happen if there were no game plan. If no one knew who was supposed to run with the ball, or who was supposed to tackle who, there would be chaos on the field. The chance of scoring any points, much less winning a game, would be slim!

The interdisciplinary care plan is the "game plan" for the health care team. The interdisciplinary care plan states the goals for the resident, and the actions that will be taken to achieve those goals. The assistance that you provide to the resident must be consistent with the planned interventions in order to help the resident achieve her goals (Fig. 12-6). Most goals on the interdisciplinary care plan have to do with helping the resident to attain or maintain her highest level of function and well-being. Sometimes we think that we are providing good care if we do everything for the resident. Since we are being paid to provide care, the more care we give, the better, right? Not

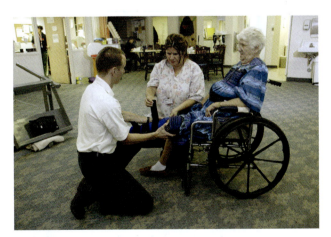

Figure 12-6
What you do for the resident must be consistent with the interventions planned by the health care team and documented on the interdisciplinary care plan. Here, the physical therapist is showing the nursing assistant how to use a piece of equipment that is to be used to help the resident.

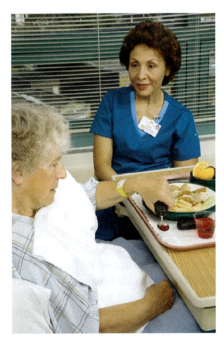

Figure 12-7
Although it may be faster or easier to just complete a task for a resident, it is important to follow the person's care plan and offer assistance only as needed. Doing too much for the resident can affect the resident's ability to attain or maintain her highest level of functioning and well-being.

necessarily. If we do everything for a resident, the resident does not have the opportunity to do things for herself. The less the resident actually does, the less she will be able to do over time, and her level of function will decline (Fig. 12-7). To ensure that you are providing care that supports the resident's goals, you must be aware of your resident's assessed needs, as well as the interdisciplinary care plan.

There are other reasons why it is important to follow each resident's interdisciplinary care plan carefully, as well. Not following the interdisciplinary care plan could result in harm to the resident. For example, let's say that Mrs. Snyder is not supposed to bear weight on her left leg as she

recovers from an injury. This limitation is noted in Mrs. Snyder's care plan. If you are not aware of this limitation, you might assist Mrs. Snyder to walk to the dining room, instead of using a wheelchair to transport her. By not providing care according to Mrs. Snyder's care plan, you would put her at risk for further injury. You could also put your facility at risk for being cited for deficiencies during a survey, and yourself at risk for losing your job! If you have questions about the interdisciplinary care plan, or are not sure that you have all the information you need, do not be afraid to ask questions. You must be sure that the care you are providing is consistent with the care that is planned for each resident.

Be Smart About Surveys!

During a survey, surveyors will be looking to see how well staff members assess the residents, develop interdisciplinary care plans based on assessed needs, and follow the care plans in the actual delivery of care. In addition to reviewing documentation in residents' medical records, surveyors will directly observe resident care to make sure that it is consistent with the interdisciplinary care plan. To help your facility remain without survey problems in this area:

- Learn about your residents' identified and potential problems so that you understand your residents' needs.

- Make sure that you are aware of the specific care plan interventions that you are responsible for carrying out. Ask for guidance if you are not sure what to do, or how to do it.

- Make sure that you carry out care according to the resident's care plan. Failure to follow the care plan can result in a negative outcome for the resident, and place the facility at risk for deficiencies during the survey.

- Be observant for any changes in the resident's condition, mood, behaviors, or need for assistance. Report these changes promptly.

- Keep the nurse informed so that he or she has a clear picture of the resident's condition, level of function, and the exact type of assistance your provide. This information helps the nurse to know when a resident may need to be reassessed, or when the interdisciplinary care plan needs to be revised.

SUMMARY

- Nursing homes in the United States are required by OBRA to complete one or both parts of the Resident Assessment Instrument (RAI) at regularly scheduled intervals, for each resident. Completion of both parts of the RAI is necessary to understand and appropriately plan for the resident's care needs.
  - The first part of the RAI, the Minimum Data Set (MDS), is a screening tool used to identify the resident's general problem areas, and the level of assistance the resident requires for care.
  - The second part of the RAI, the Resident Assessment Protocols (RAPs), guides the nurse (or other member of the health care

  team) through a more focused assessment of each problem to determine *why* the resident has the problem (or is at risk for the problem).
- Although the primary purpose of the MDS is for resident assessment, the MDS data is also used to determine reimbursement rates for care provided through government insurance programs (Medicare and Medicaid), and for monitoring the quality of care provided in the facility.
  - Accurate and timely completion of the MDS is extremely important.
  - The nursing assistant's observations help the members of the health care team to

accurately code the MDS, which helps prevent problems with reimbursement, provides support for a successful survey, and contributes to an accurate reflection of the quality of care provided by the facility.

- The interdisciplinary care plan is developed to address the resident's problems (or potential problems), as identified during the assessment process.
  - The interdisciplinary care plan states the resident's problems, the goals or expected outcomes for the resident, and the interventions that the health care team will take to help the resident achieve his goals. In addition, the interdisciplinary care plan includes an evaluation of the effectiveness of the interventions.

- OBRA requires an interdisciplinary care plan to be written (or revised) for each resident, at regular intervals.
- The nursing assistant plays a vital role in supporting assessment and the interdisciplinary care plan.
  - The nursing assistant's reports to the nurse about changes noted in the resident help the nurse and the other members of the health care team to properly identify and assess the resident's needs. Proper assessment of the resident's needs is essential for meeting OBRA's requirements for care.
  - The nursing assistant provides assistance to the resident that is consistent with the planned interventions, as noted on the interdisciplinary care plan. In this way, the nursing assistant helps the resident to achieve his or her goals.

WHAT DID YOU LEARN?

Multiple Choice

Select the single best answer for each of the following questions.

1. The assessment process in the nursing home involves the:
   a. Nurse and doctor
   b. Director of Nursing and resident
   c. Entire health care team
   d. Registered nurse assessment coordinator (RNAC)

2. The Resident Assessment Instrument (RAI) includes the:
   a. Minimum Data Set (MDS) and interdisciplinary care plan
   b. The MDS and the Resident Assessment Protocols (RAPs)
   c. The RAPs and the interdisciplinary care plan
   d. The MDS, the RAPs, and the interdisciplinary care plan

3. Who is responsible for making sure that the Minimum Data Set (MDS) is completed on time and per the requirements of the law?
   a. A registered nurse
   b. The Director of Nursing
   c. The entire health care team
   d. The doctor

4. The Minimum Data Set (MDS) is used:
   a. As a screening tool to identify resident problem areas
   b. To calculate reimbursement by government insurance programs

   c. To monitor quality of care in facilities
   d. All of the above

5. The Resident Assessment Protocols (RAPs) are used to:
   a. Confirm that the Minimum Data Set (MDS) is correct
   b. Calculate reimbursement rates
   c. Complete further assessment on identified problem areas
   d. Identify Quality Measures that are posted on Medicare's Web site

6. The nursing assistant's role in the assessment process is to:
   a. Accurately report observations about the resident's condition and provide specific information about the level and type of assistance provided
   b. Complete the activities of daily living (ADL) portion of the Minimum Data Set (MDS)
   c. Plan interventions
   d. All of the above

7. What can happen if a nursing assistant does not provide care according to the interdisciplinary care plan?
   a. The resident could be harmed
   b. The nursing assistant could lose his or her job
   c. The facility could be cited for deficiencies during the survey
   d. All of the above

STOP and Think!

- One of your co-workers, Maureen, is now assigned to care for Mrs. Preslinger, who used to be one of your assigned residents. You know that Mrs. Preslinger is recovering from a stroke. The goals of Mrs. Preslinger's interdisciplinary care plan are to help her to regain enough of her ADL skills to be able to go home and live with her daughter. While you are on break with Maureen, she is complaining about her assignment and tells you that she is very frustrated by how long it takes Mrs. Preslinger to do anything. She tells you that in order to make sure she can get her work done, she washes and dresses Mrs. Preslinger herself. Instead of assisting Mrs. Preslinger to walk to the bathroom with her walker, she transports her in a wheelchair because it is faster. She says to you that she gives more care to Mrs. Preslinger than any other nursing assistant on the unit. How should you respond? Do you think Maureen's actions are helping Mrs. Preslinger?

- You are caring for Mr. Hubert, a resident with dementia. The nurse told you that because of Mr. Hubert's dementia, he needs total assistance to bathe. She also told you that many of the other nursing assistants have reported that Mr. Hubert becomes aggressive during personal care, and that the care plan measures tried so far have not worked. Yesterday, as you began Mr. Hubert's bath, he started to yell and swing his arms, just like the nurse told you he would. You started to hum a song, and then began to sing. You noticed that Mr. Hubert stopped yelling and started to smile. You were able to finish the bath without any further behavioral problems from Mr. Hubert. This morning, when Mr. Hubert's daughter visited, you told her about the successful bath. She laughed and said, "That doesn't surprise me. My grandmother, Dad's mom, used to sing all the time. He always said he loved to hear her sing, and how much he missed it after she died." Is the information that Mr. Hubert's daughter shared with you important? Should you report this to the nurse?

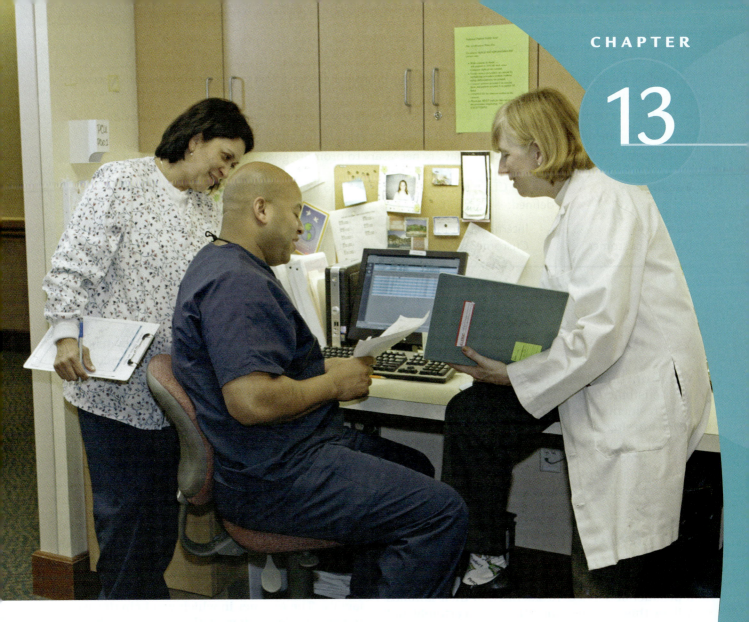

Providing Customer Service

WHAT WILL YOU LEARN?

Often, we think of customers as people who buy things. Because you are working in health care, you may not think that you need to be concerned about customers or customer service. After all, you aren't selling anything . . . or are you? In your role as a nursing assistant, you are providing a service to people that costs them a great deal of money. You *do* have customers. In this chapter, you will learn more about the importance of providing excellent customer service in the long-term care setting. When you are finished with this chapter, you will be able to:

1. Define the term *customer*, and describe who your customers are in the long-term care setting.
2. Describe common needs and expectations that customers in a long-term care setting may have.

Photo: As a nursing assistant, you have both internal and external customers. Here, a nursing assistant works with other members of the health care team to ensure quality care.

3. Define the term *customer service*, and explain why customer service efforts must extend beyond customer satisfaction.

4. Define the term *quality* and describe methods of evaluating the quality of the services you provide.

5. Describe the difficult customer and identify possible reasons for challenging behavior.

6. Describe the communication skills that are necessary to promote good customer relationships.

Vocabulary Use the CD in the front of your book to hear these terms pronounced and defined:

Customer	Internal customer	Customer need	Quality
External customer	Customer service	Customer expectation	Quality Measures

YOUR CUSTOMERS

When nursing assistants are asked to identify their customers, they often reply with the answer, "The residents and their families." While this is true, nursing assistants also have many other customers. A **customer** is *anyone* who buys or uses a product or service that you provide. As a nursing assistant, you have both external and internal customers (Fig. 13-1).

EXTERNAL CUSTOMERS

An **external customer** is a person from outside of your organization who relies on you to provide a product or service. Residents and their families fall in this category, but they are certainly not your only external customers. Other examples of external customers you may serve include:

- **Health care professionals who are not members of the facility's staff (such as doctors or pharmacists).** Health care professionals who are not a part of the regular staff, but who are involved in providing resident care, visit or call the facility and will rely on the facility staff to assist them, as needed.

- **Students who are completing the clinical portion of their training at the facility.** Students rely on the guidance and direction of the facility staff to become familiar with the layout of the facility, the facility's policies and procedures, and the residents.

- **Volunteers.** Volunteers often play a role in supporting the facility's activities program. They rely on staff members to support their efforts by helping to prepare the residents and the environment for the planned activity.

- **Surveyors.** Members of the survey team rely on staff members to provide needed information.

- **Members of the community.** Members of the community may come to the facility to visit residents, to evaluate the facility as a potential home for themselves or a loved one, or to conduct some type of business. These types of visitors will be on the units where residents live, and they will be observant of the conditions within the facility and the care provided by the staff.

For all of these external customers, the impressions that they get from observing and interacting with the staff will influence their overall opinion of the quality of care and services provided by the facility. The manner in which you help these customers can leave them with either a negative or a positive impression of your facility. A negative impression can lead to a bad reputation that can threaten future business. On the other hand, a positive impression can help a business to thrive. The saying, "You only get one chance to make a first impression" is a very important one to remember when dealing with external customers (Fig. 13-2). It is likely that you are going to encounter someone new every day, and the impression you give to that customer can help or hurt your facility's image.

INTERNAL CUSTOMERS

An **internal customer** is a person from inside your organization who relies on you to provide a product or service. In other words, your internal customers are your co-workers. This includes *everyone* in all departments. Your co-workers are your customers because they rely on you to do

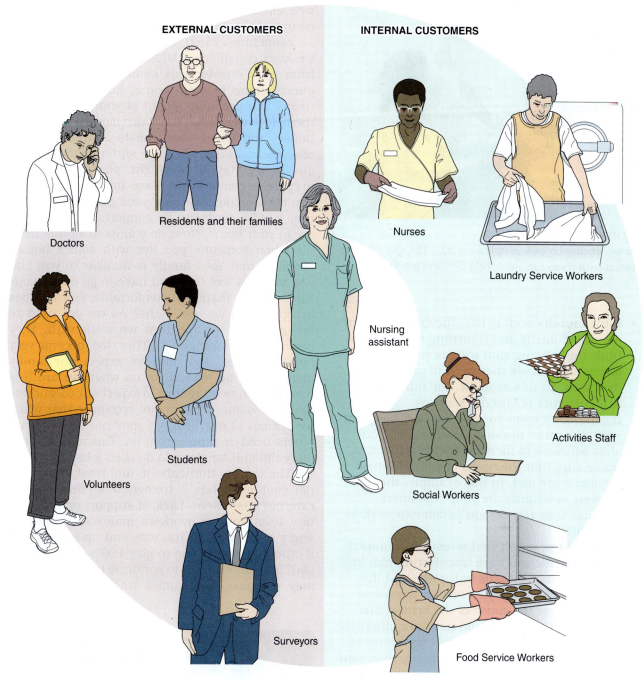

EXTERNAL CUSTOMERS   INTERNAL CUSTOMERS

Doctors

Residents and their families

Nurses

Laundry Service Workers

Nursing assistant

Volunteers

Students

Activities Staff

Social Workers

Surveyors

Food Service Workers

Figure 13-1

A customer is anyone who purchases or uses a product or service that you provide. You have both external and internal customers. External customers are those who are from outside of your organization, while internal customers are those who are part of your organization.

your job well so that they can do their jobs well. No one works in isolation. Consider these examples:

- If the nursing staff does not collect breakfast trays in a timely way for return to the kitchen, the kitchen staff will not have enough time to clean the trays and have

them ready to serve the lunch meal on time. In this example, the kitchen staff is the customer of the nursing staff (because they rely on the nursing staff to return the trays). The nursing staff is also the customer of the kitchen staff (because they rely on the kitchen staff to deliver meals on time).

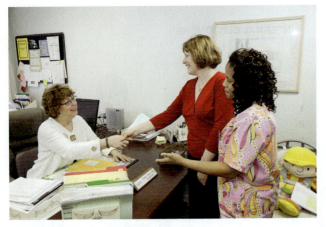

Figure 13-2
You will encounter new people every day. The way that you interact with them can either help or hurt your facility.

- If the laundry staff is not efficient in laundering soiled linens and returning them to the unit, the nursing staff will not have the clean sheets and towels they need to provide resident care. In this example, the nursing staff is a customer of laundry services.
- If you do not come to work for your assigned shift, the other nursing assistants on your shift will have to increase their workload to make sure that the needs of your assigned residents are met. In this example, the other nursing assistants are your customers, because they rely on you to come to work as scheduled.
- If you do not report that a resident bumped his arm while you were transferring him in his wheelchair into the bathroom and the resident later develops a bruise, the nurse will not know the cause of the bruise. She will spend time she would not have otherwise had to spend trying to find out the cause of the bruise. In this example, the nurse is your customer, because she benefits from a complete and accurate report from you about your resident.

In all of these examples, someone in the facility needs something from someone else in the facility in order to do his or her job safely and effectively. For your facility to provide the services necessary for your external customers, everyone in all departments must work together (Fig. 13-3). When there is a problem with service in one area, it affects the service provided in other areas. It is important to think about how the work you do affects your co-workers, in all departments. Be aware of what your co-workers need from you, as

well as how well you meet that need over the course of the day.

Sometimes when we get familiar with people, we stop considering what they need or expect from us. Consider this example. When special guests come to your home, how do you treat them? You probably go out of your way to make them feel welcome. You take care to clean the house, and when your guests arrive, you may offer them a tasty beverage and a snack. If your guests are staying overnight, you probably will prepare a comfortable place for them to sleep. You try to make sure that your guests have what they need in order to be comfortable while they are in your home. Now, do you go to all this trouble when someone you live with comes home? Probably not! Your family is familiar to you and you may not feel that you have to go out of your way to make them feel comfortable. Our families accept us as we are, right? As we get used to being around people that we work with, they become our "work family." They, too, become very familiar to us. Just like we expect our family members to be tolerant of us when we are less than perfect, we may start to expect our co-workers to do the same. We may not recognize that when we are not at our best, we may not deliver what others need or expect from us. This may make it more difficult for them to do their jobs.

The way we think about, and treat, our internal customers has a tremendous effect on our external customers. Lack of support or cooperation from your co-workers may make you feel angry or frustrated. You may end up feeling that if others are not going to give 100%, why should you? Your motivation to continue to do a good job may decrease. Sometimes unhappy employees

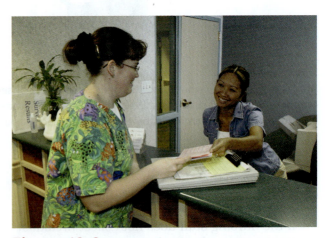

Figure 13-3
Internal customers must work together for services to flow smoothly for external customers.

speak poorly about their place of employment to others, even though this is not a professional thing to do. When internal customers show that they are not happy, external customers are not going to be happy either. Having unhappy customers, whether they are internal or external, places the entire business at risk.

DELIVERING CUSTOMER SERVICE

Customer service is all of the attention and assistance that is provided to a customer, starting with the first greeting and continuing through every point of contact thereafter. Customer service includes not only *what* you do, but also *how* you do it. Customer service (or a lack of customer service) is noticed by customers. When efforts are made to provide for positive customer experiences, good things can result. Customers who are pleased with what they experience may recommend your services to other people. On the other hand, customers who have negative experiences will probably voice their frustration to other people, which can hurt your business.

Your customers have certain basic needs and expectations. A **customer need** is a service or a product that the customer requires. A **customer expectation** is an assumption the consumer makes about the qualities or characteristics of the service or product that is being provided.

Needs and expectations will be different for each different type of customer. Table 13-1 gives examples of some of the more general needs and expectations of the customers you will be serving.

At minimum, a customer's needs and expectations must be met if the customer is going to be satisfied. For example, if you are hungry and you have limited time, you may go to a fast food restaurant to get something to eat. You need food and your expectation is that it will be fast, since that is the nature of the service at this type of restaurant. You may also have certain expectations about what the food will taste like, since you have likely eaten at this restaurant before. If you are served your sandwich quickly, and it tastes like you expect it to taste, you will probably be satisfied with your experience because your needs and expectations were met. If, however, it takes a long time for you to be served and when you receive your sandwich it is not to your liking, you will most likely be very dissatisfied with your experience. Your needs and expectations were not met.

Even if a customer's needs and expectations are met, he may not feel that anything out of the ordinary has been provided in the way of "customer service." For example, even if you were satisfied by your experience at the fast food restaurant, you probably would not go out and tell other people, "Hey, I just went to Speedy Burger. I got my hamburger quickly and it tasted just like I expected it to!" To really get customers to take notice of customer service in a positive

Table 13-1	Long-Term Care Customers' Needs and Expectations	
CUSTOMER	**NEEDS**	**EXPECTATIONS**
Resident	Housing and furnishings Food and fluids Personal assistance Medicines and treatments Support therapies	Cleanliness Comfort Competent staff Prompt care and attention to needs Courtesy and respect
Resident's family members and loved ones	Knowledge and reassurance that the resident's needs and expectations will be met Information about the resident's status	Cleanliness Comfort Competent staff Prompt care and attention to needs Courtesy and respect
Visitors	Information Assistance	Cleanliness Timely response Courtesy and respect
Co-workers	Supplies and other resources needed to perform their jobs	Clear direction Cooperation from others Courtesy and respect Acknowledgement of the job performed

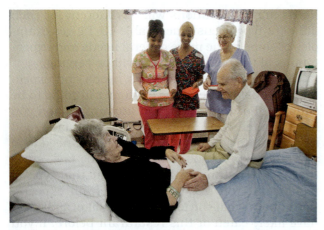

Figure 13-4
To provide truly exceptional customer service, you must go beyond simply meeting the customer's basic needs and expectations. These nursing assistants have surprised this resident and her husband by remembering and acknowledging the couple's 60th wedding anniversary!

way, you must meet their basic needs and expectations, and then go a step further. Providing something good that is unexpected is what makes the customer service you provide memorable, in a good way (Fig. 13-4). For example, Box 13-1 gives examples of different levels of service related to providing a resident with fluids. In each example, the resident has access to a beverage, but there is a significant difference in the level of service provided by the nursing assistant.

As a nursing assistant, you will have the closest contact with many of your facility's customers. How you deliver customer service can significantly impact the reputation of your facility, either in a positive or in a negative way. Customer service must be a constant effort. In a competitive market, the bar for customer service standards is constantly being raised. Customer service efforts must keep pace with what customers want. Remember, a lack of attention to customer service is still customer service. It is just bad service!

EVALUATING QUALITY

One basic expectation that most customers have is that they will receive a certain level of quality in exchange for the money they paid or the effort they put forth. **Quality** is the excellence, worth, or value of something, as perceived by the customer. Generally, the more we invest in something, the higher the level of quality we expect.

In Chapter 2, you learned about the high cost of long-term care. Remember that the average cost for nursing home care is more than $6,000.00 per month. As a result, many people spend their entire life savings on long-term care. Think about all of the hard work that goes into earning the money for a retirement "nest egg" over the course of a lifetime. For the effort it takes to earn that money, what would you be expecting in return? What level of quality care would you want for yourself, or your family member? Considering the expense and the fact that the person's quality of life is directly affected by the services provided, most of us would agree that we would want something more than just having our basic needs and expectations met. Long-term care customers want high quality and we must strive to deliver that. But what does that mean? How do we determine quality in the long-term care setting? To do this, we have to depend on feedback from our customers.

BOX 13-1 **Levels of Customer Service**

Meeting the Customer's Needs
- The nursing assistant provides a fresh pitcher of ice water at the beginning of every shift.

Meeting the Customer's Expectations
- The nursing assistant periodically checks the resident's water pitcher during the shift to see if it needs to be refilled.
- The resident uses his call light control to request a beverage and the nursing assistant brings it.

Providing Customer Service Beyond the Customer's Needs and Expectations
- The nursing assistant anticipates what the resident needs, or might like.
- The nursing assistant periodically checks the resident's water pitcher during the shift to see if it needs to be refilled.
- The nursing assistant offers the resident a favorite beverage before the resident has to ask.
- The nursing assistant is alert to the resident's usual routines and brings the resident a beverage before his favorite TV show, knowing that the resident usually asks for it at that time. The nursing assistant also offers a snack to go with the beverage, and takes the time to make sure the resident has everything he needs to enjoy his show comfortably.

OBJECTIVE EVALUATIONS OF QUALITY

You know that the government oversees long-term care to ensure that facilities deliver care according to certain standards. The government has a vested interest in the care that is provided in long-term care facilities, because the government pays for much of that care through the Medicare and Medicaid programs. Because the Centers for Medicare and Medicaid (CMS) pays for resident care, this organization is one of your customers. The CMS provides feedback to the facility on the quality of the care provided in that facility through the survey process.

Survey results help facilities to improve the quality of their services, by identifying problem areas. In addition, survey results are made available to current and potential customers through the Internet. Nursing Home Compare is a program found on the CMS web site that allows a customer to compare nursing homes according to certain indicators of quality, called **Quality Measures.** These Quality Measures are determined by analyzing the facility's resident assessment data, which is pulled from the Minimum Data Set (MDS; see Chapter 12). The data selected reflect the outcomes (results) of care provided in the facility. Generally speaking, better outcomes are associated with better practices in the delivery of care, and thus a higher level of quality.

In 2008, the government also launched a five-star rating system for the nation's nursing homes. This system is similar to the rating scales used to rate hotels and restaurants. A rating of five stars is the highest rating. A nursing home's rating is determined by reviewing its survey results, staffing numbers, and Quality Measures. Each of these areas is individually rated according to the five-star scale. In addition, an overall star rating is given as well.

Nursing Home Compare and the five-star rating scale can be helpful tools for customers. However, they do have their limitations, and nothing can replace an actual visit to the facility to form an opinion about the quality of care provided by the facility.

SUBJECTIVE EVALUATIONS OF QUALITY

Meeting the government's quality standards can be difficult, but at least these standards are specific and well defined. Meeting the quality standards of the customers we serve every day is much more complicated. While the government uses specific outcome data to measure quality, other customers use their opinions. These opinions are often based on personal experience, and sometimes even personal beliefs that may not be grounded in fact. This means that different customers will have different ideas about what determines "quality." However, when evaluating long-term care, there are some common ideas about the defining features of quality that hold true for most people. At the minimum, most people would expect a long-term care facility to deliver care according to the government's standards. In addition, many people look for evidence of personalized care and attention, which may not be reflected in the government's Quality Measures.

In your role as a nursing assistant, one of your primary responsibilities is to provide personal assistance to your residents. To begin developing standards that most people would associate with providing quality personal assistance, you can first ask yourself, "What does the customer need and expect from me, and how can I deliver what the customer needs and expects in a positive way?" Your responses may include:

- I will be well groomed and neatly dressed in a clean uniform and clean shoes.
- I will be polite, and I will address my resident in a respectful manner.
- I will ask my resident about her preferences for how care should be given, and I will honor those preferences to the best of my ability.
- I will provide my resident with all necessary and desired items for the delivery of care.
- I will protect my resident's privacy.
- I will be patient with my resident's weaknesses or disabilities, and I will not rush my resident through care.
- I will encourage and assist my resident to participate in her own care, even if I could do the task faster and easier myself.
- I will be gentle in handling my resident.
- I will help my resident look and feel her best.
- I will be careful with my resident's personal belongings.
- I will clean and straighten my resident's surroundings.
- I will make sure that my resident is safe, comfortable, and has access to the call light control before leaving the room.
- I will promptly answer any call light to respond to any resident's need.
- I will check on my resident periodically without being called to do so.

• I will always make sure that I follow proper policies and procedures to protect the safety and security of my resident.

These statements reflect standards most people would associate with providing quality personal assistance. The quality of your service can be measured by how well you meet these standards. If the customer (the resident or family) feels that you have not met these standards, the customer will probably not be satisfied. If the customer feels that you have met all of these standards, the customer may be satisfied. But if you go beyond these standards and deliver something wonderful that the customer does not expect, there is a very good chance that the customer will be extremely impressed by the quality of the care that is being provided.

Now think about the following statement:

• I will acknowledge the human value of my resident and provide caring and compassion regardless of the resident's condition or response.

Meeting this standard is often the difference between providing satisfactory customer service and providing truly exceptional customer service. This standard requires that attention be paid to the resident as a *person*. All residents, no matter their age or condition, still want to be seen and valued as unique individuals. The more you know about your residents as people, the better equipped you will be to provide care in a manner that is sensitive and personal (Fig. 13-5). When you create a caring, nurturing environment in which each resident is valued, you go beyond just meeting your customers' basic needs and expec-

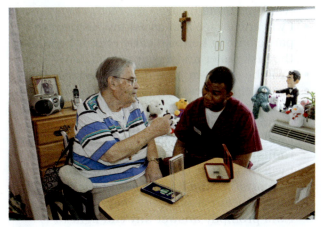

Figure 13-5
The more you know about your resident as a person, the more equipped you will be to provide personalized care.

tations. You provide customer service that is truly of the highest quality.

WHEN CUSTOMERS ARE UNHAPPY

Even if you do your very best to meet or exceed your customers' needs and expectations, not all of your customers are going to be happy. This can be upsetting, especially when you feel that you are doing your best. As you have learned, a customer's determination of quality is based largely on opinion. It is possible that different people experiencing the same service may have different opinions about the level of quality. The opinion of the customer is the reality that must be addressed. You have probably heard the expression, "The customer is always right." Good customer service is built on this concept, even if there is evidence that the customer is wrong! In the end, it is the customer's belief about his or her experience that really matters.

If you have ten customers, and nine are satisfied, but the tenth one is unhappy, you cannot disregard the tenth customer's opinion. You must be concerned about why that one customer is unhappy, because that one customer can influence a lot of other people. It is a fact that customers generally do not tell other people about an experience that was merely satisfactory. They only tell others if the service they received was remarkably good, or if they had a bad experience. So, the nine satisfied customers may never mention the service that they received, but the tenth one who is dissatisfied may tell everyone he can get to listen about his dissatisfaction! A facility can soon develop a bad reputation when negative remarks start to circulate. A bad reputation leads to the loss of customers, and threatens the ability of the facility to stay in business. Unhappy customers of long-term care facilities often file complaints with regulating agencies. Surveyors then investigate these complaints. If surveyors find that the customer complaints are valid, the facility may be found to be out of regulatory compliance. Being out of regulatory compliance can result in poor quality ratings on the government Web sites, loss of licensure, or both.

The customer who voices his complaint to someone who is in a position to improve the situation is actually of great value to any type of business. If the source of the customer's unhappiness is known, the business can take steps to remedy the situation. On the other hand, an unhappy customer who does not let the business know that he is unhappy, but instead tells other people outside of the business about the problem, is more of a danger. That organization may see a drop in business without ever understanding why.

To maintain good customer relations, businesses need to ask for feedback on how the services they provide can be improved. No complaint or comment should ever be ignored. Most long-term care facilities maintain a complaint log that lists customer complaints, the actions the facility took to investigate the complaints, and how the complaints were resolved. The complaint log helps the facility to identify areas where improvements in service are needed. It also allows the facility to monitor the number of subsequent complaints about any particular aspect of service, which is useful for tracking improvement.

DIFFICULT CUSTOMER BEHAVIORS

Some customers are difficult to please, no matter how hard we try. How do we recognize a difficult customer? When nursing assistants are asked this question, they often describe a "difficult" customer as someone who:

- Is demanding and impatient
- Complains about everything
- Constantly expresses negative thoughts and ideas
- Has no regard for the feelings or needs of others
- Is stubborn
- Will not listen
- Resists care
- Is insulting
- Is overly critical
- Has unrealistic expectations

It is a guarantee that at some time in your career, you will encounter residents, residents' family members, visitors, or even co-workers who fit this description. It is very hard to be around these kinds of people, much less to serve them and be nice while doing it. Their behaviors are a challenge to us.

Because difficult customers complain so much, we must be careful not to dismiss complaints or concerns that are actually valid. However, many times complaining about service is the difficult customer's way of dealing with a more complex issue. For example, a resident who is angry about no longer being able to live at home may find it easier to complain about everything in

the nursing home than to confront her own emotions about leaving her home. A resident who is afraid of being alone may use the call light excessively as a way of keeping people close by. You may have more patience and success with a difficult customer if you consider possible underlying reasons for the person's behavior (Box 13-2).

Even though difficult customers are "difficult," we need to be alert and attentive to the customer's discontent. If the customer's complaint is valid, we need to take steps to remedy the situation. If the difficult behaviors are a way of expressing an unmet need, we need to recognize that and make an effort to meet that need. Failure to recognize and address the person's underlying need will result in a continuation of the challenging behavior.

COMMUNICATING WITH THE UNHAPPY CUSTOMER

You have learned that communication skills are important to all aspects of health care. These skills are especially important in the delivery of customer service. You will recall that for communication to be effective, you must have a sender, a receiver, and an understood message. To provide good customer service, you must really develop your skills as a receiver. Feedback from our customers gives us important information about our customers' needs and expectations, and about the quality of our services. It is important that you hear and understand what your customers have to say. Pay attention to what your customer is saying, as well as how he is saying it.

There is no question that it is hard to respond to an unhappy customer. No one likes to hear negative comments and criticisms. Our feelings may be hurt, or we may become angry and resentful. However, it is important to remain professional and calm. To effectively handle an unhappy customer:

- **Seek a private place to have the conversation.** Providing privacy helps to regain some control over the situation. Sometimes an upset customer's behavior can get worse if an audience is present. Customer discontent can also be contagious when it is expressed in a public setting.
- **Explain to the customer that you need to step out momentarily to get your supervisor.** Do not attempt to handle an out-of-control customer alone.
- **Give the customer your undivided attention. Make full eye contact. Listen closely,**

Residents
- May not feel well
- May be upset about their health status or physical condition
- May miss their home
- May be upset about being separated from family
- May be angry with family members for bringing them to the facility
- May feel neglected
- May resent the loss of control and independence
- May be lonely and scared
- May be depressed, or grieving for recent losses
- May feel overwhelmed by being cared for by so many new people
- May not like being cared for by others
- May not like the loss of privacy

Family Members
- May be scared and uncertain about the staff's ability to meet the needs of their loved one
- May be nervous because they have heard bad things about long-term care facilities
- May feel guilty about not being able to take care of their loved one themselves
- May be over-compensating for care and attention that they did not give the resident prior to admission
- May find it difficult to watch their loved one suffer
- May be trying to maintain their loved one's sense of dignity
- May be grieving for the way their loved one used to be before the effects of age and illness
- May be in denial about the resident's condition
- May lack trust in the staff due to a previous bad experience

- May be fearful about their loved one's condition, and what it means for the future
- May be under a great deal of stress
- May have financial concerns

Visitors
- May have been given a bad first impression of the facility
- May have negative feelings about all long-term care facilities
- May feel stressed about the need to place a family member in a long-term care facility
- May not really understand the problems and conditions of the resident
- May not really understand the nature of the facility's services
- May make unrealistic comparisons to other health care settings

Co-workers
- May be unhappy about another work situation
- May be disappointed that the job did not match their expectations
- May feel a lack of support, recognition, and appreciation
- May feel that others do not work as hard
- May feel wronged by someone on staff
- May perceive unfairness among staff members
- May not be a good match for the job
- May be trying to cover up a mistake
- May feel pressured by their own job demands
- May have personal problems that are causing stress

without interrupting. It is important for you to have as complete an understanding as possible of the customer's complaint. When you give the customer your full attention, you show the customer that you care about what he is saying. Being heard and understood is vital to a customer's sense of satisfaction (Fig. 13-6). When a customer feels that he is not being heard or understood, a bad situation often becomes worse.

- **Do not try to give your view of the situation.** At this time, listening to what the customer has to say is much more important than offering your point of view.
- **Be careful not to respond negatively to what the customer is saying.** Do not

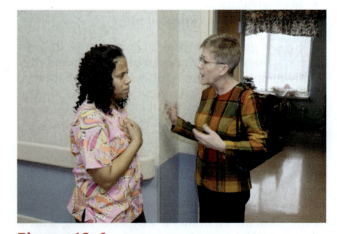

Figure 13-6
Good customer service requires good communication skills. Listening is extremely important.

become defensive, or try to convince the customer that he is wrong. Even if you do not say anything negative, your facial expression or body language could send a different message. It is important to remain calm and professional.

- **Provide appropriate feedback.** Repeat back to the customer what you have heard him say. Acknowledge the customer's complaint, as well as how the customer is feeling about it. For example, you could say, "What I am hearing is that you are very angry about the lack of attention to your mother's mouth care. Is that correct?"
- **Demonstrate empathy for the customer's point of view.** Show the customer that you can identify with, and understand, what he is going through. Examples of empathetic statements include, "I understand. If that happened to me, I would be angry, too." and "That must be very frustrating for you." These types of statements tell the customer that you understand his words, as well as his feelings.
- **Apologize for the situation.** This does not mean that you have to admit guilt, but you can certainly say, "I am so sorry that this happened." or "I am sorry that you feel that way." Keep in mind that the customer will be able to tell if your apology is sincere by your tone of voice and your body language! A sincere apology is often well received, especially

when it is followed by prompt action to correct the situation.
- **Look for a solution.** State what you will do to correct the situation, and then be sure to do it! If you are not sure what you can do, do not be afraid to ask the customer, "What can I do to make this better for you?" If you personally cannot do anything to correct the situation, be sure to put the customer in contact with someone who *can* help him. In many cases, this person will be your supervisor.
- **Make sure that the customer's concerns are communicated to all who need to know.** It is important to make sure that the same issues do not continue to occur. Customers have little tolerance for repeated occurrences of reported complaints. Make sure that your co-workers know what actions need to be taken to address the problem. Be watchful that others are doing what they are supposed to do to avoid further problems. Tactfully provide reminders when necessary, and keep your supervisor informed of any persistent problems.

Keep in mind that a dissatisfied customer can still end up being happy with the service if the problem or complaint is dealt with in a positive way. It is the way that problems are handled that is a true reflection of the facility's commitment to customer service.

SUMMARY

- As a nursing assistant, you are the closest person to many of the facility's customers. Your customer service performance will have a significant impact on the overall success of your facility.
- A customer is a person who uses a product or service. As a nursing assistant, you have external and internal customers.
  - Your external customers are people who come to your facility from the outside community, and are not part of your organization. They include your residents, their families, and all other visitors to the facility.
  - Your internal customers are your co-workers in all departments. Problems with internal customers can result in problems for the external customer. Every person's job affects someone else's job.

- Customer service is the attention and assistance that is provided to a customer. Customer service begins with the first greeting and continues through every point of contact with the customer.
  - Customer service is judged by the customer, whether or not efforts are made to provide it. If no attention is paid to customer service, the customer perceives "bad" service.
  - Meeting a customer's needs and expectations does not guarantee customer satisfaction, but failure to meet the customer's needs and expectations guarantees dissatisfaction.
  - To provide truly memorable customer service, you must strive to go beyond just meeting the customer's basic needs and expectations. In long-term care, providing

sensitive and personalized care is often the difference between merely satisfying the customer and providing a truly memorable customer service experience.

- Quality is defined by the customer. It is the customer's interpretation of the excellence, worth, or value of something for the money or energy spent.
  - The government has specific and well-defined standards for quality. Quality Measures, which come from assessment data pulled from the Minimum Data Set (MDS), are indicators of quality that are based on the outcomes of the care and services provided by the facility.
  - Individual customers are more subjective in their assessment of quality. However, many people have similar ideas about what is necessary, at minimum, to achieve quality.
- Despite your best efforts, not all of your customers are going to be happy with the service that you provide. A customer's dissatisfaction should never be disregarded, even if there is evidence that the customer is wrong.
  - Customer complaints give the business information about where efforts are needed to improve its product or service.
  - There may be many reasons for difficult customer behavior. Good communication skills, especially listening skills, are needed to really identify what is upsetting the customer.

WHAT DID YOU LEARN?

Multiple choice

Select the single best answer for each of the following questions.

1. Which of the following best defines a customer?
   a. Someone who buys a product
   b. Someone who uses a service
   c. Someone who buys or uses a product or service
   d. Someone who gets help with something

2. Which of the following people is an internal customer of a long-term care facility?
   a. A front desk receptionist
   b. A resident
   c. A physician
   d. A volunteer entertainer

3. Your co-workers are your internal customers because:
   a. they are located inside the building
   b. they depend on you to do your job effectively so that they can do their jobs effectively
   c. you get paid for serving them
   d. you are all part of the same department

4. A customer expectation is something that the customer:
   a. assumes will be provided
   b. has to have
   c. has in common with all other customers
   d. will be delighted to have

5. Customer service begins:
   a. with the first point of contact with a customer
   b. when the resident is admitted
   c. when you punch in for duty
   d. when a customer asks you for something

6. How can you determine how your customer measures quality?
   a. By reviewing the five-star rating for your facility on the Centers for Medicare and Medicaid (CMS) Web site
   b. By considering what the customer is likely to value most, with regard to the service that you are providing
   c. By noting whether or not the customer complains
   d. Quality cannot be measured

7. Which of the following communication techniques would be the least helpful in promoting a good customer relationship?
   a. Telling the customer everything that you have to do for the resident
   b. Listening carefully to what the customer is telling you
   c. Giving the customer feedback so that customer knows that you hear and understand his point of view
   d. Acknowledging the customer's emotions

STOP and Think!

- Mrs. Dempsey and Mrs. Thompson share a room in your facility. Mrs. Dempsey is a quiet, pleasant woman who rarely asks for anything and never complains. She always makes it a point to tell you how thankful she is for everything that you do for her. Mrs. Thompson is able to function much better than Mrs. Dempsey, but she complains all the time about how awful it is to be so disabled. She frequently asks for help to do things she can do herself, and when you provide help, she tells you that you are "doing it the wrong way!" What factors might explain the difference in customer satisfaction between these two roommates?

- Mrs. Stone, an 86-year-old woman, is being admitted to your facility today. She is coming from another nursing home located about 2 hours away. She had lived there for about a year because it was close to the house that she had shared with her husband. Mrs. Stone's husband passed away last month. Now Mrs. Stone's daughter is moving Mrs. Stone to your facility so that she will be able to visit her mother more frequently. Mrs. Stone arrives on your unit at about 1:15 PM, and you are assigned to help with her admission. As your customer, what does Mrs. Stone need? What do you think she would expect? Is there anything that you could do when you assist with the admission that might *delight* Mrs. Stone?

Nursing Assistants Make a Difference!

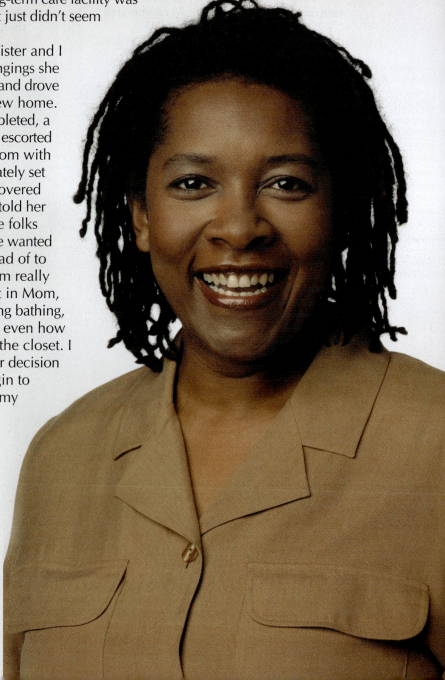

"My mother has spent her life taking care of everyone she knows. She still fusses over me and my little sister, even though we are grown now. And she took care of Dad, who couldn't even pick out the right pair of socks to wear with his slacks to church on Sunday mornings, until the day he died. She was always the first neighbor to arrive with a casserole when a new baby was born, or a pot of chicken soup when someone was sick. Now, Mom is the one who needs to be cared for.

Recently, Mom has fallen a few times. The last time, my sister found her at the bottom of the steps, where she had been lying with a broken arm for over two hours! We knew then that the time had come. Mom either needed to come live with one of us or move to a long-term care facility where she would have the help she needed.

Mom would not even discuss living with either of us, because she insisted that she would feel like a "burden," so we visited several long-term care facilities in the area. There was one that Mom liked over all the others, and we were able to make arrangements for her to move in. Although moving to a long-term care facility was Mom's choice, I still felt horribly guilty. It just didn't seem right to have strangers caring for Mom.

Soon, "Moving Day" arrived. My sister and I packed Mom and the few personal belongings she had chosen to take with her into the car, and drove to Lake View Nursing Center, Mom's new home. After the admission paperwork was completed, a nursing assistant named Anita met us and escorted us to Mom's room. It was a beautiful room with a view of the nearby lake. Anita immediately set about making Mom comfortable. She covered the bed with Mom's favorite afghan and told her that she would contact the maintenance folks to get her pictures hung up just where she wanted them. She talked to Mom directly, instead of to me and my sister, which I could tell Mom really appreciated. Anita took such an interest in Mom, asking her about her preferences regarding bathing, what types of food she liked to eat, and even how she preferred her clothes to be hung in the closet. I could tell that Mom was pleased with her decision to move to Lake View, and I cannot begin to tell you how relieved that made me and my sister feel! It's funny— in many ways, Anita has many of the same qualities as my Mom. It's nice to know that Mom will finally be able to relax and let someone care for her, in the same way that she cared for so many others."

You can listen to more stories about how nursing assistants make a difference on the CD in the front of your book.

MAINTAINING A SAFE AND COMFORTABLE ENVIRONMENT

The long-term care facility is your residents' home and your workplace. As a nursing assistant, you will play a very important role in making sure the facility environment is safe and comfortable for your residents. You will also need to take measures to keep yourself and your co-workers safe while you are at work. Maintaining a safe and comfortable environment is the focus of Unit 4.

Photo: A nursing assistant helps a resident to walk safely.

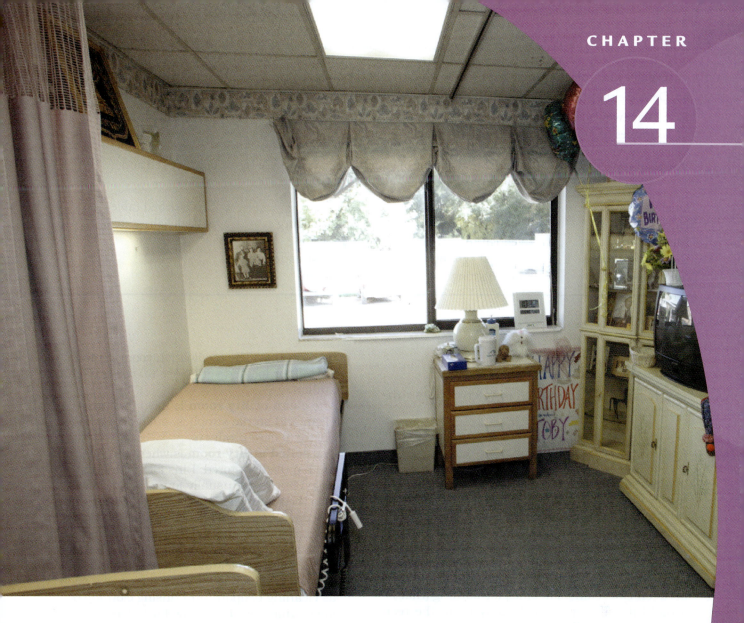

The Resident's Environment

WHAT WILL YOU LEARN?

In this chapter, we will take a closer look at the physical environment in a long-term care facility, and how that environment can affect a resident's well-being. We will also provide an overview of the standard equipment and furniture that is typically found in a resident's room. When you are finished with this chapter, you will be able to:

1. Describe the long-term care environment and the types of rooms or areas that you might find.
2. Discuss the importance of encouraging residents to have and display personal items.
3. List the Omnibus Budget Reconciliation Act (OBRA) regulations relating to the physical environment in long-term care facilities.

Photo: Residents of long-term care facilities are encouraged to make their rooms as "home-like" as possible.

4. Explain your role in helping to keep the resident's environment clean and comfortable.

5. Describe the standard equipment and furniture found in a resident's room in a long-term care facility.

6. Explain why adapting the environment to meet the individual resident's needs is important, and give examples of modifications that can be made.

Vocabulary Use the CD in the front of your book to hear these terms pronounced and defined:

Unit	Hopper	Gatches	Over-bed table
Nurses' station	Nourishment room	Trendelenburg's	Call light system
Medication room	Ventilation system	position	
Clean utility room	General lighting	Reverse Trendelenburg's	
Soiled utility room	Task lighting	position	

THE RESIDENT'S UNIT

The resident's living space is referred to as the resident's **unit.**

NURSING HOMES

In a nursing home, the term "unit" is used to refer to the individual resident rooms, which may be private or semi-private (shared with someone else), as well as common areas that are used by all of the residents as part of their living space. Resident rooms may be equipped with private bathrooms, or shared bathrooms that are located between two rooms. Facilities for bathing (that is, a bathtub, shower, or both) may be in the resident's private bathroom, or in a communal tub room located on the unit. Common areas on the unit generally include a dining room, an activity room, a television lounge, and a small living room or lounge that can be used by residents and their visitors. A shared courtyard, patio, or garden area may also be available so that residents can enjoy a pleasant outdoor setting (Fig. 14-1).

In addition to resident living spaces, the unit also includes areas for staff use:

- The **nurses' station** serves as the central base of operations for the nursing staff. Staff members use the nurses' station to complete documentation and other paperwork, receive and make telephone calls, and monitor activity on the unit. The nurses' station is usually centrally located on the unit because staff members must be able to see hallways and other resident areas from the station.
- The **medication room** is used to store medications and the supplies for administering

medications. The medication room is often part of, or located very close to, the nurses' station.

- The **clean utility room** is used to store clean and sterile supplies, such as packaged personal care products.
- The **soiled utility room** is where dirty items are handled or stored. Bins for trash and soiled linens are usually found here. This is also the room where used equipment (such as a bedside commode) is placed until it can be cleaned and disinfected. Soiled utility rooms often have a **hopper,** a sink-like fixture that flushes like a toilet and is connected to a sewer line. The hopper is used for tasks such as cleaning bedpans and rinsing clothing or linens that have been soiled with feces.

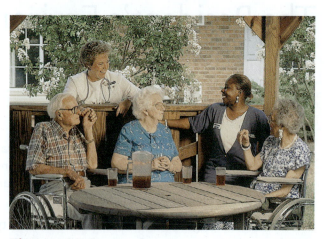

Figure 14-1

The living spaces in long-term care facilities are designed to enrich the daily lives of residents. These residents are enjoying nature and the opportunity to socialize in this pleasant outdoor space. (© *Will & Deni McIntyre/Photo Researchers, Inc.*)

- The **nourishment room** is where snacks and beverages are stored and prepared for residents. The nourishment room is equipped with a refrigerator and freezer for items like milk, juice, and ice cream. Other basic equipment usually includes a microwave, toaster, coffee maker, and ice machine. Many facilities keep a selection of fruits, cookies, crackers, cereal, and beverage supplies (such as tea bags, hot chocolate mix, and creamer) here for resident use as well. Supplies for serving snacks (such as cups, spoons, and straws) are also kept in the nourishment room.

ASSISTED-LIVING FACILITIES

In assisted-living facilities, the word "unit" usually refers to the individual resident's living quarters. Residents of assisted-living facilities often live in small apartments that have a kitchen or kitchenette, a bathroom, a living area, and a bedroom. Some units may also provide private access to a balcony or patio. As in a nursing home, bathing facilities (a tub, shower, or both) might be included in the resident's private bathroom, or they may be located down the hall and shared by many residents. Communal bathing rooms are equipped with privacy stalls or curtains to allow several residents to bathe at the same time.

Many of the same areas for staff use that are found in the nursing home setting are present in the assisted-living setting as well. However, these areas are usually not as prominent, because residents of assisted-living facilities do not require the same level of nursing and medical care. For example, while nursing homes must have a prominent nurses' station on each unit, an assisted-living facility may have only one health center or nursing office in the building.

FOSTERING A HOME-LIKE ENVIRONMENT

Have you ever moved to a new house or apartment? If so, you probably remember how strange the place felt, until you managed to get some boxes unpacked and make it your own. After you had added your own personal touch, even if it was just to hang a picture, then the place probably felt more like "home." For a person who is entering a long-term care facility, whether for a temporary stay or for the rest of his or her life, the idea of "home" takes on a whole new meaning. Suddenly, "home" may only be one room, or even half of one room, and everything the person has associated with "home" is gone, except for perhaps a few select items. Items that were never part of the person's home environment before, such as special beds and medical equipment, may now be present.

For most people, moving into a long-term care facility represents a major change. To ease the transition, residents of long-term care facilities are encouraged to furnish their rooms with one or two favorite pieces of furniture and various personal items (Fig. 14-2). Many residents bring their own bedspreads or comforters to make up the standard facility bed. They may have their own clothing, jewelry, books, and favorite wall hangings. Some residents bring a television, a stereo, or even a personal computer to their new home, and many have a private telephone line installed in their rooms so that they can keep in touch with loved ones and friends. You may see plants, drawings from grandchildren, and maybe even a small pet, such as a bird or a fish, in your residents' rooms!

Although the long-term care facility is a health care facility, it is also the resident's home. OBRA requires that the facility provide a home-like environment that reflects the individuality of each resident and minimizes the institutional nature of the setting to the best extent possible. OBRA regulations protect each resident's right to personalize his or her living space, and to have and to use personal items.

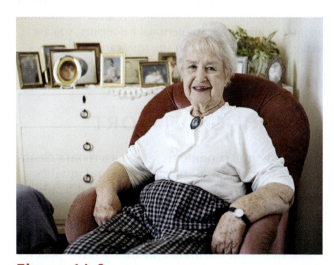

Figure 14-2
Residents are encouraged to personalize their rooms with decorative items and one or two personal pieces of furniture. This helps to foster a home-like environment.

Personal items help to create a living space that is as home-like as possible for the resident, and foster the resident's sense of independence and individuality. You should help your residents to decorate their rooms according to their own individual taste and preference, while making sure that they stay within the safety standards established by OBRA and your facility.

Helping Hands and a Caring Heart

FOCUS ON HUMANISTIC HEALTH CARE

Our homes are decorated with things that have special meaning to us. In the same way, many of the items a resident chooses to bring to a long-term care facility will hold special meaning. You can learn a lot about your residents by looking at the items they choose to display in their living spaces. You may notice items in a resident's room that represent the resident's cultural background, spiritual beliefs, or mementos from a career or a hobby. Take an interest in these things. Ask the resident to tell you about them. This lets the resident know that you care about him as an individual.

Always respect a resident's personal items as if they belonged to you. Remember that even a small scrap of paper can be very precious to a resident, especially if it is a note from someone the person loves. While you may consider a resident's personal things quite a bit of clutter, especially if you have to help keep these things neat, remember that each one of those items represents a piece of that person's life. When you show respect for, and take an interest in, a resident's personal belongings, you are letting the person know that you truly care for him.

ENSURING COMFORT

Environmental conditions, such as a room's cleanliness, temperature, noise level, and quality of light, affect how we feel. Imagine what it would be like if you were confined to bed in a dirty room, or one that smelled bad or was too hot or too noisy or too dark. To enhance the comfort and well-being of residents, long-term care facilities have policies designed to regulate the environment within the health care facility. In assisted-living facilities, state law may set policies related to the environment. In nursing homes, these policies are set by

OBRA regulations. The following aspects of the environment are regulated by OBRA:

- The size of the room
- The lighting that must be available
- The temperature at which the facility must be maintained
- The measures that must be taken to maintain air quality
- The measures that must be taken to control noise
- The types of furnishings and equipment that must be present
- The types of modifications to the room that must be present to ensure safety (such as handrails and a call light or intercom system in the bathroom)
- The minimal amount of personal space for storage of belongings that each resident is allowed to have
- The ability to provide privacy for each resident

CLEANLINESS

Cleanliness is essential for controlling the spread of infection and odors. In addition, a facility's cleanliness and overall appearance is something that residents, as well as their family members and other visitors, notice. The appearance of the facility is a reflection on the quality of service provided. To make a good impression, a facility does not need to be new or filled with state-of-the-art equipment, but it does need to be kept clean and neat.

Each member of the health care team is responsible for keeping the facility clean (Fig. 14-3). The housekeeping or custodial staff does major, routine cleaning of the facility (such as mopping floors, emptying waste containers, and cleaning bathrooms). However, if you notice something out of place, then it is your responsibility to correct the problem. For example, if you notice something spilled on the floor or a countertop, you should wipe it up. If you see a piece of trash on the floor, you should pick it up and dispose of it properly. If you notice that there is an ongoing problem, such as wastebaskets not being emptied or bathrooms not being cleaned properly, you should report this observation to the nurse, so that she can follow up with the appropriate people.

Nursing assistants are responsible for helping residents to keep their personal belongings neat and clean. We all have the tendency to accumulate things over time. Periodically, you may have to help your residents go through their belongings and either put them away neatly, or dispose of them.

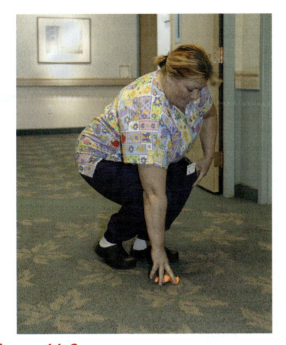

Figure 14-3
Keeping the facility neat and clean is the responsibility of each member of the health care team.

Excessive clutter makes it difficult to keep the room clean and can be a safety hazard. Residents, visitors, or staff members can trip over objects left in pathways. An excessively crowded room can also make it difficult to exit the room safely and quickly in the event of an emergency, such as a fire.

ODOR CONTROL

There are many potential sources of bad odors in a long-term care setting. The smell of urine, feces, vomit (emesis), or wound drainage can make any environment unpleasant! However, there are things you can do to help minimize odors and maintain a pleasant environment:

- Follow your facility's policy regarding the handling of waste and soiled linens.
- Keep the lids on laundry and waste receptacles closed.
- Empty and clean emesis basins, urinals, bedside commodes, and bedpans promptly.
- Use a facility-approved air freshener when appropriate.
- Assist your residents with routine personal care. Clean skin and good oral hygiene are essential for controlling odors.
- Pay attention to your personal hygiene (see Chapter 3). Scented products, such as

cologne, aftershave, or perfume, can be nice, but they must be used sparingly. If you apply too much, the scent may be overpowering, and many people are sensitive to strong scents. If you are a smoker, be aware that the odors from smoking can cling to your clothes and hair and are considered unpleasant by many people. Make sure you wash your hands after smoking and use a mint or breath freshener before continuing your resident care duties.

VENTILATION

A **ventilation system** provides fresh air and keeps air circulating. A well-functioning ventilation system is essential for carrying away unpleasant odors, for keeping the air from seeming stale, and for preventing rooms from feeling stuffy. However, good ventilation systems can also create drafts (chilly currents of air), especially near the circulation vents. Elderly people and people who are ill may become easily chilled and may require an extra blanket, a sweater, or a lap robe to stay warm (Fig. 14-4). Also, be sure to position chairs and beds so that your resident is not in a drafty area. For example, avoid placing furniture and wheelchairs right underneath a circulation vent.

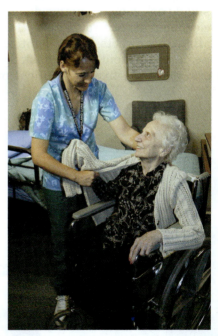

Figure 14-4
Although good ventilation is essential for health and comfort, elderly residents and residents who are ill often "catch a chill." Provide additional layers as needed, and be sure to position residents away from drafts created by the ventilation system.

ROOM TEMPERATURE

Most people prefer a room temperature that is somewhere between 68°F and 74°F. However, people who are ill, elderly, or relatively inactive may prefer a warmer room temperature. OBRA regulations require the temperature in a long-term care facility to be kept between 71°F and 81°F. Although this temperature may seem quite warm to you, especially when you are moving around and busy with your daily duties, remember that the temperature regulations are intended to ensure the comfort of the people you care for.

LIGHTING

There are two major types of lighting used in the health care setting: general lighting and task lighting. Usually, both lighting types are used in a single room. **General lighting** provides overall illumination (light), allowing a person to see and move about safely. Sunlight is one common source of general lighting. Usually the general light provided by an uncovered window is supplemented by light from a ceiling fixture. Many people prefer to have the drapes or blinds covering the windows in a room opened during the day, to allow natural light in. Some older people are very sensitive to glare, and may prefer drapes or blinds to be closed during the day. You should ask each of your residents what he or she prefers, and act accordingly (Fig. 14-5).

Task lighting directs bright light toward a specific area. In a resident's room, task lighting is usually provided by a fixture mounted over the head of the bed. Some of these fixtures provide both general and task lighting with dual switches. The resident uses task lighting for activities such as reading, needlework, or doing a crossword puzzle. You will use task lighting when providing resident care, so that you can see clearly while carrying out the procedure. The focused illumination provided by task lighting will also help you to notice changes that should be reported to the nurse, such as a change in a person's skin tone or a new rash.

Lighting helps us to orient ourselves to the time of day. If a resident prefers to have his blinds or drapes closed during the day and the overhead light fixture is in constant use, he may find it difficult to tell the difference between day and night. During the evening and night hours, overhead lights should be dimmed, and the use of bright task lighting should be kept to a minimum. These measures help residents maintain orientation to the time of day.

NOISE CONTROL

Long-term care facilities can be such busy, noisy places! Imagine that you are a resident in a nursing home. It is about 11:30 in the morning and there is a lot of activity. The telephone is ringing at the nurses' station. Here comes the man with the cart carrying the food trays up from the kitchen. You know he is coming because his cart has a squeaky wheel. A nurse and a nursing assistant are having a conversation in the hallway about what needs to be done that afternoon. A resident down the hall, who is a little bit hard of hearing, has the volume turned all the way up on his television set. He is watching a talk show, and every once in awhile, you can hear the audience clapping. Several visitors are going down the hallway and they are laughing and talking as they go. A radio is playing somewhere. You are not feeling very well, and you wonder if things will ever quiet down enough for you to get some rest!

Although a certain level of noise in a busy place is to be expected, too much noise can affect the comfort of residents. A quiet environment promotes rest and sleep and aids healing. OBRA regulations require long-term care facilities to take measures to control noise. As a nursing assistant, there are many things you can do to help minimize noise and maintain a pleasant environment:

- Encourage residents to use headsets or earphones if the volume they need to hear the radio or television is disturbing to other residents.

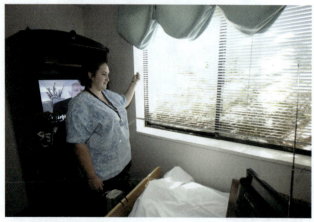

Figure 14-5
Some residents prefer to have the blinds or drapes opened during the day to let in the sunlight. Others prefer a darkened room and will want to have the blinds or drapes drawn. Always ask the resident about his or her preference.

- Answer telephones promptly.
- Report noisy equipment that needs to be adjusted or oiled.
- Be aware of the volume of your voice.

During the evening and night hours when residents are sleeping, it is especially important to take precautions to minimize noise.

FURNITURE AND EQUIPMENT

The furniture and equipment that is considered "standard" for a resident's room will differ according to the facility and to the specific needs of the resident. To ensure your own safety, as well as that of your residents, you must make sure that you know how to operate and adjust any furniture and equipment that is considered standard in the facility where you work. The furniture and equipment described in this section would be considered standard for a typical room in a nursing home. In a facility that offers specialized care (for example, a rehabilitation center or dementia care unit), items considered standard might vary from this list.

BEDS

An adjustable bed, commonly referred to as a hospital bed, is used in most health care settings (Fig. 14-6). The frame of an adjustable bed can be raised or lowered, moving the entire bed either further away from, or closer to, the floor. This helps health care workers maintain good body mechanics when performing care procedures. It also helps the resident to get into or out of the bed. The mattress platform on an adjustable bed can also be positioned in a variety of ways to keep the resident comfortable. Sometimes, the doctor will order a specific mattress position for a resident.

The mattress platforms of most adjustable beds have joints at the hips and knees, which allow the mattress to "break." These joints are called **gatches,** after Willis Gatch, the surgeon who developed the first bed that was adjustable at the hips and knees. The hip gatch raises the person's upper body to a semi-sitting position (Fowler's position). The knee gatch raises the person's knees to help prevent the person from sliding toward the end of the bed while in the Fowler's position. In addition to having hip and knee gatches, most adjustable beds permit the mattress to be "tilted" without bending the person at the waist. In **Trendelenburg's position,** the foot of the mattress is raised so that the person's head is lower than her feet. Trendelenburg's position is sometimes used for a person who has gone into shock and has a very low blood pressure, to encourage blood flow to the heart. In the **reverse Trendelenburg's position,** the head of the mattress is raised so the person's head is higher than her feet. The reverse Trendelenburg's position may be ordered for a person who is recovering from a spinal cord injury or back surgery.

Adjustable beds are adjusted either electrically, using control buttons located on or near the side rails, or manually, using a system of cranks located at the foot of the bed (Fig. 14-7). One advantage of electrically operated beds is that the control buttons are located in a place that is accessible to the resident, as well as to staff members. When using an electrically operated bed, remember that it is a piece of electrical equipment. Appropriate safety precautions should be taken when operating it to avoid electrical shock (see Chapter 17). When using a manually operated bed, remember to fold the cranks down and away under the bed after you are finished using them, so that people who are walking near the foot of the bed do not bump into them.

In addition to being adjustable, adjustable beds usually have two other features that regular beds do not—side rails and wheels (casters). The side rails on a bed are raised to help prevent a person from falling out of the bed. Some of your residents may want to have one of the side rails raised so that they can use it as an assistive device for repositioning. The resident can grab the side rail and use it to reposition himself in bed or to get up. Side rails are used according to the person's individual care plan.

Wheels make the bed easier to move from place to place, which is sometimes necessary when a resident who cannot get out of bed needs to be moved from one part of the facility to another. Wheels are also useful when it is necessary to move the bed to clean underneath it. The wheels have locking devices that are used to keep the bed steady and prevent it from rolling. Always make sure the bed's wheels are locked, unless you are moving it (Fig. 14-8)! A person could be injured while getting into or out of the bed if the bed shifts out from underneath him. Additionally, you may be injured if the bed suddenly shifts away from you while you are providing care to a resident.

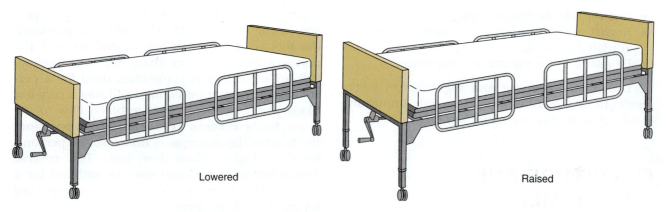

Lowered

Raised

The bed can be moved up or down in terms of distance from the floor.

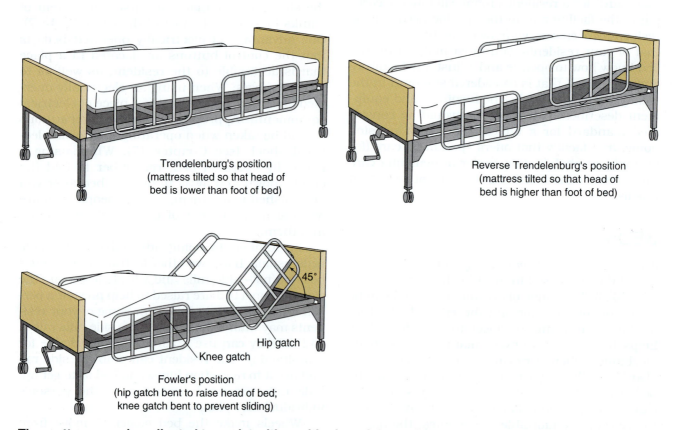

Trendelenburg's position
(mattress tilted so that head of
bed is lower than foot of bed)

Reverse Trendelenburg's position
(mattress tilted so that head of
bed is higher than foot of bed)

45°

Hip gatch

Knee gatch

Fowler's position
(hip gatch bent to raise head of bed;
knee gatch bent to prevent sliding)

The mattress can be adjusted to assist with positioning of the resident.

Figure 14-6

Most beds used in health care settings are adjustable, both in terms of their height from the floor
and the position of the mattress.

In some cases, you may care for a resident who is in a regular bed, instead of an adjustable bed. For example, some assisted-living facilities allow people to bring their own beds from home, if they prefer. When you are caring for a resident in a regular bed, you can use blocks to elevate the head of the bed. Positioning devices, such as pillows shaped to support a person in a sitting position, are available to help achieve the other positions.

CHAIRS

A resident's room should be furnished with one or two chairs. Many residents will bring a favorite chair or two from home. These chairs may recline or have a rocking action that the person finds very comfortable. Some residents with disabilities require special chairs, such as geri-chairs or chairs with special lifting devices that help the person to get in and out of the chair easily.

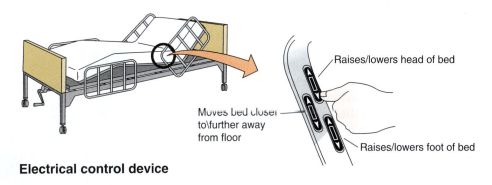

Electrical control device

Raises/lowers head of bed

Moves bed closer to\further away from floor

Raises/lowers foot of bed

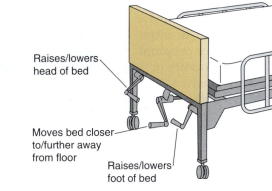

Raises/lowers head of bed

Moves bed closer to/further away from floor

Raises/lowers foot of bed

System of cranks

Figure 14-7
Adjustable beds may be adjusted electrically using a control device on the frame of the bed, or manually using a system of cranks at the foot of the bed.

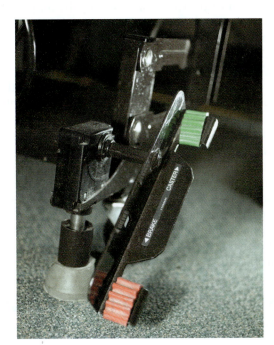

Figure 14-8
Wheel locks help to prevent unintentional movement of the bed. There are different types of wheel locks. In the type shown here, the red pedal locks the wheel, and the green pedal unlocks it.

OVER-BED TABLES

Most long-term care facilities furnish resident rooms with **over-bed tables,** which fit over the bed or a chair and can be raised or lowered as needed (Fig. 14-9). You will use the over-bed table to hold basins and other articles when providing

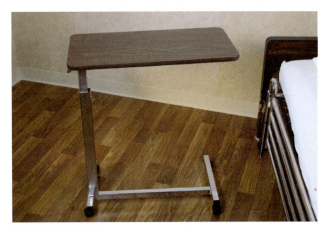

Figure 14-9
The over-bed table fits over the bed or a chair.

personal care for a resident. The resident may use the over-bed table as a surface for writing a letter, or for eating a meal or snack. The over-bed table is also an excellent place to keep a water pitcher or any other items the resident may want close by. Because the over-bed table is considered a "clean" area, items placed there should be either sterile or clean. One way to help remember this is to consider the over-bed table the resident's dining room table—you would never place dirty items, such as bedpans or soiled linens, there.

STORAGE UNITS

Various types of storage units are used to house a resident's belongings. A bedside table is often placed next to the bed and used to store personal care items. Most bedside tables have drawers or a combination of drawers and closed shelves. The person's toothpaste and toothbrush, lotion, soap, deodorant, and other personal care items are usually stored in the top drawer, while basins, bedpans, and other care equipment are stored neatly underneath in the lower drawers or shelves. The telephone, a flower arrangement, and other personal items may be placed on top of the bedside table (Fig. 14-10).

Additional storage for a resident's personal items may be provided in the form of a closet, a wardrobe, or a chest of drawers. OBRA regulations require long-term care facilities to provide each

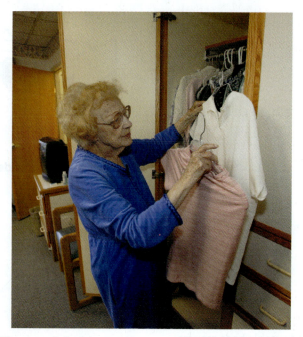

Figure 14-11
The resident's closet is considered private, personal property.

resident with enough storage space for her clothing and other personal items. The resident must have free access to this storage space and the items it contains. Because the resident's closet, wardrobe, or chest of drawers is considered private, personal property, you must have the resident's permission to remove items from it (Fig. 14-11).

Occasionally, you will need to inspect a resident's personal storage area. For example, you may suspect that a resident is keeping something in the storage area that is not permitted, such as food. Food can spoil and may attract insects and rodents. In this situation, you would be permitted to inspect the personal storage space, but first you must inform the resident of your intent to do so, and the search must be conducted in the resident's presence. If you must carry out an inspection of a resident's personal storage space, it may be a good idea to have another staff member present during the inspection to verify that you acted appropriately and within the regulations.

CALL LIGHT AND INTERCOM SYSTEMS

Residents must have a way of communicating with the health care staff at all times. Most health care facilities have a **call light system,** which residents can use to alert a staff member that they need help. Many also have an intercom

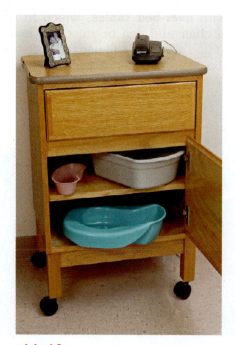

Figure 14-10
Personal care items are usually stored in the bedside table.

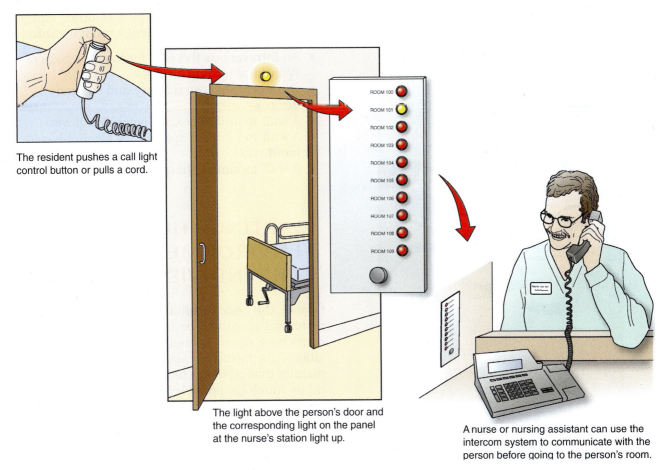

The resident pushes a call light control button or pulls a cord.

The light above the person's door and the corresponding light on the panel at the nurse's station light up.

A nurse or nursing assistant can use the intercom system to communicate with the person before going to the person's room.

Figure 14-12
Residents use the call light system to alert staff members when they need help. Staff members can use the intercom system to communicate with the resident before going to the resident's room.

system, which allows staff members to speak to a resident in his room from the nurses' station.

A call light system consists of a call light control (usually either a cord that is pulled or a hand-held button device), a light in the hall (over the doorway of the resident's room), and a panel of lights at the nurses' station or some other central location. When the resident pulls the cord or pushes the button on the call light control, the light over the doorway blinks, the light on the panel at the nurses' station lights, and a bell sounds, alerting the staff that the resident needs help. A staff member who is at the nurses' station can then use the intercom system to communicate with the resident in his room to find out what the resident needs before going to the room (Fig. 14-12). Newer systems connect the call light and intercom systems into individual headsets worn by staff members, leading to better communication between residents and staff members, as well as reduced noise levels on the unit.

When the resident is in his room, the call light control must always be within his reach,

whether he is in bed or in a chair. If the resident is seated in a common area where a call light control is not available, he should be provided with a hand bell and shown how to use it (Fig. 14-13). An unconscious resident will not be able to call for help and should be checked on very frequently. It is also important to note that a resident who is hearing impaired will have difficulty communicating with an intercom system. The resident will not be able to understand what you are saying, so remember to respond in person to a hearing-impaired resident's calls. Answer all requests for assistance promptly, even though it can be frustrating to respond to numerous requests from any particular resident, especially when you are very busy. Sometimes residents who use the call light system excessively are feeling scared and lonely. What they are really seeking is reassurance that if a problem actually does occur, someone will come quickly to their aid. Part of helping to meet a resident's safety and security needs is your quick response to a request for help.

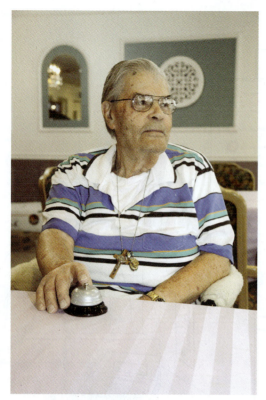

Figure 14-13
If the resident is seated in a common area where a call light control is not available, ensure that there is some other method for the resident to get your attention, such as a hand bell.

PRIVACY CURTAINS AND ROOM DIVIDERS

Each resident room will have privacy curtains (which are usually hung from the ceiling) or room dividers. The privacy curtain should be closed, or a room divider used, when you are providing care for your residents. The door to the room should also be closed, because the privacy curtains do little to keep voices and other sounds private. OBRA regulations require long-term care facilities to use privacy curtains or room dividers to protect the privacy of each resident.

Pay attention to the cleanliness of privacy curtains or room dividers. Although the privacy curtains or room dividers are cleaned routinely, they are not cleaned every day. Report any stains to the proper person so that the privacy curtain or room divider can be cleaned or replaced, as needed.

OTHER EQUIPMENT

Depending on the care the resident requires or the design of the facility, other equipment may be present in the room. Examples of other equipment you may see in a resident's room include:

- An intravenous (IV) pole for hanging bags of IV fluid or feeding formula
- Outlets for oxygen delivery and suction devices
- A wall-mounted box of disposable gloves
- A wall-mounted dispenser for alcohol-based hand rub
- A wall-mounted sharps disposal box

ADAPTING THE ENVIRONMENT TO THE INDIVIDUAL

Overall, the basic furniture and equipment in each resident's room will be the same. However, residents have many different needs. Per OBRA regulations, the facility is expected to provide care in a manner that promotes independence. Being able to do as much as possible independently helps the resident to reach the important goal of attaining (or maintaining) her highest level of function and well-being. Environmental factors can get in the way of the resident functioning at her best. The resident's environment can and should be adapted as necessary to suit the resident's individual needs and to promote independence, safety, and comfort. For example:

- The hanging rod in a closet may need to be lowered so that a resident in a wheelchair can independently remove articles of clothing from the closet.
- An elevated seat can be installed on a toilet to make it easier for a resident who has difficulty sitting down and standing up to use the toilet independently.
- For a person with visual problems, a white toilet in a bathroom with light walls and a light floor may tend to "disappear." A toilet seat in a color that contrasts with the bathroom floor and walls can help a resident with visual problems identify the toilet more easily.
- Placing signs on dresser drawers to identify the contents of each drawer can help a resident with dementia find what he is looking for without opening all of the drawers. Similarly, a picture of a toilet on the bathroom door may help the resident remain independent in toileting for a period of time.

- A "low bed" (that is, a bed that is specially designed to lower to a height that is very close to the floor) is useful for residents who may roll out of bed or get out of bed without calling for assistance when needed. For example, a resident with dementia may not remember or recognize the need to call for help. Because the bed is so low to the floor, the risk for serious injury as a result of a fall from the bed can be minimized.
- A resident who is very petite may benefit from a low bed and a chair that is lower than a standard chair, so that she can get in and out of them safely. Similarly, a pediatric (child-sized) wheelchair may be safer and more comfortable for the person.
- A resident who is very large or obese may also need special furniture and equipment to promote comfort and safety. For example, bariatric beds and wheelchairs are designed and constructed to meet the comfort and safety needs of an obese person. (*Bariatrics* is the branch of medicine that specializes in the treatment of obesity.)

As you are helping your residents with their care, it is important for you report any environmental barriers to their comfort and independence that you see. Share your observations with the nurse and other team members. Together, you may be able to find a creative solution to the resident's challenges!

Be Smart About Surveys!

Surveyors will take note of how well the environment supports the resident's ability to function at his or her best. To help your facility remain without survey problems in this area:

- Keep the environment clean and neat.
- Arrange items that the resident uses frequently in a way that allows the resident easy and convenient access to them.
- Make sure that the resident always has a call light control or other means of signaling the staff for help within easy reach. Answer calls for help promptly.
- Adjust lighting to meet the resident's needs for comfort and safety. Make sure the resident has a focused task light for close work, such as reading or needlework.
- Be alert to the special needs of residents who may have difficulty in the environment due to their size or level of function. Report your observations to the nurse so that the resident's special needs can be accommodated.

SUMMARY

- A unit is the resident's living area. In nursing homes, the "unit" includes individual resident rooms, common spaces for resident use, and work areas for the staff. In assisted-living facilities, the word "unit" is usually used to refer to the resident's private living quarters.
- Because the long-term care facility is the resident's home, it is important to foster a home-like environment. One way to do this is by encouraging residents to have and display items that have personal meaning to them. OBRA requires nursing homes that receive government funding to provide a "home-like" environment.
- The physical environment of a health care facility contributes to a resident's overall comfort, health, and well-being. Nursing homes that receive federal funding must

follow OBRA regulations concerning the physical environment of the resident's room.

- A clean environment is essential for odor and infection control. In addition, many people judge a facility according to its level of cleanliness.
  - All members of the health care team are responsible for providing a clean and comfortable environment for residents.
  - Nursing assistants are responsible for helping residents keep their rooms neat and clean.
- Odor control is achieved by promptly removing and cleaning dirty emesis basins, urinals, bedpans, and linens. Assisting residents with bathing and brushing their teeth also helps to prevent odors.

- Good ventilation helps carry away unpleasant odors and prevents stale air. It is important to protect your residents from becoming chilled as a result of the drafts created by the ventilation system.
- The temperature of a resident's room should be maintained between 71°F and 81°F.
- Adequate light must be provided for all activities that take place in a resident's room.
  - General lighting, such as that provided by sunlight or an overhead ceiling fixture, provides overall illumination.
  - Task lighting focuses bright light on one particular area.
- Efforts must be made to keep noise levels on the unit down. Too much noise interferes with a resident's ability to rest.
- Most resident rooms contain the same basic furniture and equipment.
  - All resident rooms contain a bed. In most cases, the bed will be an electrically or manually operated adjustable bed.
  - All resident rooms contain at least one chair, to accommodate a visitor and to provide a "change of scenery" for the resident. Many residents in long-term care facilities bring a favorite chair from home to furnish their rooms.
  - Over-bed tables fit over the bed to provide a work surface for both the resident and the health care worker. The over-bed table is considered a "clean" area.
  - Personal care items, such as toiletries, are usually stored in the bedside table.
  - A closet, wardrobe, or chest of drawers is used to provide private storage space for the resident's personal belongings.
  - Call light and intercom systems are used for communication.
    - The call light system allows residents to signal that they need help.
    - The intercom system allows staff members to communicate with the resident before going to the resident's room.
  - Privacy curtains or room dividers are used to help maintain a resident's privacy when care is being given.
- The environment should be adapted as necessary to help each resident remain as independent as possible, and to ensure comfort and safety.

WHAT DID YOU LEARN?

Multiple Choice

Select the single best answer for each of the following questions.

1. How should a resident's room look?
   a. Functional and sparsely decorated
   b. Like a hospital room
   c. As home-like as possible
   d. Like a hotel room
2. You show respect to a resident when you:
   a. Knock before entering his or her room
   b. Close the door and pull the privacy curtain when you are providing care
   c. Handle the person's personal belongings with care
   d. All of the above
3. The nurse tells you that Mr. Haskill's bedside table is looking a little bit disorderly, and asks you to clean it up a bit. You should:
   a. Search the shelves for hidden food and throw anything that you find away

   b. Remove the bedpan and washbasin, because these items do not belong there
   c. Straighten the items on the top of the table and on the shelves, removing any dirty items so that they can be cleaned and returned
   d. All of the above
4. Which regulations state that a resident's unit must be clean, safe, orderly, and free of obstacles in the pathway?
   a. Occupational Safety and Health Administration (OSHA) regulations
   b. Omnibus Budget Reconciliation Act (OBRA) regulations
   c. Medicare regulations
   d. Medicaid regulations

5. One of your residents has returned to the facility from the hospital following back surgery. The nurse asks you to position his bed so that the head of the bed is elevated. The resident's body needs to remain flat against the mattress. What position would the nurse tell you to put the resident in?
   a. Reverse Trendelenburg's position
   b. Fowler's position
   c. Prone position
   d. Trendelenburg's position
6. You are working in a nursing home. As you are preparing Mrs. Everly for bed, she tells you that she is feeling a bit hungry because she did not really eat much at dinner. She asks you if she can have some graham crackers and a glass of milk. Knowing that Mrs. Everly does not have any dietary restrictions, how should you respond to Mrs. Everly?
   a. You should tell Mrs. Everly that you are sorry, but the kitchen has closed for the evening. You will ask the nurse to notify the kitchen to have graham crackers available for her in the future.
   b. You should tell Mrs. Everly that you will go to the nourishment room and get a snack for her.
   c. You should tell Mrs. Everly that you will check to see what supplies are available for her snack in the clean utility room.
   d. You should tell Mrs. Everly that snacking in the room is not allowed because crumbs could attract bugs. You will be glad to assist her back to the dining room for a snack.
7. How can you help to control unpleasant odors in the workplace?
   a. Empty emesis basins promptly
   b. Assist your residents with skin care and oral hygiene
   c. Use facility-approved air fresheners, as necessary
   d. All of the above

Matching

Match each numbered item with its appropriate lettered description.

_____ 1. Side rails
_____ 2. Resident unit
_____ 3. Over-bed table
_____ 4. Task lighting
_____ 5. Bariatric bed

a. The resident's pitcher and meal trays may be placed here
b. Light source that can be directed to a specific area
c. Special bed for a very heavy person
d. The resident's living space in the long-term care facility
e. Used to prevent a person from falling out of bed and as an assistive device

STOP and Think!

- One of your residents, Mrs. Grant, is complaining that she is cold, even though you are feeling a bit too warm. What are some measures that you can take to help make Mrs. Grant more comfortable?
- Mrs. Tinetti is a new resident at the nursing home where you work. She is 86 years old, and still able to walk on her own with the help of her walker. Mrs. Tinetti is only 4'1" tall and weighs 96 pounds. You notice that she seems to have a great deal of difficulty getting out of her bed and her chair. When she is seated on either one, her feet do not touch the floor. You see her struggling to get out of bed and go over to offer her assistance. She accepts the assistance, but she snaps that this just should not be. She has always prided herself at being able to do for herself, despite her age. She does not want to lose that just because she has moved into this facility! What can be done to help Mrs. Tinetti maintain the independence that she is so proud of?

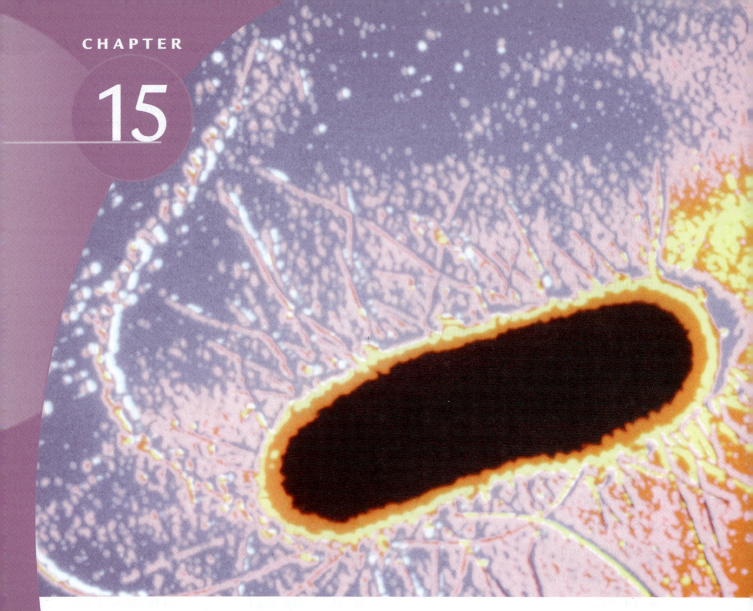

Communicable Disease and Infection Control

WHAT WILL YOU LEARN?

Communicable diseases are diseases that can be spread from one person to another. There are many factors that come together in the health care setting to make it easy for communicable diseases to spread. In this chapter, you will learn how to minimize these factors, so that you can protect yourself, your family members, your residents, and your co-workers from catching a communicable disease. You will also learn about the causes of communicable disease, and the ways communicable diseases are spread from one person to another.

Photo: Escherichia coli, *a microbe that can cause disease. Color was added to this photograph, which was taken with a special microscope (a tool that is used to see things that are not visible to the naked eye).* (© Howard Sochurek/CORBIS.)

After all, it is hard to protect yourself and others from communicable disease if you do not know what causes it or how it is spread! When you are finished with this chapter, you will be able to:

1. List the different types of "germs" (microbes) that cause disease and discuss the conditions that are essential for their survival and growth.
2. Define the terms *normal flora* and *pathogen*.
3. Explain the defense mechanisms the body uses to keep us from getting sick.
4. Define the term *infection* and describe the chain of events required for infection to occur.
5. List factors that can make a person more likely to get an infection.
6. Define the term *health care–associated infection (HAI)* and discuss ways a person could get an infection within the health care system.
7. List the four major methods of infection control.
8. List the four techniques of medical asepsis.
9. State how personal protective equipment (PPE) is used in infection control.
10. List the standard precautions that are taken with every resident.
11. Describe the three types of transmission-based precautions and explain when they are used.
12. Demonstrate proper handwashing, gloving, masking, gowning, and double-bagging technique.

Vocabulary Use the CD in the front of your book to hear these terms pronounced and defined:

Communicable disease	Methicillin-resistant	Health care–associated	Personal protective
Microbe	*Staphylococcus aureus*	infections (HAIs)	equipment (PPE)
(microorganism)	(MRSA)	Nosocomial infections	Isolation precautions
Normal (resident) flora	Vancomycin-resistant	Infection control	Standard precautions
Pathogens	enterococcus (VRE)	Cross-contamination	Transmission-based
Opportunistic microbes	Infection	Medical asepsis	precautions
Colonies	Chain of infection	Sanitization	Airborne precautions
Aerobic	Contaminated	Antisepsis	Droplet precautions
Anaerobic	Fomite	Disinfection	Contact precautions
Endospore	Vector	Sterilization	
Antibodies	Virulence	Transient flora	

WHAT IS A MICROBE?

A **microbe,** also called a **microorganism,** is a living thing that cannot be seen with the naked eye. Many (but not all) microbes consist of just one cell. (To give you an idea of how small a cell is, consider that it is estimated that the adult human body is composed of approximately 50 million cells!) Microbes are found in the air, in the soil, in water, in food, and in and on the bodies of plants and animals, including humans.

Most microbes cause no harm and are actually essential for healthy living. For example, some of the microbes that live in the human digestive tract help us to get certain vitamins from the foods that we eat. Others help to maintain an environment that is unfriendly to harmful microbes. The harmless microbes that help the human body to function properly are called **normal (resident) flora.**

Some microbes, however, can cause illness and are known as **pathogens.** Sometimes microbes can be considered normal flora in one part of the body and pathogens in another. For example, *Escherichia coli* is a microbe that normally lives in our large intestines, where it is harmless. However, when *E. coli* finds its way out of the intestine and into another part of the body where it is not normal flora, such as the bladder, it can cause an infection. These types of microbes are called **opportunistic microbes.** Given the chance, opportunistic microbes can change from harmless to pathogenic.

There are many different types of microbes that live and prosper among us. Microbes can

Table 15-1   Types of Microbes

	TYPE	EXAMPLES OF COMMONLY CAUSED INFECTIONS
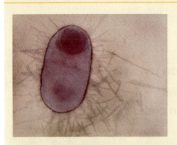	Bacteria	"Strep throat," urinary tract infections, abscesses, tuberculosis (TB), bacterial meningitis, Lyme disease, Rocky Mountain spotted fever, syphilis
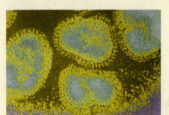	Viruses	HIV/AIDS, hepatitis, fever blisters, common cold
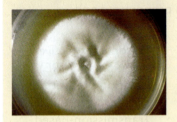	Fungi	Ringworm, "athlete's foot," vaginal yeast infections (candidiasis), oral yeast infections (thrush)
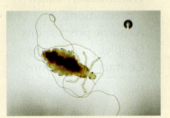	Parasites Insects	Scabies, pediculosis (lice)
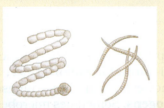	Helminths (worms)	Pinworm infestation
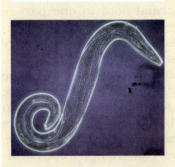	Protozoa	Malaria, amebic dysentery

Top to bottom: *Lester V. Bergman/CORBIS. © Ron Boardman; Frank Lane Picture Agency/CORBIS. © Lester V. Bergman/CORBIS. © Mike Buxton; Papilio/CORBIS. © Lloyd Birmingham/Custom Medical Stock Photo. © Lester V. Bergman/CORBIS.*

generally be classified as bacteria, viruses, fungi, or parasites (Table 15-1).

BACTERIA

Bacteria cause many of the infections you will encounter in the health care setting. Many scientists believe that bacteria lived on Earth long before any other life forms. Bacteria have been found in polar ice caps, as well as in deep cracks in the ocean floor. The ability of bacteria to adapt to all sorts of environments is proof of this life form's ability to survive.

Most bacteria consist of only one cell, and reproduce by dividing in half. Although bacteria usually consist of only one cell, they often group together to form **colonies.** Scientists classify and name bacteria in many different ways:

- By their shape
- By the way they arrange themselves in a colony
- By the way they stain (how they react to the dye scientists use to make microbes more visible under a microscope)

For example, round bacteria are called *cocci*, rod-shaped bacteria are called *bacilli*, and spiral-shaped bacteria are called *spirilla* (Fig. 15-1). Bacterial colonies may consist of pairs of bacteria (indicated by the prefix *diplo-*), chains of bacteria (indicated by the prefix *strepto-*), or grape-like clusters of bacteria (indicated by the prefix *staphylo-*). So, what would you know if you saw the word *Staphylococcus aureus* on a person's medical record? You would know that this person had an infection caused by a round bacterium (-*coccus*) that arranges itself in clusters (*Staphylo-*)! There are thousands of types of bacteria and not all of them are named using this method. However, this example illustrates how you can learn the meaning of a word that might be unfamiliar to you by taking it apart. In Appendix B, "Introduction to the Language of Health Care," you can learn about many more prefixes, suffixes, and roots that are used to form words commonly used in the health care setting.

Bacteria, like all other living things, have certain basic requirements for survival. These requirements vary, according to the type of bacteria. For example, some bacteria, called **aerobic** bacteria, need oxygen to live. Others, called **anaerobic** bacteria, die if oxygen is present. Most bacteria that can cause illness need a warm, moist, dark environment and a source of nutrition in order to grow—requirements the inside of the human body meets perfectly! Some types of bacteria can surround themselves with a hard shell, called an **endospore,** and enter a state of inactivity. If the inactive bacterium's best growing conditions become available, the bacterium will become active again. Because of their protective endospores, these types of bacteria are very difficult to kill using the standard techniques described later in this chapter. Examples of illnesses caused by bacteria that form endospores include tetanus (lockjaw) and botulism (food poisoning).

Bacteria are the most common cause of infection in the health care setting. Some common illnesses caused by bacteria include "strep throat" (caused by *Streptococcus pyogenes*), some bladder infections (such as those caused by *E. coli*), and some skin infections (such as those caused by *S. aureus*). Several types of small, rod-shaped bacteria are transmitted by ticks and fleas and cause diseases such as Rocky Mountain spotted fever and typhus. Bacteria are also responsible for some types of pneumonia and some infections of the reproductive system.

VIRUSES

Viruses, the smallest of all microbes, can only be seen using a special kind of microscope, called an electron microscope. Viruses are not even complete cells—they are just small bundles of protein. Because viruses are not complete cells, they cannot carry out normal cellular activities, such as reproduction, by themselves. Instead, they must take over a host cell, usually a plant or animal cell. Once inside the host cell, the virus uses the host cell's "machinery" to make copies of itself. Eventually, the virus and all of its copies (called *progeny*) break through the host cell's wall, killing the host cell and freeing the viruses to infect other, neighboring host cells. Many illnesses are caused by viruses, including the common cold, fever blisters (caused by herpes simplex virus), chickenpox (caused by varicella zoster virus), hepatitis, and acquired immunodeficiency

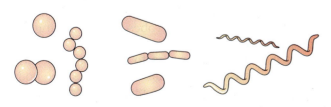

A. Cocci (spheres)   **B.** Bacilli (rods)   **C.** Spirilla (spirals)

Figure 15-1
Bacteria can be spherical, rod-shaped, or spiral-shaped.

syndrome (AIDS, caused by human immunodeficiency virus, or HIV).

FUNGI

Fungi are a group of plant-like organisms that scientists have classified together because of certain characteristics, including the make-up of their cell walls. Not all fungi are microscopic—for example, mushrooms are a type of fungus! Other types of fungi you may be familiar with include yeasts (such as the yeast that is used to make bread rise and beer foamy) and molds (such as the mildew that grows inside a shower stall or the growths that appear on bread and cheese if left too long). Many fungi help us (or, at least, do not harm us). However, some fungi are capable of causing illness. If you have ever had ringworm (caused by *Tinea corporis*), athlete's foot (caused by *Tinea pedis*), thrush (a yeast infection in the mouth), or candidiasis (a vaginal yeast infection), then you have been the victim of a fungus!

PARASITES

Parasites live in or on a host, such as a plant or animal, and use that host for food and protection. Some parasites can be transmitted from one person to another through physical contact. For example, scabies, an itchy skin condition, is caused by a mite that burrows under the skin. Pediculosis (lice) is caused by wingless insects that live on the scalp or body and feed on the host's blood. Both scabies and lice are often seen in the health care setting. Other parasites are transferred from one person to another through feces or blood.

Helminths, a type of parasite, are worm-like organisms that live in the human body (as well as the bodies of other animals). Examples of helminths include pinworms, tapeworms, and roundworms. Although the way these organisms are transmitted from one host to another varies, transmission usually involves eating or inhaling the worm eggs, which then grow in the host's digestive tract. The mature worms produce eggs or larvae of their own, which are then passed out of the host's body with the feces. Once the eggs reach the outside world again, they are free to be eaten or inhaled by another host, and the life cycle of the helminth continues.

Protozoa, another type of parasite, are said to be "animal-like" because they can take in food. Protozoa cause illnesses such as malaria (transmitted by the bite of a mosquito) and amebic

dysentery (a type of diarrhea caused by drinking water contaminated with protozoa).

DEFENSES AGAINST COMMUNICABLE DISEASE

THE IMMUNE SYSTEM

Many, many microbes share the Earth with us. If microbes are everywhere, and some of them can make us sick, then why aren't we always sick? The answer to this question lies in the body's immune system, the wonderful defense system that protects us from infection. Some of the body's defenses are non-specific, which means that they help to protect us from all pathogens. Other defenses are specific, which means that they help to protect us only from certain pathogens.

NON-SPECIFIC DEFENSE MECHANISMS

Our main non-specific defense mechanism is healthy, intact skin and mucous membranes. Skin that is without cuts, scrapes, or wounds physically prevents pathogens from entering the body. In addition, the natural lubricants on our skin contain substances that help to prevent the growth of pathogens. Mucous membranes line all of the organ systems that come in contact with the outside world (the respiratory, digestive, urinary, and reproductive systems). The special cells of the mucous membranes secrete mucus, a sticky substance that creates a physical barrier by trapping and destroying pathogens. Keeping the skin clean helps to reduce the number of pathogens on the skin. Good oral hygiene and drinking plenty of fluids helps to keep mucous membranes functioning properly. These are important measures to take for yourself, as well as for your residents. Stomach acid (which kills many of the microbes contained in the food that we eat), tears (which contain a substance that kills microbes), and the acts of coughing and sneezing (which remove inhaled microbes) are also non-specific defense mechanisms that prevent microbes from "setting up shop" in our bodies.

If a pathogen manages to get past these first lines of defense and an infection results, the body activates a general immune response that helps to fight off the infection. Blood vessels around the site of the infection dilate (widen), allowing more blood flow to the area. The increased blood flow brings more oxygen and nutrients to the tissues, along

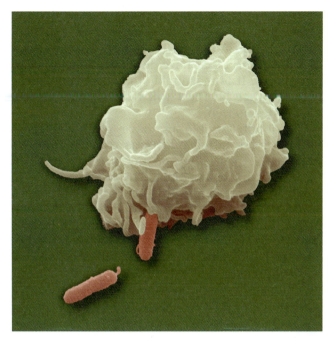

Figure 15-2
In this photograph, a white blood cell (*white*) is killing a pathogen (*red*) by eating it. This is a process called phagocytosis (*phago-* means "eat" and *cyt-* means "cell"). (*SPL/Photo Researchers, Inc.*)

with large numbers of white blood cells (leukocytes). White blood cells destroy pathogens that invade the body, either by eating them (Fig. 15-2) or by secreting substances that cause them to die. The increased blood flow causes the infected area to become red, warm, swollen, and painful (Fig. 15-3). A person who is fighting off an infection may have a high body temperature (fever). If

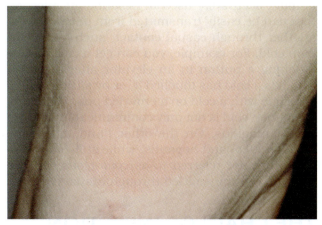

Figure 15-3
The site of infection is typically hot, red, swollen, and painful. This means the body's general immune response is at work! (*Custom Medical Stock Photo.*)

you remember, most pathogens prefer a nice, normal body temperature. The fever helps to destroy the pathogens and is a normal response for many infections.

As a nursing assistant, it is important for you to watch for signs of infection in your residents. Many residents may not be able to communicate that they do not feel well or that they have pain. Some infections, if not treated at an early stage, can be very dangerous for people. If one of your residents has signs or symptoms of an infection, the doctor may order a diagnostic test, called a *culture and sensitivity*, to find out which microbe is causing the infection and which medication is best suited to fight it. The culture and sensitivity may be performed on urine, wound drainage, or other body fluids or substances.

TELL THE NURSE

Possible signs of infection that should be reported to the nurse immediately include:

- An increase in body temperature
- A rapid pulse, a rapid respiratory rate, or changes in blood pressure
- Pain or difficulty breathing
- Redness, swelling, or pain
- Foul-smelling or cloudy urine
- Pain or difficulty urinating
- Diarrhea or foul-smelling feces
- Nausea or vomiting
- Lack of appetite
- Skin rashes
- Fatigue
- Increased confusion, disorientation, or a change in usual behavior
- Any unusual discharge or drainage from the body

Specific Defense Mechanisms

The body's non-specific defense mechanisms, including physical barriers and the general immune response, are one way our immune systems help us to prevent and fight off infections. The immune system also has the ability to develop specialized proteins called **antibodies,** which help our bodies to fight off specific pathogens. A person develops antibodies following exposure to the pathogen. This exposure may come from a previous infection with the pathogen, or through a vaccination (shot). For example, the antibodies that build up in the body following a case of measles or chickenpox are the reason most of us only get these "childhood diseases" once. Similarly, when you get your annual "flu shot," what you are getting is a dose of the virus strains that cause the flu. The viruses have been killed, so that you do not actually get sick, but the exposure is enough to cause your immune system to begin producing antibodies against those particular strains of the virus. That way, if you are exposed later, you will be immune.

ANTIBIOTICS

Many times, our immune systems can fight off invading pathogens on their own. Other times, some outside help is required. An *antibiotic* is a drug that is able to kill bacteria or make it difficult for them to reproduce and grow. The first antibiotic, penicillin, came into widespread use during World War II, and completely changed how we treat infectious disease. Today, there are many types of antibiotics, used to treat many different types of bacterial infections. Antimicrobial agents (used to treat fungal and parasitic infections) and antiviral agents (used to treat some viral infections) are other medications that we use to treat infection.

Antibiotics and other medications used to treat infection are not always effective against all infections. Bacteria, as you will recall, are very adaptable organisms that have been around since the beginning of time. As such, some bacteria have used their ability to change to develop resistance to the antibiotics used to fight them. This means that the antibiotics that used to work against these bacteria no longer work. Two types of bacteria, **methicillin-resistant Staphylococcus aureus (MRSA)** and **vancomycin-resistant enterococcus (VRE),** have become resistant to two of the most powerful antibiotics we have invented to date (methicillin and vancomycin).

S. aureus and enterococci are common microbes. *S. aureus* is often found on a person's skin and is transmitted easily through person-to-person contact. Enterococci are commonly found in a person's digestive tract and are transmitted through contact with feces. In a health care setting, these pathogens can be very dangerous because many residents do not have healthy immune systems and, therefore, are less able to fight off infection. If infection occurs, it is difficult to treat because these microbes have become resistant to the medications used to treat them in the past. MRSA and VRE are well-known examples of bacteria that have developed resistance to antibiotics. It is reasonable to expect that in the future, other bacteria will become resistant to antibiotics as well.

Although antibiotics have given us more options for treating infectious disease than we had in the past, they do not work against all pathogens all of the time. The best policy is to avoid infection in the first place. You can keep your immune system strong and healthy through proper nutrition, adequate rest, and regular exercise. You can also take steps to limit your exposure to pathogens. In the next few sections, we will look at how pathogens are spread from one person to another, and what you can do to help control their spread.

COMMUNICABLE DISEASE AND THE CHAIN OF INFECTION

An **infection** is an illness caused by a pathogen (a microbe that can cause illness). Infections can be local (affecting a small, defined area of the body), generalized (affecting a general area or an organ), or systemic (affecting the entire body). Many, but not all, infections are communicable, which means that they can be transmitted from one person to another, either directly or indirectly. Sometimes the terms *communicable* and *contagious* are used to mean the same thing, but the two terms are not truly synonymous. *Contagious* is more accurately used to describe an infection that can be easily transmitted from one person to another through casual contact, such as a common cold. For example, you can get a cold just by touching a button in an elevator after a person who has a cold has touched it, or by sitting next to someone with a cold on a crowded bus. Therefore, a common cold is not only communicable, but it is also contagious. On the other hand, infections such as AIDS and hepatitis, while still communicable, are not referred to as *contagious* because they are not transmitted through casual contact.

THE CHAIN OF INFECTION

For a person to get a communicable infection, six key conditions must be met. These six key elements are known as the **chain of infection** (Fig. 15-4).

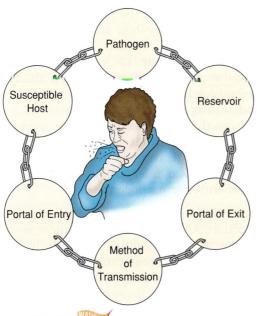

Figure 15-4
The chain of infection. For a person to get an infection, all six links in the chain must be present.

Pathogen

A *pathogen* must be present.

Reservoir

A *reservoir* must be present. A reservoir is a place where something is stored. In this case, a reservoir is a place where a pathogen can survive. Pathogens collect in the reservoir, and sometimes, they multiply there as well. Possible reservoirs include humans and other animals, food, water, milk, and objects that come in contact with an infected person's secretions or body fluids.

Portal of Exit

A *portal of exit* must be available. The word *portal* means "door." The portal of exit is the way the pathogen leaves the reservoir. The way a pathogen leaves its reservoir varies, depending on the type of pathogen and the reservoir. For example, when the reservoir is a human being, common portals of exit for pathogens include:

- The digestive tract (through feces, saliva, or vomitus)
- The respiratory tract (through mucus)
- The genitourinary tract (through urine, semen, or vaginal secretions)
- The skin (through blood, pus, or other drainage from wounds)

Method of Transmission

A *method of transmission* must be available. After the pathogen leaves its reservoir via the portal of exit, it must have a way of physically getting from one person to another. This is called the pathogen's method of transmission, and it may be direct or indirect.

- Direct transmission requires close contact between an infected and a non-infected person. Pathogens can be directly transmitted when a non-infected person touches an infected person, or inhales or ingests droplets exhaled by the infected person (for example, when that person coughs, talks, or sneezes).
- Indirect transmission occurs when a non-infected person comes into contact with a non-living object that has been **contaminated** (soiled) by pathogens. These objects are called **fomites.** For example, a water glass or a bed sheet can become a fomite if it becomes contaminated by pathogens from a person with an infection, because if a non-infected person uses the contaminated water glass or sleeps on the contaminated bed linens, he could become infected (Fig. 15-5).

Other pathogens, such as the protozoan that causes malaria, are transmitted by way of a **vector,** or a living creature (in the case of malaria, a mosquito). Some pathogens can be transmitted by more than just one method.

Portal of Entry

A *portal of entry* must be available. Now that the pathogen has left its reservoir and been successfully transmitted to another person, it must have a way of entering the new person's body. The respiratory, urinary, digestive, and reproductive

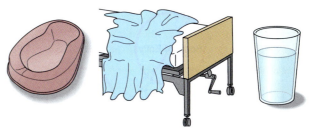

Figure 15-5
Pathogens can live on objects such as linens, bedpans, and drinking glasses. When an uninfected person touches or uses these items, he might pick up some of the pathogens on them and become sick. Non-living objects that are capable of transmitting disease are called fomites.

systems are common portals of entry. So are breaks in the skin. A pathogen can leave one person's body and be transmitted to another person, but if the pathogen is not able to enter the new person's body, infection will not occur.

Susceptible Host

Finally, a *susceptible host* must be available. Microbes that can cause infection enter the human body continuously. The defense systems of the body, both those we are born with and those we acquire (such as vaccines), can fight off most of these pathogens. However, many factors can place us at risk for infection. This is when the pathogen "makes its move." Risk factors that make a person more likely to get an infection include:

- **Very young or very old age.** The very young and the very old are more likely to get an infection. The young have not had time to develop effective defenses for fighting infections, and the elderly lose their defenses as they age.
- **Poor general health.** A person who is sick or debilitated ("worn down") is more at risk for infection because the body's defenses are already weakened by illness. Therefore, the person is not able to fight off the pathogen as easily. Additionally, certain medical treatments, such as chemotherapy or radiation

therapy, can affect the functioning of the body's immune system and put a person more at risk for infection.
- **Stress and fatigue.** Lack of rest and emotional stress can affect the body's ability to defend itself from pathogens.
- **Indwelling medical devices.** Medical devices that are placed inside the person's body, such as urinary catheters, feeding tubes, and intravenous (IV) lines, increase a person's risk of infection by providing a portal of entry for pathogens.

Many of your residents will have risk factors for infection. As you have learned, most residents of long-term care facilities are elderly people. Most have one or more chronic health conditions. Others may be recovering from an acute illness or a recent surgery. All of these conditions place them at increased risk for getting an infectious disease. A major part of your responsibility in caring for other people involves protecting them from infection.

BREAKING THE CHAIN OF INFECTION

The chain of infection can be broken by taking away just one of the six required elements (Fig. 15-6). For example, taking the right antibiotic for a bacterial

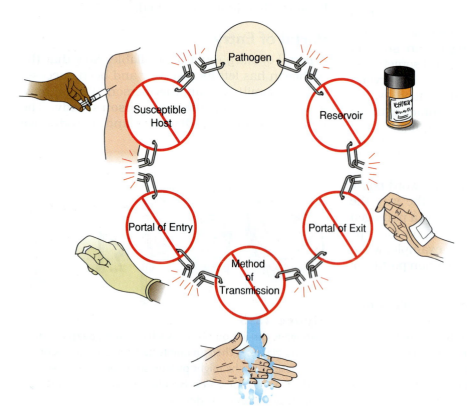

Figure 15-6
The chain of infection can be broken by removing just one of the six elements that must be present for infection to occur.

infection quickly turns a person's body into an unfriendly reservoir for bacteria. Covering an infected wound with a dressing eliminates a pathogen's portal of exit by containing the pathogen within the dressing. Washing your hands and making sure that linens, utensils, glassware, and other possible fomites are properly cleansed eliminates a method of transmission. Wearing gloves and keeping your skin healthy and intact removes one potential portal of entry available to pathogens. Receiving required immunizations and maintaining general good health make you a less susceptible host. All of these actions break a link in the chain of infection, stopping the infection from being transmitted. Other factors that determine whether or not an infection will be transmitted are the **virulence** (strength or disease-producing potential) of the pathogen and the actual number of pathogens that enter the body.

INFECTION CONTROL IN THE HEALTH CARE SETTING

Health care–associated infections (HAIs) are infections that people get while they are in the hospital or other health care setting. A patient or resident can get an HAI while she is receiving care. Or, a health care worker can get an HAI while providing care. Infections acquired by patients or residents while they are in a health care facility are also called **nosocomial infections**. The most common method of transmission for HAIs, including the very dangerous VRE, is on the hands of health care workers.

All health care facilities follow basic practices that are designed to decrease the chance that an infection will be spread from one person to another. These practices are called **infection control.** Failing to follow proper infection control procedures can lead to cross-contamination. **Cross-contamination** occurs when microbes are transferred from one person to another on the hands of a health care worker or through contact with a fomite. For example, cross-contamination can occur when equipment shared by more than one resident is not cleaned properly between uses, or when personal care products are used for more than one resident.

There are four major methods of infection control—medical asepsis, surgical asepsis, barrier methods, and isolation precautions.

MEDICAL ASEPSIS

Medical asepsis involves physically removing or killing pathogens, and is primarily achieved through processes involving soap, water, antiseptics, disinfectants, or heat. The goal of medical asepsis is to remove pathogens from surfaces, equipment, and the hands of health care workers.

Four Techniques of Medical Asepsis

There are four techniques that make up the practice of medical asepsis: sanitization, antisepsis, disinfection, and sterilization (Fig. 15-7):

- **Sanitization** is the word we use to describe practices associated with basic cleanliness, such as handwashing, cleansing of eating utensils and other surfaces with soap and water, and providing clean linens and clothing. Sanitization practices physically remove microbes, thereby preventing their spread. General guidelines for maintaining a sanitary environment are given in Guidelines Box 15-1.
- **Antisepsis** takes sanitization one step further, by actually killing microbes or stopping them from growing. An antiseptic is a chemical that is capable of killing a microbe, or preventing it from growing. Antiseptics can be used on the skin or other surfaces to kill pathogens. Rubbing alcohol and iodine are common antiseptics used on the skin to prevent infection. Many soaps used in the health care setting now contain an antiseptic agent as well.
- **Disinfection** involves the use of stronger chemicals to kill microbes. The chemicals used for disinfection are too strong to be used on the skin. Instead, disinfectants are used to clean non-living objects that come in contact with body fluids or substances such as bedpans, urinals, and tray tables.
- **Sterilization** is the most thorough method of killing microbes. Sterilization is used on objects that must be completely free of any pathogens, such as surgical instruments, hypodermic needles, or intravenous (IV) catheters. These objects must be sterilized because they are placed in the patient's or resident's body. Therefore, they can act as portals of entry for microbes. Items are sterilized either by placing them in an autoclave (a machine that uses pressurized steam heat to kill pathogens) or by soaking them in chemicals that destroy all microbes. Although covering items in boiling water will kill most microbes, boiling is not an effective method of sterilization.

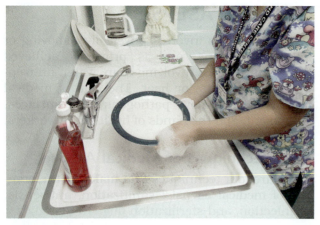

A. Sanitization

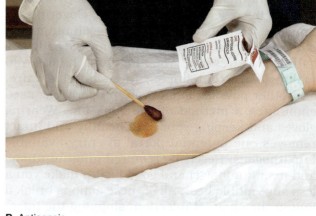

B. Antisepsis

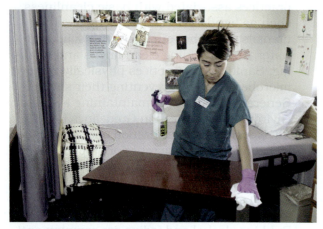

C. Disinfection

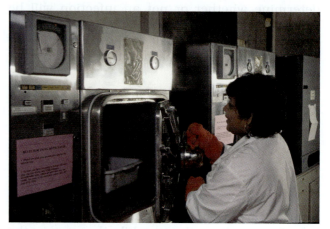

D. Sterilization

Figure 15-7

There are many approaches to medical asepsis, a general term used to describe techniques used to remove or kill microbes. **(A)** Sanitization is physically removing microbes from surfaces. **(B)** Antisepsis involves the use of agents that kill microbes or slow down their growth, such as iodine (Betadine) or rubbing alcohol. **(C)** Disinfection also involves the use of agents that kill microbes. Because disinfectants are strong chemicals, disinfection is used only to clean non-living objects. **(D)** Sterilization involves the use of pressurized steam heat or very strong chemicals to kill microbes. (**D**, © Wedgwood/Custom Medical Stock Photo.)

Before disinfecting or sterilizing an object, the object must be cleaned first using basic sanitization methods. The chemicals used to disinfect or sterilize an object cannot work properly unless the surface to be disinfected or sterilized is clean and free of any organic material (material from a living organism such as blood, urine, or feces). Organic materials contain fats and proteins that coat the surface of the object, much like an egg yolk coats the surface of a plate. If the plate is not washed with detergent and warm water before the egg yolk dries, the hardened yolk becomes very difficult to remove. The same principle applies to dirty bedpans, urinals, and other pieces of equipment—if the piece of equipment is not washed first using

soap and water, any organic material that is present can harden, making it difficult for the disinfectant or sterilization agent to kill the microbes underneath the dried material. Therefore, equipment must be properly cleaned using basic sanitization methods before moving on to disinfection or sterilization.

Handwashing

As a nursing assistant, the technique of medical asepsis that you will use most frequently is handwashing. According to the Centers for Disease Control and Prevention (CDC), *handwashing is the single most important method of preventing the*

Guidelines Box   15-1   Guidelines for Maintaining a Sanitary Environment and Preventing Cross-Contamination

WHAT YOU DO	WHY YOU DO IT
Wash your hands after contact with any body fluid or substance, whether it is your own or another person's. Examples of body fluids and substances include blood, saliva, vomitus, urine, feces, vaginal discharge, semen, wound drainage, pus, mucus, and respiratory secretions.	Pathogens often leave the body through the gastrointestinal tract, genitourinary tract, respiratory tract, or breaks in the skin. In addition, some pathogens are transmitted in blood and other body secretions, such as breast milk.
Wash your hands frequently, especially after using the bathroom; before handling food, drink, or eating utensils; and before and after any contact with a resident.	Frequent handwashing eliminates a method of transmission for microbes.
Cover your mouth or nose with a tissue when you cough or sneeze, and teach your residents to do the same. Dispose of tissues properly by placing them in a waste container.	Some microbes are transmitted in particles of saliva or sputum. Covering your nose or mouth with a tissue contains these particles and helps to prevent the spread of infection.
Provide each resident with his or her own personal care items (such as toothbrushes, combs, and brushes) and personal care supplies (such as toothpaste, soap, and deodorant). Make sure each resident's personal care items and supplies are labeled with the resident's name and room number. Never share personal care items or supplies among residents.	These items can act as fomites. Therefore, it is better to limit their use to one person.
Keep contaminated or dirty items, such as soiled linens, away from your uniform.	Microbes can be transferred from the dirty item to your uniform, which can then act as a fomite.
When cleaning, take care not to stir up dust. For example, wiping dusty surfaces with a damp cloth or mop helps prevent the movement of dust and lint into the air. Do not shake linens when making beds.	Dust can act as a fomite and carry microbes from one area to another.
Dispose of trash properly.	If not disposed of properly, trash can provide an ideal environment for microbial growth, especially if the trash contains food or other materials susceptible to rotting.
Follow established procedures for preparing dirty linens and clothing for the laundry.	Soiled linens and clothing act as fomites and must be handled in a way that will lessen the chance of someone else coming in contact with the contaminated item.
Maintain good personal hygiene, and help your residents to do the same. Bathing, washing hair, brushing teeth, and wearing clean clothing are all grooming practices that help prevent the spread of infection.	Personal grooming practices help to reduce the number of microbes present on the skin.

spread of infection. This is true in the "real world," as well as in the health care setting. However, in the health care setting, handwashing takes on a special importance because the chance of picking up a pathogen and passing it on to someone else is greater than in normal, everyday life. In addition, many of the people who are in health care facilities are less able to handle an infection, should they get one. The easiest way to protect yourself, your residents, and your co-workers is to be conscientious about washing your hands!

Before you move from one resident's room to another, you must always wash your hands. In the process of taking care of your residents, you will collect microbes on your hands. These microbes could then be easily transferred to the next resident you care for, a co-worker, yourself, or one of your family members. Failing to wash your hands before giving care to a resident could even be considered abuse.

There are two main types of microbes found on a person's hands. Earlier in this chapter, you learned about the first type, normal (resident) flora. These are the microbes that normally live on a person's skin and usually do not cause infections. Normal flora lives deep in the pores of the skin and cannot be totally removed. The other type of microbe typically found on a person's hands is called **transient flora.** Transient flora is picked up from touching contaminated objects or people who have an infectious disease. Most nosocomial infections are caused by transient flora—the hands of the health care worker serve as the method of transmission from one person to another. Transient flora lives on the surface of the skin and is easily removed by proper handwashing.

There are differences in opinion about handwashing techniques, such as the time required, the type of cleaning agents that should be used, and the frequency with which handwashing should occur. Certain situations may require specific handwashing techniques. Procedure 15-1 describes the basic handwashing procedure. Although the specifics of how handwashing is performed vary from setting to setting, one aspect of handwashing always remains the same—it must be performed thoroughly, properly, and consistently. At the minimum, wash your hands:

- When you first arrive at your facility
- Before entering a resident's room
- Before entering a "clean" supply room
- Before obtaining clean linen from a linen cart
- Before handling a resident's meal tray
- Before and after you go on break and before you leave your shift

- Before and after drinking, eating, or smoking
- Before and after inserting contact lenses
- After using the bathroom
- After coughing, sneezing, or blowing your nose
- After touching anything that may be considered dirty—especially objects contaminated with blood or other body fluids or substances
- After picking an object up from the floor
- After removing disposable gloves, including those times when you are replacing a torn glove
- After handling your hair or applying make-up or lip balm

When washing your hands, make sure you clean those areas that microbes love to hide, under and around the fingernails and between the fingers. As you learned in Chapter 3, long fingernails do not really have a place in the nursing assistant's professional life. Long fingernails trap microbes underneath them and therefore are harder to clean. Nail polish cracks and peels, providing many places for transient microbes to hide. False nails, acrylics, and wraps often lift, creating an excellent breeding ground for microbes. Many health care facilities ban the use of these types of nail treatments by anyone involved in providing hands-on care for patients or residents.

It is also not a good idea to wear rings and bracelets while on the job. Many health care workers think that by removing their jewelry before washing their hands, they can remove any microbes trapped underneath the jewelry. But, think about this: Even if you remove your jewelry before you wash your hands, the jewelry itself is still dirty, so you will be putting dirty jewelry back onto your clean hands. For the sake of efficiency and cleanliness, it is best to keep your fingernails short and unpolished, and to leave your jewelry at home when performing your duties as a nursing assistant.

A good lather of soap and the physical motion of rubbing your hands together removes skin oils and lotions, which can harbor microbes. Rinsing thoroughly removes microbes, along with the dirt and lather. Because frequent handwashing can cause the skin to become excessively dry, leading to cracking, applying a lotion or hand cream after washing is recommended. Remember, your own intact skin is important to help protect you from infection too.

While nothing can replace the effectiveness of good handwashing to remove visible dirt, blood, or other body fluids or substances, the CDC issued guidelines in October 2002, recommending the use of alcohol-based hand rubs for routine hand decontamination. Alcohol-based hand rubs work by reducing the number of bacteria on the hands. Alcohol-based hand rubs have several advantages:

- Using an alcohol-based hand rub is quicker than washing your hands at the sink, which means that during duties that require frequent handwashing, using an alcohol-based hand rub can save time.
- Alcohol-based hand rubs are gentler on the skin than soap and water.
- Alcohol-based hand rubs are used without water, so they can be used anywhere. In many facilities, alcohol-based hand rubs can be dispensed at the resident's bedside, saving many trips back and forth to the sink. Many even come in containers small enough to carry in your uniform pocket.

It is very simple to use an alcohol-based hand rub. The label on the product will tell you how much product to use. Apply this amount to one of your palms and rub your hands together, covering your hands and fingers (front and back) with the product. Continue rubbing your hands together until your skin is dry. That is all there is to it!

Remember, if your hands are visibly soiled with dirt, blood, or other body fluids or substances, you must wash them at the sink, using soap and water. You must also wash your hands with soap and water if you have been caring for someone with an infection caused by *Clostridium difficile* (also known as "*C. diff*"). *C. difficile* is a type of bacteria that can cause severe diarrhea and inflammation of the large intestine (colitis). *C. difficile* has a protective endospore, which makes alcohol-based hand rubs less effective against this type of bacteria. In situations other than those mentioned here, it is acceptable to use an alcohol-based hand rub to decontaminate your hands.

SURGICAL ASEPSIS

Surgical asepsis is used for procedures that involve entering a person's body. Examples of procedures that require surgical asepsis include inserting urinary catheters, giving injections, and starting intravenous (IV) lines. Because these procedures disrupt the body's natural protective barriers, all instruments and equipment used must be sterile, or totally free from microbes. In most states, performing procedures that require surgical asepsis is not within a nursing assistant's scope of practice. However, some facilities will provide extra training in this area if performing procedures that require surgical asepsis is part of your job description.

BARRIER METHODS

In addition to medical asepsis and surgical asepsis, barrier methods are used to control infection in the health care setting. A *barrier* is an object that physically prevents microbes from reaching a health care worker's skin or mucous membranes. Examples of barriers used in infection control, called **personal protective equipment (PPE)**, include disposable gloves, gowns, masks, and protective eyewear. While in use, the barrier becomes contaminated with microbes and must be removed in a way that prevents transmission of the microbes onto the skin of the health care worker.

Gloves

Gloves are the most commonly used barrier method. Gloves are worn in the following situations:

- When there is a possibility that you will come in contact with body fluids or substances
- When you are performing or assisting with perineal care (cleaning of the area between the legs)
- When you are performing or assisting with mouth care
- When you have a cut or abrasion on your hands
- When you are shaving a resident
- When you are performing care on a resident who has an open wound or other break in the skin

To effectively prevent contamination of your hands, gloves must be intact (without holes or tears), and they must fit properly. Gloves that are too tight are uncomfortable. Gloves that are too loose will not stay on your hands. Many people are allergic or sensitive to latex, the material that is most commonly used to make disposable gloves. If you or someone you are caring for is sensitive to latex, then you should use gloves made from another synthetic material, such as vinyl. Health care facilities must provide non-latex barrier methods for people who are sensitive to latex.

The most common error made by people who wear gloves for barrier protection is becoming too comfortable with the fact that they are protecting themselves, and forgetting to protect others! If you are wearing gloves and you touch a surface that is contaminated, then your gloves become contaminated. If you then touch another surface, such as the side rail, light switch, or doorknob, with your contaminated gloves, the pathogens will be transferred from your gloves to that surface. The next person who touches the surface

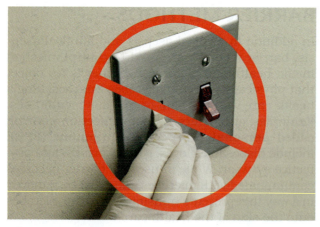

Figure 15-8

Do not make this mistake! By touching the light switch with her gloved hands, this nursing assistant has transferred whatever microbes were on her gloves onto the light switch, where they could be easily transferred onto the hands of the next person who turns on the light.

could then pick up the pathogens you deposited there with your dirty gloves (Fig. 15-8). Gloves that become contaminated with material that may contain pathogens should be removed before touching any other surface. You may need to change gloves several times during one procedure to prevent the transfer of pathogens from dirty areas to clean areas (for example, when cleaning feces from a person who has soiled himself, or changing soiled

sheets). Always wash your hands after removing your gloves. Procedure 15-2 describes the proper way to remove gloves.

Gowns

A gown (fabric or paper) should be used when it is likely that your uniform will be soiled with body fluids or substances. Many gowns that are used for PPE are fluid-resistant. The use of the gown prevents contamination of your uniform. Each gown is worn only once. Any gown, fabric or paper, is considered contaminated if it becomes wet. Procedures 15-3 and 15-4 describe how to put on and take off a gown, respectively.

Masks

Masks prevent you from breathing in pathogens through your nose or mouth, and are worn when there is a chance that you will be exposed to pathogens that are transmitted through the air or in droplets of saliva. For example, the pathogens that cause measles and tuberculosis (TB) are airborne pathogens, and the pathogens that cause pneumonia, strep throat, and meningitis are transmitted in droplets of saliva. You could be exposed to these pathogens when a person with one of these diseases talks, coughs, or sneezes.

Surgical masks are most commonly used, but if you are caring for a person with TB, you may be required to wear a special high-filtration mask

---

Be Smart About Surveys!

Practicing good infection control is essential for maintaining the safety and well-being of your residents. One of the ways surveyors evaluate the quality of care provided by a facility is by monitoring the number of health care–associated infections (HAIs) that occur within the facility. In addition, during the survey, surveyors will pay close attention to make sure that you are following proper infection control practices, consistently. To help your facility remain without survey problems in this area:

- Make good infection control practices part of your normal routine so that these habits become second nature to you.
- Be aware of the most common breaks in infection control that occur in long-term care facilities, and make it a point to avoid falling into these bad habits:
  - Failing to wash hands
  - Failing to change gloves

- Failing to remove gloves immediately after caring for a resident or handling a soiled item
- Placing dirty linens on the floor
- Carrying unused clean linens from one resident's room to another resident's room
- Failing to provide each resident with his or her own personal care items and supplies
- Failing to appropriately label each resident's personal care items and supplies
- Storing basins on bathroom floors
- Storing bedpans and urinals inappropriately
- Never hesitate to speak up if you see a co-worker practicing poor infection control. Find a time when you can speak to the person privately about your concerns. If necessary, share your concerns with the nurse.

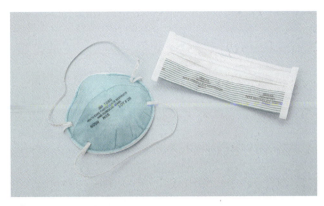

Figure 15-9
Masks cover your nose and mouth and protect you from inhaling pathogens that are transmitted in the air or in saliva. (*Left*) A high-filtration respirator mask, worn when caring for people with tuberculosis (TB). (*Right*) A surgical mask.

(Fig. 15-9). Surgical masks are "one size fits all," but high-filtration masks are available in various sizes and you must be fitted for them in advance. All masks are used only once. You must discard and replace your mask if it becomes wet or soiled. Procedure 15-5 explains how to put on and take off a mask.

Protective Eyewear

Goggles, face shields, and other types of protective eyewear are used to protect your eyes from substances that may splash (Fig. 15-10). Blood and other body fluids, as well as the fluid used to clean wounds, may contain pathogens, which can enter your body through your eyes. Goggles fit close to your face and can be worn over prescription eyeglasses. Face shields may be attached to a mask, or to an elastic band that fits around

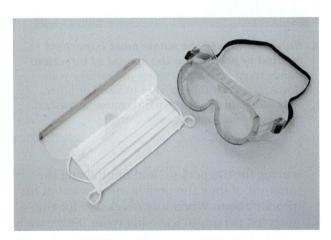

Figure 15-10
Face shields (*left*) and goggles (*right*) are used to protect your eyes from substances that may splash.

the head. Your employer is required to provide you with appropriate protective eyewear.

Putting on and Taking off Multiple Articles of Personal Protective Equipment

In many situations, you may need to wear more than one article of PPE. The best sequence for putting these items on is as follows: gown, mask, protective eyewear, gloves. The order is reversed when it is time to remove the PPE. Procedure 15-6 describes how to remove PPE when more than one article is being used. After use, PPE is considered contaminated. Removal of PPE in the correct sequence helps to protect you from infection. For instance, you would not want to remove your mask first, because this would mean that you would have to touch your face with your contaminated gloves.

ISOLATION PRECAUTIONS

The last major method of controlling the spread of infection throughout a health care facility is by using isolation precautions. **Isolation precautions** are guidelines, based on a pathogen's method of transmission, that we follow to contain the pathogen and limit others' exposure to it as much as possible.

Standard Precautions

Standard precautions are precautions that health care workers take with every patient or resident to protect themselves from pathogens that are transmitted in blood. Standard precautions involve the use of barrier methods, as well as certain environmental control methods, to protect the health care worker (Box 15-1). *For these methods to be effective, they must be used consistently.*

Transmission-based Precautions

Transmission-based precautions are used when a person is known to have a disease that is transmitted a certain way, for example, via the air, in droplets, or by direct contact. When transmission-based precautions are being used with a resident, equipment that is used for routine care (such as a stethoscope or thermometer) will often be left in the resident's room and used only for that resident while the transmission-based precautions are in effect. When it is no longer necessary to use transmission-based precautions with the resident, the equipment is properly cleaned and disinfected before being put back into general use.

BOX 15-1   Standard Precautions

1. Gloves must be worn if the *possibility* exists that the hands could come in contact with blood or other body fluids. Gloves must also be worn when touching any surface or linen that could be contaminated with infected materials. Remember that you cannot see a virus with the naked eye.

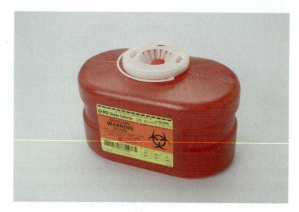

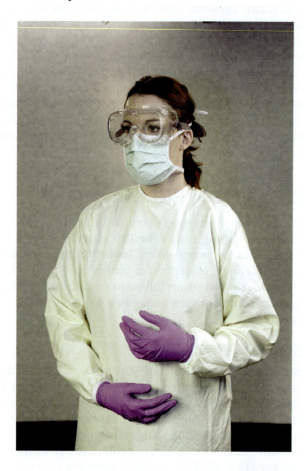

2. A waterproof (impervious) gown must be worn if the *possibility* exists that your clothes could become soiled with blood or other body fluids.

3. A mask, face shield, and eye goggles must be worn if the *possibility* exists that blood or other body fluids could splash or spray.

4. Sharps, such as used needles, razors, or broken glass, must be disposed of properly in labeled, OSHA-approved containers. Contaminated, broken glass items should not be handled, even with gloved hands. They should be swept or vacuumed up for disposal.

5. Spills of blood or other body fluids must be cleaned up promptly with an approved viricidal cleaning agent or a solution of 1 part household bleach to 10 parts water. Personal protective equipment (PPE), such as gloves and a gown, should be worn while cleaning up spills.

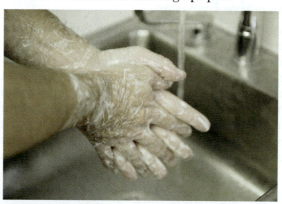

6. ***Handwashing is the single most important method of preventing the spread of infection!*** Hands must be washed when you remove your gloves. If accidental exposure to blood or other body substances occurs, hands must be washed thoroughly and immediately.

- **Airborne precautions** are used when caring for people infected with pathogens that can be transmitted through the air. Airborne pathogens enter the respiratory tract of people breathing the same air as the infected person. Therefore, airborne precautions include placing the person in a private room with the door closed, wearing a mask when caring for the person, and minimizing the amount of time the person spends out of his private room. When it is necessary for the infected person to leave his room, he wears a mask. Diseases caused by pathogens that can be transmitted in the air include TB, chickenpox, and measles. Airborne precautions are listed in Box 15-2.

BOX 15-2 Airborne Precautions

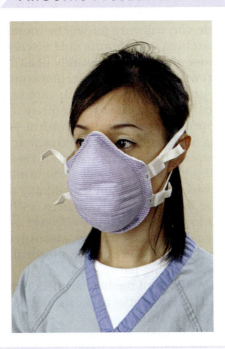

1. Residents known or suspected to be infected with an airborne pathogen are to be placed in private rooms with special ventilation systems.
2. Health care workers should wear masks when caring for residents with known or suspected tuberculosis (TB). If the health care worker has not been exposed to measles or chickenpox (and is therefore not immune), then he is at risk for these diseases, and a mask should be worn when caring for residents with measles or chickenpox. If the health care worker is immune to measles or chickenpox, a mask is not necessary.
3. A surgical mask should be placed over the resident's face if she must be transported from one location to another. Transport of the resident should be kept to a minimum.
4. All precautions for preventing transmission of TB should be implemented if the resident is known or suspected to have TB.

- **Droplet precautions** are used when caring for people with diseases caused by pathogens that are transmitted by direct exposure to droplets released from the mouth or nose (for example, when the person coughs, sneezes, or talks). Droplet precautions must also be taken when performing procedures that involve contact with an infected person's mouth or nose. Diseases caused by pathogens that can be transmitted in droplets include mumps, influenza, whooping cough, strep throat, scarlet fever, rubella, meningitis, pneumonia, diphtheria, and epiglottitis. Droplet precautions are the same as airborne precautions, except that it is usually only necessary to wear a mask when you are within 3 feet of the infected person.
- **Contact precautions** are used when caring for people with diseases caused by pathogens that are transmitted directly (by touching the person) or indirectly (by touching fomites). Diseases that can be transmitted by contact include skin and wound infections, digestive tract infections, and some respiratory tract infections. Contact precautions involve using barrier methods whenever you must touch the infected person or items contaminated with wound drainage or body substances. Contaminated linen and waste materials must be contained and disposed of properly. Procedure 15-7 describes how to transfer contaminated items out of a person's room when contact precautions are being followed.

Helping Hands and a Caring Heart

FOCUS ON HUMANISTIC HEALTH CARE

When caring for a person with a communicable disease, it is very important to remember the person. We work hard to follow all of the procedures that help to prevent the spread of infection, and this is a very important part of providing care. However, sometimes it is easy to forget about how the person with the infection might feel. A person with a communicable disease often feels dirty or unwanted. Think about it—how would you feel if a health care worker had to wear gloves or a mask every time he or she came near you? When airborne or droplet precautions are in effect, the person with the communicable disease may feel isolated and lonely, and desperately miss the company of other people. Friends and family members may avoid visiting the person. When you are caring for a resident with a communicable disease, checking on the person frequently and taking the time to talk with the person when you are providing care can help to make the person feel better.

SUMMARY

- A huge variety of microbes share our planet.
  - Major types of microbes include bacteria, viruses, fungi, and parasites.
  - Some cause disease, and are called pathogens, while others are harmless. Harmless microbes that live in and on our bodies are called normal flora.
- Our immune systems help us to fight off infections.
  - The human immune system's non-specific defense mechanisms include the physical barriers provided by the skin and mucous membranes, and the general immune response.
  - The human immune system's specific defense mechanisms include antibodies.
- Health care facilities provide the perfect environment for the spread of infection.
  - The chain of infection describes the elements that must be present in order for infection to occur. The six elements of the chain of infection are pathogen, reservoir, portal of exit, method of transmission, portal of entry, and susceptible host.
  - Breaking just one link in the chain of infection stops the spread of infection from one person to another.
- Some of the people you will care for will be receiving health care because they have a serious communicable disease. Others may have a serious communicable disease and not even know it. In addition, many of the people you will care for will be more at risk for catching a communicable disease because they are not entirely healthy to begin with. Therefore, infection control is very important in the health care setting.
  - Health care workers take many approaches to infection control. As a nursing assistant, it is your ethical and legal responsibility to protect your residents from infectious disease. You must also protect yourself and your family members. The techniques used to help control the spread of infection are effective only if performed properly and consistently.
- Medical asepsis involves physically removing or killing pathogens.
  - Methods of medical asepsis include sanitization, antisepsis, disinfection, and sterilization.
  - Handwashing, a form of medical asepsis, is the single most important method of controlling the spread of infection.
- Surgical asepsis is required for procedures that involve entering a person's body.
- Barrier methods prevent a pathogen from gaining access to a health care worker's body. Commonly used barrier methods include gloves, gowns, masks, and protective eyewear.
- Isolation precautions are based on a pathogen's mode of transmission (blood, air, droplet, direct contact).

WHY YOU DO IT   Handwashing is the most important method of preventing the spread of infection.

1. Gather needed supplies, if not present at the handwashing area: *soap or the cleansing agent specified by your facility, hand lotion* (optional), *paper towels, a nailbrush* (optional), *an orange stick* (optional).

2. Stand away from the sink, so that your uniform does not touch the sink. Push your sleeves up your arms 4 to 5 inches; if you are wearing a watch, push it up too.

3. Use a clean paper towel to turn on the faucet, adjusting the water temperature until it is warm. Dispose of the paper towel in a facility-approved waste container.

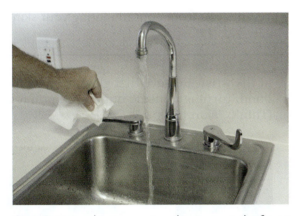

Step 3 Use a clean paper towel to turn on the faucet.

4. Wet your hands, keeping your fingers pointed down. This will cause the water to run off your fingertips and into the sink. Do not allow water to run up your forearms.

5. Press the hand pump or step on the foot pedal to dispense the cleaning agent into one cupped hand.

6. Lather well, keeping your fingers pointed down at all times. Make sure the lather extends at least 1 inch past your wrists.

7. Rub your hands together in a circular motion, washing the palms and backs of your hands. Interlace your fingers to clean the spaces between your fingers. Continue for at least 15 seconds.

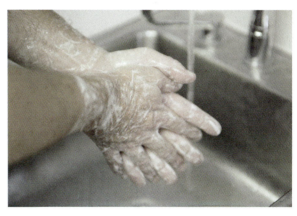

Step 7 Interlace your fingers.

8. Rub the fingernails of one hand against the palm of the opposite hand to force soap underneath the tips of the fingernails, *or* clean underneath the tips of the fingernails with the blunt edge of an orange stick or a nailbrush.

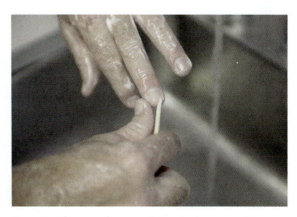

Step 8 Clean under your fingernails.

9. Rinse your hands, keeping your fingers pointed down at all times.

(continued)

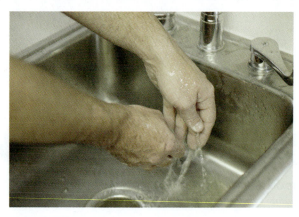

Step 9 Always point your fingertips down.

10. Dry your hands thoroughly with a clean paper towel. Dispose of the paper towel in a

facility-approved waste container, being careful not to touch the container.

11. With a new paper towel, turn off the faucet. Carefully dispose of the paper towel.

12. As you leave the handwashing area, if there is a doorknob, open the door by covering the doorknob with a clean paper towel. If there is no doorknob, push the door open with your hip and shoulder to avoid contaminating your clean hands.

13. After leaving the handwashing area, apply a small amount of hand lotion to keep your skin supple and moist.

PROCEDURE 15-2

Removing Gloves

WHY YOU DO IT   Removing your gloves properly prevents you from contaminating your skin or uniform.

---

1. With one gloved hand, grasp the other glove at the palm and pull the glove off your hand. Keep the glove you have removed in your gloved hand. (Think, "glove to glove.")

at the wrist. Remove that glove from your hand, turning it inside-out as you pull it off. (Think, "skin to skin.")

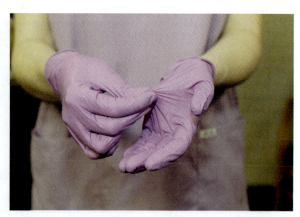

Step 1 "Glove to glove."

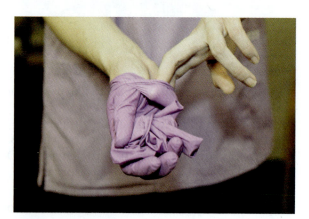

Step 2 "Skin to skin."

3. Dispose of the soiled gloves in a facility-approved waste container.

4. Wash your hands.

2. Slip two fingers from the ungloved hand underneath the cuff of the remaining glove,

PROCEDURE 15-3

Putting on a Gown

WHY YOU DO IT   Putting on a gown properly prevents your uniform from becoming soiled with body fluids.

1. Gather needed supplies: *a gown, gloves.*

2. Remove your watch and place it on a clean paper towel or in your pocket. (If you are wearing jewelry, remove that as well.) Roll up the sleeves of your uniform so that they are about 4–5 inches above your wrists.

3. Wash your hands.

4. Put on the gown by slipping your arms into the sleeves.

5. Secure the gown around your neck by tying the ties in a simple bow or by fastening the Velcro™ strips.

6. Reach behind yourself and overlap the edges of the gown so that your uniform is completely covered. Secure the gown at your waist by tying the ties in a simple bow or by fastening the Velcro™ strips.

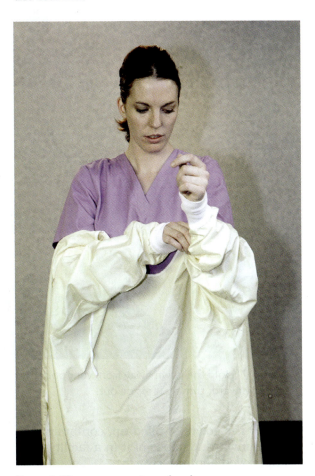

Step 4 Slip your arms into the sleeves.

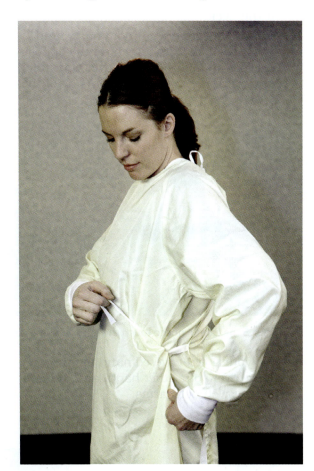

Step 6 Overlap and tie.

7. Put on the gloves. The cuffs of the gloves should extend over the cuffs of the gown.

PROCEDURE 15-4

Removing a Gown

WHY YOU DO IT   Removing a gown properly prevents you from contaminating your skin or uniform.

1. Untie the waist ties (or undo the Velcro™ strips at the waist).

2. Remove and dispose of your gloves, as described in Procedure 15-2.

3. Untie the neck ties (or undo the Velcro™ strips at the neck). Be careful not to touch your neck or the outside of the gown.

4. Grasping the gown at the neck ties, loosen it at the neck.

5. Slip the fingers of your dominant hand under the cuff of the gown on the opposite sleeve, and pull the sleeve over your hand. Be careful not to touch the outside of the gown with either hand.

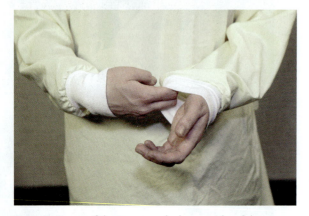

Step 5 Be careful not to touch the outside of the gown.

6. Use your gown-covered hand to pull the sleeve over your other hand, and then pull the gown off both arms.

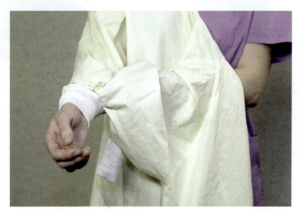

Step 6 Use your gown-covered hand to pull the sleeve over your other hand.

7. Holding the gown away from your body, roll it downward, turning it inside out as you go. Take care to touch only the noncontaminated side of the gown.

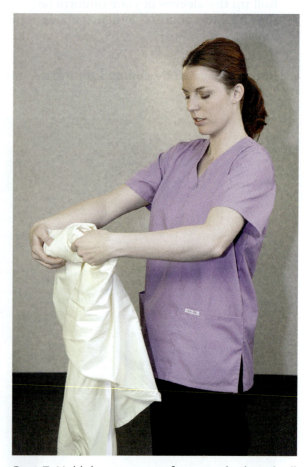

Step 7 Hold the gown away from your body and roll it downward, turning it inside out.

8. After the gown is rolled up, contaminated side inward, dispose of it in a facility-approved container.

9. Wash your hands.

PROCEDURE 15-5

Putting on and Removing a Mask

WHY YOU DO IT Putting on a mask properly prevents pathogens that are transmitted through the air or in droplets from entering your nose and mouth. Removing a mask properly prevents you from contaminating your skin or uniform.

Putting on a Mask

1. Gather needed supplies: *a mask.*
2. Wash your hands.
3. Place the mask over your nose and mouth, being careful not to touch your face with your hands.

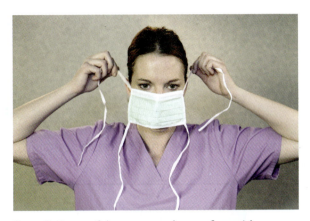

Step 3 Be careful not to touch your face with your hands.

4. Tie the top strings of the mask securely behind your head.

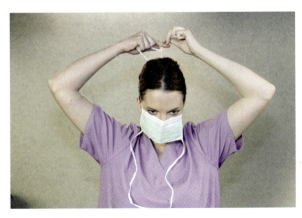

Step 4 Tie the top strings securely.

5. Tie the bottom strings of the mask securely behind your neck. Make sure that the mask fits snugly around your face. You want to breathe through the mask, not around it.

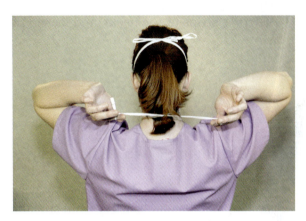

Step 5 Tie the bottom strings securely.

Removing a Mask

1. Wash your hands. (You do not want to touch your face with dirty hands.)
2. Untie the bottom strings first, and then untie the top strings.
3. Remove the mask by holding the top strings. Dispose of the mask, holding it by its ties only, in the facility-approved container located inside the resident's room.
4. Wash your hands.

PROCEDURE 15-6

Removing More Than One Article of Personal Protective Equipment (PPE)

WHY YOU DO IT   Removing PPE in the proper order helps to prevent you from contaminating your skin or uniform.

1. Untie the gown's waist ties (or undo the Velcro™ strips at the waist).
2. Remove and dispose of your gloves, as described in Procedure 15-2.
3. Remove your protective eyewear.
4. Untie the gown's neck ties (or undo the Velcro™ strips at the neck), and loosen the gown at the neck. Remove and dispose of the gown, as described in Procedure 15-4.
5. Remove and dispose of the mask as described in Procedure 15-5.
6. Wash your hands.

PROCEDURE 15-7

Double-Bagging (Two Assistants)

WHY YOU DO IT   Double-bagging helps to keep any pathogens that may be on the outside of the bag from spreading to other places.

1. The nursing assistant inside the person's room places the contaminated items into an isolation bag (usually a color-coded plastic bag) and secures the bag with a tie.
2. Another nursing assistant, referred to as the "clean" nursing assistant, stands outside of the person's room, holding a plastic bag cuffed over her hands. The cuff at the top of the bag protects the "clean" nursing assistant's hands.
3. The nursing assistant inside the isolation unit deposits the bag of contaminated items into the bag held by the "clean" nursing assistant.
4. The "clean" nursing assistant secures the top of the plastic bag tightly and disposes of the double-bagged items according to facility policy.

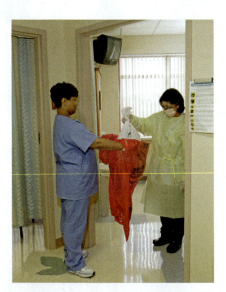

Step 3 The assistant inside the room places the bag of contaminated items in the bag held by the nursing assistant outside of the room.

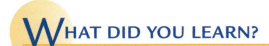

WHAT DID YOU LEARN?

Multiple Choice

Select the single best answer for each of the following questions.

1. When you wash your hands, you should:
   a. Use the hottest water possible
   b. Scrub with a brush for 3 minutes
   c. Rinse with your fingers pointed up
   d. Rinse with your fingers pointed down

2. When should you wash your hands?
   a. When you wake up in the morning and before you go to bed at night
   b. Before and after contact with a resident
   c. When the charge nurse tells you to
   d. Only when they are visibly soiled

3. You have been told to follow contact precautions with one of your residents. Therefore, this resident's soiled linen should be:
   a. Thrown away
   b. Bagged prior to removing it from the room
   c. Taken directly to the laundry
   d. Placed in the linen hamper

4. Which of the following procedures best destroys all bacteria?
   a. Sterilizing
   b. Washing with bleach
   c. Soaking in alcohol
   d. All of the above

5. Bacteria may enter the body through:
   a. The mouth
   b. The nose
   c. Cuts in the skin
   d. All of the above

6. Which statement about the handwashing procedure is correct?
   a. As long as soap is used, the temperature of the water does not matter
   b. The faucet is clean and may be touched during handwashing
   c. Wash at least 1 inch above the wrist
   d. All of the above

7. Pathogens can be spread by:
   a. Looking at a person with a communicable disease
   b. Coughing or sneezing
   c. Touching a person with a communicable disease
   d. Both "b" and "c"

8. Which one of the following statements about protective gowns is true?
   a. The outside is considered the "clean" side
   b. The gown opens in the front
   c. A gown may be used more than once
   d. A gown is considered contaminated when wet

9. Which one of the following could be a fomite?
   a. A water glass that has been used
   b. A mosquito
   c. Linens that have just come back from the laundry
   d. A cut in the skin

10. Which one of the following must be present in order for infection to spread?
    a. A nursing assistant
    b. An indwelling medical device
    c. A susceptible host
    d. A patient or resident who looks ill

11. When are goggles a necessary part of personal protective equipment (PPE)?
    a. Whenever blood is present
    b. Whenever blood may splash or spray
    c. Whenever you are taking care of a person with tuberculosis (TB)
    d. Goggles are not really a necessary part of PPE

12. For health care workers, which of the following is the most important method of preventing the spread of infection?
    a. Standard precautions
    b. Handwashing
    c. Wearing gloves
    d. Wearing gowns and goggles

13. Personal protective equipment (PPE) refers to:
    a. Sterilization and disinfection
    b. Security personnel
    c. Disposable gloves, face masks, gowns, and eye protection
    d. Isolation precautions

Matching

Match each numbered item with its appropriate lettered description.

_____ **1.** Communicable disease

_____ **2.** Pathogen

_____ **3.** Leukocyte

_____ **4.** Opportunistic microbe

_____ **5.** Fomite

_____ **6.** Aerobic

_____ **7.** Health care–associated infection (HAI)

_____ **8.** Vector

_____ **9.** Anaerobic

_____**10.** Antibody

a. Describes bacteria that need oxygen to survive

b. Special proteins that help fight specific pathogens

c. Can be transferred from one person to another

d. Microbe that can cause illness

e. Non-living object that is contaminated

f. White blood cell

g. Can change from harmless to pathogenic, given a chance

h. Infection gotten in the health care setting

i. A living creature that transmits disease

j. Describes bacteria that die if oxygen is present

STOP and Think!

● Several residents in your care have come down with a nasty intestinal virus that causes diarrhea. One resident, Mrs. Grande, is so weak that she was unable to get out of bed in time and soiled her clothing and bedding.

Where is the most likely portal of exit for this pathogen? What steps should you take when cleaning up Mrs. Grande that will help to keep this virus from being spread to other residents, your co-workers, and you?

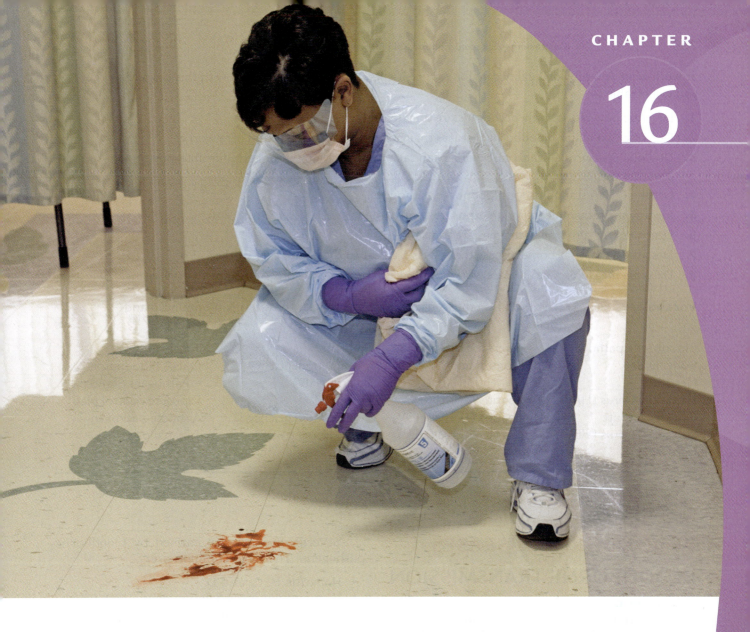

Bloodborne and Airborne Pathogens

WHAT WILL YOU LEARN?

As a nursing assistant, you will have close contact with residents, some of whom will have life-threatening communicable diseases. Although your risk of getting these diseases is real, there are things you can do to minimize that risk. In this chapter, you will learn about some of the communicable diseases that pose the most risk to health care workers, and how these diseases are transmitted. You will learn what you can do to minimize your risk of getting one of these infections. In addition, we will review the standards that have been developed by the Occupational Safety and Health Administration (OSHA) with the goal of protecting you

Photo: Following standard precautions, such as wearing personal protective equipment (PPE) whenever contact with blood or other body fluids is likely, helps to protect you from bloodborne pathogens.

at work while you provide quality care for your residents. When you are finished with this chapter, you will be able to:

1. Describe how bloodborne pathogens are transmitted.
2. Describe two major bloodborne diseases that pose a threat to the health care worker.
3. Describe measures a health care worker can take to protect himself or herself from exposure to bloodborne pathogens.
4. List the OSHA standards for bloodborne pathogens.
5. Identify the requirements for an exposure control plan.
6. Describe how airborne pathogens are transmitted.
7. Describe a major airborne disease that poses a threat to the health care worker.
8. Describe measures a health care worker can take to prevent the spread of airborne pathogens.

Vocabulary Use the CD in the front of your book to hear these terms pronounced and defined:

Bloodborne pathogen	Centers for Disease	Human	T cell
Body fluids	Control and	immunodeficiency	OSHA Bloodborne
Hepatitis	Prevention (CDC)	virus (HIV)	Pathogens Standard
Hepatitis A virus (HAV)	Hepatitis C virus (HCV)	Acquired	Exposure control plan
Oral–fecal route	Hepatitis D virus (HDV)	immunodeficiency	Airborne pathogen
Hepatitis B virus (HBV)	Hepatitis E virus (HEV)	syndrome (AIDS)	Tuberculosis (TB)
Carrier			

BLOODBORNE DISEASES

BLOODBORNE TRANSMISSION

A **bloodborne pathogen** is a disease-producing microbe that is transmitted to another person through blood or other body fluids. **Body fluids** are liquid or semi-liquid substances produced by the body such as blood, urine, feces, vomitus, saliva, drainage from wounds, sweat, semen, vaginal secretions, tears, cerebrospinal fluid, amniotic fluid, and breast milk. For a bloodborne pathogen to be transmitted from one person to another, blood or body fluids from an infected person must enter the bloodstream of a person who is not infected. There are several ways this could occur in the workplace:

- Needlesticks (puncture wounds caused by dirty hypodermic needles)
- Cuts from contaminated, broken glass (such as that from a broken blood tube)
- Direct contact between infected blood and broken skin, mucous membranes, or the eyes

Additionally, bloodborne pathogens can be transmitted via sexual intercourse, or through blood transfusions.

Several diseases are caused by bloodborne pathogens. The most common are:

- Hepatitis B, C, and D
- Human immunodeficiency virus (HIV), which causes acquired immunodeficiency syndrome (AIDS)
- Malaria
- Syphilis
- Ebola

Of these, hepatitis and HIV pose the greatest occupational risk to the health care worker.

HEPATITIS AND HIV/AIDS

Hepatitis

Hepatitis is inflammation of the liver, the organ that removes toxic substances from the bloodstream (Fig. 16-1). Hepatitis is most commonly caused by a viral infection, but it may also be caused by chemicals, drugs, or drinking alcohol. Some infections with a hepatitis virus are mild, producing no lasting effects on the liver. Others are chronic and affect the liver's ability to function over time. If the liver failure is severe, the person will die unless she receives a liver transplant.

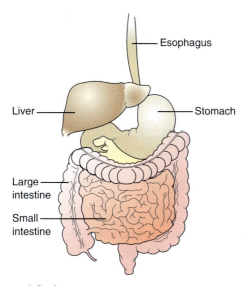

Figure 16-1
Hepatitis is inflammation of the liver, the organ that removes toxic substances from the blood.

Currently, five types of hepatitis virus have been identified: the hepatitis A, B, C, D, and E viruses.

Hepatitis A Virus (HAV)

Hepatitis A virus (HAV) is not a bloodborne pathogen. This virus is transmitted through the **oral–fecal route,** which means that the virus lives in the digestive tract of an infected person and leaves the person's body through the feces. The feces can contaminate food or water. Then, when a person eats or drinks the contaminated food or water, he becomes infected. (*Oral* means mouth. In this case, the infection is transmitted by taking contaminated food or water into the mouth.) For example, HAV can be passed on when a food service worker who has the virus uses the restroom but fails to wash her hands properly before returning to work and handling a customer's food (Fig. 16-2). Hepatitis A outbreaks are also found in areas where raw sewage comes into contact with bodies of water where shellfish, such as oysters, live. The virus infects the shellfish and is then passed on to unsuspecting people who eat the contaminated shellfish raw. Fortunately, the illness caused by HAV (commonly referred to as *infectious hepatitis*) is usually acute and the person usually recovers fully. An effective vaccine against this virus is available and recommended for the general public.

Hepatitis B Virus (HBV)

Hepatitis B virus (HBV), a bloodborne pathogen, is a serious threat for the health care worker. The virus is found in blood, as well as in other body fluids, such as semen and vaginal secretions. This means that HBV can be transmitted through

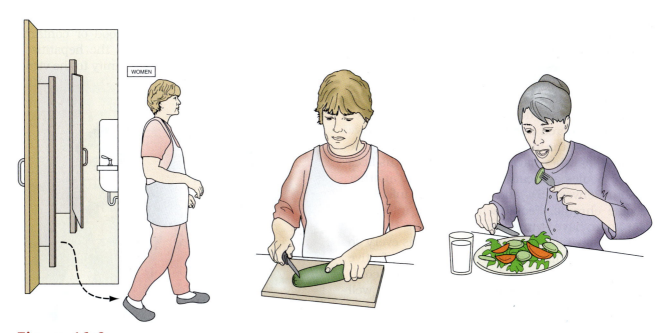

Figure 16-2
Hepatitis A virus (HAV) is transmitted via the oral–fecal route. The virus lives in an infected person's digestive tract and leaves the body in the feces. If the person's hands become contaminated with feces and then the person handles food, the infection could be passed on to the person who eats the contaminated food.

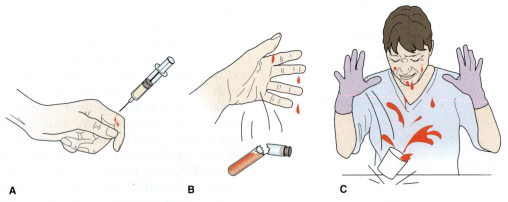

Figure 16-3

In the workplace, hepatitis B virus (HBV) can be transmitted by **(A)** a needlestick injury, **(B)** cuts from contaminated glass, or **(C)** direct contact with blood, for example, through a blood splash to the face.

transfusion of infected blood or blood products, across the placenta from mother to infant, and through unprotected sexual intercourse (both heterosexual and homosexual). Health care workers are at risk for getting HBV through:

- Needlestick injuries
- Cuts from contaminated objects
- Exposure of broken skin or mucous membranes to contaminated blood or other body fluids (Fig. 16-3)

In addition to blood, semen, and vaginal secretions, body fluids known to carry high amounts of HBV include wound drainage and cultures, cerebrospinal fluid, amniotic fluid, and breast milk. Other body secretions do not typically have high viral counts unless there is visible blood present.

Infection with HBV causes an acute illness in most people, but some people can be infected by the virus and never develop symptoms. These people are considered **carriers.** Carriers do not have symptoms of the disease and therefore may be unaware that they have it. However, the virus lives in their bodies and can be transmitted to another person. Between 5% and 10% of HBV infections become chronic. People with chronic infections may never have symptoms and become carriers. Or, they may have flare-ups of symptoms every so often, resulting in months of disability. An effective vaccination against HBV is available and is recommended by OSHA for health care workers, as well as the general public (Fig. 16-4).

Health care workers who have any direct contact with residents can be exposed to body fluids that contain HBV. Although the virus is not known to be transmitted in saliva, the gums of people with periodontal (gum) disease may bleed during oral care and tooth brushing, exposing the health care

worker to potentially contaminated blood. There is always the risk of nicking a resident with the razor during shaving, and residents may fall and injure themselves, resulting in wounds that bleed. A used hypodermic needle could be lost in the bed linens or accidentally tossed in the trash, placing an unsuspecting health care worker at risk for a puncture injury. Because of these occupational risks, the **Centers for Disease Control and Prevention (CDC)**—the government agency that provides statistics about health conditions and diseases, monitors for disease outbreaks, and implements prevention strategies—recommends that all health care workers who have even the slightest potential for being exposed to blood or contaminated body fluids should receive the hepatitis B vaccination, which provides immunity to the virus.

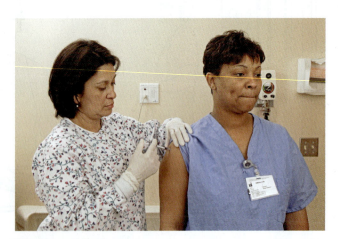

Figure 16-4

A vaccine against hepatitis B virus (HBV) is available. The Occupational Safety and Health Administration (OSHA) requires employers to make the vaccine available to nursing assistants, and other workers at risk, free of charge.

OSHA requires employers to offer this vaccine to employees, free of charge.

Hepatitis C Virus (HCV)

Hepatitis C virus (HCV) is also a bloodborne pathogen. The most common mode of transmission is through contaminated blood transfusions, although some needlestick exposures have caused infection. Although the mode of HCV transmission is mainly bloodborne, in more than 40% of people who are diagnosed with HCV, no obvious route of transmission is found. The illness that results from infection with HCV tends to be more chronic and serious than that resulting from infection with HBV. As many as 85% of people with hepatitis C develop chronic disease, and of these, 20% go on to develop end-stage cirrhosis (a fatal liver disease), liver failure, or liver cancer. Hepatitis C is the leading cause for liver transplantation in the United States. Currently, no vaccine against HCV is available.

Hepatitis D Virus (HDV)

Hepatitis D virus (HDV), also a bloodborne pathogen, is found only in people who are already infected with HBV. Vaccination against HBV protects against HDV.

Hepatitis E Virus (HEV)

Hepatitis E virus (HEV) is not a bloodborne type of hepatitis. Like HAV, HEV is spread through the oral–fecal route of transmission. HEV infection is most common in countries with poor sanitation controls. There is no vaccination for this virus.

HIV/AIDS

Human immunodeficiency virus (HIV) is the virus that causes **acquired immunodeficiency syndrome (AIDS).** HIV is a bloodborne pathogen, and is transmitted in the same way as HBV. Its effect on the body, however, is very different.

As described in Chapter 15, the human immune system recognizes and destroys pathogens (microbes that can enter the body and cause illness). One way the immune system does its job is through **T cells,** special white blood cells (leukocytes) that play a role in the immune response to invading pathogens. There are two main types of T cells. One type of T cell recognizes cells that are foreign to the body, such as those infected by viruses, and kills them by producing substances that cause the foreign cells to burst. The other type of T cell produces substances that help other cells in the immune system to defend the body against pathogens.

T cells are the main target of HIV (Fig. 16-5). The virus invades the T cell. But, instead of

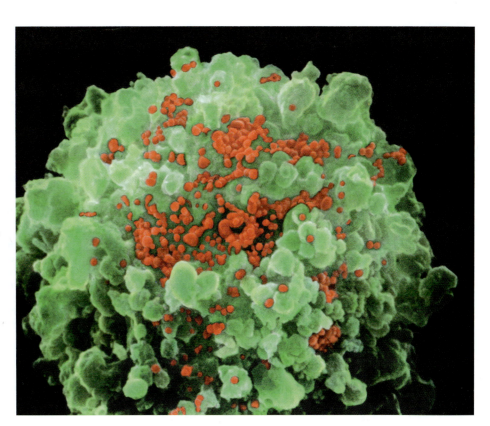

Figure 16-5
This photograph was taken by a special microscope, and color was added to enhance it. It shows a T cell (*green*) that is infected with the human immunodeficiency virus (HIV), shown in *red*. Infection with HIV can lead to the development of acquired immunodeficiency syndrome (AIDS), a fatal disease. (*NIBSC/Photo Researchers, Inc.*)

killing the T cell immediately, it uses the T cell to make copies of itself and increase its numbers. Eventually, the virus kills the T cell, and then the virus (and all of its copies) move on to repeat the process in other T cells. This process, over time, results in an increase in the virus count and a decrease in the T cell count.

In addition to invading and killing T cells, HIV invades the cells that form new T cells. This causes the body to produce T cells that cannot recognize pathogens. The body then becomes unable to recognize and fight off infections, leading to the condition known as AIDS. People with AIDS do not die from the virus itself. They die from infections that the body is no longer able to fight. To date, there is no cure for AIDS and no vaccine for HIV.

PROTECTING YOURSELF FROM BLOODBORNE DISEASES

Standard Precautions

Bloodborne pathogens, such as HIV and HBV, pose an occupational risk to the health care worker (Table 16-1). Because of the type of work you do, you will come in contact with substances that carry these viruses. Additionally, in many cases, you will not be able to easily identify residents who have these diseases. For example, HIV can be present in the blood of an infected person for a long time without causing symptoms or being detected using the diagnostic tests that are currently available. Similarly, the viruses that cause hepatitis B and hepatitis C can live in a person's body without causing signs or symptoms. For these reasons, you must treat each resident you have contact with as if he may be infected with a bloodborne pathogen. This is why standard precautions (see Chapter 15, Box 15-1) are taken with each resident. *For standard precautions to be effective, they must be used consistently with every resident.*

It is important to remember that although those who choose to work in the health care field place themselves at risk for exposure to substances that can cause disease, the risk of encountering these substances outside of the workplace also exists. In fact, your behavior outside of the workplace could put you at much higher risk for getting one of these diseases. For example, having unprotected sexual intercourse is the most common way of getting HBV and HIV, and the rate of new hepatitis B and AIDS cases is growing fastest among young, heterosexual men and women. Your job exposes you to risks, such as needlesticks, that people in other professions

Table 16-1	Comparison of Hepatitis B Virus (HBV) and Human Immunodeficiency Virus (HIV)	
	HEPATITIS B VIRUS (HBV)	**HUMAN IMMUNODEFICIENCY VIRUS (HIV)**
Virus's ability to live outside of the body	HBV can live on a dry surface in the form of dried blood or body fluid for as long as **7 days.**	HIV can live for up to **24 hours** on a dry surface.
Virus content per cc/mL of blood*	**1,000,000,000 (1 billion)** virus particles per cc/mL of blood	**1,000 (1 thousand)** virus particles per cc/mL of blood
Risk of getting virus from a needlestick injury	**6%–30%**	**Less than 0.1%**[†]
Modes of transmission	Not transmitted by casual contact. Outside of the health care profession, HBV can be transmitted by having unprotected sexual intercourse or sharing needles used to inject drugs. It can also be transmitted to a fetus across the placenta or following exposure to the mother's blood during birth.	Not transmitted by casual contact. Outside of the health care profession, HIV can be transmitted by having unprotected sexual intercourse or sharing needles used to inject drugs. It can also be transmitted to a fetus across the placenta or following exposure to the mother's blood during birth.
Associated annual death rate among health care workers	Approximately 250 health care workers die each year from HBV	Statistic not available

*One cc/mL of blood is equal to approximately one large drop of blood. Therefore, even minor cuts can be significant in terms of their ability to expose the health care worker to bloodborne pathogens.
[†]97.7% of occupational exposures do not result in HIV infection.

BOX 16-1   OSHA Bloodborne Pathogens Standard

- People working in an area where exposure to bloodborne pathogens is possible must receive training on the risks associated with bloodborne pathogens and on the methods they can use to safeguard themselves. Proof of initial training (at orientation) is to be on file in the employee's records, and training must be updated annually.
- Employers must make the hepatitis B vaccine available to workers who are at risk, free of charge. If an employee refuses the vaccination, a disclaimer signed by the employee must be kept on file. If the employee decides to accept the vaccine at a later date, the employer must provide it.
- The employer must provide adequate personal protective equipment (PPE), as required by the employee's duties. This includes gloves (non-latex, if the employee has allergies), face and eye protection, gowns and aprons, and scrub attire. It is the employee's responsibility to use the PPE consistently and conscientiously.

- Environmental control methods must be used to protect both the employees and the residents. Environmental control methods include special ventilation systems to keep the air clean, procedures for the disposal of liquid waste, the availability of sharps disposal containers, and procedures for handling contaminated linen and trash. Housekeeping and cleaning methods must also meet OSHA's standards.
- Each health care facility must have an **exposure control plan** in place in case an employee is exposed to blood or other body fluids from a resident. The exposure control plan states what actions must be taken if an employee is exposed to blood or other body fluids while on the job. This plan must be up to date, available in written form, and available to all employees. It is the employee's responsibility to report any exposure incidents so that the employer can arrange for appropriate medical tests and treatment.

do not need to worry about. But, if you follow the standard precautions, your risk of getting a bloodborne disease in the workplace will probably be lower than your risk of getting a bloodborne disease outside of it!

OSHA Bloodborne Pathogens Standard

Your safety in the workplace is a shared responsibility. You are responsible for following the standard precautions. Your employer is responsible for making sure that you have the equipment and training you need to maintain your safety in the workplace. To help employers to meet their responsibilities toward their employees, OSHA has created certain standards that all employers must follow, called the **OSHA Bloodborne Pathogens Standard** (Box 16-1).

Any health care facility that does not follow the OSHA standards for bloodborne pathogens may risk heavy fines and serious penalties, such as closure of the facility. For health care workers who do not follow standard precautions, the penalty can be even greater—a deadly illness. Additionally, if you have an exposure accident and were not following the recommended precautions, you may not be covered by worker's compensation if you become sick as a result of the exposure. The consequences of not following proper procedures in the workplace are not worth the risk.

AIRBORNE DISEASES

AIRBORNE TRANSMISSION

Airborne pathogens are disease-producing microbes that are transmitted through the air. When an infected person coughs or sneezes, the pathogens leave the body through particles of saliva or sputum (Fig. 16-6). As these particles spray through the air, they dry out and remain in the air for a long time (much like particles of dust

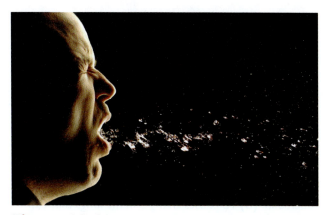

Figure 16-6

A typical sneeze sends several thousand droplets of microbe-containing mucus and saliva into the air. (*Getty Images/William Radcliffe.*)

caught in a shaft of sunlight). Like dust, the dried-out droplets containing pathogens are in the air we breathe and on the surfaces we touch. Infection spreads when a person breathes the air containing the suspended pathogens. Infections that are transmitted in this way include measles, chickenpox, and tuberculosis (TB). Although vaccines are available to prevent measles and chickenpox, there is currently no vaccine against TB.

TUBERCULOSIS (TB)

Tuberculosis (TB) is an infection caused by a bacterium that usually infects the lungs, but may also infect the kidneys or bones. The bacteria are present in the sputum of an infected person and are spread by airborne droplets when the person coughs, sneezes, speaks, or sings. People who have close, frequent contact with a person who has TB are most likely to get the disease. A person infected with TB may have the disease for years before she shows any symptoms.

In the early 1900s, TB caused many deaths. It was often called "consumption" because the disease progressed slowly and caused a wasting effect on the person. (In other words, the person grew very thin, and appeared to be eaten, or "consumed," by the disease). During this time, people with TB were usually sent to special hospitals called *sanitoriums,* which offered treatment and also served as a way of limiting the spread of the disease, by keeping people with TB away from others. In the early 1950s, the development of antibiotics that worked against the bacterium that causes TB resulted in a decrease in the number of people with the disease. However, TB is still a public health concern today for the following reasons:

- Strains of the bacterium that cause TB have become resistant to the antibiotics used to treat the infection, making the antibiotics less effective.
- People with immunodeficiency syndromes, such as AIDS, are more at risk for infections, such as TB, and the number of people with immunodeficiency syndromes has increased.
- More people are traveling to developing nations, where TB is still common.
- People who are poor or who live in crowded urban areas (for example, homeless people and illegal immigrants) are at increased risk for TB.

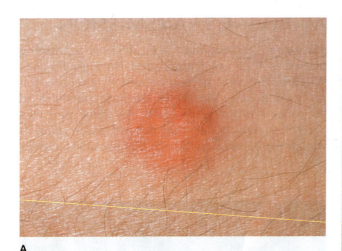

A

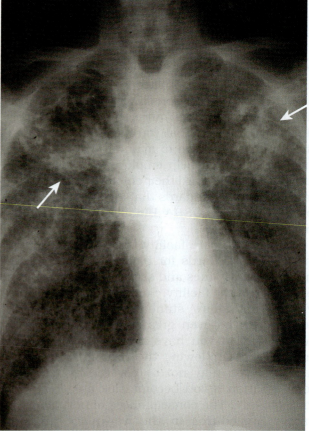

B

Figure 16-7

Health care facilities and agencies routinely screen employees for tuberculosis (TB). **(A)** A simple skin test is used to screen for exposure to TB. A person who has been exposed to the bacterium that causes TB will develop redness and swelling in the area (*shown here*). A person who has not been exposed will not have any reaction to the tuberculin. **(B)** TB causes changes in the lungs that can be seen on a chest x-ray (*arrows*). The chest x-ray of a person with a TB infection in the upper part of the lungs is shown here. (*A, Dr. P. Marazzi, Photo Researchers, Inc.; B, B. Bates M.D./Custom Medical Stock Photo.*)

People who get TB need to be treated for a long time, with many different antibiotics. Unfortunately, the people who are most likely to get the disease are least likely to complete the course of treatment for it because they lack money, a stable home, or both.

Because TB may go undiagnosed, a very real potential for exposure to TB in the workplace exists. Generally, a resident of a long-term care facility who is found to have active TB will be transferred to a hospital to receive the proper treatment. However, it is still important that you have knowledge of this disease and how it is spread. You will still be at risk until that transfer is made.

Because health care workers are at risk for getting TB from residents, long-term care facilities regularly screen employees for TB using a simple skin test. A small amount of test material, called *tuberculin*, is placed under the skin on the arm using a needle or tines. In a few days, the area is checked. A person who has been exposed to the bacterium that causes TB will develop redness and swelling in the area (Fig. 16-7A). A person who has not been exposed will not have any reaction to the tuberculin. Testing positive on a skin test does not mean that you have TB, just that you have been exposed to it. Additional tests, such as a chest x-ray, are necessary to determine if a person actually has TB (Fig. 16-7B).

PROTECTING YOURSELF FROM AIRBORNE DISEASES

If a patient or resident is known or suspected to have an airborne disease, such as TB, airborne precautions (see Chapter 15, Box 15-2) are taken.

SUMMARY

- Hepatitis B virus (HBV), hepatitis C virus (HCV), hepatitis D virus (HDV), and human immunodeficiency virus (HIV) are bloodborne pathogens that a health care worker may be exposed to. These viruses cause serious, possibly even life-threatening, diseases.
  - For a bloodborne pathogen to be transmitted from one person to another, blood or body fluids from an infected person must enter the bloodstream of a non-infected person.
    - Needlesticks, cuts from contaminated glass, and splashes and sprays of contaminated blood can put a health care worker at risk for a bloodborne disease.
    - Bloodborne diseases can also be transmitted through sexual intercourse and through blood transfusions.
    - A person who is infected with a bloodborne pathogen may not appear to be ill.
  - You and your employer share the responsibility for maintaining your safety in the workplace.
    - Employers must follow the standards outlined by the Occupational Safety and Health Administration (OSHA) to ensure that the work environment is safe (the OSHA Bloodborne Pathogens Standard).

  - Employees must follow the recommended precautions for preventing the spread of disease (standard precautions). Following the recommended standard precautions, at all times, is the single most important thing you can do to ensure your own safety.
  - A vaccine against HBV is available and offers protection against HDV, as well. Currently, there is no vaccine available for HCV or HIV.
- Tuberculosis (TB) is caused by an airborne pathogen. The pathogen that causes TB is spread when an infected person coughs, sneezes, speaks, or sings.
  - A person with TB may not appear to be ill.
  - Although antibiotics are available to treat TB, treatment is difficult, time-consuming, and expensive. There is currently no vaccine available for TB.
- You will face exposure to many infections, some life-threatening, while caring for others. Learning about these infections and how they are transmitted, as well as staying well informed about new developments and treatments for these diseases, will allow you to provide quality care to those you are responsible for.

WHAT DID YOU LEARN?

Multiple Choice

Select the single best answer for each of the following questions.

1. Hepatitis B virus (HBV), a bloodborne pathogen, can be found in all of the following body fluids except:
   a. Blood
   b. Semen
   c. Wound drainage
   d. Sweat

2. Human immunodeficiency virus (HIV) can be transmitted through all of the following means except:
   a. Blood splash to mucous membrane
   b. Sexual intercourse
   c. Sharing needles
   d. A mosquito bite

3. A vaccination against which one of the following bloodborne diseases is available?
   a. Lyme disease
   b. AIDS
   c. Hepatitis C
   d. Hepatitis B

4. Hepatitis B is a viral disease of the:
   a. Spleen
   b. Liver
   c. Blood
   d. Heart

STOP and Think!

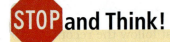

- You are walking past the TV room of the nursing facility where you work. You hear a call for help. As you enter the room, you see that Mr. Torres has a pretty bad nosebleed. There is blood on his hands and clothes, and some has puddled on the floor. What should you do as you rush to help Mr. Torres? How will you clean up the blood afterward?

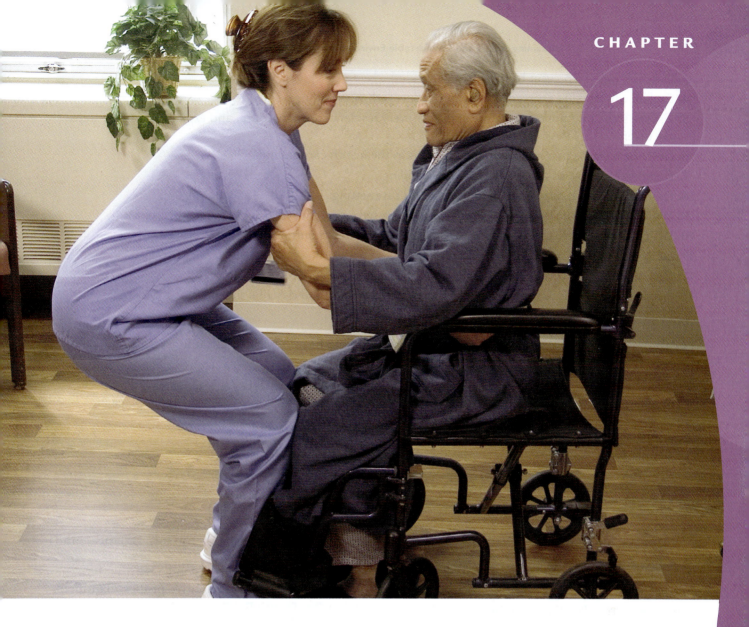

Workplace Safety

WHAT WILL YOU LEARN?

As you have learned in Chapters 15 and 16, the risk of infectious disease is a work-related hazard faced by all people in the long-term care setting—residents, family members and visitors, and health care workers. Although minimizing the spread of infectious disease is a major safety concern for health care workers, it is not the only one. In this chapter, we will explore other threats to the safety of people who work or live in a long-term care facility, and the measures you can take to minimize these threats. When you are finished with this chapter, you will be able to:

1. Define the term *body mechanics* and demonstrate actions that make the body more effective when working.
2. Demonstrate the use of good body mechanics when lifting.

Photo: A nursing assistant uses good body mechanics to protect herself from injury while assisting a resident to stand.

3. Describe ways to prevent back injury.

4. Explain why nursing assistants follow procedures when providing resident care.

5. List the steps that are taken before and after every resident care procedure, and explain why these steps are taken.

6. Describe hazards that increase the risk of falls in the health care setting.

7. Demonstrate how to assist a person who is falling.

8. Describe chemical hazards found in the health care setting.

9. Discuss electrical hazards found in the health care setting and ways to avoid them.

10. List the elements necessary for a fire to start and continue to burn.

11. Describe the RACE fire response plan.

12. Demonstrate how to use a fire extinguisher.

13. List disaster situations that may affect a health care facility, and describe the focus of a disaster preparedness plan in a long-term care facility

Vocabulary Use the CD in the front of your book to hear these terms pronounced and defined:

Body mechanics	Procedure	Materials Safety Data	Disaster
Alignment	Pre-procedure actions	Sheet (MSDS)	Shelter in place
Balance	Post-procedure	Grounded	
Coordinated body	actions	RACE fire response plan	
movement			

PROTECTING YOUR BODY

Performing the same action over and over again places stress on the body—for example, think of the stress on a baseball catcher's knees as he squats, then stands, then squats again hundreds of times throughout a single game. In addition, moving a large, awkward, or heavy object also places strain on the body and can lead to injury. As a nursing assistant, you will place stress on your body as you lift, push, pull, stoop, and bend repeatedly, on a daily basis. In addition, in many cases, you will need to move a person or piece of equipment that is larger and heavier than you are. There is no doubt about it—being a nursing assistant is extremely physically demanding! Fortunately, by practicing good body mechanics and learning proper lifting techniques, you can minimize your risk for physical injury.

THE "ABCs" OF GOOD BODY MECHANICS

The efficient movement and use of the body is accomplished through good **body mechanics.** The basic components (the "ABCs") of good body mechanics are **A**lignment, **B**alance, and **C**oordinated movement.

Alignment is simply good posture. For the body to work most efficiently, proper alignment is necessary to ensure that no excess strain is placed on the joints and muscles. The back is held in a "neutral" position, with the natural curvature of the lower back intact. Imagine that you are looking at a person who is holding her body in proper alignment (Fig. 17-1). On the side view, you would be able to draw a straight line connecting the person's ear, shoulder, hip, knee, and ankle. From the front view, you would be able to draw a straight line that connected the nose, the sternum (breastbone), and the navel, and then continued between the legs, dividing that space equally in half.

Balance is stability produced by the even distribution of weight. Balance involves holding your center of gravity, or area of largest mass, close to your base of support. For example, when you are standing, your base of support is your feet (which are placed squarely on the floor), and your center of gravity is your torso, the heaviest part of your body. The larger your base of support, and the closer the heaviest part of your body is to that base of support, the more balanced you will be.

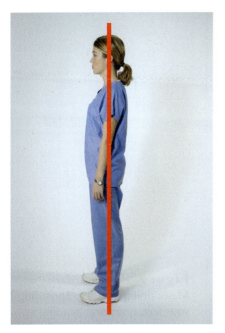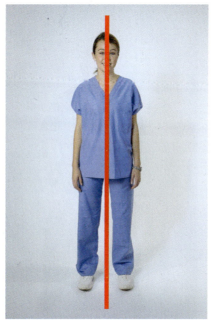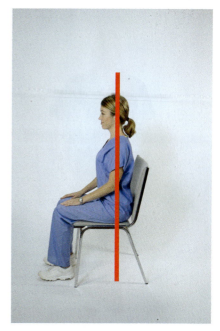

Figure 17-1
When the body is held in proper alignment, the back is in a "neutral" position, with the curve of the lower spine intact. Holding the body in proper alignment prevents strain on the joints and muscles.

How, then, can you stabilize your body and maximize your ability to remain balanced? There are two ways:

- You can increase your base of support by spreading your feet further apart.
- You can bring your center of gravity closer to your base of support by bending at the knees and hips, so that your torso is closer to your feet.

Imagine that you are standing with your legs together and your ankles touching. If someone pushed you, you might lose your balance and fall. Now, imagine that you are standing with your feet about shoulder-width apart. The same shove might not cause you to lose your balance. And, if you were then to lower your body into a squat, it would be even harder to push you over! Increasing your base of support by standing with your feet apart, and positioning yourself so that your center of gravity (your torso) is close to your base of support (your feet) improves your balance and is a very important part of practicing good body mechanics (Fig. 17-2).

Coordinated body movement involves using the weight of your body to help with movement. For example, when moving a person up in bed, you stand facing the bed, with your feet apart. As you step sideways to move the person's head and shoulders up, you transfer your weight from one foot to the other and the momentum helps you to move the person (Fig. 17-3).

LIFTING AND BACK SAFETY

Practicing good body mechanics is important, especially when you must lift heavy equipment or move people who have trouble moving on their own. Lifting is a required task for nursing assistants who provide direct care to residents. Therefore, it is important to learn proper technique. Failure to use good body mechanics when lifting something or someone can result in back injuries. Back injuries are the most common work-related injury in the nursing field. Injuries of the back range from muscle strains and soreness to ruptured vertebral discs (a condition that may require surgery and a long recovery period). Back injuries are painful and costly (in terms of medical care and missed work), and can be serious enough to end your career and prevent you from participating in other activities that you enjoy. If you do not take precautions to prevent back injuries, you could find yourself in the position of being a patient instead of a care provider!

If you have ever watched the weightlifting event in the Olympics, you know that competitive weightlifters can lift more than 500 pounds. The

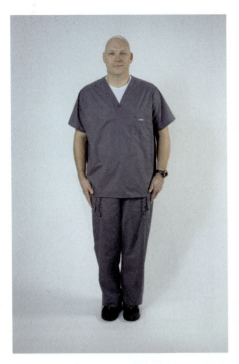 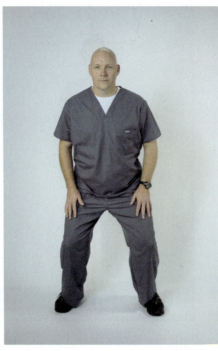

Figure 17-2
Maintaining balance. Spreading your feet apart and bending at the hips and knees improves your ability to stay balanced.

weightlifter's lifting technique is an excellent example of good body mechanics being used. The athlete squats low to the ground, using his arms and shoulders to pull the weight close to his body at chest level. He then uses his hips and legs to stand up with the weight. After becoming upright,

he widens his base of support by moving one foot ahead of the other. These maneuvers allow the large, strong muscles of the body to do the work of lifting and also protect the back from injury.

The muscles of the arms and legs are attached to the long bones in our limbs. The muscle contracts by pulling against the bone it is attached to. This allows us to move and to lift weight. In contrast, the muscles of the back are flat and fan-like, and are not designed to lift weight. When the competitive weightlifter lifts his weights, he uses his leg muscles, not his back muscles. As he raises himself out of the squat, he uses the powerful muscles in his buttocks, hips, and thighs to move himself, and the weight, upward. Although you will not be required to practice competitive weightlifting at work, you should try to imitate the professionals with your technique! For example, if you had to move a resident from the bed to a chair, you would bend your knees and hold the person close to the center of your body. Then, you would use the muscles in your thighs and hips to lift and move the person from the bed to the chair. Proper lifting technique is summarized in Figure 17-4.

Some health care facilities and agencies require employees who must lift to wear back supports. When used appropriately and correctly, a back support will remind you to hold your body in proper alignment when lifting. Bending at the waist with a tight back support around you is

Figure 17-3
Coordinated body movement involves using the weight of your body to help with movement. When the nursing assistant steps sideways, shifting her weight from her left foot to her right, the momentum of her body helps to move the person up in bed.

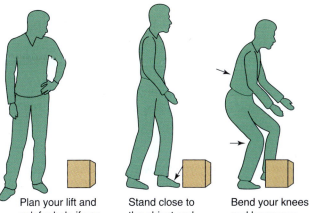

Plan your lift and ask for help if you need it.

Stand close to the object and widen your base of support.

Bend your knees and keep your back straight.

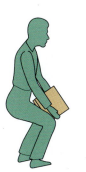

Tighten your stomach muscles.

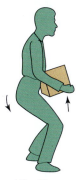

Lift with your leg muscles.

Figure 17-4
Proper lifting technique.

body mechanics and apply them consistently, both at work and at home.

FOLLOWING PROCEDURES

To ensure that the care you provide is safe and correct, you will follow specific **procedures.** A procedure is a series of steps followed in a particular order. Following the recommended steps of a procedure helps to protect the person you are caring for, and it protects you.

Certain steps, called **pre-procedure actions,** are followed before performing any procedure on a resident. In this book, we call these actions "Getting Ready" steps (Guidelines Box 17-2). The "Getting Ready" steps promote efficiency, safety, courtesy, and respect of the resident's rights. Similarly, there is a group of actions that are routinely performed at the end of each procedure, called **post-procedure actions.** In this book, we call these actions "Finishing Up" steps (Guidelines Box 17-3). The "Finishing Up" steps promote comfort, safety, and communication among members of the health care team. As you review the procedure boxes throughout this book, you will see references to these "Getting Ready" and "Finishing Up" steps in each of them. You must learn these steps and perform them before and after every procedure.

PREVENTING FALLS

Nursing assistants work hard and have many duties that must be completed during a shift. Being in too much of a hurry can increase your risk of falling. Even in an emergency situation, when you need to move quickly, be aware of your surroundings and move only as fast as you are safely able. You are not a help in an emergency if you fall and hurt yourself!

Wet floors also increase your risk of falling. Helping residents with showers and baths often results in water on the floor. A resident who is incontinent can leave a puddle of urine in the hallway that you could slip in, especially if you are in a hurry. If you see water or other fluids or substances on the floor, immediately stop what you are doing and dry the area (Fig. 17-5). If the floor is left wet from cleaning, be sure that a "Caution: Wet Floor" sign is put in place.

Be aware of objects in your path that could cause you to trip. Electrical cords can pose a

very uncomfortable! However, if your facility requires you to wear a back support when lifting, make sure you have been properly trained in its correct use. Improper or prolonged use of a back support can actually weaken the back muscles. In addition, using a back support may give you a false sense of security, leading you to attempt to lift more than you are actually capable of lifting.

Because of the risk of injury that is associated with lifting, many long-term care facilities are starting to adopt "no lift" policies. This means that health care workers are being encouraged to use mechanical lifts for lifting residents, and to avoid the practice of manual lifting, whenever possible. You will learn more about the use of mechanical lifts in Chapter 20.

Guidelines for protecting yourself from injury as a result of the physical nature of your job are summarized in Guidelines Box 17-1. To protect your health, remember the principles of good

Guidelines Box 17-1 Guidelines for Protecting Yourself From Physical Injury

WHAT YOU DO	WHY YOU DO IT
Make a habit of practicing good posture.	Keeping the body in proper alignment, regardless of the activity, reduces stress and fatigue to the muscles and joints.
Create a solid base of support by moving your feet apart, either by widening your stance or by placing one foot in front of the other.	A solid base of support improves your balance, reducing the chance that you will injure yourself during the maneuver.
Allow the weight of your own body to assist in pulling or pushing heavy objects.	Using coordinated body movement to move something minimizes the stress on your body while making the task you are trying to accomplish easier.
When moving or lifting people or objects, place your body as close as possible to the object being moved.	Bringing your body's center of gravity closer to the object improves your balance and allows the strong muscles of the shoulders and upper arms to assist in the move.
Squat, do not lean over, to lower your center of gravity when lifting.	Lowering your center of gravity improves your balance. However, this lowering should be accomplished by squatting, rather than leaning over. Squatting allows you to use the strong muscles of your lower body to move yourself, and the weight, upward. Leaning over while lifting weight strains the back joints and muscles.
Use the large, strong muscles of the hips, buttocks, and thighs to do the lifting.	Using the strong muscles of the legs to move yourself upward is preferable to placing strain on the muscles of the back, which are not meant to be used to lift substantial amounts of weight.
Do not lift heavy objects from a position higher than your head. Use a step stool or a short safety ladder to raise your entire body closer to the desired level.	Attempting to lift a heavy object from an awkward position (for example, with your arms raised above your head) interferes with your ability to balance and places you at risk for injury.
If an object is very heavy, do not attempt to lift it. Instead, pull, push, or roll the object.	Pushing, pulling, or rolling a heavy object places less strain on your body because you can use your body weight to help you accomplish the task. In other words, you can use the principle of coordinated movement.
Use assistive devices whenever possible to make the job easier.	Hand carts and dollies permit the easy movement of objects by placing them on wheels. Gait belts, draw sheets, and mechanical lifts (discussed in detail in Chapter 20) help make moving people easier.

(continued)

WHAT YOU DO	WHY YOU DO IT
Ask for help when lifting or moving heavy people or objects. You should also get help when you need to move a person who cannot offer any assistance, or is combative.	Heavy or awkward loads increase your risk of injury (and, if you are attempting to lift a person, increase that person's risk of injury as well.) A person who is "dead weight" or uncooperative is both heavy and awkward.
Keep your body in good physical condition by exercising regularly, eating nutritious foods, and getting enough rest.	Your body can be compared to an automobile. It must be properly maintained in order to provide you with years of solid performance.

tripping hazard. Try to position furniture so that the electrical cords for lamps and other appliances are close to the outlet. If the beds in your facility are manually operated, remember to fold the cranks down and away under the bed after you are finished using them so that they do not pose a tripping hazard for people who are walking near the foot of the bed.

Make sure that you can see clearly. Nightlights positioned near the floor are useful in a health care setting. They allow you to see where you are going without disturbing the resident by turning on the overhead light.

Helping a very weak, unsteady, or uncooperative person to walk or transfer from one place to another without help can cause both of you to fall. You may not want to ask a busy co-worker for help, but resist the temptation to "go it alone."

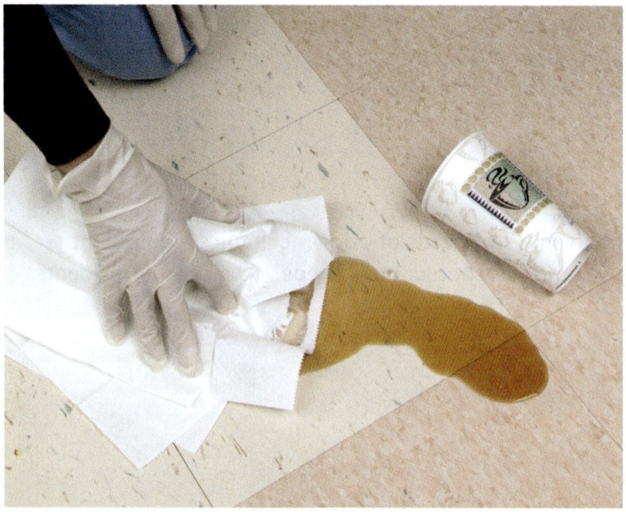

Figure 17-5
Mopping up spills is an important safety measure. Failing to do so can lead to falls.

If the resident you are attempting to help falls, she will take you with her, potentially resulting in serious injury to you both. Attempting to prevent a resident from falling can also result in a back injury for you. Please ask for help whenever you feel you need it, in order to safely continue. If you are assisting a person who begins to fall, follow the steps in Box 17-1 to minimize the risk of injury for everyone involved.

PREVENTING CHEMICAL INJURIES

Health care facilities use many chemicals on a daily basis (for example, cleaning and sanitizing agents and floor care products). Many of these chemicals can be harmful if they are inhaled, swallowed, absorbed through the skin, or splashed in the eyes. Some chemicals are relatively harmless alone but can become dangerous if accidentally mixed with another product.

The Occupational Safety and Health Administration (OSHA) requires all employers to maintain a list of the chemicals that are used in the facility, from household cleaners to highly toxic solutions, and to inform and educate all workers about the chemicals that are in use in their workplace. One way of communicating information about chemicals to employees is through a **Materials Safety Data Sheet (MSDS)**, which the manufacturer of the chemical is required to supply. The MSDS for each chemical in use must be kept on file and be readily available in each unit of the health care facility. The manufacturer must renew the MSDS every 3 years (or sooner, if there is a change in the product). The MSDS summarizes key information about the chemical such as what it is made from,

Guidelines Box 17-2   Guidelines for Getting Ready (Pre-procedure Actions)

WHAT YOU DO	WHY YOU DO IT
WASH your hands. Apply gloves and follow standard precautions if contact with blood or body fluids is possible.	Washing your hands and taking standard precautions prevents the spread of infection.
GATHER needed supplies.	Having everything you need before you start promotes efficiency.
KNOCK on the door and identify yourself by name and title to the person.	Knocking before you enter protects the person's right to privacy. Identifying yourself respects the person's right to know who is providing care.
IDENTIFY the person, and greet him or her by name. Methods of identifying residents will vary depending on where you work. Common methods of identifying people in health care facilities include wrist bands and photographs.	Identifying the person ensures that the procedure is being done on the correct resident. Greeting the person by name is courteous.
EXPLAIN the procedure and encourage the person to participate as appropriate.	Explaining the procedure lets the person know what to expect and helps him to understand how he can help.
PROVIDE PRIVACY by showing any visitors where they may wait, if necessary, until you have completed the procedure. Close the door and the curtain. Drape the person for modesty as appropriate.	Asking visitors to leave the room, closing the door and curtain, and draping the person for modesty protects the person's right to privacy.
SEE TO SAFETY. Take safety precautions by following standards of body mechanics, equipment use, and infection control. In procedures that involve getting a person out of bed, lower the bed to its lowest position. This decreases the distance between the bed and the floor, should the person fall. In procedures that involve providing care while the person remains in bed, raise the bed to a comfortable working height. This protects your back.	Following standards of body mechanics, equipment use, and infection control keeps you and your residents safe.

Guidelines Box 17-3 — Guidelines for Finishing Up (Post-procedure Actions)

WHAT YOU DO	WHY YOU DO IT
CONFIRM that the person is comfortable and in good body alignment.	Proper body alignment is most comfortable for the person. It relieves strain on the muscles and joints, promotes good heart and lung function, and helps prevent contractures and pressure ulcers.
LEAVE the call light control, telephone, and fresh water within easy reach of the person.	Having necessary items nearby promotes independence and helps to prevent falls.
SEE TO SAFETY. Return the bed to the lowest position, lock the wheels, and raise the side rails (if side rails are in use).	Lowering the bed, locking the wheels, and raising the side rails (if side rails are in use) helps to prevent falls.
OPEN the curtain and door if desired by the resident, and inform visitors that they may return to the room.	Opening the curtain and door and letting visitors know that they can return helps to prevent feelings of isolation.
WASH your hands. If gloved, remove and discard the gloves following facility policy, and then wash your hands.	Washing your hands prevents the spread of infection.
REPORT AND RECORD actions as required by your facility.	Reporting lets the nurse know that you have completed the task and allows you to update the nurse about any changes in the resident's status. Recording formally documents the care that was provided and ensures that all members of the health care team have the same information about the resident's status and care.

which exposures may be dangerous, what to do if an exposure occurs, and how to clean up spills. Container labels also provide information about the chemicals in the container, and all containers must be clearly labeled. As a nursing assistant, it is your responsibility to be familiar with the chemicals that you may come in contact with in your facility, and to know the proper, safe way to handle each chemical in use.

Many times, chemicals are supplied in large containers. It may be more efficient for health care workers who use the chemical to have smaller containers of the chemical in their immediate work areas. When this is the case, there is usually a person in the facility who is responsible for transferring chemicals to smaller containers, and labeling the smaller containers. The contents of the smaller container must be clearly

Minimizing the Risk of Injury as a Result of a Fall

1. If the person complains of dizziness or seems unsteady, help him to sit in a chair. If a chair is not close by, help the person to sit on the floor. Stay with the person and call for assistance. This action can prevent a fall completely.

2. If a fall cannot be avoided, place your body behind the person and place your arms around his torso, pulling him close to your body. Do not grab the person's arm in an attempt to prevent the fall, because doing so may actually cause more extensive injuries in elderly people, who may have brittle bones and fragile skin.

3. With the person's body pulled close to yours, widen your base of support by placing one foot behind the other, and allow the person to slide down your body toward the floor.

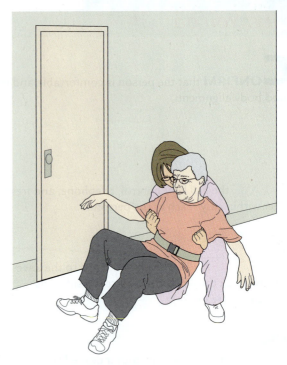

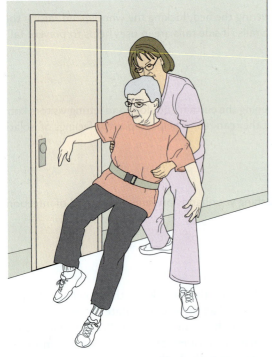

4. As the person slides down, squat while still supporting his body and gently lower him to the floor. Lower yourself to the floor and assume a sitting position with the person's head in your lap.

5. Stay with the person and call for assistance.

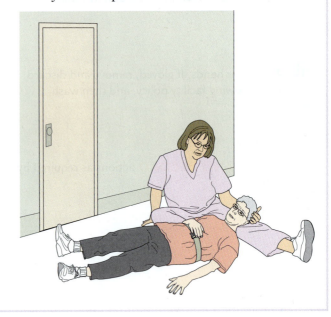

marked on the container. If the chemical is accidentally spilled or swallowed (for example, by a confused resident), it is important to know what the chemical is! If the container is unmarked, a great deal of time could be wasted trying to identify the chemical, with potentially very serious results.

PREVENTING ELECTRICAL SHOCKS

Many electrical appliances are used in the long-term care setting, from electrically controlled beds to the common hair dryer. Knowing how to

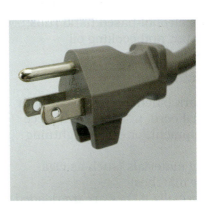
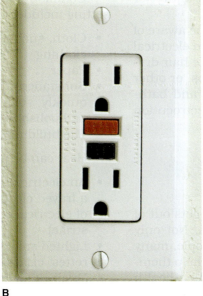
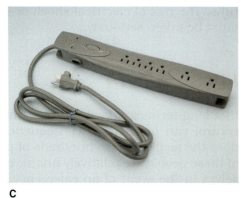

A   B   C

Figure 17-6
(A) Three-prong plugs, **(B)** outlets with ground-fault breakers, and **(C)** power strips help to reduce the risk of electrical shock and fire.

safely operate and maintain electrical equipment in the workplace helps to create a safe working environment for you and a safe living environment for your residents.

Precautions, such as using grounded appliances and power strips, help to minimize the risk of electrical shock. Most electrical equipment used in the health care setting is **grounded.** This means that it has a way of returning stray electrical current to the outlet so that the risk of electrical shock is reduced. Grounding may be achieved through a three-prong plug (Fig. 17-6A) or a safety outlet with a ground-fault breaker (Fig. 17-6B). The use of extension cords is not recommended and outlets should not be overloaded. If more than two items must be plugged into an outlet, a facility-approved power strip should be used (Fig. 17-6C).

As a nursing assistant, you must be alert for electrical items that pose potential shock or fire hazards. Residents often bring small electrical items with them to furnish their rooms such as radios, televisions, and table lamps. Most facilities require items like these to be inspected by the maintenance department before the resident can use them. However, if you should notice anything unsafe about an electrical appliance that is being used, such as frayed wires or loose plugs, you should remove the appliance from use immediately. This is true of facility-owned equipment

as well, such as electrically controlled beds and call light controls. Most health care facilities have a system for tagging defective items and equipment and sending them for repair (Fig. 17-7). (This system also usually applies to equipment that is not electrically operated, such as wheelchairs.) Follow your facility's policy. Failure to remove a defective item or piece of equipment from service could put the next person who uses the item or

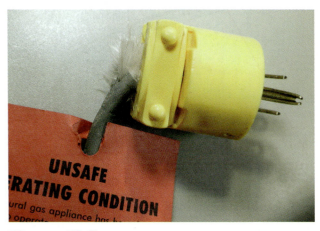

Figure 17-7
If you notice that a piece of equipment is malfunctioning or presents a safety hazard, follow your facility's policy for removing it from use and getting it repaired.

piece of equipment at risk for serious injury, or even death.

When using electrical equipment, be aware of the safety hazard posed by operating an electrical appliance around water. Do not operate hair dryers, electric razors, curling irons, radios, or other electrical appliances around showers and bathtubs. The risk of electrical shock or electrocution must be taken seriously.

FIRE SAFETY

In a long-term care facility, a fire that gets out of control can have tragic consequences. Not only does the facility house hundreds of people, many of these people are relatively unable to help themselves in the event of an emergency. As a health care worker, you must know how to prevent fires in the workplace, and what to do in the event that a fire does occur. General guidelines for fire safety are given in Guidelines Box 17-4.

PREVENTING FIRES

For a fire to occur, three elements must be present: fuel (something that burns), heat (something to ignite the fuel), and oxygen (Fig. 17-8).

Common sources of fuel in the health care setting include:

- Cloth, such as bed linens, mattresses, and clothing
- Paper
- Substances that easily catch fire and burn quickly, such as alcohol-based hand rubs, nail polish remover, and cooking oil
- The building itself

Heat can be provided by:

- An electrical spark (such as may occur with a frayed electrical cord, a "short" in a piece of electrical equipment, or even a lightning strike)
- Lighted smoking materials (such as cigarettes, cigars, or matches)
- Dryer units (especially if they are overloaded, or have full lint traps)
- Heating elements (such as radiators or furnaces)
- Lamps
- Stoves

Oxygen is found in the air around us, and generally, the better the air supply, the better a fire will burn. Some residents receive oxygen therapy, which increases the content of the oxygen in the air in the immediate area. Safety precautions that are used to prevent fires are extremely important when oxygen therapy is in use (see Guidelines Box 17-4). Caution signs are used to alert people in the facility that extra precautions are needed when oxygen therapy is in use (Fig. 17-9). Caution signs are also posted where oxygen is stored.

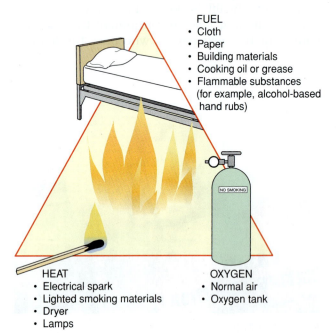

FUEL
- Cloth
- Paper
- Building materials
- Cooking oil or grease
- Flammable substances (for example, alcohol-based hand rubs)

HEAT
- Electrical spark
- Lighted smoking materials
- Dryer
- Lamps

OXYGEN
- Normal air
- Oxygen tank

Figure 17-8
Three things must be present for a fire to occur: fuel, heat, and oxygen.

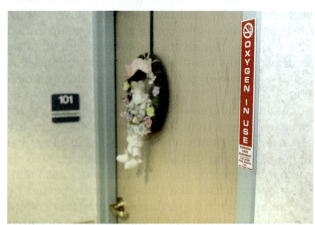

Figure 17-9
"Oxygen In Use" signs are posted to warn residents and their visitors that extra precautions are needed when oxygen therapy is in use.

Guidelines Box 17-4   Guidelines for Fire Safety

WHAT YOU DO	WHY YOU DO IT
Know your facility's fire safety plan and your role and responsibilities should a fire occur.	Knowing exactly what you are supposed to do in the event of a fire will allow you to take immediate action and remain calm.
Promptly investigate smoke or smells of anything burning. Be aware of the location of fire alarms and fire extinguishers and know how to activate and use them.	Early discovery and quick action can contain a fire before it gets out of control.
Know all emergency routes and exits.	If a fire does occur, you may need to evacuate residents. Knowing the location of emergency routes and exits helps the process go more quickly and more smoothly.
Make it a point to minimize clutter, and keep walking paths in rooms and hallways clear. Do not block emergency exits with carts or equipment.	Clutter just adds fuel in a fire situation. Should a fire break out, traffic areas need to be clear to allow easy exit from the area.
Report any malfunctioning smoke detectors immediately.	A smoke detector is the best early fire detection device available, but only if it is functioning.
Be alert to the location of sprinkler heads. Do not obstruct them, or stack linens or other items higher than allowed.	Items must be stored enough distance away from the sprinkler for the water spray to be effective. If burning items are above the sprinkler head, the spray will not be able to douse the flames.
Make sure that fire doors are not propped open.	Fire doors are designed to prevent a fire from spreading from one area of the building to another. They are wired to automatically close when a fire alarm sounds. Propping the door open disables this safety function and allows the spread of fire.
Know your facility's smoking policies and be sure that you, your residents, and their visitors adhere to them.	Smoking policies are in place to minimize the risk of fire resulting from the use of smoking materials.
If smoking is permitted in the facility, make sure that all smoking occurs only in designated smoking areas.	Designated smoking areas have ashtrays for properly extinguishing lit smoking materials. They are also located in a part of the building that is a safe distance away from where oxygen is stored or used.
Do not allow any resident to smoke in bed. (Although long-term care facilities prohibit smoking in resident rooms, some people may forget or disregard the rules.)	Smoking in bed brings together all three elements necessary for fire (fuel = bed linen, heat = lit match or cigarette, and oxygen = surrounding air). Smoking in bed is especially dangerous because the person is likely to fall asleep with the smoking material still lit.

(continued)

Guidelines Box 17-4   Guidelines for Fire Safety (continued)

WHAT YOU DO	WHY YOU DO IT
Appropriately supervise residents who are smoking. Be alert for residents who are confused or seem drowsy.	A confused or sleepy resident will not be attentive to the lit smoking material, which increases the chance a fire will start.
Keep smoking materials, lighters, and matches in a place where confused residents cannot access them. Let family members know that if they bring in these materials for a resident's use, they should give them to someone on the nursing staff so that they can be stored safely.	A confused resident cannot use these materials responsibly on his own, and should be supervised while smoking. Even if the resident who smokes is not confused, these materials should still be stored safely to prevent other residents who may be confused from gaining access to them.
Be especially alert to fire safety wherever oxygen is used or stored. Be sure caution signs are used in these areas to alert all staff, residents, and visitors that extra precautions must be taken. Do not provide residents who are receiving oxygen therapy with wool or mohair blankets, or anything else that could generate a spark.	Oxygen is a highly combustible gas. Any spark could easily ignite a fire, and because of the presence of oxygen, the fire would burn much more rapidly.
Handle flammable substances (such as alcohol-based hand rubs) safely and clean up any spills immediately. Do not use flammable substances near a heat source, such as a hair dryer or heater, or while smoking.	These substances will ignite easily and burn quickly. If they come in contact with a heat source, a fire is likely to start.
Keep all electrical equipment in good working order.	A spark from a frayed wire, an improperly grounded plug, or an electrical "short" can start an electrical fire.

REACTING TO A FIRE EMERGENCY

Sometimes, despite taking precautions, a fire will occur. In some cases, the fire will be small and can be dealt with rather easily if the situation is addressed promptly and correctly. For example, imagine a fire that begins in a resident's room because a visitor drops a half-lit cigarette in a wastebasket full of paper, or a stovetop fire that begins in the facility's kitchen. In both of these situations, an alert person who knew what to do could control the fire and it is possible that others outside of the immediate area would not even be aware of the disturbance. However, sometimes a fire can begin on a much larger scale, for example, as a result of faulty electrical wiring in the walls of the building, a gas leak, or even a terror-

ist attack. In situations like these, a large-scale evacuation (removal) of those in the facility will most likely be necessary.

The general actions that are taken in the event of a fire emergency are known as the **RACE fire response plan** (Fig. 17-10):

Remove any residents who are in immediate danger to safety. Escort residents who can walk. Use wheelchairs for unsteady residents. To prevent a confused or disoriented resident from accidentally wandering back into the fire area, assign another, alert resident or a visitor to attend to the person. Residents who cannot get out of bed should be moved in their beds, if possible. If the bed cannot be moved out of the room, or if stairs

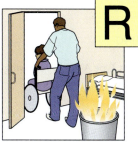

Remove

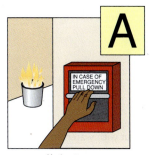

Activate

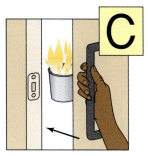

Contain

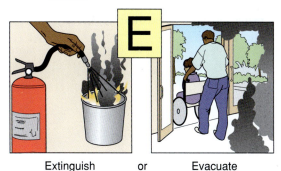

Extinguish   or   Evacuate

Figure 17-10
The RACE fire response plan.

must be used, the resident can be pulled to safety using the linens from the bed (Box 17-2). Some facilities will train you in special techniques that are used to carry a person to safety.

Activate the alarm, if the alarm has not been sounded. Follow your facility's policy for

---

BOX 17-2	**Using Bed Linens to Evacuate a Bedridden Person**

1. Loosen the bottom sheet from the foot of the person's bed.
2. Make sure that the bed is lowered to its lowest position and that the wheels are locked.
3. Grasp the top of the bottom sheet near the person's head and shoulders. Have a co-worker grasp the bottom sheet at the foot of the bed. Using the sheet, gently lower the person to the floor, feet first.
4. Pull the sheet, with the person cradled in it, toward the nearest exit.
5. If it is necessary to move the person down stairs, support the person's upper body by pulling up on the sheet and proceed down the steps backward. Do not allow the person's body to bump against the steps.

reporting a fire. For example, you may be required to pull the fire alarm, or use the intercom or telephone system.

Contain the fire by closing doors and windows. This action helps to slow the spread of the fire.

Extinguish the fire if possible (a general rule is to only consider extinguishing the fire yourself if the fire is no higher than your knee), or . . .

Evacuate, if the fire is large or spreading quickly. Follow your facility's evacuation procedures or the directions of emergency personnel. It may not be necessary to evacuate the entire building. In some cases, it may only be necessary to move residents to another area of the building that is not in danger.

Extinguishing Fires

As you know, there are three elements that must be present for a fire to continue burning—fuel, heat, and oxygen. If you remove just one of these elements, you can put out (extinguish) the fire. Not all fires are alike. Fires are classified as either "A" type, "B" type, or "C" type fires (Table 17-1). This classification determines the best way to put them out.

A commonly used tool for putting out fires is a fire extinguisher (Fig. 17-11). There are fire extinguishers that are specific for each type of fire, but the most common type of fire extinguisher, an ABC extinguisher, can be used for all types of fires. ABC fire extinguishers use carbon dioxide to remove the oxygen from the fire. This smothers

Table 17-1   Types of Fires

TYPE	DESCRIPTION	METHOD OF EXTINGUISHING
A	Fueled by ordinary material such as wood, paper, cloth, leaves, and grass	Water effectively extinguishes a Type A fire by removing the heat.
B	Fueled by a petroleum product (for example, gasoline, automotive oil), cooking oil, or grease	Do not try to put these fires out with water! Instead, smother the fire by sprinkling powder (such as baking soda) on it or by using a fire extinguisher made for a Type B fire. A stovetop fire that starts in a pan can be extinguished by covering the pan and removing it from the heat source.
C	An electrical fire	Attempting to put an electrical fire out with water can result in shock or electrocution. Use a fire extinguisher that is specific to an electrical fire instead.

the fire, putting it out. All health care facilities must have easily accessible fire extinguishers, in case a fire should occur. You are responsible for knowing where fire extinguishers are kept in your facility. During your orientation, you will be trained in the use of your facility's fire extinguishers, and these instructions will be reviewed with you each year. In the event of a small fire, you should be able to use a fire extinguisher to put the fire out safely and effectively. When using a fire extinguisher, remember the word **PASS**:

Pull the safety pin out.
Aim the hose toward the base of the fire.
Squeeze the handle.
Spray the contents of the fire extinguisher at the base of the fire, sweeping from side to side.

Evacuating the Building

If a large, uncontrollable fire breaks out, you will need to know how to get your residents and

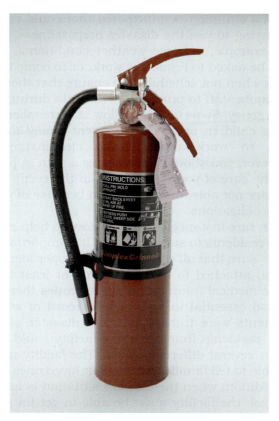

Figure 17-11
An ABC fire extinguisher is effective against all types of fires.

yourself to safety. Health care facilities must regularly practice and evaluate fire safety plans. You should take these fire drill exercises seriously so that if a fire emergency should occur, your actions will be almost second nature. By knowing what to do and acting calmly, you will increase the efficiency of the evacuation and help to calm those around you.

DISASTER PREPAREDNESS

A **disaster** is a sudden, unexpected event that causes injury to many people, major damage to property, or both. Disasters can be caused by acts of nature (such as tornadoes, earthquakes, hurricanes, floods, blizzards, or ice storms), or they may be the result of explosions, accidents, or acts of war or terrorism. Acts of terrorism can easily be targeted at vulnerable areas, such as health care facilities and schools. These acts could include the use of explosives, the release of chemicals (for example, nerve gas agents), or the release of biological agents (such as anthrax).

Helping Hands And A Caring Heart

FOCUS ON HUMANISTIC HEALTH CARE

Imagine, for a minute, what it would be like to be a resident in the midst of an emergency situation. You are alone in your room and you smell smoke, or the weather is severe and you see damage to your surroundings. No one seems to hear your cries for help. Residents are not in a position to protect themselves, and they may become very fearful knowing that they must depend on someone else to help them to safety. You can help by providing calm reassurance to those around you, even those you cannot get to right away. Your words may help to keep residents calm, which will make everyone's job a little easier. During an emergency situation, our focus must be on maintaining safety—but it is also important to be sensitive to human needs and responses.

Your facility will have a disaster preparedness plan to direct the actions of the health care team in the event of such an occurrence. The focus of a long-term care facility's disaster preparedness plan is on protecting residents and staff and continuing with care and services under emergency conditions (such as during bad weather or the temporary loss of power or water). The devastation that occurred with Hurricane Katrina in 2005 also showed us

Caring For Those With Dementia

In an emergency situation, residents with dementia may become particularly frightened. They may sense that there is a serious emergency occurring, but they may not understand what it is or how to respond. They may believe that their children or other family members are lost or in danger. As a result, they may put themselves in more danger by trying to get to safety on their own, or by trying to find or reach someone else. To help your residents with dementia during an emergency situation:

- Make sure that each resident with dementia is partnered with a staff member who can stay with the resident and keep her safe.

- If the resident has a special item that brings her comfort (such as a stuffed animal), make sure that the item is brought along with the resident.

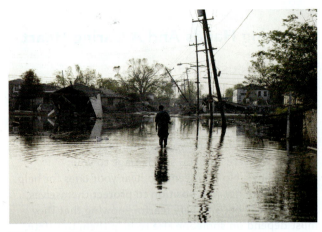

Figure 17-12

Disaster conditions may make it difficult for emergency personnel and supplies to reach the facility, or for people in the facility to leave. Disaster preparedness plans should include plans for "sheltering in place" that will allow the facility to be self-sufficient for several days, in the event that help is delayed. (*AP Photo/Christopher Morris/VII*)

that disaster preparedness plans need to include the ability to "shelter in place" when the disaster affects the entire community (Figure 17-12). To **shelter in place** means that the facility has the ability to be self-sufficient for several days, in the event that help from emergency or support services is delayed (Box 17-3).

If a situation is anticipated that could result in having to use the disaster preparedness plan (for example, extreme weather conditions), you may be asked to remain at work, or to come in to work when not scheduled, to ensure that there is adequate staff to provide for residents during the emergency. Some facilities allow staff members to bring children or other dependent family members to work under these circumstances. However, you should always have a plan in place for the care of your own family in the event that you are not able to be with them because of your work obligations.

In rare instances, you may have to help evacuate residents to safer quarters. It is important to make sure that all residents have proper identification attached to them, and that at least their basic medical information accompanies them. It is also essential to maintain a record of where residents were transferred. In a disaster situation, residents from the same facility could end up in several different places. The facility must be able to tell families where their loved ones are. In addition, when the disaster situation is under control, the facility must be able to get its residents back.

Just as you will be required to participate in fire drill exercises, you will be required to participate in disaster drill exercises. Participating in these exercises will help you to remain calm if a

---

BOX 17-3   Disaster Preparedness: Sheltering in Place

In the event of a large disaster, moving or evacuating residents to another place may not be desirable, or even possible. Moving elderly, frail residents through disaster conditions may be too risky. In addition, roads may be closed or blocked. Plans for "sheltering in place" include procedures for providing for residents and staff when conditions prevent:

- Transport of residents out of the facility
- Emergency response crews from reaching the facility
- Relief staff from getting to work, and staff on duty from leaving
- The arrival of delivery trucks with food, water, and other supplies

Plans for "sheltering in place" generally address:

- Alternate sources for power and light (such as generators and battery-powered devices)
- Emergency food supplies, and plans for meal preparation and distribution
- Emergency water supplies, and plans for how water is to be used
- Emergency communication systems
- Plans for how available medications, medical supplies, and equipment are to be distributed among residents and staff (staff members may have priority status for use of what is available, because if staff members become unable to perform their duties due to lack of medication or treatment, they will not be able to care for residents)
- Work/rest schedules and accommodations for available staff

Be Smart About Surveys!

Surveyors will be very interested in making sure that staff members take responsibility for workplace safety. They will watch what you do, and they may ask you questions to make sure that you are knowledgeable about your facility's fire and disaster preparedness plans. To help your facility remain without survey problems in this area:

- Routinely practice good body mechanics in your daily routines.

- Follow your facility's policies and procedures closely. These are designed to protect you, your residents, and your co-workers.

- Be alert to potentially unsafe situations in the workplace (such as spills, loose handrails, or broken floor tile) and take immediate action to correct them. If you cannot correct the situation yourself, post a caution sign to block off the problem area, and notify the correct person or department of the need for their services.

- Do not use broken or unsafe equipment. Follow your facility's procedure for tagging the item for repair,

and take it out of circulation so no one else will use it. Help to keep equipment in good working order by using it and storing it correctly.

- Keep all chemicals and solutions in their original, labeled containers.

- Use caution in all areas where oxygen is used or stored. Make sure "Oxygen in Use" signs are posted in these areas.

- Know your facility's policies and procedures for fire safety and disaster response. Take part in practice drills, and review the manuals, as necessary, to keep the information fresh in your mind. Be prepared to answer a surveyor's questions.

- Know the locations of fire alarms and extinguishers and how to use them.

- Know the locations of all emergency exits and evacuation routes. Make it a daily practice to make sure that clutter, supplies, and equipment do not block access to exits and evacuation routes.

---

disaster actually occurs, because you will know what you are supposed to do. Read and review all of your facility's emergency policies and procedures as often as you need to in order to keep them fresh in your mind. The worst time to read the manual to find out what to do is during an actual emergency! Your preparation is crucial for the protection of those around you, especially your residents who are dependent on you for their safety and well-being.

SUMMARY

- There are many factors that contribute to workplace safety and there are many people that the safety of the workplace affects.
  - It is your responsibility to help make your workplace safe, both for yourself and others, by following the guidelines for safety and by reporting any unsafe conditions to the appropriate person.
  - The Occupational Safety and Health Administration (OSHA) oversees safety regulations in all types of workplaces and addresses everything from safe lifting techniques to the control of hazardous materials.

  - OSHA mandates that employers inform workers of all safety risks that are present in their workplace.
  - OSHA requires employers to provide regular training about the safety risks in the work environment, and how injury is to be avoided. Your employer must keep records of any training you have received that meets OSHA regulations.

- Practicing good body mechanics allows you to use your body effectively when lifting and moving residents and equipment, and helps to protect you from injury as you perform your daily duties.

- The "ABCs" of good body mechanics are alignment, balance, and coordinated movement.
  - Learning proper lifting technique is especially critical to preventing back injuries.
- Following procedures when providing resident care helps to ensure that the care you provide is safe and correct.
  - Pre-procedure actions ("Getting Ready" steps) are taken before every resident care procedure. These actions promote efficiency, safety, and respect of the resident's rights.
  - Post-procedure actions ("Finishing Up" steps) are taken after every resident care procedure. These actions promote comfort, safety, and communication among members of the health care team.
- Falling poses a risk to both the health care worker and the resident. Asking for assistance and knowing how to properly assist a person who is falling can help to prevent injuries to everyone involved.
- Most health care facilities use many chemicals in their daily operation. Information about how to respond to a chemical exposure is found on the Materials Safety Data Sheet (MSDS), which each chemical manufacturer must supply, and on the labeled container.
- Malfunctioning electrical appliances, or electrical appliances that are used improperly,

can lead to electric shock, electrocution, and electrical fires.
- A fire in a long-term care facility can have tragic consequences because many of the people who live there are unable to move independently or quickly in the event of a fire.
  - Three elements are necessary to start a fire and keep it burning: fuel, heat, and oxygen.
  - The RACE fire response plan describes the general actions that are to be taken in the event of a fire emergency: **R**emove people in the immediate area, **A**ctivate the alarm, **C**ontain the fire, and **E**xtinguish or **E**vacuate as indicated by the situation.
- In long-term care facilities, disaster preparedness plans focus on protecting residents and staff and continuing with care and services under emergency conditions caused by severe weather, accidents, or acts of war or terrorism.
  - Know your facility's disaster plan, including your particular duties and responsibilities.
  - Be prepared to stay or return to the facility to care for residents in the event of an emergency. This includes having a plan for care of your own family if you cannot be with them.

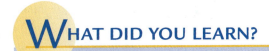

WHAT DID YOU LEARN?

Multiple Choice

Select the single best answer for each of the following questions.

1. In the event of a fire in a resident's room, your first action should be to:
   a. Remove the resident to a safe place
   b. Get the fire extinguisher
   c. Sound the fire alarm
   d. Notify the head nurse

2. When lifting, remember to use the large muscles of your:
   a. Chest
   b. Hips, buttocks, and thighs
   c. Back
   d. Shoulders

3. You accidentally knock over a water pitcher, spilling water on the floor of a resident's room. What should you do?
   a. Call housekeeping
   b. Continue with your assignment and make a mental note to wipe up the spill later
   c. Place a towel over the spill to absorb the liquid and alert others to be careful
   d. Wipe the spill up immediately

4. While you are walking with Mrs. Davis in the hallway, she complains of dizziness. Your first response should be to:
a. Assist Mrs. Davis back to her bed as quickly as possible
b. Assist Mrs. Davis to the floor and call for help
c. Ask Mrs. Davis to breathe deeply and reassure her that everything will be fine
d. Encourage Mrs. Davis to continue walking because she needs the exercise

5. The fire alarm begins sounding in the facility just before the change of shift. All of the staff members begin to follow procedures, clearing the hallways and shutting doors. You notice that Mrs. Pratt, who has dementia, has come out into the hall. She appears frightened and confused in all of the chaos. To ensure Mrs. Pratt's safety, you should:
a. Tell Mrs. Pratt to go back into her room and stay there until you return.
b. Apply a restraint to Mrs. Pratt until the fire drill is over.
c. Bring Mrs. Pratt to the nurses' station so that the nurse who is there can watch Mrs. Pratt to make sure that Mrs. Pratt does not try to leave.
d. Put Mrs. Pratt in the television room with the other residents, and then complete your emergency duties.

6. Using good body mechanics to lift an object off the floor means that you would:
a. Use a mechanical lift
b. Kneel down to get the broadest base of support and lift up
c. Squat and lift with your legs
d. Lean over at the waist, keeping your back flat

7. Unsafe conditions in a health care facility can be caused by:
a. Health care workers who allow residents to get out of bed
b. Health care workers who stop doing an assigned task to clean up a spill
c. Overloaded outlets and extension cords
d. Residents who smoke in "smoking only" areas

8. All of the following actions could cause a fire except:
a. Using a three-prong plug
b. Emptying an ashtray into a wastebasket
c. Smoking in a room where a person is receiving oxygen therapy
d. Placing a stack of linens on a heating unit to warm them

9. Where should you direct the foam when using a fire extinguisher to put out a fire?
a. At the base of the fire
b. In a circle around the fire, to prevent the fire from spreading
c. At the top of the fire
d. Anywhere in the general area of the fire

10. What are the "ABCs" of good body mechanics?
a. Assess, Balance, Complete
b. Assign, Begin, Complete
c. Alignment, Balance, Coordinated movement
d. Attempt, Brace, Change

11. You need to disinfect the over-bed table in a resident's room. Where can you find out information about the chemical product you are to use?
a. The care plan
b. The Material Safety Data Sheet (MSDS)
c. The Occupational Safety and Health Administration (OSHA)
d. The Minimum Data Set (MDS)

12. Following pre-procedure and post-procedure actions before and after each procedure is important to:
a. Prevent the resident from becoming confused
b. Ensure that the care you give is safe and correct
c. Make the nurse happy
d. Pass the certification exam

13. Which one of the following is a pre-procedure ("Getting Ready") step?
a. Report and record
b. Identify the person
c. Confirm that the person is comfortable and in good body alignment
d. Open the curtain or door

14. How do you "see to safety" before and after performing a procedure?
a. Use good body mechanics
b. Use equipment properly
c. Practice infection control
d. All of the above

15. During a disaster emergency in your long-term care facility, it is most likely that you will be involved in:
a. Admitting and discharging multiple residents
b. Protecting and caring for residents according to the disaster preparedness plan
c. Evacuating residents to another place
d. Helping rescue workers to find their way around the building

STOP and Think!

- You work on the second floor of a long-term care facility. As you are walking down the hall toward the nurses' station, you hear one of your residents, Miss Verna, call for help. When you look into her room, you see that her wastebasket is on fire. What should you do? Is it possible to accomplish more than one step of the RACE plan at once?

- You are a nursing assistant employed by a local nursing home. The weather forecast is calling for a major ice storm to hit your area tomorrow. Emergency officials in your area report that there is likely to be loss of electrical power, and the roads may be impassable for a day or two. As a result, the facility's disaster preparedness plan will be put into effect. What will be expected of you as a nursing assistant in this situation?

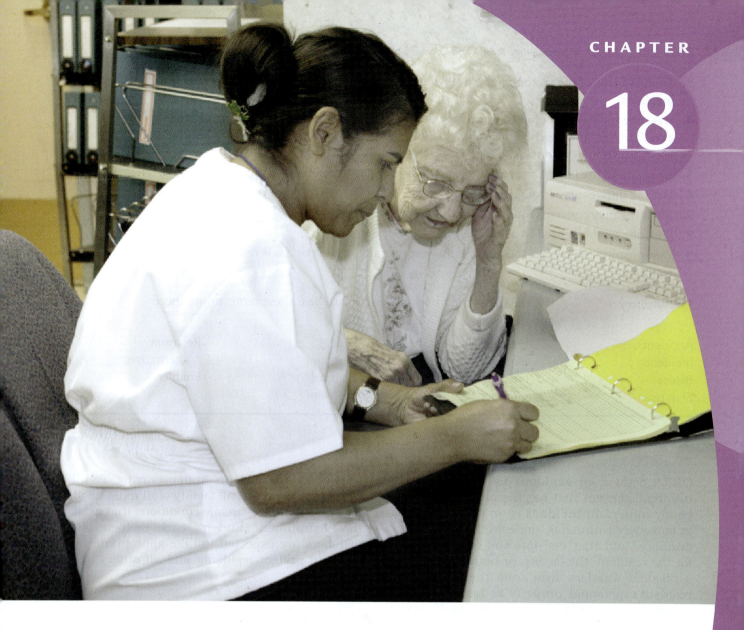

Resident Safety

WHAT WILL YOU LEARN?

As you remember from Chapter 7, safety is a basic human need. If we feel safe, we can relax and rest and we feel secure and comfortable. The previous chapters have explained principles and procedures designed to help keep you safe while you perform your duties as a nursing assistant. In this chapter, we will focus on what you need to know to help keep those you care for safe. When you are finished with this chapter, you will be able to:

1. Define the terms *accident* and *incident*, and discuss how each can threaten resident safety.
2. Discuss the OBRA requirements related to accidents and incidents.

Photo: As a nursing assistant, you will play an important role in keeping your residents safe. Here, a resident with dementia sits with a nursing assistant at the nurses' station while she completes paperwork. The nursing assistant is able to make sure the resident stays safe, and the resident enjoys the nursing assistant's company.

3. Discuss some of the factors that place residents of long-term care facilities at risk for accidents and incidents.

4. Describe the most common types of accidents and incidents that occur among residents of long-term care facilities, and describe measures the nursing assistant can take to help prevent these accidents and incidents from occurring.

5. Understand the importance of reporting and recording accidents and incidents.

6. List the different types of restraints.

7. Identify safety concerns associated with the use of restraints.

8. Describe methods used to avoid the need for restraints.

9. Demonstrate the proper application of a vest restraint, a wrist or ankle restraint, and a lap or waist (belt) restraint.

Vocabulary Use the CD in the front of your book to hear these terms pronounced and defined:

Accident	Entrapment	Physical	Restraint
Incident	Elopement	restraint	alternatives
Bruise	Incident (occurrence)	Chemical	Enabler
Skin tear	report	restraint	

OBRA defines an **accident** as an unexpected, unintended event that has the potential to cause bodily injury. An **incident** is an occurrence that is considered unusual, undesired, or out of the ordinary, and that disrupts the normal routine for the resident, the facility, or both (for example, a resident wanders away from the facility, or a resident's personal property is lost). Accidents and incidents can involve residents, staff, or visitors to the facility.

All accidents are considered incidents. For example, if a resident trips and falls, an accident has occurred because the fall was unintended, and could cause injury to the resident. An incident has also occurred, because the fall is an undesired event that disrupts the normal routine. On the other hand, not all incidents are accidents. For example, if a resident becomes angry with another resident and hits him, an accident has not occurred, because the angry resident intended to hit the other resident. However, an incident has occurred, because the action is undesired, out of the ordinary, and disrupts the normal routine.

Because accidents and most incidents threaten the safety and welfare of the residents, OBRA requires the facility to maintain an environment that lowers the risk of accidents and incidents to the greatest extent possible. In addition, OBRA requires that all residents receive the supervision and assistance needed to prevent accidents and incidents from occurring. To fulfill those requirements, all facility staff must be alert for any potentially unsafe conditions that exist in the environment, and for each resident. Staff members are expected to take appropriate measures to protect residents and all others in the facility.

FACTORS THAT INCREASE A RESIDENT'S RISK FOR ACCIDENTS AND INCIDENTS

Recognizing the factors that can increase a resident's risk of experiencing an accident or an incident can help you to minimize the chance that one of these events will occur.

PHYSICAL CHANGES OF AGING

Most of your residents will be elderly. The normal physical changes that occur with aging can affect a resident's ability to be safe. For example:

- **Neurological changes.** It takes an older person longer to regain balance if she starts to fall, or to change course to avoid running into another person or tripping over an object in her path.

- **Sensory changes.** Vision, hearing, taste, and smell decrease with age. These changes can make it more difficult for an older person to detect and respond to dangerous situations.
- **Musculoskeletal changes.** Loss of muscle tissue causes an older person to become weaker, which means the person becomes fatigued during physical activity more easily. When a person is fatigued, he is at increased risk for accidents, such as falling.
- **Urinary changes.** The amount of urine the bladder is able to hold before the person feels the urge to urinate decreases with age, leading to urinary frequency (the need to urinate more often). Rushing to the bathroom or failing to take necessary safety measures (such as waiting for help, using a walker, or turning on a light) can put the person at higher risk for falls.
- **Respiratory changes.** With age, lung capacity decreases. This can cause an older person to feel short of breath and weak during physical activity, putting the person at risk for falls.

EFFECTS OF MEDICAL CONDITIONS OR TREATMENTS

Most of your residents will have chronic health conditions. The health condition, its treatment, or both can increase the resident's risk for accidents or incidents. For example, diabetes can decrease a person's sense of touch, putting the person at risk for burns and other injuries. Pain and stiffness from arthritis can affect a person's mobility, putting the person at increased risk for falling. Neurological disorders, such as stroke or Parkinson's disease, can cause a person to shuffle her feet when she walks, increasing the person's risk for tripping and falling. An irregular heartbeat can cause a person to suddenly lose consciousness and fall. An incontinence accident can cause the person to slip and fall in urine or feces on the floor.

Many of your residents will take one or more medications to treat their chronic health conditions. These medications can affect a person's ability to be safe. For example, a medication that affects blood pressure can cause a person to become dizzy if he stands up quickly, leading to a fall. Some medications cause confusion in the elderly, especially if they are not taken properly.

ENVIRONMENTAL CONDITIONS

The risk for accidents and incidents is also increased simply by the nature of the long-term care environment itself. Consider the following points:

- Something as simple as a change in living environment (such as a move to a long-term care facility) can cause a new resident to become confused or disoriented, increasing the resident's risk for an accident or incident.
- In a long-term care facility, there are many residents living under the same roof, each with varying degrees of mental disability, physical disability, or both. Each resident needs a different level of supervision and assistance to remain safe.
- Long-term care facilities are very busy places. The hustle and bustle of people and equipment creates an environment where accidents and incidents are likely to occur.
- Environmental hazards (such as clutter, slippery surfaces, poor lighting, and sun glare) can also affect resident safety.

As you can see, there are many factors that can affect a resident's safety. When several of these risk factors are combined, complex safety issues can result (Fig. 18-1). As a nursing assistant, you must evaluate each resident and situation individually so that you can provide a safe environment for those you care for.

COMMON ACCIDENTS AND INCIDENTS

Many accidents and incidents can be prevented, especially if you are knowledgeable about the factors that put a resident at risk for experiencing them, and strategies for preventing them.

ACCIDENTS

Bruises and Skin Tears

A **bruise** is discoloration of the skin caused by rupture of the blood vessels beneath the skin's surface. The skin is not broken. A new bruise is usually purple or blue. As the bruise begins to heal, the color changes to yellow, brown, or green. Bruises are often tender to the touch, and may be swollen.

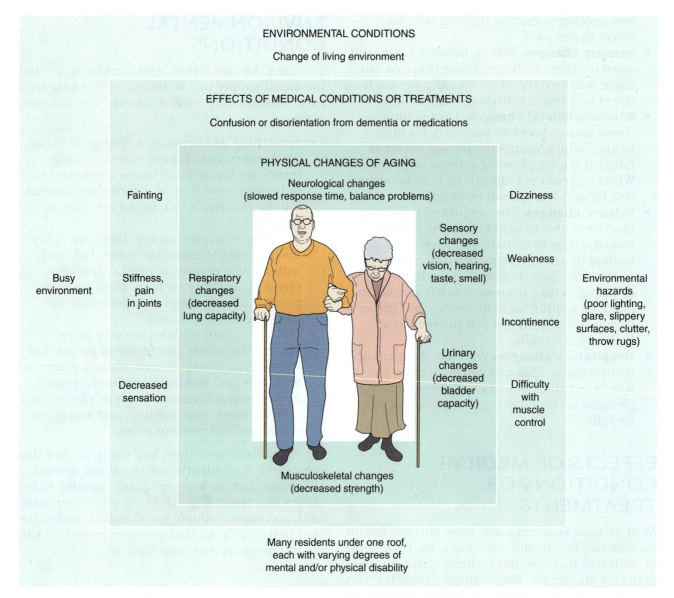

Figure 18-1

The normal physical changes of aging, the effects of medical conditions or treatments, and environmental conditions can all combine to significantly increase a resident's risk for an accident or an incident.

A **skin tear** is an injury that occurs when the top layer of the skin is separated from the bottom layers. The top layer of skin usually looks like a "flap" that fits over the open wound (Fig. 18-2). Sometimes, however, the flap may completely tear away, leaving a large open wound. Because the skin is torn or missing, the person is at risk for infection.

Risk factors

Elderly people are at very high risk for experiencing bruises and skin tears, often during routine care. In older people, the blood vessels become more fragile, which increases the tendency to bruise. In addition, an older person's skin is very thin, dry, and fragile. These changes can cause the skin to tear very easily. Residents who are very dependent on the staff for care are at the highest risk for bruises and skin tears, because they require the most "hands-on" care.

Prevention

To help prevent bruises or skin tears, always take care to handle residents gently when you are assisting them with care. Bruises and skin tears often occur during activities such as

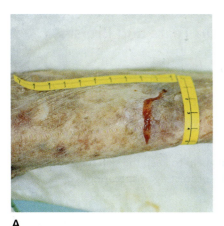
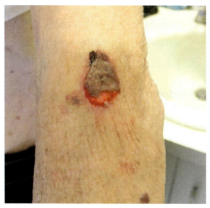
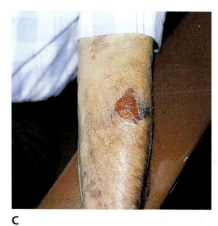

A   **B**   **C**

Figure 18-2

Because skin becomes thin and fragile with age, elderly residents are at high risk for experiencing skin tears during routine care. (Used with permission from Baranoski, S. and Ayello, E.A. [2008]. *Wound Care Essentials Practice and Principles* [2nd ed., p. C2]. Philadelphia: Lippincott Williams & Wilkins.)

helping a resident change position in bed, helping a resident to get out of bed or a wheelchair, assisting a resident on or off a bedpan, helping a resident to walk, and even helping a resident to dress. When assisting a resident with care, always follow the proper procedure, and use a gentle touch.

It is also important to look at the furnishings in the room and the equipment that the resident uses. Padding hard edges can help to prevent bruises and skin tears. For example, the footrests of wheelchairs often cause bruises and skin tears on the lower legs. Padding the footrests while the resident is in the wheelchair and removing the footrests during transfers can help to prevent injuries.

The resident's skin can also be "cushioned" to help prevent trauma. Residents who are prone to skin tears should wear long-sleeved tops and long pants. Alternatively, elastic tube-like coverings for the arms and legs that are made of cushioned, soft material may be used (Fig. 18-3).

General guidelines for preventing bruises and skin tears are given in Guidelines Box 18-1.

Falls

Among all the types of accidents that can occur in a long-term care setting, falls are the most common. Many residents who fall will experience bruises, skin tears, or broken bones (fractures, discussed in Chapter 32). Some will die, either as a result of the fall itself, or because of complications resulting from injuries caused by the fall. Remember that many residents have medical conditions that affect the body's ability

to heal and can make recovering from injuries caused by a fall difficult. Falls are the leading cause of accidental death among elderly people.

In addition to causing physical injury, falls also affect the person emotionally. A fear of falling again can make the person afraid to move. The resulting immobility leads to decreased strength and further increases the person's risk for falling. In addition, the fear of falling again can lead to mental health problems, such as anxiety and depression. As a result, the person may stop interacting with others and participating in activities. This negatively affects the person's quality of life.

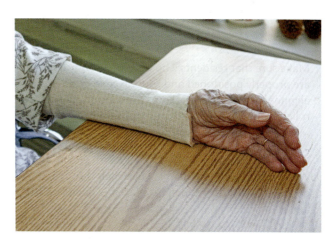

Figure 18-3

Care needs to be taken to protect older skin from skin tears. The arms and hands are frequently involved in skin tear injuries. Extra protection for the skin can be provided by the use of specially designed padded sleeves, or tubes.

Guidelines Box 18-1 Guidelines for Preventing Skin Tears and Bruises

WHAT YOU DO	WHY YOU DO IT
Use soapless cleanser ("no-rinse soap") as ordered.	Soap can be drying to the skin. Dry skin is more likely to tear.
Apply lotion or cream to the resident's skin at least twice a day, or as ordered.	Lotions and creams help to keep the skin moist and soft, which helps to protect against tearing.
Ensure that the resident is receiving enough fluids by encouraging fluid intake at meals and offering beverages of choice between meals. Offer fluids during the night if the resident is awake.	Providing sufficient fluids to maintain good hydration helps to keep the skin from drying out, thus decreasing the risk for tearing.
Encourage the resident to wear long sleeves and long pants.	Covering the arms and legs provides an additional layer of protection to the skin.
Never use force when assisting a resident to dress. If a resident's clothing is too tight or is too difficult to put on the resident, report this to the nurse so that the family can be asked to provide clothing that is easier to put on.	Forcing a resident's arm or leg through a sleeve or pant leg increases the resident's risk for skin trauma. Replacing clothing with items that are easier to put on the resident may prevent unnecessary skin injury.
Pad hard surfaces in the environment that the resident is likely to bump into (for example, leg and arm rests on wheelchairs, side rails, the edges of furniture).	Cushioning hard edges helps to prevent trauma to the skin.
Use a lift sheet (draw sheet) when moving the resident up in bed. Use transfer belts when assisting the resident to transfer as ordered.	The more you have to handle a resident, the greater the risk for skin tears and bruising. Minimizing handling of the resident's arms and legs decreases the chance that trauma will occur.
Make sure that residents who have poor body control are properly positioned and supported in good body alignment, and that their limbs are supported with rolled blankets, pillows, or other positioning devices.	If not properly supported, residents with poor body control often slump to the side, and unsupported limbs fall and dangle over the arm or leg rests of the chair. This significantly increases the person's risk for bruising and skin tears.
When pushing a resident in a wheelchair through a doorway, assist the resident to place her hands on her lap.	You may accidentally misjudge the space needed to clear the doorway with the wheelchair. Having the resident place her hands in her lap helps to prevent injuries to the hands or arms should the wheelchair bump into the edge of the door on the way through.

Risk factors

Because of age or disability, all residents should be considered at risk for falls, but some are at higher risk than others are. Risk factors for falling are listed in Box 18-1. The more risk factors a resident has, the greater the likelihood that the resident is going to fall. In addition, one fall puts the resident at very high risk for another fall in the future.

Helping Hands and a Caring Heart

FOCUS ON HUMANISTIC HEALTH CARE

Many residents who need assistance with mobility resist calling for help because they have the emotional need to try to maintain their sense of independence. Not calling for help puts the resident at very high risk for falling, and can be very frustrating for staff members who are trying to keep the resident safe. However, it is important for you to understand how the resident feels, and to recognize and respect the resident's need for independence. Take care not to give safety instructions to the resident as if he were a child, and avoid scolding the resident for not calling for help. For example, instead of saying, "Mr. Jeffries, are you OK? Why didn't you call for help like I told you to? I warned you that you could fall if you tried to get to the bathroom alone! You have to call me before you get up. If you don't follow instructions, you are really going to get hurt one of these days, and then you will have to have help for everything!" you could say, "Mr. Jeffries, are you OK? I know that it must be difficult for you to have to call somebody every time you want to go to the bathroom, but it is important to me that you get to the bathroom safely. I would like to keep you walking as long as possible. I would much rather you call me, than have you fall and break a hip! That kind of injury could make things really difficult for you." This response acknowledges the resident's feelings and need for independence, while gently reminding him of his long-term goal (to keep walking as long as possible). When you recognize and acknowledge a resident's emotional needs, as well as his physical needs, you are truly providing humanistic health care.

Prevention

Identifying each resident's specific risk factors for falls is essential for maintaining the resident's safety. The nurse, with input from other members of the health care team, completes a fall risk assessment when the resident is admitted, and at regular intervals throughout the resident's stay

---

BOX 18-1 Risk Factors For Falls

Normal Changes of Aging
- Decreased muscle strength
- Decreased endurance
- Decreased vision
- Decreased balance
- Slowed response time
- Decreased hearing

Medical Conditions and Treatments
- Heart disorders (dizziness or fainting; decreased endurance with physical exercise)
- Blood and circulatory disorders (increased fatigue, shortness of breath, decreased endurance, dizziness, complications such as sores or amputation of lower limbs)
- Respiratory disorders (shortness of breath, decreased endurance)
- Neurological disorders (loss of muscle control, abnormal movement or loss of movement, slowed reaction time, loss of feeling, dizziness)
- Joint disorders (pain with movement, limited range of motion)
- Bone disorders (bones may break with pressure of standing or walking)
- Bowel and bladder disorders (hurrying to the bathroom, loss of bowel or bladder control on the way to the bathroom)
- Diabetes (change in mental status due to high or low blood glucose levels, nerve damage leading to loss of feeling in feet, loss of vision)
- Eye disease (loss of vision)
- Dementia and psychiatric disorders (confusion, lack of awareness or misinterpretation of surroundings)
- Medication effects (dizziness, sedation or drowsiness, increased need to urinate)

Environmental Conditions
- Poor lighting
- Uneven surfaces
- Clutter
- Lack of access to assistive devices or handrails
- Slippery surfaces
- Chairs or beds that are too high for the resident
- The need to bend or reach for belongings

(Fig. 18-4). Measures that need to be taken to help prevent falls are then included in the resident's care plan. Some facilities place a picture of a "falling leaf" or a "falling star" next to the resident's room number (on the sign next to the resident's door) or over the resident's bed. In this way, even staff members who do not have access to the resident's care plan can be made aware of

RESIDENT FALL RISK SCORES					Resident Score		
					TIME		
PARAMETERS	**4**	**3**	**2**	**1**			
Age	—	80+	70 to 79	—			
Mental status	Intermittent confusion or impulsiveness (or both)	—	Confused (baseline)	—			
Elimination	Can't wait or won't wait	Independent and incontinent	Needs assistance	Indwelling catheter			
History of falling	History of multiple falls (3 or more)	—	Has fallen 1 or 2 times	—			
Gait and balance	Unsteady or poor balance standing or walking	Orthostatic hypotension	—	Needs supervision or assistance with equipment			
Medications (By drug class below)	3 or more drug classes	2 drug classes	1 drug class	—			
TOTAL RISK SCORES							

Drug classes:
1. **Cardiovascular** (antihypertensives, vasodilators, antiarrhythmics, nitrates)
2. **Psychoactive** (sedatives, hypnotics, barbiturates, anxiolytics, antihistamines, anticonvulsants, antidepressants)
3. **Pain** (narcotics, patient-controlled analgesia, epidural)
4. **Diuretics and cathartics**
5. **Anesthetics** (first 24 hours post-op)

Total risk scores:
9 to 20 = extremely high risk
5 to 8 = high risk
0 to 4 = low risk
If score is >4, falls prevention protocol should be implemented.

DATE	TIME	NAME

Figure 18-4

Many long-term care facilities use a form like this one to assess a new resident's risk of falling. Once the risk factors are known, precautions can be taken to decrease the resident's risk of falling.

the resident's risk for falling, so that extra precautions can be taken.

As a nursing assistant, you will play a very important role in helping to prevent falls by following each resident's care plan carefully. General guidelines for preventing falls are given in Guidelines Box 18-2.

Care of a person following a fall

Despite the measures you will take to prevent falls from occurring, a resident may experience a fall. If you discover that a resident has fallen, do not try to move her. If the resident has broken a bone as a result of the fall, moving her could cause more harm. Instead, call the nurse so that the nurse can assess the resident before moving her.

Burns

Burns are injuries to the skin and underlying tissues, caused by contact with heat, chemicals, or electricity. Burns can be minor, causing only slight redness or pain, or they can be very severe.

Risk factors

Older people are at high risk for burns. Normal age-related changes and chronic health conditions (such as stroke or diabetes) can affect the person's ability to feel temperatures that are too hot. As a result, a burn can occur without the person even being aware of it. In addition, as you have learned, the skin becomes thinner and more fragile as we age. As a result, in an older person, a burn can occur very rapidly, and it may be more severe because the skin is so thin and fragile.

Prevention

Water temperatures that are too hot can put a resident at risk for severe burns during bathing or showering. Always check the water temperature

Guidelines Box 18-2   Guidelines for Preventing Falls

WHAT YOU DO	WHY YOU DO IT
Check the resident's clothing and shoes. Clothing should fit properly. Shoes should provide good foot support and have nonskid soles.	Long or loose clothing (such as a robe) or shoes that provide inadequate foot support or have slippery soles could lead to tripping.
Encourage the resident to use rails along hallways and stairways while walking.	The additional support offered by rails may be all that is needed to allow a resident to move about safely and independently.
Observe the resident for signs of unsteadiness and offer physical assistance as needed.	Offering assistance as needed allows the resident to remain as independent as possible, while minimizing the risk of falls.
Observe the resident's ability to use walking aids, such as canes and walkers, and correct incorrect use.	Using a piece of equipment improperly can be just as hazardous as not using it at all.
Check equipment, such as walkers and wheelchairs, to ensure that it is in good condition. Nonskid tips should be intact on walkers. Wheelchair wheel locks should function properly.	Malfunctioning or broken equipment increases a resident's risk for accidents.
Make sure a resident who needs glasses or hearing aids is wearing them when she is out of bed.	Being able to see and hear clearly promotes safety by increasing the resident's awareness of her surroundings. A resident who cannot see clearly could trip over an obstacle in her pathway. A resident who cannot hear well may not be able to hear words of caution.
Remove any clutter or obstacles from walkways and provide adequate lighting.	Proper lighting enhances the ability to see. Removal of obstructions is an easy way to minimize falls.
Keep beds in the lowest position. Keep bed wheels locked.	Keeping the bed in the lowest position minimizes the distance from the bed to the floor, should the resident fall out of bed. Keeping the wheels on the bed locked prevents the bed from rolling. A rolling bed could result in injury to the nursing assistant, the resident, or both.
Keep side rails up or down, according to the care plan for that particular resident.	Side rails can prevent a resident from falling out of bed. Because side rails are considered a form of restraint, they should always be lowered, unless the resident's medical condition is such that he needs the protection that is offered by having the side rails raised.

(continued)

Guidelines Box 18-2 Guidelines for Preventing Falls (continued)

WHAT YOU DO	WHY YOU DO IT
Always make sure the call light control is within easy reach of the resident. Answer call lights promptly, and offer to help the resident with toileting frequently.	Many falls are the result of a resident trying to make it to the bathroom without assistance.
Allow the resident time to adjust to changes in position when getting out of the bed or a chair.	A resident may experience changes in blood pressure that cause dizziness when moving from a lying position to a seated position, or from a seated position to standing. Allowing the resident some extra time to adjust to the change in position allows the resident's blood pressure to stabilize, and reduces the risk of the falling.
Wipe up any spills immediately. Make sure caution signs are posted when the floor is wet.	Wet surfaces may not be obvious (especially to people with some degree of visual impairment) and greatly increase the risk of slipping.
Keep residents who are disoriented and at risk for falling close to the nurses' station or involved in supervised activities. Offer frequent assistance with walking.	Keeping a resident who is disoriented and at risk for falling close to the nurses' station or involved in a supervised activity allows staff to "keep an eye" on the resident, and also minimizes the chance that a resident who feels lonely will try to get up to look for company. A resident who is offered help with walking on a regular basis is less likely to try to get up on his own, thereby minimizing the chance of a fall.
Orient a newly admitted resident to the unit and her room.	Falls and other accidents often occur when a resident is unfamiliar with her surroundings.

using a bath thermometer before assisting the resident into the tub or spraying the shower. The water temperature should be between 105°F (40.5°C) and 115°F (46°C). Although many modern tub and shower units have controls that preset the water temperature, you should still double-check the water temperature with a bath thermometer before assisting the resident into the tub or shower. Equipment malfunctions can, and do, occur. Also, be sure to teach residents who will be bathing themselves to check the water temperature with a bath thermometer or a hand or wrist before getting into the bathtub or shower.

Meal time is another time when the risk for burns is increased. The routine can become very hectic at meal time, as staff members hurry to serve residents their meals in a timely way. Hot foods or liquids can easily cause a burn if they are spilled on someone. When delivering meal trays or hot beverages, move efficiently, but carefully. Be aware of others around you, or obstacles in your path that could cause you to trip. Warn the resident that a food or beverage is hot before giving it to him. Also, make sure that the resident can safely handle a cup or other container holding hot liquid. Some residents may need a cup with a lid for their coffee or tea if weakness or unsteadiness puts them at risk for spilling.

Electrical appliances can be another source of burn injuries. All electrical appliances should be checked for safety before use, and used in accordance with the safety precautions described in Chapter 17. When using electrical appliances that produce heat (such as curling irons, hair dryers, and heating pads), use the lowest heat setting and monitor the person closely. Any application of heat to a resident's skin should be done with extreme care. You will learn more about heat applications in Chapter 27.

Entrapment

The resident's bed has side rails, which can be raised to help prevent the resident from falling out of bed. Some residents may also use a raised side rail as an assistive device for repositioning themselves in bed, or for getting up. Although the use of side rails is often ordered to help protect the resident or to promote independence, the use of side rails can also put the resident at risk for **entrapment.** Entrapment occurs when a person becomes trapped in the side rail, or between the

side rail and the mattress (Fig. 18-5). Severe injury, or even death, can occur, especially if the person's head, neck, or chest becomes trapped.

Risk factors

Any time the side rails are in use, there is a risk for entrapment. Residents who are confused (for example, as a result of medications or dementia) and those with physical disabilities (such as a lack of muscle control) are at the highest risk for entrapment.

Prevention

To help lower a resident's risk for entrapment, always use the side rails as ordered in the resident's care plan. If the use of side rails has been ordered, check on the resident frequently,

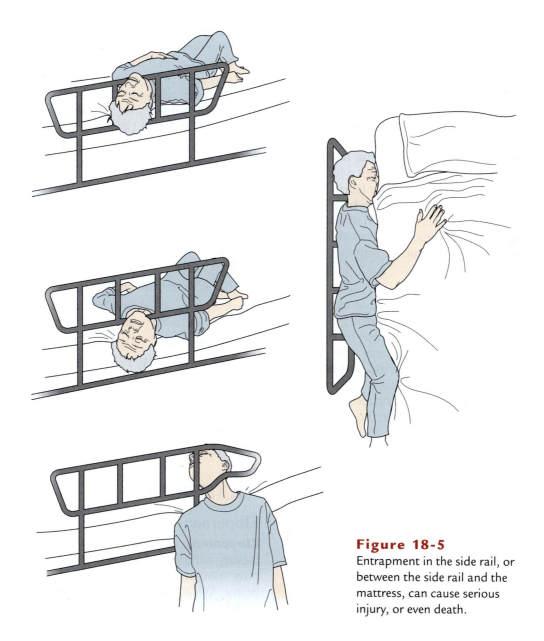

Figure 18-5

Entrapment in the side rail, or between the side rail and the mattress, can cause serious injury, or even death.

especially if the resident has risk factors for entrapment. Devices that are designed to reduce the risk for entrapment by covering open spaces between the side rails or between the side rail and the mattress are available. If the resident's care plan specifies that these devices should be used, make sure the devices are properly in place.

Poisoning and Other Injuries Resulting From Exposure to Harmful Substances

Think of all of the different chemical products used in the long-term care setting. There are personal care products, such as soaps and lotions. There are cleaning products, such as disinfectants and air fresheners. Medications, including ointments, creams, pills, and liquids, are also plentiful! All of these items serve a useful purpose, but if they are not handled properly, they can easily cause harm to the resident. Almost any substance can cause harm if enough of it is swallowed, inhaled, or applied, or if it is misused.

Risk factors

Poor eyesight and confusion (for example, as a result of dementia) are risk factors for accidental poisoning and other injuries resulting from exposure to harmful substances. A resident who cannot see well may not be able to read the label identifying the contents of a container, or the instructions for its use. A resident who is confused may swallow substances that are not meant to be swallowed, or misuse the product in some other way.

Prevention

As you learned in Chapter 17, special care needs to be taken when handling and storing the various chemical products that are used in the facility. Always make sure containers are clearly labeled, and return cleaning agents and personal care supplies to their proper place after you are finished using them. As a nursing assistant, you must be alert to potentially dangerous situations, and take the appropriate action to protect your residents, as well as others in the facility.

Special precautions also need to be taken when handling and storing medications. Staff members who administer medications (that is, nurses and certified medication assistants) must always take care to lock the medication cart when it is unattended. Usually, residents are not permitted to keep medications in their rooms. If the doctor has written a specific order allowing a resident to keep medications in his room, the medications must be stored in a secure place (to prevent other residents from gaining access to them).

Be Smart About Surveys!

During the survey, surveyors will take note of staff members' attention to ensuring resident safety. Surveyors will also pay attention to how staff members respond to potentially unsafe situations. To help your facility remain without survey problems in this area:

- Be aware of each resident's risk factors for accidents and injuries. Ask the nurse about residents on your assignment who are prone to falls, skin tears, and bruising. Listen to report to identify other residents who are at risk.
- Be aware of the safety interventions listed on each resident's care plan, and be sure to carry them out. If you have questions, ask the nurse.
- Be alert to potentially unsafe situations in the environment (such as spills, loose handrails, broken floor tile, malfunctioning equipment, or light bulbs that need to be replaced) and take immediate action to correct them. If you cannot correct the situation yourself, post a caution sign to block off the problem area, and notify the correct person or department of the need for their services.
- Properly secure all supplies when you are finished using them.
- Make sure each resident's footwear and clothing fits well and does not affect the resident's ability to walk safely.
- Keep pathways clear of clutter and equipment. Make sure residents have clear access to the handrails.
- Check walkers for proper tips.
- Make sure all residents have a call light control or hand bell within reach.
- Respond promptly to all call lights and alarms.
- Know your facility's policies and procedures for reporting an accident or incident. Be prepared to answer a surveyor's questions about policies and procedures related to accidents and incidents.

INCIDENTS

Elopement

Elopement occurs when a resident leaves the facility without the knowledge of facility staff. You may also hear this referred to as the resident being AWOL, or "away without leave." ("Leave" means permission.) A confused resident may leave the facility by accident, simply by exploring the various doors in the facility. Some residents leave the facility on purpose. Residents at highest risk for elopement are those who have dementia or psychiatric problems, and those who resist the need for long-term care.

Residents who leave the facility unaccompanied are at risk for serious harm. These residents usually travel on foot, because their access to other forms of transportation is often limited. If the resident is confused, she may not be properly dressed for the weather, and she may encounter danger in the form of other environmental hazards (such as a busy highway, a body of water, or a heavily wooded area). The resident can easily get lost, or fall victim to crime. The resident may go without food or water for an extended period of time.

Many facilities use an alarm system, called a wanderer monitoring system, to help prevent elopement. The resident wears a small sensor around the wrist or ankle. If the resident tries to leave the facility, an alarm will sound, alerting the staff so that the resident can be gently and safely led back inside. These sensors work the same way as anti-shoplifting devices in shopping malls work.

Behavioral Incidents

Emotional distress, anger, or frustration can cause a resident to act aggressively or violently toward another resident, a staff member, or even herself, resulting in physical harm. Often the residents who are involved in behavioral incidents have dementia, but this is not always the case. In a long-term care setting, there are many factors that could cause a resident to experience emotional distress, anger, or frustration. For example, many people who are basically strangers to one another must learn to live together under one roof. This is not an easy thing to do. Disagreements can easily occur. It may also be difficult for residents to constantly adjust to the different caregivers who are involved in their care.

As a nursing assistant, you must be alert to any change in a resident's appearance or behavior that could indicate that the person is experiencing emotional distress or frustration that could lead to aggression. For example, a firm set to the person's mouth or furrowed brows may indicate that the person is getting angry. As anger increases, the person may gesture others to stay away. If you see these changes when you are caring for a resident, give the resident some space until the resident calms down. If you see these changes when a resident is interacting with another resident, take steps to separate the residents. You may need to ask a co-worker for help.

Caring For Those With Dementia

Residents with dementia are at increased risk for injury because they have difficulty understanding and responding to the environment. To help promote safety for your residents with dementia:

- Make sure that all exit doors are closed, monitored, and/or alarmed as per your facility's policy.
- Secure all potentially harmful substances.
- Use non-toxic products for arts and crafts activities.
- Provide periods of rest for a resident who paces.
- Make sure that the person wears proper footwear and uses a walker if one is needed.
- Keep the resident in an area where he can be more easily supervised, such as near the nurses' station, or in a structured activity.
- Taking time to talk with the resident before providing care may calm the resident and lessen resistive behavior.

Also, remember that it is easiest to remove the resident who is being threatened from the area (as opposed to trying to remove the resident who is angry and upset).

All behavioral incidents must be reported immediately. Be sure to report exactly what you saw, what you heard, and what was happening before the incident occurred. These observations can help the nurse identify the trigger for the outburst.

REPORTING ACCIDENTS AND INCIDENTS

Accidents and incidents will happen despite the precautions taken by even the most conscientious of health care workers. When an accident or incident occurs, you must know and follow your facility's procedures for reporting and documenting the occurrence. Residents who are involved in an accident or incident must be monitored for a period of time following the occurrence. This is necessary to ensure that the resident has not developed any problems as a result of the accident or incident that were not noticeable at the time of the occurrence. The monitoring period is usually specified by facility policy.

All accidents and incidents are to be verbally reported immediately to the nurse. In addition, a written report called an **incident (occurrence) report** must be completed. You may need to complete a preprinted document like the one shown in Fig. 18-6, or you may need to enter the necessary information into a computer. Some facilities will require your supervisor to complete the incident (occurrence) report, based on your input. Information about the accident or incident should be provided in a straightforward and factual manner, without opinion or blame.

The completed incident (occurrence) report is used by the person in the facility who is responsible for quality assurance, and is very important for follow-up. For example, consider a situation where an accident has occurred because a wheelchair's brakes did not hold properly. The completed incident (occurrence) report may help the person responsible for quality assurance identify a trend that could help prevent accidents like this from happening in the future. For example, the quality assurance review might reveal that several similar accidents have occurred with wheelchairs of the same type, or after repairs from the same shop, or on the same shift of work scheduling.

Some health care workers hesitate to report an accident or incident because they feel responsible for it, or are afraid that they will be blamed for what occurred. Other times, they know that a co-worker was careless, and they do not want to get the person in trouble by reporting the person's error to a supervisor. As described in Chapter 3, the nursing assistant must be honest and dependable in carrying out her duties. Reporting accidents and incidents promptly helps to protect your residents, your facility, and you.

RESTRAINTS

Restraints are used to restrict a person's freedom of movement, or to prevent a person from reaching parts of his body. In some very specific situations, restraints may be used to maintain a resident's safety. However, there are many dangers associated with restraint use (Box 18-2). Current standards of care set forth by The Joint Commission and the Centers for Medicare and Medicaid Services (CMS) require that health care facilities minimize their use of restraints. Today, many health care facilities, especially long-term care facilities, are almost restraint-free. Although restraints are rarely used in long-term care, it is important for you to understand what they are, the dangers associated with their use, and how to use them properly if their use is ordered. It is also important for you to know about the many alternatives to restraints that are available.

Restraints can be either physical or chemical. A **physical restraint** is a device that is attached to or near a person's body to limit the person's freedom of movement or access to her body, and which cannot be easily or purposefully removed by the person (Fig. 18-7). Physical restraints confine a person to a bed or a chair or prevent movement of a specific body part. Physical restraints can be applied to parts of the body, such as the wrists, ankles, chest, waist, or elbows. Additionally, some types of chairs or attachments to chairs can act as restraints. So can the side rails of beds or tightly tucked sheets. Not permitting a person free access to other rooms or parts of the facility is also considered a form of physical restraint.

A **chemical restraint** is any medication that alters a person's mood or behavior, such as a sedative or tranquilizer. There is a fine line between using medications to help calm an anxious, combative (physically aggressive), or agitated resident and using medications for staff convenience (that is, to sedate the resident so that the staff does not have to worry about difficult behaviors). These medications should assist in the control of anxiety, combative behavior, or agitation. They should not be used in so high a dose as to make the resident sleepy or unable to function in a normal fashion.

The use of restraints is clearly defined in guidelines issued by OBRA. The *Resident Rights* portion of OBRA addresses a resident's right to be free from physical and chemical restraints. According to OBRA, the improper use of restraints can be considered holding a resident against his or her will, or false imprisonment.

RESTRAINT ALTERNATIVES

Although the use of physical or chemical restraints is not forbidden by any regulating agency, measures must be taken to avoid their use. In other words, **restraint alternatives** must be sought and used. The measures taken to avoid the use of restraints on a resident must be documented and proven to be unsuccessful before resorting to the use of restraints to protect the resident's safety.

INCIDENT (OCCURRENCE) REPORT

EMPLOYEE INVOLVED:

Name:_____

Address:_____

Phone:_____

Employee: _____
        (RN, PT, Aide, etc.)

RESIDENT INVOLVED:

Name:_____

Address: _____

Phone: _____

FID #: _____

OTHERS INVOLVED: Name: _____ Phone:_____

        Address: _____ Relationship: _____

- -

Date of incident:_____ Time of incident:_____

Location of incident: _____

Incident reported to: _____ Time:_____ Date:_____

DESCRIPTION OF INCIDENT: (Complete Workers Comp. form if on-job injury)

_____
Employee Signature

FOLLOW UP:

Family aware of incident: _____

Physician aware of incident:_____

Action taken:

Follow-up/Supervisor's comments:

Figure 18-6

An incident (occurrence) report like this one must be completed if an accident or incident occurs. The report provides information that might help to prevent a similar accident or incident from happening again.

BOX 18-2   Complications of Restraint Use

- **Strangulation** (cutting off the resident's air supply) can occur if a vest restraint is improperly applied or if the restraint gets tangled in a piece of furniture.
- **Bruises, skin trauma,** and **nerve damage** can result if a restrained resident pulls at the restraint, or if the restraint is applied too tightly.
- **Permanent tissue damage** as a result of impaired blood flow can occur if a restraint is placed incorrectly or too tightly. All of the tissues of the body require oxygen to live, and oxygen is carried to the tissues in the blood. If something stops blood from flowing to a certain part of the body, the affected tissues can be permanently damaged from lack of oxygen.
- **Broken bones** and **other serious injuries** can occur if a restrained resident tries to get out of the restraints. For example, a resident restrained in a chair may still try to get up, which could

result in injury if the chair overturns. Similarly, a resident who is improperly restrained in a bed could slide between the bed and the side rails, or attempt to climb over the side rails, actions that could lead to injury or death if the restraint gets caught in the side rails.
- **Pneumonia, pressure ulcers,** and **blood clots** (complications of immobility) can occur if a resident is left in a restraint for too long.
- **Incontinence** can occur if the resident is not taken to the bathroom regularly.
- **Loss of independence** can occur when decreased mobility from restraint use leads to a decrease in bone and muscle strength, affecting the resident's ability to stand, transfer, and walk.
- **Mental effects** (such as agitation, increased confusion, humiliation, embarrassment, and depression) are associated with the use of restraints and can be serious.

Examples of alternatives to restraint are described in Table 18-1.

Helping Hands and a Caring Heart
FOCUS ON HUMANISTIC HEALTH CARE

Physically and emotionally, restraints have a very negative impact on a person's quality of life. Imagine how you would feel if you had to be "tied down." You might feel embarrassed, frightened, or humiliated. As a nursing assistant, there are many things you can do that may eliminate or reduce the need for restraints. These things require planning and effort, but the effort is considered part of the quality, individualized care that should be given to each resident.

PROPER USE OF RESTRAINTS

Restraints are never used as punishment or for the staff's convenience. They are used in very specific situations to provide postural support, to protect the resident from harm, and/or to protect the staff from harm (in the case of a combative or violent resident). Restraints are to be used only if all alternatives to restraint have failed and the resident is considered to be a danger to herself or

others if restraints are not applied. Examples of situations where the use of restraints may be appropriate include, but are not limited to:

- A confused resident repeatedly attempts to remove or pull out tubing necessary for medical treatment
- A resident does not have the ability to walk, but repeatedly tries to get out of the bed or chair due to mental status changes or dementia
- A resident cannot control body movements or maintain proper posture due to a medical condition (for example, a nervous system disorder)
- A resident is demonstrating combative behavior that poses a serious threat to the welfare and safety of that resident, other residents, or staff

Before deciding that restraint use is appropriate for a resident, the health care team must perform a thorough assessment. As part of this assessment, there must be evidence that less restrictive measures have been tried and proven unsuccessful in meeting the resident's needs. In addition, the health care team must carefully consider the risks and benefits of restraint use, and agree that in this particular situation, the benefits of restraint use outweigh the risks. For example:

- Mrs. Burgess requires intravenous (IV) antibiotic therapy for a serious infection. She

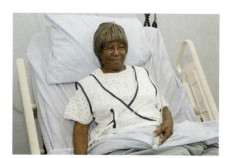

A. Vest restraint

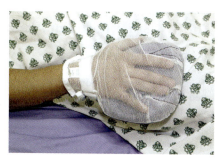

D. Mitt restraint

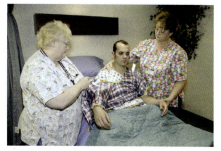

B. Jacket restraint

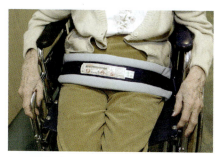

E. Seat belt

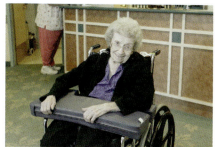

F. Lap buddy

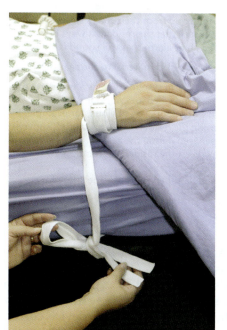

C. Wrist restraint

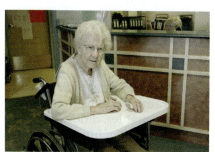

G. Chair with a tray table

Figure 18-7
Physical restraints are attached on or near a person's body. They limit freedom of movement. Some examples of physical restraints are shown here. **(A)** A vest restraint. **(B)** A jacket restraint. **(C)** A wrist restraint. **(D)** A mitt restraint. **(E)** A seat belt, **(F)** a lap buddy, and **(G)** a chair with a tray table are considered restraints if the resident cannot remove the seat belt, lap buddy, or tray table independently.

is agitated and disoriented, and she repeatedly tries to remove the IV line from her arm. The team may determine that in this situation, the benefits of using a restraint to ensure that the IV line stays in place and Mrs. Burgess receives the necessary medication outweigh the risks of using the restraint.

• Mr. Miller is a resident with dementia who cannot focus on his meal. He constantly

wanders away without eating, and as a result is at risk for weight loss and perhaps dehydration. Mr. Miller may benefit from being temporarily confined to his chair with a tray table during meals. Being confined to the chair helps Mr. Miller focus on the food in front of him so that he can finish his meal before getting up to walk around. In this way, he will be able to better meet his

Table 18-1   Restraint Alternatives

RESIDENT'S BEHAVIOR	ALTERNATIVES TO RESTRAINT USE TO TRY
The resident tries to get out of bed but is not able to stand up or walk safely independently.	• Use a low bed or place the mattress on the floor to reduce the distance that the resident could potentially fall. • Place cushioned mats on the floor to prevent injury if the resident should fall.
The resident rolls out of bed.	• Use a special mattress that has a "dip" in the center. This will make it more difficult for the resident to roll out of bed because he will have to roll "uphill." • Place a pressure-sensitive pad on the mattress that sounds an alarm if the resident gets out of bed.
The resident tries to get out of a chair but is not able to stand up or walk safely independently.	• Place the resident in or close to the nurses' station so that staff members are more easily able to supervise the resident. • Provide the resident with structured, supervised activities to do. The resident will be supervised during the activity, and being involved in the activity reduces boredom and may divert the resident's attention away from attempting to get out of the chair. • Include the resident in a daily exercise program. The resident will be supervised during the activity, and exercise meets the resident's need to move and helps to maintain the resident's independence. • Call on volunteers, other residents, and staff members to provide company for the resident. Residents who are comforted by the presence of others may be less likely to try to get up on their own. • Frequently check on the resident and address the resident's needs. Address physical needs (such as hunger, thirst, and the need to use the bathroom) and offer gentle words of reassurance. Residents who are comfortable and feel secure are less likely to try to get up from their chairs to seek a different environment. • Make sure that the resident always has a way of calling the staff when he needs help. • Use a chair alarm that will sound if the resident tries to get up.
The resident slides out of the chair.	• Apply non-skid material to the seat of the chair to prevent sliding.
The resident frequently wanders, or the resident tries to deliberately leave the unit or facility.	• Use an alarm system, such as a wanderer monitoring system, or individual door alarms that sound when an exit door is opened. • Make exit doors less obvious, for example, by painting them to look like the walls. • Provide the resident with structured, supervised activities to do. The resident will be supervised during the activity, and being involved in the activity reduces boredom and may divert the resident's attention away from wandering or attempting to leave the facility. • Schedule supervised "outside" time for the resident when the weather permits.

nutrition and hydration needs. Although the chair with a tray table is being used as a restraint, in this situation it is also being used as an **enabler,** a device that helps to support a higher level of functioning for Mr. Miller.

If it is determined that use of a restraint is appropriate, the doctor must write an order for the restraint. The order must specify the type of device, why it must be used, and when it is to be used. As a nursing assistant, you may be responsible for applying the restraint, and you will be responsible for providing care for the resident while he is restrained. If a doctor orders a restraint for one of your residents, always follow the doctor's order exactly. If one of the residents in your care has orders to use restraints, you must be sure to:

• Know exactly what type of restraint device is to be used, when it is to be used, and when it is to be removed
• Know how to apply the ordered restraint device correctly
• Check on the resident every 15 minutes
• Attend to the resident's needs for nutrition, hydration, toileting, and general comfort
• Release the restraint device at least every 2 hours, and provide range-of-motion exercises and repositioning to prevent loss of mobility and skin breakdown
• Provide for the resident's emotional needs, as well as his physical needs

All care that you give to a restrained resident must be recorded promptly. In addition to providing and recording care, you will also be responsible for observing the resident's response to the restraint and reporting any signs of trouble to the nurse immediately.

TELL THE NURSE ❗

Each time you attend to a person who is wearing a restraint, you should be alert to signs and symptoms related to the use of the restraint. Tell the nurse immediately if:

- The person complains of, or shows any signs of, shortness of breath or difficulty breathing

- The hand or foot beyond the restraint is swollen, pale, blue, or cold

- The person complains of pain, numbness, or tingling at or below a restrained body part

- The skin beneath a restraint device is red, blistered, broken, or bruised

- The person has become more confused, disoriented, or agitated

---

Any restraint that is tied should be tied with a "quick-release" knot (Fig. 18-8). A quick-release knot, or slipknot, will hold tightly if the restrained person pulls against it, but can be undone quickly by pulling on its "tails." The use of a quick-release knot will allow you to free a resident from a restraint quickly in the event of an emergency.

Each health care facility has policies and procedures detailing the use of restraints for residents. As a nursing assistant, you must understand your facility's policies and your responsibilities regarding the use of restraints. Failure to follow these policies can result in a situation that is dangerous for your resident. Additionally, failure to follow these policies can leave you and your facility open for litigation. General guidelines for the use of restraints are given in Guidelines Box 18-3. Information about applying specific types of restraints is given in the sections that follow.

Applying a Vest Restraint

A vest restraint is applied to a person's chest to protect the person from falling out of bed or a chair. The person's arms are placed through the armholes of the vest, and the flaps of the vest are crossed over each other, across the person's chest. A vest restraint should never be put on backwards (that is, with the back of the vest on the person's chest and the flaps crossed across her back). Putting the vest on backwards can cause the person to strangle if she slides down against the improperly placed restraint, because the back of the restraint is higher than the front. The procedure for applying a vest restraint is given in Procedure 18-1.

A jacket restraint is similar to a vest restraint, in that it is applied to the chest, but a jacket restraint has sleeves and closes in the back.

Applying Wrist or Ankle Restraints

In some cases, wrist or ankle restraints are applied to keep a person from moving his arms, legs, or both. The doctor specifies the number

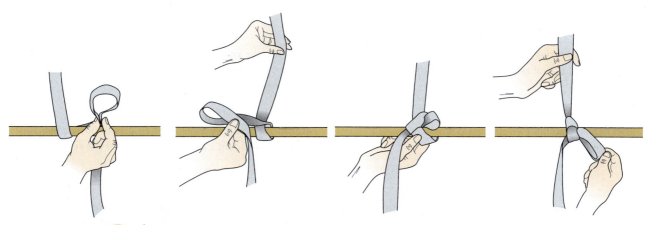

Figure 18-8
To make a quick-release knot, make a regular overhand knot, but slip a loop (instead of the end of the strap) through the first loop.

Guidelines Box 18-3 Guidelines for Using Restraints

WHAT YOU DO	WHY YOU DO IT
Do not use a restraint without a written doctor's order that states the reason for the restraint.	OBRA and state laws protect residents from being unnecessarily restrained.
Never use a restraint to "punish" a resident, or for your own convenience.	Physically and emotionally, the use of restraints has a very negative impact on the resident's quality of life. Therefore, restraints are only used when absolutely necessary, after all other methods of ensuring the resident's safety have failed.
Use the least restrictive restraint for the least amount of time.	Minimizing the use of restraints is important to preserve the resident's quality of life.
Follow the manufacturer's instructions, nurse's direction, and facility policy for applying restraints.	Improper application of restraints can lead to serious medical complications, injury, or even death.
Use a restraint that is the correct size and in good condition.	If the restraint is too large, the resident may be able to remove it, either completely or partially. This puts the resident at risk for falling and strangulation. If the restraint is too small, complications such as restriction of blood supply to areas beyond the restraint can result. If the restraint is in poor condition, it may not properly restrain the resident, or the resident may be injured when the restraint is applied.
Use commercial restraints. Do not use makeshift restraints, such as bed sheets or locks.	Using anything other than a commercial restraint to restrain a resident is unprofessional and dangerous.
Restraints are always applied over clothing, pajamas, or a gown.	Clothing offers a layer of protection between the restraint and the resident's skin.
Restraints with ties are tied in simple, quick-release knots placed out of reach of the resident's hands.	Quick-release knots must be used in case a resident needs to be released from the restraint quickly due to an emergency (for example, choking).
Ensure that you have enough help when applying a restraint.	Attempting to apply a restraint to an uncooperative, combative resident can lead to injury of the resident, you, or both.
Check on the restrained resident every 15 minutes to make sure that the restraint is correctly positioned and that feeling and blood flow are normal in any restrained extremity (arm or leg).	Checking on the resident regularly helps to prevent him from feeling abandoned, and ensures his safety. The resident may manage to shift the restraint to an unsafe position. Also, a restraint that is applied too tightly can lead to poor blood flow, which in turn can lead to permanent tissue or nerve damage.

WHAT YOU DO	WHY YOU DO IT
Completely remove the restraint every 2 hours, for a total of 10 minutes.	Releasing the restraint allows you to reposition the resident. All residents should be repositioned at least every 2 hours, whether they are restrained or not.
Record any care given to a restrained resident promptly and according to your facility's policy.	In a litigation situation, any action not recorded is considered not done. You can provide the best care possible, but if you do not record it, your effort will not protect you or your facility if legal action is taken.
Use restraints only if you have been properly trained in their use.	**Incorrect use of restraints can result in death!**

of extremities that are to be restrained. For example, a two-point restraint would involve two extremities (for example, both wrists), a three-point restraint would involve three extremities, and a four-point restraint would involve all four extremities. The procedure for applying wrist or ankle restraints is given in Procedure 18-2.

APPLYING LAP OR WAIST (BELT) RESTRAINTS

Lap restraints are used to prevent a person from sliding out of a chair. Waist (belt) restraints can be used to secure a person in a chair or in a bed. The procedure for applying a lap or waist (belt) restraint is given in Procedure 18-3.

SUMMARY

- Safety is a basic human need.
  - If we feel safe, we can relax and rest because we feel secure and comfortable.
  - Nursing assistants are responsible for helping to ensure the safety of those they care for.
- Accidents and incidents will occur in the long-term care setting, and they threaten the safety of residents.
  - Accidents are unexpected, unintended events that have the potential to cause bodily injury.
  - Incidents are events that are considered unusual, undesired, or out of the ordinary, and that disrupt the normal routine for the resident, the facility, or both.
  - OBRA requires the facility to maintain an environment that lowers the risk of accidents and incidents to the greatest extent possible.

- Residents are at increased risk for accidents and incidents as a result of normal age-related changes, medical conditions, and their treatments. These factors, especially when combined with environmental conditions, increase the likelihood that accidents will happen.
- Common accidents and incidents that can occur in a long-term care facility include bruises and skin tears, falls, burns, exposure to harmful substances, elopement, and behavioral incidents.
- Staff members play a very important role in minimizing the number of accidents and incidents that occur in a long-term care facility.
  - Providing for the safety of those we care for is a never-ending process.
  - A nursing assistant must be continuously aware, observing residents and their environment for safety risks. Nursing assistants

must also perform their duties in accordance with specified policies and procedures that have been established for safety.

- If an accident or incident does occur, it should be reported immediately and an incident (occurrence) report should be completed promptly. Proper reporting and recording of accidents helps to protect your residents, your facility, and you.

- Restraints are sometimes necessary to help ensure a resident's safety. Because the use of restraints can be associated with complications (and possibly even death), restraints are used only when all other measures to ensure a resident's safety have failed.

- Restraints are never used to punish a resident, or for the convenience of the staff.

- Physically and emotionally, restraints have a very negative impact on a resident's quality of life. The use of restraints requires extra care on the part of the nursing assistant to protect the resident's safety and dignity.

PROCEDURE 18-1

Applying a Vest Restraint

WHY YOU DO IT A vest restraint is applied to a person's chest to prevent the person from falling out of bed or a chair.

Getting Ready WCKIEPS

1. Complete the "Getting Ready" steps.

Supplies

- vest restraint in proper size

Procedure

2. Get help from a nurse or another nursing assistant, if necessary.

3. Assist the person to a sitting position by locking arms with her.

4. Support the person's back and shoulders with one arm while slipping the person's arms through the armholes of the vest using your other hand. Apply the restraint according to the manufacturer's instructions. The vest should cross in the front, across the person's chest.

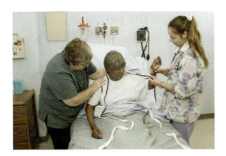

Step 4 Support the person's back and shoulders while slipping her arms through the armholes of the vest.

5. Make sure there are no wrinkles across the front or back of the restraint.

6. Bring the ties through the slots.

7. Help the person to lie or sit down.

8. Make sure the person is comfortable and in good body alignment.

9. If the person is in a chair, thread the straps *between* the seat and the armrest or *between* the back of the seat and the back of the chair, according to the manufacturer's directions. If the person is in bed, attach the straps to the bed frame, never the side rails. Always use the quick-release knot approved by your facility.

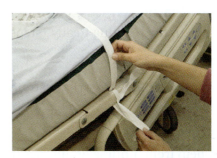

Step 9 Attach the straps to the bed frame, never the side rails.

10. Make sure the restraint is not too tight. You should be able to slide a flat hand between the restraint and the person. Adjust the straps if necessary.

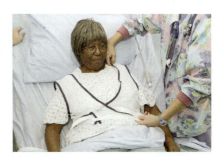

Step 10 Check to make sure the restraint is not too tight.

(continued)

Finishing Up CLSOWR

11. Complete the "Finishing Up" steps.

12. Check on the restrained person every 15 minutes.

13. Release the restraint every 2 hours and:

   a. Reposition the person.

   b. Meet the person's needs for food, fluids, and elimination.

   c. Give skin care and perform range-of-motion exercises.

14. Reapply the restraint.

15. Report and record the procedure, noting the type of restraint used, the time the restraint was applied, and the person's response to the restraint. Include any other relevant observations and sign the chart. Be sure to include your title as well as your name.

PROCEDURE 18-2

Applying Wrist or Ankle Restraints

WHY YOU DO IT   Wrist or ankle restraints are applied to keep a person from moving his arms, legs, or both.

Getting Ready WGKIEpS

1. Complete the "Getting Ready" steps.

Supplies

● appropriate number of wrist restraints, ankle restraints, or both

Procedure

2. Get help from a nurse or another nursing assistant, if necessary.

3. Apply the wrist or ankle restraint following the manufacturer's instructions. Place the soft part of the restraint against the skin.

4. Secure the restraint so that it is snug, but not tight. You should be able to slide two fingers under the restraint.

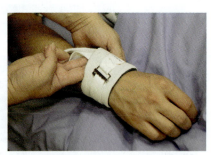

Step 4 You should be able to slip two fingers between the person's wrist and the restraint.

5. Attach the straps to the bed frame. Always use the quick-release knot approved by your facility.

6. If applying more than one restraint, repeat steps 3 through 5.

Finishing Up CLSOWR

7. Complete the "Finishing Up" steps.

8. Check on the restrained person every 15 minutes.

9. Release the restraint every 2 hours and:

   a. Reposition the person.

   b. Meet the person's needs for food, fluids, and elimination.

   c. Give skin care and perform range-of-motion exercises.

10. Reapply the restraint.

11. Report and record the procedure, noting the type of restraint used, the time the restraint was applied, and the person's response to the restraint. Include any other relevant observations and sign the chart. Be sure to include your title as well as your name.

PROCEDURE 18-3

Applying Lap or Waist (Belt) Restraints

WHY YOU DO IT   Lap restraints are used to prevent a person from sliding out of a chair. Waist (belt) restraints can be used to secure a person in a chair or in a bed.

Getting Ready WORKSTEPS

1. Complete the "Getting Ready" steps.

Supplies

- lap or waist restraint in proper size

Procedure

2. Get help from a nurse or another nursing assistant, if necessary.

3. If the person is in a chair, assist him to a proper sitting position, making sure that the person's hips are as far back against the back of the chair as possible. (If the person is in a wheelchair, make sure the brakes are locked first, and position the footrests to support the person's feet.)

4. Wrap the restraint around the person's abdomen, crossing the straps behind the person's back.

5. Bring the ties through the loops at the sides of the restraint, according to the manufacturer's directions.

6. Make sure the person is comfortable and in good body alignment.

7. Thread the straps between the chair arm and the chair back before securing the straps out of the person's reach, at the back of the chair. Always use the quick-release knot approved by your facility.

8. Secure the restraint, making sure it is not too tight. You should be able to slide a flat hand between the restraint and the person.

Finishing Up CLOSURE

9. Complete the "Finishing Up" steps.

10. Check on the restrained person every 15 minutes.

11. Release the restraint every 2 hours and:

   a. Reposition the person.

   b. Meet the person's needs for food, fluids, and elimination.

   c. Give skin care and perform range-of-motion exercises.

12. Reapply the restraint.

13. Report and record the procedure, noting the type of restraint used, the time the restraint was applied, and the person's response to the restraint. Include any other relevant observations and sign the chart. Be sure to include your title as well as your name.

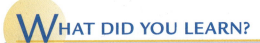WHAT DID YOU LEARN?

Multiple choice

Select the single best answer for each of the following questions.

1. Which of the following is a requirement of OBRA with regard to resident safety?
   a. Residents must receive the supervision and assistance they need to remain safe, and efforts must be made to eliminate environmental safety hazards
   b. All accidents and incidents must be prevented for the protection of the residents
   c. Residents who are at the greatest risk for accidents or incidents must be restrained
   d. The resident's right to freedom of movement is most important

2. Mrs. Chang's vision is clouded by cataracts. She shuffles her feet when she walks and frequently stumbles on uneven surfaces. Which of the following actions will help her to remain safe in the long-term care facility?
   a. Providing good lighting
   b. Assisting Mrs. Chang to put on proper footwear
   c. Removing the throw rug from Mrs. Chang's bathroom
   d. All of the above

3. Which of the following best describes a skin tear injury?
   a. A blister breaks open
   b. A top layer of skin is separated from a lower layer
   c. An abrasion occurs along the top layer of skin
   d. The skin breaks open from pressure

4. What is entrapment?
   a. The resident cannot leave the facility without the knowledge of the staff
   b. A type of restraint alternative
   c. The resident becomes trapped in the side rail or between the side rail and the mattress
   d. A type of physical restraint

5. After applying a restraint to a resident:
   a. Try to ignore the resident's complaints; he just wants attention
   b. Check the restraint every 6 hours
   c. Change the restraint once a day
   d. Remove the restraint at least every 2 hours

6. Vest restraints are applied so that the flaps:
   a. Cross in the back
   b. Cross in the front
   c. Are left open
   d. Are wrapped tightly around the person's chest

7. What is the leading cause of accidental death among elderly people?
   a. Burns
   b. Falls
   c. Poisonings
   d. Drowning

8. You enter Mr. Watkins' room to help him with his morning care, and you find him on the floor. He is conscious and complaining that his ankle hurts. He says he was trying to get to the bathroom and his foot got caught in the bed covers. What should you do first?
   a. Call the nurse to come and assess Mr. Watkins
   b. Help Mr. Watkins to a comfortable position in bed so that the nurse can assess him more easily
   c. Fill out an incident report
   d. Remind Mr. Watkins that he was not supposed to get up without help

9. Why is a restraint used?
   a. To make caregiving easier for the staff
   b. To punish residents who refuse to follow the rules
   c. To protect a resident from harming himself or others, when all other methods of keeping the resident safe have failed
   d. All of the above

10. One of your residents receives all of her nutrition and hydration through a gastrostomy tube (a tube inserted through the skin directly into the stomach). The resident keeps trying to pull the gastrostomy tube out. What should you do to prevent the resident from removing the feeding tube?
    a. Apply a mitt restraint
    b. Report your observations to the nurse
    c. Explain to the resident that she has to leave the tube alone
    d. Use a sensor alarm

11. In which situation would a seat belt on a wheelchair *not* be considered a restraint?
   a. The seat belt can easily be removed by the staff
   b. The seat belt is filled to the resident snugly, but it is not tight
   c. The resident is able to unfasten the seat belt when you ask her to
   d. The resident unfastens the seat belt by accident while playing with it

12. What do you need to know before applying a restraint to a resident?
   a. The type of restraint the doctor has ordered
   b. When the restraint is supposed to be used
   c. How the restraint is used
   d. All of the above

STOP and Think!

- Mr. Lovell, one of the residents with dementia at the long-term care facility where you work, has become very agitated. He is prone to falling and should not get up without help. However, today, he is refusing to stay in his bed or his wheelchair. You get him situated, and then as soon as you leave the room, he tries to get up again. This has happened twice, and you are only in the first hour of your shift. You are very concerned that Mr. Lovell will fall and hurt himself, but you cannot stay with him all day because you have other residents to attend to. Describe some things that you could do to help protect Mr. Lovell.

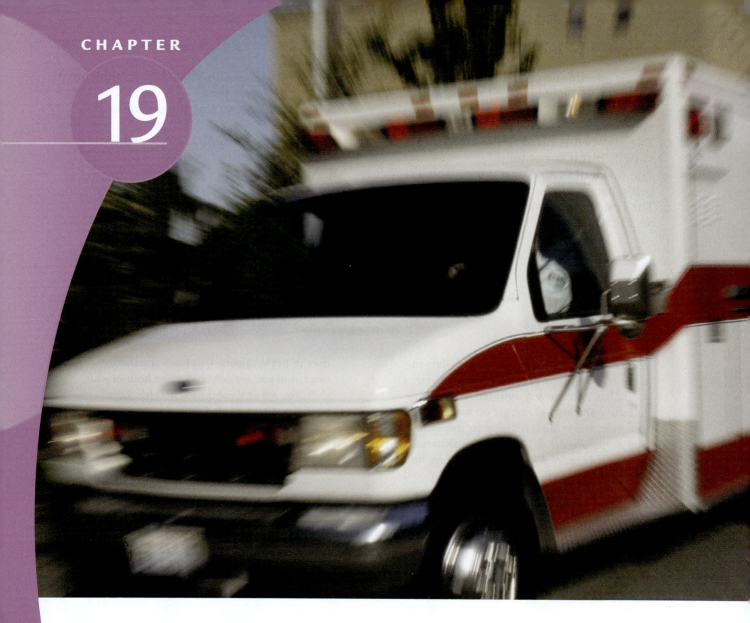

Basic First Aid and Emergency Care

WHAT WILL YOU LEARN?

Any condition that requires immediate medical attention to prevent a person from dying or having a permanent disability is an **emergency.** An emergency can occur as a result of an accident (such as a fall) or as a result of a medical condition (such as a heart attack or stroke). Emergency situations can occur anywhere, even in a health care setting. As a nursing assistant, you must be prepared to provide safe, compassionate care for a person in an emergency situation. When you are finished with this chapter, you will be able to:

1. Discuss your role in an emergency situation.
2. Define terms used to describe a person's condition in an emergency situation.
3. Describe changes in a person's behavior that may suggest delirium, and explain why it is important to report these changes to the nurse right away.

Photo: An ambulance speeds through the streets to aid a person in need.

4. List and discuss the ABCs of emergency care.

5. List some of the organizations that offer approved training in first aid and basic life support (BLS) measures.

6. List the signs and symptoms of a "heart attack" and describe the actions that a nursing assistant would take to assist a person with these signs and symptoms.

7. List the signs and symptoms of a stroke.

8. Describe how you would assist a person who complains of feeling faint, or who has fainted.

9. Describe how you would assist a person who is having a seizure.

10. Describe how you would assist a person who is bleeding uncontrollably (hemorrhaging).

11. Describe some of the types and causes of shock, and describe how you would assist a person who is in shock.

12. Demonstrate how to clear the airway of a choking adult or child older than 1 year by using abdominal or chest thrusts.

13. Describe the steps of the chain of survival.

Vocabulary Use the CD in the front of your book to hear these terms pronounced and defined:

Emergency	Respiratory arrest	Automated external	Shock
Oriented to person,	Cardiac arrest	defibrillator (AED)	Cardiogenic shock
place, and time	Clinical death	Syncope	Hemorrhagic shock
Disoriented	Biological death	Grand mal seizure	Septic shock
Unresponsive	Basic life support (BLS)	Petit mal (absence)	Anaphylactic shock
Delirium	Rescue breathing	seizure	Aspiration
Emergency medical	Cardiopulmonary	Hemorrhage	Chain of survival
services (EMS) system	resuscitation (CPR)	Pulse points	
First aid			

RESPONDING TO AN EMERGENCY

As you learned in Chapter 5, the nature of your daily duties will bring you in close and frequent contact with your residents. This unique relationship gives you insight that others might not have. Through your interactions with your residents, you become aware of their individual qualities, personalities, and habits. For example, you know that Mrs. Smith typically has an above-average blood pressure reading, even though she is taking medication. You know that Mr. Martin complains about his arthritis, especially in the morning. You know that Mr. Allen always says that he is starving after eating a full meal. You know which of your residents are "morning people," and which are slow until after they have had their first cup of coffee.

Your familiarity with your residents makes you more likely to notice when something is not quite right. For example, the first sign of a stroke is often just a slight slurring of speech or a small change in a person's personality. Heart attacks may be signaled by complaints of fatigue or indigestion. Other emergency situations are recognized by changes in vital signs (such as respiratory rate, heart rate, and blood pressure) or behavior. By conscientiously reporting signs or symptoms that seem unusual or give you cause for alarm to the nurse, you may prevent an emergency situation from worsening (Fig. 19-1).

The people you care for will have varying levels of ability and awareness, and you will come to learn what is normal for each person. A change in a person's usual abilities or level of awareness (sometimes called level of consciousness, or LOC) can be a sign that something is wrong. A person who is usually alert and **oriented to person** (able to tell you who he is and who you are), **place** (able to tell you where he is), and **time** (able to tell you the year, the day of the week, and the time of day) can suddenly become **disoriented,** or unable to

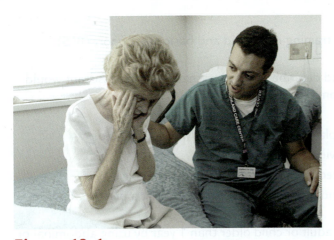

Figure 19-1
Being able to recognize an impending emergency is a life-saving skill.

answer those basic questions. A person is said to be **unresponsive** if she is unconscious and cannot be aroused, or conscious but not responsive when spoken to or touched. Either of these conditions should be reported to the nurse immediately.

Delirium (a temporary state of confusion) can be a sign of a serious medical crisis, especially in an older person. It may also be a side effect of medication. Once the underlying disorder is treated or the medication is stopped, the delirium goes away. In some cases, the person may die if the underlying cause of the delirium is not identified and treated.

TELL THE NURSE

As a nursing assistant, you may be the first to notice changes in a resident's behavior that may suggest delirium. If you notice any of the following in a person who is normally alert and oriented, report your observations to the nurse immediately:

- The person is hallucinating (seeing or hearing something that you know cannot possibly be true, such as mice crawling all over the bed)

- The person does not recognize someone familiar, or mistakes a stranger for a close family member or friend

- The person is very restless, especially at night

- The person seems confused

- The person talks frequently about events from the past, but cannot remember events that occurred recently (such as a meal eaten 2 hours ago)

- The person gets lost and wanders the halls aimlessly, even through the person knows his way around the facility

---

In an emergency situation, your responsibilities as a nursing assistant are clear. You should:

1. **Recognize that an emergency exists.** Use your observation skills and familiarity with the resident to detect changes in behavior or physical condition.

2. **Decide to act.** Stay calm and organize your thoughts. Check the scene to make sure that you are not entering a situation that is potentially dangerous for you, or for other members of the health care team. For example, you could be entering an area that is contaminated with hazardous materials or gases. Acting hastily can make the problem worse in some situations. For example, someone who has fallen may have injuries to the spinal column that would be made worse if the person were moved.

3. **Check for consciousness.** If it is safe to do so, gently shake the person and call to him. The person may have just fainted ("passed out"), in which case you will need to call the nurse for help. Keep the person lying down, and stay with the person until the nurse arrives. The nurse will make sure that no other injuries are present and work to find out why the person fainted. If the person does not respond when you gently shake his arm and call to him, then you will need to. . .

4. **Activate the emergency medical services (EMS) system.** An **EMS system** is a network of resources (including people, equipment, and facilities) that is organized to respond to an emergency. Make sure you know your facility's procedure for activating the EMS system, and your responsibilities. For example, you may just be required to notify the nurse of the emergency. Or, you may be responsible for dialing "911" or some other emergency telephone number. Early activation of the EMS system allows a person in an emergency situation to get advanced medical care as soon as possible. This greatly increases the person's chances of survival. When you call, be prepared to give accurate information about your location and the condition of your resident (Box 19-1). The information you provide will be very helpful for the EMS personnel who respond to your call.

5. **Provide appropriate care until the EMS personnel arrive.** Provide **first aid** (the care given to an injured or sick person while waiting for more advanced help to arrive) according to the situation and your level of training. (As in any situation, you should

Information To Provide When Activating the Emergency Medical Services (EMS) System

Information About your Location
- The name and address of your facility, including the name of the building (if you are on a campus with many buildings)
- The entrance to the campus and/or to the building that the EMS personnel should use (it can help to save time if the EMS personnel know exactly where to come)
- The unit or floor, and directions to your specific location (for example, "Turn right when you get off the elevator on the 4th floor.")

Information About your Resident's Condition
- Whether or not the resident is responsive or unresponsive

- If the resident is responsive, the resident's level of alertness
- Vital sign measurements and characteristics (for example, "Pulse is 92, weak and irregular.")
- Other significant signs or symptoms (for example, changes in skin color, excessive perspiration, complaints of nausea)

Information About the Environment
- Anything unusual in the surrounding area (such as broken furniture, a peculiar odor, or an open medication container) that may offer clues about what caused the emergency (especially important if the resident is not responsive)

---

perform only those procedures that you have been trained to do and that are within your scope of practice.) Speak gently and calmly to the person, and reassure him that more help is on the way.

6. **Report and record the care you provided.** As always when you provide care, you must accurately report and record your observations and the care that you provided, per your facility's policy.

Helping Hands and a Caring Heart

FOCUS ON HUMANISTIC HEALTH CARE

An emergency can be very frightening for the person experiencing it. Although you will be focused on the person's physical needs, try not to forget about the other needs that the person and his or her family members have. Remain calm. Reassure the person and family members that more help is on the way. While the situation may be too serious to say something like, "Everything will be OK," you can certainly tell the person that you will "do everything you can to help." Make an effort to provide as much privacy for the person as you are able. Whenever there is an emergency, others in the area have a tendency to want to see what is going on. Politely ask others who are not immediately involved in the situation to leave the area. If it is possible to shield the area with privacy curtains or panels, please do so. These measures help to maintain the person's dignity and right to privacy.

BASIC LIFE SUPPORT (BLS) MEASURES

Emergency situations often result when something occurs that affects breathing or circulation. The body's cells need oxygen to live. When we inhale, we take air, which contains oxygen, into our lungs. Once in the lungs, the oxygen in the air passes from the tiny air sacs of the lungs (called the *alveoli*) into the blood in the blood vessels that surround the alveoli. Each time the heart beats, the oxygen-containing blood is sent to all of the cells in the body.

Any process that affects our ability to take air into our lungs or to send oxygen-containing blood to the cells of the body is an emergency. Without oxygen, the cells of the body begin to die. Humans can live for days without food and water but only for a few minutes without oxygen.

Respiratory arrest means that breathing has stopped (*arrest* means "stop"). When breathing stops, the oxygen content of the blood decreases, and there is not enough oxygen for the cells of the body to function properly. Soon, key organs such as the brain and the heart stop functioning. A person who is in respiratory arrest may have a heartbeat initially, but if breathing is not started again soon, his heart will stop beating. The condition is called **cardiac arrest.** A person who has no pulse or is not breathing is said to be *clinically dead.* **Clinical death** can sometimes be reversed with prompt emergency treatment that restarts the heart and breathing. However, if clinical death is not promptly reversed, allowing oxygen-

BOX 19-2   The ABCs of Emergency Care

"A" is for "airway." Open the person's airway by tilting her head back and lifting her chin. This prevents the person's tongue from falling backward against the back of the throat, blocking the flow of air to the lungs.

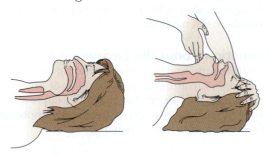

"B" is for "breathing." Check to see if the person is breathing by leaning close and placing your ear over her mouth and nose. Listen for the sounds of breathing, feel the person's breath moving against your cheek, and look for the rise and fall of the person's chest. The person is not breathing unless there is air movement as well as chest movement!

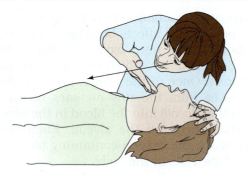

- If the person is breathing, keep her airway open or position her on her side. Continue to monitor the person's condition closely while waiting for assistance.
- If the person is not breathing, start rescue breathing according to your training. Remember that if an airway is not established and oxygen is not sent to the person's lungs, the person will not survive the incident, no matter what additional measures are taken.

"C" is for "circulation." Check the person's pulse. You can feel an adult's or child's pulse by placing your fingers on either side of the Adam's apple, over the carotid artery in the neck. An infant's pulse is felt over the brachial artery, in the upper arm. A person in an emergency situation may have a rapid, weak, erratic (irregular), or very slow pulse. A person with no pulse is in cardiac arrest and needs immediate CPR.

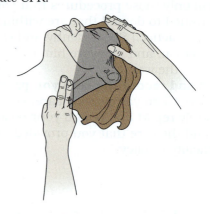

containing blood to reach the brain and the heart, **biological death** soon follows. Biological death is not reversible.

Basic life support (BLS) measures are taken in response to respiratory arrest, cardiac arrest, or both. The ABCs of emergency care (Box 19-2) are used to determine whether a person needs BLS measures. If the person is already in respiratory or cardiac arrest, BLS is used to keep the person alive until advanced medical assistance arrives. BLS measures include rescue breathing, cardiopulmonary resuscitation (CPR), and the use of an automated external defibrillator.

- In **rescue breathing,** the rescuer blows air into the person's mouth to perform the function of breathing for the person until the person begins breathing again on her own.

- In **cardiopulmonary resuscitation (CPR),** the rescuer uses a combination of rescue breathing and chest compressions to sustain breathing and circulation for a person who has gone into respiratory or cardiac arrest.

- An **automated external defibrillator (AED)** is a small, portable device that automatically detects a person's heart rhythm and delivers an electrical shock to the heart to stop fast, abnormal heartbeats and restore the heart's normal rhythm. If the facility where you work has an AED, you should know exactly where it is located. Often, the AED is stored in a closet or on a cart with other emergency equipment. In the event of a cardiac emergency, it is important to get the AED to the person as quickly as possible. The person's chances of survival decrease with every minute that passes without its use.

Your facility may require first aid and BLS training as a requirement for employment. In some states, first aid and BLS training are provided as part of nursing assistant training. However, because improvements are periodically made in the way some of these techniques, such as CPR, are taught, we have not provided specific instructions for all first aid and BLS techniques in this text. If training in first aid and BLS is not included as part of your nursing assistant training course, you can learn these techniques in courses offered by organizations such as the American Red Cross (ARC), the National Safety Council (NSC), and the American Heart Association (AHA). The programs offered by these organizations are taught by certified instructors, using approved teaching methods (Fig. 19-2). This additional training will allow you to be better prepared for emergency situations that may arise in your workplace, home, or community.

If you are trained in BLS measures and you find one of your residents in a state of respiratory or cardiac arrest, be sure you know the person's wishes for resuscitation before beginning BLS. For example, a person who is terminally ill may not want to be resuscitated if she goes into respiratory or cardiac arrest. In this case, the person's chart would carry a no-code or do not resuscitate (DNR)

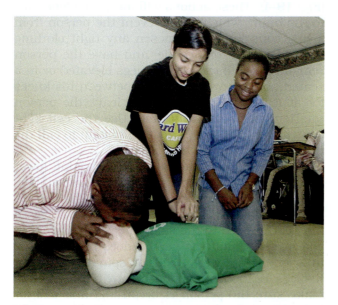

Figure 19-2
Students practice rescue breathing and cardiopulmonary resuscitation (CPR) on a mannequin during a basic life support (BLS) training course. (*AP Photo/The Commercial Dispatch, Kelly Tippett.*)

order (see Chapter 28). If a person is on DNR status, follow your facility's policy accordingly.

EMERGENCY SITUATIONS

Many different emergency situations can occur, both in the home and community and in the health care setting. In this section, we will review some of the most common emergency situations, as well as what you should do to help a person in one of these situations.

"HEART ATTACKS" AND STROKES

Both heart attacks and strokes can occur suddenly. These are life-threatening situations that require emergency care.

Myocardial Infarction ("Heart Attack")

Perhaps the classic emergency situation is that of a "heart attack," or myocardial infarction (MI). The myocardium is the muscular wall of the heart. An infarction occurs when blood flow to a part of the body is blocked, depriving the cells of oxygen and causing them to die. So when a person has a myocardial infarction (MI), blood flow to the muscular wall of the heart is blocked, and part of the heart muscle dies. As a result, the heart is unable to pump blood effectively throughout the body, creating an emergency situation. If the damaged area of the heart is large enough, cardiac arrest can occur.

TELL THE NURSE

The signs and symptoms of a heart attack can vary greatly from one person to the next. Any of the following could be signs and symptoms of a heart attack and should be reported to the nurse immediately:

- Pain or tightness in the chest, which may extend to the neck, back, or arm

- Pale or grayish skin

- Excessive sweating

- Trouble breathing

- Nausea or heartburn-like pain

Although chest pain is the "classic" sign of a heart attack, older people often do not experience chest pain with a heart attack. Instead, an older person may experience other symptoms, such as nausea or heartburn. Be sure to alert the nurse if a resident is experiencing these symptoms.

If you observe that a person is having signs or symptoms of a heart attack, have the person lie down. Raise the person's head to help make breathing easier, and call the nurse or activate the EMS system immediately. Prompt medical intervention can help to minimize damage to the heart muscle. If the person goes into respiratory or cardiac arrest, you will need to begin BLS (unless the person is on DNR status).

Stroke

A stroke, also known as a cerebrovascular accidents (CVA), is also caused by blocked blood flow to a body part. In the case of a stroke, the affected body part is the brain, rather than the heart. Like a heart attack, a stroke can cause different signs and symptoms in different people. For example, a stroke might cause only mild physical changes in some people. In others, it might cause loss of consciousness or a coma.

TELL THE NURSE

Signs and symptoms of a stroke could include any of the following:

- The person is unconscious or difficult to arouse from sleep
- The person suddenly seems confused or disoriented
- The person slurs his or her speech or is unable to speak clearly
- The person is drooling
- One of the person's eyelids or the corner of the mouth is drooping
- The person complains of the sudden onset of a severe headache
- The person complains of weakness, paralysis, tingling, or numbness of an arm or leg or the side of the face
- There is a change in the person's vital signs, especially the blood pressure or pulse

Figure 19-3 shows two very common signs of stroke, facial droop and arm weakness. If you think that a person is having or has had a stroke,

report your observations to the nurse and activate the EMS system. Keep the person lying down and watch for signs of respiratory arrest until advanced care arrives. New advances in the treatment of stroke have resulted in improved outcomes for some people, when treatment is started early.

FAINTING (SYNCOPE)

The medical word for fainting is **syncope.** Fainting occurs when the blood supply to the brain suddenly decreases, resulting in a loss of consciousness. Although fainting may be an early sign of a serious medical condition, such as a heart problem, it can also be the result of hunger ("low blood sugar"), pain, extreme emotion, fatigue, medication side effects, a "stuffy" room (poor ventilation), excessive heat, or standing for a long time. Fainting is not life-threatening in and of itself, but because a person who faints is at risk for injury from falling, it is important to act quickly if you believe a person is about to faint. A person who is about to faint may complain of dizziness or a temporary loss of vision. His skin may be pale and clammy, and he may sweat excessively. He may breathe shallowly, and his pulse may be weak.

If you think that a person is about to faint, have the person lie down on his back and elevate his legs 12 inches, or ask him to sit down and bend forward, placing his head between his knees (Fig. 19-4). These actions will increase blood flow to the brain, which may prevent the person from losing consciousness. Loosen any tight clothing (such as a belt or necktie) and have the person remain on his back with his legs elevated or in a seated position with his head between his knees for at least 5 minutes. Do not leave the person unattended during this time. Use the call light control or staff communication system to call the nurse, or call out for assistance.

If a person you are assisting does faint, lower him to the floor or other flat surface, remembering to use good body mechanics (see Chapter 17, Box 17-1). Position the person on his back with his head turned to the side, in case he vomits. If you are sure that the person does not have any injuries to the head, neck, or spinal cord, raise his legs 12 inches, and loosen any tight clothing. Make sure the person is breathing, and call for help. Then check the person's vital signs. Even if the person recovers from the episode quickly, have him continue to lie down until the nurse arrives.

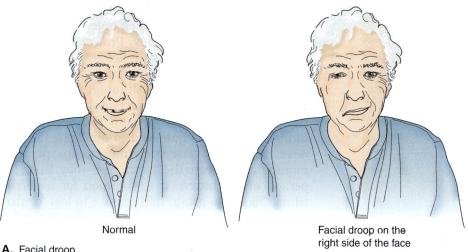

Normal

Facial droop on the right side of the face

A. Facial droop

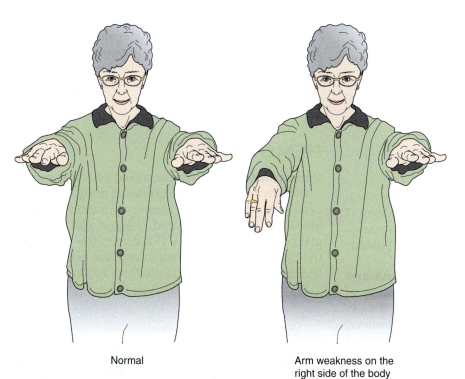

Normal

Arm weakness on the right side of the body

B. Arm weakness

Figure 19-3
Two very common signs of stroke include **(A)** facial droop and **(B)** arm weakness.

TELL THE NURSE ❗

Because fainting may be a sign of a serious medical condition, it is important to report and record the following for the nurse:

- What time the person fainted
- Whether there was a change in the person's level of consciousness (LOC), and if so, how long this change lasted
- Whether the person vomited
- The person's appearance at the time of the incident (for example, overheated, pale, sweaty)
- Whether the person complained of anything before the incident (for example, loss of vision, dizziness, nausea)
- The actions you took to assist the person

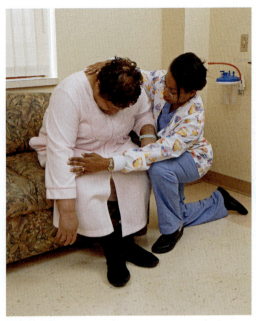

Figure 19-4

Having a person sit with her head between her knees increases blood flow to the brain and may prevent a fainting episode.

SEIZURES

Seizures, also known as *convulsions*, occur when brain activity is interrupted. Seizures can result from head injuries (either recent or past), strokes, infections, high fevers, low blood sugar, poisonings, brain tumors, and epilepsy.

The severity of a seizure can vary. **Grand mal seizures** are characterized by violent jerking of the muscles all over the body. A person who is having a **petit mal (absence) seizure,** however, may simply stop speaking in mid-sentence and stare into space.

Grand mal seizures cause a loss of consciousness and, because of the violent jerking of the muscles, place the person who is having the seizure at risk for injuring herself. If a person is standing or sitting when a seizure begins, she could be injured when she falls as the result of losing consciousness. A person who is having a grand mal seizure is also at risk for injuring herself by striking nearby objects or by severely biting her own tongue and lips. A grand mal seizure may last for just a few seconds, or it may go on for as long as 5 to 10 minutes.

First aid for a person having a grand mal seizure involves protecting the person until the seizure is over, and keeping the airway open during the period of unconsciousness afterwards. If a person is standing or sitting when a grand mal seizure begins, gently help the person to the floor and move furniture or other objects that might cause injury out of the way. Protect the person's head by placing a pillow or folded towel underneath it and call for help while allowing the seizure to run its course. Although in the past, it was common practice to insert a tongue blade into the person's mouth to prevent the person from biting her own tongue, you should not do this. Never attempt to place anything in the person's mouth or between the teeth. You may hurt the person or get bitten. It is common for a person who is having a grand mal seizure to lose control of her bladder or bowels. Because the gag reflex may also be temporarily lost, saliva may pool in the mouth. After the seizure is over, turn the person to her side (place her in the recovery position) and allow any secretions to drain from her mouth to prevent choking. Provide warmth and a quiet environment (Fig. 19-5). A person who has just had a grand mal seizure may be very disoriented, tired, or both, and she may have no memory of the episode at all.

HEMORRHAGE

Hemorrhage (severe, uncontrolled bleeding) can be caused by trauma to a blood vessel or by certain illnesses, such as gastric ulcers. Ordinarily, when a blood vessel wall is injured, a blood clot forms to prevent the loss of blood. However, if the trauma to the blood vessel wall is major, or if the person lacks the clotting factors needed to form blood clots, the

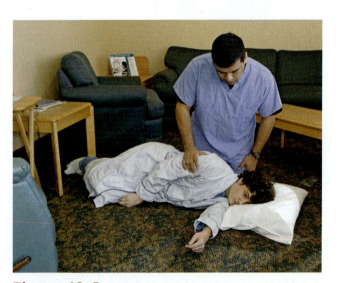

Figure 19-5

After the seizure has passed, place the person in the recovery position and allow secretions to drain from the mouth.

bleeding will not stop. People who are taking medications to prevent blood clotting are also at high risk for hemorrhage, because the medication decreases the body's normal clotting response.

Hemorrhage can be either external (plainly visible) or internal (occurring within the body). Internal hemorrhage may be hidden unless the person vomits blood or passes blood through the rectum. Hemorrhage can be either venous or arterial, depending on the type of blood vessel that is injured. Venous hemorrhage flows steadily. Arterial hemorrhage spurts or pulses with the heartbeat. If hemorrhage is not controlled quickly, death will result.

If a person is hemorrhaging, call for help and make sure the person is lying down. Take standard precautions to protect yourself from exposure to bloodborne pathogens. Apply firm, steady pressure directly to the wound using a clean towel, gauze pads, or whatever else is clean and available for use as a compress. Continue to apply pressure to the wound until more advanced medical help comes. If the direct pressure does not stop or slow the flow of blood, raise the affected body part (if it is an arm or leg) and apply pressure to a pulse point above the wound. **Pulse points** are the points where large arteries run close enough to the surface of the skin to be felt as a pulse (see Chapter 22, Fig. 22-8). At these points, the artery can be compressed against a bone by applying direct pressure, helping to slow blood loss from a wound. A tourniquet is a device that is placed tightly around an arm or leg to cut off nearly all blood supply. A tourniquet is only used as a last resort to control bleeding, and should always be applied by a specially trained emergency responder.

SHOCK

Shock results when the organs and tissues of the body do not receive enough oxygen-containing blood. There are many different causes and types of shock. For example:

- **Cardiogenic shock** can occur when the heart is unable to pump enough blood throughout the body to meet the tissues' need for oxygen.
- **Hemorrhagic shock** results from massive blood loss, which means that there is not enough blood in the vessels to supply the tissues of the body.
- **Septic shock** is caused by severe bacterial infections that involve the entire body. The toxins produced by the bacteria cause the blood vessels to dilate (widen), leading to

pooling of blood away from the heart and poor circulation.
- **Anaphylactic shock** is caused by a severe allergic reaction (for example, to medications, bee stings, or certain foods, such as nuts) As in septic shock, widening of the blood vessels occurs, causing the blood to pool away from the heart. In addition, the tiniest tubes in the lungs (called bronchioles) close off, preventing the oxygen in the air from passing into the lungs and reaching the blood.

To treat shock, the underlying cause of the shock must be addressed. For example, if a person is in shock because of hemorrhage, the bleeding must be stopped and the fluid replaced intravenously to prevent death. If the pumping action of the heart is too weak or erratic to circulate blood to the organs and tissues, the heart's ability to pump must be restored through medications or other measures, such as the implantation of a pacemaker.

A person entering a state of shock will have low blood pressure that continues to decrease. His pulse will be rapid and weak. His skin will be cool, clammy, and pale. He will be confused or disoriented. He will breathe rapidly, and if he is conscious, he may complain of thirst. Make sure that advanced emergency medical care has been called and keep the person warm and calm. The treatment for anaphylactic shock is the immediate administration of a medication called epinephrine (adrenaline). People who know that they are allergic to something that could cause them to go into anaphylactic shock (for example, bee stings) often carry this medication with them (Fig. 19-6). If a person who is in anaphylactic shock is unable to give himself this medication, someone else will need to do this for him.

AIRWAY OBSTRUCTIONS ("CHOKING")

Foreign material, such as food or vomitus, can become lodged in the airway ("windpipe"), blocking the flow of air to the lungs. The accidental inhalation of foreign material into the airway is called **aspiration.**

Aspiration is very common during meal times. Residents with poorly fitting dentures or who are missing teeth cannot chew their food properly, which puts them at risk for aspiration. Residents who have had strokes may have difficulty chewing and swallowing, and as a result are also at risk

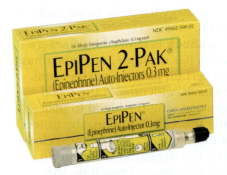
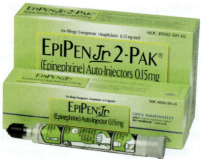

Figure 19-6

The EpiPen Auto-Injector, a self-injectable cartridge of epinephrine, is used to treat anaphylactic shock. The yellow EpiPen is for adults. The green one is for children. (*Photo courtesy of Dey, L.P.*)

for aspiration. In addition, talking or laughing with food in the mouth can lead to aspiration.

Vomiting (in a person who is unconscious or who has weak coughing or swallowing reflexes as a result of paralysis or the effects of a medication) can also lead to aspiration. This is why, when you are assisting a person who is vomiting or at risk for vomiting and who may not be able to keep his airway clear on his own, you turn the person's head to the side to help keep the airway clear.

Types of Airway Obstructions

An airway obstruction can be either partial or complete. In a partial airway obstruction, the object is not totally blocking the airway and some air can pass through. A person who is coughing strongly and has good skin color most likely has a partial airway obstruction with good air exchange (that is, an adequate ability to breathe). Stay with the person and allow him to continue to cough. If the person is not already sitting up, help him to sit up to make breathing easier. If the person does not quickly cough up the object, call for help because advanced emergency medical assistance may be necessary to remove the item. Also, there is the risk that the item will move and totally obstruct the airway, in which case the person will need immediate assistance.

A partial airway obstruction with poor air exchange (that is, an inadequate ability to breathe) is demonstrated by a weak, ineffective coughing effort; high-pitched, "crowing" sounds as the person tries to breathe; and a bluish skin color (cyanosis). A person with this type of airway obstruction needs immediate help.

A complete airway obstruction is one that totally blocks all airflow to the lungs. The person cannot cough, speak, or breathe and will lose consciousness quickly if the object that is blocking airflow is not removed. The person will be frightened, and will usually grab his throat in

what is considered the universal choking sign (Fig. 19-7).

Clearing the Airway

Abdominal thrusts (called the *Heimlich maneuver* in the past, after the man who invented the technique) are used to clear an obstructed airway in a person who is choking. The thoracic (chest) cavity, which contains the heart and

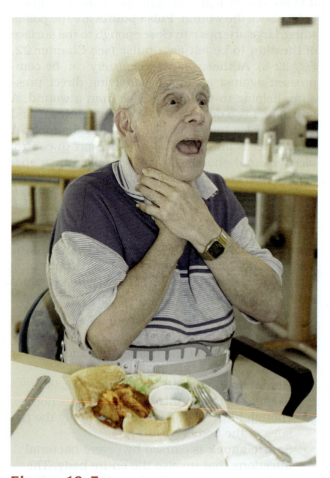

Figure 19-7

Grasping the throat is the universal sign for "I'm choking!"

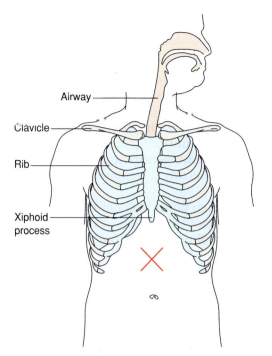

Figure 19-8
Applying pressure to the abdominal cavity (red X) forces the air out of the lungs, which in turn forces the object out of the person's airway.

lungs, is separated from the abdominal cavity, which contains the stomach and other organs, by the diaphragm, a flat muscle. In abdominal thrusts, the area beneath the diaphragm (the abdominal cavity) is compressed, forcing the air out of the lungs. This dislodges the object that is blocking the airway (Fig. 19-8). The procedure for performing abdominal thrusts on a person who is conscious is given in Procedure 19-1. The procedure for clearing the airway of a person who is unconscious is given in Procedure 19-2.

In very heavy people or pregnant women, chest thrusts, rather than abdominal thrusts, are used. This is because in these situations, giving abdominal thrusts would be either impossible or dangerous. In the case of a very heavy person, it is too hard to get your arms around the person. In the case of a pregnant woman, applying pressure to the abdomen could harm the baby. Procedure 19-3 explains how to give chest thrusts.

When a person is choking, the EMS system should be activated as soon as possible. While you wait for help, perform abdominal or chest thrusts repeatedly, until the airway is open again and the person starts breathing on his own. If the person does not start breathing on his own, perform rescue breathing after the airway is cleared. You may need to start CPR if the person goes into cardiac arrest.

THE CHAIN OF SURVIVAL

A person's ability to survive an emergency, and to survive it without any permanent damage, relies on a series of events called the **chain of survival:**

1. Someone must recognize that an emergency situation exists, and activate the EMS system.
2. First responder care (basic first aid, including BLS if applicable) must be given by able people at the scene of the emergency.
3. Medical intervention, such as that provided by an emergency medical technician (EMT), a paramedic, a nurse, or a doctor, must be provided as soon as possible.
4. After the immediate crisis passes, hospital care may be needed to help the person survive. As the person's condition improves, she may be transferred to a sub-acute care unit or return to the long-term care facility for further recovery.
5. Rehabilitation, the final step in the chain of survival, focuses on improving the general health status of the person. One goal of rehabilitation may be to help the person to recover abilities that may have been lost as a result of the emergency. For example, a person who has had a stroke may need to relearn skills such as walking or speaking. Another goal of rehabilitation may be to help the person learn how to prevent further progression of a disease. For example, a person who has had a heart attack may be taught new diet management skills, and started on an exercise program.

As a nursing assistant, you can play a vital role in helping to see a person through the immediate crisis (steps 1 and 2). You may also care for someone who is in the recovery phase (steps 4 and 5).

SUMMARY

- Any situation in which a person needs immediate medical attention to prevent death or permanent disability is considered an emergency. Emergencies can result from medical conditions (such as a heart attack or stroke) or from an accident (such as a fall).
  - Your knowledge of your resident's usual condition may allow you to recognize a potential emergency situation. By communicating what you have observed to the nurse, you may be able to prevent the emergency from getting worse.
  - In an emergency situation, you will be responsible for (1) recognizing that an emergency exists, (2) deciding to act, (3) checking for consciousness, (4) activating the facility's emergency response system, (5) providing appropriate care per your training and scope of practice until the emergency personnel arrive, and (6) recording your observations and the care you provided.
- The ABCs of emergency care involve maintaining the person's airway, making sure that the person is breathing, and checking the person's pulse to make sure that the heart is beating and blood is circulating throughout the body.
  - Basic life support (BLS) measures support the ABCs: airway, breathing, and circulation. BLS measures include rescue breathing, cardiopulmonary resuscitation (CPR), and the use of an automated external defibrillator (AED).

- Training in first aid and BLS measures, whether required by your employer or not, will prepare you for emergency situations that may arise in your workplace, home, or community.
- Common emergency situations include fainting, seizures, hemorrhage, shock, and choking.
  - Although fainting is not life threatening, it could put the person at risk for injury from falling. If a person complains of feeling faint, have her lie down or place her head between her knees to increase blood flow to the brain.
  - First aid for a person who is having a seizure involves protecting the person from injury during the seizure and keeping the airway open after the seizure.
  - Hemorrhage is controlled by applying direct pressure to the wound or to a pulse point above the wound.
  - Shock results when the organs and tissues of the body do not receive enough oxygen-rich blood. Keep a person who is in shock warm and calm until emergency personnel arrive.
  - Airway obstructions block the flow of oxygen into the lungs and can quickly result in death if the obstruction is not cleared.
- Receiving skilled first aid, along with early medical intervention, increases a person's chance of surviving an emergency and minimizes the person's chances of having permanent disabilities as a result of the incident.

Relieving An Obstructed Airway in Conscious Adults and Children Older Than 1 Year

WHY YOU DO IT   If the object is not removed from the airway, allowing air to get to the lungs, the person will die.

1. Check the person's ability to breathe and speak by tapping him or her on the shoulder and saying, "Are you okay? Can you talk? I can help you." A person who cannot breathe or speak needs immediate help.

2. If the person starts to cough, wait and see whether the coughing will dislodge the object. If the person's cough is weak and ineffective, or if the person is in obvious distress, continue with step 3.

3. Stay with the person and call for help. Have the person who is helping you activate the facility's emergency response system.

4. Stand behind the person with the obstructed airway and wrap your arms around her waist.

5. Make a fist with one hand and place the thumb of the fist against the person's abdomen, just above the navel and below the sternum (breastbone). Grasp your fist with the other hand.

6. Being careful not to put pressure on the person's ribs or sternum with your forearms, press your fist inward and pull upward, using quick thrusting motions, until the object is expelled, the person begins to cough forcefully, or the person loses consciousness. (In a child, less force is applied to the abdomen to avoid injuring the child's ribs, sternum (breastbone), and internal organs.)

   a. If the object is expelled, stay with the person, and follow the nurse's directions.

   b. If the person begins to cough, wait and see whether the coughing results in expulsion of the object. If it does not, continue giving abdominal thrusts.

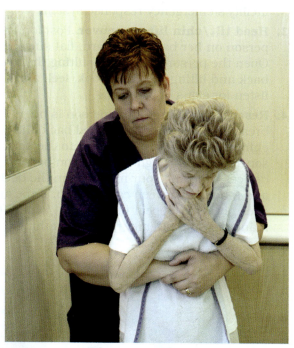

Step 5 Place your fist just above the person's navel and below the sternum.

   c. If the person loses consciousness, lower the person to the floor and begin Procedure 19-2, beginning with step 3.

7. The person should be evaluated by a doctor following the choking incident.

8. Record your observations and actions according to facility policy.

PROCEDURE 19-2

Relieving An Obstructed Airway in Unconscious Adults and Children Older Than 1 Year

WHY YOU DO IT   If the object is not removed from the airway, allowing air to get to the lungs, the person will die.

1. Check the person's state of consciousness by gently shaking or tapping her. An unresponsive person needs immediate help.

2. Stay with the person and call for help. Have the person who is helping you activate the facility's emergency response system.

3. **Head tilt/chin lift maneuver.** Position the person on her back on a hard, flat surface. Open the person's airway by tilting the head back and lifting the chin. Look, feel, and listen for signs of breathing.

4. **Rescue breathing.** If the person is not breathing, keep her head tilted back and the chin lifted. Blow two breaths into the person's mouth through a ventilation barrier device, removing your mouth from the device and inhaling between each breath. If the air does not go in, repeat the head tilt/chin lift maneuver and attempt rescue breathing once again.

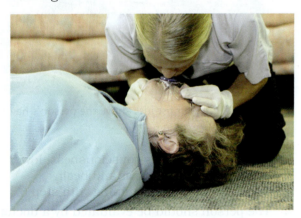

Step 4 Rescue breathing.

5. **Object check.** If no air enters the person's lungs after the second attempt, perform an object check. Kneel beside the person's head and open the airway using the head tilt/chin lift maneuver. Look for the object. If you see the object, remove it. If you cannot see the object, continue to step 6.

6. Repeat the head tilt/chin lift maneuver. Blow two slow breaths into the person's mouth through a ventilation barrier device, removing your mouth from the device and inhaling between each breath. If the air does not go in, repeat the head tilt/chin lift maneuver and attempt rescue breathing once again.

7. **Chest compressions.** If no air enters the person's lungs after the second attempt, begin chest compressions. To give chest compressions to an unconscious person:

   a. Kneel beside the person.

   b. Place the heel of your hand closest to the person's head on her sternum (breastbone) and place your other hand on top and interlock your fingers.

   c. Position your body forward so that your shoulders are over the center of the person's chest and your arms are straight. You will want to compress straight down and up. Do not rock back and forth.

   d. Compress the chest 1½ to 2 inches on an adult (1 to 1½ inches on a child) quickly at a rate of 100 compressions per minute for 30 compressions.

8. Perform an object check.

9. Repeat the head tilt/chin lift maneuver. Blow two breaths into the person's mouth through a ventilation barrier device, removing your mouth from the device and inhaling between each breath. If the air does not go in, repeat the head tilt/chin lift maneuver and attempt rescue breathing once again.

10. Repeat the chest compression–object check–rescue breathing sequence until the object is expelled, rescue breathing is successful, or other trained personnel arrive and take over.

11. The person should be evaluated by a doctor following the choking incident.

12. Record your observations and actions according to facility policy.

PROCEDURE 19-3

Performing Chest Thrusts on an Obese or Pregnant Person

WHY YOU DO IT   If the object is not removed from the airway, allowing air to get to the lungs, the person will die.

1. Stand behind the person and place your arms under the person's armpits and around her chest.

2. Make a fist with one hand and place the thumb of the fist against the center of the person's sternum. Be sure that your thumb is centered on the sternum, not on the lower tip of the sternum (the xiphoid process) and not on the ribs.

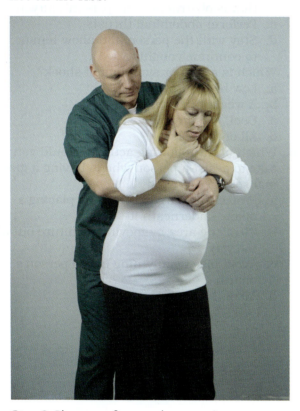

Step 2 Place your fist over the person's sternum.

3. Give up to five quick chest thrusts by grasping your fist with your other hand and pressing inward five times. Each thrust should compress the chest 1½ to 2 inches.

4. Continue to give chest thrusts until the object is expelled, the person begins to cough forcefully, or the person loses consciousness.

   a. If the object is expelled, stay with the person, and follow the nurse's directions.

   b. If the person begins to cough, wait and see whether the coughing results in expulsion of the object. If it does not, continue giving chest thrusts in groups of five.

   c. If the person loses consciousness, lower the person to the floor and follow the steps to Procedure 19-2.

5. The person should be evaluated by a doctor following the choking incident.

6. Record your observations and actions according to facility policy.

WHAT DID YOU LEARN?

Multiple Choice

Select the single best answer for each of the following questions.

1. A person with an airway obstruction will usually:
   a. Have a seizure
   b. Vomit
   c. Be able to speak and breathe normally
   d. Clutch at his or her throat

2. The first step in the chain of survival is:
   a. Rehabilitation
   b. Recognizing that an emergency exists and calling for help
   c. Giving first aid
   d. Initiating basic life support (BLS) measures

3. In the ABCs of emergency care, the "C" stands for:
   a. Cardiac
   b. Consciousness
   c. Circulation
   d. Check for bleeding

4. You are helping to prepare a holiday dinner at your mother's house, when suddenly your sister misses the vegetable she is trying to slice and cuts deeply into her finger instead. Blood is spurting from the cut, which indicates to you that your sister:
   a. Is hemorrhaging internally
   b. Has cut a vein
   c. Has cut an artery
   d. Requires the application of a tourniquet

5. Where do you place your fist while clearing an obstructed airway in a conscious adult?
   a. On the person's back
   b. Above the person's navel
   c. On the person's chest
   d. Below the person's navel

6. If a person is coughing but able to breathe, you should:
   a. Administer oxygen
   b. Use a finger sweep to remove the object that is obstructing the person's airway
   c. Perform abdominal thrusts
   d. Stay with the person and allow him or her to continue coughing

7. Which is a sign or symptom of shock?
   a. Low blood pressure
   b. A weak, rapid pulse
   c. Cool, clammy, pale skin
   d. All of the above

8. Which of the following actions should you take to assist a person who is having a grand mal seizure?
   a. Protect the person's head by placing a pillow underneath it
   b. Clear the area by moving furniture out of the way
   c. Avoid placing anything in the person's mouth
   d. All of the above

Matching

Match each numbered item with its appropriate lettered description.

_____ **1.** Emergency medical services (EMS) system

_____ **2.** First aid

_____ **3.** Basic life support (BLS)

_____ **4.** Clinical death

_____ **5.** Respiratory arrest

_____ **6.** Cardiac arrest

_____ **7.** Grand mal seizure

_____ **8.** Petit mal (absence) seizure

_____ **9.** Anaphylactic shock

_____**10.** Fainting (syncope)

a. Occurs when the blood supply to the brain suddenly decreases, resulting in a loss of consciousness

b. Occurs when a person has no pulse or is not breathing

c. Breathing has stopped

d. A potentially deadly allergic reaction (for example, to a bee sting or certain foods, such as nuts)

e. Heart has stopped

f. Care given to an injured person before more advanced medical assistance arrives

g. A network of resources, including people, equipment, and facilities, that is organized to respond to an emergency

h. The person stares off into space or stops speaking for a moment

i. Measures taken to prevent respiratory arrest, cardiac arrest, or both

j. Generalized and violent contraction and relaxation of the body's muscles

STOP and Think!

- As a nursing assistant, one of your responsibilities is to check on the residents while the nurses are attending the change-of-shift report. You enter Mrs. Oblonsky's room and find her on the floor. She has no roommate, so no one witnessed what happened. It does not appear that Mrs. Oblonsky fell out of bed. Her color is pale, and her lips are turning blue. What should you do first?

- One of your responsibilities is to oversee the residents of the long-term care facility where you work while they are in the recreation room. Today, the residents are gathered and getting ready for an activity. Everyone is busy talking, selecting teams, and generally having fun. Everyone, that is, except for Mr. Grant. Normally outgoing and friendly, today Mr. Grant is just sitting in his wheelchair, staring into space without moving. You speak to Mr. Grant and notice that he seems confused and is having difficulty forming his words. The left side of his mouth looks droopy and he is drooling a bit. These observations may be signs of what emergency situation? What should you do?

- One day, you go to the room of one of your residents, Mrs. Craven, to answer her call light. When you enter the room, Mrs. Craven cries out to you in a frightened voice, "Get them out of here! Get them out of here now!" You don't know what she is talking about—you don't see anybody or anything in the room. You ask Mrs. Craven to explain what she means, and she tells you that there are spiders crawling all over the walls. Normally, Mrs. Craven is alert and oriented, but today, she definitely seems "out of it." What do you think is wrong with Mrs. Craven? What should you do?

Nursing Assistants Make a Difference!

*"**I am the Director of Nursing** at Spanish Moss Manor, a long-term care facility in Mississippi. We are located right on the coast of the Gulf of Mexico, and last September, we found ourselves directly in the path of a hurricane. In preparation for the coming storm, we put our disaster preparedness plan into effect— all staff members were asked to report to work to assist with storing water and food and moving the residents to the center of the building. As the storm came closer, flooding was predicted for the lower-lying areas of our community, and we received word that our sister facility to the west had been ordered to evacuate all staff and residents to a safer facility on higher ground. We opened our doors and our arms to 50 additional residents that day, and I heard not one word of complaint from my staff. The storm hit hard in the middle of the night and we lost all power, except for the emergency generators. As the winds howled around us, some of the residents became frightened but were quickly reassured and comforted by the nursing assistants and other staff members. Some assistants could even be heard singing softly to the residents in the dark.*

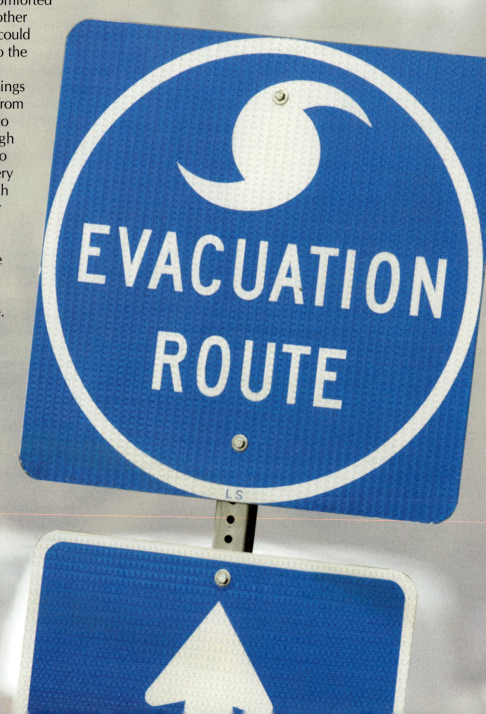

Forty-eight hours later, things settled down and the residents from our sister facility were able to return to their home. Although short on sleep and anxious to return to their own homes, every single staff member at Spanish Moss stayed to clean up after the storm and put the rooms back in order. Not one of my nursing assistants asked to leave until after the very last resident had been tucked into a freshly made bed and was comfortable. Those days during and after the storm showed me how truly dedicated our nursing assistants are to ensuring the welfare of those in their care. I couldn't be prouder of them!"

You can listen to more stories about how nursing assistants make a difference on the CD in the front of your book.

*Photo credit: Don Farrall
Photodisc Green/Getty Images*

5

BASIC RESIDENT CARE

Y ou may have chosen to pursue a career as a nursing assistant for many reasons, but chances are good that at least one of those reasons had to do with a desire to help and care for others. As a nursing assistant, you will have the chance to fulfill this desire many times over! In Unit 5, we will explore the skills and responsibilities that form the basis for the daily care you provide for your residents.

Photo: Taking blood pressures is a skill you will use every day.

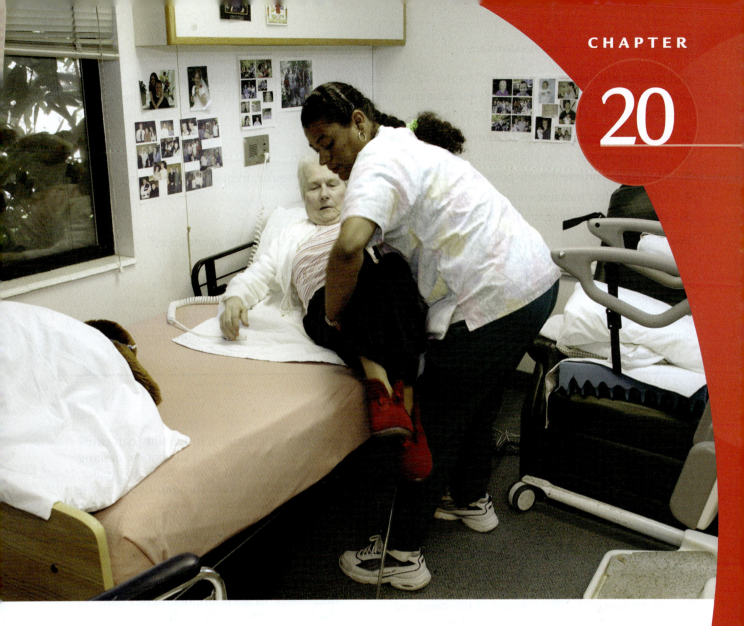

Positioning, Lifting, and Transferring Residents

WHAT WILL YOU LEARN?

Have you ever been awakened from sleep because the position you were in was uncomfortable? If so, you probably rolled over, found a more comfortable position, and went back to sleep. Can you imagine what it would be like to be unable to change position on your own? The ability to change position is important for our comfort, as well as for our physical health. In a nursing home setting, most of the residents will need help changing their position in bed or in a chair. Many will also need your help "transferring," or getting out of their bed or chair.

Repositioning, lifting, and transferring people is a major part of the nursing assistant's daily routine. You will do this many times a day. By following the guidelines for body mechanics

Photo: A nursing assistant helps a resident to transfer out of bed.

and back safety that you learned in Chapter 17, you can protect yourself from fatigue and injury. In this chapter, you will learn how to keep your residents safe while assisting them with movement. When you are finished with this chapter, you will be able to:

1. Explain the complications of immobility.
2. Describe proper body alignment, and explain why it is important.
3. Identify the different body positions and explain the purpose of regular, frequent repositioning.
4. Discuss safety measures related to lifting and transferring people.
5. Demonstrate techniques of safe lifting and transfer.

Vocabulary 🎧 Listen & Learn   Use the CD in the front of your book to hear these terms pronounced and defined:

Pressure ulcers	Fowler's position	Prone position	Transfer
Body alignment	Semi-Fowler's (low	Sims' position	Weight bearing
Supportive devices	Fowler's) position	Shearing	Transfer belt (gait belt)
Supine (dorsal	High Fowler's position	Friction	Ambulate
recumbent) position	Lateral position	Logrolling	

POSITIONING RESIDENTS

There are many reasons why a person may not be able to shift positions without help, such as painful or swollen limbs, paralysis, or weakness (as a result of age or illness). A person who is unconscious or in a coma will also need help with repositioning.

The inability to change positions regularly can lead to discomfort and, potentially, serious complications (Fig. 20-1). Some of the most serious complications affect the skin, bones, muscles, lungs, and heart:

- **Integumentary system (skin).** The most common complication of immobility is pressure ulcers. **Pressure ulcers,** also known as *decubitus ulcers* or *bed sores,* form when bony areas press against the mattress. The pressure slows down blood flow to the tissues that are pressed between the bone and the mattress. This results in a sore, which can be very difficult to heal and might even be fatal. Pressure ulcers are discussed in detail in Chapter 31.
- **Musculoskeletal system (bones and muscles).** Contractures, discussed in detail in Chapter 10, occur when a joint is held in the same position for too long a time. Contractures cause stiffness and shortening of the tendons, leading to loss of motion of the joint that may be permanent. Long-term immobility can also cause loss of muscle mass

and strength. Finally, immobility can cause the loss of calcium from the bones, making the bones brittle and more likely to break.
- **Respiratory system (lungs).** Lying in one position for a long period of time can prevent the lungs from completely filling with air when the person breathes. This causes the small air sacs in the lungs, called *alveoli,* to close. As a result, the person's ability to get oxygen into his or her bloodstream is decreased. In addition, decreased filling of the lungs with air allows fluids and mucus to collect in the lungs. This fluid and mucus creates an environment that is favorable for the types of bacteria that cause pneumonia.
- **Cardiovascular system (heart).** When we walk, the large muscles in our legs contract. Contraction of the leg muscles squeezes the veins, helping to move blood from the legs back up to the heart. People who must stay in bed are not using their leg muscles. Therefore, the blood flow from the legs back up to the heart becomes slow. This situation can lead to the formation of blood clots in the lower legs.

BASIC POSITIONS

Proper positioning is necessary for proper **body alignment.** A person in proper body alignment is positioned so that his spine is not twisted or crooked. To check for alignment, imagine a line that connects the person's nose, breastbone

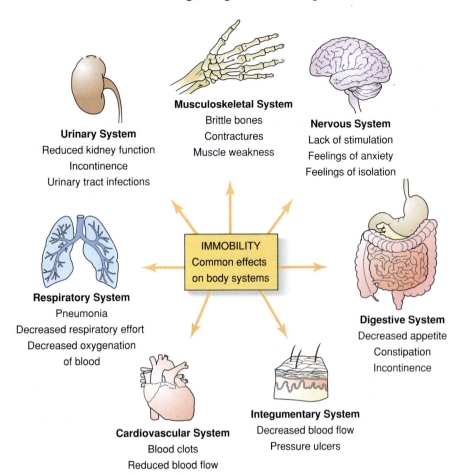

Figure 20-1

Immobility can cause complications in almost every body system.

(sternum), and pubic bone, and then continues between the person's knees and ankles. This imaginary line should be straight whether the person is lying on his back, side, or abdomen (Fig. 20-2). If the person's legs are spread apart, each leg should be the same distance from the imaginary line. When helping to position one of your residents, imagine yourself in that particular position and remember how your body is most comfortable.

Proper body alignment is most comfortable for the resident. It relieves strain on muscles and joints, promotes good heart and lung function, and helps prevent contractures and pressure ulcers. Sometimes **supportive devices,** such as pillows; rolled sheets, towels, or blankets; and devices designed specifically for the purpose of offering support (Fig. 20-3), are needed to keep the person in proper body alignment. Learning to position these supports correctly is essential. Proper use of supportive devices helps to keep your residents both safe and comfortable. The nurse or physical therapist can show you how to

properly place any supportive devices that are being used for your residents.

There are several basic positions that are used when a person must stay in bed or seated for long periods of time (Fig. 20-4). As you work as a nursing assistant, you may see variations or restrictions on these positions for reasons specific for your resident. Refer to the person's care plan or ask the nurse if there are any limitations or special positioning needs that the person may have.

Supine (Dorsal Recumbent) Position

When a person is in the **supine (dorsal recumbent) position,** she is lying on her back. The bed is flat and the person's head is supported by a pillow. Sometimes, pillows are placed to support the arms and hands as well. Some people may be more comfortable with a pillow under their knees and calves to take strain off the lower back. Others may ask for a small pillow under the lower back. In an older person, the supine position can lead to skin breakdown on the heels, which puts

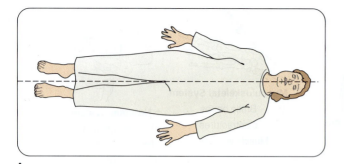

A

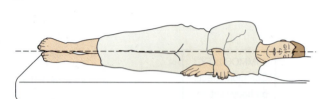

B

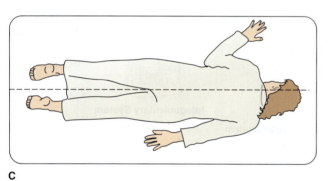

C

Figure 20-2

When a person is in proper body alignment, an imaginary straight line can be drawn connecting the person's nose, breastbone (sternum), and pubic bone. **(A)** Proper body alignment for a person who is lying on her back in bed (supine). **(B)** Proper body alignment for a person who is lying on her side in bed (lateral). **(C)** Proper body alignment for a person who is lying on her stomach in bed (prone).

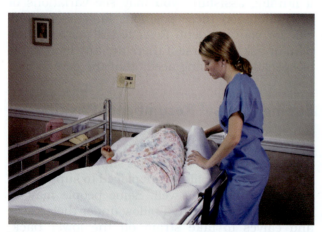

Figure 20-3

Some people require extra support to maintain proper body alignment. This support can be achieved by using pillows; a rolled-up towel, sheet, or blanket; or a supportive device made especially for this purpose.

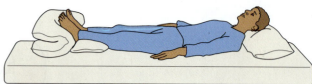

A Supine (dorsal recumbent) position

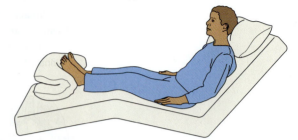

B Fowler's position

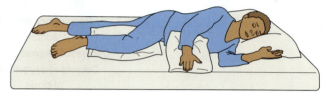

C Lateral position

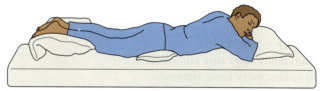

D Prone position

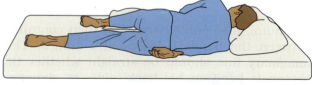

E Sims' position

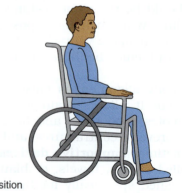

F Seated position

Figure 20-4

There are several basic positions that are used when a person must remain in bed or seated for a long period of time.

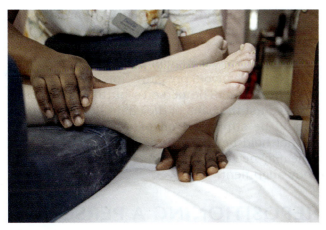

Figure 20-5
"Floating" the person's heels above the surface of the bed when the person is in the supine position helps to prevent skin breakdown on the heels.

the person at risk for developing pressure ulcers. To prevent this complication, "float" the person's heels above the surface of the bed by placing a pillow underneath the person's calves (from the knees to the ankle). You should be able to slide your hand in the space between the mattress and the person's heels (Fig. 20-5).

Fowler's Position

A variation of the supine position is **Fowler's position,** in which the head of the bed is elevated to between 45 and 60 degrees. In **semi-Fowler's (low Fowler's) position,** the head of the bed is elevated approximately 30 to 45 degrees. In **high Fowler's position,** the head of the bed is elevated approximately 60 to 90 degrees (Fig. 20-6). The knee-gatch area of the bed may be bent or a pillow may be placed under the person's knees and calves. Pillows may also support the arms and hands.

The semi-Fowler's position is comfortable for people who are resting in bed and want to read, watch television, or talk with visitors. It is also the most comfortable position for a person who has trouble breathing when lying flat. Some medical conditions, such as hiatal hernia with reflux, and some treatments, such as tube feedings, require the person to be positioned in the semi-Fowler's position. High Fowler's position is useful when a person is eating a meal in bed, and during grooming procedures.

Lateral Position

A person who is in the **lateral position** is lying on his side. When documenting the lateral position, the side of the person that is on the bed is used as the descriptor. For example, a person lying with his left side down on the mattress is in "left lateral position." The person's lower leg is straight and his upper leg is slightly bent at the knee, so that the knees are not pressed together. Pillows are placed under the person's head and neck, between the legs, and under the upper arm to keep the spine in alignment. A small pillow or rolled sheet may be placed close against the back to keep the person from rolling backward.

A variation of the lateral position may be used to keep pressure off the side of the hip. In the semi–side-lying position, pillows are placed either against the person's back and hip or along the front of her body. The pillows cause the person to lie either a little more forward or a little more toward the back. When the pillows are placed along the person's back and hip, she will lie a little more on her back, leaning toward the pillows. When the pillows are placed along the person's front, she will lie a little more on her abdomen.

The lateral position is part of the cycle of positions for people who are unable to reposition

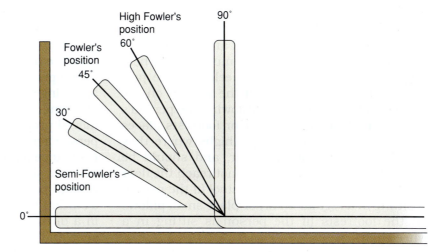

Figure 20-6
In Fowler's position, the head of the bed is elevated. Variations of Fowler's position include semi-Fowler's (low Fowler's) position and high Fowler's position.

themselves—the person is moved from the supine position to the lateral position, then back to the supine position, and then to the lateral position on the other side at least every 2 hours, routinely. The lateral position is also often used for people with back pain to relieve pressure on the spine.

Prone Position

A person who is in the **prone position** is lying on his abdomen with his head turned to one side. A small pillow is placed under the person's head. Another small pillow is placed under the lower abdomen and pelvis to allow room for the chest to expand when the person breathes. (Alternatively, a rolled towel can be placed under each of the person's shoulders to reduce pressure on the chest.) A pillow is also placed under the person's shins to keep the feet in proper position. The person's arms are bent at the elbows and his hands are placed on either side of the head, palms facing down. Many people, especially elderly people, are not comfortable in the prone position. Make sure you check with the nurse before placing a person in this position.

Sims' Position

Sims' position is an extreme side-lying position that is almost prone. The person's head is turned to one side and her knee on that side is bent sharply and supported by a pillow. The corresponding arm is bent at the elbow with the hand in front of the face, palm down, resting on a pillow. The lower leg is straight, the lower arm extends out from the side with the hand down near the hips, and the palm turned upward. Sims' position is used for people who are receiving enemas, and to relieve pressure on areas that may be prone to developing pressure ulcers, such as the coccyx (the "tailbone") and the greater trochanter of the femur (the "hip bone").

Seated Position

Positioning and body alignment are important for everyone, not just people who must stay in bed. When seated in a chair or wheelchair, the person's feet should rest flat on the floor or on the footrests of the wheelchair. Allowing the person's feet to dangle above the floor or footrests places pressure on the back of the thighs where they rest on the edge of the chair, and should be avoided. If the person's feet do not reach the floor or the footrests, provide a footstool (if the person is sitting in a regular chair) or place small pillows on the footrests (if the person is sitting in a wheelchair).

The person's knees are bent at approximately 90 degrees and the calves do not touch the chair. If the person is seated in a wheelchair, it may be necessary to place a small pillow behind the person's calves to avoid pressure from the leg rests of the wheelchair. The person's buttocks and back rest against the back of the chair. Paralyzed arms should be supported on pillows. A person who cannot hold her body upright for long periods of time may need postural supports to assist in good body alignment.

REPOSITIONING A PERSON

At minimum, a person should be repositioned every 2 hours. Some of your residents may require repositioning as frequently as every hour. Each time you reposition a person, you should be alert to signs and symptoms of complications related to immobility.

TELL THE NURSE

Possible signs and symptoms of complications related to immobility that should be reported to the nurse immediately include:

- Reddened skin, especially over bony areas, that does not return to its normal color after gentle massage of the surrounding tissue

- Pale, white, or shiny skin over a bony area

- Tears, scrapes, or skin that looks burned

- Hot, reddened, painful areas in the lower legs (do not rub these areas because doing this could dislodge a blood clot, which could then move to a vital organ such as the heart, lungs, or brain)

- New occurrence of urinary or bowel incontinence

- New complaints of pain on movement

To assist a person who is in bed into a new position, you will need to know how to lift and turn the person without causing injury to yourself or the person you are trying to move. People who are being moved in bed are particularly at risk for shearing and friction injuries if they are not moved properly. **Shearing** is caused by pulling a person across a sheet or other surface that offers resistance (for example, if you try to pull a person who has slid down in the bed or chair back into an upright position). When a person is pulled against a surface that offers resistance, the skin is dragged in a direction opposite that of the underlying tissues and muscles, injuring the blood vessels and connective tissue under the skin and starting the process of skin breakdown. **Friction** occurs when two surfaces, such as a sheet and the person's skin, rub against each other. The rubbing action can injure the skin and contribute to skin breakdown. The risk of shearing and friction can be minimized by rolling or lifting, instead of pulling or dragging, a person who needs to be moved. Guidelines for repositioning a person are given in Guidelines Box 20-1.

Moving a Person to the Side of the Bed

There are many reasons why you may need to reposition a person so that he is lying on one side of the bed or the other. For example, if you want to turn a person, you would first want to move the person to the side of the bed so that when the turn is completed, he is in the middle of the bed (not on one side). You might also need to move a person to the side of the bed before performing a personal care procedure, so that the person is closer to you during the procedure. Depending on the situation, you may be able to move the person to the side of the bed by yourself (Procedure 20-1), or you may need help (Procedure 20-2). Generally speaking, you should get help from a co-worker if the person is large, seriously ill or injured, or uncooperative.

Helping a Person to Move up in Bed

People who are sitting up in bed tend to slide down, toward the foot of the bed, over time (Fig. 20-7). This can lead to discomfort and an inability to breathe easily. To keep a person who is sitting in bed comfortable and in proper body alignment,

you must help him with moving up in the bed periodically. Some residents will be able to move themselves up in bed with the aid of a trapeze. Others will require your assistance (Procedures 20-3 and 20-4).

Raising a Person's Head and Shoulders

Often, you will need to lift a person's head and shoulders away from the bed. For example, you may need to do this to help a person with drinking or to rearrange the pillow. Procedure 20-5 explains how to lift a person's head and shoulders away from the bed safely.

Turning a Person Onto His or Her Side

Helping a person to roll over in bed helps to keep the person comfortable. It also helps to prevent many of the complications associated with remaining in a single position for a long period of time. The person may be turned away from you (Procedure 20-6) or toward you, depending on the situation. Make sure that the side rail on the opposite side of the bed is raised whenever you are turning a person away from you.

Logrolling a Person

Logrolling is performed whenever it is necessary to move a person who has had back surgery or an injury to the spine. In the long-term care facility, logrolling is most frequently used to reposition a person when there is a possibility that the person's spine has been injured (for example, as the result of a fall). In logrolling, the person is rolled in one fluid motion so that the head, torso, and legs move as one unit and the body (the "log") is kept in

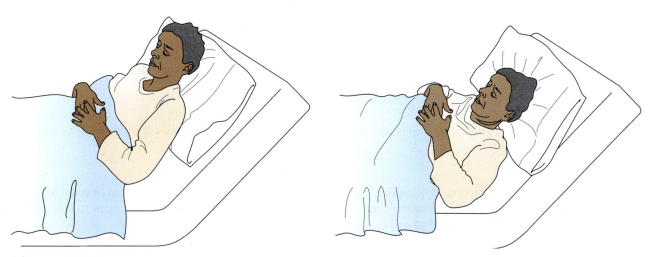

Figure 20-7

Gravity causes a person who is sitting in bed to slide down over time, leading to discomfort and interfering with the person's ability to breathe.

Guidelines Box 20-1 Guidelines for Repositioning a Person

WHAT YOU DO	WHY YOU DO IT
Plan how you will reposition the person and get help from others if necessary.	Depending on the person's medical condition or size, extra equipment or people may be necessary. Planning ahead helps to ensure that the procedure will be carried out efficiently, and with the most consideration for the person's safety and comfort.
Know the specific positioning guidelines for each person in your care. Refer to the person's care plan or ask the nurse as necessary.	Depending on the person's medical condition, some positions may be required and others may not be allowed. Failure to follow your resident's specific positioning guidelines can cause the person injury or discomfort.
Reposition the person at least every 2 hours, or according to the person's care plan.	Regular repositioning is necessary to prevent complications of immobility, such as pressure ulcers.
Explain the procedure to the person, even if he is unconscious.	Understanding how the procedure is done builds trust and helps the person feel like an active participant. Although an unconscious person will not be able to assist in the procedure, the person may still be aware that he is being moved. Telling the person what you are doing as you are doing it helps to reassure the person.
Make sure that you allow the person to assist in the repositioning to the full extent of her ability.	Being able to assist with one's own repositioning promotes feelings of independence and lessens the embarrassment some people may feel over having to rely on someone else for assistance.
Provide for the person's modesty by keeping his body covered.	Keeping the person's body covered preserves his dignity.
Take care to protect any tubes or drains from being pulled out while the person is being moved.	Dislodging tubes or drains is painful for the person. In addition, if tubes or drains become dislodged, it is necessary to reinsert them, which can cause additional discomfort.
Use good body mechanics when helping to reposition a person.	Using good body mechanics will protect you, as well as the resident, from injury.
Use a gentle touch to avoid injury to delicate skin and fragile bones. Use a lift sheet to reposition the person whenever possible. (A lift sheet, also called a draw sheet, is a small sheet that is placed over the bottom sheet so that it extends from the person's shoulders to below her buttocks. Lift sheets are discussed in detail in Chapter 21.)	A lift sheet allows you to lift the person (instead of dragging her across the sheets). This helps to prevent shearing and friction injuries.

WHAT YOU DO	WHY YOU DO IT
Avoid moving or lifting someone by holding onto his arm or leg.	The skin of an older person is very fragile. Holding onto an older person's arm or leg could cause the skin to tear. You could also pull the arm or leg out of its socket, or stretch the joint beyond its range of motion.
After repositioning a person, make sure that the bed linens are free of wrinkles, and that the person's clothing is not twisted or wrinkled up underneath the person.	Lying on wrinkled bed linens or clothing can lead to skin breakdown. Skin breakdown increases the person's risk of getting a pressure ulcer.
Gently move the person's clothing aside to check the person's skin, especially on the part of the body the person was just lying on.	Reddened or pale skin can be a sign that a pressure ulcer is starting.

alignment. Two or three assistants, plus a lift sheet, are usually necessary to logroll a person. Procedure 20-7 explains how to logroll a person safely.

TRANSFERRING RESIDENTS

To **transfer** means to move from one place to another. As a nursing assistant, you will help people with transfers many times each day. For example, residents transfer from the bed to a chair and back again, or from a wheelchair to a dining chair or commode and back again. Some residents are able to transfer from one place to another with little or no help, but many will require a lot of help. The assistance you offer will vary from just providing a steadying hand to totally lifting a person from one place to another.

A resident's ability to assist with her own transfers may be affected by the resident's ability to bear weight. **Weight bearing** refers to a person's ability to stand on one or both legs. A limited ability to bear weight could be caused by injury to the hip, leg, or foot; pain; weakness; or paralysis. Some people with paraplegia have learned to transfer themselves by using their arms to support the weight of their body as they move from one surface to another.

A **transfer belt** is a webbed or woven belt with a buckle that is used to assist a weak or unsteady person with standing, walking, or transferring. (When used to help a person walk, a transfer belt is called a **gait belt**.) The belt is approximately

1.5 to 2 inches wide, and it is 54 to 60 inches long. Many health care facilities require nursing assistants to use a transfer belt when helping people to stand, walk, or transfer. The transfer belt is applied around the person's waist (Procedure 20-8), giving the nursing assistant a place to grasp and support the person (other than by the person's arms or ribcage). When using a transfer belt, remember:

- Some residents may have medical conditions that make it dangerous to use a transfer belt on them. For example, a transfer belt should not be applied to a person who is recovering from abdominal surgery. Transfer belts are also not used with people with certain heart disorders. If you are in doubt about using a transfer belt on a resident, check the person's care plan or ask the nurse for specific directions.
- A transfer belt is only an assist device and should never be used to "lift" a person who is unable to bear weight. A person who is unable to bear weight should be moved with a mechanical lift device.

Before beginning a transfer, advance planning is always necessary. Ask the nurse or physical therapist about any specific limitations the resident has and what the recommended method of transfer is. Many care plans will also have this information. Gather any needed equipment (for example, a mechanical lift or wheelchair) and make sure the equipment is in good working condition. If necessary, move the furniture in the room to make space for a safe transfer. Finally, ask others for help as necessary.

It is important that you learn safe transfer techniques to protect yourself and your residents. Accidents are common during the act of transferring, for both the nursing assistant and the person being transferred. Regardless of the particular type of transfer, the safety measures summarized in Guidelines Box 20-2 should always be followed. Specific procedures for various types of transfers are described in the sections that follow.

Guidelines Box 20-2 Guidelines for Assisting a Person with Transferring	
WHAT YOU DO	**WHY YOU DO IT**
Plan how you will transfer the person and get help from others if necessary.	Depending on the person's medical condition or size, extra equipment or people may be necessary. Planning ahead helps to ensure that the procedure will be carried out efficiently, and with most consideration for the person's safety and comfort.
Explain the procedure to the person, even if he is unconscious.	Understanding how the procedure is done builds trust and helps the person feel like an active participant. Although an unconscious person will not be able to assist in the procedure, the person may still be aware that he is being moved. Telling the person what you are doing as you are doing it helps to reassure the person.
Use good body mechanics. Keep your body close to the person and bend at the knees. Use a transfer belt.	Using good body mechanics will protect you, as well as the resident, from injury.
Make sure that beds are lowered to their lowest position and wheels are locked on beds, stretchers, and wheelchairs.	Lowering the bed to the lowest position makes it easier and safer for the person to transfer, because the lowest position allows the person to put his feet on the floor. Locking the wheels on equipment prevents the equipment from moving out from under the person as he transfers.
Check the person's clothing and shoes. Clothing should fit. Shoes should provide good foot support and have non-skid soles.	Long or loose clothing and shoes that do not provide enough support or have slippery soles could lead to tripping.
Plan the transfer so that the person is leading with her strongest side, if possible.	Doing so allows the person to bear weight in the direction she is going.
Do not allow a person to hold onto you around your neck. Instead, have an unsteady person grasp the arm of the chair or your arm for support.	If the person stumbles or falls while grasping you around the neck, you could be injured.
Do not place your hands under a person's arms to help support him.	If the person stumbles or falls, he may be injured when you lift up as he is falling down.

TRANSFERRING A PERSON TO AND FROM A WHEELCHAIR OR CHAIR

Wheelchairs present some specific safety issues. Wheelchairs, like any other piece of equipment, need to be checked before use to ensure safety. Check to make sure that there are no broken or missing parts, that the wheels turn smoothly, that any safety straps are secure, and that the brakes hold well. Trying to transfer a person into or out of a wheelchair with unlocked or poorly locked wheels is a common cause of accidents. Procedure 20-9 describes how to transfer a person into a wheelchair or chair by yourself. Procedure 20-10 describes how to transfer a person into a wheelchair or chair with assistance. Procedure 20-11 explains how to transfer a person from a wheelchair or chair to a bed.

TRANSFERRING A PERSON TO AND FROM A STRETCHER

In the long-term care facility, stretchers are primarily used to transport residents to or from an ambulance. Procedure 20-12 describes how to transfer a person from a bed to a stretcher. Procedure 20-13 describes how to transfer a person from a stretcher to bed.

TRANSFERRING A PERSON USING A MECHANICAL LIFT

In the past, mechanical lifts were used primarily to move very heavy or completely dependent residents. However, because using a mechanical lift is safer for both the resident and the staff, many facilities encourage the use of these devices for all transfers (Fig. 20-8). Before using a mechanical lift, always make sure the person you need to transfer weighs less than the weight limit specified on the lift. Some facilities require two staff members to operate the mechanical lift. Make sure you know your facility's policy. Procedure 20-14 describes one method of transferring a person using a mechanical lift. Because lifts from different manufacturers may vary greatly in their procedures for use, do not use a mechanical lift until you have been taught specifically how to use that lift.

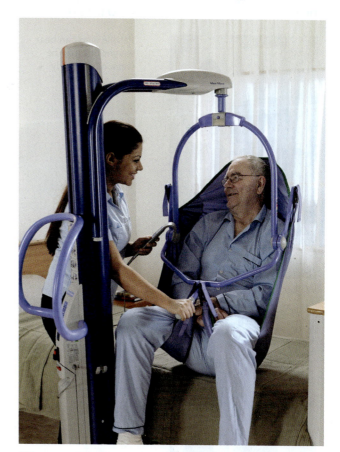

Figure 20-8

A mechanical lift helps to make transfers safer for both the resident and the nursing assistant. There are many different types of mechanical lifts in use. You should be trained to operate the lift at the facility where you work before using it. (*Photo courtesy of ARJO.*)

ASSISTING A PERSON WITH WALKING (AMBULATING)

Some residents may be able to transfer without using a wheelchair or stretcher, if they are offered assistance with ambulating. To **ambulate** means to walk. It is important to encourage people who are able to walk (either with or without assistance) to do it on a regular basis. Walking helps to preserve mobility, improves heart and lung function, and promotes digestion. In addition, walking helps the person to remain as independent as possible for as long as possible. A person who feels weak or unsteady benefits, both physically and emotionally, from being encouraged to walk with assistance.

Sitting on the edge of the bed, also called "dangling," is the first step for someone who is going to get out of bed and walk. Procedure 20-15 explains how to help a person to sit on the edge of the bed. When a person has been resting in bed, especially for a long time, sitting up and then standing causes blood to flow to the legs and away from the head. This can lead to dizziness and fainting. Dangling allows time for the heart and blood vessels to make up for the change in position. This reduces the person's risk of falling due to dizziness or loss of consciousness.

There are many different devices people use to help them walk (Table 20-1). These devices are specially fitted to the individual and, therefore, should not be shared.

Table 20-1   Assistive Devices for Walking (Ambulating)

DEVICE	WHO USES IT	HOW IT IS USED
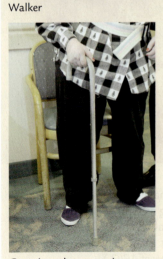 Walker	People who can bear weight but may be weak or unsteady	**Proper fit:** Handgrips level with the person's hips **Proper technique:** • *For rolling walker (pictured).* The person grasps the top of the frame. The person propels the walker forward as he or she walks. The walker is not lifted from the floor. Placing plastic tips or tennis balls over the back legs of the walker helps the walker to glide across the floor more easily. • *For standard walker.* The person grasps the top of the frame, lifts the walker up, and places it squarely on the ground 10 to 18 inches in front of his or her body. The tips of the walker are placed flat on the floor. Using the top of the frame for support, the person moves one leg forward and then the other, stepping into the frame of the walker. The process is then repeated. The person can use the top of the frame for support between steps if necessary.
Cane (may have one tip, three tips, or four tips)	People who can bear weight but are weak on one side	**Proper fit:** Handle level with the person's hip **Proper technique:** The person holds the cane on his or her strong side, placing it in front of the body and using it to support his or her weight while moving. The tip of the cane is placed flat on the floor. If the person is using a three- or four-tipped cane, all of the tips are placed flat on the floor at the same time. The weaker leg is moved forward first, followed by the stronger leg. The nursing assistant stands slightly behind and to the side of the person, on the person's weak side.

Guidelines Box	20-3	Guidelines for Assisting a Person With Walking (Ambulating)

WHAT YOU DO	WHY YOU DO IT
Use good body mechanics.	Using good body mechanics will protect you, as well as the resident, from injury.
Use a transfer belt on the person according to your facility policy and the person's care plan.	The transfer belt gives you a safe place to grasp and support the person.
Watch the person for fatigue or discomfort.	A person who is tired or uncomfortable is at greater risk for tripping or fainting.
Check the person's clothing and shoes. Clothing should fit. Shoes should provide good foot support and have non-skid soles.	Long or loose clothing and shoes that do not provide enough support or have slippery soles could lead to tripping.
Check ambulation devices to ensure that they are in good condition. Robber tips on canes and standard walkers should not be cracked, worn, or missing. Rolling walkers should have plastic tips or other modifications (such as tennis ball covers) on the back legs.	The rubber tips on canes and standard walkers provide traction. If they are cracked or worn, they can slip, causing the person to fall. The plastic tips or other modifications on the back legs of a rolling walker help the walker to glide across the floor easily.
Request help from a co-worker as necessary when you must assist a weak, unsteady, or uncooperative person with walking.	A person who is weak, unsteady, or uncooperative is likely to fall, injuring both of you. Having help from a co-worker makes a fall less likely.
Allow the person to "dangle" for the specified amount of time before assisting the person to stand up.	Allowing a person time to "dangle" before getting out of bed reduces the person's risk of falling due to dizziness or loss of consciousness.
Ensure that the person is using ambulation devices correctly.	Using an ambulation device correctly reduces the person's risk of slipping and falling.

Procedure 20-16 describes how to assist a person with walking. Be alert to potential problems and be sure to report these to the nurse. Safety guidelines for assisting a person with walking are summarized in Guidelines Box 20-3.

TELL THE NURSE

Each time you assist a person with a transfer, tell the nurse immediately if:

- The person complains of dizziness, shortness of breath, chest pain, a rapid heartbeat (palpitations), or sudden head pain

- The person complains of pain when he tries to bear weight, and this is new

- You observe any changes in the person's usual grip, strength, or ability

- A usually cooperative person refuses to participate ("I just don't feel like it today")

- The equipment is not working properly or is broken

SUMMARY

- For many different reasons, residents in a long-term care facility may be unable to reposition themselves without assistance.
  - The resulting immobility can cause serious complications, including pressure ulcers, contractures, pneumonia, and the formation of blood clots in the legs.
  - Preventing the complications of immobility, through frequent repositioning and transferring, is a major responsibility of the nursing assistant.
    - Some people will have conditions that require frequent, regular repositioning, as often as every hour, but at least every 2 hours.
    - There are several basic positions that are used when a person must remain in bed for extended periods of time: the supine (dorsal recumbent), Fowler's, lateral, prone, and Sims' positions. Proper positioning helps to ensure proper body alignment, which relieves strain on the muscles and joints, promotes good heart and lung function, and helps to prevent contractures and pressure ulcers. It is essential for comfort.
    - When repositioning a person, it is important to take care to prevent shearing and friction injuries to the skin.
- Nursing assistants also help people to transfer from one place to another many times throughout the day.
  - Advance planning and proper technique help to ensure a safe transfer.
  - Some patients and residents may be able to walk on their own, with help. Encouraging and assisting patients and residents to walk enhances their quality of life by providing both physical and emotional benefits.

Moving a Person to the Side of the Bed (One Assistant)

WHY YOU DO IT   Moving a person to the side of the bed is a necessary first step in many procedures, such as the procedures for turning a person onto his or her side, assisting a person to sit on the edge of the bed, or assisting a person to get out of bed.

Getting Ready   WORKIEPS

1. Complete the "Getting Ready" steps.

Procedure

2. Make sure that the bed is positioned at a comfortable working height (to promote good body mechanics) and that the wheels are locked.

3. Place the pillow at the head of the bed, on its edge against the headboard. This gets the pillow out of the way.

4. If the side rails are in use, lower the side rail on the working side of the bed. The side rail on the opposite side of the bed should remain up. Lower the head of the bed so that the bed is flat (as tolerated). Fanfold the top linens to the foot of the bed.

5. Stand at the side of the bed with your feet spread about 12 inches apart and with your knees slightly bent to protect your back.

6. Gently slide your hands under the person's head and shoulders and move the person's upper body toward you.

7. Gently slide your hands under the person's torso and move the person's torso toward you.

8. Gently slide your hands under the person's hips and legs and move the person's lower body toward you.

9. Now, position the person as planned (for example in the prone or lateral position).

10. Reposition the pillow under the person's head and straighten the bottom linens. Draw the top linens over the person. Raise the head of the bed as the person requests.

11. Make sure that the bed is lowered to its lowest position and that the wheels are locked. If the side rails are in use, return them to the raised position.

Finishing Up   CLSOWR
12. Complete the "Finishing Up" steps.

PROCEDURE 20-2

Moving a Person to the Side of the Bed (Two Assistants)

WHY YOU DO IT This method of moving a person to the side of the bed is safer for both you and the person if the person is large, very ill or injured, or uncooperative. Using a lift sheet also helps to prevent shearing and friction injuries.

Getting Ready WORKIEPS

1. Complete the "Getting Ready" steps.

Supplies

- lift sheet (if one is not already on the bed)

Procedure

2. Make sure that the bed is positioned at a comfortable working height (to promote good body mechanics) and that the wheels are locked.

3. Place the pillow at the head of the bed, on its edge against the headboard. This gets the pillow out of the way.

4. If the side rails are in use, lower the side rails. Lower the head of the bed so that the bed is flat (as tolerated). Fanfold the top linens to the foot of the bed.

5. If the lift sheet is already on the bed, make sure that it is positioned so that it is under the person's shoulders and hips. (If a lift sheet is not already on the bed, position one under the person's shoulders and hips.)

6. Stand at the side of the bed, opposite your co-worker, with your feet spread about 12 inches apart and with your knees slightly bent to protect your back.

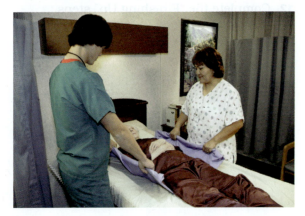

Step 6 Stand opposite your co-worker.

7. Grasp the edge of the lift sheet and roll it over as close to the person's body as possible. This will provide for a better grip. (Your co-worker does the same.)

8. Grasp the rolled edge of the lift sheet with both hands, palms and fingers facing down. One hand should be level with the person's shoulders and the other should be level with his or her hips.

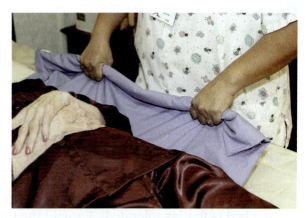

Step 8 Grasp the rolled lift sheet with both hands, palms and fingers facing down.

9. On the count of "three," slowly and carefully lift up on the lift sheet in unison and move the person to the side of the bed.

10. Now, position the person as planned (for example, in the prone or lateral position).

11. Reposition the pillow under the person's head and straighten the bottom linens. Draw the top linens over the person.

12. Make sure that the bed is lowered to its lowest position and that the wheels are locked. If the side rails are in use, return them to the raised position.

Finishing Up CLSOWR

13. Complete the "Finishing Up" steps.

PROCEDURE 20-3

Moving a Person up in Bed (One Assistant)

WHY YOU DO IT   Gravity causes a person who is sitting in bed to slide down over time, leading to discomfort and interfering with the person's ability to breathe. Helping the person to move up in bed promotes comfort and makes it easier for the person to breathe.

Getting Ready WGKIEpS

1. Complete the "Getting Ready" steps.

Procedure

2. Make sure that the bed is positioned at a comfortable working height (to promote good body mechanics) and that the wheels are locked.

3. If the side rails are in use, lower the side rail on the working side of the bed. The side rail on the opposite side of the bed should remain up. Fanfold the top linens to the foot of the bed.

4. Place the pillow at the head of the bed, on its edge against the headboard. This gets the pillow out of the way. It also pads the headboard in case you move the person up a little too much or too fast!

5. **Method "A":**

   a. Face the head of the bed. Position your outside foot (that is, the foot that is farthest away from the edge of the bed) 12 inches in front of the other foot and bend your knees slightly to protect your back.

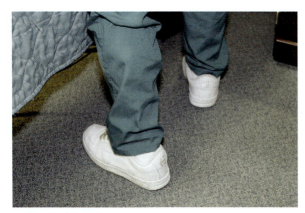

Step 5 Position your outside foot 12 inches in front of your inside foot.

   b. Place your arm that is nearest the head of the bed under the person's head and shoulders. Lock your other arm with the person's arm that is closest to you.

   c. Have the person bend her knees.

   d. Tell the person that on the count of "three," she is to lift her buttocks and press her heels into the mattress as you lift her shoulders. On the count of "three," help the person to move smoothly toward the head of the bed.

6. **Method "B":**

   a. Have the person grasp the head of the bed or a trapeze, if there is one.

   b. Face the head of the bed. Position your outside foot (that is, the foot that is farthest away from the edge of the bed) 12 inches in front of the other foot and bend your knees slightly to protect your back.

   c. Place your hands under the person's back and buttocks.

   d. Have the person bend his knees.

   e. Tell the person that on the count of "three," he is to lift his buttocks and press his heels into the mattress. On the count of "three," help the person to move smoothly toward the head of the bed.

7. Reposition the pillow under the person's head and straighten the bottom linens. Draw the top linens over the person. Raise the head of the bed as the person requests.

8. Make sure that the bed is lowered to its lowest position and that the wheels are locked. If the side rails are in use, return them to the raised position.

Finishing Up CLSOWR

9. Complete the "Finishing Up" steps.

PROCEDURE 20-4

Moving a Person up in Bed (Two Assistants)

WHY YOU DO IT   This method of moving a person up in bed is safer for both you and the person if the person is large, very ill or injured, or uncooperative. Using a lift sheet also helps to prevent shearing and friction injuries.

Getting Ready WORKIEDS

1. Complete the "Getting Ready" steps.

Supplies

- lift sheet (if one is not already on the bed)

Procedure

2. Make sure that the bed is positioned at a comfortable working height (to promote good body mechanics) and that the wheels are locked.

3. Place the pillow at the head of the bed, on its edge against the headboard. This gets the pillow out of the way. It also pads the headboard in case you move the person up a little too much or too fast!

4. If the side rails are in use, lower the side rails. Lower the head of the bed so that the bed is flat (as tolerated). Fanfold the top linens to the foot of the bed.

5. If the lift sheet is already on the bed, make sure that it is positioned so that it is under the person's shoulders and hips. (If a lift sheet is not already on the bed, position one under the person's shoulders and hips).

6. Stand at the side of the bed, opposite your co-worker, with your feet spread about 12 inches apart and with your knees slightly bent to protect your back.

7. Grasp the edge of the lift sheet and roll it over as close to the person's body as possible. This will provide for a better grip. (Your co-worker does the same.)

8. Grasp the rolled edge of the lift sheet with both hands, palms and fingers facing down. One hand should be level with the person's shoulders and the other should be level with his or her hips.

9. On the count of "three," slowly and carefully lift up on the lift sheet in unison and move the person toward the head of the bed. Avoid dragging the person across the bottom linens.

10. Reposition the pillow under the person's head and straighten the bottom linens. Draw the top linens over the person. Raise the head of the bed as the person requests.

11. Make sure that the bed is lowered to its lowest position and that the wheels are locked. If the side rails are in use, return them to the raised position.

Finishing Up CLOSWR

12. Complete the "Finishing Up" steps.

PROCEDURE 20-5

Raising a Person's Head and Shoulders

WHY YOU DO IT Raising the person's head and shoulders away from the bed is necessary when you need to adjust the pillow and during some care procedures, such as dressing. Knowing how to perform this procedure safely prevents injury to you and your resident.

Getting Ready WGKIEPS
1. Complete the "Getting Ready" steps.

Procedure
2. Make sure that the bed is positioned at a comfortable working height (to promote good body mechanics) and that the wheels are locked.
3. Place the pillow at the head of the bed, on its edge against the headboard. This gets the pillow out of the way.
4. If the side rails are in use, lower the side rail on the working side of the bed. The side rail on the opposite side of the bed should remain up. Fanfold the top linens to the foot of the bed.
5. Face the head of the bed. Position your outside foot (that is, the foot that is farthest away from the edge of the bed) 12 inches in front of the other foot, and bend your knees slightly to protect your back.
6. Slide one hand under the person's shoulder that is nearest to you.
7. Slide the other hand under the person's upper back.
8. On the count of "three," slowly and carefully lift the person's head and shoulders.
9. Reposition the pillow under the person's head and straighten the bottom linens. Draw the top linens over the person. Raise the head of the bed as the person requests.
10. Make sure that the bed is lowered to its lowest position and that the wheels are locked. If the side rails are in use, return them to the raised position.

Finishing Up CLSOWR
11. Complete the "Finishing Up" steps.

PROCEDURE 20-6

Turning a Person Onto His or Her Side

WHY YOU DO IT The lateral position is part of the cycle of positions for people who are unable to reposition themselves. The person is moved from the supine position to the lateral position, then back to the supine position, and then to the lateral position on the other side.

Getting Ready WGKIEPS
1. Complete the "Getting Ready" steps.

Supplies
- additional pillows (if not already in the room)

Procedure
2. Make sure that the bed is positioned at a comfortable working height (to promote good body mechanics) and that the wheels are locked.
3. Place the pillow at the head of the bed, on its edge against the headboard. This gets the pillow out of the way.
4. If the side rails are in use, lower the side rail on the working side of the bed. The side rail on the opposite side of the bed should remain up. Lower the head of the bed so that

(continued)

the bed is flat (as tolerated). Fanfold the top linens to the foot of the bed.

5. Stand at the side of the bed with your feet spread about 12 inches apart and with your knees slightly bent to protect your back.

6. Move the person to the side of the bed nearest you.

7. Cross the person's arm that is nearest to you over the person's chest.

8. Bend the person's leg that is nearest to you, placing the foot on the bed. (Or, cross the person's leg that is nearest to you over her other leg.)

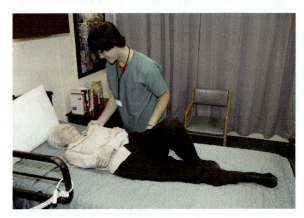

Step 8 Bend the person's leg that is nearest to you, placing the foot on the bed.

9. Roll the person onto her side. If the person is able to assist, guide the person's hand that is nearest to you to the side rail so that the person can help to pull herself over as you roll the person's hips.

   a. **To roll the person away from you:** Place one of your hands on the person's shoulder that is nearest to you, and place your other hand on the person's hip that is nearest to you. Gently roll the person away from you, toward the opposite side of the bed.

   b. **To roll the person toward you:** Raise the side rail and move to the other side of the bed. Lower that side rail. Place one hand on the person's shoulder that is farthest away from you, and place your other hand on the person's hip that is farthest away from you. Gently roll the person toward you.

10. Reposition the pillow under the person's head and straighten the bottom linens. Support the person by placing a pillow lengthwise between the person's legs. The person's lower leg should be straight, and the upper leg should be slightly bent at the knee. Place additional pillows under the person's upper arm, and behind her back. Draw the top linens over the person.

11. Make sure that the bed is lowered to its lowest position and that the wheels are locked. If the side rails are in use, return them to the raised position.

Finishing Up CLOSWR

12. Complete the "Finishing Up" steps.

PROCEDURE 20-7

Logrolling a Person (Two Assistants)

WHY YOU DO IT Logrolling is done when it is necessary to move someone while keeping the spine in alignment. The person is rolled in one fluid motion so that the head, torso, and legs move as one unit and the body is kept in alignment.

Getting Ready WCKIEpS

1. Complete the "Getting Ready" steps.

Supplies

- lift sheet (if one is not already on the bed)

Procedure

2. Make sure that the bed is positioned at a comfortable working height (to promote good body mechanics) and that the wheels are locked.

3. Place the pillow at the head of the bed, on its edge against the headboard. This gets the pillow out of the way.

4. If the side rails are in use, lower the side rail on the working side of the bed. The side rail on the opposite side of the bed should remain up. Lower the head of the bed so that

the bed is flat (as tolerated). Fanfold the top linens to the foot of the bed.

5. Stand with the other assistant on the side of the bed with the lowered side rail. Stand facing the bed with your feet spread about 12 inches apart and with your knees slightly bent to protect your back. One assistant is aligned with the person's head and shoulders; the other is aligned with the person's hips.

6. Place your hands under the person's head and shoulders while your co-worker places his or her hands under the person's hips and legs (or vice versa). Lifting in unison, gently move the person toward the side of the bed closest to you.

7. Place a pillow lengthwise between the person's legs and fold the person's arm so that it will be on top of his chest when he is turned.

8. Raise the side rail and make sure that it is secure.

9. Go to the opposite side of the bed and lower the side rail.

10. Working with the other assistant, turn the person onto his side.

   a. If a lift sheet is being used, turn the person by reaching over him and grasping the lift sheet. One assistant should place one hand on the lift sheet at the level of the person's shoulder and the other hand at the level of the person's hip; the other assistant should place one hand on the liftsheet at the level of the person's hip and the other at the level of the person's calves.

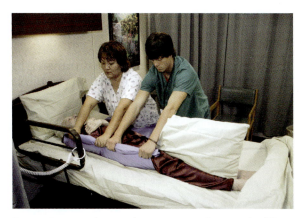

Step 10a Reach over the person and grasp the lift sheet.

   b. If a lift sheet is not being used, one assistant should position his or her hands on the person's shoulders and hips and the other assistant should place his or her hands on the person's thigh and calves.

11. On the count of "three," roll the person toward the side on which you are standing in a single movement, being sure to keep the person's head, spine, and legs aligned.

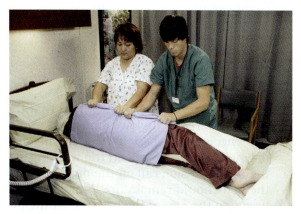

Step 11 On the count of "three," roll the person in one fluid movement.

12. Reposition the pillow under the person's head and straighten the bottom linens. Support the person by bolstering his back with pillows. The pillow between the person's legs should remain in place, and additional pillows or folded towels should be used to support the person's arms. Draw the top linens over the person.

13. Make sure that the bed is lowered to its lowest position and that the wheels are locked. If the side rails are in use, return them to the raised position.

Finishing Up CLOSWR

14. Complete the "Finishing Up" steps.

PROCEDURE 20-8

Applying a Transfer (Gait) Belt

WHY YOU DO IT   The transfer belt gives you a safe place to grasp and support the person when assisting the person with standing, transferring, or walking.

Getting Ready WORKIEPS

1. Complete the "Getting Ready" steps.

Supplies

- transfer belt

Procedure

2. If the person is in bed, make sure that the bed is lowered to its lowest position and that the wheels are locked. If the side rails are in use, lower the side rail on the working side of the bed. The side rail on the opposite side of the bed should remain up. Fanfold the top linens to the foot of the bed. Assist the person to sit on the edge of the bed.

3. Apply the belt around the person's waist, over his or her clothing. Buckle the belt in the front by threading the tongue of the belt through the side of the buckle that has "teeth" first, and then placing the tongue of the belt through the other side of the buckle.

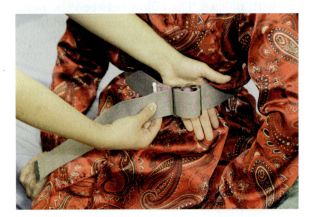

Step 3 Thread the tongue of the belt through the side of the buckle that has "teeth" first.

4. Before tightening the belt, turn it so that the buckle is off-center in the front or to the side.

5. Tighten the belt and check for fit. The belt should be snug, but you should be able to slip your fingers between the belt and the person's waist. When applying a transfer belt to a woman, make sure that her breasts are not trapped underneath the belt.

6. Use an underhand grasp when holding the belt to provide greater safety.

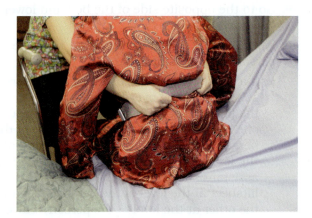

Step 6 Use an underhand grasp to hold the belt.

Finishing Up CLSOWR

7. When the person has finished transferring and is ready to return to bed, reverse the procedure.
8. Complete the "Finishing Up" steps.

PROCEDURE 20-9

Transferring a Person From a Bed to a Wheelchair (One Assistant)

WHY YOU DO IT Wheelchairs are used to transport people who have trouble walking. Using proper technique helps to keep both you and the person safe during the transfer from bed to wheelchair.

Getting Ready WORKIEDS

1. Complete the "Getting Ready" steps.

Supplies

- wheelchair
- lap blanket (optional)
- person's robe
- person's slippers or shoes
- transfer belt

Procedure

2. Determine the person's strongest side, and then place the wheelchair alongside the bed. Position the wheelchair so that the person will move toward the chair "strong side first." Whenever possible, position the wheelchair so that it is against a wall or a solid piece of furniture so that it will not slide backward during the transfer.

3. Lock the wheelchair wheels, and either remove the footrests or swing them to the side.

4. Fanfold the top linens to the foot of the bed.

5. Make sure that the bed is lowered to its lowest position and that the wheels are locked. Raise the head of the bed as tolerated.

6. Help the person to move toward the side of the bed where the wheelchair is located.

7. Assist the person to dangle.

8. Allow the person to rest on the edge of the bed. The person should be sitting squarely on both buttocks, with her knees apart and both feet flat on the floor (to offer a broad base of support). The person's arms should rest alongside her thighs. Watch for signs of dizziness or fainting. Position yourself in front of the person so that you can offer assistance in case she loses balance.

9. Help the person to put her shoes or slippers on. If the person is in nightwear or a hospital gown, help her to put on a robe. Apply a transfer belt.

10. Help the person to stand.
    a. Stand facing the person.

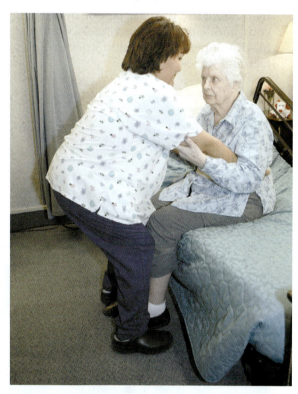

Step 10 Help the person to stand. Brace the person's knees with your knees, and the person's feet with your feet.

    b. Have the person put her hands on the edge of the bed, alongside each thigh.
    c. Make sure the person's feet are flat on the floor.
    d. Have the person lean forward.
    e. Grasp the transfer belt at each side, using an underhand grasp. (If you are not using a transfer belt, pass your arms under the person's arms and rest your hands on her upper back.)
    f. Position your feet alongside the person's feet, flexing your knees. Place your shins

(continued)

against the person's shins to block the person's feet and keep her knees from buckling as she stands up.

g. Have the person push down on the bed with her hands and stand on the count of "three." Assist the person into a standing position by pulling on the transfer belt as you straighten your knees. (If you are not using a transfer belt, assist the person into a standing position by gently pulling her up and forward as you straighten your knees.) Remember to keep your back straight.

11. Support the person in the standing position by holding the transfer belt or by keeping your hands on her upper back. Continue to block the person's feet and knees with your feet and knees.

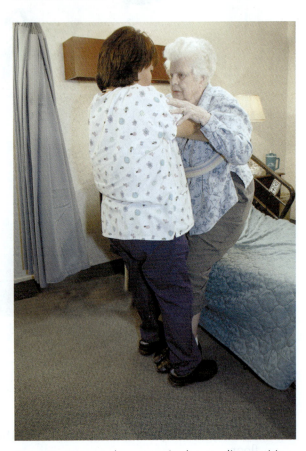

Step 11 Support the person in the standing position.

12. Help the person to turn by pivoting on the stronger leg toward the chair. This will allow the person to grasp the far arm of the wheelchair.

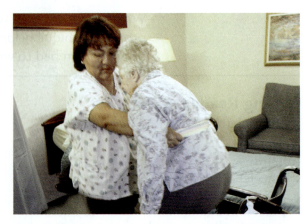

Step 12 Help the person to turn so that she can grasp the arms of the wheelchair and sit down.

13. Continue to assist the person with turning until she is able to grasp the other armrest. The backs of the person's legs should touch the edge of the chair.

14. Lower the person into the wheelchair by bending your hips and knees.

15. Make sure the person's buttocks are at the back of the chair. Make sure the person is comfortable and in good body alignment.

16. Remove the transfer belt.

17. Position the person's feet on the footrests of the wheelchair. Buckle the wheelchair safety belt (if ordered) and cover the person's lap and legs with a lap blanket, if desired. Make sure that the lap blanket does not drag on the floor.

Finishing Up CLSOWR

18. Position the wheelchair according to the person's preference.

19. Complete the "Finishing Up" steps.

PROCEDURE 20-10

Transferring a Person From a Bed to a Wheelchair (Two Assistants)

WHY YOU DO IT   Wheelchairs are used to transport people who have trouble walking. Using proper technique helps to keep both you and the person safe during the transfer from bed to wheelchair.

Getting Ready WGKIEpS

1. Complete the "Getting Ready" steps.

Supplies
- wheelchair
- lap blanket (optional)
- person's robe
- person's slippers or shoes

Procedure

2. Place the wheelchair alongside the bed, facing the foot of the bed.

3. Lock the wheelchair wheels and either remove the footrests or swing them to the side.

4. Fanfold the top linens to the foot of the bed.

5. Make sure that the bed is positioned at a comfortable working height (to promote good body mechanics) and that the wheels are locked. Raise the head of the bed as tolerated.

6. Help the person to move toward the side of the bed where the wheelchair is located.

7. Help the person to put his shoes or slippers on, and help him get into a robe.

8. Stand by the side of the bed, behind the wheelchair. Standing behind the person, pass your arms under the person's arms and grasp his forearms. The other assistant grasps the person's thighs and calves.

9. Working in unison with the other assistant, lift the person from the bed and bring him toward the wheelchair on the count of "three." Lower the person into the wheelchair.

10. Make sure the person's buttocks are at the back of the chair. Make sure the person is comfortable and in good body alignment.

11. Position the person's feet on the footrests of the wheelchair. Buckle the wheelchair safety belt (if ordered) and cover the person's lap and legs with a lap blanket, if desired. Make sure that the lap blanket does not drag on the floor.

Finishing Up CLSOWR

12. Position the wheelchair according to the person's preference.

13. Complete the "Finishing Up" steps.

PROCEDURE 20-11

Transferring a Person From a Wheelchair to a Bed

WHY YOU DO IT   Wheelchairs are used to transport people who have trouble walking. Using proper technique helps to keep both you and the person safe during the transfer from wheelchair to bed.

Getting Ready WGKIEpS

1. Complete the "Getting Ready" steps.

Supplies
- transfer belt

Procedure

2. Make sure that the bed is lowered to its lowest position and that the wheels are locked. Raise the head of the bed, fanfold the top linens to the foot of the bed, and raise the opposite side rail.

(continued)

3. Position the wheelchair close to the side of the bed so that the person's strong side is next to the bed. Lock the wheelchair wheels and either remove the footrests or swing them to the side.

4. Remove the person's lap blanket (if one was used) and release the wheelchair safety belt, if in use. Apply a transfer belt.

5. Stand facing the person with your feet spread about 12 inches apart and with your knees slightly bent to protect your back. With your back straight, slide the person to the front of the wheelchair seat.

6. Grasp the transfer belt (or pass your arms under the person's arms, placing your hands on her upper back). Position your feet alongside the person's feet, flexing your knees. Place your shins against the person's shins to block the person's feet and keep her knees from buckling as she stands up.

7. Have the person rest her hands on your arms and assist her to stand by pulling on the transfer belt as you straighten your knees. (If you are not using a transfer belt, assist the person into a standing position by gently pulling her up and forward as you straighten your knees.) Remember to keep your back straight. Alternatively, a person who requires less assistance can place her hands on the wheelchair arms for support and "push off" while you offer support.

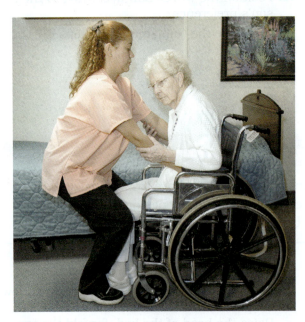

Step 7 Help the person to stand.

8. Slowly help the person to turn toward the bed by pivoting on her strong leg. Help the person to sit on the edge of the bed.

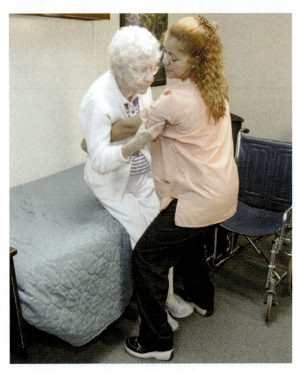

Step 8 Help the person to sit on the edge of the bed.

9. Remove the person's robe and slippers, if appropriate.

10. Move the wheelchair out of the way.

11. Place one of your arms around the person's shoulders and one arm under her legs. Swing the person's legs onto the bed.

12. Help the person to move to the center of the bed and position her comfortably.

13. Straighten the bottom linens and make sure the person is comfortable and in good body alignment. Draw the top linens over the person.

14. If the side rails are in use, return them to the raised position.

Finishing Up CLOSWR

15. Complete the "Finishing Up" steps.

PROCEDURE 20-12

Transferring a Person From a Bed to a Stretcher (Four Assistants)

WHY YOU DO IT   Using proper technique helps to keep both you and the person safe during the transfer from bed to stretcher.

Getting Ready ᴡ₵ᴋᴵᴇᴅˢ

1. Complete the "Getting Ready" steps.

Supplies

- stretcher
- lift sheet (if one is not already on the bed)
- blanket

Procedure

2. Raise the bed to its highest level. (The stretcher should be slightly lower than the bed.) Lower the head of the bed so that the bed is flat. Make sure that the bed wheels are locked. Lower the side rails. Fanfold the top linens to the side of the bed opposite the stretcher.

3. If the lift sheet is already on the bed, make sure that it is positioned so that it is under the person's shoulders and hips. (If a lift sheet is not already on the bed, position one under the person's shoulders and hips.)

4. Position the stretcher alongside the bed. Lock the stretcher wheels and move the stretcher safety belts out of the way.

5. Two assistants stand at the side of the bed facing their co-workers, who are positioned along the outside edge of the stretcher.

6. Grasp the edge of the lift sheet and roll it over as close to the person's body as possible. This will provide for a better grip. (Your co-workers do the same.)

7. On the count of "three," all four assistants slowly and carefully lift up on the lift sheet in unison and move the person to the side of the bed.

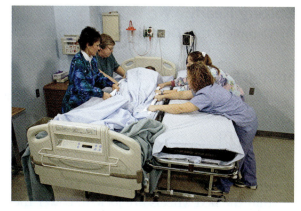

Step 5 Stand at the side of the bed facing your co-worker, who is positioned along the outside edge of the stretcher. Another pair of assistants does the same.

8. On the count of "three," all four assistants slowly and carefully lift up on the transfer sheet in unison and move the person to the side of the stretcher.

9. Position the person on the stretcher and make sure he or she is in good body alignment. Reposition the pillow under the person's head and cover the person with a blanket for modesty and warmth. Buckle the stretcher safety belts across the person and raise the side rails on the stretcher. Raise the head of the stretcher as the person requests.

Finishing Up ₵ᴸˢᴼᵂᴿ

10. Transport the person to the appropriate site. A person on a stretcher should always be transported "feet first." Remain with the person; never leave someone alone on a stretcher.

11. Complete the "Finishing Up" steps.

PROCEDURE 20-13

Transferring a Person From a Stretcher to a Bed (Four Assistants)

WHY YOU DO IT   Using proper technique helps to keep both you and the person safe during the transfer from stretcher to bed.

Getting Ready WORK STEPS

1. Complete the "Getting Ready" steps.

Supplies

- lift sheet (if one is not already on the stretcher)

Procedure

2. Raise or lower the bed so that it is slightly lower than the stretcher. Lower the head of the bed so that the bed is flat. Make sure that the bed wheels are locked. Lower the side rails. Fanfold the top linens to the side of the bed opposite the stretcher.

3. If the lift sheet is already on the stretcher, make sure that it is positioned so that it is under the person's shoulders and hips. (If a lift sheet is not already on the stretcher, position one under the person's shoulders and hips.)

4. Unbuckle the stretcher safety belts and lower the side rails on the stretcher.

5. Position the stretcher against the bed and lock the stretcher wheels.

6. Two assistants stand at the far side of the bed facing their co-workers, who are positioned along the outside edge of the stretcher. (Some facilities allow the assistants on the far side of the bed to kneel on the bed to complete the transfer; follow your facility's policy.)

7. Grasp the edge of the lift sheet and roll it over as close to the person's body as possible. This will provide for a better grip. (Your co-workers do the same.)

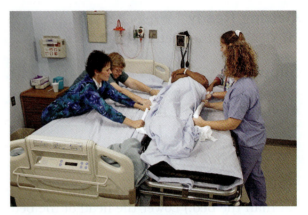

Step 6 Stand at the side of the bed facing your co-worker, who is positioned along the outside edge of the stretcher. Another pair of assistants does the same.

8. On the count of "three," all four assistants slowly and carefully lift up on the lift sheet in unison and move the person to the bed. Move the stretcher away from the bed.

9. Help the person to move to the center of the bed and, if desired, remove the lift sheet by turning the person first to one side, then the other. Position the person comfortably.

10. Straighten the bottom linens and make sure the person is comfortable and in good body alignment. Draw the top linens over the person.

11. Make sure the bed is lowered to its lowest position and that the wheels are locked. If the side rails are in use, return them to the raised position.

Finishing Up CLOSURE

12. Complete the "Finishing Up" steps.

PROCEDURE 20-14

Transferring a Person Using a Mechanical Lift (Two Assistants)

WHY YOU DO IT   Using a mechanical lift to transfer a person is safer for both you and the person, especially if the person is helpless or very heavy.

Getting Ready WGK Steps

1. Complete the "Getting Ready" steps.

Supplies

- wheelchair
- mechanical lift
- sling in proper size
- lap blanket (optional)
- lap restraint (if ordered)

Procedure

2. Make sure that the bed is positioned at a comfortable working height (to promote good body mechanics) and that the wheels are locked.

3. If the side rails are in use, lower the side rails.

4. Fanfold the top linens to the foot of the bed.

5. Center the sling under the person. (To get the sling under the person, move the person as if you were making an occupied bed.) The lower edge of the sling should be positioned underneath the person's knees.

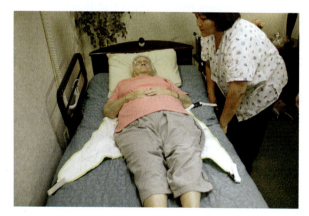

Step 5 Center the sling under the person.

6. Raise the head of the bed as tolerated.

7. Move the release valve on the lift to the closed position.

8. Raise the lift so that it can be positioned over the person.

9. Spread the legs of the lift to provide a solid base of support. The legs must be locked in this position, or the lift could tip over, injuring you, the person you are trying to transfer, or both.

10. Move the lift into position over the person.

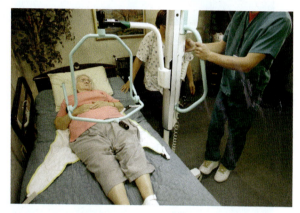

Step 10 Move the lift into position over the person.

11. Fasten the sling to the straps or chains of the lift. Make sure the hooks face away from the person.

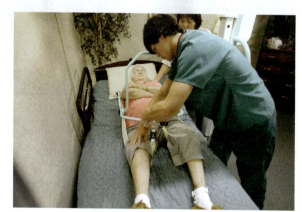

Step 11 Fasten the sling to the lift according to the manufacturer's instructions.

12. Attach the sling to the swivel bar with the short side attached to the top of the sling and the long side attached to the bottom of the sling.

13. Cross the person's arms across her chest. The person may hold onto the straps, but do not let her hold onto the swivel bar.

(continued)

14. Raise the lift until the person and the sling are clear of the bed.

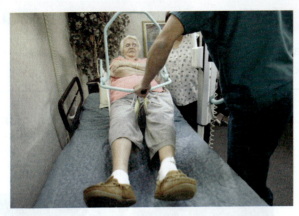

Step 14 Raise the lift until the person and the sling are clear of the bed.

15. Place the wheelchair alongside the bed, facing the foot of the bed. Lock the wheelchair wheels.

16. Have your co-worker support the person's legs as you move the lift into position over the wheelchair.

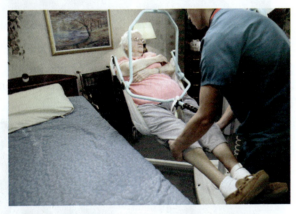

Step 16 A co-worker supports the person's legs as you move her into position over the wheelchair.

17. Turn the person so that she is facing the mast of the lift and is centered over the base. (The person's back should be facing the wheelchair.)

18. Move the lift so that the person is over the seat of the wheelchair.

19. Slowly open the release valve on the lift. Gently lower the person into the wheelchair. Make sure the person's buttocks are at the back of the chair.

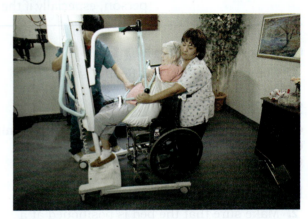

Step 19 Gently lower the person into the wheelchair.

20. Lower the swivel bar so that you can unhook the sling. Leave the sling under the person.

21. Make sure the person's buttocks are at the back of the chair. Make sure the person is comfortable and in good body alignment.

22. Position the person's feet on the footrests of the wheelchair. Buckle the wheelchair safety belt (or place a lap restraint, if ordered). Cover the person's lap and legs with a lap blanket, if desired. Make sure that the lap blanket does not drag on the floor.

Finishing Up CLSOWR

23. Position the wheelchair according to the person's preference.

24. Follow the "Finishing Up" steps.

25. When the person is ready to return to bed, reverse the procedure.

PROCEDURE 20-15

Assisting a Person With Sitting on the Edge of the Bed ("Dangling")

WHY YOU DO IT   Allowing a person time to "dangle" before getting out of bed reduces the person's risk of falling due to dizziness or loss of consciousness.

Getting Ready WORKSTEPS

1. Complete the "Getting Ready" steps.

Procedure

2. Make sure that the bed is lowered to its lowest position and that the wheels are locked.

3. If the side rails are in use, lower the side rail on the working side of the bed. The side rail on the opposite side of the bed should remain up. Raise the head of the bed as tolerated. Fanfold the top linens to the foot of the bed.

4. **Method "A":**

   a. Stand at the side of the bed with your feet spread about 12 inches apart and with your knees slightly bent to protect your back.

   b. Have the person bend her knees and plant her feet on the bed.

   c. Gently slide one arm behind the person's upper back. Slide the other arm under her knees and rest your hand on the side of her thigh.

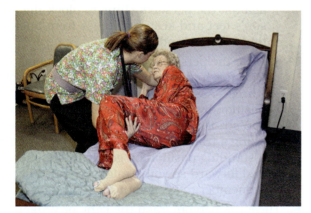

Step 4c Slide one arm behind the person's upper back. Slide the other arm under her knees.

   d. With a single smooth movement, slide the person's legs over the side of the bed while moving her head and shoulders upward so that she is sitting on the edge of the bed.

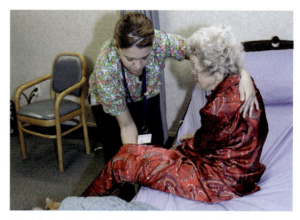

Step 4d Help the person to sit on the edge of the bed.

5. **Method "B":**

   a. Help the person to move toward the side of the bed.

   b. Have the person roll over onto her side, facing the side of the bed. Have the person flex her knees and bend the arm she is lying on in preparation for using it to prop her upper body up. Have the person bend her top arm so that her hand is in a position that will enable her to push off the bed.

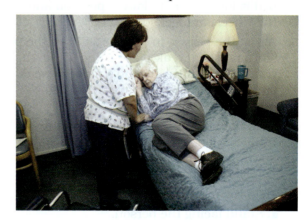

Step 5b Have the person roll onto her side, facing the side of the bed.

   c. Instruct the person to rise to a sitting position by using the elbow of her bottom arm to raise her upper body while pushing against the mattress with her other hand.

(continued)

Advise the person to allow her legs to swing over the edge of the bed while you help to guide her into an upright position.

6. Have the person put her hands on the edge of the bed, alongside each thigh, for support. Watch for signs of dizziness or fainting. If the person feels faint, help her to lie down and call for the nurse.

7. Allow the person to "dangle" her legs over the side of the bed for the specified period of time, and then either take her vital signs (if indicated), help her to lie back down, or assist her to a standing position. Stay with her during the entire time.

Finishing Up CLSOWR

8. Complete the "Finishing Up" steps.

PROCEDURE 20-16

Assisting a Person With Walking (Ambulating)

WHY YOU DO IT Assisting a person to ambulate regularly helps to meet the person's need for exercise and helps prevent complications of immobility. It also helps to keep a person as independent as possible for as long as possible.

Getting Ready WCKIEpS

1. Complete the "Getting Ready" steps.

Supplies

- transfer belt
- cane or walker (if indicated)
- person's robe
- person's slippers or shoes (non-skid soles)

Procedure

2. If the person is in bed, make sure that the bed is lowered to its lowest position and that the wheels are locked.

3. Assist the person to "dangle." Check the person's pulse; a weak pulse could lead to light-headedness. If the person's pulse is weak, stay with her and alert the nurse before attempting ambulation.

4. Help the person put her shoes or slippers on. If the person is in nightwear or a hospital gown, help her to put on a robe. Apply a transfer belt.

5. Help the person to stand.

   a. Stand facing the person.

   b. Have the person put her hands on the edge of the bed, alongside each thigh.

   c. Make sure the person's feet are flat on the floor.

   d. Have the person lean forward.

   e. Grasp the transfer belt at each side, using an underhand grasp. (If you are not using a transfer belt, pass your arms under the person's arms and rest your hands on her upper back.)

   f. Position your feet alongside the person's feet, flexing your knees. Place your shins against the person's shins to block the person's feet and keep her knees from buckling as she stands up.

   g. Have the person push down on the bed with her hands and stand on the count of "three." Assist the person into a standing position by pulling on the transfer belt as you straighten your knees. (If you are not using a transfer belt, assist the person into a standing position by gently pulling her up and forward as you straighten your knees.) Remember to keep your back straight.

6. Have the person grasp the cane or walker, if she is using one, in order to maintain balance. The person should hold the cane on her strong side.

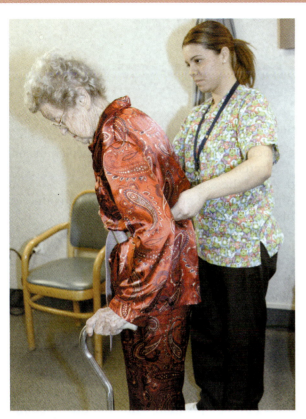

Step 7 Grasp the transfer belt with an underhand grip from the back.

7. Help the person to walk. Stand slightly behind the person on her weaker side. Grasp the transfer belt with an underhand grip from the back. If the person is using an ambulation device, make sure she is using it correctly.

8. After returning to the person's room, help her back into bed or a chair.

Finishing Up CLOSUR

9. Complete the "Finishing Up" steps.

WHAT DID YOU LEARN?

Multiple Choice

Select the single best answer for each of the following questions.

1. Which of the following describes good standing posture when helping to reposition or transfer a person?
   a. Feet 12 inches apart
   b. Abdominal muscles relaxed
   c. Arms out straight
   d. Feet close together

2. When assisting a person to move to the head of the bed, you should:
   a. Face the head of the bed
   b. Unlock the bed wheels
   c. Place a pillow under the person's head
   d. Place the foot that is farthest away from the bed edge behind the other foot

3. Which person is likely to need help moving and turning in bed?
   a. A person who is ambulatory
   b. A confused person
   c. A sleeping person
   d. A person paralyzed on the right side from a stroke

4. To transfer a person correctly from a bed to a stretcher, you must:
   a. Use a mechanical lift
   b. Get help from at least five co-workers
   c. Use good body mechanics
   d. Raise the far side rail of the stretcher first

5. When moving and positioning people, you should:
   a. Avoid friction and shearing
   b. Use good body mechanics
   c. Use pillows and rolled towels to maintain the position
   d. All of the above

6. Sitting a person on the side of the bed is called:
   a. Semi-sitting
   b. Proning
   c. Supining
   d. Dangling

7. When transferring a person from one place to another, you should:
   a. Use a transfer belt (unless the person has a condition that prevents the use of a transfer belt)
   b. Adjust the bed to the lowest possible height

   c. Lock the brakes of the bed, wheelchair, or stretcher
   d. All of the above

8. A person in the prone position is lying on his:
   a. Right side
   b. Left side
   c. Abdomen
   d. Back

9. When moving a person by yourself and the person is wearing a transfer belt:
   a. Lift from the side
   b. Use an underhand grasp
   c. Use an overhand grasp
   d. Stand behind the person

10. A nurse asks you to place a resident in the semi-Fowler's position while his tube feeding is running. You know the head of the bed should be elevated:
    a. 90 degrees
    b. 60 degrees
    c. 30 degrees
    d. 15 degrees

11. A mechanical lift can be used to:
    a. Move a resident who is very heavy
    b. Move a resident who is very weak
    c. Help a nursing assistant carry out her duties without injuring herself
    d. All of the above

12. When transferring a person from a bed to a stretcher, you should position the bed:
    a. At its lowest level
    b. At its highest level
    c. In the high Fowler's position
    d. In the supine position

13. A person who cannot reposition himself independently is at risk for developing:
    a. Pressure ulcers
    b. Blood clots
    c. Pneumonia
    d. All of the above

14. What is it called when a joint is held in one position for too long, and the tendons shorten?
    a. A pressure ulcer
    b. A bed sore
    c. A contracture
    d. A shearing injury

15. Why is it important to ensure that your residents are in good body alignment every time you reposition them?
   a. Good body alignment is most comfortable for the resident
   b. Good body alignment helps prevent complications, such as pressure ulcers and contractures
   c. Good body alignment helps the person to breathe easier and improves blood flow to tissues
   d. All of the above

16. Mrs. Rosen has fallen and the nurse suspects an injury to her spine. What technique would be used to move Mrs. Rosen for transport to the hospital?
   a. Logrolling
   b. A mechanical lift
   c. Dangling
   d. Turning

STOP and Think!

- Cynthia, a new nursing assistant, has been assigned to take care of Mrs. Adkins. Mrs. Adkins weighs more than 250 pounds and has had a stroke, so she is paralyzed completely on her left side. Cynthia has to transfer Mrs. Adkins from her bed to a wheelchair so she can go to the shower room. What steps should Cynthia take to help ensure a safe transfer for Mrs. Adams?

- You have been assigned to the north hall and have five residents you must assist to the dining room for breakfast. Mr. Clark is recovering nicely from a fractured hip and is eager to walk to the dining room with the aid of his new walker. What words of advice can you give Mr. Clark to help him use his walker more efficiently?

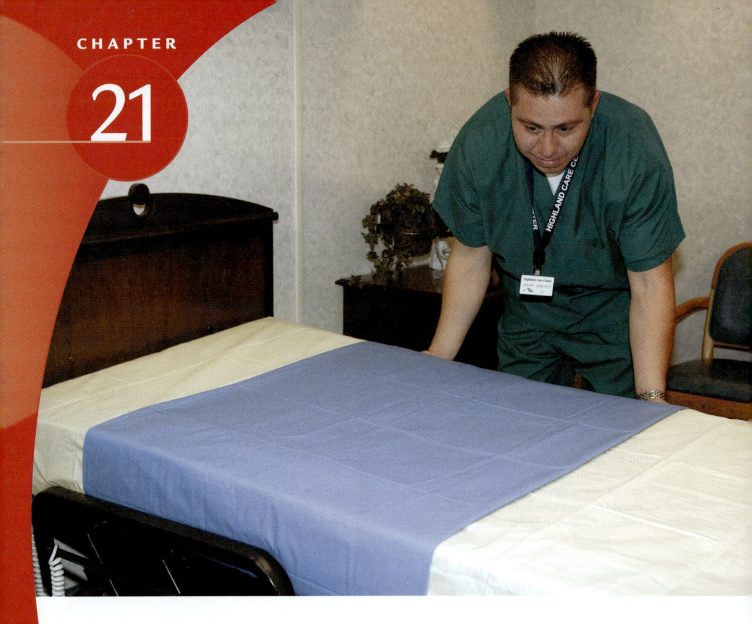

Bedmaking

WHAT WILL YOU LEARN?

For someone who is tired or ill, nothing is quite as comforting as clean, crisp linens on the bed. Clean linens are essential not only for your resident's comfort, but also for infection control and the prevention of skin breakdown and pressure ulcers. A neat, well-made bed is a sign that the facility provides capable, competent care to its residents. When you are finished with this chapter, you will be able to:

1. Describe ways that a properly made bed can increase a person's comfort and well-being.
2. List the different types of linens and their uses.
3. Demonstrate the proper way to handle and care for linens.
4. Explain the infection control measures that are used during bedmaking.

Photo: A well-made bed is essential to a person's mental and physical well-being. Here, a nursing assistant tucks in a draw sheet.

5. Demonstrate techniques of proper bedmaking, including making a closed bed, opening a bed, preparing a surgical bed, and making an occupied bed.

Vocabulary Use the CD in the front of your book to hear these terms pronounced and defined:

Draw sheet	Pressure-relieving	Mitered corner	Surgical bed
Lift sheet	mattress	Closed bed	Occupied bed
Bed protector	Bed cradle	Fanfolded	Toe pleat
Bath blanket	Footboard	Open bed	

LINENS AND OTHER SUPPLIES FOR BEDMAKING

LINENS

Many types of linens are used to make a bed. On your bed at home, you probably have a mattress pad, a bottom (or fitted) sheet, a top (or flat) sheet, a pillow covered in a pillowcase, and a bedspread or comforter. If you live in a cold climate, you may add a blanket to your bed during the winter months to provide extra warmth. In a long-term care facility, all of these basic linens are used, and some special ones may be added, depending on the needs of the resident. Linens that you may see in use in a long-term care facility include the following.

Mattress Pads

A mattress pad is a thick layer of padding that is placed on the mattress to help make the bed more comfortable for the resident, and to protect the mattress from moisture and soiling. The mattress pad may be "fitted." In this case, it will have elasticized sides that wrap around and underneath the mattress, holding the pad securely to the mattress. Or, the mattress pad may be "flat" (non-fitted).

Often, in health care facilities, the mattress has a rubber coating that helps to keep the mattress dry. When no mattress pad is used, and a bottom sheet is placed directly on the rubberized mattress, the person may become very warm and start to sweat because the rubber retains the person's body heat. The bottom sheet becomes damp and stays damp, because the rubberized mattress does not absorb the extra moisture. Lying on a damp sheet is uncomfortable for the resident. In addition, lying on a damp sheet can cause the skin to become reddened and irritated, which can lead to skin breakdown and pressure ulcers. Therefore, when a rubberized mattress is in use, a mattress pad may be used to help pull moisture away from the person's skin.

Bottom and Top Sheets

The sheets used to make a bed may be white or colored, plain or print. Regardless of their other characteristics, however, sheets need to be clean and wrinkle-free. A bed is made with two sheets, a bottom sheet and a top sheet. Some facilities use flat, or non-fitted, sheets as bottom sheets, or the bottom sheet may be fitted. When you are using a flat sheet as the bottom sheet, it is important to tuck the sheet tightly so that movement does not cause the sheet to loosen and wrinkle underneath the person. Wrinkled sheets are uncomfortable and can create areas of pressure on a person's skin, which can lead to skin breakdown.

The top sheet is a flat sheet.

Draw Sheets

A **draw sheet** is a small, flat sheet that is placed over the middle of the bottom sheet, covering the area of the bed from above the person's shoulders to below the buttocks (Fig. 21-1). When a rubberized mattress is in use, a draw sheet may be used instead of a mattress pad to form a protective, moisture-absorbing barrier between the person's body and the rubberized mattress. Some facilities use rubberized or plastic draw sheets to protect the mattress from soiling. If a rubberized draw sheet is used, it is always covered with a cotton draw sheet to protect the person's skin from contact with the rubber. The sides of the draw sheet are tucked tightly under the mattress to prevent wrinkling.

A **lift sheet** is simply a draw sheet that is used to help lift or reposition a person who needs assistance with moving in bed (see Chapter 20). A

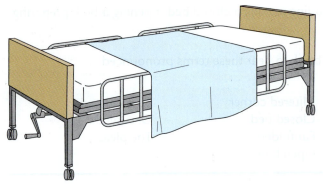

Figure 21-1
A draw sheet is a small sheet that is placed over the middle of the bottom sheet to absorb extra moisture when a mattress pad is not used. Sometimes, draw sheets are used to assist with turning or lifting a person. When a draw sheet is used for this purpose, it is called a "lift sheet."

draw sheet or a lift sheet can be made easily by folding a flat sheet in half. Make sure that the seams are folded toward the inside so that they do not rub against the person's skin. If a folded flat sheet is being used as a lift sheet, the folded edge of the sheet is positioned above the person's shoulders and the loose ends are positioned below the buttocks. When a draw sheet is to be used as a lift sheet, the sides are usually allowed to hang free, although some facilities may require you to tuck the sides of the lift sheet under the mattress after lifting or repositioning the person, to reduce wrinkling.

Bed Protectors

A **bed protector** is a square of quilted absorbent fabric backed with waterproof material. The bed protector measures approximately 3 feet by 3 feet. Bed protectors may be disposable, or they may be laundered and reused.

Some facilities may call bed protectors "incontinence pads," "soaker pads," or "chux." In addition to being used for people who are incontinent, bed protectors are often used for people with draining wounds. The urine, feces, or wound drainage is pulled away from the person's body by the absorbent layers of the bed protector, and the waterproof layer keeps the liquid from soiling the rest of the linens on the bed. Sometimes, only the bed protector needs to be changed, resulting in more efficient and economical care.

Blankets

Blankets are used to provide warmth and should be available as requested by a person for his or her comfort. Residents of long-term care facilities

sometimes bring favorite blankets from home. Blankets and other types of bedding brought from home must be checked to make sure that the articles are flame-retardant (treated with chemicals that make it harder for the fabric to catch fire and burn) before the resident can be allowed to use them.

Blankets provided by a facility are usually woven cotton, but blankets may also be made of wool or synthetic fibers. Because wool blankets can create static and sparks, they should be used with caution if the resident is receiving supplemental oxygen. Electric blankets should be checked for faulty wiring or plugs and may not be safe to use if the person is incontinent or unable to adjust the controls independently. Electric blankets should only be used according to facility policy.

Bedspreads

A bedspread adds the finishing touch to a well-made bed and can add a decorative touch to a person's room. Many residents of long-term care facilities bring a favorite bed covering along with them when they move to the facility. Allowing a person to use her bedspread from home is one way to foster a sense of independence and individuality among residents.

Pillows and Pillowcases

Pillows are used for comfort and to aid in positioning. They may be available in many sizes and are made from a variety of materials. Some pillows are covered with waterproof material or treated with a waterproofing substance to protect them from moisture and to aid with cleaning. Pillows are always covered with clean pillowcases. Care for pillows that become wet or soiled will vary according to facility.

Bath Blankets

A **bath blanket** is a lightweight cotton blanket or flannel sheet that is used to provide modesty and warmth during a bed bath or a linen change. A flat sheet may also be used for this purpose if the facility does not provide a special bath blanket. The bath blanket is not made into the bed, but because it is used during bed baths and linen changes, it is gathered along with the other linens.

OTHER BEDMAKING SUPPLIES

Occasionally, other equipment or supplies are used on a person's bed, depending on the specific needs of the resident. Some of the items used include the following.

- A **pressure-relieving mattress** (or "overlay") may be placed on top of the regular mattress to help prevent skin breakdown in residents who must stay in bed for long periods of time. Thin foam pads that resemble the inside of an egg carton, called "egg crate mattresses," were used in the past to help relieve pressure, but now they are used only for comfort. Use of foam pads is decreasing because the foam is difficult to keep clean and dry, especially if the person is incontinent. Newer versions of pressure-relieving mattresses may be filled with air, water, or gel and are made out of a material that is easily cleaned. Special beds used to prevent skin breakdown are described in Chapter 31.
- A **bed cradle** is a metal frame that is placed between the bottom and top sheets to keep the top sheet, the blanket, and the bedspread away from the person's feet (Fig. 21-2). Bed cradles are used for people who are at risk for developing pressure ulcers on their feet. Lifting the weight of bedding materials from the feet relieves pressure from the feet, thus protecting the skin.
- A **footboard** is a padded board that is placed upright at the foot of the bed (Fig. 21-3). The person's feet rest flat against the footboard, helping to keep the feet in proper alignment. A footboard is used to prevent foot drop, a condition that can affect people who must stay in bed for prolonged periods of time. In foot drop, the toes point downward as if the foot has "dropped." If

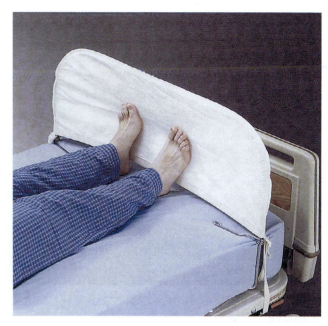

Figure 21-3
A footboard is placed against the end of the bed to keep the person's feet in proper alignment. (*Courtesy of the Posey Company.*)

foot drop is not prevented, the person may lose the ability to stand and walk because he will lose the ability to place the soles of his feet flat on the floor.

HANDLING OF LINENS

The types of linens used for bedmaking will vary, depending on the facility and the needs of the resident. During your employee orientation, you will learn which linens to use to make the beds. Additional information specific to each resident will be provided on the care plan.

No matter which linens are used in your facility, you should always collect the linens in the order that they will be used—mattress pad, bottom sheet, draw sheet, top sheet, blanket, bedspread, pillowcases. Once you have collected your stack of linens, flip the stack over so that the item you will need first is on the top of the stack (Fig. 21-4). Collecting linens in the order that they will be put on the bed helps you to remember which linens you need to collect. In addition, because the linens will be arranged in order of use, you will be able to make the bed more efficiently, without searching through the stack for the proper item.

Always remember that linens can act as fomites, or objects capable of spreading infection.

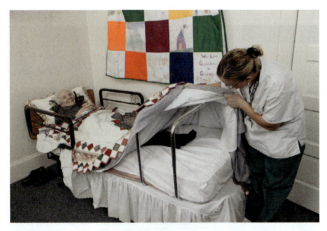

Figure 21-2
A bed cradle is used to keep the top sheet, the blanket, and the bedspread off the resident's feet. The linens are tucked in at the end of the bed and along the sides to keep the person from getting cold.

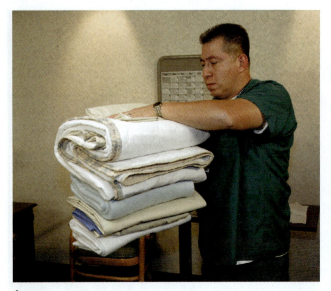
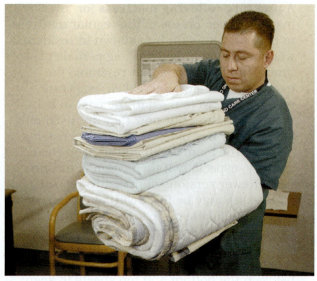

A   B

Figure 21-4

Handling linens. **(A)** First, collect the linens in the order that they will be used. Here, the nursing assistant has gathered a mattress pad, a bottom sheet, a draw sheet, a top sheet, a blanket, a bed-spread, and two pillowcases. The mattress pad is on the bottom of the stack and the pillowcases are on the top. Note that the nursing assistant is holding the linens away from his body. **(B)** Next, flip the stack of linens over so that the item you will need first is on top. Now the pillowcases are on the bottom of the stack and the mattress pad is on top, ready to be put on the bed.

For this reason, you should always use infection control practices when handling linens. Always wash your hands before collecting clean linens, and avoid letting clean linens come into contact with dirty surfaces, such as your uniform or the floor. When removing used linens from the bed, wear gloves, and roll the linens toward the center of the bed (down from the top and up from the bottom) to confine any soiled areas on the inside (Fig. 21-5). You may be required to place the used linen in a linen bag as it is removed from the bed to help prevent the spread of pathogens. The linen bag is then removed from the room and taken to a designated area. If a linen bag is not used, then the used linens are placed in the linen hamper immediately, as per your facility's policy. Never place dirty linens on the floor, or hold them against your uniform.

Guidelines Box 21-1 summarizes some general guidelines for the handling of linens.

STANDARD BEDMAKING TECHNIQUES

Routine bedmaking is usually done in the morning, before visiting hours, while your residents are bathing or dressing. How often the linens on a person's bed are changed will vary according to the type of health care facility and the person's needs. For example, in a hospital, the policy may be to change each person's linens completely on a daily basis. In a long-term care facility, the policy may call for less frequent linen changes. However, a person's bed must be remade each time any of the linens become soiled or excessively wrinkled,

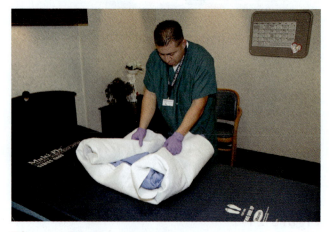

Figure 21-5

Gloves are worn to remove linens from the bed, because the linens may be soiled with body fluids. The soiled area is rolled toward the center of the bed.

Guidelines Box 21-1   Guidelines for Handling Linens

WHAT YOU DO	WHY YOU DO IT
Always wash your hands before collecting clean linens.	Washing your hands prevents microbes on your hands from being transferred to the clean linens.
Do not hold linens, clean or dirty, against your uniform.	If you hold clean linens against your uniform, microbes on your uniform could be transferred to the linens. If you hold dirty linens against your uniform, then microbes from the dirty linens could be transferred to your uniform.
When collecting linens, collect only those that you will need for that person's bed. For example, if a draw sheet is not needed, do not collect one.	Extra linens brought into a person's room are considered soiled, and therefore must not be returned to the clean linen cart or used for another person. These linens must now be laundered, which costs the facility extra money and manpower and creates additional wear on the linens, shortening their lifetime of use.
Collect linens in the order that they will be used. Once you have collected your stack of linens, flip the stack over so that the item you will need first is on the top of the stack.	Collecting linens in the order that they will be put on the bed helps you to remember which linens you need to collect. In addition, because the linens will be arranged in order of use, you will be able to make the bed more efficiently, without searching through the stack for the proper item.
Place clean linens on a clean surface in the room, such as the over-bed table or a chair. Do not place clean linens on the floor.	Clean linens can become contaminated with microbes if you place them on a "dirty" surface, such as the floor.
Wear gloves when removing used linens from a bed. Roll the linens toward the center of the bed to confine the soiled area inside.	Any item contaminated with blood or other body substances is a potential source of exposure to pathogens for the health care worker. Following the standard precautions and wearing proper personal protective equipment (PPE) will help to minimize your exposure. Confining the soiled area to the inside of the linens helps to ensure that other people, such as the people in the laundry, do not come in contact with the potentially infectious material.
If body fluids or substances leak through the linens to the mattress or bed frame, the mattress or bed frame should be wiped with an appropriate cleaning solution before placing clean linens on the bed. Remove your gloves and wash your hands before handling the clean linens.	These infection control methods help to prevent the clean sheets from becoming contaminated.
After removing the dirty linens from the bed, place them in the linen hamper immediately. Your facility may require you to place dirty linens in a plastic bag or pillowcase before placing them in the linen hamper. Do not place dirty linens on the floor or on any other surface.	Placing the dirty linens in the linen hamper immediately helps to control the spread of infection.

Guidelines Box 21-2 Guidelines for Bedmaking

WHAT YOU DO	WHY YOU DO IT
Always place linens on the bed so that the seams of the sheets face away from the person's skin.	The seams of the sheets can rub the person's skin, causing irritation and leading to skin breakdown.
Linens must be pulled tightly to avoid wrinkling. Layering should be kept to a minimum.	The wrinkles and extra layers of linens can cause skin breakdown and contribute to the formation of pressure ulcers.
Linens should be changed whenever they become soiled or wet, regardless of the time of day.	Besides causing discomfort, soiled or wet sheets can cause skin breakdown and contribute to the formation of pressure ulcers.
Do not shake linens when placing them on the bed.	Dust is a transport mechanism for microbes. Shaking linens stirs up dust from the floor. The dust then settles on surfaces in the room and can be easily transferred onto eating utensils or into a wound, causing an infection.
When you need to change the linens on a person's bed with the person still in the bed, always be sure to explain what you are doing throughout the procedure. Talk reassuringly to the person, even if the person is unconscious and you think that the person cannot hear you. Close the door, pull the privacy curtain, and keep the person covered at all times.	Having the bed linens changed while still in the bed can be a frightening experience for a bedridden person, particularly if the person is unconscious. Even if the person is conscious, movement may cause pain, and incontinence (the involuntary loss of urine or feces) can be embarrassing if it occurs. If the person is mentally impaired, he or she may become combative. Explaining what you are doing and taking care to preserve the person's modesty during the procedure will make the procedure more pleasant for the person.
Check the bed linens for personal items before removing the linens from the bed.	Personal items, such as dentures, eyeglasses, or jewelry, may become lost in the bed linens. If these linens are removed from the bed, bundled up, and sent to the laundry, the mislaid personal items may not be discovered and they could be damaged in the wash cycle, or they may be lost altogether. Personal items may be expensive and inconvenient to replace. If they hold sentimental value, they may be irreplaceable.

regardless of the time of day. Soiling of the sheets can occur as a result of spilled food or drink or as a result of excessive sweating, vomit, urine, feces, wound drainage, or leakage from a feeding tube. In each of these instances, a linen change would be required. Change as many of the bed linens as necessary to ensure a clean, dry, wrinkle-free bed

for your resident. General guidelines for bedmaking are given in Guidelines Box 21-2.

To make a bed, you will need to know how to make a **mitered corner** (Fig. 21-6). Mitering is a way of folding and tucking the sheet so that it lies flat and neat against the mattress. When a flat sheet is used as the bottom sheet, the mitered

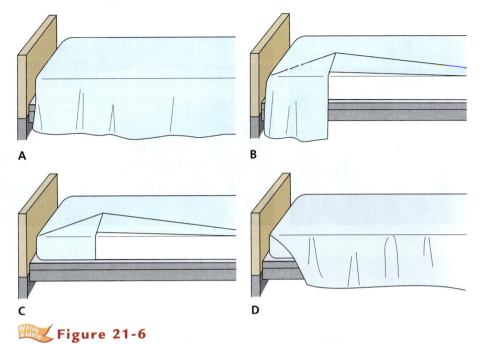

Figure 21-6

How to make a mitered corner. Here, a mitered corner is being made on a top sheet. **(A)** The bottom of the sheet has been tucked under the end of the mattress. The side of the sheet is hanging over the side of the bed. **(B)** Grasp the edge of the sheet about 12 inches from the foot of the bed and lift it up, forming a triangle. Lay the triangular fold on the top of the bed, and smooth the hanging portion of the sheet against the side of the mattress. **(C)** Tuck the hanging portion of the sheet underneath the mattress, while holding the triangular fold taut against the top of the bed. **(D)** Bring the triangular fold back down over the edge of the mattress, and leave the side hanging loose.

corners are made at the top of the bed to help secure the sheet to the mattress. Mitered corners are made at the foot of the bed to hold the top sheet, blanket, and bedspread in place.

CLOSED (UNOCCUPIED) BEDS

A **closed bed** is an empty bed (Fig. 21-7A). A bed that is unoccupied because the previous resident has been discharged from the facility and a new resident has yet to arrive is considered a closed bed. Similarly, a bed that is unoccupied because the resident is simply not in it at the moment (and is not expected back any time soon) is also considered a closed bed. For example, many long-term care facilities make closed beds each day for residents who are not bedridden. Procedure 21-1 explains how to make a closed bed.

When the top sheet, blanket, and bedspread of a closed bed are turned back, or **fanfolded,** the closed bed becomes an **open bed,** or a bed ready to receive a resident. For example, you would open a bed in preparation for a new admission, or after you have changed the linens while the resident is bathing. Because the resident would be expected to return to the bed shortly, you would fanfold the linens back in anticipation of his return. Similarly, in some long-term care facilities, the linens on the beds of residents who are not bedridden are folded back in the evening, before the residents return to their rooms. To open a closed bed, you first grasp the bedspread, blanket, and top sheet and fold them back to the foot of the bed, creating a fanfold (Fig. 21-7B). Finish by making sure that the bed is in the lowest position and the bed wheels are locked. Place the call light control near the head of the bed, clipping it to the bottom sheet.

A **surgical bed** is a closed bed that has been opened to receive a resident who will be arriving by stretcher. When preparing a surgical bed, instead of folding the top sheet, blanket, and bedspread to the foot of the bed, you loosen these linens from the foot of the bed and fold them toward the side of the bed, leaving one side open and ready to receive the person (Fig. 21-7C). After folding the linens to the side, raise the bed so that the stretcher will be slightly higher than the bed. Make sure that the bed wheels are locked, and ensure a clear path by moving any furniture away from the bed.

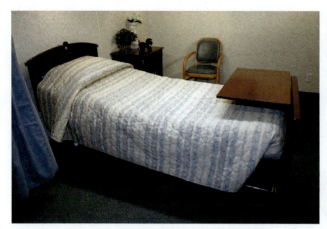

A

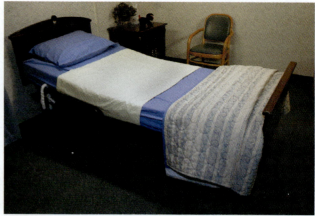

B

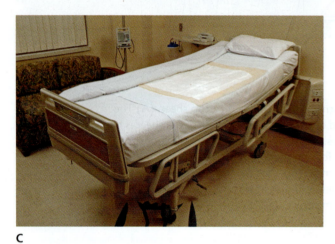

C

Figure 21-7

Types of beds. **(A)** A closed bed is an unoccupied bed. **(B)** When a closed bed is "opened," the top sheet, blanket, and bedspread are "fanfolded" to the foot of the bed. **(C)** A surgical bed is a closed bed that has been "opened" to receive a person on a stretcher. The top linens are fanfolded to the side of the bed.

OCCUPIED BEDS

Some conditions make it difficult or impossible for a person to get out of bed for a linen change. When this is the case, it is necessary to change the linens while the person is still in the bed. This is called making an **occupied bed** (Procedure 21-2). In most facilities, this procedure is carried out on a routine basis after the person has been bathed. However, as always, if the linens become wet or soiled in between scheduled linen changes, then they must be changed. Because it can be frightening for a bedridden person to have the linens changed while she is still in the bed, remember to explain to the person what you are doing throughout this procedure. Keep the privacy curtain and the door closed during the procedure, to help maintain the person's modesty. If the linens you are removing from the bed are soiled with blood or other body substances, you must wear

gloves. Remember to remove the soiled gloves and put on clean ones before handling the clean linens.

Helping Hands and a Caring Heart

FOCUS ON HUMANISTIC HEALTH CARE

All of us can probably remember a time when we were really sick and someone came and freshened us up and changed our sheets. Think about how loved and well-cared-for you felt! That is how your residents will feel when you replace their hot, wrinkled, soiled linens with cool, pressed, clean ones. When a complete linen change is not necessary, the simple act of pulling the wrinkles out of the linens and plumping up the pillow can be very comforting to a resident.

SUMMARY

- A well-made bed is essential to a person's mental and physical well-being.
  - Clean, dry, wrinkle-free linens help make a person who is ill feel cared for and more comfortable.
  - Clean, dry, wrinkle-free linens help to prevent complications, such as pressure ulcers. Dampness contributes to skin breakdown and wrinkled sheets can cause friction, both of which are factors in the development of pressure ulcers.
  - Clean, dry linens are important for odor and infection control.
- A variety of linens are used to make a bed. Facility policy and the resident's particular needs dictate which linens are used to make the bed.
- Special devices, such as pressure-relieving mattresses and bed cradles, are used to improve the resident's comfort and to prevent the development of complications related to spending long periods of time in bed, such as pressure ulcers.
- Because linens can act as fomites if they are not handled properly, it is important to use good infection control practices when handling them.
  - Never hold dirty linens against your uniform, or place them on the floor or other surface in the room. Dirty linens must be placed in the linen hamper or linen bag immediately.
  - Always wear gloves when it is possible you will be handling linens soiled with body fluids or other substances.
  - Always wash your hands before handling clean linens. Never hold clean linens against your uniform, or place them on the floor. Clean linens may be placed on a clean surface in the room, such as the over-bed table.
  - Once clean linens are brought into a resident's room, they are considered soiled and should not be returned to the linen cart or used to make another resident's bed.
  - A bed is either unoccupied ("closed") or occupied. A closed bed may be "opened" in anticipation of receiving a resident by fan-folding the sheets to allow easier access.

PROCEDURE 21-1

Making an Unoccupied (Closed) Bed

WHY YOU DO IT   Clean, dry, wrinkle-free linens promote comfort, help to prevent complications (such as pressure ulcers), and are important for odor and infection control.

Getting Ready WGKIEPS

1. Complete the "Getting Ready" steps.*

Supplies

- mattress pad
- bottom sheet
- lift (draw) sheet (if necessary)
- bed protector (if necessary)
- top sheet
- blanket
- bedspread
- pillowcase

Procedure

2. Place the linens on a clean surface close to the bed (for example, the over-bed table).

3. Make sure that the bed is positioned at a comfortable working height (to promote good body mechanics) and that the wheels are locked.

4. Lower the side rails and move the mattress to the head of the bed (it may have shifted toward the foot of the bed if the occupant of the bed had the head of the bed elevated).

   Note: The mattress pad, bottom sheet, and draw sheet are positioned and tucked in on one side of the bed before moving to the other side to complete these actions. This is most efficient in terms of energy and time.

5. Place the mattress pad on the bed and unfold it so that only one vertical crease remains. Make sure that this crease is centered on the mattress. If the mattress pad is fitted, carefully pull the corners of the near side over the corners of the mattress and smooth down the sides. If the mattress pad is flat, make sure the top of the pad is even with the head of the mattress. Open the mattress pad across the bed, taking care to keep it centered.

6. Place the bottom sheet on the bed. If the bottom sheet is fitted, carefully pull the corners of the near side over the corners of the mattress and smooth down the sides. If the bottom sheet is flat:

   a. Place the sheet so that when you unfold it, the wide hem will be at the head of the bed and the hem stitching will be against the mattress, away from the person who will be occupying the bed.

   b. Unfold the sheet so that only one vertical crease remains. Make sure that this crease is vertically centered on the mattress.

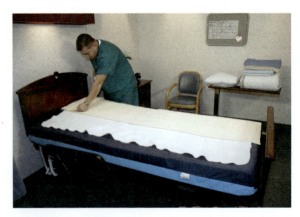

Step 6b Unfold the sheet so that only one vertical crease remains.

---

*It is assumed that the dirty linens have been removed from the bed, and the mattress and bed frame have been cleaned, as per facility policy, prior to beginning this procedure.

c. Open the sheet across the bed, taking care to keep it centered. The same length of sheet (approximately 12 to 18 inches) should hang over each side of the bed. Make sure that the lower edge of the sheet is even with the foot of the mattress.

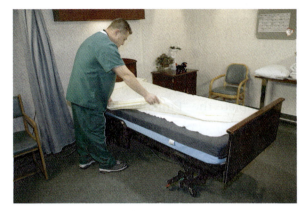

Step 6c Open the sheet across the bed, taking care to keep it centered.

d. Tuck the sheet under the mattress at the head of the bed and miter the corner.

e. Tuck the near side of the sheet underneath the mattress, working from the head of the bed toward the foot. As you tuck, make sure there are no wrinkles in the sheet and that the mattress pad remains smooth and in place.

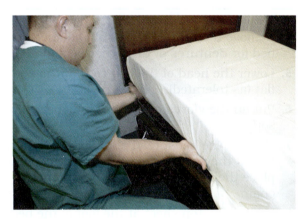

Step 6e After mitering the corner at the head of the bed, tuck the side of the sheet underneath the mattress.

7. Place the lift sheet on the bed so that the top of the sheet is approximately 12 inches from the head of the mattress. If you are using a plastic or rubberized lift sheet, place a cotton lift sheet on top of it. Smooth the lift sheet across the bed and tuck the near side under the mattress.

8. Now, move to the other side of the bed and repeat the process of aligning the mattress pad, mitering the corner, and tucking in the bottom sheet and lift sheet.

9. Place the top sheet on the bed so that when you unfold it, the wide hem will be at the head of the bed and the hem stitching will be facing upward, away from the person who will be occupying the bed.

a. Unfold the sheet so that only one vertical crease remains. Make sure that this crease is centered vertically on the mattress.

b. Open the sheet across the bed, taking care to keep it centered. The same length of sheet (approximately 12 to 18 inches) should hang over each side of the bed. Make sure that the top edge of the sheet is even with the head of the mattress. Pull the bottom of the sheet over the foot of the bed, but do not tuck it in yet (it will be tucked in with the blanket and bedspread).

10. Place the blanket on the bed and unfold it in the same manner as the sheet, keeping the center crease in the center of the bed. The same length of blanket (approximately 12 to 18 inches) should hang over each side of the bed. Make sure that the top edge of the blanket is approximately 6 to 8 inches from the head of the mattress. Fold the top edge of the sheet back over the top edge of the blanket, creating a cuff. Pull the bottom edge of the blanket over the sheet at the foot of the bed, but do not tuck anything in yet.

11. Place the bedspread on the bed and unfold it in the same manner as the sheet, keeping the center crease in the center of the bed. The sides of the bedspread should be even and cover all of the other bed linens. Make sure that the top of the bedspread is even with the head of the mattress, unless the pillow is to be tucked under the bedspread (in which case you will need to allow more length at the top). Pull the bottom of the bedspread over the blanket and sheet at the foot of the bed.

12. Together, tuck the bedspread, the blanket, and the top sheet under the foot of the mattress. Make a mitered corner at the foot of the bed on both sides.

13. Fold the top of the bedspread back over the blanket to make a cuff.

(continued)

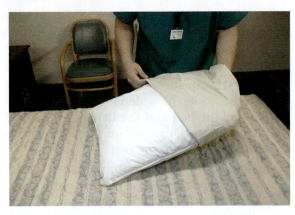

Step 14 Grasp the pillow through the pillowcase and pull the pillowcase down over the pillow.

14. Rest the pillow on the bed. Grasping the closed end of the pillowcase, turn the pillowcase inside out over your hand and arm. Grasp the pillow through the pillowcase and pull the pillowcase down over the pillow. Make sure any tags or zippers are on the inside of the pillowcase.

15. Place the pillow on the bed with the open end of the pillowcase facing away from the door.

Finishing Up CLOSER

16. Complete the "Finishing Up" steps.

PROCEDURE 21-2

Making an Occupied Bed

WHY YOU DO IT   Clean, dry, wrinkle-free linens promote comfort, help to prevent complications (such as pressure ulcers), and are important for odor and infection control.

Getting Ready WORKIEPS

1. Complete the "Getting Ready" steps.

Supplies

- gloves
- bath blanket
- mattress pad
- bottom sheet
- lift (draw) sheet
- bed protector (if necessary)
- top sheet
- blanket
- bedspread
- pillowcase

Procedure

2. Place the linens on a clean surface close to the bed (for example, the over-bed table).

3. Make sure that the bed is positioned at a comfortable working height (to promote good body mechanics) and that the wheels are locked.

4. Remove the call light control and check the bed for dentures or any other personal items.

5. Lower the head of the bed so that the bed is flat (as tolerated).

6. Put on the gloves (the linens may be wet or soiled).

7. Remove the bedspread and blanket from the bed. If they are to be reused, fold them and place them on a clean surface, such as a chair.

8. Loosen the top sheet at the foot of the bed and spread a bath blanket over the top sheet (and the person).

9. If the person is able, have her hold the bath blanket. If not, tuck the corners under the

person's shoulders. Remove the top sheet by pulling it out from underneath the bath blanket, being careful not to expose the person.

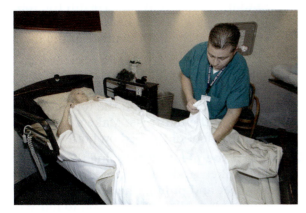

Step 9 Remove the top sheet by pulling it out from underneath the bath blanket.

10. Place the top sheet in the linen hamper or linen bag.

11. If the side rails are in use, lower the side rail on the working side of the bed. The side rail on the opposite side of the bed should remain up. Turn the person onto her side so that she is facing away from you. Reposition the pillow under the person's head, and adjust the bath blanket to keep the person covered.

12. Loosen the lift sheet, bottom sheet, and (if necessary) the mattress pad.

13. Fanfold the bottom linens toward the person's back, tucking them slightly underneath her.

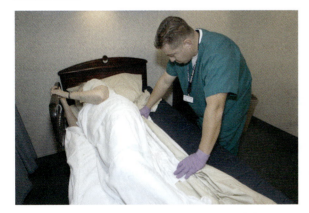

Step 13 Fanfold the bottom linens toward the person's back.

14. Straighten the mattress pad (if it is not being changed). If the mattress pad is being changed, place the clean mattress pad on the bed and unfold it so that only one vertical crease remains. Make sure that this crease is centered vertically on the mattress. If the

mattress pad is fitted, carefully pull the corners of the near side over the corners of the mattress and smooth down the sides. If the mattress pad is flat, make sure the top of the pad is even with the head of the mattress. Fanfold the opposite side of the mattress pad close to the resident.

15. Place the clean bottom sheet on the bed. If the bottom sheet is fitted, carefully pull the corners over the corners of the mattress and smooth down the sides. If the bottom sheet is flat:

a. Place the sheet so that when you unfold it, the wide hem will be at the head of the bed and the hem stitching will be against the mattress, away from the person who will be occupying the bed.

b. Unfold the sheet so that only one vertical crease remains. Make sure that this crease is centered vertically on the mattress.

c. Open the sheet across the bed, taking care to keep it centered. The same length of sheet (approximately 12 to 18 inches) should hang over each side of the bed. Make sure that the lower edge of the sheet is even with the foot of the mattress. Fanfold the opposite side of the sheet close to the patient or resident.

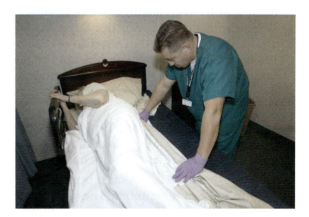

Step 15c Open the sheet across the bed, taking care to keep it centered.

d. Tuck the sheet under the mattress at the head of the bed and miter the corner.

e. Tuck the near side of the sheet underneath the mattress, working from the head of the bed toward the foot. As you tuck, make sure there are no wrinkles in the sheet and that the mattress pad remains smooth and in place.

(continued)

16. Place the lift sheet on the bed so that the top of the sheet is approximately 12 inches from the head of the mattress. If you are using a plastic or rubberized lift sheet, place a cotton lift sheet on top of it. Fanfold the opposite side of the lift sheet close to the patient or resident. Smooth the lift sheet across the bed and tuck the near side under the mattress.

17. Raise the side rail on the working side of the bed. Help the person to roll toward you, over the folded linens. Reposition the pillow under the person's head and adjust the bath blanket to keep the person covered.

18. Move to the other side of the bed and lower the side rail.

19. Loosen and remove the soiled bottom linens and place them in the linen hamper or linen bag. Change your gloves if they become soiled.

20. Now, repeat the process of aligning the mattress pad, mitering the corner, and tucking in the bottom sheet and lift sheet.

21. Help the person to move to the center of the bed and position her comfortably. Raise the side rail on the working side of the bed.

22. Change the pillowcase and place the pillow under the person's head.

23. Place the clean top sheet over the person (who is still covered with the bath blanket), being careful not to cover her face. The sheet should be placed so that when you unfold it, the wide hem will be at the head of the bed and the hem stitching will be facing upward, away from the person who will be occupying the bed.

   a. Unfold the sheet so that only one vertical crease remains. Make sure that this crease is centered vertically on the mattress.

   b. Open the sheet across the bed, taking care to keep it centered. The same length of sheet (approximately 12 to 18 inches) should hang over each side of the bed.

   c. If the person is able, have her hold the top sheet. If not, tuck the corners under her shoulders. Remove the bath blanket by pulling it out from underneath the top sheet, being careful not to expose the person. Place the bath blanket in the linen hamper or linen bag.

24. Place the blanket and then the bedspread over the top sheet. Together, tuck the bedspread, the blanket, and the top sheet under the foot of the mattress. Make a mitered corner at the foot of the bed on both sides.

25. Make a **toe pleat** by grasping the top sheet, the blanket, and the bedspread over the person's feet and pulling the linens straight up. The toe pleat allows the person to move her feet and helps to relieve pressure on the feet from tightly tucked linens.

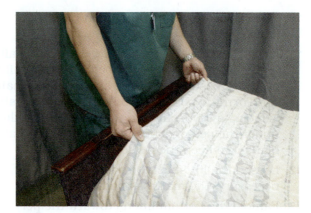

Step 25 Make a toe pleat by pulling straight up on the top linens.

26. Lower the bed to its lowest position and make sure that the wheels are locked. Raise the head of the bed as the person requests.

27. Remove your gloves and dispose of them in a facility-approved waste container.

Finishing Up   CLOSUR

28. Complete the "Finishing Up" steps.

WHAT DID YOU LEARN?

Multiple Choice

Select the single best answer for each of the following questions.

1. What is a draw sheet?
   a. A fitted bottom sheet
   b. A half-sized sheet that is placed over the middle of the bottom sheet and has varied uses, including protecting the mattress from soiling
   c. A half-sized sheet that is placed over the middle of the top sheet and used to make toe pleats
   d. A sheet used to add a decorative touch to the person's room
2. Mrs. Smith is in bed. How would you describe her bed?
   a. An open bed
   b. A closed bed
   c. A surgical bed
   d. An occupied bed
3. A bed that has the top linens fanfolded to the side has been prepared for what type of resident?
   a. A resident who is paraplegic
   b. A resident who is incontinent
   c. A resident who will be arriving on a stretcher
   d. A resident who will be returning to bed in the evening
4. When you are handling linens, always remember to:
   a. Shake the bedspread to remove dust
   b. Place the dirty linens on the floor, to get them out of your way
   c. Hold the linens away from your body
   d. All of the above
5. What do you call a metal frame that is placed between the bottom and top sheets to keep the bed linens from resting on the person's feet?
   a. A bed board
   b. A pressure-relieving mattress
   c. A bed cradle
   d. A footboard
6. What personal protective equipment (PPE) should be worn when removing used bed linens?
   a. Gloves
   b. A gown
   c. Eye goggles
   d. No PPE is necessary
7. When are bed linens changed?
   a. When they become wet or soiled
   b. According to facility policy
   c. When they become excessively wrinkled
   d. All of the above

STOP and Think!

- You are making an occupied bed. There is no linen hamper in the room, and you have already removed the soiled linens from the bed. What should you do with the soiled linens until you can take them to the linen room or hallway hamper? Mrs. O'Shea, the resident, is lying on her side in the bed, covered with a bath blanket.
- Barbara is a nursing assistant on 3 West. She has already changed the bed linens twice during her shift for one of her residents, Mrs. Bridges. Mrs. Bridges is receiving an antibiotic, and one of the side effects of the medication is diarrhea. Now Mrs. Bridges' call light is on again. When Barbara goes to check on her, she discovers that Mrs. Bridges has soiled the bed again. Barbara tells Mrs. Bridges she will be right back, and leaves to go get supplies from the linen closet. What are some items Barbara should collect, along with clean sheets?

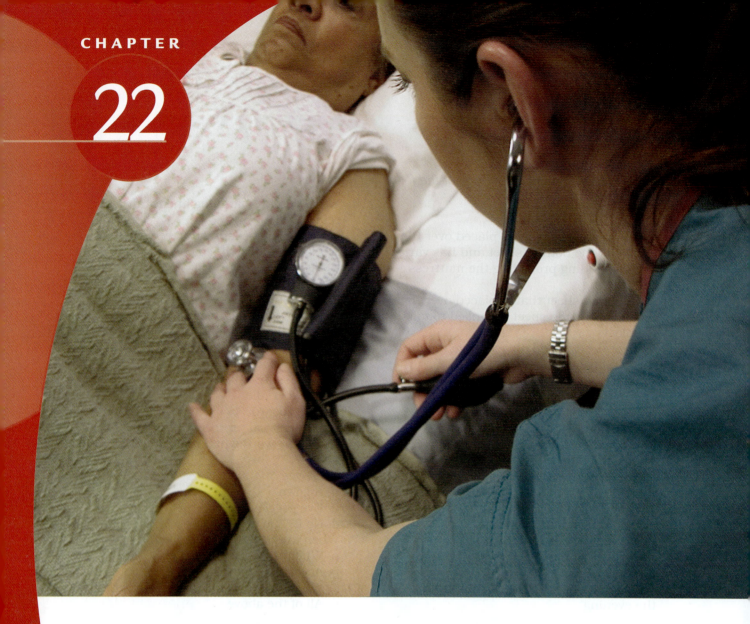

Vital Signs, Height, and Weight

WHAT WILL YOU LEARN?

The word "vital" means "necessary to life." This is why those in the health care field refer to certain key measurements that provide essential information about a person's health as **vital signs.** When we evaluate a person's vital signs, we look at the person's body temperature, heart beat (pulse), breathing (respirations), and blood pressure. One of the many important duties you will perform as a nursing assistant will be to routinely measure and record your residents' vital signs. A person's height and weight, although not technically vital signs, also provide insight into a person's overall health status. Therefore, you will also be responsible for obtaining and recording these measurements (although not as frequently as the vital sign measurements). Because a change in a person's normal vital sign measurements can be a sign of illness, your ability to detect a change and report this to the nurse promptly is essential to the well-being of your residents. When you are finished with this chapter, you will be able to:

Photo: A nursing assistant takes a resident's blood pressure.

1. Define the term *vital signs* and discuss how the vital signs reflect changes in a person's medical condition.

2. Understand the importance of accurately measuring and recording vital signs, and of reporting any changes to the nurse.

3. Describe the factors affecting a person's body temperature.

4. Discuss various terms used to describe an abnormal body temperature.

5. List common sites used for measuring a person's body temperature, and the advantages and disadvantages associated with each site.

6. Demonstrate the proper use of a glass thermometer, an electronic thermometer, and a tympanic thermometer.

7. Define the term *pulse* and describe factors that may affect a person's pulse.

8. Describe the different qualities of the pulse that a nursing assistant should be aware of when taking a person's pulse.

9. List common sites used for taking a person's pulse.

10. Diagram the parts of the stethoscope and explain how this tool is used.

11. Demonstrate the proper way to measure and record a radial pulse and an apical pulse.

12. Describe the factors that may affect a person's respirations.

13. Explain the terms used to describe a person's respirations.

14. Demonstrate the proper way to measure and record a person's respirations.

15. Define the term *blood pressure* and describe factors that may affect a person's blood pressure.

16. Discuss various terms used to describe an abnormal blood pressure.

17. Discuss the various methods used to measure a person's blood pressure.

18. Explain how a sphygmomanometer works, and demonstrate how to use this tool to measure a person's blood pressure.

19. List and describe the Korotkoff sounds, which are heard while taking a person's blood pressure.

20. Discuss factors that can lead to a change in a person's weight.

21. Demonstrate the proper way to measure a person's height and weight using an upright scale.

22. Demonstrate the proper way to measure a person's weight using a chair scale.

23. Demonstrate the proper way to measure a person's height when the person is in bed.

Vocabulary Use the CD in the front of your book to hear these terms pronounced and defined:

Vital signs	Diaphragm	Depth of	Diastolic pressure
Body temperature	Bell	respiration	Pulse pressure
Metabolism	Pulse deficit	Eupnea	Orthostatic blood
Febrile	Tachycardia	Tachypnea	pressures
Pulse	Bradycardia	Bradypnea	Sphygmomanometer
Pulse rate	Inhalation	Dyspnea	Korotkoff sounds
Pulse rhythm	(inspiration)	Hyperventilation	Hypertension
Dysrhythmia	Exhalation (expiration)	Hypoventilation	Hypotension
Pulse amplitude	Respiratory rate	Blood pressure	Orthostatic
Stethoscope	Respiratory rhythm	Systolic pressure	hypotension

WHAT DO VITAL SIGNS TELL US?

Vital signs reflect functions that are regulated automatically by the body, such as:

- How fast the heart beats
- The internal temperature of the body
- The rate at which a person breathes

Because the body is always trying to maintain a state of balance, "control centers" (located mostly in the brain) regulate what is going on inside the body and make adjustments, as necessary, to keep things within the range of normal. Therefore, a change in a vital sign may indicate that something has put the body out of balance, and the body is trying to get that balance back.

There are many factors that can cause changes in a person's vital sign measurements. A person's vital sign measurements may vary over the course of a day (for example, in response to emotional or physical stress or a change in position), while still staying within the range of "normal." However, a major or a long-lasting change in one or more of a person's vital sign measurements may be a response to illness or injury. As you read this chapter, pay attention to the ranges that are considered "normal" for each vital sign. Knowing these ranges will allow you to quickly recognize measurements that are not within the range of normal. Also, remember that your definition of "normal" will vary according to the person. For example, you may come to know that Ms. Goldblum's blood pressure tends to be at the low end of the normal range, while Mr. Hanson's tends to be a little bit higher than average. Your knowledge of your resident will allow you to know whether the vital sign measurements you have obtained are normal readings for that person.

MEASURING AND RECORDING VITAL SIGNS

Vital signs are measured and compared with normal values (as well as the values that are considered normal for the individual) under many different circumstances. Residents of a long-term care facility may have their vital signs taken routinely once daily, once weekly, or perhaps only once monthly. The care plan, the physician orders, or both will specify how often each of your resident's vital signs are to be measured and recorded.

It may also be necessary to check a resident's vital signs:

- Before and after certain medications are given
- Before, during, and after a diagnostic procedure
- In an emergency situation
- If the resident complains of not feeling well, or does not seem to be looking or acting like he normally does
- After an incident or accident, such as a fall

If a resident has been participating in an activity that may affect her vital signs (for example,

walking, drinking, eating) you should give the resident a few minutes to sit and relax before taking her vital signs.

Facilities will have different policies regarding how vital signs are recorded. Some facilities will record vital sign measurements on one flow (graphic) sheet for the unit, which lists the names of all of the residents on a particular unit. Other facilities will use one flow sheet per resident. This flow sheet may be kept in the resident's medical record, or in a designated binder at the nurses' station. If you take a resident's vital signs and get a measurement that is abnormal (either higher or lower than normal for that particular person), you should take the measurement again for the sake of accuracy and then report your findings to the nurse immediately.

The skills you will use to measure a person's vital signs may seem difficult when you are first learning them, but practice will make you more comfortable with taking vital sign measurements. Timely and accurate measurement and recording of vital signs is critical because many people rely on this information to make important decisions about the resident's care. In addition, a problem may go unnoticed if a vital sign is measured or

Be Smart About Surveys!

Surveyors will be checking to make sure that each resident's vital signs, height, and weight are measured and recorded as scheduled, and that any changes are promptly recognized and followed up on by the staff. To help your facility remain without survey problems in this area:

- Always complete vital sign, height, and weight measurements when you are assigned to do them.
- Always follow proper procedure to ensure accuracy of measurements. Do not take shortcuts.
- Be sure to document all of your measurements accurately and promptly.
- Be aware of what is normal for each resident so that you can recognize significant changes.
- If you have any difficulties measuring a resident's vital signs, height, or weight, ask for help from the nurse. Accurate measurements are a must!
- Report abnormal measurements as early in the shift as possible to allow the nurse enough time to evaluate and act on them. They may indicate a change in the resident's condition.

recorded inaccurately. Always ask for assistance, either from another nursing assistant or from a nurse, if you are having difficulty when checking a person's vital signs. Asking for help when you need it is not a sign of failure or an inability to do your job—rather, it demonstrates that you are responsible and interested in seeing that your resident receives the best possible care.

BODY TEMPERATURE

The **body temperature** is simply how hot the body is. When we measure someone's body temperature, what we are measuring is the difference between the heat produced by the person's body and the heat lost by the person's body. The human body produces heat as a normal process of **metabolism.** Metabolism is the word used to describe the physical and chemical changes that occur when the cells of the body change the food that we eat into energy. Muscle movement also produces heat. This is why we become hotter when we exercise, and why we shiver when we are cold (shivering moves the muscles, producing heat). Heat loss occurs normally through the skin, through the passing of urine and feces, through the process of breathing, and is increased by bodily responses, such as sweating. The body temperature is regulated by a "control center" that is located in the brain.

FACTORS AFFECTING THE BODY TEMPERATURE

Although a healthy person's body temperature is usually fairly constant, small changes may occur as a result of physical or emotional stress, the environmental temperature, or even the time of day. For example, it is typical for a person's body temperature to be lower in the morning and increase slightly throughout the day, probably from an increase in activity levels. Stress causes the release of hormones that increase metabolism and the heart rate, readying the body to respond to the source of the stress. This response, called the "fight-or-flight" response, is discussed in detail in Chapter 37. The increase in metabolism and heart rate can lead to an increase in body temperature as well. Finally, exposure to either very hot or very cold environmental temperatures can cause changes in a person's body temperature.

A person's age and gender also play a role in determining body temperature. Elderly people are more sensitive to environmental temperature changes. In addition, an elderly person's body may not produce as much heat as it did in younger years, due to muscle loss as a result of normal aging. A woman's body temperature tends to change more frequently than a man's body temperature, because of the hormonal changes that occur with the menstrual cycle and during pregnancy and menopause.

MEASURING THE BODY TEMPERATURE

The body temperature can be measured from several different areas of the body:

- The mouth (an *oral temperature*)
- The rectum (a *rectal temperature*)
- The armpit (an *axillary temperature*)
- The ear (a *tympanic temperature*)
- The forehead (a *temporal temperature*)

Where the body temperature is measured depends on facility policy and the needs of the resident. Because the method used to measure the temperature affects the accuracy of the measurement, you should note which method was used when you record the temperature, as per your facility's policy. For example, many facilities use "O" for oral, "R" for rectal, "T" for tympanic, and "A" for axillary. The body temperature is measured in either degrees Fahrenheit (°F) or degrees Celsius (°C), using a clinical thermometer.

Types of Thermometers

There are many different types of thermometers in use.

Glass thermometers

When most of us think of a thermometer, we think of a glass thermometer (Fig. 22-1). Glass

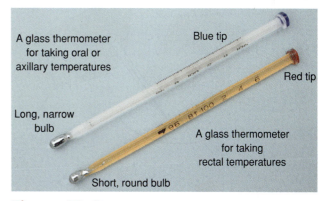

A glass thermometer for taking oral or axillary temperatures

Blue tip

Red tip

Long, narrow bulb

A glass thermometer for taking rectal temperatures

Short, round bulb

Figure 22-1
Glass thermometers may vary slightly in appearance depending on their intended use.

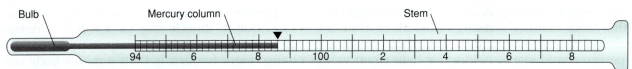

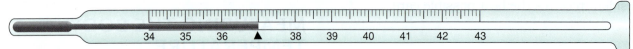

A **Fahrenheit (F°) thermometer** is scaled from 94°F to 108°F. Each long line indicates 1 degree and each short line indicates $2/10$ (0.2) of a degree. This thermometer is reading 98.6°F.

A **Celsius (C°) thermometer** is scaled from 34°C to 43°C. Each long line indicates 1 degree and each short line indicates $1/10$ (0.1) of a degree. This thermometer is reading 37°C.

Figure 22-2
Temperature scales on glass thermometers.

thermometers consist of a glass bulb attached to a thin glass tube that is marked with a temperature scale and filled with mercury (a metallic substance). The mercury inside the thermometer expands with heat and moves up the glass tube, showing the temperature on the scale. The Fahrenheit thermometer is scaled from 94°F to 108°F, while the Celsius thermometer is scaled from 34°C to 43°C (Fig. 22-2). Before you use a glass thermometer, the mercury must be "shaken down" to below the 94° mark on a Fahrenheit thermometer, or the 34° mark on a Celsius thermometer (Fig. 22-3). To read a glass thermometer, hold it horizontally by the stem at eye level and rotate it until the line of mercury becomes visible (Fig. 22-4).

Because glass thermometers are not disposable, they must be cleaned properly after each use, according to facility policy. Sometimes, a clear plastic cover called a *sheath* is used to cover the thermometer; after the sheath is used, it is discarded. The thermometer is washed with warm water and soap (never hot water, which can cause the thermometer to shatter), rinsed with cool water, and placed in a disinfectant solution. The amount of time that the thermometer must soak in the disinfectant will vary, depending on the type of disinfectant solution used. If a glass thermometer breaks while you are cleaning it (or at any other time), avoid touching the mercury and the broken glass, and prevent others from doing so as well. Call the nurse immediately. Mercury is toxic and must be cleaned up according to facility policy.

Because of the dangers associated with breakage and spilled mercury, many facilities have stopped using glass thermometers. Some facilities still use glass thermometers, but have switched to using newer models, which contain a substance that behaves the same way as mercury but is less toxic.

Electronic thermometers

Because glass thermometers can break, posing a danger to both the resident and the health care

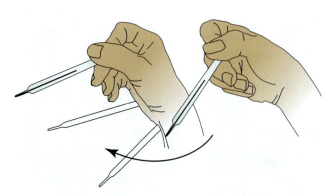

Figure 22-3
A glass thermometer is "shaken down" before use by holding the thermometer firmly by the stem and snapping your wrist downward.

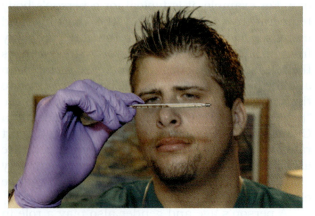

Figure 22-4
To read a glass thermometer, hold it horizontally by the stem at eye level.

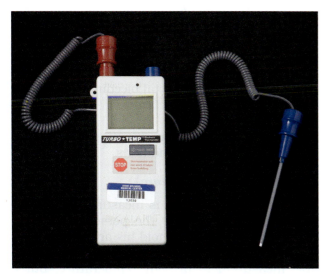

Figure 22-5
A battery-operated electronic thermometer.

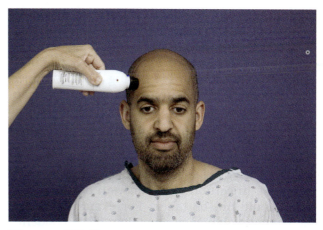

Figure 22-7
A temporal artery thermometer is placed on the middle of the person's forehead and swept toward the ear, stopping in front of the ear.

worker, more and more facilities are using electronic thermometers instead (Fig. 22-5). Electronic thermometers are powered by batteries, and the temperature is displayed on a screen on the front of the instrument. A probe, covered with a disposable sheath, is placed in the resident's mouth, rectum, or armpit to measure the temperature. A blue probe is used for taking oral or axillary temperatures. A red probe is used for taking rectal temperatures. After the probe is used, the disposable sheath is discarded.

Tympanic thermometers

A tympanic thermometer (Fig. 22-6) is used to measure the body temperature in the ear. The probe of this battery-operated instrument is inserted into the ear canal, where it rests near the eardrum (tympanic membrane). The person's

temperature is displayed on a screen after a few seconds.

Temporal artery thermometers

The temporal artery thermometer represents the latest development in thermometer technology (Fig. 22-7). Remember how your mother used to place her cool hand on your hot forehead to check for a fever? The temporal artery thermometer is simply a "high-tech" version of Mom's gesture. As the device is passed over a person's forehead, it detects the body temperature at numerous points. It then performs a series of calculations on the readings to arrive at the person's peak body temperature. The temporal artery thermometer is even more accurate than a tympanic thermometer, and it is considered the least invasive of all of the thermometers available (because it does not have to be inserted into any body opening).

Sites for Measuring Body Temperature
Mouth (oral temperature)

Measuring a person's body temperature by placing the thermometer in his or her mouth is simple and causes the person minimal discomfort. Because the thermometer is being placed in the mouth, which is not an entirely enclosed space, the temperature reading may not be as accurate as with some of the other methods. For example, measuring the temperature in the rectum or ear gives a more accurate reading, because the thermometer is placed into a tightly closed space. However, many times, the reading provided by placing the thermometer in the mouth is accurate

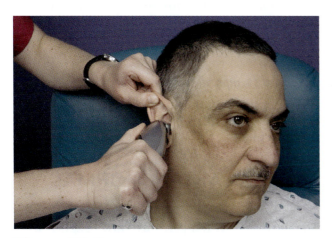

Figure 22-6
A tympanic thermometer is inserted into the ear canal.

enough. An oral temperature may be measured using a glass thermometer or an electronic thermometer (Procedure 22-1).

If a person eats, drinks, smokes, or chews gum within 15 minutes of having an oral temperature taken, the measurement may not be accurate. If one of your residents has done any of these things shortly before you intend to take his temperature orally, then you must either use a different method or wait for a period of time as specified by your facility's policy (usually 15 to 30 minutes). In certain situations, an oral temperature should not be taken. For example, an oral temperature should not be taken if the resident:

- Is unconscious
- Is unable to keep his mouth closed (necessary in order to keep the thermometer in place)
- Is unable to breathe through his nose
- Is likely to bite the oral thermometer (for example, a confused or disoriented resident, or a resident with a history of seizures)
- Is coughing or sneezing
- Has recently had mouth surgery or an injury to the mouth
- Is receiving oxygen by a face mask (because the oxygen may cause the temperature measurement to be inaccurate)

Rectum (rectal temperature)

Measuring a person's body temperature by placing the thermometer in the rectum provides a more accurate measurement of the person's body temperature because the thermometer is placed in an enclosed space. However, placing the thermometer rectally is also the most risky method of taking a temperature, and it can be uncomfortable and embarrassing for the resident.

A rectal temperature may be obtained using a glass thermometer or an electronic thermometer (Procedure 22-2). The thermometer must be lubricated and inserted carefully into the rectum, not more than 1 inch in an adult.

When you are taking a temperature rectally, it is important that you stay with the person during the entire procedure, both to hold the thermometer in place and to make sure that the person is all right. The thermometer could stimulate the vagus nerve, an important nerve that begins in the brain and sends branches to the heart, lungs, stomach, and rectum. Stimulation of the vagus nerve may temporarily decrease the person's heart rate and blood pressure, which can be dangerous. The person could also roll onto his back, pushing the thermometer too high into the rectum, or causing the thermometer to break. In either case, serious injury could result. A different method of measuring the temperature should be used if the person:

- Has hemorrhoids, rectal bleeding, or a disease involving the rectum
- Has diarrhea
- Has had rectal surgery
- Has certain heart conditions

Armpit (axillary temperature)

An axillary temperature is measured by placing the thermometer under the person's arm and then having the person hold his arm close to his body. The axillary method provides the least reliable measurement of body temperature, but if the oral and rectal methods are not safe, and a tympanic or temporal thermometer is not available, then the axillary method can be used. The axillary temperature may be taken using a glass thermometer or an electronic thermometer (Procedure 22-3). If the person has just washed under her arms, or applied deodorant or antiperspirant, then you must wait for at least 15 minutes before taking the axillary temperature. Also, if the person has recently had chest or breast surgery, and it is necessary to take the person's temperature using the axillary method, then the thermometer should be placed on the unaffected side of the body.

Ear (tympanic temperature)

Because a tympanic thermometer measures the temperature of the blood in the small vessels in the eardrum, the temperature it gives is very accurate. Because the tympanic method allows the temperature to be measured in a safe, quick, and relatively painless manner, it is often a good choice for residents with dementia who are comfortable having the thermometer placed in the ear. Procedure 22-4 describes how to take a tympanic temperature.

Forehead (temporal temperature)

A temporal artery thermometer is swept across a person's forehead to obtain a body temperature measurement.

NORMAL AND ABNORMAL FINDINGS

The normal body temperature varies slightly from person to person. In fact, a person's normal body temperature may be anywhere from 0.5°F to 1°F

Table 22-1	Normal Adult Temperature Ranges	
METHOD USED TO OBTAIN TEMPERATURE	**FAHRENHEIT (°F)**	**CELSIUS (°C)**
Oral	97.6 to 99.6	36.5 to 37.5
Rectal	98.6 to 100.6	37 to 38.1
Axillary	96.6 to 98.6	36 to 37
Tympanic	98.6	37
Temporal	98.6	37

higher or lower than the range generally considered normal. The normal range also varies according to what method is used to measure the body temperature (Table 22-1).

A person who has an increased body temperature is said to have a fever, or be **febrile.** Fever is a common finding with illness and is the body's normal response to infection. However, an elderly person's temperature may actually decrease, or only slightly increase, in response to illness or infection. For this reason, even a very slight change in an older person's temperature should be reported to the nurse.

TELL THE NURSE ❗

Changes in a person's temperature can be a sign that something is wrong. Be sure to report the following observations to the nurse immediately:

- The person's temperature is higher than normal

- The person's temperature is lower than normal

- You have difficulty taking or reading the person's temperature

PULSE

Each time the heart beats, it sends a wave, or **pulse,** of blood through the arteries. The arteries are the blood vessels that carry oxygen-containing blood away from the heart to all of the tissues of the body. The pulse, a throbbing sensation just underneath the skin, can be felt (palpated) by placing your fingers gently over an artery that runs close to the surface of the skin, such as the carotid artery in the neck or the radial artery in the wrist (Fig. 22-8). Although we can only feel

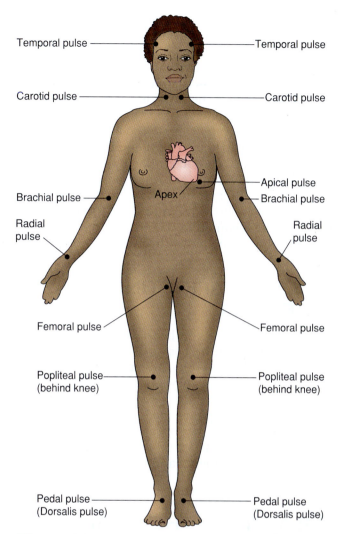

Figure 22-8
The pulse points are places where the arteries run close to the surface of the skin, allowing the pulse to be felt. When taking a person's pulse, it is common to place your fingers on the radial artery (in the wrist). An apical pulse can be taken by placing a stethoscope on the person's chest, over the apex of the heart.

the pulse in a few of the body's arteries (those that run closest to the surface of the skin), all of the arteries in the body have a pulse. The pulse tells us many things:

- By feeling for and counting the pulse, we are able to measure the **pulse rate,** or the number of pulsations that can be felt in 1 minute. The pulse rate tells us the heart rate, or how fast the heart is beating.

- In addition to measuring the pulse rate, we can detect the **pulse rhythm,** or the pattern of the pulsations and the pauses between them. Normally, the pulse rhythm is smooth and regular, with the same amount of time in between each pulsation. In other words, the heart is beating at regular intervals. An irregular pulse rhythm is called a **dysrhythmia** (*dys-* means "bad" or "difficult"), and indicates that the heart is beating in an irregular manner.

- Finally, we can evaluate the force or quality of the pulse, known as the **pulse amplitude** or the pulse character. Each pulsation should be strong, and easy to feel. Pulses that are difficult to feel may be described as "weak" or "thready." A weak or thready pulse usually means that the heart is having trouble circulating blood throughout the body.

FACTORS AFFECTING THE PULSE

The rate at which the heart beats is controlled automatically by the body's central nervous system. When the nervous system senses that the tissues need more oxygen and nutrients (for example, when a person is exercising), it increases the heart rate so that blood reaches the tissues faster. A person's heart rate will also increase during times of anger and anxiety, illness, pain, fever, and excitement, and when taking certain medications.

MEASURING THE PULSE

Radial Pulse

One common way of measuring the pulse rate is by placing the middle two or three fingers over the radial artery, which is located on the inside of the wrist, and counting the number of pulses that occur in either 30 seconds or 1 minute. The thumb is not used to palpate the artery because the thumb has its own pulse. You may end up counting your own pulse if you mistake the sensation you feel in your thumb for the resident's pulse! Although the pulse may be taken at other pulse points, taking the pulse at the radial artery is easiest for the resident. The carotid or femoral arteries may be used to assess the pulse during an emergency situation when cardiopulmonary resuscitation (CPR) is being administered. Procedure 22-5 describes how to take a radial pulse.

Apical Pulse

The apical pulse is measured by listening (auscultating) over the apex of the heart with a stetho-

scope. The apex of the heart (that is, the lower tip of the heart) is located approximately 2 inches below the level of the left nipple (Fig. 22-8). An apical pulse is taken when a person has a weak or irregular pulse that may be difficult to feel in the radial artery. An apical pulse may also be used to measure the heart rate in people with known heart disease, and before administering certain medications for heart conditions.

A **stethoscope,** a device that makes sound louder and transfers it to the listener's ears, is used to take an apical pulse. The stethoscope allows you to hear, rather than feel, each beat of the person's heart. The stethoscope has the following parts (Fig. 22-9):

- Earpieces, which are placed in your ears
- A brace and binaurals, which connect the earpieces to the rubber or plastic tubing that conducts the sound

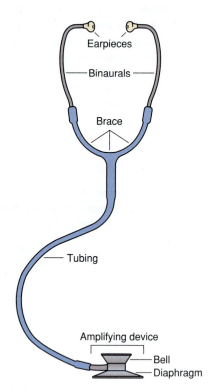

Figure 22-9

A stethoscope is used to listen to the heartbeat (when taking an apical pulse) or blood moving through the arteries (when taking a blood pressure). The sound is made louder by the amplifying device and transmitted by the rubber tubing to the earpieces, which fit snugly in the user's ear canals. The brace and binaurals, which are usually made of metal, connect the rubber or plastic tubing to the earpieces and prevent it from twisting or kinking, which could distort the sound. The rubber or plastic tubing may be single (as shown) or double.

- An amplifying device, which makes the sound louder

The amplifying device, which is the part of the stethoscope that is placed against the person's skin, is usually two-sided. One side, called the **diaphragm,** is a large flat surface that is used to hear loud, harsh sounds like an apical pulse, blood rushing through the arteries, or respiratory sounds. The other side, called the **bell,** is a small rounded surface that is designed to pick up faint sounds like heart murmurs or difficult-to-hear blood pressures. The amplifying device rotates so that the sound comes from either the diaphragm or the bell, but not both at the same time.

Before using a stethoscope, clean both the earpieces and the diaphragm or bell by wiping them with alcohol wipes. Place the earpieces in each ear canal. You will know that the earpieces are placed correctly when they fit snugly, yet comfortably, and block out any outside sound. Next, tap lightly on the diaphragm. You should be able to hear the tapping. If you cannot hear the tapping, rotate the amplifying device and tap again. When you can hear the tapping, you are ready to go! Procedure 22-6 describes how to take an apical pulse using a stethoscope.

When taking an apical pulse, the stethoscope must be placed under the person's clothing, directly on the person's skin. Be sure to protect the person's modesty during the procedure. Pull the privacy curtain, or, if the person is not in his room, take him to a private place before proceeding with the procedure.

The apical pulse rate and the radial pulse rate should be the same in any single person. Occasionally, however, the heart does not pump strongly enough to send enough blood through the arteries with each beat. This means that while each beat of the heart may be heard over the apex of the heart using a stethoscope, it may not be felt in the wrist. This difference between the apical pulse rate and the radial pulse rate is known as the **pulse deficit.** The pulse deficit is measured by having one member of the nursing team take the person's apical pulse while another team member takes the person's radial pulse. The two counts are then compared to determine the pulse deficit. For example, if the apical pulse is 84 beats/min and the radial pulse is 80 beats/min, the difference between the apical pulse and the radial pulse (that is, the pulse deficit) is 4 beats/min (84 – 80 = 4). The apical pulse rate will always be higher than the radial pulse rate, because it is easier to hear a heartbeat at the source than to feel it.

NORMAL AND ABNORMAL FINDINGS

The accepted normal pulse rate for an adult is 60 to 100 beats/min. **Tachycardia** is a rapid heart rate, or a pulse rate of more than 100 beats/min for an adult (*tachy-* means "fast" and *cardia* means "heart"). A heart rate that is slower than normal (that is, a pulse rate of less than 60 beats/min in an adult) is called **bradycardia** (*brady-* means "slow"). Certain illnesses, conditions, and medications can cause tachycardia or bradycardia.

TELL THE NURSE

Changes in a person's pulse rate, rhythm, or amplitude can be a sign that something is wrong. Be sure to report the following observations to the nurse immediately:

- The person's pulse rate is higher than normal
- The person's pulse rate is lower than normal
- The person's pulse rhythm is irregular
- The person's pulse is weak or "thready"
- You have difficulty taking the person's pulse

RESPIRATION

Respiration is the process of breathing. To live, we must have oxygen. We must also get rid of waste products that are created as a result of normal cellular function (metabolism). One of these waste products is carbon dioxide.

When we inhale, we take oxygen-containing air into the body. Once in the lungs, the oxygen in the air passes across a thin membrane into the bloodstream, where it is carried by the red blood cells to all of the cells in the body by the action of the heart, which pumps the oxygen-rich blood throughout the body. As the body's cells use the oxygen and nutrients delivered to them by the blood, they give off carbon dioxide, which the blood takes back to the lungs. There, the carbon dioxide crosses the same thin membrane, moving from the blood into the air still remaining in the lungs. When we exhale, we breathe out the carbon dioxide in the lungs. So, the process of breathing performs two vital functions—it brings oxygen, a substance necessary for life, into the body, and it removes carbon dioxide, a waste product that is not necessary for life, from the body.

During the **inhalation (inspiration)** phase of respiration, the chest expands (rises) as air is brought into the lungs. During the **exhalation (expiration)** phase of respiration, the chest deflates (falls) as air moves out of the lungs. When we measure a person's respirations, we look at the person's:

- **Respiratory rate,** or the number of times the person breathes in 1 minute (one breath is both an inhalation and an exhalation)
- **Respiratory rhythm,** or the regularity with which the person breathes
- **Depth of respiration,** or the quality of each breath (for example, is it deep or shallow?)

We also listen for any abnormal sounds, such as wheezing or congestion.

FACTORS AFFECTING RESPIRATION

As with other vital functions, the process of breathing is controlled mainly by the central nervous system, in a part of the brain called the medulla. Control centers, called chemoreceptors, are located in the medulla and in some of the major arteries. These control centers monitor the carbon dioxide and oxygen content of the blood and adjust the rate and depth of breathing accordingly. For example, exercise increases the body's use of oxygen as well as its production of carbon dioxide and will increase both the rate and depth of a person's respirations. Other factors that may affect respiration rate, depth, and regularity include anxiety, pain, fear, fever, infections and diseases of the heart and lungs, stroke or head injury, and certain medications.

In addition to being controlled automatically by the nervous system, breathing can also be controlled to a certain extent by the individual (for example, when we "hold our breath" while swimming). In this respect, breathing is different from the other vital signs.

MEASURING RESPIRATION

The respiratory rate is easily determined by watching the rise and fall of a person's chest and counting the number of breaths that occur in either 30 seconds or 1 minute. (Remember that one breath consists of both an inhalation and an exhalation.) Usually, the rise and fall of the chest can be easily observed by standing beside the person, or by watching her back. In some situations, you may need to stand slightly behind the person while she is seated and look down at her chest to detect the movement. Or, you can place your hand near the person's collarbone or on the person's side to feel her breathing if the rise and fall of the chest is not easily seen. Some older adults use their abdominal muscles to assist with breathing. In these people, breathing can be easily seen by watching the abdomen move instead of the chest.

Because a person can consciously control her respirations if she is aware that she is being observed, a more accurate measurement may be obtained if you measure the respiratory rate right after you take the person's pulse, with your fingers still on the person's wrist as if you were still counting the pulse. It is also easy to count a person's respirations while she sleeps, before you have awakened her to measure other vital signs. This is the one instance where it is acceptable to carry out a task without telling the resident exactly what you are doing! Procedure 22-7 describes how to measure a person's respiratory rate.

NORMAL AND ABNORMAL FINDINGS

In an adult, the normal respiratory rate is 16 to 20 breaths/min. A normal respiratory rate is called **eupnea.** (The prefix *eu-* means "good" and the suffix *-pnea* means "breathing.") A respiratory rate that is higher than normal (greater than 24 breaths/min in an adult) is called **tachypnea,** while a respiratory rate that is lower than normal (less than 10 breaths/min in an adult) is called **bradypnea.** (Recall that *tachy-* means "fast," and *brady-* means "slow.")

Normally, the chest should rise and fall evenly, in a regular rhythm. Breathing should be quiet and easy. Labored or difficult respirations are termed **dyspnea** (recall that *dys-* means "bad" or "difficult"). Other notable respiratory patterns are **hyperventilation** (increased rate and depth of breathing) and **hypoventilation** (decreased rate and depth of breathing).

TELL THE NURSE ❗

Changes in a person's respiratory rate, respiratory rhythm, or depth of respirations can be a sign that something is wrong. Be sure to report the following observations to the nurse immediately:

- The person's respiratory rate is greater than 24 breaths/min

- The person's respiratory rate is less than 10 breaths/min

- The person's respiratory rhythm is irregular

- The person's breaths are either very deep or very shallow

- The person's breathing is difficult or painful

- The person's chest does not rise equally on both sides

- The person's respirations are noisy, with wheezing sounds or congestion

BLOOD PRESSURE

The force of the blood pushing against the arterial walls is known as the **blood pressure.** There are two pressure levels that are measured when taking a person's blood pressure measurement. The first, known as the **systolic pressure,** is the pressure that is caused by the blood when the heart muscle contracts, sending a wave of blood through the artery. The second, known as the **diastolic pressure,** occurs when the heart muscle relaxes. Although the heart is relaxed, there is still pressure as the blood flows through the arteries.

Blood pressure is measured in millimeters of mercury (mm Hg) and is recorded as a fraction. The systolic pressure, which is higher, is recorded first, followed by the diastolic pressure, which is lower. For instance, if a person's systolic measurement is 110 mm Hg and his diastolic measurement is 72 mm Hg, then the blood pressure would be recorded as 110/72 mm Hg. The difference between the systolic and diastolic pressures is known as the **pulse pressure,** which in this case would be 38 mm Hg (110 − 72 = 38).

Blood pressure is considered a vital sign because it gives us important information about a person's health and risk for disease. Adequate blood pressure is necessary to keep blood flow constant to all of the tissues of the body. A blood pressure that is too low is a bad sign because it means the tissues of the body are not receiving enough oxygen and nutrients. On the other hand, a blood pressure that is too high forces the heart to do extra work, which, over time, damages the heart. High blood pressure also places stress on the kidneys, which can lead to kidney failure, and the blood vessels, which can lead to stroke. Blood pressure measurements allow health care workers to monitor existing problems and possibly prevent future ones.

For some residents, you may be asked to take **orthostatic blood pressures** (a series of blood pressure measurements, usually taken first with the person lying down, then sitting, then standing). Facility policy will state the order of the blood pressure measurements when a series of measurements is needed. The health care team uses orthostatic blood pressure measurements to evaluate how well the person's body adapts to changes in position, and to assess the person's risk for falling.

FACTORS AFFECTING BLOOD PRESSURE

The pressure that the blood puts on the arterial walls is controlled by three factors:

- **Cardiac output.** The cardiac output is the amount of blood that the heart is able to pump with each beat. If the heart is able to pump more blood into the vessel with each beat, then blood flow increases, leading to an increase in blood pressure. On the other hand, if the cardiac output is weak, then blood flow decreases, leading to a decrease in blood pressure.

- **Blood volume.** The amount of blood in the vessels at any given time influences the blood pressure. If the blood volume is low, for example, as a result of dehydration (see Chapter 25) or hemorrhage (see Chapter 19), then the blood pressure will decrease. Similarly, an increase in blood volume leads to an increase in blood pressure. In some people, a salty meal is enough to increase blood pressure, because the salt causes the body to store water, which increases the blood volume.

- **Resistance to blood flow.** Resistance is how hard it is for the blood to flow through the vessels. If the vessels are narrowed (for example, as a result of arteriosclerosis ["hardening of the arteries"]), then the resistance will be high and so will the blood pressure. Resistance is also increased when the blood is thick.

Blood pressure is also influenced by certain factors that we cannot do anything about, such as age, gender, and race:

- **Age.** Young people tend to have lower blood pressures than older people. Aging causes a decrease in the elasticity of the blood vessels (that is, the blood vessels' ability to stretch and bounce back as the blood pulses through). Decreased elasticity results in increased resistance and a higher blood pressure.

- **Gender.** Women tend to have lower blood pressures than men.
- **Race.** People of certain races (for example, African Americans) tend to have higher blood pressures than people of other races.

MEASURING BLOOD PRESSURE

Manual Sphygmomanometers

Measuring and recording a person's blood pressure is a routine task for nursing assistants. There are many ways to measure a person's blood pressure. The most common method is by using a manual **sphygmomanometer** and a stethoscope. (*Sphygmo-* is from the Greek word for "pulse," and *-manometer* means "a flat instrument used to measure pressure.") A manual sphygmomanometer consists of:

- A cuff (a flat, cloth-covered inflatable pouch)
- A bulb, which is squeezed or pumped to fill the cuff with air
- A manometer (the device that measures the air pressure in the inflatable pouch)

Cuffs come in various sizes. The cuff must fit the person properly, or the blood pressure measurement will not be accurate. To find out what size cuff to use, measure around the person's upper arm, halfway between his elbow and shoulder. Cuff sizes are given in Table 22-2.

Two tubes are attached to the pouch within the cuff—one is attached to the bulb used to inflate the pouch, and the other is attached to the manometer. The manometer may be either aneroid or mercury (Fig. 22-10). An aneroid manometer is a small, round dial with a needle that indicates the pressure. A mercury manometer is a column of mercury that may be mounted on a wall or placed on a table. The manometer measures the pressure of the air in the cuff in millimeters of mercury (mm Hg). Long dashes mark increments of 10 mm Hg and the short dashes in between mark increments of 2 mm Hg.

The most common place to measure a person's blood pressure is in the brachial artery of the upper arm. However, the popliteal artery (which can be felt at the back of the person's knee) can be used as well. Measuring a blood pressure is quite simple, once you have had some

Table 22-2	Blood Pressure Cuff Sizes
ARM MEASUREMENT (cm)	**NAME OF CUFF TO USE**
13 to 20	Child
24 to 32	Adult
32 to 42	Large Adult
42 to 50	Thigh

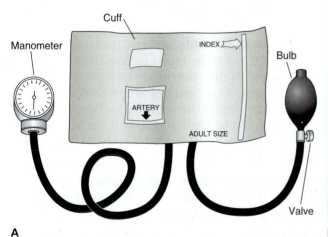
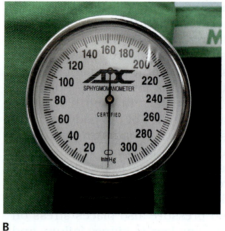
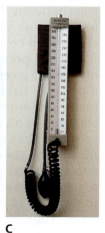

Figure 22-10
(A) A manual sphygmomanometer consists of a cuff, a bulb, and a manometer. The manometer may be either aneroid or mercury. The tubes attach the inflatable pouch inside the cuff to the bulb and to the manometer. **(B)** An aneroid manometer. **(C)** A mercury manometer.

practice. The cuff is wrapped around the person's upper arm where the brachial artery is located. You can feel the brachial artery pulse in the antecubital space (the inner bend of the elbow) by straightening the person's arm and placing your fingers across the inside of the joint. After positioning the cuff, place the diaphragm of your stethoscope directly over where you felt the brachial artery in the antecubital space, and close the valve on the pumping bulb by turning it clockwise. Do not close the valve too tightly, or it will be difficult to release the air when you are ready. As you pump the bulb, air will enter the pouch in the cuff and you will see the needle (on an aneroid manometer) or the column of mercury (on a mercury manometer) move, indicating that the pressure of the air in the cuff is increasing.

Remember that you have two pressures that are measured within an artery, the systolic pressure (when the heart pumps) and the diastolic pressure (when the heart relaxes). When the pressure within the cuff becomes higher than the systolic pressure in the artery, it will cut off the circulation and not allow any blood to flow through the brachial artery past the cuff. Continue pumping the bulb until the pressure in the cuff is 30 mm Hg higher than the systolic pressure. There are two ways to do this:

- Place the stethoscope over the brachial artery, and inflate the cuff slowly. After you have inflated the cuff a bit, you will start to hear the pulse through your stethoscope. Continue inflating the cuff until you hear the pulse stop (this is the person's systolic pressure) and continue inflating the cuff 30 mm Hg more.
- Or, with your fingers on the person's radial pulse, you can inflate the cuff until you no longer can feel the pulse. The reading on the manometer will indicate the person's systolic pressure. Continue inflating the cuff 30 mm Hg more.

When the pressure in the cuff is 30 mm Hg higher than the systolic pressure, open the valve slightly (by turning it counter clockwise). Opening the valve slightly allows the slow release of air from the cuff, which lowers the pressure in the cuff. Under normal conditions, you may not be able to hear the brachial pulse, but under pressure, you will be able to hear the pulse through the stethoscope. As the pressure in the cuff falls (as indicated by the needle on the aneroid dial or the column of mercury), you listen for sounds, called **Korotkoff sounds** (Box 22-1), through the stethoscope. When the pressure in the cuff is equal to or slightly lower than the systolic pressure in the

---

BOX 22-1 Korotkoff Sounds

In some people, you will only be able to hear the beginning and ending sounds while auscultating the blood pressure, but in others, all of these sounds will be distinct.

Phase I: Faint but clear tapping sounds that gradually become louder. The first tapping sound is the systolic pressure.
Phase II: Muffled or swishing sounds that may actually disappear if a person has significant hypertension.
Phase III: Distinct, loud tapping sounds as the blood begins to flow more freely through the artery.
Phase IV: The sound may abruptly become muffled and soft. Keep listening.*
Phase V: The last sound heard before a period of continuous silence. This is the diastolic pressure.

---

*Occasionally, the tapping sounds of the pulse will be heard all the way down to zero. In this case, listening for the abrupt softening of phase IV will give you an approximate diastolic reading.

---

artery, blood will suddenly begin to flow through the brachial artery and you will start hearing the pulse. When you hear the first sound of the pulse, note the reading on the manometer. This is your systolic pressure. Now, continue to listen to the pulse. When the pressure inside the cuff is less than the lowest arterial pressure, or diastolic pressure, the sound of the pulse will stop, because the artery is no longer under pressure. The last sound that you hear is the diastolic pressure, and is shown by the reading on the manometer.

Procedure 22-8 summarizes how to take a blood pressure. Guidelines for taking a blood pressure are given in Guidelines Box 22-1. Learning to take blood pressures takes time and practice. At first, you will need to concentrate on how to operate the equipment and control the rate at which the air leaves the cuff. Next, you will need to become familiar with the sounds that you will hear as the cuff deflates, and learn to recognize the beginning and ending sounds. Each person's blood pressure will sound slightly different. In some people, the blood pressure is easy to measure. In others, measuring the blood pressure will challenge even the most experienced nursing assistant. A good rule of thumb is if a person's brachial or radial pulse feels stronger in one arm over the other, you will have an easier time taking the blood pressure in the arm with

Guidelines Box 22-1 Guidelines for Taking a Person's Blood Pressure

WHAT YOU DO	WHY YOU DO IT
Allow the person time to relax prior to taking the blood pressure.	Recent exercise and emotions (such as fear) can cause a blood pressure reading to be falsely elevated.
Make sure the manometer is properly calibrated (that is, it reads "0" when there is no air in the cuff).	A manometer that is not properly calibrated will not give an accurate pressure reading.
Use a cuff that is properly sized for the resident.	A cuff that does not fit will not allow you to accurately measure the person's blood pressure. A cuff that is too small will result in a high reading, while a cuff that is too large will result in a low reading.
Make sure the cuff fits snugly around the person's arm before inflating it.	A cuff that is too loose can cause the skin to "pinch" under the cuff when the cuff is inflated, damaging the skin.
Do not place the cuff over a person's clothing.	Clothing will distort the Korotkoff sounds.
Do not take a blood pressure on an arm where an intravenous (IV) line is placed, or on an arm that is injured or in a cast.	Inflating the cuff can cause pain and swelling, and it may dislodge an IV line if one is present.
In a person who has had a mastectomy, do not take a blood pressure on the arm that is on the same side of the body as the breast that was removed.	Some people who have mastectomies also have the lymph nodes in the armpit removed, which disrupts fluid flow from the tissues in the hand and lower arm. This can lead to an inaccurate blood pressure reading.
Do not partially deflate the cuff and then reinflate it while taking a blood pressure measurement. If you make a mistake, release all of the air from the cuff and wait at least 30 seconds before trying again.	Partially deflating and then reinflating the cuff is uncomfortable for the resident, and it will result in an inaccurate reading.
If you are unable to hear the Korotkoff sounds, make sure the room is quiet and check your equipment: ● Make sure the diaphragm of the stethoscope is active by gently tapping on it. ● Make sure the diaphragm of the stethoscope is placed directly over the brachial pulse. ● Make sure the earpieces of the stethoscope are seated properly in your ears.	Most difficulties with measuring blood pressure result from operator error. However, if you have checked your equipment and you still cannot hear the Korotkoff sounds, notify the nurse immediately. The person may have severe hypotension.

the stronger pulse. Do not get discouraged if taking blood pressures is difficult at first. The more you practice, the more competent and confident you will become. As with any skill you will learn, if you have difficulty taking a person's blood pressure or if you are unsure of a reading you get, always ask for a second opinion or help from another nursing assistant or a nurse. Your responsibility to the people you care for takes priority over your pride.

Automated Sphygmomanometers

Your facility may use automated (electronic) sphygmomanometers instead of manual ones. Some automated models feature automatic inflation and deflation of the cuff, while others require the cuff to be manually inflated but will deflate it automatically. The blood pressure is displayed digitally.

NORMAL AND ABNORMAL FINDINGS

In an adult, the normal blood pressure range is 100 to 140 mm Hg systolic and 60 to 90 mm Hg diastolic. Normally, a person's blood pressure moves up and down within the range of normal during the course of a day. For example:

- Blood pressure readings are usually lowest in the morning, and can increase by as much as 10 mm Hg later in the day.
- Blood pressure is generally lower when a person is lying down, as compared to when he is sitting or standing.
- Blood pressure readings are usually slightly higher after a meal, especially a meal with a high salt content.
- Exercise will temporarily increase the systolic blood pressure.
- Stress, anxiety, fear, and pain will also temporarily raise a person's blood pressure.

When you are taking a person's blood pressure, it is important to allow that person time to relax or rest for a bit so that the blood pressure reading reflects the person's normal pressure, and not the changes that can occur from exertion or being emotionally upset. Also, as a nursing assistant, you must learn to recognize the range of blood pressure measurements that can be considered "normal" for each of your residents so that you will be able to recognize any changes. A person's blood pressure could rise or fall 20 to 30 mm Hg and still be within the range of what is considered normal for that person. However, a change in a person's blood pressure that is that large should be recognized and reported immediately to the nurse.

TELL THE NURSE !

Changes in a person's blood pressure can be a sign that something is wrong. Be sure to report the following observations to the nurse immediately:

- The person's blood pressure is higher than normal
- The person's blood pressure is lower than normal
- You have difficulty measuring the person's blood pressure

Hypertension

If an adult has a blood pressure that is consistently higher than 140 mm Hg (systolic) and/or 90 mm Hg (diastolic), then that person is said to have **hypertension** (high blood pressure). To diagnose a person with hypertension and start treatment for this condition, the person's blood pressure measurements must be taken and recorded over a period of time to show a pattern of constant elevation. Medications that are taken for hypertension should be taken as ordered. If the person stops taking the medication or does not take it according to the prescribed schedule, the person's hypertension will usually return. Hypertension is often called the "silent killer" because a person with this condition does not feel ill, yet is at great risk for complications (and possibly even death) as a result of it.

Hypotension

An adult who has a blood pressure that is consistently lower than 90 mm Hg (systolic) and/or 60 mm Hg (diastolic) is said to have **hypotension** (low blood pressure). Some people may have **orthostatic hypotension,** which is a sudden decrease in blood pressure that occurs when a person stands up from a sitting or lying position. When a person is sitting or lying down, the heart does not need to work as hard to pump blood throughout the body and the blood vessels are relaxed, so resistance is low. However, when the person stands up, the body needs to make up for the change in position. The heart pumps harder and the vessels constrict to bring the blood pressure back up to a normal level.

Until the body manages to make up for the sudden change in position, the person may feel lightheaded and faint. Some medications and aging can increase the time the body needs to adjust. The lack of blood flow to the brain can cause the person to feel dizzy. This is why, when you are assisting a person to "dangle" (see Chapter 20), you must give the person a minute to adjust before proceeding. Always remind your residents to first sit for a moment before standing up, to allow time for the body to adjust. Helping a person who experiences orthostatic hypotension to remember to take those extra few moments for the body to adjust can help prevent a fall.

HEIGHT AND WEIGHT

Although height and weight are not technically vital signs, these measurements are taken periodically while a person is receiving care. The relationship of a person's weight to his height can provide insight into the person's overall health and nutritional status. In some cases, a change in a person's height or weight can indicate that a person's condition is getting worse, or that it is getting better. For these reasons, it is useful to obtain a "baseline" height and weight for each resident, and to measure the resident's height and weight periodically thereafter.

A resident's height is measured on admission, and each time the Minimum Data Set (MDS) is completed for an annual assessment or to assess a significant change in the resident's condition. Although you might think that an adult's height would stay the same, some older people may actually lose height in the presence of bone disease, such as osteoporosis. A resident's weight is measured on admission and at regular intervals throughout the resident's stay in the long-term care facility. A resident's weight is rechecked periodically for various reasons:

- Weight is an indicator of nutritional status.
- Weight is an indicator of heart and kidney function. If the heart or kidneys are not functioning well, the person will retain fluid, which will cause an increase in weight.
- Changes in weight can be a sign of disease. For example, one of the signs of some types of cancer is major, unexplained weight loss. Unexplained weight loss can also be a sign of undiagnosed or poorly controlled diabetes.
- Some medications are prescribed according to body weight. If a person gains or loses a great deal of weight, it may be necessary to adjust the person's medication dosages.

MEASURING HEIGHT AND WEIGHT

Height is measured in feet (') and inches (") or in centimeters (cm). Weight is measured in pounds (lbs) or kilograms (kg).

The type of scale you will use to measure a person's weight will depend on the person's ability to get out of bed and stand. Common types of scales include upright scales, chair scales, and sling scales.

Scales may be mechanical or digital. If you are using a mechanical scale to measure a person's weight, you must slide weights along a bar by hand until the bar is balanced (Fig. 22-11). If

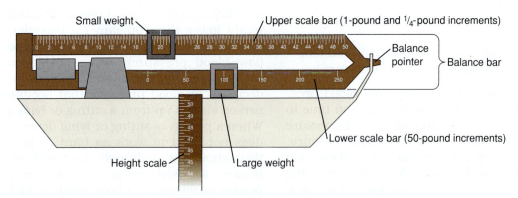

Figure 22-11

A mechanical scale. The *balance bar* has two scale bars and two weights. The *large weight* slides along the *lower scale bar*, which is marked off in 50-pound increments. The *small weight* slides along the *upper scale bar*, which is marked off in quarter-pound and pound increments. The *balance pointer* is centered between the two scale bars when the weight on the scale bars equals the person's weight.

Guidelines Box 22-2   Guidelines for Measuring Weight

WHAT YOU DO	WHY YOU DO IT
Know the person's previous weight before measuring the new weight.	If you know the person's previous weight, you will be able to recognize immediately if there is a significant change. This will allow you to remeasure the weight to check for accuracy right away. If you get the same weight again, you will be able to report the change to the nurse more promptly.
Have the person wear approximately the same amount of clothing each time he or she is weighed.	Clothing can make a difference in the person's weight measurement (for example, a sweat suit and tennis shoes weigh more than a nightgown and slippers). Weighing the person in the same amount of clothing each time results in more consistent measurements. Consistency helps the nurse properly evaluate changes in the person's weight.
Weigh the person at approximately the same time of day each time you measure the person's weight.	A person's weight can change throughout the day. Weighing the person at approximately the same time of day each time results in more consistent measurements. Consistency helps the nurse properly evaluate changes in the person's weight.
Weigh the person using the same scale each time.	Different scales may result in different weights. Using the same scale for the person each time results in more consistent measurements. Consistency helps the nurse properly evaluate changes in the person's weight.
Make sure that the scale is balanced to "0" before measuring the person's weight.	A scale that is not balanced to "0" will not give an accurate weight.
Use the correct type of scale to weigh the person.	If the person requires the use of a specific scale for safety reasons, use of a different scale could result in injury to the person.

you are using a digital scale, you simply turn the scale on. The digital scale measures the person's weight automatically and displays it on a screen. Guidelines for measuring a person's weight are given in Guidelines Box 22-2.

Measuring Height and Weight Using an Upright Scale

An upright scale is used to obtain height and weight measurements for a person who is able to stand on her own. Procedure 22-9 describes how to use an upright scale to measure a person's height and weight.

Measuring Weight Using a Chair Scale

A chair scale (Fig. 22-12) is used to obtain a weight measurement for a person who cannot stand independently, but is able to get out of bed. One type of chair scale is for use with a wheelchair. The wheelchair is first weighed without the

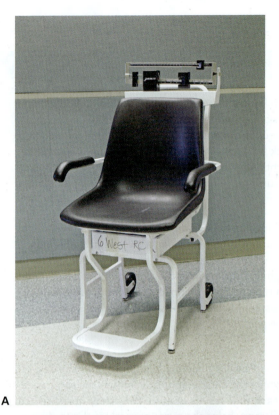

A

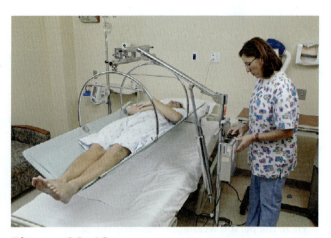

Figure 22-13
A sling scale is used to obtain weight measurements for a person who cannot get out of bed.

person in it to determine its weight. Next, the wheelchair, with the person in it, is rolled onto the scale. The weight of the empty wheelchair is subtracted from the weight of the wheelchair with the person in it to determine the person's weight. The other type of chair scale is simply a chair-like device that allows the person to sit while having his weight measured. Procedure 22-10 describes how to use a chair scale.

Measuring Height and Weight Using a Tape Measure and a Sling Scale

If a person is unable to get out of bed at all, the person will have to be weighed in bed. Some facilities have beds with built-in scales. If this type of bed is not available where you work, then you will have to weigh the person using a sling scale (Fig. 22-13). The person's height is measured using a tape measure. Procedure 22-11 describes how to obtain height and weight measurements using a tape measure and a sling scale. Because sling scales from different manufacturers may vary greatly in their procedures for use, do not attempt to use a sling scale unless you have been trained in its use.

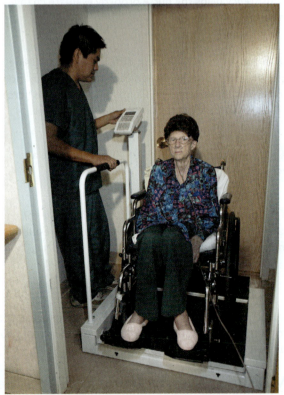

B

Figure 22-12
A chair scale is used to obtain weight measurements for a person who cannot stand up independently but is able to get out of bed. **(A)** A chair scale. **(B)** A chair scale for use with a wheelchair.

Caring For Those With Dementia

Measuring the vital signs of a person who has dementia can be very challenging. The changes that occur in the brain may make it difficult for the person to understand what you are trying to do, or why you need to do it. The person may feel that you are invading his personal space by touching him, and become upset. Having a thermometer inserted in the mouth (or worse yet, the rectum!) can also be very upsetting for a person with dementia, causing the person to react with resistance or aggression. To make these procedures less threatening for your residents with dementia:

- Take some time to talk with the person before beginning the procedure to help him feel more comfortable with you.

- Explain exactly what you need to do, and how you need to do it. Asking the person "Will you let me...?" instead of saying "I need to...." can help you to gain the person's cooperation.

- Be sure to provide for privacy during the procedure.

- Use distraction techniques as appropriate to take the person's attention away from what you are doing.

For example, giving the person a favorite item to hold may be enough to distract his attention away from the procedure. Sometimes, having another nursing assistant distract the person while you perform the procedure can be helpful. However, it is important to avoid making the person feel like he is being outnumbered by staff members.

- Try to use newer equipment featuring more advanced technology, when possible. Newer equipment is often faster and less invasive.

- If possible, try to count respirations before approaching the person, so that the person is unaware of what you are doing. The person's respirations may increase if he becomes upset by your presence.

- You may be able to count the person's pulse by gently holding the person's wrist in a comforting way, without the person being aware of what you are doing.

- If the person becomes upset, report your difficulty to the nurse and try again later. Do not persist if the person is resistant or combative.

SUMMARY

- Vital signs provide essential information about a person's health.
  - The vital signs are body temperature, pulse, respirations, and blood pressure. A person's height and weight, although not technically vital signs, also provide insight into a person's overall health.
  - Measuring and recording vital signs is a routine part of a nursing assistant's daily duties.
    - Vital signs must be measured and recorded accurately because many people rely on this information to make decisions about the person's care. In addition, a change in vital signs can be an important early sign that something is wrong.
    - Nursing assistants must be familiar with accepted normal ranges for all of the vital signs. In addition, nursing assistants must come to recognize what is "normal" for each of the residents in their care.
    - Learning the skills associated with taking vital signs takes practice. With practice, comes confidence.

- Body temperature is a measure of how hot the body is.
  - The body temperature can be measured using a number of devices in a number of places.
    - Types of thermometers include glass (mercury) thermometers, electronic thermometers, tympanic thermometers, and temporal artery thermometers.
    - A person's temperature may be measured in the mouth, rectum, ear, armpit, or forehead.
  - A temperature that is higher or lower than normal may be a sign of infection in an elderly person. Changes in the environmental temperature can also affect a person's body temperature.
- The pulse reflects the rate, rhythm, and strength of the heartbeat, and therefore is a vital sign.
  - The pulse can be measured by feeling the radial artery (in the wrist) or by listening to the apical pulse (in the chest) with a stethoscope.

- Tachycardia is an excessively rapid heartbeat. Bradycardia is an excessively slow heartbeat.
- The respiratory rate, rhythm, and depth are a reflection of how well the person is breathing.
  - The respiratory rate is measured by counting the number of times the person inhales and exhales in 30 seconds (or 1 minute, if the respirations are irregular).
    - The chest rises with each inhalation and falls with each exhalation.
    - One respiration = one inhalation + one exhalation.
  - Dyspnea is labored breathing. Tachypnea is a respiratory rate that is too fast, and bradypnea is a respiratory rate that is too slow.
- The blood pressure reflects the force the blood exerts against the arterial walls. Cardiac output, blood volume, and resistance affect the blood pressure.
  - Blood pressure is most often measured in the brachial artery using a sphygmomanometer and a stethoscope.
  - Korotkoff sounds are the sounds the blood makes as it rushes through the artery.
    - Phase I Korotkoff sounds signal the systolic pressure, or the pressure when the heart beats.

- Phase V Korotkoff sounds signal the diastolic pressure, or the pressure when the heart relaxes.
- Listening for and interpreting the Korotkoff sounds takes practice.
- Hypertension, or a consistently high blood pressure, can have serious long-term consequences if not treated.
- Orthostatic hypotension, or low blood pressure on changing positions, affects many people and is the reason people are encouraged to sit for a minute before standing up from a lying position.
- Height and weight are measured when a person enters a long-term care facility, and at regular intervals throughout the person's stay.
  - Significant weight loss or gain can be an early sign of disease. In addition, some medication dosages are calculated according to a person's body weight.
  - A variety of devices, including upright scales, chair scales, and sling scales, can be used to measure a person's weight, depending on the person's situation.
  - Following your facility's policies and procedures when weighing a resident helps to ensure accurate measurements and helps to keep the resident safe.

PROCEDURE 22-1

Measuring an Oral Temperature (Glass or Electronic Thermometer)

WHY YOU DO IT   A change in a person's normal temperature may be a sign of illness. Taking an oral temperature is fast and causes the resident minimal discomfort.

Getting Ready WGKIEpS

1. Complete the "Getting Ready" steps.

Supplies

If using a glass thermometer:
- paper towels
- tissues
- thermometer sheath
- oral glass thermometer

If using an electronic thermometer:
- probe sheath
- electronic thermometer with oral (blue) probe

Procedure

2. Ask the person if he or she has eaten, consumed a beverage, chewed gum, or smoked within the last 15 minutes. If so, wait 15 to 30 minutes before proceeding (or follow facility policy).

3. Prepare the thermometer.

   a. **Glass thermometer:** Run cool water over the thermometer to rinse away the disinfectant. Dry the thermometer with a paper towel and inspect it for cracks or chips. Carefully shake down the glass thermometer so that the indicator material is below the 94° mark (if using a Fahrenheit thermometer) or the 34° mark (if using a Celsius thermometer). Cover the end of the glass thermometer with the thermometer sheath.

   b. **Electronic thermometer:** Cover the electronic probe with the probe sheath. Turn the thermometer on and wait until the "ready" sign appears on the display screen.

4. Ask the person to open his or her mouth. Slowly and carefully insert the thermometer, placing the tip under the person's tongue and to one side.

5. Ask the person to gently close his or her mouth around the thermometer without biting down. If necessary, hold the thermometer in place. Ask the person to breathe through his or her nose.

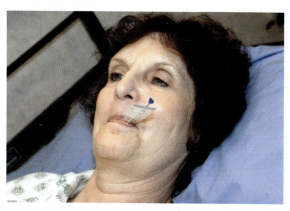

Step 5 The person breathes through her nose while holding the thermometer in her mouth.

6. Leave the thermometer in place for the specified amount of time:

   a. **Glass thermometer:** 3 to 5 minutes (or follow facility policy)

   b. **Electronic thermometer:** until the instrument blinks or beeps (usually just a few seconds)

7. Ask the person to open his or her mouth. Remove the thermometer from the person's mouth.

8. Read the temperature measurement.

   a. **Glass thermometer:** Using a tissue, remove the thermometer sheath from the glass thermometer, being careful not to touch the bulb end of the thermometer. Dispose of the tissue and the thermometer sheath in a facility-approved waste

(continued)

container. Hold the thermometer horizontally by the stem at eye level while facing a light source. Rotate the thermometer until you can see the level of the indicator material. Read the temperature.

b. Electronic thermometer: Read the temperature on the electronic thermometer's display screen. Remove the probe sheath from the probe by pushing the button on the top of the probe. Direct the probe sheath into a facility-approved waste container.

9. Prepare the thermometer for its next use.

a. Glass thermometer: Shake down the glass thermometer, clean it according to facility policy, and return it to its disinfectant-filled case.

b. Electronic thermometer: Replace the probe into the electronic thermometer.

(Always read the temperature before placing the probe in the instrument because this action clears the display screen.) Turn the instrument off if it does not automatically turn itself off. Place the thermometer in its charger.

10. Record the person's name, the time, the temperature, and the method according to facility policy. Place an "O" (or the notation designated by your facility) next to the measurement to indicate that the measurement was taken orally. Report an abnormal temperature to the nurse immediately.

Finishing Up   CLOSOWR

10. Complete the "Finishing Up" steps.

PROCEDURE 22-2

Measuring a Rectal Temperature (Glass or Electronic Thermometer)

WHY YOU DO IT   A change in a person's normal temperature may be a sign of illness. The rectal temperature measurement is a very accurate measurement of the body's temperature.

Getting Ready   WGKIEDS

1. Complete the "Getting Ready" steps.

Supplies
- gloves
- paper towels
- tissues
- lubricant jelly

If using a glass thermometer:
- thermometer sheath
- rectal glass thermometer

If using an electronic thermometer:
- probe sheath
- electronic thermometer with rectal (red) probe

Procedure

2. Make sure that the bed is positioned at a comfortable working height (to promote good body mechanics) and that the wheels are locked.

3. Prepare the thermometer.

a. Glass thermometer: Run cool water over the thermometer to rinse away the disinfectant. Dry the thermometer with a paper towel and inspect it for cracks or chips. Carefully shake down the glass thermometer so that the indicator material is below the 94° mark (if using a Fahrenheit thermometer) or the 34° mark (if using a Celsius thermometer). Cover the end of the glass thermometer with the thermometer sheath.

b. Electronic thermometer: Cover the electronic probe with the probe sheath. Turn the thermometer on and wait until the "ready" sign appears on the display screen.

4. Place the thermometer on a clean paper towel on the over-bed table. Open the lubricant package and squeeze a small amount of

lubricant onto the paper towel. Lubricate the tip of the thermometer to ease insertion.

5. If the side rails are in use, lower the side rail on the working side of the bed. The side rail on the opposite side of the bed should remain up. Lower the head of the bed so that the bed is flat (as tolerated).

6. Ask the person to lie on his or her side, facing away from you, in Sims' position. Help the person into this position, if necessary.

7. Fanfold the top linens to below the person's buttocks. Adjust the person's clothing as necessary to expose the person's buttocks.

8. Put on the gloves.

9. With one hand, raise the person's upper buttock to expose the anus. Suggest that the person take a deep breath and slowly exhale as the thermometer is inserted. Using your other hand, gently and carefully insert the lubricated end of the thermometer into the person's rectum (not more than 1 inch for adults). Never force the thermometer into the rectum. If you are unable to insert the thermometer, stop and call the nurse.

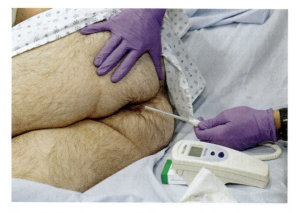

Step 9 Gently and carefully insert the lubricated end of the thermometer into the person's rectum.

10. Hold the thermometer in place for the specified amount of time:

   a. **Glass thermometer:** 3 to 5 minutes (or follow facility policy)

   b. **Electronic thermometer:** until the instrument blinks or beeps (usually just a few seconds)

11. Remove the thermometer from the person's rectum. Wipe the person's anal area with a tissue to remove the lubricant, and adjust the person's clothing as necessary to cover the buttocks.

12. Read the temperature measurement.

   a. **Glass thermometer:** Using a tissue, remove the thermometer sheath from the glass thermometer, being careful not to touch the bulb end of the thermometer. Dispose of the tissue and the thermometer sheath in a facility-approved waste container. Hold the thermometer horizontally by the stem at eye level while facing a light source. Rotate the thermometer until you can see the level of the indicator material. Read the temperature.

   b. **Electronic thermometer:** Read the temperature on the electronic thermometer's display screen. Remove the probe sheath from the probe by pushing the button on the top of the probe. Direct the probe sheath into a facility-approved waste container.

13. Remove your gloves and dispose of them according to facility policy. Wash your hands.

14. Record the person's name, the time, the temperature, and the method according to facility policy. Place an "R" (or the notation designated by your facility) next to the measurement to indicate that the measurement was taken rectally. Report an abnormal temperature to the nurse immediately.

15. Help the person back into a comfortable position, straighten the bottom linens, and draw the top linens over the person. Raise the head of the bed, as the person requests.

16. Make sure that the bed is lowered to its lowest position and that the wheels are locked. If the side rails are in use, return the side rails to the raised position.

17. Prepare the thermometer for its next use.

   a. **Glass thermometer:** Shake down the glass thermometer, clean it according to facility policy, and return it to its disinfectant-filled case.

   b. **Electronic thermometer:** Replace the probe into the electronic thermometer. (Always read the temperature before placing the probe in the instrument because this action clears the display screen.) Turn the instrument off if it does not automatically turn itself off. Place the thermometer in its charger.

Finishing Up CLSOWR

18. Complete the "Finishing Up" steps.

PROCEDURE 22-3

Measuring an Axillary Temperature (Glass or Electronic Thermometer)

WHY YOU DO IT   A change in a person's normal temperature may be a sign of illness. The axillary method is used when other methods cannot be used.

Getting Ready WGKIEpS

1. Complete the "Getting Ready" steps.

Supplies

- paper towels
- tissues

If using a glass thermometer:
- thermometer sheath
- oral glass thermometer

If using an electronic thermometer:
- probe sheath
- electronic thermometer with oral (blue) probe

Procedure

2. Ask the person if he or she has bathed or applied deodorant or antiperspirant within the last 15 minutes. If so, wait 15 to 30 minutes before proceeding (or follow facility policy).

3. Prepare the thermometer.

   a. **Glass thermometer:** Run cool water over the thermometer to rinse away the disinfectant. Dry the thermometer with a paper towel and inspect it for cracks or chips. Carefully shake down the glass thermometer so that the indicator material is below the 94° mark (if using a Fahrenheit thermometer) or the 34° mark (if using a Celsius thermometer). Cover the end of the glass thermometer with the thermometer sheath.

   b. **Electronic thermometer:** Cover the electronic probe with the probe sheath. Turn the thermometer on and wait until the "ready" sign appears on the display screen.

4. Assist the person with removing his or her arm from the sleeve of his or her clothing.

5. Pat the axilla (underarm area) gently with a paper towel.

6. Ask the person to lift his or her arm slightly. Position the tip of the thermometer in the center of the axilla and ask the person to hold the thermometer in place by holding his or her arm close to the body (or by grasping the arm with the opposite hand).

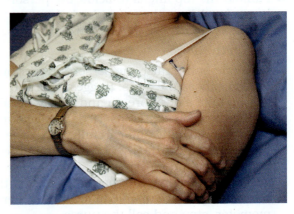

Step 6 The person holds the thermometer in place by grasping her arm with the opposite hand.

7. Leave the thermometer in place for the specified amount of time:

   a. **Glass thermometer:** 10 minutes (or follow facility policy)

   b. **Electronic thermometer:** until the instrument blinks or beeps (usually just a few seconds)

8. Ask the person to lift his or her arm slightly. Remove the thermometer.

9. Read the temperature measurement.

   a. **Glass thermometer:** Using a tissue, remove the thermometer sheath from the glass thermometer, being careful not to touch the bulb end of the thermometer. Dispose of the tissue and the thermometer sheath in a facility-approved waste container. Hold the thermometer horizontally by the stem at eye level while facing a light source. Rotate the thermometer until you can see the level of the indicator material. Read the temperature.

   b. **Electronic thermometer:** Read the temperature on the electronic thermometer's display screen. Remove the probe sheath from the probe by pushing the button on the top of the probe. Direct the probe sheath into a facility-approved waste container.

10. Record the person's name, the time, the temperature, and the method according to facility policy. Place an "A" (or the notation designated by your facility) next to the measurement to indicate that the measurement was taken in the axilla. Report an abnormal temperature to the nurse immediately.

11. Help the person back into his or her clothing.

12. Prepare the thermometer for its next use:

    a. **Glass thermometer:** Shake down the glass thermometer, clean it according to

facility policy, and return it to its disinfectant-filled case.

    b. **Electronic thermometer:** Replace the probe into the electronic thermometer. (Always read the temperature before placing the probe in the instrument because this action clears the display screen.) Turn the instrument off, if it does not automatically turn itself off. Place the thermometer in its charger.

Finishing Up   CLSOWR

13. Complete the "Finishing Up" steps.

PROCEDURE 22-4

Measuring a Tympanic Temperature (Tympanic Thermometer)

WHY YOU DO IT   A change in a person's normal temperature may be a sign of illness. Taking a tympanic temperature is fast and causes the resident minimal discomfort.

Getting Ready   WCKIEPS

1. Complete the "Getting Ready" steps.

Supplies

- tympanic probe
- sheath (cover)
- tympanic thermometer

Procedure

2. If the person wears a hearing aid, remove it carefully and wait 2 minutes before taking the person's temperature.

3. Inspect the ear canal for excessive cerumen (ear wax). If you see excessive wax build-up in the ear canal, gently wipe the ear canal with a warm, moist washcloth.

4. Cover the cone-shaped end of the thermometer with the probe sheath. Turn the thermometer on and wait until the "ready" sign appears on the display screen.

5. To straighten the ear canal (which will ease insertion of the thermometer), grasp the top portion of the person's ear and gently pull up and back.

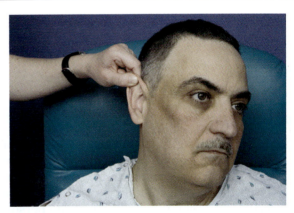

Step 5 Grasp the top portion of the person's ear and gently pull up and back to insert the thermometer.

6. Insert the covered probe into the person's ear canal, pointing the probe down and toward the front of the ear canal (pretend that you are aiming for the person's nose). This will seal off the ear canal by seating the probe properly, leading to a more accurate temperature reading.

7. To take the temperature, press the button on the instrument. Keep the button depressed

(continued)

and the probe in place until the instrument blinks or beeps (usually 1 second).

8. Remove the probe and read the temperature on the display screen.

9. Remove the probe sheath from the probe by pushing the button on the side of the instrument. Direct the probe sheath into a facility-approved waste container.

10. Record the person's name, the time, the temperature, and the method according to facility policy. Place a "T" (or the notation designated by your facility) next to the measurement to indicate that the measurement

was taken in the ear (that is using a tympanic thermometer). Report an abnormal temperature to the nurse immediately.

11. If your facility requires a tympanic temperature to be taken in both ears, repeat the procedure, using a clean probe cover for the other ear.

12. Turn the instrument off if it does not automatically turn itself off. Place the thermometer in its charger.

Finishing Up CLSOWR

13. Complete the "Finishing Up" steps.

PROCEDURE 22-5

Taking a Radial Pulse

WHY YOU DO IT   A change in a person's normal pulse rate, rhythm, or amplitude may be a sign of illness. Taking the pulse at the radial artery is easiest for the resident.

Getting Ready WGKIEPS

1. Complete the "Getting Ready" steps.

Supplies

- watch with second hand

Procedure

2. Rest the person's arm on the over-bed table, on the bed, or on her lap if she is seated in a chair. Locate the radial pulse in the person's wrist using your middle two or three fingers. (TIP: The radial pulse will be on the person's "thumb" side.)

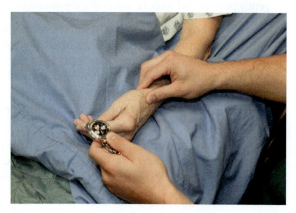

Step 2 Locate the radial pulse in the person's wrist using your middle two or three fingers.

3. Note the strength and regularity of the pulse. Look at your watch and wait until the second hand gets to the "12" or "6." When the second hand reaches the "12" or the "6," begin counting the pulse.

   a. If the pulse rhythm is regular, count the number of pulses that occur in 30 seconds and multiply the result by 2 to arrive at the pulse rate.

   b. If the pulse rhythm is irregular, count the number of pulses that occur in 60 seconds. Counting each pulse that occurs over the course of 1 full minute is the only way to obtain a truly accurate pulse rate when the pulse is irregular.

4. Record the person's name; the time; and the pulse rate, rhythm, and amplitude according to facility policy. Report an abnormal pulse rate, rhythm, or amplitude to the nurse immediately.

Finishing Up CLSOWR

5. Complete the "Finishing Up" steps.

PROCEDURE 22-6

Taking an Apical Pulse

WHY YOU DO IT   An apical pulse is taken when a person has a weak or irregular pulse that may be difficult to feel in the radial artery. An apical pulse may also be used to measure heart rate in people with known heart disease.

Getting Ready   WORKIEPS

1. Complete the "Getting Ready" steps.

Supplies
- alcohol wipes
- dual-sided stethoscope
- watch with second hand

Procedure

2. Help the person to a sitting position by raising the head of the bed.

3. Using alcohol wipes, clean the earpieces, the diaphragm, and the bell of the stethoscope. Place the earpieces in your ears.

4. Place the diaphragm of the stethoscope under the person's clothing, on the apical pulse site (located approximately 2 inches below the person's left nipple). The diaphragm or bell must be placed directly on the person's skin because clothing will distort the sound.

5. Using two fingers, hold the diaphragm firmly against the person's chest. Look at your watch and wait until the second hand gets to the "12" or "6." When the second hand reaches the "12" or the "6," begin counting the heartbeat.

6. Count the number of heartbeats that occur in 60 seconds. Each time the heart beats, you will hear two sounds, best described as a "lubb" and a "dupp." Both sounds make up one beat of the heart and should be counted as such.

7. After 60 seconds, remove the diaphragm of the stethoscope from the person's chest. Adjust the person's clothing as necessary and help the person back into a comfortable position. Lower the head of the bed, as the person requests.

8. Record the person's name; the time; the pulse rate, rhythm, and amplitude; and the method according to facility policy. Place an "a" (or the notation designated by your facility) next to the measurement to indicate that the measurement was taken apically. Report an abnormal pulse to the nurse immediately.

9. Using alcohol wipes, clean the earpieces, the diaphragm, and the bell of the stethoscope.

Finishing Up   CLSOWR

10. Complete the "Finishing Up" steps.

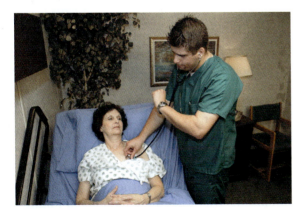

Step 5 Hold the diaphragm firmly against the person's chest.

PROCEDURE 22-7

Counting Respirations

WHY YOU DO IT   A change in a person's normal respiratory rate, rhythm, or depth of breathing may be a sign of illness.

Getting Ready WGKIEPS

1. Complete the "Getting Ready" steps.

Supplies

- watch with second hand

Procedure

2. Look at your watch and wait until the second hand gets to the "12" or "6." When the second hand reaches the "12" or the "6," look at the person's chest (or place your hand near the person's collarbone or on his or her side) and begin counting each rise and fall of the chest as one breath.

   a. If the respiratory rhythm is regular, count the number of breaths that occur in 30 seconds and multiply the result by 2 to arrive at the respiratory rate.

   b. If the respiratory rhythm is irregular, count the number of breaths that occur in 60 seconds. Counting each respiration that occurs over the course of 1 full minute is the only way to obtain a truly accurate respiratory rate when the person's breathing is irregular.

3. Record the person's name, the time, and the respiratory rate according to facility policy. Report abnormal respirations to the nurse immediately.

Finishing Up CLSOWR

4. Complete the "Finishing Up" steps.

PROCEDURE 22-8

Measuring Blood Pressure

WHY YOU DO IT   Blood pressure measurements allow health care workers to monitor existing problems and possibly even prevent future ones.

Getting Ready WGKIEPS

1. Complete the "Getting Ready" steps.

Supplies

- alcohol wipes
- sphygmomanometer
- stethoscope

Procedure

2. Assist the person into a sitting or lying position. Position the person's arm so that the forearm is level with the heart and the palm of the hand is facing upward. Assist the person with rolling up his or her sleeve so that the upper arm is exposed.

3. Using alcohol wipes, clean the earpieces, the diaphragm, and the bell of the stethoscope.

4. Stand no more than 3 feet away from the manometer. If it is not mounted on the wall, stand a mercury manometer upright on a flat surface, at eye level. Lay an aneroid manometer on a flat surface directly in front of you or leave it attached to the blood pressure cuff.

5. Squeeze the cuff to empty it of any remaining air. Turn the valve on the bulb clockwise to close it; this will cause the cuff to inflate when you pump the bulb.

6. Locate the person's brachial artery in the antecubital space by placing your fingers at the inner aspect of the elbow.

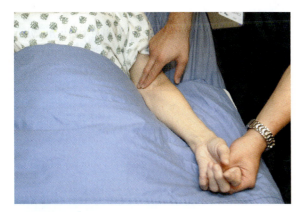

Step 6 Locate the person's brachial artery in the antecubital space (inner aspect of the elbow).

7. Place the arrow mark on the cuff over the brachial artery. Wrap the cuff around the person's upper arm so that the bottom of the cuff is at least 1 inch above the person's elbow. The cuff must be even and snug.

8. Place the stethoscope earpieces in your ears.

9. Pump the bulb until the pressure in the cuff is 30 mm Hg higher than the systolic pressure. There are two ways to do this:

   Method "A." Hold the bulb in one hand and position the diaphragm of the stethoscope over the brachial artery with the other hand. Inflate the cuff until you hear the pulse stop and then inflate the cuff 30 mm Hg more.

   Method "B." Hold the bulb in one hand and feel for the person's radial pulse (in his or her wrist) with the other hand. Inflate the cuff until you are no longer able to feel the radial pulse and then inflate the cuff 30 mm Hg more.

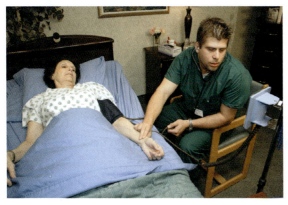

Step 9 Hold the bulb in one hand and feel for the person's radial pulse (in the wrist) with the other hand.

10. Position the diaphragm of the stethoscope over the brachial artery (or continue to hold it there if you used method "A" to inflate the cuff).

11. Turn the valve on the bulb slightly counterclockwise to allow air to escape from the cuff slowly.

12. Note the reading on the manometer where the first Korotkoff sound is heard. This is the systolic reading.

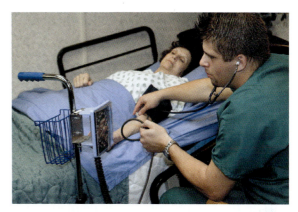

Step 12 With the diaphragm of the stethoscope over the person's brachial artery, allow the air to leave the cuff slowly while listening for the beginning and ending sounds of the brachial pulse and watching the manometer.

13. Continue to deflate the cuff. Note the reading on the manometer where the last Korotkoff sound is heard. This is the diastolic reading.

14. Deflate the cuff completely and remove it from the person's arm. Remove the stethoscope from your ears.

15. Record the person's name, the time, and the blood pressure according to facility policy. Report an abnormal blood pressure to the nurse immediately.

16. Return the sphygmomanometer to its case or wall holder.

17. Using alcohol wipes, clean the earpieces, the diaphragm, and the bell of the stethoscope.

Finishing Up CLSOWR

18. Complete the "Finishing Up" steps.

PROCEDURE 22-9

Measuring Height and Weight Using an Upright Scale

WHY YOU DO IT   An upright scale is used to measure the height and weight of a person who can stand independently. A change in a person's weight might indicate that the person's condition is getting worse or that it is getting better.

Getting Ready WGKIEPS

1. Complete the "Getting Ready" steps.

Supplies

- upright scale

Procedure

2. Ask the person to urinate. If necessary, assist the person to the bathroom or offer the bedpan or urinal.

3. Move the weights all the way to the left of the balance bar.

4. Help the person onto the scale platform so that she is facing the balance bar. Once the person is on the scale platform, do not allow her to hold on to you or to the scale.

5. Move the large weight on the lower scale bar to the right to the weight closest to the person's prior weight. For example, if the person weighed 155 pounds the last time you weighed her, you would move the large weight to the "150" mark.

6. Move the small weight on the upper scale bar to the right until the balance pointer is centered between the two scale bars.

7. Read the numbers on the upper and the lower scale bars where each weight has settled and add these two numbers together. This is the person's weight.

8. Have the person carefully turn around to face away from the scale bar. Slide the height scale up so that you can pull out the height rod, which extends from the top of the height scale. Be careful not to hit the person in the head with the height rod.

9. Slide the height rod down so that it lightly touches the top of the person's head. Read the number at the point where the height rod meets the height scale. This is the person's height.

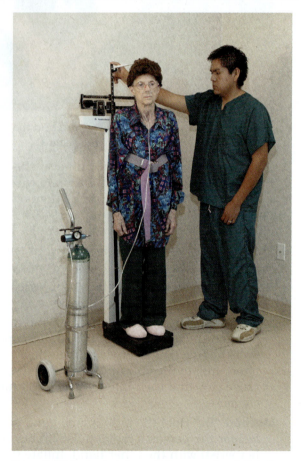

Step 9 Slide the height rod down so that it lightly touches the top of the person's head.

10. Hold the height rod in your hand, and help the person step down from the scale.

11. Assist the person back to her room.

12. Record the person's name, the time, and the weight and height according to facility policy. Report a change in the person's weight or height to the nurse.

Finishing Up CLSOWR

13. Complete the "Finishing Up" steps.

PROCEDURE 22-10

Measuring Weight Using a Chair Scale

WHY YOU DO IT   A chair scale is used to measure the weight of a person who cannot stand independently but is able to get out of bed. A change in a person's weight might indicate that the person's condition is getting worse or that it is getting better.

Getting Ready WCKIEPS

1. Complete the "Getting Ready" steps.

Supplies

● transfer belt   ● wheelchair*

Procedure

2. Ask the person to urinate. If necessary, assist the person to the bathroom or offer the bedpan or urinal.

3. Assist or wheel the person to the scale, using a transfer belt, a wheelchair, or both.

4. Reset the scale to "0" by turning it on.

5. Help the person onto the scale.

   a. If a regular chair scale is being used, help the person to sit in the chair on the scale. Make sure the person is seated properly, with his or her buttocks against the back of the chair and feet on the footrests.

   b. If a wheelchair scale is being used, roll the occupied wheelchair onto the platform and lock the wheels.

6. Read the weight on the display screen. If a wheelchair scale is being used, you must subtract the weight of the unoccupied wheelchair from this figure to determine the person's weight.

---

*If you will be using a wheelchair scale to weigh the person, take the empty wheelchair to the wheelchair scale and weigh it before taking it to the person's room. Be sure to write down the weight of the empty wheelchair.

Step 6 Read the weight on the display screen.

7. Help the person off of the scale.

   a. If a regular chair scale is being used, assist the person out of the chair and back into a wheelchair if one was used for the transfer.

   b. If a wheelchair scale is being used, unlock the wheels and roll the wheelchair off the platform.

8. Assist the person back to his or her room.

9. Record the person's name, the time, and the weight according to facility policy. Report a change in the person's weight to the nurse.

Finishing Up CLSOWR

10. Complete the "Finishing Up" steps.

PROCEDURE 22-11

Measuring Height and Weight Using a Tape Measure and a Sling Scale

WHY YOU DO IT   A tape measure and a sling scale are used to obtain a person's height and weight when the person cannot get out of bed at all. A change in a person's weight might indicate that the person's condition is getting worse or that it is getting better.

Getting Ready WGKIEDS

1. Complete the "Getting Ready" steps.

Supplies

- sling scale
- tape measure

Procedure

2. Ask the person to urinate. If necessary, assist the person to the bathroom or offer the bedpan or urinal.

3. Position the sling scale next to the bed. Make sure that the bed is positioned at a comfortable working height (to promote good body mechanics) and that the wheels are locked. If the side rails are in use, lower the side rail on the working side of the bed. The side rail on the opposite side of the bed should remain up.

4. Fanfold the top linens to the foot of the bed.

5. Center the sling under the person. (To get the sling under the person, move the person as if you were making an occupied bed.

6. Position the person in the supine position, or according to the manufacturer's instructions.

7. Move the release valve on the sling scale to the closed position.

8. Raise the sling scale so that it can be positioned over the person.

9. Spread the legs of the sling scale to provide a solid base of support. The legs must be locked in this position, or the scale could tip over, injuring you, the person you are trying to weigh, or both.

10. Move the scale into position over the person.

11. Fasten the sling to the straps or chains of the scale. Make sure the hooks face away from the person.

12. Cross the person's arms over her chest.

13. Slowly raise the sling until the person is clear of the bed.

14. Read the weight on the display screen. Record the person's name, the time, and the weight according to facility policy. Report a change in the person's weight to the nurse.

15. Gently lower the person to the bed and remove the sling by gently rolling the person first to one side, then the other.

16. Position the person in the supine position, with her arms by her sides and her legs straight.

17. Using a pencil, make a small mark on the bottom sheet at the top of the person's head. Make another small mark at her heels.

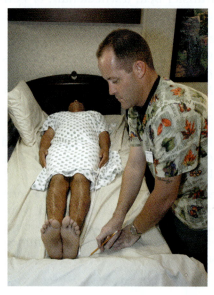

Step 17 Using a pencil, mark the bottom sheet at the top of the person's head and at his heels.

18. Using the tape measure, measure the distance between the pencil marks. This is the person's height.

19. Record the person's name, the time, and the height according to facility policy.

20. Make sure that the bed is lowered to its lowest position and that the wheels are locked. If the side rails are in use, return the side rails to the raised position.

Finishing Up CLSOWR

21. Complete the "Finishing Up" steps.

WHAT DID YOU LEARN?

Multiple Choice

Select the single best answer for each of the following questions.

1. A stethoscope is used to determine the:
   a. Brachial pulse rate
   b. Carotid pulse rate
   c. Apical pulse rate
   d. Popliteal pulse rate

2. Which one of the following is the pressure exerted by the blood flowing through the arteries when the heart muscle relaxes?
   a. Diastolic pressure
   b. Pulse pressure
   c. Pulse deficit
   d. Systolic pressure

3. The most common site for counting the pulse is the:
   a. Brachial artery
   b. Radial artery
   c. Carotid artery
   d. Apex of the heart

4. When counting respirations, you should:
   a. Have the person exercise first to get a true reading
   b. Count five respirations and then check your watch
   c. Avoid telling the person what you are going to do
   d. Have the person count respirations while you take her pulse

5. You are using a glass Fahrenheit thermometer. When you shake it down, the mercury should be below the:
   a. 98.6°F mark
   b. Arrow
   c. 100°F mark
   d. 94°F mark

6. Which of the following can cause an inaccurate oral temperature reading?
   a. The person exercised 10 minutes prior to having his temperature taken
   b. The nursing assistant failed to shake down the mercury thermometer
   c. The person drank a cup of hot coffee 15 minutes prior to having his temperature taken
   d. All of the above

7. One of your residents, Mrs. Jones, has a temperature of 98.8°F, a pulse rate of 80 beats/min, and a respiratory rate of 30 breaths/min. Which finding should be reported to the nurse immediately?
   a. Mrs. Jones' respiratory rate
   b. Mrs. Jones' pulse rate
   c. Mrs. Jones' temperature
   d. None of these findings needs to be reported to the nurse

8. What should you observe when taking a person's pulse?
   a. The rhythm and regularity of the pulse
   b. The number of beats per minute
   c. The strength of the pulse
   d. All of the above

9. If you notice a significant change in a person's vital signs, what should you do?
   a. Record the change with a special notation to indicate that the reading was different
   b. Mention the change to the nurse at the end of your shift
   c. Tell the resident about the change
   d. Report the change to a nurse immediately

10. Which instrument is used to measure blood pressure?
    a. A temporal artery thermometer
    b. A sphygmomanometer
    c. An upright scale
    d. A watch with a second hand

11. Which one of the following conditions would prevent you from taking an oral temperature?
    a. The person has diarrhea
    b. The person has just had a mastectomy
    c. The person is very elderly
    d. The person is confused and disoriented

12. You must obtain Mrs. Gulden's monthly weight. Why is it important to know Mrs. Gulden's weight from last month before you complete this assignment?
    a. You will be able to tell Mrs. Gulden if she is closer to achieving her goal of gaining 5 pounds.
    b. You will be able to recognize a change in Mrs. Gulden's weight that would need to be reported to the nurse immediately.
    c. You will be able to tell if you have performed the weight measurement correctly.
    d. None of the above

13. Which of the following is true regarding height measurements?

a. Accurate height measurements are necessary for medication dosage adjustments.

b. Height can decrease as a result of bone disease.

c. Height does not change once a person has reached adulthood.

d. Height should be measured in kilograms.

STOP and Think!

- Mrs. Tinetti's vital signs are due this morning. After you have finished taking her blood pressure, Mrs. Tinetti says, "You know, they started giving me pills for my blood pressure, but I don't think I need them. I feel fine, and my blood pressure is normal, right?" Her blood pressure measurement is in the normal range. How would you respond to Mrs. Tinetti? Would you report her comments to the nurse? Why or why not?

- The nurse tells you that one of your residents, Mr. Vincent, is in active left-sided heart failure. The doctor has written orders for weights to be measured daily. Why is obtaining accurate weights important for Mr. Vincent? What will you do to ensure that the weights you obtain are as accurate as possible? What other things are important for you to consider when obtaining Mr. Vincent's weight measurements?

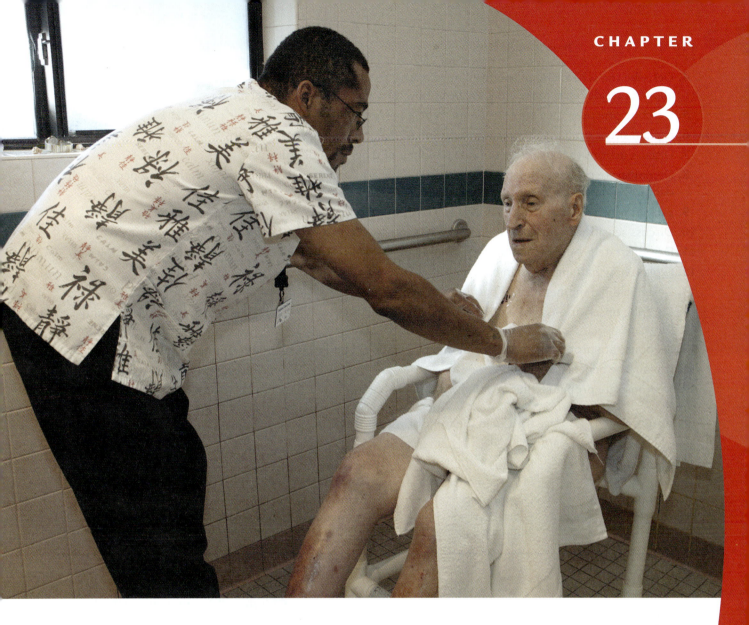

Cleanliness and Hygiene

WHAT WILL YOU LEARN?

In Chapter 3, you learned about how important good personal hygiene (cleanliness) is for both physical and emotional health. In this chapter, you will learn how to assist your residents with keeping their skin and mouths clean, two activities that are key to maintaining personal hygiene. When you are finished with this chapter, you will be able to:

1. List the practices that make up personal hygiene.
2. Understand the importance of good hygiene in relation to a person's physical and emotional well-being.
3. Understand the importance of allowing residents to participate in their own self-care to the greatest extent possible.

Photo: A nursing assistant assists a resident in the tub room, following a shower.

415

4. Describe the scheduling of routine care in a long-term care facility, and explain the importance of allowing residents to make choices about how and when they receive personal care.

5. Describe practices that are considered to be a part of oral care.

6. Explain situations that may require a person to need more frequent oral care.

7. Discuss actions that promote the safe handling of a person's dentures.

8. Demonstrate proper technique for providing oral care for a person with natural teeth, for a person with dentures, and for an unconscious person.

9. Explain why perineal care is an essential aspect of daily hygiene.

10. Discuss sensitivity issues that a nursing assistant should be aware of when assisting with perineal care.

11. Demonstrate proper technique for providing perineal care for males and for females.

12. Explain how bathing and skin care benefit a person's health.

13. Describe different methods of bathing a person.

14. Describe observations that a nursing assistant should make while assisting a person with bathing and skin care.

15. Demonstrate proper technique for bathing a person (in bed or in a shower or bathtub).

16. Explain the benefits of massage.

17. Demonstrate proper technique for giving a back massage.

Vocabulary Use the CD in the front of your book to hear these terms pronounced and defined:

Early morning care	Rounds	Gingivitis	Barrier cream or ointment
Morning (AM) care	PRN (as-needed) care	Periodontitis	Circumcision
Afternoon care	Diaphoretic	Edentulous	Foreskin
Evening (hour of sleep, hs) care	Dental caries	Perineal care (peri-care)	Deodorant
	Halitosis	Perineum	Antiperspirant

Personal hygiene (cleanliness) helps to promote both physical and emotional health. The practices associated with personal hygiene—skin care (including bathing and moisturizing) and oral care (including brushing and flossing the teeth)—keep the skin and the mucous membranes of the mouth healthy. As you will remember from Chapter 15, the skin and mucous membranes of the body act as the first line of defense against infection. Caring for the skin and the mouth helps to prevent conditions such as rashes, dry skin, and cracked lips, which interrupt the body's first line of defense by creating a portal of entry for microbes. In addition, keeping the skin and mouth clean helps to reduce the number of microbes on these surfaces, which also helps to minimize the risk of infection.

In addition to promoting physical health, good personal hygiene promotes emotional health by helping a person to feel relaxed and well cared for. A person who feels relaxed and comfortable is able to rest better. Being clean and refreshed also helps a person meet his or her need for self-esteem (see Chapter 7) by preventing body and breath odors and helping the person feel attractive to others.

When assisting a resident with personal care, it is important to allow the resident to do as much for himself as possible, even if it takes longer to complete the task. Provide assistance, as needed, to fill in for what the resident is not able to do. Participating in self-care helps the resident to attain or maintain his highest level of function and well-being. This is important for the resident's self-esteem, and also for meeting OBRA requirements.

SCHEDULING OF ROUTINE PERSONAL CARE

The scheduling of routine personal care promotes efficiency and allows the nursing staff to plan these activities around other scheduled activities, such as meals, treatments, visiting hours, and social events. However, as a result of the culture change movement that is happening in long-term care right now, many facilities are changing their policies to allow residents to have more control over their daily lives. Residents are asked about their preferences for care, and these preferences are accommodated as much as possible within the daily routines of the facility.

Routine personal care is provided throughout the day:

- **Early morning care** is provided after a resident wakes up to prepare him for breakfast or other early morning activities. The resident is assisted with using the toilet, washing the face and hands, brushing the teeth or inserting dentures, and brushing or combing the hair. If the resident will be eating breakfast in the dining room, the resident is assisted to dress in appropriate clothing.
- **Morning (AM) care** is provided between breakfast and lunch. During morning care, the resident is assisted with oral care, toileting, shaving, bathing, dressing, and putting on make-up (if desired). In some facilities, the morning bath is followed by a back massage. General housekeeping duties, such as tidying the person's room and changing the bed linens, are also performed during morning care.
- **Afternoon care** is care that is provided before and after lunch and dinner. During afternoon care, the resident is assisted with preparing for the afternoon and evening meals and activities (for example, receiving visitors, attending a group activity, or napping). Before each meal, the resident is assisted with using the toilet, washing the face and hands, and oral care. After each meal, the resident is again assisted with these activities. In addition, the resident is assisted with changing clothes as necessary (for example, to replace an article of clothing that was soiled during the meal, or to ensure that the resident is wearing clothing that is appropriate for planned activities).
- **Evening (hs, hour of sleep) care** is provided in preparation for sleep. During evening care, the resident is assisted with toileting, washing the face and hands, brushing the teeth (or cleaning and soaking the dentures), and changing into nightwear. Many residents prefer to bathe in the evening instead of in the morning, so a bath or a shower may be

part of evening care. Other bedtime preparations include turning down the bed linens and fluffing the pillows. "Extras" such as soft music, a back massage, or reading in bed for a while before turning out the light can help a person fall into a restful sleep. Allowing for these "extras" when providing evening care to your residents shows a caring and compassionate attitude, because you are considering the person's preferences and honoring these wishes, whenever possible.

Helping Hands and a Caring Heart

FOCUS ON HUMANISTIC HEALTH CARE

If you had always bathed in the evening, before bed, and then after entering a nursing home were told you had to bathe in the morning, how would you feel? To provide truly humanistic care, ask your residents about their preferences for care, and then accommodate those preferences as much as possible. Allowing residents to make choices about care shows that you care about them as individuals, helps them to maintain a sense of familiarity in an otherwise changed life, and helps them to maintain their satisfaction with their quality of life.

In addition to care that is provided at routinely scheduled times, care is provided whenever a resident needs it. **Rounds** are routinely done, usually at least every 2 hours, throughout the 24-hour time period. During rounds, nursing assistants check on each of their assigned residents to provide toileting assistance or incontinence care, assist with turning and positioning, offer fluids, and take care of any other needs the resident may have. **PRN (as-needed) care** is personal hygiene care that is provided whenever a resident needs it, throughout the day or night. For example, a person in a coma needs frequent mouth care because he tends to breathe through his mouth and he cannot take food or liquids orally, situations that put him at risk for a dry mouth. An incontinent person requires perineal care (pericare), or cleansing of the genital and anal region, each time she loses control of her bowel or bladder. If her clothing or bedding is wet or soiled, these items will need to be changed as well. A person who is **diaphoretic** (that is, a person who has a medical condition that causes him to sweat a great deal) may need partial sponge baths, fresh linens, and a change of clothes frequently throughout the day. Any situation or condition that causes wetness or soiling of the skin, clothing, or bedding needs immediate attention.

ASSISTING WITH ORAL CARE

Keeping the mouth and teeth clean and healthy is an important part of personal hygiene. A clean, healthy mouth feels good and makes food taste better, and contributes to overall health. **Dental caries** (cavities) and **halitosis** (bad breath that does not go away) are caused by poor oral hygiene. Poor oral hygiene can also cause **gingivitis** (inflammation of the gums), which can lead to **periodontitis** (infection and inflammation of the soft tissue and bones that support the teeth). Periodontitis is the main cause of tooth loss in people older than 35 years, and it may be associated with other serious health problems as well, such as heart disease. Assisting your residents with regular oral care is an important responsibility because healthy teeth and gums are important for a person's overall health and well-being.

A person who has lost one or more natural teeth may have dental implants (prosthetic teeth that are surgically placed in the jawbone), dentures (prosthetic teeth that can be taken in and out), or a combination of these. A person may have a partial denture or a full denture. Partial dentures are used when only some teeth are missing. Full dentures are used when a person is missing all of his top teeth or all of his bottom teeth. A person who has no teeth at all is said to be **edentulous** (without teeth).

Oral care is usually provided on awakening, after meals, and before bed. People who are unable or not allowed to take food or fluids by mouth will need oral care as often as every 1 or 2 hours to keep their mouths fresh and moist. Some residents will be able to manage their own oral care with minimal assistance from you, but many will require a great deal of assistance. Because the gums sometimes bleed during routine oral care, it is important to practice standard precautions when assisting with brushing and flossing the teeth or cleaning dentures. Droplet precautions should be taken if the resident is known to have an infection that could be spread by exposure to droplets released from the mouth or nose.

Helping your residents with oral care presents many opportunities for observation.

TELL THE NURSE

While assisting a person with oral care, pay attention to the following:

- Dry, red, cracked, or bleeding lips, gums, or mucous membranes
- Cold sores on the lips or mucous membranes
- Red, irritated, swollen, or bleeding gums
- Cracked, chipped, or broken teeth; loose teeth; blackened teeth
- Chipped, cracked, or poorly fitting full or partial dentures
- Red sores or canker sores inside the mouth, white spots inside the mouth, or any areas of pus or infection
- Bad breath that does not improve after oral care
- Fruity-smelling breath (possibly a sign of diabetes mellitus)
- A red or swollen tongue or a white coating on the tongue
- Complaints of pain or sensitivity

PROVIDING ORAL CARE FOR A PERSON WITH NATURAL TEETH

Natural teeth are best cleaned with a toothbrush and toothpaste, followed by flossing. Because bacteria in the mouth do the most damage to the teeth and gums after eating, the best time to brush is after meals. Brushing alone is not enough to remove food that lodges between the teeth, so flossing once a day is recommended as part of good oral hygiene. Many people like to use a mouthwash after brushing to complete their oral care routine. The use of mouthwash can further reduce harmful bacteria in the mouth.

Toothbrushes should have soft bristles and be small enough to reach all of the teeth. Electric toothbrushes are simple to use and can be effective, especially for people who have limited strength or use of their hands. The toothbrush (or the disposable brush head of an electric toothbrush) should be replaced on a regular basis, as the bristles lose their shape.

Procedure 23-1 describes how to assist a person with brushing and flossing the teeth.

PROVIDING ORAL CARE FOR A PERSON WITH DENTURES

Dentures take the place of a person's natural teeth, allowing the person to chew food properly. Dentures that do not fit properly or that hurt the mouth when worn are not very useful for chewing. Proper care of the gums and dentures helps to keep the dentures fitting properly and comfortably.

Some people wear their dentures all of the time. Others may leave their dentures out at night or only wear them for meals. Personal preference for wearing dentures is to be respected. Remember that people are more likely to wear their dentures if they are kept clean.

A denture brush (or a toothbrush) and denture cleaner (or toothpaste) are used to clean all surfaces of the denture. Some people use a denture adhesive to help keep the denture in place better. Be sure to remove all of the adhesive material when cleaning the denture. Rinse the denture with lukewarm water. Hot water should not be used because it can damage the dentures.

General guidelines for providing oral care for a person with dentures are given in Guidelines Box 23-1. Procedure 23-2 describes how to provide oral care for a person who wears dentures.

Guidelines Box 23-1   Guidelines for Providing Oral Care for a Person with Dentures

WHAT YOU DO	WHY YOU DO IT
Handle a person's dentures with care.	Dentures are expensive and difficult to replace.
When a person is not wearing his or her dentures, store them in a denture cup filled with lukewarm water or a denture solution.	The water or solution prevents the dentures from drying out and warping. If the dentures warp, they will not fit properly.
When cleaning dentures, use lukewarm (not hot) water.	Hot water can damage the dentures.
When cleaning dentures, line the sink with a washcloth or paper towels.	The washcloth or towels help to prevent breaking or chipping of the denture if you accidentally drop it into the sink.
Have the person rinse his or her dentures after eating.	Rinsing the dentures after eating removes food trapped between the gums and dentures. Trapped food can cause discomfort and promotes the growth of bacteria.
Before placing the dentures in the person's mouth, allow the person to rinse with water or mouthwash or use a moist, foam-tipped applicator to clean the surfaces inside the person's mouth. Wet the dentures before placing them in the person's mouth.	Placing dentures inside the mouth is more difficult when the mouth and dentures are dry. In addition, the moisture helps to create the suction that is needed to hold the dentures in place.
Label the person's denture cup with the person's name and room number.	Putting the person's name and room number on the denture cup helps prevent the dentures from being misplaced.

PROVIDING ORAL CARE FOR AN UNCONSCIOUS PERSON

A person who is unconscious needs frequent mouth care to keep the mucous membranes of the mouth moist and healthy. An unconscious person breathes with her mouth open, which causes secretions to thicken and dry on the lips and in the mouth. These dried secretions, along with the intake of air through the mouth, can lead to cracking of the lips and tongue. Cracked, dry lips are very uncomfortable and they create a portal of entry for microbes.

Natural teeth are gently brushed with either a small amount of toothpaste or saline (salt water). If the person is edentulous, the gums, tongue, and inside of the cheeks are cleaned using a sponge-tipped swab moistened with saline or mouthwash. The mouth can be rinsed with a small amount of saline or water to clean out dried secretions. You may need to place a padded tongue blade between the upper and lower back teeth to keep the mouth open during oral care (Fig. 23-1). General guidelines for providing oral care for a person who is unconscious are given in Guidelines Box 23-2. Procedure 23-3 describes how to provide oral care for a person who is unconscious.

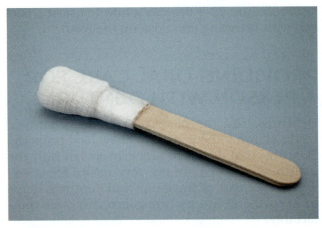

Figure 23-1

It may be necessary to use a padded tongue blade to keep an unconscious person's mouth open while providing oral care. A padded tongue blade is made by folding a gauze square around two wooden tongue blades and taping the gauze in place.

ASSISTING WITH PERINEAL CARE

Perineal care (peri-care) is the cleaning of the **perineum** and associated structures (Fig. 23-2). In women, the perineum extends from the bottom of

Guidelines Box 23-2	Guidelines for Providing Oral Care for a Person Who Is Unconscious
WHAT YOU DO	**WHY YOU DO IT**
Turn the person on his or her side (or turn the person's head to the side) so that fluids run out of the mouth, not back toward the throat.	Turning the person onto his or her side (or turning the head to the side) helps to prevent aspiration (the accidental inhalation of foreign material into the airway). Aspiration can lead to complications such as choking or pneumonia.
Never place your fingers in the person's mouth.	An unconscious person may bite down involuntarily and without warning.
Explain what you are doing throughout the procedure, even though the person may not seem to be able to hear you or respond to you.	The person may be aware on some level that someone is doing something to him or her. Telling the person what you are doing reassures the person and helps the person to feel safe.
Apply lip lubricant to the person's lips as needed.	This helps to prevent drying and cracking of the lips, which is uncomfortable for the person and can lead to infection.

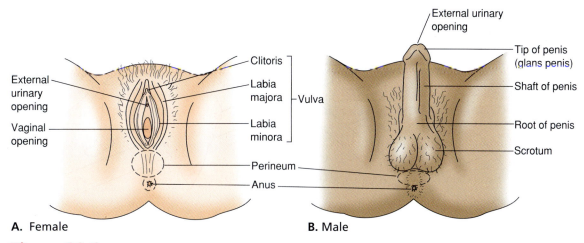

External
urinary
opening

Vaginal
opening

Clitoris

Labia
majora

Labia
minora

Perineum

Anus

Vulva

External urinary
opening

Tip of penis
(glans penis)

Shaft of penis

Root of penis

Scrotum

A. Female

B. Male

Figure 23-2

Perineal care refers to care of the perineum and associated structures. **(A)** The female perineum and associated structures. **(B)** The male perineum and associated structures.

the vagina to the anus. In men, the perineum extends from the root of the penis to the anus. When nurses talk about "providing perineal care," they mean cleaning the perineum and anus, as well as the vulva (in women) and the penis (in men).

Making sure that the perineum, the vulva (in women), and the penis (in men) are clean is important for two main reasons:

- **Prevention of infection.** Inadequate hygiene in the perineal area puts the person at risk for infection. Because many microbes live in our digestive tracts and are passed from the body in the feces, there are always large numbers of microbes in and around the anus. The perineal area provides the perfect environment to support the growth of these microbes, because it is warm, dark, and moist. Because the perineum is close to the vulva (in women) and the penis (in men), these microbes can easily enter the vagina or urethra, causing infection.
- **Prevention of skin breakdown and odor.** The perineum, vulva, and penis are delicate, with many folds of skin. Feces, urine, and other body fluids can become trapped in these folds, leading to skin irritation and odor if they are not properly removed.

Perineal care is routinely performed at least once daily, as part of the bath. Residents with diarrhea or who are incontinent of urine or feces will need perineal care performed more frequently. For these residents, a **barrier cream or ointment** may be applied after perineal care to help protect the skin from contact with urine or

feces. Women with vaginal bleeding or discharge will also need more frequent perineal care.

Any person who can manage her own perineal care should be encouraged to do so to the best of her ability. You may need to provide specific instructions. A person who is unable to provide for her own self-care will need your help. When helping your residents with perineal care, be aware of signs and symptoms that could indicate a health problem.

TELL THE NURSE ❗

Tell the nurse immediately if you observe any of the following signs when providing perineal care for one of your residents:

- Any unusual redness, inflammation, skin rashes, or skin breaks in the perineal area
- Any unusual discharge from the vagina or penis
- Any bleeding from the vagina (especially in a post-menopausal woman) or the anus
- Any abnormal odor

Before assisting a resident with perineal care, you must make the resident aware of what you are going to do. If the resident can understand and respond to you, explain what you are about to do and ask the person's permission to continue. Make sure to explain the procedure completely and professionally, using words that are understandable to the resident (such as "crotch,"

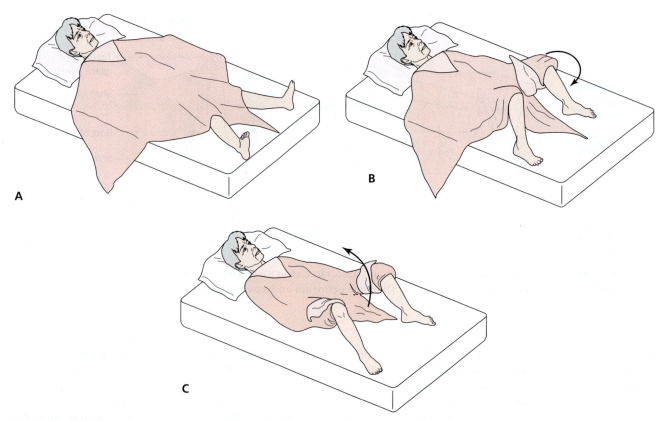

Figure 23-3
A bath blanket is used to preserve the person's modesty during perineal care. **(A)** The bath blanket is placed over the person's body so that one corner is pointing toward the person's head and the other is between the person's legs, covering the perineum. The other two corners are to the right and to the left, respectively. **(B)** The right corner is brought under and around the person's right leg, and then the same is done on the left. **(C)** The top corner is lifted up to expose only the perineal area.

"privates," "bottom," or "the area between your legs"). For a resident with dementia, you may need to use body language or gestures to get your message across. If the resident speaks a foreign language, you may need an interpreter.

For many reasons (such as cultural or religious beliefs, or a history of physical abuse), some people may object strongly to being touched by a member of the opposite sex, or even by a member of the same sex. Please respect your resident's wishes and work to find a suitable compromise, if at all possible. Perineal care can be embarrassing, both for the person receiving it and for the person providing it. Draping the resident's body with a bath blanket so that only the area to be cleaned is exposed helps to preserve the resident's sense of modesty (Fig. 23-3). Be aware that a male resident may become aroused during perineal care, simply from stimulation of the penis during washing. Acting in a profes-

sional, competent manner and using a gentle touch will help to ease embarrassment on the part of the resident. Guidelines for providing perineal care are given in Guidelines Box 23-3.

Helping Hands and a Caring Heart

FOCUS ON HUMANISTIC HEALTH CARE

Having to help another person with perineal care may seem very unpleasant or embarrassing to you. But think of it this way—what if you were sick or injured to the point that you had wet yourself or had a bowel movement in the bed? Think of how wonderful it would feel to have someone clean you up, help you change your clothes, and give you fresh bed linens. You would feel clean and cared for.

Guidelines Box 23-3	Guidelines for Providing Perineal Care
WHAT YOU DO	**WHY YOU DO IT**
Explain the procedure to the person, even if he or she is unconscious.	Many people find being touched in an intimate area by a stranger embarrassing, frightening, or even offensive. Explaining the procedure in a professional way helps to put the person at ease and reassures the person that he or she will be treated with respect.
Take care to protect the person's modesty.	Receiving perineal care can be very embarrassing. Properly draping the person may help to relieve some of the person's discomfort and feeling of being "exposed."
Always check the temperature of the water using a bath thermometer. The water temperature should be between 110°F (43.3°C) and 115°F (46.1°C).*	Water that is too cold is uncomfortable, and water that is too hot could scald the person. A bath thermometer provides *objective* information. Testing the water with your hand provides *subjective* information. (In other words, water that "feels all right" to your touch may, in reality, be much too hot or too cold. The only way to know that the water temperature is within the safe range is to measure it.)
Follow standard precautions when providing perineal care.	Providing perineal care places you at risk for exposure to urine, feces, and other body substances (for example, blood, vaginal secretions, semen).
Perineal care is the last part of a person's bathing routine. Washcloths, towels, and the water in the wash basin (if a bed bath is being given) are discarded and not used on any other body parts after the perineal care is completed.	The anus is a source of microbes and the perineum provides an environment that supports their growth. To prevent spread of these microbes to other parts of the body, where they may gain access and cause infection, the perineal area is washed last.
The vulva (in women) or the penis (in men) is cleaned before the perineum.	Because the anus opens onto the perineum, the perineum is often contaminated with microbes from the digestive tract. Therefore, this area is washed last to prevent microbes from the digestive tract from being introduced into the vagina or urethra, where they can cause infection.
Rinse the skin thoroughly to remove all soap.	The skin of the perineum and surrounding structures is delicate. Soap is drying and can irritate the skin if not rinsed away.
Gently pat the skin dry. Do not rub vigorously. Dry the skin thoroughly.	The skin of the perineum and surrounding structures is delicate. Vigorously rubbing the skin with a towel is uncomfortable for the person and can create friction, which in turn can cause skin breakdown. Moisture in areas where skin comes in contact with skin can also lead to skin breakdown.

(continued)

Guidelines Box **23-3**	Guidelines for Providing Perineal Care (continued)
WHAT YOU DO	**WHY YOU DO IT**
Apply a barrier cream or ointment if the person is incontinent, according to the person's care plan.	The barrier cream or ointment helps to protect the skin from contact with urine or feces. Prolonged contact with urine or feces can lead to skin breakdown.
Remove your gloves and wash your hands before touching clean clothing or linens.	Gloves worn while providing perineal care are considered contaminated.

*The water in the basin can be slightly hotter [110°F (43.3°C)] than the water in a tub or shower [105°F (40.5°C)] because it cools off quickly and the person will not be immersed in it.

PROVIDING PERINEAL CARE FOR FEMALE RESIDENTS

Procedure 23-4 describes how to assist a female resident with perineal care.

PROVIDING PERINEAL CARE FOR MALE RESIDENTS

Male residents may be circumcised or uncircumcised (Fig. 23-4). **Circumcision** is a procedure involving the removal of the **foreskin,** the fold of loose skin that covers the head of the penis. Male infants are often circumcised for religious or cultural reasons. When you are assisting an uncircumcised man with perineal care, it is important

to pull the foreskin back so that the head of the penis can be cleaned thoroughly. After cleaning and rinsing the penis, always remember to pull the foreskin back up over the head of the penis. If the foreskin is not pulled back into place, it can create a band around the penis, causing pain and swelling. Procedure 23-5 describes how to assist a male resident with perineal care.

ASSISTING WITH SKIN CARE

BATHING

Bathing serves many purposes. The act of bathing:

- Cleans the skin and eliminates body odors
- Helps a person feel relaxed and refreshed
- Exercises muscles that might otherwise not be used
- Simulates blood flow to the skin (through touching and massaging of the skin), which helps to prevent skin breakdown
- Helps the resident meet the needs of love and belonging and self-esteem
- Gives the nursing assistant an opportunity to observe for skin problems and to communicate and bond with the resident

The frequency and method of bathing are determined by many factors, including:

- Personal choice
- Cultural or religious beliefs
- The person's state of health

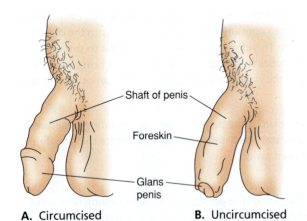

A. Circumcised **B. Uncircumcised**

Figure 23-4
Male patients or residents may have a circumcised or uncircumcised penis. **(A)** A circumcised penis. **(B)** An uncircumcised penis.

- The person's ability to care for himself
- The facility's policy (for example, in a long-term care facility, residents may receive complete baths or showers two or three times weekly, with partial baths on days in between)

A complete bath, or one that involves the entire body, is not always necessary. A partial bath provides many of the same health benefits and achieves the same goals of odor and infection control. During a partial bath, only the face, hands, axillae (armpits), back, buttocks, and perineal area are washed. A partial bath can be done at the sink or, if the person cannot get out of bed, at the bedside.

A resident may ask to skip his or her bath for many reasons. For example, the resident may tell you, "I'm tired and I want to sleep," "I feel a cold coming on," or "I just don't feel up to it today." You could insist that the person bathe, creating tension and causing the person to feel unappreciated and disrespected. Or, you could offer to help the person "just freshen up a bit instead" and achieve the goal of bathing in a different manner. For example, you could assist the person with a partial bath at the sink instead of a complete bath in a tub or shower. With this approach, the person is clean but was allowed to refuse his or her bath (so to speak), and you have fulfilled your responsibility, while also respecting the person's wishes. You should always report any refusal of care to the nurse, along with a description of what care you were able to provide. If a resident refuses personal hygienic care consistently, the decision may be made to bathe the person against his or her wishes out of respect for the person's health.

Helping Hands and a Caring Heart

FOCUS ON HUMANISTIC HEALTH CARE

When assisting a resident with bathing, think about how you would feel if you were in that person's situation. You might feel embarrassed because you have to rely on someone else to help you with one of life's most basic tasks. You might also feel exposed because another person (possibly of the opposite sex) is seeing and touching your body. Acknowledge your resident's feelings by providing as much privacy as possible during the procedure and by maintaining a professional attitude at all times.

Supplies for Bathing

Various supplies are used for bathing and skin care:

- **Soap,** available in liquid or cake form, is used to clean the skin. The lather lifts away dirt, oil, microbes, and sweat. Because soap is drying to the skin, it is important to rinse it away completely.
- **Soapless cleanser ("no-rinse soap")** is often used instead of soap to cleanse fragile, dry skin (such as the skin of elderly people). Soapless cleanser cleans, moisturizes, and protects the skin. Many soapless cleansers do not need to be rinsed away. Often, these products are supplied on pre-moistened disposable cloths. Some of these products are for use specifically in the perineal area.
- **Lotions** and **creams,** which may be perfumed or unscented, are applied to skin that is still slightly damp to create a moisture barrier that helps to prevent drying and chapping. Lotions and creams are an especially important part of skin care for elderly people, because with aging, the skin secretes a reduced amount of natural oil, resulting in dryness and a loss of elasticity.
- **Bath oils** are added to the bath water to scent and moisten the skin. Because bath oils make the surface of the bathtub slippery, these products are not generally recommended for use with older people. If bath oils are used, they should be used with extreme caution.
- **Body powder** can help absorb moisture and sweat and reduces friction between skin surfaces that touch. Powder should only be applied to skin that has been dried thoroughly. When using powder, sprinkle a small amount into the palm of your hand and then gently pat it onto the person's skin. Avoid big clouds of powder—too much powder can irritate the skin, and if the person inhales it, then it can irritate the airways too. In addition, powder spilled on the floor can be very slippery.
- **Deodorants** and **antiperspirants** are often applied after bathing to help prevent body odor. **Deodorants** are products that cover or mask odor. **Antiperspirants** contain ingredients that stop or slow sweating. Most antiperspirant products also contain a deodorant. Application of an antiperspirant or deodorant should be included as part of a person's personal care routine if the person requests it.

Most people are particular about the skin care products they use. Some people are sensitive or allergic to ingredients commonly used in skin care products. If you notice that one of your residents develops itching, redness, or a rash after using a skin care product, please report this observation to the nurse and stop use of that particular product until the source of the skin irritation has been determined. Always ask new residents if they have particular preferences in skin care products, or if there are any products that cause problems for them.

In addition to skin care products, a variety of linens are used for bathing. Bath blankets are used to preserve a person's modesty during a bed bath and when providing perineal care. A washcloth is wrapped around the hand to form a "mitt" for cleansing the body (Fig. 23-5). A towel is used to dry the body, and can also be used to help preserve the person's modesty. A clean change of clothes should be available for the person to put on after the bath.

Standard Bathing Techniques

General guidelines for assisting residents with bathing are given in Guidelines Box 23-4. The amount of assistance each resident will need to bathe will vary. For people who can bathe themselves, you will only need to see that they have bathing supplies and clean clothes. Some people will only need your help to clean hard-to-reach areas, such as the back or feet. Others will need your help throughout the bath.

Assisting your residents with bathing provides an excellent opportunity for you to observe the resident's skin and body for any changes in condition that should be reported to the nurse.

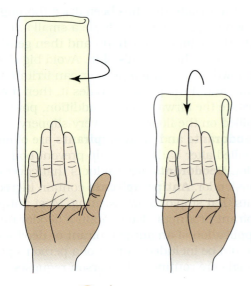

Figure 23-5
Making a bath mitt from a washcloth.

Because you will be caring for the person regularly, you will be more likely to notice changes that might go unnoticed by others.

TELL THE NURSE !

Tell the nurse immediately if you observe any of the following signs or symptoms while assisting a person with his or her bath:

- New rashes, bruises, broken skin, bleeding, or unusual odors
- Areas that are red, pale, or have a bluish cast (cyanosis)
- Areas that are swollen or tender
- Any complaints of burning or itching
- New hair loss (anywhere on the body, not just on the head)
- A flaking, itchy, or sore scalp or the presence of nits (head lice)
- Redness or yellow discoloration of the sclera (that is, the whites of the eyes)
- Yellowing or thickening of the fingernails or toenails
- Changes in mental status and alertness (for example, disorientation, confusion)

Showers and tub baths

Taking a shower or bathing in a bathtub are ways of cleansing the body that are familiar to all of us. In many long-term care facilities, residents are taken to a shower or tub room down the hall to shower or bathe (Fig. 23-6). In some long-term care facilities, there is a shower or bathtub in the bathroom attached to the resident's room.

Showers in many long-term care facilities have stalls that are large enough for a shower chair to fit inside, allowing a weak or unsteady person to sit down while taking a shower (Fig. 23-7). Padding the shower chair with towels and placing a footstool under the resident's feet can help the resident feel more comfortable and secure in the chair.

Most long-term facilities have whirlpool tubs that stimulate blood flow and relax muscles by the action of the water (Fig. 23-8). These tubs usually have chair-lift devices to allow for easy and safe transfer of residents into and out of the tub. The lift devices also allow residents who are in a coma or who are severely physically disabled to receive the comfort and benefit of a whirlpool

Guidelines Box 23-4   Guidelines for Bathing

WHAT YOU DO	WHY YOU DO IT
Follow the care plan or the nurse's directions for bathing the person	A person's medical condition may dictate the type of bath he or she can have. For example, a person with a spinal injury may not be permitted to have a whirlpool bath, while for a person with poor skin circulation, a whirlpool bath may be considered a type of therapy.
Before beginning the bath, explain to the person how the bathing procedure will be carried out (and how the person can assist in the process). In addition, explain the benefits of bathing (such as comfort, healthy skin).	Explaining the details of the bathing process may help to relieve the person's fears (for example, about potential exposure), and will help the person to see how he or she can participate in the process. Explaining the procedure is particularly important for people with memory problems, who may find the bathing experience frightening because they cannot remember what bathing is or why it is important.
Collect all necessary equipment, linens, bath products, and clothing before beginning the bath. Check the tub room for cleanliness and prepare the tub before bringing the person into the room.	Being prepared and having all necessary supplies and equipment at hand will allow the bath to proceed efficiently. Efficiency is necessary to protect the person's modesty and to prevent chills.
Close all doors and windows in the room, and make sure the blinds are down or the curtains are drawn.	Closing doors and windows eliminates drafts in the room, which could cause the person to become chilled. In addition, closing doors and covering the windows protects the person's modesty and privacy.
Ensure the resident's physical and emotional comfort. For example, make sure the room is warm enough, and pad the frame and seat of the shower chair with rolled towels. Having the person rest his feet on a foot stool while he is seated in a shower chair can help him feel more secure. Keep the resident covered with a robe or bath blanket, as much as possible.	Taking steps to make bath time as comfortable and pleasant as possible for the person can help overcome resistance to taking a bath or shower.
Place a non-skid mat in the bathtub or on the shower floor. Encourage the person to use handrails. Provide a shower chair for people who are weak or unsteady.	These measures help to protect the person from falling.
Never lock the bathroom door.	Because you should never leave a person alone in the bathtub or shower, if you need help for any reason, you will have to call for someone to come to you. This person will need to be able to access the bathroom without your help.

(continued)

Guidelines Box 23-4 Guidelines for Bathing (continued)

WHAT YOU DO	WHY YOU DO IT
Always check the temperature of the water using a bath thermometer. The water temperature should be between 105°F (40.5°C) and 115°F (46.1°C).	Water that is too cold is uncomfortable, and water that is too hot could scald the person. A bath thermometer provides *objective* information. Testing the water with your hand provides *subjective* information. (In other words, water that "feels all right" to your touch may, in reality, be much too hot or too cold. The only way to know that the water temperature is within the safe range is to measure it.)
When assisting a person to and from the tub room, always make sure that he or she is adequately covered.	The person's privacy and modesty must be protected at all times.
Always help the person into and out of the bathtub or shower.	A wet bathroom floor can be slippery, and can place the person at risk for falling.
Follow standard precautions when bathing a person.	Bathing a person places you at risk for coming into contact with non-intact skin or body fluids.
Wash from the cleanest to the dirtiest areas.	This approach prevents contamination of clean areas.
Touch the person's body gently yet deliberately, using long, firm strokes.	A gentle yet firm touch conveys to the person that this is a routine procedure being carried out by a professional, ensures that the skin is properly cleaned, and stimulates skin circulation.
Rinse the skin thoroughly to remove all soap.	Soap is drying and can irritate the skin if not rinsed away.
Gently pat the skin dry. Do not rub vigorously. Dry the skin thoroughly, especially in areas where skin touches skin (for example, underneath the breasts, between the legs).	The skin, especially that of elderly people, is fragile. Vigorously rubbing the skin with a towel is uncomfortable for the person and can create friction, which in turn can cause skin breakdown. Moisture in areas where skin comes in contact with skin can also lead to skin breakdown.

bath. Most tubs have a shower attachment so that hair can be washed during the bath.

Many modern tub and shower units have controls that pre-set the water temperature, ensuring that it is not too hot or too cold. After each use, the tub or shower stall (and the shower chair, if one was used) is disinfected. This is important to prevent the spread of infection. Facility policy will state who is responsible for cleaning and disinfecting the bathing equipment.

Procedure 23-6 describes how to assist with a tub bath or shower.

Bed baths

Some residents are simply too weak or ill to take a shower or tub bath, or taking a shower or tub

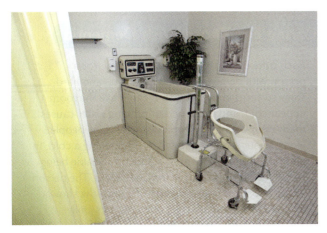

Figure 23-6
"Home-like" touches, such as soothing paint colors, hanging plants, and colorful shower curtains, help residents to feel more comfortable in the shower or tub room.

bath is a source of too much stress. In these situations, bath supplies and a basin of warm water are brought to the bedside, and the person is assisted with bathing in bed (Fig. 23-9). A complete or partial bed bath is given, depending on the needs of the resident (Procedures 23-7 and 23-8, respectively).

An alternative to the traditional bed bath is the use of a "bag bath." "Bag baths" are very comfortable and refreshing for a resident, and they are

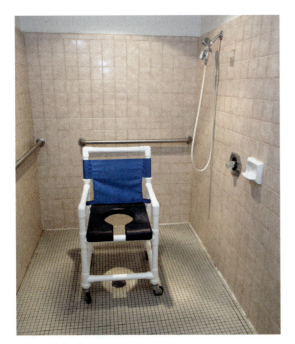

Figure 23-7
A shower chair is used to reduce the resident's risk of falling in the shower.

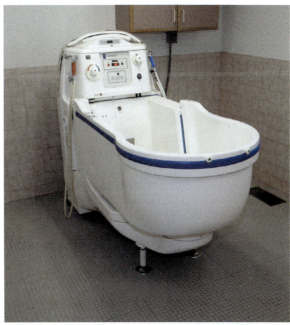

A

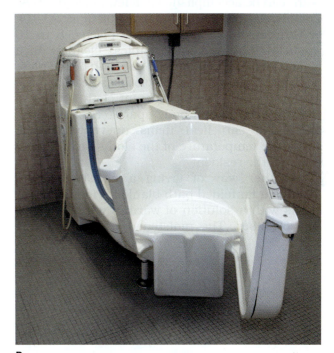

B

Figure 23-8
(A) Many long-term care facilities have whirlpool tubs, which help to stimulate circulation and massage the skin. **(B)** On this model, the front of the tub swings open to make it easier for the resident to get into and out of the tub.

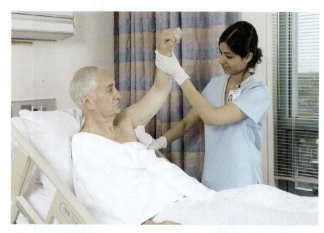

Figure 23-9
When a shower or tub bath is not possible, a bed bath can be given.

efficient and effective for the nursing staff. A "bag bath" can be accomplished in a few different ways. Commercial bag baths are available (Fig. 23-10), or you can make your own by placing 8 to 10 washcloths soaked in a soapless cleanser in a plastic bag. The commercial bag bath or the plastic bag containing the washcloths is heated in the microwave, and then a different cloth is used to clean each main body part. Because the microwave can heat items unevenly, always check the temperature of the cloths before using them on the resident.

Another way of giving a bag bath is to moisten a fanfolded bath blanket and two washcloths with a solution of warm water and soapless cleanser. The moistened bath blanket is

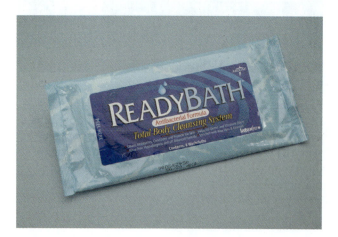

Figure 23-10
Many facilities use "bag baths" as a quick and efficient alternative to a traditional bed bath.

Caring For Those With Dementia

Bath time can be a very upsetting time for a person with dementia. The bright lights and hard, shiny surfaces in the tub room can make the room appear cold, and the sound of running water causes many people with dementia distress. Many people worry about slipping and falling or catching a cold. In addition, most people are very uncomfortable being naked (or nearly naked) in front of others. The person might also be physically uncomfortable—the shower chair is hard, and the large, open room is chilly!

To help bath time go more smoothly for your residents with dementia:

- Try to make the room feel warm and inviting. Fill the tub ahead of time, and make sure the room is warm. Soft music can also be soothing.

- Keep the resident covered with a robe or bath blanket as much as possible.

- Pad the frame of the shower chair with rolled towels and place a folded towel on the seat for comfort. Using a footstool to support the resident's feet may help the resident to feel more secure in the chair.

- Put off shampooing the resident's hair until the end of the bath or shower if getting the head wet is upsetting to the resident. Using a wet washcloth to wet the resident's hair might be less upsetting for the resident than using the shower spray.

- Keep your focus on the resident, not the task.

placed over the resident while the resident is in bed, and then covered with a dry bath blanket. The resident's body is massaged through the blanket layers to clean the skin. The washcloths are used to cleanse the resident's face and the perineal area. You will need to check the temperature of the bath blanket and washcloths before using them on the resident to make sure that they are not too hot or too cold.

MASSAGE

Illness, disability that results in loss of mobility, and aging all contribute to a loss of blood flow (circulation) to the skin. A person who sits in a chair or wheelchair for long periods of time or who must remain in bed is at an increased risk for developing pressure ulcers (see Chapter 31), as a result of that lack of blood flow. Massaging the skin regularly helps to stimulate the circulation. It is also very relaxing for the resident. A back massage is usually performed after a person's bath while rubbing lotion or cream into the skin, when repositioning a helpless person, or as a part of evening care to promote relaxation and sleep. Some studies have shown that slow, gentle massage can be very calming for people with dementia.

An effective back massage takes approximately 4 to 6 minutes to complete and can be performed with the person in either the prone or the lateral position. The extra minutes spent massaging a resident's back are well worth the effort and are beneficial for both physical and emotional health. While performing a back massage, you have an excellent opportunity to observe the person's skin for potential problems.

TELL THE NURSE

Skin breakdown can lead to pressure ulcers. Tell the nurse immediately if you observe any of the following early signs of skin breakdown:

- Reddened or darkened skin, especially over a bony area, that does not return to its normal color after pressure is relieved

- Pale, white, or shiny skin over a bony area

- Areas of skin that are hot to the touch

- Areas of skin that are painful or tender

As with any personal care procedure, always check with a nurse or read the person's care plan before beginning—a back massage should not be performed on a person with fractured ribs or a back injury, nor should it be performed on a person who has recently had back surgery. Procedure 23-9 describes how to give a back massage.

SUMMARY

- Cleanliness of the body is essential for a person's physical and emotional well-being.
  - Healthy skin and mucous membranes help protect the body from being invaded by infection-causing microbes.
  - Feeling clean also improves a person's self-esteem and increases comfort.
- Allowing people to participate in their own self-care helps to maintain independence, but assisting, as necessary, helps to ensure that hygiene is performed thoroughly. Assisting a person with personal hygiene activities provides many opportunities for observation.
- Activities associated with personal hygiene are usually carried out at scheduled times throughout the day.
  - When possible, adjustments are made to the schedule to accommodate personal preferences (for example, bathing in the evening versus the morning).
  - Assistance with personal hygiene is provided any time that a resident's condition warrants it. Wet or soiled skin, clothing, or bedding requires immediate attention.
- Oral care involves caring for the teeth, gums, lips, and mucous membranes of the mouth.

A clean, healthy mouth makes food taste better, provides a line of defense against infection, and allows a person to chew food properly.
  - Natural teeth should be brushed and flossed daily.
  - Dentures must be handled with care because they are expensive.
  - Standard precautions should be taken when providing oral care because contact with body fluids is possible. Droplet precautions should be taken if the resident is known to have an infection that is spread by exposure to droplets released from the mouth or nose.
- Perineal care involves cleansing of the perineum, the anus, the vulva (in women), and the penis (in men).
  - Inadequate hygiene in the perineal area places a person at risk for infection and skin breakdown, and can lead to unpleasant odors.
  - Because receiving assistance with perineal care is embarrassing for most people, take extra care to preserve the person's modesty. Having a professional attitude when assisting a person with perineal care also demonstrates competence and helps to ease embarrassment on the part of the resident.

- Standard precautions should be taken when providing perineal care because contact with body fluids is likely.
- Always wash toward the anus, away from the urethra. This helps to prevent the spread of microbes from the anus and perineum into the urethra or vagina, where they could cause infection.

- Skin care involves keeping the skin clean and moisturized. Skin care may also involve massage to enhance blood flow to the skin.

- Bathing may be accomplished in a bathtub or shower, at the sink, or in bed.
- During a partial bath, only the face, hands, axillae, back, buttocks, and perineum are washed.
- A back massage is relaxing for the resident and helps to prevent the development of pressure ulcers.

Brushing and Flossing the Teeth

WHY YOU DO IT   Brushing and flossing the teeth helps to keep the teeth and gums healthy, makes the mouth feel better and food taste better, and prevents bad breath.

Getting Ready WORK STEPS

1. Complete the "Getting Ready" steps.

Supplies

- gloves
- mask (if necessary)
- goggles (if necessary)
- paper towels
- straw (optional)
- paper cups
- emesis basin
- toothbrush
- toothpaste
- dental floss
- lip lubricant (optional)
- mouthwash (optional)
- towel

Procedure

2. Cover the over-bed table with paper towels. Place the oral care supplies on the over-bed table. Fill a paper cup with water.

3. Make sure that the bed is positioned at a comfortable working height (to promote good body mechanics) and that the wheels are locked.

4. If the side rails are in use, lower the side rail on the working side of the bed. The side rail on the opposite side of the bed should remain up.

5. Raise the head of the bed as tolerated. Place a towel under the person's chin.

6. Put on the mask, goggles, or both, if necessary. Put on the gloves.

7. Wet the toothbrush. Put a small amount of toothpaste on the toothbrush.

8. Brush the person's teeth as follows:

    a. Position the toothbrush at a 45° angle to the gums, against the outer surface of the top teeth. Starting at the back of the mouth, brush the outer surface of each tooth using a gentle circular motion.

Repeat for the lower teeth. Allow the person to spit toothpaste into the emesis basin as necessary.

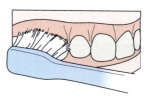

Step 8a Clean the outer surfaces of the teeth.

b. Position the toothbrush at a 45° angle to the gums, against the inner surface of the top teeth. Starting at the back of the mouth, brush the inner surface of each tooth using a gentle circular motion. Repeat for the lower teeth.

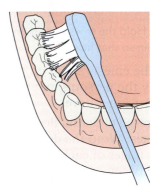

Step 8b Clean the inner surfaces of the teeth.

c. Brush the chewing surfaces of the upper and lower teeth using a gentle circular motion.

(continued)

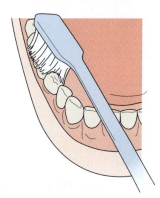

Step 8c Clean the chewing surfaces of the teeth.

d. Brush the tongue.

9. Offer the person the cup of water (and a straw, if allowed) and ask him to rinse his mouth completely. Hold the emesis basin underneath the person's chin so that he can spit the water into the basin.

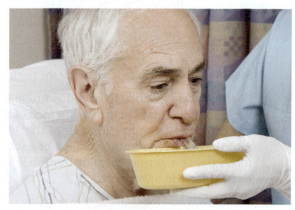

Step 9 Hold the emesis basin underneath the person's chin so that he can spit.

10. Place the emesis basin on the over-bed table and dry the person's mouth and chin thoroughly using a towel.

11. Cut a piece of dental floss measuring about 18 inches. Wrap the dental floss around the middle finger of each hand. Hold the dental floss between your thumb and index finger on each hand and stretch it tight.

12. Insert a segment of dental floss between two teeth, starting with the back upper teeth. Move the floss up and down gently, and then remove the dental floss from the person's mouth. Advance the floss a bit by releasing it from one middle finger and wrapping it around the other, and move on to the next two teeth. Use a new strand of

dental floss as necessary. Offer the person the glass of water (and the straw, if allowed) to rinse as necessary. Floss all of the person's teeth.

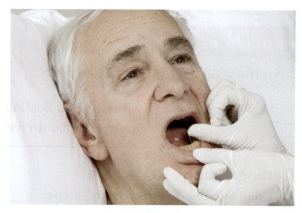

Step 12 Insert the dental floss between two teeth and move it up and down gently.

13. Offer the person the cup of water (and the straw, if allowed) and ask him to rinse his mouth completely. Hold the emesis basin underneath the person's chin so that he can spit the water into the basin.

14. Place the emesis basin on the over-bed table and dry the person's mouth and chin thoroughly using a towel.

15. Pour a small amount of mouthwash (approximately ¼ cup) into another paper cup and help the person to rinse, as the person requests.

16. Apply lip lubricant to the lips, as the person requests.

17. If the side rails are in use, return the side rails to the raised position. Lower the head of the bed as the person requests. Make sure that the bed is lowered to its lowest position and that the wheels are locked.

18. Gather the soiled linens and place them in the linen hamper or linen bag. Dispose of disposable items in a facility-approved waste container. Clean equipment and return it to the storage area.

19. Remove your gloves (and goggles and mask, if using) and dispose of them in a facility-approved waste container.

Finishing Up CLOSWR

20. Complete the "Finishing Up" steps.

PROCEDURE 23-2

Providing Oral Care for a Person With Dentures

WHY YOU DO IT   Proper care of the gums and dentures helps to keep the mouth healthy and the dentures fitting properly and comfortably. It also makes the mouth feel better and food taste better and prevents bad breath.

Getting Ready WGKIEPS

1. Complete the "Getting Ready" steps.

Supplies

- gloves
- mask (if necessary)
- goggles (if necessary)
- paper towels
- gauze squares (4″ × 4″)
- straw (optional)
- foam-tipped applicators (optional)
- emesis basin
- paper cups
- denture cup
- denture brush or toothbrush
- denture cleaner or toothpaste
- denture solution (optional)
- mouthwash (optional)
- lip lubricant (optional)
- towel
- washcloth

Procedure

2. Cover the over-bed table with paper towels. Place the oral care supplies on the over-bed table. Fill a paper cup with water.

3. Make sure that the bed is positioned at a comfortable working height (to promote good body mechanics) and that the wheels are locked. Raise the head of the bed as tolerated. Place a towel under the person's chin.

4. Put on the mask, goggles, or both, if necessary. Put on the gloves.

5. Ask the person to remove his dentures and place them in the emesis basin. If the person needs assistance with removing his dentures:

   a. Ask the person to open his mouth.

   b. Holding a gauze square between your thumb and index finger, grasp the upper denture, moving it up and down slightly to break the seal. Ease the denture down, forward, and out of the mouth. Place the denture in the emesis basin.

   c. Holding a gauze square between your thumb and index finger, grasp the lower denture. Turn the denture slightly, lifting it out of the mouth. Place the denture in the emesis basin.

6. Take the emesis basin, the washcloth, the denture cup, the denture brush or toothbrush, and the denture cleaner or toothpaste to the sink. Line the sink with the washcloth to provide extra cushioning. Fill the sink partially with lukewarm water. Do not place the dentures in the sink.

7. Wet the denture brush or the toothbrush. Put a small amount of toothpaste or denture cleaner on the denture brush or toothbrush. Working with one denture at a time, hold the denture in the palm of your hand and brush it on all surfaces until it is clean. Rinse the denture thoroughly under lukewarm running water and place it in the denture cup. Repeat with the other denture.

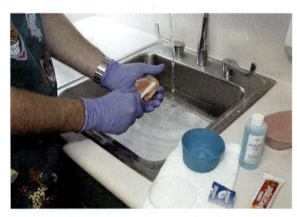

Step 7 Hold the denture in the palm of your hand, and brush it on all surfaces until it is clean.

8. If the dentures are to be stored, fill the denture cup with lukewarm water, a mixture of one part mouthwash to one part lukewarm water, or a denture solution so that the dentures are covered. Put the lid on the denture cup. Return the denture cup to the person's bedside table, making sure that it is within easy reach.

(continued)

9. If the dentures are to be reinserted in the person's mouth, take the emesis basin, the denture cup, and the toothbrush to the over-bed table. If the side rails are in use, lower the side rail on the working side of the bed. The side rail on the opposite side of the bed should remain up.

   a. Offer the person the cup of water (and a straw, if allowed) and ask him to rinse his mouth completely. Some people may wish to use mouthwash instead of water. Hold the emesis basin under-neath the person's chin so that he can spit the water or mouthwash into the basin.

   b. Place the emesis basin on the over-bed table and dry the person's mouth and chin thoroughly using a face towel.

   c. Gently clean the person's gums and tongue and the insides of the cheeks with the toothbrush or a foam-tipped applicator moistened with water or mouthwash. Use fresh applicators as needed.

   d. Ask the person to insert his dentures. If the person needs assistance with inserting his dentures:
      - Ask the person to open his mouth.
      - Gently lift the person's upper lip up. Grasp the upper denture between your thumb and index finger and insert it in the person's mouth. Press gently on the

   denture to be sure that it is seated properly.
      - Gently pull the person's lower lip down. Grasp the lower denture between your thumb and index finger and insert it in the person's mouth.

   e. Return the denture cup to the person's bedside table, making sure that it is within easy reach.

10. Dry the person's mouth and chin thoroughly using a towel. Apply lip lubricant to the lips, as the person requests.

11. Reposition the person comfortably and lower the head of the bed if necessary. If the side rails are in use, return the side rails to the raised position. Make sure that the bed is lowered to its lowest position and that the wheels are locked.

12. Gather the soiled linens and place them in the linen hamper or linen bag. Dispose of disposable items in a facility-approved waste container. Clean equipment and return it to the storage area.

13. Remove your gloves (and goggles and mask, if using) and dispose of them in a facility-approved waste container.

Finishing Up CLSOWR

14. Complete the "Finishing Up" steps.

PROCEDURE 23-3

Providing Oral Care for an Unconscious Person

WHY YOU DO IT   An unconscious person breathes through the mouth, causing the lips and mucous membranes to dry out. Frequent mouth care keeps the mucous membranes of the mouth moist and healthy and promotes comfort.

Getting Ready WGKIEpS

1. Complete the "Getting Ready" steps.

Supplies

- gloves
- paper towels
- sponge-tipped applicators
- padded tongue blade
- paper cups
- emesis basin
- toothbrush and toothpaste (if the person has natural teeth)
- lip lubricant
- saline (optional)
- mouthwash (optional)
- towels

Procedure

2. Cover the over-bed table with paper towels. Place the oral care supplies on the over-bed table. Fill the paper cup with water.

3. Make sure that the bed is positioned at a comfortable working height (to promote good body mechanics) and that the wheels are locked. If the side rails are in use, lower the side rail on the working side of the bed. The side rail on the opposite side of the bed should remain up.

4. Raise the head of the bed as tolerated. Turn the person's head to the side facing you. If it is difficult to keep the person's head turned to the side, roll the person onto his or her side.

5. If the person's condition permits, gently lift the person's head and place a towel on the pillow. Place the emesis basin on the towel, level with the person's chin.

6. Put on the gloves.

7. Open the person's mouth using the padded tongue blade. Be gentle; do not force the mouth open. Insert the tongue blade between the upper and lower teeth at the back of the mouth to hold the person's mouth open.

8. Clean the inside of the mouth:

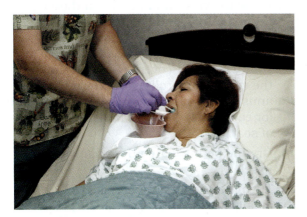

Step 8 Clean the inside of the person's mouth, using a padded tongue blade to keep the mouth open.

   a. If the person has natural teeth, they should be gently brushed as described in Procedure 23-1.

   b. If the person is edentulous, gently clean the person's gums and tongue and the insides of the cheeks with the toothbrush or a foam-tipped applicator moistened with water, saline, or mouthwash. Use fresh applicators as needed.

9. Dry the person's mouth and chin thoroughly using a towel. Apply lip lubricant to the lips. Reposition the person comfortably.

10. If the side rails are in use, return the side rails to the raised position. Lower the head of the bed. Make sure that the bed is lowered to its lowest position and that the wheels are locked.

11. Gather the soiled linens and place them in the linen hamper or linen bag. Dispose of disposable items in a facility-approved waste container. Clean equipment and return it to the storage area.

12. Remove your gloves and dispose of them in a facility-approved waste container.

Finishing Up CLSOWR

13. Complete the "Finishing Up" steps.

PROCEDURE 23-4

Providing Female Perineal Care

WHY YOU DO IT   Proper perineal care helps to prevent skin breakdown (which can lead to pressure ulcers), infection, and odor.

Getting Ready WCKIEpS

1. Complete the "Getting Ready" steps.

Supplies

- gloves
- paper towels
- bed protector
- bath thermometer
- wash basin
- bedpan
- soap
- bath blanket
- washcloths
- towel
- clean clothing
- clean linens (if necessary)
- barrier cream or ointment (if ordered)

Procedure

2. Cover the over-bed table with paper towels. Place the wash basin, toiletries, clean clothing, and clean linens on the over-bed table.

(continued)

3. Make sure that the bed is positioned at a comfortable working height (to promote good body mechanics) and that the wheels are locked.

4. Put on the gloves.

5. Because bathing often stimulates the urge to urinate, offer the bedpan. If the person uses the bedpan, empty and clean it before proceeding with the perineal care. Remove your gloves and dispose of them in a facility-approved waste container. Wash your hands and put on a clean pair of gloves.

6. Lower the head of the bed to a flat position (as tolerated).

7. Fill the wash basin with warm water [110°F (43.3°C) to 115°F (46.1°C) on the bath thermometer]. Place the basin on the over-bed table.

8. If the side rails are in use, lower the side rail on the working side. The side rail on the opposite side of the bed should remain up.

9. Spread the bath blanket over the top linens (and the person). If the person is able, have her hold the bath blanket. If not, tuck the corners under the person's shoulders. Fanfold the top linens to the foot of the bed.

10. Assist the person with undressing.

11. Ask the person to open her legs and bend her knees, if possible. If she is not able to bend her knees, help her spread her legs as much as possible.

12. Position the bath blanket over the person so that one corner can be wrapped under and around each leg.

13. Position the bed protector under the person's buttocks to keep the bed linens dry.

14. Lift the corner of the bath blanket that is between the person's legs upward, exposing only the perineal area.

15. Form a mitt around your hand with one of the washcloths. Wet the mitt with warm, clean water and apply soap.

16. Using the other hand, separate the labia. Clean the vulva by placing your washcloth-covered hand at the top of the vulva and stroking downward to the anus. Use a different part of the washcloth for each stroke. Repeat until the area is clean.

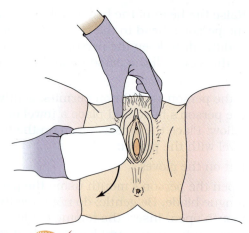

Step 16 📐 Clean the vulva by placing your washcloth-covered hand at the top of the vulva and stroking downward to the anus.

17. Rinse the vulva and perineum thoroughly. Form a mitt around your hand with a clean, wet washcloth. Using the other hand, separate the labia. Rinse the vulva by placing your washcloth-covered hand at the top of the vulva and stroking downward to the anus. Use a different part of the washcloth for each stroke. Repeat until the area is free of soap.

18. Dry the perineal area thoroughly using a towel.

19. Turn the person onto her side so that she is facing away from you. Help the person toward the working side of the bed so that her buttocks are within easy reach. Adjust the bath blanket to keep the person covered.

20. Form a mitt around your hand with one of the washcloths. Wet the mitt with warm, clean water and apply soap.

21. Using the other hand, separate the buttocks. Place your washcloth-covered hand at the front of the body and stroke toward the back. First clean one side, then the other side, and finally the middle, using a different part of the washcloth each time, until the anal area is clean.

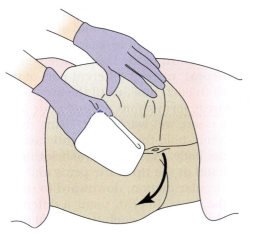

Step 21 Clean the anal area by placing your wash-cloth-covered hand at the front of the body and stroking toward the back.

22. Rinse and dry the anal area thoroughly.

23. Apply a barrier cream or ointment to the perineal area as ordered.

24. Remove the bed protector from underneath the person.

25. Remove your gloves and dispose of them in a facility-approved waste container. Put on a clean pair of gloves.

26. Assist the person into the supine position. Reposition the pillow under her head. Remove the bath blanket and help the person into the clean clothing.

27. If the bedding is wet or soiled, change the bed linens.

28. If the side rails are in use, return the side rail to the raised position. Raise the head of the bed as the person requests. Make sure that the bed is lowered to its lowest position and that the wheels are locked.

29. Gather the soiled linens and place them in the linen hamper or linen bag. Dispose of disposable items in a facility-approved waste container. Clean equipment and return it to the storage area.

30. Remove your gloves and dispose of them in a facility-approved waste container.

Finishing Up CLOSUR

31. Complete the "Finishing Up" steps.

PROCEDURE 23-5

Providing Male Perineal Care

WHY YOU DO IT   Proper perineal care helps to prevent skin breakdown (which can lead to pressure ulcers), infection, and odor.

Getting Ready WORKEPS

1. Complete the "Getting Ready" steps.

Supplies

- gloves
- paper towels
- bed protector
- bath thermometer
- wash basin
- bedpan or urinal
- soap
- bath blanket
- washcloths
- towel
- clean clothing
- clean linens (if necessary)
- barrier cream or ointment (if ordered)

Procedure

2. Cover the over-bed table with paper towels. Place the wash basin, toiletries, clean clothing, and clean linens on the over-bed table.

3. Make sure that the bed is positioned at a comfortable working height (to promote good body mechanics) and that the wheels are locked.

4. Put on the gloves.

5. Because bathing often stimulates the urge to urinate, offer the bedpan or urinal. If the person uses the bedpan or urinal, empty and clean it before proceeding with the perineal care. Remove your gloves and dispose of them in a facility-approved waste container. Wash your hands and put on a clean pair of gloves.

6. Lower the head of the bed to a flat position (as tolerated).

7. Fill the wash basin with warm water [110°F (43.3°C) to 115°F (46.1°C) on the bath

(continued)

thermometer]. Place the basin on the over-bed table.

8. If the side rails are in use, lower the side rail on the working side. The side rail on the opposite side of the bed should remain up.

9. Spread the bath blanket over the top linens (and the person). If the person is able, have him hold the bath blanket. If not, tuck the corners under the person's shoulders. Fanfold the top linens to the foot of the bed.

10. Assist the person with undressing.

11. Ask the person to open his legs and bend his knees, if possible. If he is not able to bend his knees, help him spread his legs as much as possible.

12. Position the bath blanket over the person so that one corner can be wrapped under and around each leg.

13. Position the bed protector under the person's buttocks to keep the bed linens dry.

14. Lift the corner of the bath blanket that is between the person's legs upward, exposing only the perineal area.

15. Form a mitt around your hand with one of the washcloths. Wet the mitt with warm, clean water and apply soap.

16. Using the other hand, hold the penis slightly away from the body.

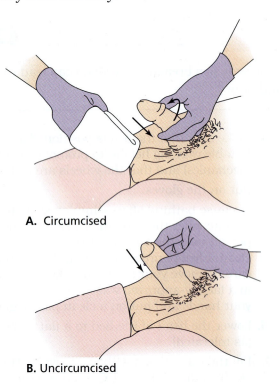

A. Circumcised

B. Uncircumcised

Step 16 To wash the penis, pass the washcloth in a circular motion, moving from the tip of the penis to the base. **(A)** circumcised penis; **(B)** uncircumcised penis.

a. **If the person is circumcised:** Place your washcloth-covered hand at the tip of the penis and wash in a circular motion, downward to the base of the penis. Repeat, using a different part of the washcloth each time, until the area is clean. To rinse, form a mitt around your hand with a clean, wet washcloth. Using the other hand, hold the penis slightly away from the body. Place your washcloth-covered hand at the tip of the penis and wipe in a circular motion, downward to the base of the penis. Repeat, using a different part of the washcloth each time, until the area is rinsed. Dry the tip and the shaft of the penis thoroughly.

b. **If the person is uncircumcised:** Retract the foreskin by gently pushing the skin toward the base of the penis. Place your washcloth-covered hand at the tip of the penis and wash in a circular motion, downward to the base of the penis. Repeat using a different part of the washcloth each time until the area is clean. Rinse and dry the tip and shaft of the penis thoroughly before gently pulling the foreskin back into its normal position.

17. Form a mitt around your hand with one of the washcloths. Wet the mitt with warm, clean water and apply soap. Wash the scrotum and perineum. Rinse and dry the scrotum and perineum thoroughly.

18. Turn the person onto his side so that he is facing away from you. Help the person toward the working side of the bed so that his buttocks are within easy reach. Adjust the bath blanket to keep the person covered.

19. Form a mitt around your hand with one of the washcloths. Wet the mitt with warm, clean water and apply soap.

20. Using the other hand, separate the buttocks. Place your washcloth-covered hand at the front of the body and stroke toward the back. First clean one side, then the other side, and finally the middle, using a different part of the washcloth each time, until the anal area is clean.

21. Rinse and dry the anal area thoroughly.

22. Apply a barrier cream or ointment to the perineal area as ordered.

23. Remove the bed protector from underneath the person.

24. Remove your gloves and dispose of them in a facility-approved waste container. Put on a clean pair of gloves.

25. Assist the person into the supine position. Reposition the pillow under the person's head. Remove the bath blanket and help the person into the clean clothing.

26. If the bedding is wet or soiled, change the bed linens.

27. If the side rails are in use, return the side rail to the raised position. Make sure that the bed is lowered to its lowest position and that the wheels are locked.

28. Gather the soiled linens and place them in the linen hamper or linen bag. Dispose of disposable items in a facility-approved waste container. Clean equipment and return it to the storage area.

29. Remove your gloves and dispose of them in a facility-approved waste container.

Finishing Up CLSOWR

30. Complete the "Finishing Up" steps.

PROCEDURE	23-6

Assisting With a Tub Bath or Shower

WHY YOU DO IT   Cleansing of the skin helps to prevent skin breakdown (which can lead to pressure ulcers), infection, and odor.

Getting Ready WGKIEPS

1. Prepare the tub room. Place a non-skid mat on the floor of the tub or shower. If the person will be taking a tub bath, fill the tub halfway with warm water (105°F [43.3°C] to 115°F [46.1°C] on the bath thermometer). Obtain a shower chair if necessary and place it in the shower. Place a towel on the chair in the tub room where the person will sit while drying off.

2. Complete the "Getting Ready" steps.

Supplies

- gloves
- bath thermometer
- soap
- washcloths
- towels
- lotion (optional)
- powder (optional)
- deodorant or antiperspirant (optional)
- clean clothing

Procedure

3. Ask the person if she needs to use the bathroom before bathing.

4. Assist the person to the tub room.

5. If the person will be taking a tub bath, check the temperature of the water and make sure the non-skid mat is secure. If the person will be taking a shower, turn on the water and adjust the temperature until the water is comfortable.

6. Assist the person with undressing. Assist the person into the bathtub or shower.

7. If the person is able to bathe herself, either partially or completely:

  a. Place bathing supplies within easy reach.

  b. Many facilities require you to remain in the room while the person bathes or showers. If facility policy permits you to leave the room, explain how to use the call light control and ask the person to signal when bathing is complete or when she has done as much as she can on her own and needs help completing the bath. Stay nearby and check on the person every 5 minutes. The person should not remain in the bathtub or shower for longer than 20 minutes. Return when the person signals. Remember to knock before entering.

8. If the person is unable to bathe herself or requires assistance:

  a. Put on the gloves and form a mitt around your hand with one of the washcloths.

  b. If necessary, ask the person what parts of the body were not washed. Assist the person as needed with completing the bath. Wash the cleanest areas first and the dirtiest areas last:

    ● **Eyes.** Wet the mitt with warm, clean water. Ask the person to close her eyes. Place your washcloth-covered hand at

(continued)

the inner corner of the eye and stroke gently outward, toward the outer corner. Use a different part of the washcloth for each eye.

- **Face, neck, and ears.** Ask the person if you should use soap on the face. Rinse the washcloth and apply soap, if requested. Wash the face, neck, and ears, moving from the top of the head to the bottom (so that the nose and mouth are washed last). Rinse thoroughly.
- **Arms and axillae (armpits).** Rinse the washcloth and apply soap. Place your washcloth-covered hand at the shoulder and stroke downward, toward the hand, using long, firm strokes. Wash the hand. If necessary, assist the person with raising her arm so that you can wash the axilla. Repeat for the other arm and axilla.
- **Chest and abdomen.** Using long, firm strokes, wash the person's chest and abdomen.
- **Legs and feet.** Place your washcloth-covered hand at the top of the thigh and stroke downward, toward the foot, using long, firm strokes. Wash the foot. Repeat for the other leg.
- **Back and buttocks:** Wash the person's back and buttocks, moving from top to bottom and using long, firm strokes.
- **Perineal area:** Complete perineal care.

9. Make sure that soap is thoroughly rinsed from all parts of the body.

10. Remove your gloves and dispose of them in a facility-approved waste container. Put on a clean pair of gloves.

11. If the person is taking a tub bath, drain the water and carefully assist the person out of the tub and into the towel-covered chair. If the person is taking a shower, turn the water off and assist the person into the towel-covered chair.

12. Wrap a towel around the person. Using another bath towel, help the person to dry off, patting the skin dry. Take care to ensure that areas where "skin meets skin" are dried thoroughly (for example, in between the toes and underneath the breasts).

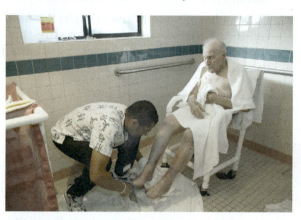

Step 12 Help the person to dry off, taking extra care to dry areas where "skin meets skin."

13. Help the person to apply lotion, powder, deodorant, antiperspirant, or other personal care products, as the person requests.

14. Help the person into the clean clothing. If the person is wearing nightwear, help her into a robe. Help the person into her slippers.

15. Remove your gloves and dispose of them in a facility-approved waste container.

16. Assist the person back to her room.

Finishing Up CLSOWR

17. Complete the "Finishing Up" steps.

18. Gather the soiled linens and place them in the linen hamper or linen bag. Dispose of disposable items in a facility-approved waste container. Clean equipment and return it to the storage area.

19. Clean the tub room and shower chair (if used), if housekeeping is not responsible for this task at your facility.

PROCEDURE 23-7

Giving a Complete Bed Bath

WHY YOU DO IT   Cleansing of the skin helps to prevent skin breakdown (which can lead to pressure ulcers), infection, and odor. A bed bath is given when a shower or tub bath is not possible.

Getting Ready CLSOWR

1. Complete the "Getting Ready" steps.

Supplies

- gloves
- paper towels
- bed protectors
- oral hygiene supplies (see Procedures 23-1 through 23-3)
- bath thermometer
- wash basin
- bedpan or urinal
- soap
- lotion (optional)
- powder (optional)
- deodorant or antiperspirant (optional)
- washcloths
- towels
- bath blanket
- clean clothing
- clean linens (if necessary)

Procedure

2. Cover the over-bed table with paper towels. Place the wash basin, toiletries, clean clothing, and clean linens on the over-bed table.

3. Make sure that the bed is positioned at a comfortable working height (to promote good body mechanics) and that the wheels are locked.

4. Put on the gloves.

5. Because bathing often stimulates the urge to urinate, offer the bedpan or urinal. If the person uses the bedpan or urinal, empty and clean it before proceeding with the bath. Remove your gloves and dispose of them in a facility-approved waste container. Wash your hands and put on a clean pair of gloves.

6. Assist the person with oral care.

7. Remove the bedspread and blanket from the bed. If they are to be reused, fold them and place them on a clean surface, such as the chair.

8. Spread the bath blanket over the top linens (and the person). If the person is able, have her hold the bath blanket. If not, tuck the corners under the person's shoulders. Fanfold the top linens to the foot of the bed.

9. Assist the person with undressing.

10. Lower the head of the bed so that the bed is flat (as tolerated). Position the pillow under the person's head.

11. Fill the wash basin with warm water [110°F (43.3°C) to 115°F (46.1°C) on the bath thermometer]. Place the basin on the over-bed table.

12. If the side rails are in use, lower the side rail on the working side of the bed. The side rail on the opposite side of the bed should remain up.

13. Place a towel over the person's chest to keep the bath blanket dry.

14. To keep the bath water from becoming soapy too quickly, you can use two washcloths-one with soap, for washing; and one without soap, for rinsing. Form a mitt around your hand with one of the washcloths. Wet the mitt with warm, clean water. Ask the person to close her eyes. Place your washcloth-covered hand at the inner corner of the eye and stroke gently outward, toward the outer corner. Use a different part of the washcloth for each eye. Using a towel, dry the person's eyes.

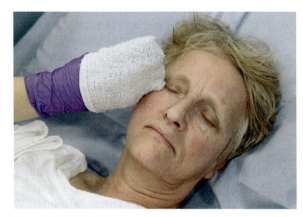

Step 14 Wash the person's eyes, moving from the inside corner toward the outer corner.

(continued)

15. Ask the person if you should use soap on the face. Rinse the washcloth and apply soap, if requested. Wash the face, neck, and ears, moving from the top of the head to the bottom (so that the nose and mouth are washed last). Using the clean washcloth, rinse thoroughly, and pat the person's face, neck, and ears dry with a towel.

16. Place a bed protector under the person's far arm, to keep the linens dry. Form a mitt around your hand with the washcloth. Wet the mitt and apply soap. Place your washcloth-covered hand at the shoulder and stroke downward, toward the hand, using long, firm strokes. Wash the hand. If necessary, assist the person with raising her arm so that you can wash the axilla. Rinse thoroughly, and pat the person's arm, hand, and axilla dry with a towel. Remove the bed protector from underneath the person's arm.

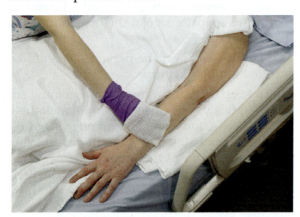

Step 16 Wash the person's arm, moving from the shoulder to the wrist.

17. Repeat for the other arm.

18. Place a towel horizontally across the person's chest. (The person is now covered with both a bath blanket and a towel.) With the towel in place, fold the bath blanket down to the person's waist. Wet the mitt and apply soap. Reach under the towel and wash the person's chest, using long, firm strokes. Using the clean washcloth, rinse thoroughly, and pat the person's chest dry with a towel.

19. With the towel still in place, fold the bath blanket down to the pubic area. Form a mitt around your hand with the washcloth. Wet the mitt and apply soap. Reach under the towel and wash the person's abdomen, using long, firm strokes. Rinse thoroughly and pat the person's abdomen dry with a towel.

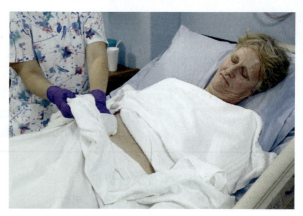

Step 19 Wash the person's abdomen.

20. Replace the bath blanket by unfolding it back over the towel and the person's body. Slide the towel out from underneath the bath blanket.

21. Change the water in the wash basin if it is cool or soapy. (If the side rails are in use, raise the side rails before leaving the bedside.)

22. Fold the bath blanket so that the far leg is completely exposed. Place a bed protector under the person's far leg to keep the linens dry. Wet the mitt and apply soap. Place your washcloth-covered hand at the top of the thigh and stroke downward, toward the foot, using long, firm strokes. Rinse thoroughly and pat the person's leg dry with a bath towel.

23. Put the wash basin on the bed protector and place the person's foot in the basin. Wash the entire foot, including between the toes, with the soapy washcloth. Rinse thoroughly and pat the person's foot dry with a towel. Be sure to dry between the toes. Remove the wash basin. Remove the bed protector from underneath the person's leg.

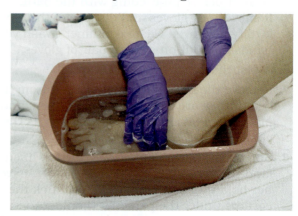

Step 23 Put the wash basin on the bed protector and place the person's foot in the basin.

24. Repeat for the other leg and foot.

25. Change the water in the wash basin. (If the side rails are in use, raise the side rails before leaving the bedside.)

26. Turn the person onto her side so that she is facing away from you. Help the person toward the working side of the bed so that her back is within easy reach. Adjust the bath blanket to keep the front of the person covered (exposing only the back and buttocks). Place a bed protector on the bed alongside the person's back to keep the linens dry.

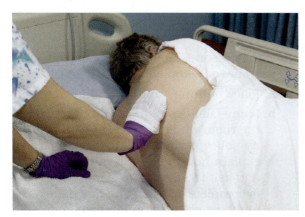

Step 26 Wash the person's back and buttocks using long, firm strokes.

27. Form a mitt around your hand with the washcloth. Wet the mitt and apply soap. Wash the person's back and buttocks, moving from top to bottom and using long, firm strokes. Rinse thoroughly and pat the person's back and buttocks dry using a bath towel. At this point, a back massage may be given.

28. If the person is able to perform perineal care, assist the person into Fowler's position and adjust the over-bed table so that the bathing supplies are within easy reach. Place the call light control within easy reach and ask the person to signal when perineal care is complete. If the person is unable to perform perineal care, assist the person onto her back and complete perineal care.

29. Remove your gloves and dispose of them in a facility-approved waste container. Put on a clean pair of gloves.

30. Help the person to apply lotion, powder, deodorant, antiperspirant, or other personal care products as the person requests.

31. Help the person into the clean clothing.

32. If the bedding is wet or soiled, change the bed linens.

33. Carry out range-of-motion exercises as ordered.

34. If the side rails are in use, return the side rails to the raised position. Raise or lower the head of the bed as the person requests. Make sure that the bed is lowered to its lowest position and that the wheels are locked.

35. Gather the soiled linens and place them in the linen hamper or linen bag. Dispose of disposable items in a facility-approved waste container. Clean equipment and return it to the storage area.

36. Remove your gloves and dispose of them in a facility-approved waste container.

Finishing Up CLSOWR

37. Complete the "Finishing Up" steps.

PROCEDURE 23-8

Giving a Partial Bed Bath

WHY YOU DO IT   Cleansing of the skin helps to prevent skin breakdown (which can lead to pressure ulcers), infection, and odor. A partial bed bath is given on days when a complete bath or shower is not scheduled, or when a resident does not feel up to a complete bath or shower.

Getting Ready CLSOWR

1. Complete the "Getting Ready" steps.

Supplies

- gloves
- paper towels
- bed protectors
- oral hygiene supplies (see Procedures 23-1 through 23-3)
- bath thermometer
- wash basin
- bedpan or urinal
- soap
- lotion (optional)
- powder (optional)
- washcloths
- towels
- bath blanket
- clean clothing
- clean linens (if necessary)

Procedure

2. Cover the over-bed table with paper towels. Place the wash basin, toiletries, clean clothing, and clean linens on the over-bed table. Put on the gloves.

3. Because bathing often stimulates the urge to urinate, offer the bedpan or urinal. If the person uses the bedpan or urinal, empty and clean it before proceeding with the bath. Remove your gloves and dispose of them in a facility-approved waste container. Wash your hands and put on a clean pair of gloves.

4. Assist the person with oral hygiene. Remove your gloves and dispose of them in a facility-approved waste container. Wash your hands.

5. Fill the wash basin with warm water (110°F [43.3°C] to 115°F [46.1°C] on the bath thermometer). Place the basin on the over-bed table.

6. If the person will be bathing independently, make sure that the bed is lowered to its lowest position and that the wheels are locked. If you will be assisting the person with bathing, make sure that the bed is positioned at a comfortable working height (to promote good body mechanics) and that the wheels are locked. If the side rails are in use, lower the side rail on the working side. The side rails on the opposite side of the bed should remain up.

7. The bath may either be carried out with the person in Fowler's position, or the person can be assisted to sit on the edge of the bed. Help the person to undress as necessary.

8. If the person is able to bathe herself, either partially or completely:

    a. Place bathing supplies within easy reach.

    b. Many facilities require you to remain in the room while the person bathes. If facility policy permits you to leave the room, explain how to use the call light control and ask the person to signal when bathing is complete or when she has done as much as she can on her own and needs help completing the bath. Stay nearby and check on the person every 5 minutes. Return when the person signals. Remember to knock before entering.

9. If the person is unable to bathe herself, or requires assistance:

    a. Put on the gloves and form a mitt around your hand with one of the washcloths.

    b. If necessary, ask the person what parts of the body were not washed. Assist the person as needed with completing the bath. Wash the cleanest areas first and the dirtiest areas last:

    - **Face, neck, and ears.** Ask the person if you should use soap on the face. Rinse the washcloth and apply soap, if requested. Wash the face, neck, and ears, moving from the top of the head to the bottom (so that the nose and mouth are washed last). Rinse thoroughly, and pat the person's face, neck, and ears dry with a towel.
    - **Hands.** Wash the hand. Rinse thoroughly, and pat the hand dry with a towel. Repeat for the other hand.
    - **Axillae (armpits).** If necessary, assist the person with raising her arm so that you can wash the axilla. Rinse

thoroughly, and pat the axilla dry with a towel. Repeat for the other axilla.

- **Back and buttocks.** Rinse the washcloth and apply soap. Wash the person's back and buttocks, moving from top to bottom and using long, firm strokes. Rinse thoroughly, and pat the back and buttocks dry with a towel.
- **Perineal area.** Complete male or female perineal care.

10. Remove your gloves and dispose of them in a facility-approved waste container. Put on a clean pair of gloves.

11. Help the person to apply lotion, powder, deodorant, antiperspirant, or other personal care products as the person requests.

12. Help the person into the clean clothing.

13. If the bedding is wet or soiled, change the bed linens.

14. Carry out range-of-motion exercises as ordered.

15. If the side rails are in use, return the side rails to the raised position. Raise or lower the head of the bed as the person requests. Make sure that the bed is lowered to its lowest position and that the wheels are locked.

16. Gather the soiled linens and place them in the linen hamper or linen bag. Dispose of disposable items in a facility-approved waste container. Clean equipment and return it to the storage area.

17. Remove your gloves and dispose of them in a facility-approved waste container.

Finishing Up   CLSOWR

18. Complete the "Finishing Up" steps.

PROCEDURE 23-9

Giving a Back Massage

WHY YOU DO IT   A back message promotes comfort and relaxation. Massage also stimulates blood flow to the skin, which helps to prevent pressure ulcers.

Getting Ready   CLSOWR

1. Complete the "Getting Ready" steps.

Supplies

- gloves (if contact with broken skin is likely)
- wash basin
- lotion
- bath blanket
- towel

Procedure

2. Fill the wash basin with warm water. Place the bottle of lotion in the basin of warm water to warm it.

3. Make sure that the bed is positioned at a comfortable working height (to promote good body mechanics) and that the wheels are locked.

4. Lower the head of the bed so that the bed is flat (as tolerated). If the side rails are in use, lower the side rail on the working side of the bed. The side rail on the opposite side of the bed should remain up.

5. Help the person into the prone position, or turn the person onto her side so that she is facing away from you.

6. Reposition the pillow under the person's head and adjust the bath blanket to keep the person covered, exposing only the back and buttocks.

7. Put on the gloves if contact with broken skin is likely.

8. Pour some lotion into your cupped palm and rub your hands together to distribute the lotion onto both palms.

9. Apply the lotion to the person's back with the palms of your hands. Massage the lotion into the person's skin, using long, gliding strokes (*effleurage*), moving up the center of the back from the buttocks to the shoulders, and then back down along the outside of the back. Do not directly rub any reddened areas. Repeat four times.

(continued)

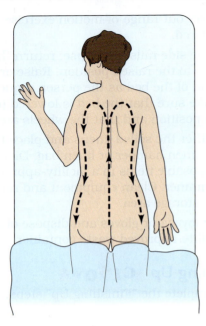

Step 9 Move up the center of the back from the buttocks to the shoulders, and then back down along the outside of the back.

10. For the next set of strokes, move up the center of the back from the buttocks to the shoulders and then back down along the outside of the back. On the downstroke, massage the person's shoulders and back using a small circular motion. Repeat four times.

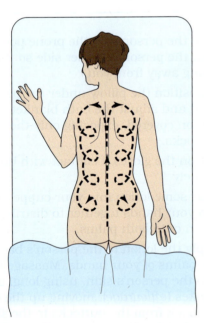

Step 10 For the next set of strokes, massage the person's shoulders and back using a small circular motion on the downstroke.

11. For the next set of strokes, move up the center of the back from the buttocks to the

shoulders, and then back down along the outside of the back. On the downstroke, massage the person's shoulders, back, and buttocks using a small circular motion, paying special attention to the area at the base of the spine. Repeat four times.

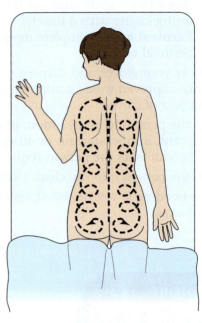

Step 11 For the final set of strokes, massage the person's shoulders, back, and buttocks using a small circular motion on the downstroke.

12. Finish with long, gliding strokes (*effleurage*), moving up the center of the back from the buttocks to the shoulders and then back down along the outside of the back. Repeat four times.

13. Remove your gloves and dispose of them in a facility-approved waste container.

14. If the back massage is being given as part of a bath, assist the person onto his or her back and continue with the bath. If the back massage is being given before bed or at any other time, help the person back into his or her pajamas, nightgown, or hospital gown.

15. If the side rails are in use, return the side rails to the raised position. Make sure that the bed is lowered to its lowest position and that the wheels are locked.

16. Gather the soiled linens and place them in the linen hamper or linen bag. Dispose of disposable items in a facility-approved waste container. Clean equipment and return it to the storage area.

Finishing Up CLSOWR

17. Complete the "Finishing Up" steps.

WHAT DID YOU LEARN?

Multiple Choice

Select the single best answer for each of the following questions.

1. As a safety measure, when you give mouth care to an unconscious person, you should position the person in which position?
   a. Semi-Fowler's position with head turned to side
   b. Supine position
   c. Fowler's position
   d. Prone position

2. Why do you line the sink with a washcloth when cleaning a person's dentures?
   a. To ensure that you always have a wet washcloth handy when you need one
   b. To protect the sink from scratches
   c. To guard against breaking the dentures
   d. To prevent contamination of the dentures

3. Which one of the following is within the range of appropriate temperatures for bath water?
   a. 98°F (36.6°C)
   b. 212°F (100°C)
   c. 120°F (48.9°C)
   d. 105°F (40.5°C)

4. When giving a complete bed bath, you should:
   a. Position yourself on one side of the bed and stay there
   b. Use the same water throughout the bath to minimize trips to the sink
   c. Avoid washing the person's perineal area because the person may be embarrassed
   d. Keep the person covered as much as possible

5. When assisting a man with perineal care, you should always:
   a. Hold the penis at a 90° angle to the body
   b. Wash from the base of the penis toward the tip
   c. Retract the foreskin if the man is uncircumcised
   d. Clean the scrotum first

6. When assisting a person with a shower, you should:
   a. Use a bath blanket to prevent falls
   b. Run the water until the temperature reaches 125°F (51.6°C)
   c. Wear waterproof personal protective equipment (PPE) to protect yourself from getting wet
   d. Use a shower chair if the person is weak or unsteady

7. Which one of the following actions must be taken to keep the skin healthy?
   a. Apply generous amounts of lotion after the bath
   b. Rinse the skin well and dry it thoroughly, especially in areas where "skin meets skin"
   c. Apply generous amounts of powder after the bath
   d. Rub the skin vigorously with the washcloth

8. How are natural teeth brushed?
   a. Using a circular motion
   b. For at least 10 minutes on each side
   c. Using an "up and down" motion
   d. All of the above

9. When assisting a woman with perineal care, you should always:
   a. Gently yet thoroughly dry the perineal area and vulva
   b. Clean the rectal area last
   c. Move the washcloth in a downward direction, from the urethra to the anus
   d. All of the above

10. What is the first thing you should do before assisting a person with a tub bath?
    a. Gather the necessary supplies
    b. Make sure the tub is clean
    c. Check the temperature of the water
    d. Check the care plan to make sure the person is allowed to have a tub bath

11. Which of the following observations made while assisting with mouth care would you report to the nurse?
    a. Lips that are dry, cracked, swollen, or blistered
    b. Irritations, sores, or white patches in the mouth or on the tongue
    c. Bleeding, swelling, or redness of the gums
    d. All of the above

12. How long should a back massage last?
    a. 2 minutes
    b. 1 minute
    c. 4 to 6 minutes
    d. 15 minutes

Matching

Match each numbered item with its appropriate lettered description.

_____ **1.** Perineal care (peri-care)

_____ **2.** Evening (hour of sleep, hs) care

_____ **3.** Gingivitis

_____ **4.** PRN (as-needed) care

_____ **5.** Antiperspirant

_____ **6.** Edentulous

a. Without teeth

b. Care that is provided at any time of the day or night, when the person's condition warrants it

c. Inflammation of the gums, caused by poor oral hygiene

d. Stops or slows secretion of sweat

e. Care that is routinely provided at bedtime

f. Cleaning of the perineum, the anus, and the vulva or penis

STOP and Think!

- Mrs. Davis is a resident at your facility, which specializes in caring for people with Alzheimer's disease. As Mrs. Davis's disease has progressed, she has become progressively more lax about matters related to personal hygiene. She dislikes bathing, and if you do not remove her soiled clothes from her room, she will continue to wear them every day. Today Mrs. Davis is scheduled to have a shower, and as you might have predicted, she tells you that she "will not take a shower today." What should you do?

- You need to give Mrs. Burland, a new resident, a bed bath, and you can tell that she is very embarrassed at the prospect. What can you do to make the situation more comfortable for Mrs. Burland?

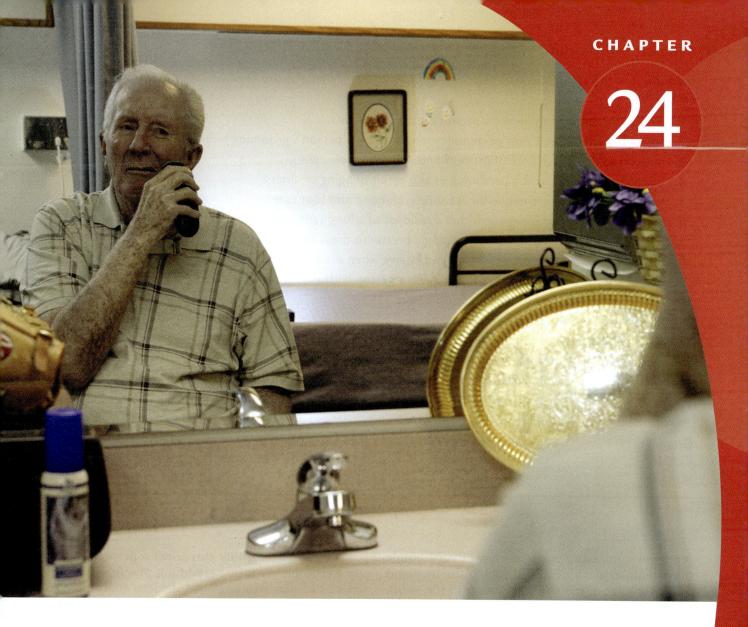

Grooming

WHAT WILL YOU LEARN?

The routine care of the hands and feet (including the nails), shampooing and styling of the hair, the application of make-up, and shaving are all **grooming** practices that help us to maintain a neat and attractive appearance. Imagine that you are a resident, and you are unable to complete your regular grooming activities. Your hair is uncombed, you have not applied make-up (if you are a woman) or shaved (if you are a man), and you are not dressed for visitors, yet company arrives anyway. How would you feel? Would you be able to fully enjoy your guests, or would you be worried about your appearance? Helping your residents with "putting their best face forward,"

Photo: Grooming practices help people to feel more attractive and confident.

the subject of this chapter, is part of providing holistic care. When you are finished with this chapter, you will be able to:

1. Describe factors that influence a person's grooming habits.
2. Explain the effect that illness or disability may have on a person's grooming habits.
3. Understand the importance of proper hand and foot care.
4. List changes that occur in a person's feet as a result of aging or illness.
5. Demonstrate proper technique for assisting with hand and foot care.
6. Discuss the various dressing needs that a resident of a long-term care facility may have.
7. Demonstrate proper technique for helping a person to dress and undress.
8. Discuss disorders a nursing assistant may observe when assisting with hair care.
9. Describe the different methods used to assist a person with shampooing his or her hair.
10. Describe methods used to style a person's hair.
11. Demonstrate proper technique for shampooing a bedridden person's hair and combing a person's hair.
12. Describe the tools and supplies used for shaving.
13. Demonstrate how to safely shave a man's face.
14. Explain how the use of make-up can affect a person's sense of well-being.

Vocabulary Use the CD in the front of your book to hear these terms pronounced and defined:

Grooming	Tinea pedis	Tinea capitis	Alopecia
Cuticle	Podiatrist	Seborrheic dermatitis	Pediculosis capitis
Hangnail	Dandruff	(cradle cap)	Nits

A person's grooming practices may be very simple (for example, washing and combing the hair and applying a bit of moisturizing lotion to the skin). Or they may be very complex (for example, styling the hair with a blow dryer and curlers, applying make-up, wearing perfume or cologne, and polishing the nails). Think for a moment about the routine grooming practices that you perform each day before you leave home to face the world. Have you ever overslept and had to go to school or work without your routine grooming accomplished? How did you feel? Did it affect your self-esteem?

Residents have personal grooming routines that help them to feel attractive and self-confident, just as you do. Like your grooming practices, your residents' grooming practices are influenced by cultural and religious beliefs, upbringing, age, attention to fashion, and feelings about sexuality. For example, a woman may feel more feminine if she is wearing lipstick and has polished nails, while a man may feel more masculine after he shaves and applies cologne or aftershave. Grooming helps us to maintain our sense of identity. As always, it is important to find out each resident's preferences, and to accommodate these preferences as much as possible.

Illness or disability can affect a person's ability to complete routine grooming practices. Many residents can use assistive devices to complete grooming tasks independently. However, some residents will need your help to complete their

Helping Hands and a Caring Heart

FOCUS ON HUMANISTIC HEALTH CARE

As a nursing assistant, you must provide humanistic, holistic care for your residents. This means looking after their physical needs, as well as their emotional needs. Helping a person to complete routine grooming practices meets many of the person's emotional needs, as well as some physical ones. When you take the time and make the effort to style a person's hair attractively, polish her nails, or help apply make-up as part of morning care, you make that person feel extra special. Your actions help the person to meet the needs of love and belonging, because she feels cared for as the unique individual that she is. You also help the person to meet her need for self-esteem. Not only is she clean and comfortable, but she feels attractive too.

grooming routine. As with any aspect of care, check with the nurse or check the person's care plan to find out about any limitations or specifics related to grooming.

ASSISTING WITH HAND AND FOOT CARE

CARE OF THE HANDS

Soft, smooth skin and trimmed, filed fingernails are important for overall health and comfort. Dryness and chapping of the skin on the hands is uncomfortable and creates a portal of entry for microbes. Poorly cared for fingernails can become long and rough, placing the person at risk for injury. For example, a person who is disoriented can scratch himself if his fingernails are not kept short and smooth. For people who are alert and oriented, fingernail length is a personal choice, but the edges should be kept smooth.

A simple care routine is used to keep the skin of the hands healthy and the fingernails neat (Procedure 24-1). Even if a resident can care for her own hands and fingernails, getting a manicure from someone else can really lift the resident's spirits, especially if the resident is not feeling her best (Fig. 24-1). Helping a resident with hand and nail care also gives you the chance to observe for signs of health. In a healthy person, the nail bed is pink. There is no gap between the nail and the nail bed. When viewed from the side, the nail is convex (it curves slightly). The **cuticle** (the skin along the edges of the nail) is smooth and unbroken.

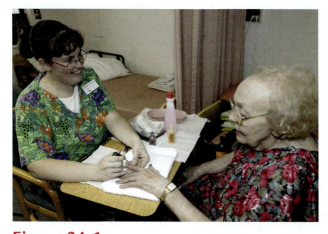

Figure 24-1
Giving a resident a manicure gives you the opportunity to spend "quality time" with the person.

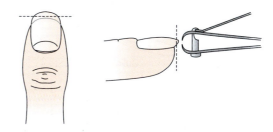

Figure 24-2
Nails are cut using nail clippers. Cut the nails straight across, being careful not to cut too close to the skin. Always make sure that it is within your scope of practice to trim a resident's fingernails or toenails. In many facilities, a nurse must perform this task.

Nail care is usually easiest to perform on nails that have been soaked for a short time in warm water. During or immediately following a bath is an ideal time to perform nail care because the water makes the nails soft and flexible. When nail care is to be provided at a time other than bath time, the nails can be softened by soaking the ends of the fingers for a short time in a small basin of warm water.

Fingernails are trimmed with clippers, not scissors, to a length no shorter than even with the ends of the fingers (Fig. 24-2). In some states and facilities, trimming a resident's fingernails is outside of the scope of practice for nursing assistants, so be sure to follow the policy at the facility where you work. After trimming, the nails are filed into an oval shape using an emery board. Pain or tenderness can result from **hangnails** (broken pieces of cuticle). Hangnails may need to be trimmed using cuticle scissors so that they do not rub or snag on clothing or linens. Torn hangnails can cause bleeding and inflammation of the cuticle.

The blunt end of an orange stick (Fig. 24-3) or the edge of a washcloth is used to gently push the cuticles back, and then the orange stick is used to clean underneath the tips of the nails.

Some people like to use nail polish. If nail polish is not used, then the surfaces of the nails can be lightly buffed to give them shine. Applying hand cream helps to seal in moisture and prevent dryness of the skin and cuticles.

CARE OF THE FEET

Care of the feet is essential for good grooming as well as for good health. The feet tend to sweat, especially when slippers or shoes and socks are worn, leading to odors and a warm, moist environment that encourages the growth of microbes.

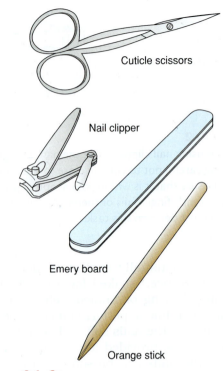

Figure 24-3
Tools used during hand and foot care.

For example, the disorder commonly known as "athlete's foot" **(tinea pedis)** is a fungal infection of the skin and nails. ("Pedis" comes from the Latin word for foot, *pedalis*.) Toenails that are allowed to grow too long can make wearing footwear uncomfortable, and the nails may become ingrown (a condition where the nail curves down and back into the skin, causing injury and pain).

The feet are at risk for injury—how many times have you had your foot stepped on, stubbed your toes against a piece of furniture, or developed a blister as a result of shoes that did not fit properly? Injuries such as cuts and blisters are painful for a person with normal blood flow to the feet and toes. For a person with poor blood flow (for example, as a result of the normal aging process, a heart problem, or diabetes mellitus), a cut or a blister might develop into a life-threatening condition. Because the wounded area is not receiving the normal amount of blood, the area receives less oxygen and nutrients and fewer infection-fighting white blood cells. Healing is delayed, and the risk of infection is increased. In addition, people with poor blood flow often have reduced sensation as well. While you would certainly notice if a new pair of shoes made a blister on your heel, a person with reduced blood flow and sensation might not be aware of the blister,

and a small blister could quickly become a dangerous infection. Helping a person with foot care allows you to observe the person's feet for small blisters, cracks in the skin, peeling of the skin between the toes or on the soles of the feet, ingrown toenails, and other problems. Discolored or tender areas should also be reported to the nurse immediately.

Like hand care, foot care is a grooming task that is easily added to the bathing routine. If foot care is to be done at a time other than bath time, the feet should first be bathed, rinsed, and dried thoroughly (especially between the toes). Prolonged soaking is not recommended. In most facilities, nursing assistants are not allowed to trim the toenails of residents, because a small injury could cause a life-threatening infection. This task is usually performed by a nurse or a **podiatrist,** a doctor who specializes in the care of the feet. The attention of a podiatrist is especially necessary when the toenails are thick and difficult to trim (as a result of aging or poor blood flow; Fig. 24-4). If you are allowed to trim your residents' toenails, use clippers and cut the toenails straight across. Never try to trim or file corns or calluses.

After the toenails are trimmed, they are filed to remove rough edges. Applying foot powder or lotion to dry feet is refreshing and comforting. Cotton socks help to keep the feet warm and will absorb sweat. (Be careful when helping an elderly person to put on socks—roll the cuff of the sock down before putting it on the person's foot and

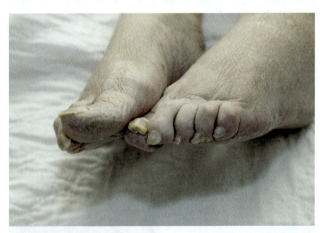

Figure 24-4
Many elderly people have thick, yellowed toenails as a result of age or poor circulation. Because thickened toenails may be difficult to trim and an accidental injury can have serious consequences, many health care facilities require that a nurse or a podiatrist trim residents' toenails.

take care not to accidentally scratch the person with your fingernails or jewelry when pulling the sock up over the heel). Encourage your residents to wear appropriate footwear. Well-fitting, supportive shoes with non-skid soles help to protect the feet and make walking safer by helping to prevent falls and slipping. To help prevent blisters or sores from occurring, check the inside of the person's shoes for stray objects or rough spots before helping the person to put them on.

Procedure 24-2 describes how to assist a resident with foot care.

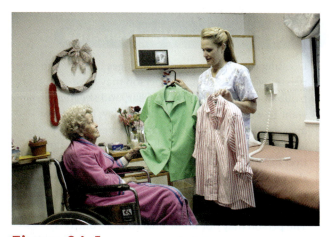

Figure 24-5
Whenever possible, a person should be permitted to choose which articles of clothing he or she will wear.

TELL THE NURSE ❗

While providing hand and foot care, always be aware of potential signs and symptoms of illness or infection. Tell the nurse if you observe any of the following:

- Nail beds that are either very pale or blue, or bruised
- Nails that are unusually yellow or white
- Nails that are unusually thick
- Nails that are broken or have been cut too short (especially if there is also bleeding or tenderness)
- Nails that are ingrown
- Cuticles that are torn, red, or swollen
- Skin that is blistered, tender, or discolored (especially on the feet)
- Skin that is cracked or peeling
- Any unusual rashes or odors

ASSISTING WITH DRESSING AND UNDRESSING

As a nursing assistant, you will be responsible for helping your residents to change their clothes, possibly several times a day. Dressing is usually a routine part of morning and evening care. However, clothing should be changed any time that it becomes wet or soiled. The type of clothing worn by residents of long-term care facilities differs according to the type of facility and the abilities of the person. If a resident is able to be out of bed during the day, he will probably wear street clothes during the day and nightwear at night. Procedure 24-3 describes how to assist a person with dressing in street clothes and nightwear. A resident who has a specific disability or medical

condition may wear a hospital gown or nightwear day and night. Procedure 24-4 describes how to change a hospital gown.

As with other personal care routines, the amount of help that each resident needs for dressing will vary. Some residents will be able to dress themselves and may only need help from you to zip a back zipper or tie shoelaces. Others will need a lot of assistance with every part of the process, from selecting clothes to putting them on. Allowing a resident to choose the clothing he or she wishes to wear is a top priority when assisting with dressing (Fig. 24-5). When a resident is unable to choose his own clothes, use good taste and common sense when choosing items for the person to wear. Assisting a resident to dress appropriately for the day's activities and with consideration for the season and environment is important for the resident's comfort. If a resident chooses an item of clothing that is not appropriate for the weather or the day's planned activities, gently suggest a more appropriate choice. Remember that many elderly people chill easily. As a result, many residents will need a sweater or jacket, especially if there is air conditioning.

Comfort and ease of dressing help determine clothing choices for many residents. Remember that we are responsible for helping our residents to attain or maintain their highest level of function and well-being. Clothes that are easy to take on and off may be easier for residents to manage independently. In addition, many assistive devices are available to make dressing easier. For example, clothing that closes with a Velcro™ fastener instead of zippers or buttons allows a person with limited use of his fingers to manage dressing and toileting with little or no assistance (Fig. 24-6A).

Caring For Those With Dementia

Dressing can present many challenges for a person with dementia. The person may have trouble selecting an outfit to wear, and she may want to wear the same outfit every day. Because of apraxia, the person may put her clothes on in the wrong order (for example, she may put her bra on over her blouse). Apraxia can also make it difficult for the person to figure out how to put on an article of clothing (for example, does it go over my head? Do I step into it? Which is the right and which is the left?) The person may not know how to work buttons, snaps, or zippers. To help dressing go more smoothly for your residents with dementia:

- Ask family members to provide several identical outfits for the person. This way, the person can wear the same outfit several days in a row if she wants to!

- Let family members know that clothing without fasteners (for example, dresses, tops, and sweaters that slip on over the head; pants with elastic waistbands) may be easier for the person to manage independently. Clothing and shoes with Velcro™ fasteners are also often easier for the person to manage on her own.

- When helping the resident to select an outfit, provide limited choices. For example, ask, "Would you like to wear the red dress, or the blue dress?" Limiting choices helps to prevent the resident from becoming overwhelmed.

- Provide articles of clothing to the resident in the order that they will be put on (for example, underwear before pants).

- Provide step-by-step directions to guide the resident through the process of dressing. (For example, "OK, Mrs. Lyons, put this leg through this opening. Now, put the other leg through the other opening. Pull the pants up . . .")

Long-handled shoehorns and graspers allow a person to put on her own socks and shoes (Fig. 24-6B). The use of these assistive devices can allow a person to maintain a large amount of personal independence, in spite of disabilities.

Some situations present special challenges related to dressing and undressing, such as:

- An extremity (an arm or a leg) that is weak, paralyzed, in a cast, or splinted
- Recent surgery on an arm or a leg
- An intravenous (IV) line

Good planning on your part can help you to meet these challenges. For example, if you place the garment's sleeve or leg onto the affected extremity first, dressing becomes much easier. (When it comes time to remove the garment, reverse the procedure—work with the strong arm or leg first and undress the affected arm or leg last.) If the resident has an IV line, bring the IV bag and tubing through the sleeve first and then follow with the arm (Fig. 24-7). You should not remove an IV line from an infusion pump or disconnect IV tubing when assisting a resident to dress or undress. If you are unsure about how to manage an IV line while helping a resident to dress or undress, ask a nurse for assistance.

ASSISTING WITH HAIR CARE

Routine care is necessary to keep the hair clean and neat. For many people, the appearance of their hair affects how they feel about themselves. Have you ever had a "bad hair day?" Did you feel like you would rather walk around with a paper bag on your head than have other people see your hair dirty or poorly styled? Helping with hair care is an essential part of providing care for those who need you.

Routine grooming of the hair involves daily brushing, combing, and styling. Residents should be encouraged to participate in caring for their own hair to their fullest ability. For example, a resident with a paralyzed arm can be encouraged to brush her hair on her "strong" side, and then you can complete the job on the other side (Fig. 24-8). Usually, the hair is brushed or combed during early morning care, and styled after a shampoo. Additional grooming may be necessary throughout the day, for example, after napping or before visiting times. Many long-term care facilities have on-site salons and barbershops where residents can have their hair cut, washed, and professionally styled (Fig. 24-9).

The texture and length of the hair affect how a person cares for it. Hair that is straight and fine can be as hard to manage as hair that is curly and coarse. The hair of elderly people tends to be fragile. Personal preferences regarding hairstyle and the products used when grooming the hair vary and should be respected, whenever possible. Asking a resident about his or her usual hair care routine and preferred products will provide you with much useful information.

When assisting with grooming of the hair, it is important to observe the hair and scalp for any

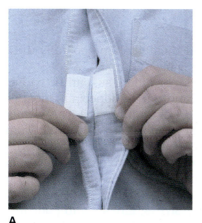

A

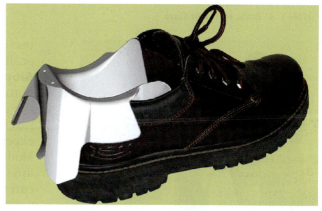

B

Figure 24-6

Assistive devices are available to help people with disabilities dress themselves independently.
(A) Velcro™ fasteners on this shirt replace buttons or a zipper, which require more use of the
fingers to manage. **(B)** A shoehorn makes it easier to put on shoes. (*Photos courtesy of Sammons
Preston Rolyan, Bolingbrook, IL.*)

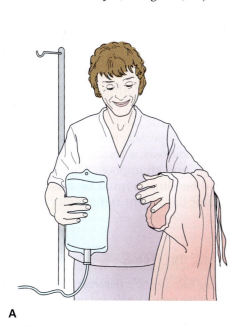

A

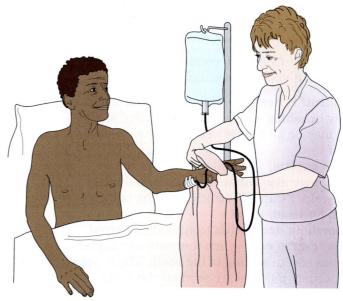

B

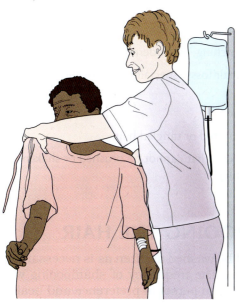

C

Figure 24-7

Helping a person who has an intravenous (IV) line in place get
dressed is not as difficult as it may seem. **(A)** Put the IV bag and
tubing through the sleeve of the gown first, and place the IV bag
on the hook. **(B)** Gently thread the sleeve down the tubing and
gently bring the person's arm through the sleeve of the gown.
(C) Bring the gown across the person's chest and guide the other
arm through the other sleeve.

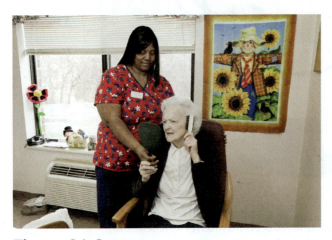

Figure 24-8
To foster independence and self-esteem, encourage your residents to do as much as possible for themselves, while you stand by ready to offer assistance, as needed.

abnormalities. Common conditions of the hair and scalp that you may see include the following.

- **Dandruff** is itching and flaking of the scalp. Daily brushing and using a medicated shampoo may be all that is needed to control dandruff.
- **Tinea capitis,** a fungal infection of the scalp, may also cause itching and flaking of the scalp. ("Capitis" comes from the Latin word for head, *caput*.)
- **Seborrheic dermatitis** (commonly referred to as **"cradle cap"** when it occurs in infants) causes severe scaling of the scalp. Thick, yellow, crusty patches are seen on the scalp. The nurse may ask you to help the person

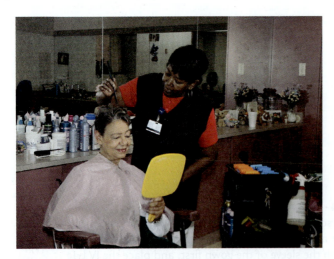

Figure 24-9
Many long-term care facilities have on-site salons and barbershops for the convenience of residents.

use a medicated shampoo daily until the scaling is cleared up.

- **Alopecia,** or baldness, can be caused by many conditions. Alopecia is most commonly the result of an inherited trait in men and is rarely seen in women, although women may experience thinning of the hair with aging. Medications used to treat cancer (chemotherapy) and certain forms of radiation treatment can cause total baldness in both men and women. Stress, illness, and poor nutrition can also cause the hair to thin.
- **Pediculosis capitis** is head lice. Lice are very small parasitic insects that feed on the blood of the host, or the person who is infected. The insects lay their eggs (called **nits**) on the hair shaft, near the root. The nits look like dandruff flakes or small pieces of lint, but cannot be brushed or shaken off the hair. Head lice are transmitted from person to person by direct contact with an infected person's hair. They may also be transmitted indirectly, through contact with clothing, bed linens, brushes and combs, and cloth-covered furniture (for example, the back of a sofa or chair where an infected person has rested his or her head). Pediculosis is treated with medicated creams and shampoos. The person's clothing and bed linens must be washed in very hot water to prevent reinfection.

TELL THE NURSE

When providing hair care, it is important to observe the condition of the person's hair and scalp. Make sure to report any of the following findings to the nurse immediately:

- Flaking, crusting, or scaling of the scalp
- Redness, itching, or tenderness of the scalp
- Unusual hair loss, especially if it is occurring in patches
- A foul smell
- Severely matted or tangled hair
- Nits ("flakes" that cannot be brushed or shaken off the hair)

SHAMPOOING THE HAIR

Hair should be washed as often as is necessary to keep it clean. The frequency of shampooing will vary according to personal preference and health status. Residents who are feverish or who have been sweating may welcome a non-scheduled shampoo to help them feel fresh and clean. Other residents may only need their hair washed once or twice a week.

Some residents can shampoo their own hair when they bathe. Others will need help. Many bathtubs and showers have hand-held shower-heads that make it easy to shampoo the hair during a person's bath. When a person cannot get out of bed, a shampoo trough is used to wash the hair (Procedure 24-5), or a shampoo cap containing a dry shampoo product may be used instead (Fig. 24-10).

There are many different types of shampoos and conditioners to choose from. (Conditioners are used by many people to improve the hair's texture and reduce tangles.) Respecting personal preference in products is important. Before shampooing a resident's hair, always check the person's care plan to find out necessary details such as the frequency of shampoos, the method used, and the products preferred.

STYLING THE HAIR

After the hair has been washed and towel dried, the hair is dried and styled according to the person's wishes (Fig. 24-11). If a resident is not able to tell you how she prefers to have her hair styled, choose a style that is age appropriate. Child-like hairstyles and ornaments are not appropriate for older adults. The time and attention you spend helping your residents style their hair helps to make those in your care feel and look attractive, which certainly has a positive effect on their well-being. Stop and think for a moment how you felt

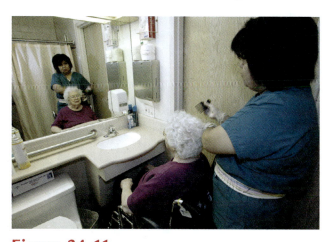

Figure 24-11
After shampooing, some people may like to have their hair dried and styled.

the last time you had your hair professionally done, or a friend offered to wash and style your hair. That is how well cared for and pampered your residents will feel when you provide these services for them!

Most men and some women with shorter hair may prefer to allow their hair to air dry. Others may want to have their hair styled and dried with a blow dryer, or they may want their hair rolled on curlers and dried under a salon-style dryer. If you are using electric appliances to dry and style a person's hair, be sure to follow the safety precautions related to the use of electrical items, as described in Chapter 17—for example, check for frayed cords and never use an electrical appliance near water. Be very careful not to burn the person's scalp with the dryer or curling iron. It is best to use a low-heat setting.

PREVENTING TANGLES

Regular brushing and combing of the hair helps to keep hair soft and tangle free. The scalp produces oil that keeps the hair shiny and soft. Brushing distributes this oil throughout the hair. Hair that is long or curly may need to be braided after it is brushed to help prevent tangling (Fig. 24-12). Many African American people have curly hair and a very dry scalp. African American hair may require braiding and the application of a moisturizing product to keep the hair soft and pliable. Before braiding a resident's hair, be sure to obtain the resident's permission. The use of barrettes, headbands, and clips can be both functional (by keeping hair out of the face) and decorative.

Sometimes the hair becomes tangled, especially if the person has been restricted to bed for

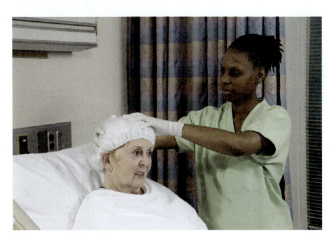

Figure 24-10
Shampoo caps contain a product that cleans the hair and scalp without water.

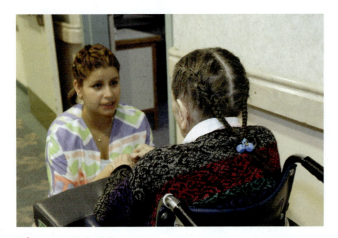

Figure 24-12
Braiding helps to prevent tangles in hair that is long or curly.

a period of time. To remove tangles from the hair, use a wide-tooth comb and start at the ends of the hair, one section at a time, gently working up toward the scalp (Procedure 24-6). Hair that is very tangled or matted may need to be cut, but the nurse must first obtain permission from the resident or his health care agent to cut the hair.

ASSISTING WITH SHAVING

ASSISTING MEN

Shaving is a routine grooming practice among most men. Shaving a man's face should be a part of either morning or evening care, depending on the man's preference (some men prefer to shave before going to bed). Prior to shaving, the face

should be cleaned and the beard softened, making bath time an ideal time to complete the shave. The frequency of shaving depends on how fast the beard grows and personal preference.

The type of shaving tool used also varies (Fig. 24-13). Many men prefer to use a safety razor, which may be disposable or have a changeable blade unit. Blades that are dull pull at the beard and do not cut the hair smoothly and should be changed. Disposable razors are used once and then discarded. Used blades and disposable razors should always be disposed of in a sharps container, not in a wastebasket. When using a safety razor, the beard is softened with warm water and a shaving cream or gel is applied to retain the moisture and reduce the friction of the blade against the skin. Some men may prefer to use shaving soap instead of a shaving cream or gel. In this case, a shaving brush is used to lather the soap and apply it to the beard. Procedure 24-7 describes how to shave a man's face using a safety razor and shaving cream, gel, or soap.

Other men like to use electric razors. Residents who are taking medications that decrease the blood's ability to form a clot should always use an electric razor, because electric razors are less likely to cut or nick the skin. If an electric razor is being used, a pre-shave lotion is applied to soften the beard and allow the razor to glide smoothly across the face. The usual safety precautions that are taken with all electrical appliances should be taken when using an electric razor. The electric razor is cleaned after each use.

If a resident is able, he should be encouraged to do his own shaving. You should provide whatever assistance is necessary, which may range

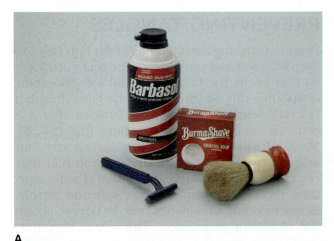

A

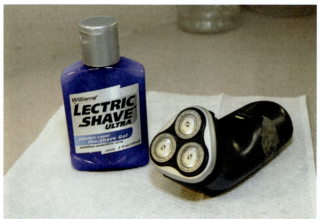

B

Figure 24-13
Shaving supplies. **(A)** A safety razor is used with shaving cream or gel or shaving soap. **(B)** An electric razor is used with a pre-shave lotion. An electric razor carries less risk of cuts or nicks, and therefore is preferred for a person who is taking medications that affect the blood's ability to clot.

from placing a chair and a mirror near the sink or bringing supplies and water to the bedside, to completing the shave in full. When shaving a resident, always remember to wear gloves because a cut or a nick will put you at risk for exposure to bloodborne pathogens. Always ask the nurse or check the care plan to determine if there are any limitations or special instructions for a person's shave.

A man may prefer to have a beard or mustache instead of being clean shaven. Beards and mustaches need routine grooming care also. They must be kept clean and free of food and drink and will need to be combed or brushed and trimmed regularly. Never shave off a person's beard or mustache unless the person requests that you do so. Be careful when shaving near the mustache or beard to avoid accidentally shaving part of the facial hair off.

Be Smart About Surveys!

As surveyors walk through the facility, they will pay attention to how the residents look. The physical appearance of the residents helps the surveyors to form an opinion about the care provided in the facility, and gives them an indication of the amount of attention the staff pays to maintaining the respect and dignity of those in their care. To help your facility remain without survey problems in this area:

- Make sure each resident's hands and feet are cared for. The nails should be clean, with smooth, filed edges. Cuticles should be smooth and unbroken. The skin should be soft, without dryness or chapping.

- Make sure each resident is dressed in clothing that fits properly and is clean, neat, and in good repair (no rips, holes, or missing buttons).

- Make sure each resident is wearing clothing that is appropriate for the environmental temperature and for the resident's activities.

- When assisting a resident to dress, be sure to give the resident the opportunity to select what he or she wants to wear.

- Make sure each resident's hair is clean, neatly combed, and styled in an age-appropriate style. If the resident is male, his hair should be neatly trimmed.

- Make sure each male resident is clean shaven or has neatly trimmed and well-cared for facial hair, according to his preference.

ASSISTING WOMEN

Shaving the legs, underarms, or both makes many women feel feminine and attractive. In addition, some women experience the growth of coarse facial hair as they age and may request your help with removing this unwanted hair. If a woman is unable to shave her legs, armpits, or face and wants to do so, you should help her, as necessary.

Many of the same principles used when assisting men to shave apply to women as well. The hair should be softened with warm water first, making bath time the ideal time to shave. A safety razor or an electric razor may be used. If a safety razor is used, shaving cream or gel should be applied first. Like men, many women will have clear preferences regarding the type of razor and shaving products that are used, and respecting the person's preferences is important. A woman's face is shaved in the same manner as a man's face. When shaving the armpits, it is best to move in the direction of hair growth. When shaving the legs, start at the ankle and move upward, against the direction of hair growth. Many women shave their legs only below the knee, while others may shave the thigh as well.

ASSISTING WITH THE APPLICATION OF MAKE-UP

Many women, and some men, wear make-up because it helps them to feel more confident and attractive. A person's culture, religion, age, and feelings about his or her own sexuality all contribute to that person's feelings about, and use of, make-up. Many times, the types of make-up a person likes and the way she applies them are influenced by the time in that person's life when she felt most attractive. For example, many of your elderly ladies will like to wear dark lipstick and heavy face powder because that was the style that was popular during their younger years.

Helping a resident to continue with her normal personal grooming routine has an enormous impact on the resident's continued well-being. For some people, wearing make-up increases their self-esteem and feelings of self-worth. When you help a person who likes to wear make-up to complete this part of her grooming routine, the person will feel that you take special care of her and that you value her as the unique human being that she is. This idea is at the heart of humanistic care.

SUMMARY

- Caring for the hands and feet (especially the fingernails and toenails), selecting an outfit to wear, shampooing and styling the hair, shaving, and applying make-up are grooming practices that people may engage in to make themselves feel more attractive and confident.
  - Grooming contributes to a person's emotional health, as well as his or her physical health.
  - Personal grooming practices are highly variable and are influenced by many factors, including culture, religion, upbringing, age, fashion preferences, and a person's feelings about his or her own sexuality. Respecting your resident's personal preferences is an important part of providing holistic care.
- Care of the hands and feet focuses on keeping the skin and nails clean and healthy.
  - Assisting with hand and foot care gives the nursing assistant the chance to observe for potential health problems, including poor blood flow and fungal infections.
  - Poor blood flow to the feet is associated with many health problems, including decreased sensation and an increased risk for a life-threatening infection. Poor blood flow may be caused by heart disease, diabetes mellitus, or the normal aging process.
  - Trimming a person's toenails is usually beyond the nursing assistant's scope of practice. Instead, a nurse or a podiatrist performs this task.
- Dressing daily is necessary for warmth and modesty, and it gives residents a sense of purpose.
- For many people, dressing is a way of expressing themselves. Therefore, a person's preferences regarding outfit selection should be followed, whenever possible.
- Wet or soiled garments must be exchanged for dry, clean ones as often as necessary.
- Assistive devices, such as Velcro™ fasteners, shoehorns, and graspers, increase a disabled person's independence. With increased independence, comes increased self-esteem.
- Certain conditions (for example, a weak, paralyzed, or injured arm or leg or an IV line) can make dressing more challenging but by no means impossible.
- Most people feel best when their hair is clean, free of tangles, and styled in a familiar style.
  - Assisting with hair care gives the nursing assistant a chance to observe for conditions of the scalp and hair, including dandruff, tinea capitis, seborrheic dermatitis (cradle cap), alopecia, and pediculosis capitis (head lice).
  - Hair may be shampooed as part of a tub or shower bath, or in bed using a shampoo trough or shampoo cap.
  - Styling tools include blow dryers, curling irons, hot curlers, and salon-style hairdryers. Caution must be used when operating these electrical appliances.
  - Regular brushing and combing keeps the hair shiny and tangle free.
- Most men shave their faces daily, either completely or partially. Many women shave their legs, their underarms, or both.
- Many women, and some men, consider the application of make-up to be an essential grooming activity.

PROCEDURE **24-1**

Assisting With Hand Care

WHY YOU DO IT   Soft, smooth skin and trimmed, filed fingernails are important for overall health and comfort

Getting Ready   WCKIEPS

1. Complete the "Getting Ready" steps.

Supplies

- gloves (if contact with broken skin is likely)
- paper towels
- orange stick
- nail clippers
- emery board (nail file)
- bath thermometer
- emesis basin
- soap
- lotion
- nail polish remover (optional)
- nail polish (optional)
- cotton balls (optional)
- washcloth
- towel

Procedure

2. Make sure that the bed is lowered to its lowest position and that the wheels are locked.

3. Cover the over-bed table with paper towels. Pour some liquid soap into the emesis basin and fill the basin with warm water (100°F [37.7°C] to 115°F [46.1°C] on the bath thermometer). Place the emesis basin on the over-bed table, along with the nail care supplies and clean linens.

4. If the side rails are in use, lower the side rail on the working side of the bed. The side rail on the opposite side of the bed should remain up.

5. Help the person to transfer from the bed to a bedside chair, assist the person to sit on the edge of the bed, or raise the head of the bed as tolerated.

6. Put on the gloves if contact with broken skin is likely.

7. If the person is wearing nail polish and wants it removed, remove the nail polish by putting a small amount of nail polish remover on a cotton ball and gently rubbing each nail.

8. Help the person to position the tips of his or her fingers in the basin to soak. Let the person soak his or her fingers for about 5 minutes.

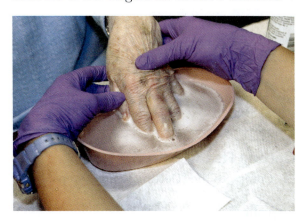

Step 8 Soak the nails to soften them.

9. Working with one hand at a time, lift the person's hand out of the basin and wash the entire hand, including between the fingers, with the soapy washcloth. Use the orange stick to gently clean underneath the person's fingernails. Rinse thoroughly and pat the person's hand dry with a towel. Be sure to dry between the fingers. Repeat with the other hand.

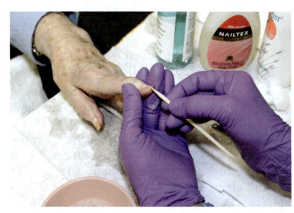

Step 9 Clean under the person's nails using the orange stick.   *(continued)*

10. Remove the emesis basin and dry the person's hands thoroughly. If facility policy allows it, gently push the cuticles back with the orange stick.

11. If facility policy allows it, use the nail clippers to cut the person's fingernails. If the person's nails need to be trimmed but this task is outside of your scope of practice, report this need to the nurse.

12. Use the emery board to file the fingernails into an oval shape and smooth the rough edges.

13. Apply lotion to the person's hands and gently massage it into the skin.

14. Apply nail polish as the person requests.

15. If necessary, help the person return to bed. If the side rails are in use, return the side rails to the raised position. Lower the head of the bed as the person requests.

16. Gather the soiled linens and place them in the linen hamper or linen bag. Dispose of disposable items in a facility-approved waste container. Clean equipment and return it to the storage area.

17. Remove your gloves and dispose of them in a facility-approved waste container.

Finishing Up CLSOWR

18. Complete the "Finishing Up" steps.

PROCEDURE 24-2

Assisting With Foot Care

WHY YOU DO IT   Soft, smooth skin and trimmed, filed toenails are important for overall health and comfort.

Getting Ready WGKIEPS

1. Complete the "Getting Ready" steps.

Supplies

- gloves (if contact with broken skin is likely)
- paper towels
- bed protector
- orange stick
- nailbrush
- nail clippers
- emery board (nail file)
- wash basin
- bath thermometer
- soap
- lotion
- nail polish remover (optional)
- nail polish (optional)
- cotton balls (optional)
- washcloth
- towels

Procedure

2. Make sure that the bed is lowered to its lowest position and that the wheels are locked.

3. Cover the over-bed table with paper towels. Pour some liquid soap into the wash basin and fill the basin with warm water (100°F [37.7°C] to 115°F [46.1°C] on the bath thermometer). Place the wash basin on the over-bed table, along with the nail care supplies and clean linens.

4. If the side rails are in use, lower the side rail on the working side of the bed. The side rail

on the opposite side of the bed should remain up.

5. If the person is able to get out of bed, help the person to transfer from the bed to a bedside chair. If the person is not able to get out of bed, raise the head of the bed as tolerated. Fanfold the top linens to the foot of the bed.

6. Put on the gloves if contact with broken skin is likely.

7. If the person is wearing nail polish and wants it removed, remove the nail polish by putting a small amount of nail polish remover on a cotton ball and gently rubbing each nail.

8. Place a bed protector on the floor in front of the chair (if the person is out of bed) or on the bottom sheet (if the person is in bed). Place the wash basin on the bed protector.

9. Help the person to position his or her feet in the basin to soak. Let the person soak his or her feet for about 5 minutes.

10. Working with one foot at a time, lift the person's foot out of the basin and wash the entire foot, including between the toes, with the soapy washcloth. Apply soap to the nailbrush and gently scrub any rough areas. Use the orange stick to gently clean underneath

the person's toenails. Rinse thoroughly and pat the person's foot dry with a towel. Be sure to dry between the toes. Repeat with the other foot.

11. If facility policy allows it, use the nail clippers to cut the person's toenails. If the person's nails need to be trimmed but this task is outside of your scope of practice, report this need to the nurse.

12. Use the emery board to smooth the rough edges of the toenails.

13. Apply lotion to the person's feet and gently massage it into the skin.

14. Apply nail polish as the person requests.

15. If necessary, help the person return to bed. If the side rails are in use, return the side rails to the raised position. Lower the head of the bed as the person requests.

16. Gather the soiled linens and place them in the linen hamper or linen bag. Dispose of disposable items in a facility-approved waste container. Clean equipment and return it to the storage area.

Finishing Up CLOSURE

17. Complete the "Finishing Up" steps.

PROCEDURE 24-3

Assisting a Person With Dressing

WHY YOU DO IT   Residents who are able to be out of bed during the day usually wear regular clothing during the day and nightwear at night. Getting dressed in the morning helps residents to feel better about themselves. Clothing must be changed every time it becomes wet or soiled.

Getting Ready WORK STEPS

1. Complete the "Getting Ready" steps.

Supplies

- gloves (if contact with broken skin is likely)
- bath blanket
- clean clothing

Procedure

2. Make sure that the bed is positioned at a comfortable working height (to promote good body mechanics) and that the wheels are locked.

3. Lower the head of the bed so that the bed is flat (as tolerated). If the side rails are in use, lower the side rail on the working side of the bed. The side rail on the opposite side of the bed should remain up.

4. Put on the gloves if contact with broken skin is likely.

5. Spread the bath blanket over the top linens (and the person). If the person is able, have him or her hold the bath blanket. If not, tuck the corners under the person's shoulders. Fanfold the top linens to the foot of the bed.

6. Assist the person with undressing:

a. **Garments that fasten in the back.** Undo any fasteners, such as buttons, zippers, snaps, or ties. Gently lift the person's head and shoulders and gather the garment around the person's neck. Working with the person's strongest side first, gently remove the arm from the garment by sliding the garment down the arm. Repeat with the other arm. (If it is not possible to lift the person's head and shoulders, roll the person onto his or her side facing away from you. Working with the person's strongest side first, gently remove the arm from the garment. Roll the person onto his or her other side, facing you and remove the other arm from the garment.) Remove the garment completely by lifting it over the person's head.

b. **Garments that fasten in the front.** Undo any fasteners, such as buttons, zippers, snaps, or ties. To remove the top, gently lift the person's head and shoulders. Working with the person's strongest side first, gently remove the arm from the

(continued)

garment by sliding the garment over the shoulder and down the arm. Gather the garment behind the person and remove the garment completely by sliding the other sleeve over the weak shoulder and arm. To remove the bottoms, undo any fasteners, such as buttons, zippers, or snaps. Ask the person to lift his or her buttocks off the bed and gently slide the pants down to the ankles and over the feet. (If the person cannot raise his or her buttocks off the bed, help the person to roll first to his or her strong side, allowing you to pull the bottoms down on the weak side. Then roll the person to his or her weak side and finish pulling the bottoms down.)

7. Assist the person with putting on his or her undergarments:

   a. **Underpants.** Facing the foot of the bed, gather the underpants together at the leg opening and at the waistband. Working with one foot at a time, slip first one foot and then the other through the waistband and into the leg openings. Slide the underpants up the person's legs as far as they will go, and then ask the person to lift his or her buttocks off the bed. Gently slide the underpants up over the buttocks. (If the person cannot raise his or her buttocks off the bed, help the person to roll first to his or her strong side, allowing you to pull the underpants up on the weak side. Then roll the person to his or her weak side and finish pulling the underpants up.) Adjust the underpants so that they fit comfortably.

   b. **Bra.** Working with the person's weak side first, slip the arms through the straps and position the straps on the shoulders so that the front of the bra is covering the person's chest. Adjust the cups of the bra over the person's breasts. Raise the person's head and shoulders and help the person to lean forward so that you can fasten the bra in the back.

   c. **Undershirt.** Facing the head of the bed, gather the top and the bottom of the undershirt together at the neck opening. Place the undershirt over the person's head. Working with the person's weak side first, slip the arms through the arm openings. Raise the person's head and shoulders and help the person to lean forward

so that you can pull the undershirt down, smoothing out any wrinkles.

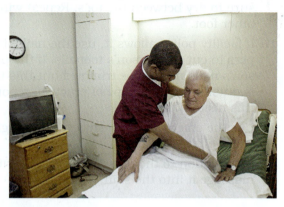

Step 7c Help the person lean forward and pull the undershirt down, smoothing out any wrinkles.

8. Assist the person with putting on his or her outerwear:

   a. **Pants.** Assist the person with putting on his or her pants by following the same procedure as that used for putting on underpants (see step 7a). Fasten any buttons, zippers, snaps, or ties.

   b. **Shirts and sweaters that fasten in the front.** Facing the head of the bed, place your hand and arm through the wristband of the garment. Working with the person's weak side first, grasp the person's hand and slip the garment off of your hand and arm, gently guiding the person's arm into the sleeve. Pull the sleeve up, adjusting it at the shoulder. Raise the person's head and shoulders and help the person to lean forward so that you can bring the other side of the garment around the back of the person's body. Guide the person's strong arm into the sleeve of the garment. Fasten any buttons, zippers, snaps, or ties.

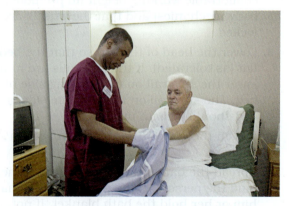

Step 8b Grasp the person's hand and slip the sleeve of the garment onto the person's arm.

c. **Sweatshirts and pullover sweaters.** Assist the person with putting on a sweatshirt or pullover sweater by following the same procedure as that used for putting on an undershirt (see step 7c). Fasten any buttons, zippers, snaps, or ties.

d. **Blouses that fasten in the back.** Facing the head of the bed, place your hand and arm through the wristband of the garment. Working with the person's weak side first, grasp the person's hand and slip the garment off of your hand and arm, gently guiding the person's arm into the sleeve. Pull the sleeve up, adjusting it at the shoulder. Repeat for the other side. Raise the person's head and shoulders and help the person to lean forward so that you can bring the sides of the garment around to the back. Fasten any buttons, zippers, snaps, or ties.

9. Assist the person with putting on footwear:
   a. **Socks or knee-high stockings.** Gather the sock or stocking, bringing the toe area and the opening together. With the toe area facing up, slip the sock or stocking over the person's foot. Smooth the heel of the sock or stocking over the person's heel, and pull the sock or stocking up into position. Adjust the sock or stocking so that it fits comfortably. Repeat for the other foot.

   b. **Shoes or slippers.** If the shoe has laces, loosen them completely to make it easier to slip the shoe onto the foot. Guide the person's foot into the shoe or slipper. A shoehorn may be used to help ease the person's heel into the shoe. Make sure that the foot is seated properly in the shoe. Socks or stockings should not be bunched at the toe. If necessary, tie the shoe or fasten the Velcro™ fasteners securely.

10. If the person will be remaining in bed and the side rails are in use, return the side rails to the raised position. Raise the head of the bed as the person requests.

11. Gather the soiled garments and place them in the linen hamper or linen bag.

12. Remove your gloves and dispose of them in a facility-approved waste container.

Finishing Up

13. Complete the "Finishing Up" steps.

PROCEDURE 24-4

Changing a Hospital Gown

WHY YOU DO IT   People who are too ill to get out of bed may wear a hospital gown. The gown must be changed every time it becomes wet or soiled.

Getting Ready

1. Complete the "Getting Ready" steps.

Supplies

- gloves (if contact with broken skin is likely)
- clean hospital gown

Procedure

2. Make sure that the bed is positioned at a comfortable working height (to promote good body mechanics) and that the wheels are locked.

3. Lower the head of the bed so that the bed is flat (as tolerated). If the side rails are in use, lower them on the working side of the bed. The side rails on the opposite side of the bed should remain up.

4. Put on the gloves if contact with broken skin is likely.

5. Have the person turn onto his or her side facing away from you so that you can untie the gown at the neck and waist. Assist the person back into the supine position. If the person cannot turn onto his or her side, reach under the person and untie the gown.

6. Loosen the gown from around the person's body.

(continued)

7. Unfold the clean gown and lay it over the person's chest.

8. Working with the person's strongest side first, remove one sleeve at a time, leaving the old gown draped over the person's body.

9. Working with the person's weakest side first, slide the arm through the sleeve of the clean gown. Repeat for the other arm.

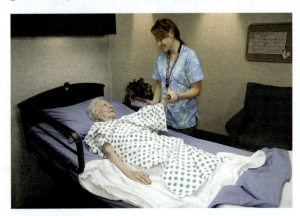

Step 9 Slide the person's arm through the sleeve of the clean gown.

10. Remove the soiled gown from underneath the clean gown and place it in the linen hamper or linen bag.

11. Have the person turn onto his or her side, facing away from you, so that you can tie the gown at the neck and waist (or reach under the person and tie the gown). Adjust the gown so that it fits comfortably.

12. If the side rails are in use, return the side rails to the raised position. Raise the head of the bed as the person requests.

13. Remove your gloves and dispose of them in a facility-approved waste container.

Finishing Up CLSOWR

14. Complete the "Finishing Up" steps.

PROCEDURE 24-5

Shampooing a Person's Hair in Bed

WHY YOU DO IT   Clean hair helps a person to look and feel attractive and is important for a person's self-esteem.

Getting Ready WCKIEPS

1. Complete the "Getting Ready" steps.

Supplies

- gloves (if contact with broken skin is likely)
- paper towels
- bed protector
- wash basin
- water pitcher
- bath thermometer
- shampoo trough
- comb
- brush
- blow dryer (optional)
- shampoo
- conditioner (optional)
- towels

Procedure

2. Make sure that the bed is positioned at a comfortable working height (to promote good body mechanics) and that the wheels are locked.

3. Fill the water pitcher with warm water (100°F [37.7°C] to 115°F [46.1°C] on the bath thermometer).

4. Cover the over-bed table with paper towels. Place the hair care supplies and clean linens on the over-bed table.

5. Raise the head of the bed as tolerated. Comb the person's hair to remove snarls and tangles.

6. Lower the head of the bed so that the bed is flat (as tolerated). If the side rails are in use, lower the side rail on the working side of the bed. The side rail on the opposite side of the bed should remain up.

7. Put on the gloves if contact with broken skin is likely.

8. Gently lift the person's head and shoulders and reposition the pillow under the person's shoulders. Cover the head of the bed and the pillow with the bed protector. Position the shampoo trough at the head of the bed. Help the person to rest his head on the shampoo trough. Place a towel across the person's shoulders and chest.

9. Place the wash basin on the floor to catch the water as it drains from the shampoo trough.

10. Holding the water pitcher in one hand, slowly pour water over the person's hair until the hair is completely wet. Use your other hand to help direct the flow of water away from the person's eyes and ears.

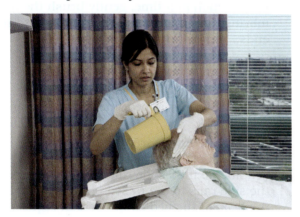

Step 10 Wet the person's hair, being careful to keep the water out of his eyes.

11. Apply a small amount of shampoo to the wet hair. Lather the hair and massage the scalp to help stimulate the circulation.

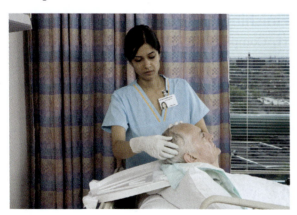

Step 11 Apply a small amount of shampoo and work it into a lather.

12. Using the water pitcher, rinse the hair thoroughly.

13. Apply conditioner, as the person requests. Rinse the hair thoroughly.

14. Gently lift the person's head and shoulders and remove the shampoo trough and bed protector. Wrap the person's hair in a towel.

15. Raise the head of the bed as tolerated. Gently pat the person's face, neck, and ears dry and finish towel drying the hair.

16. Replace any wet or soiled linens. (If the side rails are in use, raise the side rails before leaving the bedside to get the necessary replacement linens.)

17. Comb the person's hair to remove snarls and tangles.

18. Dry and style the hair with the brush and blow dryer, as the person requests. Use the cool setting and take care not to burn the person's scalp or face.

19. Reposition the pillow under the person's head and straighten the bed linens. If the side rails are in use, return the side rails to the raised position. Lower the head of the bed as the person requests.

20. Gather the soiled linens and place them in the linen hamper or linen bag. Dispose of disposable items in a facility-approved waste container. Clean equipment and return it to the storage area.

21. Remove your gloves and dispose of them in a facility-approved waste container.

Finishing Up   CLOSWR

22. Complete the "Finishing Up" steps.

PROCEDURE 24-6

Combing a Person's Hair

WHY YOU DO IT Combing the hair helps to prevent tangles and gives the hair a neat appearance.

Getting Ready WORKSTEPS

1. Complete the "Getting Ready" steps.

Supplies

- paper towels
- wide-toothed comb or pick
- brush
- mirror
- hair accessories (optional)
- detangler or leave-in conditioner (optional)
- towels

Procedure

2. Make sure that the bed is positioned at a comfortable working height (to promote good body mechanics) and that the wheels are locked.

3. Cover the over-bed table with paper towels. Place the hair care supplies and clean linens on the over-bed table.

4. Raise the head of the bed as tolerated. Gently lift the person's head and shoulders and cover the pillow with a towel. Drape another towel across the person's back and shoulders.

5. If the side rails are in use, lower the side rail on the working side of the bed. The side rail on the opposite side of the bed should remain up.

6. If the hair is tangled, work on the tangles first. Put a small amount of detangler or leave-in conditioner on the tangled hair. Begin at the ends of the hair and work toward the scalp. Hold the lock of hair just above the tangle (closest to the scalp) and use the wide-tooth comb to gently work through the tangle.

7. Using the brush and working with one 2-inch section at a time, gently brush the hair, moving from the roots of the hair toward the ends.

8. Secure the hair using barrettes, clips, or pins or braid the hair, as the person requests. Offer the person the mirror to check his or her appearance when you are finished.

9. Remove the towels, reposition the pillow under the person's head, and straighten the bed linens. If the side rails are in use, return the side rails to the raised position. Lower the head of the bed as the person requests.

10. Gather the soiled linens and place them in the linen hamper or linen bag. Dispose of disposable items in a facility-approved waste container. Clean equipment and return it to the storage area.

Finishing Up CLOSURE

11. Complete the "Finishing Up" steps.

PROCEDURE 24-7

Shaving a Person's Face

WHY YOU DO IT   Shaving removes unwanted hair and is a routine grooming practice for many residents.

Getting Ready WORKSTEPS

1. Complete the "Getting Ready" steps.

Supplies

- gloves
- paper towels
- safety razor
- shaving cream/ gel/soap
- shaving brush (if using shaving soap)
- aftershave lotion (optional)
- wash basin
- bath thermometer
- mirror
- washcloth
- towels

Procedure

2. Make sure that the bed is lowered to its lowest position and that the wheels are locked.

3. Fill the wash basin with warm water (100°F [37.7°C] to 115°F [46.1°C] on the bath thermometer).

4. Cover the over-bed table with paper towels. Place the wash basin, shaving supplies, and clean linens on the over-bed table.

5. If the side rails are in use, lower the side rail on the working side of the bed. The side rail on the opposite side of the bed should remain up.

6. Help the person to transfer from the bed to a bedside chair, assist the person to sit on the edge of the bed, or raise the head of the bed as tolerated.

7. Place a towel across the person's shoulders and chest.

8. Put on the gloves.

9. Wet the washcloth with warm, clean water. Soften the beard by holding the washcloth against the person's face for 2 to 3 minutes.

10. Apply shaving cream, gel, or soap to the beard.

11. Shave the person's cheeks:
    a. Stand facing the person.
    b. Gently pull the skin tight and shave downward, in the direction of hair growth (that is, toward the chin). Use short, even strokes, rinsing the razor frequently in the wash basin. Repeat until all of the lather on the cheek has been removed.
    c. Repeat for the other cheek.

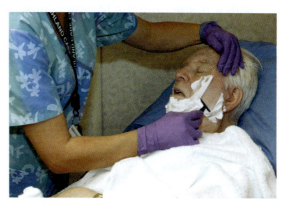

Step 11 Shave downward, in the direction of hair growth.

12. Shave the person's chin:
    a. Ask the person to "tighten the chin" by drawing the lower lip over the teeth.
    b. Shave the chin using short, even, downward strokes. Repeat until all of the lather on the chin has been removed, rinsing the razor frequently in the wash basin.

13. Shave the person's neck:
    a. Ask the person to tip his head back.
    b. Gently pull the skin tight and shave upward, in the direction of hair growth (that is, toward the chin). Use short, even strokes, rinsing the razor frequently in the wash basin. Repeat until all of the lather on the neck has been removed.

14. Shave the area between the person's nose and upper lip:
    a. Ask the person to "tighten his upper lip" by drawing the upper lip over the teeth.
    b. Shave the area between the nose and the upper lip using short, even downward strokes. Repeat until all of the lather has been removed, rinsing the razor frequently in the wash basin.

(continued)

15. Change the water in the wash basin. (If the side rails are in use, raise the side rails before leaving the bedside.) Form a mitt around your hand with the washcloth and wet the mitt with warm, clean water. Wash the person's face and neck. Rinse thoroughly and pat the person's face, neck, and ears dry with the face towel.

16. Apply aftershave lotion, as the person requests.

17. If you have accidentally nicked the skin and the person is bleeding, apply direct pressure with a tissue until the bleeding stops. Report the incident to the nurse.

18. If necessary, help the person return to bed. If the side rails are in use, return the side rails to the raised position.

19. Gather the soiled linens and place them in the linen hamper or linen bag. Dispose of disposable items in a facility-approved waste container. Clean equipment and return it to the storage area.

20. Remove your gloves and dispose of them in a facility-approved waste container.

Finishing Up CLOSURE

21. Complete the "Finishing Up" steps.

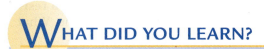

WHAT DID YOU LEARN?

Multiple Choice

Select the single best answer for each of the following questions.

1. You are a nursing assistant in a long-term care facility. Which one of the following procedures may be beyond your scope of practice?
   a. Assisting a resident with bathing
   b. Polishing a female resident's fingernails
   c. Trimming the toenails of a resident with diabetes
   d. Assisting a resident with oral hygiene

2. When helping a person to dress, which item of clothing would you put on first?
   a. Underpants
   b. Socks
   c. Slacks
   d. Sweater

3. Mrs. Dinksley, one of your residents, had a stroke that caused her left side to become weak. You are helping Mrs. Dinksley put on a cardigan sweater. Which arm should you put in the sleeve first?
   a. The left arm
   b. The right arm
   c. Either arm; it makes no difference
   d. Neither arm; Mrs. Dinksley should wear a hospital gown

4. Mr. Bush has just been admitted to the long-term care facility where you work. When you tell Mr. Bush that baths are routinely scheduled on Monday, Wednesday, and Friday mornings, Mr. Bush looks worried. He says that he always bathes and shaves before he goes to bed, and he likes to do this every night. How do you react to this?
   a. You tell Mr. Bush that you're sorry, but he has to follow facility policy.
   b. You tell Mr. Bush "OK" but then schedule him for a bath every Monday, Wednesday, and Friday morning, just like everyone else.
   c. You respect Mr. Bush's choice and ask the nurse if you can schedule him for a bath and a shave as part of evening care, every evening.
   d. You report Mr. Bush to the nurse because he is being difficult.

5. Brushing the hair is important to:
   a. Make it grow faster
   b. Keep it soft and shiny and prevent tangles
   c. Keep it clean
   d. Keep it free from lice

6. When shaving a man's face with a safety razor and shaving cream, you should:
   a. Soften the beard with warm water before applying the shaving cream
   b. Apply aftershave lotion after the shave is complete, if the man requests it
   c. Give the man a mirror so that he can check his appearance when you are finished
   d. All of the above

7. When shaving a man's face, you should:
   a. Apply shaving cream sparingly
   b. Use upward strokes when shaving the cheeks
   c. Apply an antiseptic to any cuts or nicks
   d. Use downward strokes to shave the chin

8. Which one of the following statements about nail care is true?
   a. Scissors are used to trim the nails.
   b. Elderly people do not need nail care because their nails do not grow as fast.
   c. Providing nail care allows you to examine the hands and feet for signs of health and disease.
   d. Nail care is an activity that can be skipped if there is not enough time.

9. Which one of the following benefits does a resident enjoy when you shampoo his or her hair?
   a. Improved circulation (blood flow) to the scalp
   b. A clean, neat appearance
   c. Increased feelings of well-being
   d. All of the above

10. Which one of the following statements about helping a resident to dress is true?
    a. Residents like staff members to decide what they are going to wear.
    b. Residents are used to being dressed in front of others.
    c. Residents care about how they look.
    d. Residents who are disabled do not need to dress in street clothes.

11. One of your residents, Mrs. Ament, has diabetes. Why is providing foot care an important part of caring for Mrs. Ament?
    a. The circulation to her feet is likely to be poor, which puts her at risk for infection and other complications.
    b. Diabetes makes the toenails grow faster.
    c. People with diabetes usually do not take good care of their feet.
    d. All of the above

12. You must remove a soiled gown from a resident who has an intravenous (IV) line. What is the best way to do this?
    a. Remove the gown from the arm with the IV first.
    b. Ask the nurse to disconnect the bag and tubing before beginning.
    c. Disconnect the bag and tubing before beginning.
    d. Remove the opposite arm from the gown first.

Matching

Match each numbered item with its appropriate lettered description.

_____ 1. Pediculosis

_____ 2. Alopecia

_____ 3. Podiatrist

_____ 4. Tinea pedis

_____ 5. Tinea capitis

a. A fungal infection of the scalp
b. Loss of hair
c. A fungal infection of the feet
d. Head lice
e. A doctor who specializes in care of the feet

STOP and Think!

• Today, you are helping Mrs. Wiseman get dressed. She is especially excited this morning, because it is Saturday and her son is coming to visit. Since her son's favorite color is blue, Mrs. Wiseman has picked out a lightweight blue blouse to wear. You know that Mrs. Wisemen tends to chill easily, and you don't think she is going to be comfortable wearing the blouse that she has picked out.

You suggest a different blouse, but Mrs. Wiseman tells you that she would rather wear the blouse that she picked out originally. How can you provide Mrs. Wiseman with her choice of clothing and still make sure that she is warm enough? What other grooming tasks can you help Mrs. Wiseman with so that she feels presentable for her son's visit?

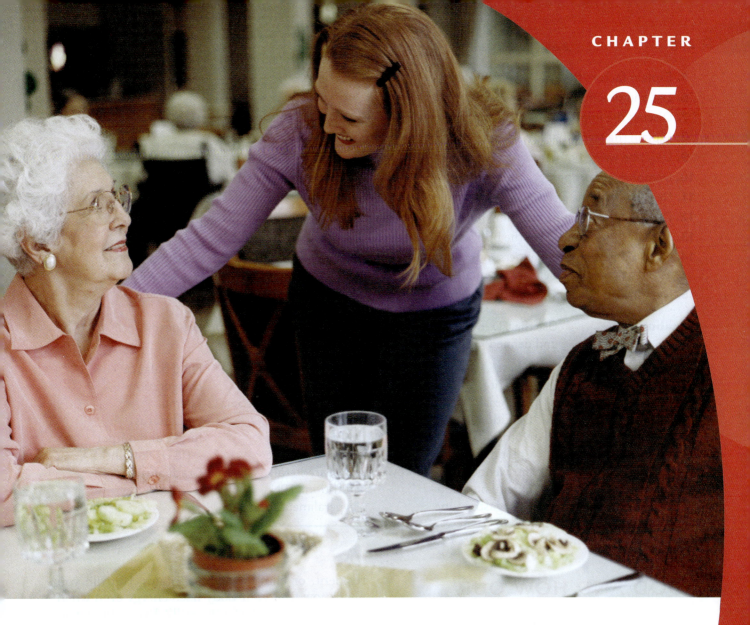

Basic Nutrition

WHAT WILL YOU LEARN?

Few things are more satisfying than a good meal—you know, one that is made up of your favorite foods, all cooked to perfection, just like Mom's home cooking. Eating meets many needs for people, both emotionally and physically. In this chapter, you will learn about what we need to eat to keep our bodies healthy. You will also learn how to help your residents to meet their own nutritional needs. When you are finished with this chapter, you will be able to:

1. Define the term *nutrition* and explain why our bodies need adequate nutrition.
2. List the general types of nutrients and describe how the body uses them.
3. Discuss how MyPyramid can be used to help plan and provide better nutrition for a person.
4. Explain factors that influence a person's food preferences and eating habits.

Photo: Meal time is as much about socializing as it is about eating. (Punchstock)

475

5. Explain factors that can affect an older person's food intake.

6. List and describe common special diets.

7. Discuss the importance of making meals attractive and the dining experience pleasant.

8. Explain the steps that are taken to help prepare a resident for meal time.

9. Describe ways that a nursing assistant may need to help a resident during meal time.

10. Demonstrate proper technique for feeding a resident who cannot feed herself.

11. Describe how the amount of solid food eaten is recorded.

12. Discuss other ways of providing nutrition for residents who are unable to take food by mouth.

13. Explain the fluid needs of the body and factors that affect the body's fluid balance.

14. List reasons why an older person might be at risk for dehydration, and describe measures a nursing assistant can take to ensure adequate fluid intake.

15. Demonstrate methods used to measure and record fluid intake and output.

Vocabulary Use the CD in the front of your book to hear these terms pronounced and defined:

Nutrients	Obese	Nasointestinal tube	Fluid balance
Nutrition	Appetite	Gastrostomy tube	Dehydration
Ingestion	Anorexia	Percutaneous endoscopic	Edema
Digestion	Dentition	gastrostomy (PEG)	NPO status
Absorption	Nutritional supplement	tube	Intake and output
Glucose	Calorie count	Jejunostomy tube	(I&O) flow sheet
Amino acids	Intravenous (IV) therapy	Total parenteral	Graduate
Fat-soluble	Enteral nutrition	nutrition (TPN,	
Water-soluble	Nasogastric tube	hyperalimentation)	

FOOD AND HOW OUR BODIES USE IT

All living things eat. The food that we take into our bodies is broken down into essential elements, called **nutrients.** The body uses these nutrients to grow, to repair itself, and to carry out processes essential for living. **Nutrition,** or the process of taking in and using food, involves the following steps:

- **Ingestion,** the intake of food
- **Digestion,** the breaking down of food into simple elements (nutrients)
- **Absorption,** the transfer of these nutrients from the digestive tract into the bloodstream
- **Metabolism,** the process that occurs in cells to convert the nutrients into energy

To function, the body needs a continuous supply of energy, which it gets from the metabolism of food. You know that your body uses energy when you run to catch a bus, reposition a resident, or climb a flight of stairs. But did you also know that your body uses energy even when you are sitting perfectly still? Every time you blink, your heart beats, or your lungs expand to take in air, you are using energy. The energy to power our bodies comes from food, especially food that is high in carbohydrates, protein, or fat. Energy is measured in units called kilocalories, more commonly known as **calories.**

In addition to providing us with energy, food provides us with other substances our bodies need to function properly. Other substances found in food that benefit us include vitamins and minerals, fiber, and water:

- **Vitamins** and **minerals** are small molecules that help to regulate body processes and form structures within the body. For example, vitamin K helps the blood to clot, and calcium, a mineral, helps to build strong bones. Table 25-1 lists some of the common vitamins and minerals and describes how they benefit the body.
- **Fiber** is found in fruits, vegetables, and whole grain cereals and breads. Fiber may be

Table 25-1 **Vitamins and Minerals**

NUTRIENT	SOURCES	FUNCTION
VITAMINS		
Vitamin A	Liver, carrots, egg yolks, fortified milk	Helps us to see in dim light Keeps skin and mucous membranes healthy
Vitamin B_1 (thiamin)	Pork, liver, whole and enriched grains, legumes	Helps produce energy from glucose Assists with nerve function
Vitamin B_2 (riboflavin)	Milk, organ meats (for example, brain, kidneys, liver), enriched grains, green vegetables	Assists with the metabolism of carbohydrates, protein, and fat
Vitamin B_3 (niacin)	Kidneys, grains, lean meats, nuts	Assists with the metabolism of carbohydrates, protein, and fat
Vitamin B_{12}	Meat (including organ meats), eggs, milk, cheese	Assists with the formation of hemoglobin (the molecule that carries oxygen throughout the body) and red blood cells
Folic acid	Green leafy vegetables, meats, and whole grains	Assists with protein metabolism and the formation of red blood cells
Vitamin C (ascorbic acid)	Citrus fruits, broccoli, green peppers, strawberries, green leafy vegetables	Assists with tissue healing, building red blood cells, and iron absorption
Vitamin D	Sunlight, fortified milk, fish liver oils	Assists with the absorption of calcium and phosphorus to strengthen bones
Vitamin E	Vegetable oils, wheat germ, whole grains	Assists with the formation of red blood cells Assists with the reproductive system
Vitamin K	Vegetable oils, wheat germ, whole grains, liver, green leafy vegetables, eggs	Assists with metabolism of the proteins necessary for normal blood clotting
MINERALS		
Calcium	Milk, cheese, canned fish with bones, green leafy vegetables	Keeps the teeth and bones strong Assists with blood clotting Assists with nerve function and contraction of the heart and skeletal muscles
Phosphorus	Milk, soft drinks, meat, nuts, peas, beans	Keeps the teeth and bones strong Assists with the metabolism of carbohydrates, protein, and fat
Iron	Liver, lean meats, enriched and whole-grain breads, cheese, green leafy vegetables	Used to produce hemoglobin (the molecule that carries oxygen throughout the body)
Iodine	Table salt and seafood	Used by the thyroid gland to produce hormones for cell metabolism
Sodium	Table salt	Assists with fluid balance, nerve function, and contraction of the heart and skeletal muscles
Potassium	Whole grains, fruits, green leafy vegetables	Assists with fluid balance, nerve function, and contraction of the heart and skeletal muscles

soluble, which means that it can be broken down (digested). Or it may be insoluble, which means that it cannot be digested. Insoluble fiber helps to prevent problems with bowel movements by adding bulk to the feces.

- **Water,** which will be discussed in more detail later in this chapter, plays many important roles in helping the body to function well.

TYPES OF NUTRIENTS

There are six general types of nutrients. Three of these nutrient types (carbohydrates, proteins, and fat) supply energy. The remaining three (minerals, vitamins, and water) regulate body processes.

Carbohydrates

Foods containing carbohydrates form the basis of many diets throughout the world because these foods tend to be plentiful and inexpensive. Carbohydrates are found in bread, cereal, rice, fruit, vegetables, and table sugar. Carbohydrates are the source of the body's most basic type of fuel, **glucose.** Glucose, sometimes called "blood sugar," is carried in the blood and rapidly absorbed by every cell in the body. The cells use the glucose to "run," much like your car uses gas. Glucose is a simple carbohydrate, or sugar, which means that it passes quickly from the digestive tract into the bloodstream. Other carbohydrates, known as complex carbohydrates, or starches, must be broken down into simple sugars before the body can use them. Extra carbohydrates that are not used immediately as fuel are either stored in the liver or converted to fat and stored elsewhere in the body. Each gram of carbohydrate provides the body with 4 calories, or energy units.

Protein

Protein is found in foods such as milk and cheese, meat, poultry, fish, eggs, nuts, and dried peas and beans. Proteins contain **amino acids,** small molecules that are the "building blocks" of all of the body's cells. Foods containing protein help the body to rebuild tissue that breaks down from normal use and to grow new tissue after illness or injury. In addition to providing amino acids, protein is a source of fuel. Like carbohydrates, protein provides the body with 4 calories per gram.

Fats (lipids)

Fats are found in butter, cooking oils, whole milk, cheese, meat, egg yolks, nuts, shortening, and lard. Fats make food taste better and satisfy the appetite longer because they take longer to digest than most other food sources. Although a "lowfat" diet is recommended for most people to maintain health, not all fats are bad. In fact, the body requires a certain amount of dietary fat to function properly. For example, some vitamins will dissolve only in fat, not water (that is, they are **fat-soluble**). This means that fat must be present in order for the body to use the vitamins. Fat also protects our organs and helps us to stay warm. Finally, fats are the most concentrated source of energy, providing 9 calories per gram.

Vitamins

Vitamins, as described earlier and in Table 25-1, play a key role in many body processes. Vitamins are classified as water-soluble or fat-soluble. **Water-soluble** vitamins dissolve in water. Water-soluble vitamins (vitamin C and the B-complex vitamins) are absorbed directly from the digestive tract into the bloodstream. The body cannot store water-soluble vitamins. Instead, any extra amounts of these vitamins are passed from the body in the urine. This means that water-soluble vitamins must be replenished daily for use by the body.

Fat-soluble vitamins (vitamins A, D, E, and K) are absorbed and stored in the body's fat, where they can be used as needed. Unlike water-soluble vitamins, fat-soluble vitamins are not easily passed from the body. For this reason, consuming too much of a fat-soluble vitamin can be as harmful as not consuming enough, because the vitamin builds up in the body. In some cases, this build-up may actually be harmful.

Minerals

Minerals help provide structure within the body. For example, fluoride strengthens the teeth and calcium strengthens the bones. Minerals also regulate body processes. For example, red blood cells need iron to do their job of carrying oxygen to all of the cells in the body. Key minerals that the body needs to function properly are summarized in Table 25-1.

Water

Water is provided in the diet in the form of beverages such as juice, soda, milk, coffee, tea, and, of course, water! Water is also found in many foods, such as fruits and vegetables. Water provides no calories or nutrition, but may be more essential to life than food. You can live for quite a long time without food, but only for 3 to 7 days without water. Every cell in your body contains water, which is why water accounts for approximately 50% to 60% of your body weight! Water does the following things for our bodies:

- The nutrients found in food must be dissolved in fluid and circulated throughout the body. Water forms the basis for this fluid.
- Water transports waste products out of the body, by way of the urine and feces.
- Water keeps us cool when it evaporates from our skin in the form of sweat.
- Water keeps the mucous membranes moist.
- Water forms the basis of the fluid that helps our joints to move smoothly.

A BALANCED DIET

For the best health, you must follow a diet that provides your body with a balanced amount of the essential nutrients. Two tools are available to help you achieve this goal—MyPyramid and the nutrition labels on food.

MyPyramid

In the United States, the number of children and adults who are overweight or **obese** (extremely overweight) is increasing every year. Unhealthy eating habits, combined with a lack of physical activity, are the primary reasons we are seeing an increase in obesity. As a result, we are also seeing a significant increase in health problems related to being overweight or obese, such as cardiovascular disease and diabetes.

To help Americans plan a healthy diet, the United States government developed MyPyramid (Fig. 25-1). MyPyramid emphasizes the importance of getting enough physical activity and eating a healthy, balanced diet. Some foods contain many nutrients that our bodies need to remain healthy, but other foods have little or no nutritional value. The best way to get the nutrients you need is to eat a variety of healthy food every day. MyPyramid describes a healthy diet as one that:

- Emphasizes fruits, vegetables, whole grains, and fat-free or low-fat milk products
- Includes lean meats, poultry, fish, beans, eggs, and nuts
- Is low in saturated fats, *trans* fats, cholesterol, salt (sodium), and added sugars

In general, the recommendations in MyPyramid apply for all healthy people older than 2 years of age. However, nutritional requirements vary at different times throughout a person's life. For example:

- Infants and young children have an increased need for calories and iron because they are growing rapidly.
- Teenagers experiencing "growth spurts" have increased caloric and nutritional needs.
- Women who are pregnant or breast-feeding need more protein and calcium.
- People who are recovering from physical trauma, such as that caused by burns or surgery, have different nutritional requirements than healthy people. Similarly, some illnesses change the nutritional requirements of the body, including chronic conditions such as diabetes, kidney disease, or alcoholism.
- Older people have different nutritional requirements because of the physical changes that occur with normal aging. Older people do not need as many calories as younger people because they are usually less active. They also may not feel thirsty as often, although the need for water and other fluids increases with age.

Food Labels

There is a second tool available to help you plan a balanced diet—the nutrition labels that appear on most foods offered for sale at the grocery store. Education about proper nutrition and diet planning is one of the most effective ways of promoting health and helping to prevent some illnesses. In recognition of this fact, the United States Congress passed the Nutritional Labeling and Education Act in 1990, which requires that the labels of all packaged foods include information about the food's nutritional value, approximate serving size, and any related health claims (Fig. 25-2). By reading the nutrition label, you can see how the food can help you to achieve your nutrition goals for the day.

FACTORS THAT AFFECT FOOD CHOICES AND EATING HABITS

MyPyramid and food labels help us to make wise food choices. However, factors other than the nutritional content of a food often affect the choices we make about what we eat and when we eat it. Some people prefer a hot, hearty breakfast to start the day while others may want only a bowl of cereal or coffee and toast. Some people like a light meal at lunch time while others eat their main meal at mid-day. Dinner may consist of a light snack for some, while others routinely have a seven-course meal. Listed below are some of the factors that affect a person's food choices and eating habits. Think about your own eating habits and food likes and dislikes. Are any of your personal preferences related to the factors listed here?

- **Religion.** Dietary restrictions are a part of many religions. Some of these restrictions are specific to certain days (for example, the Roman Catholic custom of avoiding meat on Fridays during Lent, or the Jewish tradition of avoiding flour-based foods during Passover). Other dietary restrictions are in effect all of the time (for example, Jewish people who follow kosher dietary laws do not eat pork or shellfish, and they do not serve meat and dairy dishes at the same meal).

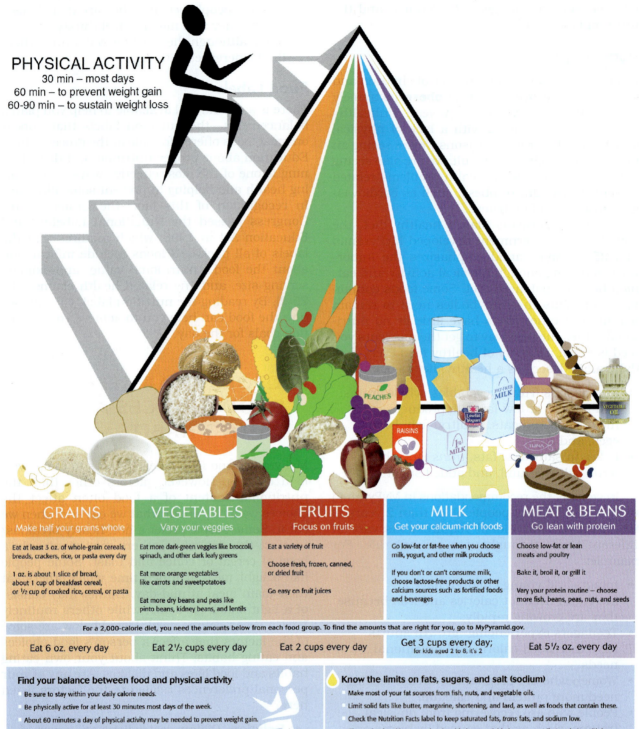

PHYSICAL ACTIVITY
30 min – most days
60 min – to prevent weight gain
60-90 min – to sustain weight loss

GRAINS	VEGETABLES	FRUITS	MILK	MEAT & BEANS
Make half your grains whole	Vary your veggies	Focus on fruits	Get your calcium-rich foods	Go lean with protein
Eat at least 3 oz. of whole-grain cereals, breads, crackers, rice, or pasta every day 1 oz. is about 1 slice of bread, about 1 cup of breakfast cereal, or ½ cup of cooked rice, cereal, or pasta	Eat more dark-green veggies like broccoli, spinach, and other dark leafy greens Eat more orange vegetables like carrots and sweetpotatoes Eat more dry beans and peas like pinto beans, kidney beans, and lentils	Eat a variety of fruit Choose fresh, frozen, canned, or dried fruit Go easy on fruit juices	Go low-fat or fat-free when you choose milk, yogurt, and other milk products If you don't or can't consume milk, choose lactose-free products or other calcium sources such as fortified foods and beverages	Choose low-fat or lean meats and poultry Bake it, broil it, or grill it Vary your protein routine – choose more fish, beans, peas, nuts, and seeds

For a 2,000-calorie diet, you need the amounts below from each food group. To find the amounts that are right for you, go to MyPyramid.gov.

Eat 6 oz. every day	Eat 2½ cups every day	Eat 2 cups every day	Get 3 cups every day; for kids aged 2 to 8, it's 2	Eat 5½ oz. every day

Find your balance between food and physical activity

- Be sure to stay within your daily calorie needs.
- Be physically active for at least 30 minutes most days of the week.
- About 60 minutes a day of physical activity may be needed to prevent weight gain.
- For sustaining weight loss, at least 60 to 90 minutes a day of physical activity may be required.
- Children and teenagers should be physically active for 60 minutes every day, or most days.

Know the limits on fats, sugars, and salt (sodium)

- Make most of your fat sources from fish, nuts, and vegetable oils.
- Limit solid fats like butter, margarine, shortening, and lard, as well as foods that contain these.
- Check the Nutrition Facts label to keep saturated fats, *trans* fats, and sodium low.
- Choose food and beverages low in added sugars. Added sugars contribute calories with few, if any, nutrients.

Figure 25-1

MyPyramid was developed by the U.S. government to help Americans plan a healthy diet. MyPyramid recommends balancing food intake and physical activity, and choosing foods that have high nutritional value.

Nutrition Facts
Serving Size 1 1/2 oz (40 g/about 5 dried plums)
Servings Per Container About 9

Amount Per Serving

Calories 100   Calories from Fat 0

	% Daily Value*
Total Fat 0 g	**0**%
Saturated Fat 0 g	**0**%
Cholesterol 0 mg	**0**%
Sodium 5 mg	**0**%
Potassium 290 mg	**8**%
Total Carbohydrate 24 g	**8**%
Dietary Fiber 3 g	**11**%
Soluble Fiber 1 g	
Insoluble Fiber 1 g	
Sugars 12 g	
Protein 1 g	

Vitamin A 10% (100% as beta carotene)

Vitamin C 0%   •   Iron 2%

Calcium 2%

*Percent Daily Values are based on a 2,000 calorie diet. Your daily values may be higher or lower depending on your calorie needs:

	Calories:	2,000	2,500
Total Fat	Less than	65 g	80 g
Sat Fat	Less than	20 g	25 g
Cholesterol	Less than	300 mg	300 mg
Sodium	Less than	2,400 mg	2,400 mg
Potassium		3,500 mg	3,500 mg
Total Carbohydrate		300 g	375 g
Dietary Fiber		25 g	30 g

INGREDIENTS: PITTED CALIFORNIA DRIED PLUMS (PRUNES), NATURAL AND ARTIFICIAL FLAVOR, POTASSIUM SORBATE AS A PRESERVATIVE.
PACKED BY: SUNSWEET GROWERS INC. YUBA CITY, CA 95993-9370 U.S.A.
® SUNSWEET and THE SMART SNACK are Registered Trademarks of Sunsweet Growers Inc. in the U.S. and Other Countries
© SUNSWEET GROWERS INC.
FOR QUESTIONS OR COMMENTS CALL:
1-800-417-2253, 9 A.M.-6 P.M. (E.T.), MON.-FRI.
OR VISIT OUR WEB SITE: WWW.SUNSWEET.COM

Look for the Sun to See
Sunsweet Dried Plums Healthy Facts

Exchange: 1 1/2 fruit. Exchange calculations based on the Exchange Lists for Meal Planning. © 1995 The American Dietetic Association, the American Diabetes Association.

Figure 25-2
The law requires all packaged foods to have a nutrition label like this one. (*Courtesy of Sunsweet Growers, Inc.*)

- **Culture and geography.** People often like certain foods because they are associated with their culture, or the area where they grew up. For example, a person who was raised in the southern United States may have grown up eating "grits" (corn mush) for breakfast instead of oatmeal. Now imagine that this person has moved to a long-term care facility in the Northeast to be closer to a son or daughter, where the typical "northern" dish of oatmeal is served for breakfast.

Although the person might like oatmeal just fine, she might prefer grits because they are familiar and they remind her of home. Cultural preferences are a combination of heritage, religion, geography, and all of the characteristics that make a person unique. Some people are willing to try new foods, while others prefer to stay with what they know. This desire for familiar foods is one reason why chain restaurants are so popular in the United States.

- **Finances.** Food can be expensive. People who are on a fixed income, especially disabled or elderly people, may find it difficult to afford foods that supply good nutrition. Often, fresh fruits and vegetables and lean cuts of meat are among the most expensive items in the grocery cart. Milk and cheese, which are also nutritious, may also be out of many people's price range. Instead, people in the lower economic levels often rely on cheaper foods that are high in calories and carbohydrates, but low in many nutrients. Fortunately, a small food budget does not necessarily make it impossible to eat healthy foods. With information and planning, it is possible to afford nutritionally sound food, even on a fixed income.

- **Kitchen skills.** People who do not know how to cook, do not like to cook, or do not have time to cook may choose to eat in restaurants more often. They may also rely on convenience foods and packaged foods.

- **Individual taste.** Some people find certain foods delicious while others could barely swallow a bite. Some people may not like a certain food because of its texture, or the degree of spiciness. Others will avoid a food because of the way it looks or smells. Many people are unable to eat certain foods, no matter how much they love them, because of food allergies. As you certainly know from your own experience, individual tastes vary greatly, even among people who belong to the same culture (or the same family)!

FACTORS THAT CAN AFFECT NUTRITION IN AN OLDER PERSON

Many factors (both physical and emotional) can put an older person at risk for poor nutrition and weight loss.

LOSS OF APPETITE

Appetite is simply the desire for food. Appetite is both physically driven (by the feeling of hunger) and emotionally driven. Have you ever seen a commercial for some type of food, where the food looked so good you actually started to feel hungry? You may not have actually been physically hungry, but the sight of the food and the thought of how it would taste stimulated your appetite. The opposite can be true as well. For example, a person who is ill or under emotional stress may be physically hungry, but have no appetite for food. This loss of appetite is called **anorexia.**

An older person may experience anorexia, or loss of appetite, for many different reasons:

- **Illness.** Older people often have one or more chronic health conditions. These chronic health conditions can affect how well a person feels on any given day. When a person is not feeling well, his interest in food generally decreases. You can probably relate to this yourself. Think about a time when you did not feel well. Most likely, you did not have interest in food, and you probably ate less than usual.
- **Medications.** Most older people take a number of different medications. Some medications (or combination of medications) can cause a decrease in appetite.
- **Decreased taste and smell.** Together, the senses of taste and smell have a very powerful effect on appetite. You have probably noticed for yourself how the wonderful smell of food cooking can stimulate your appetite. As we age, our senses of taste and smell become less intense. When these senses are decreased, the enjoyment we get from eating is decreased, which can affect appetite.
- **Depression.** Even though depression is not a normal part of aging, it is very common among older people as a result of the many changes and losses they experience. Depression often causes a disinterest in usual activities, including eating.

FUNCTIONAL PROBLEMS

Some older people experience changes in their physical function as a result of aging or illness. For example, a person with Parkinson's disease may have difficulty feeding himself because the disease causes his hand to shake, making it difficult to keep the food on the fork or spoon until it gets to the mouth. Someone who has had a stroke may need to learn how to eat using her non-dominant hand. Some people of advanced age may just become too tired or weak from the effort that it takes to eat. As a result, they may stop eating before the meal is finished. A person with functional problems may need to be fed by a member of the nursing staff. For some people, having to be fed by another person is emotionally upsetting, which can also lead to decreased intake.

CHEWING PROBLEMS

Dentition refers to the type of teeth a person has, how many teeth, and the arrangement of those teeth in the mouth. Problems with dentition affect the person's ability to chew and can make eating difficult or painful. Most people do not want to eat much if doing so is painful or uncomfortable. In addition, chewing difficulties increase the energy that it takes to eat, which can cause a person to tire more easily during the meal. Finally, problems with dentition and chewing may make it difficult for the person to enjoy favorite foods (such as a chewy roast beef sandwich), which can take some of the pleasure out of eating.

Many older people have problems chewing food as a result of missing, broken, loose, or decayed teeth. Missing teeth may be replaced with a partial denture or a bridge. (A *bridge*, like a partial denture, replaces missing teeth, but it is permanently fixed in the mouth and is not removable like a denture.) A denture that does not fit properly can affect the person's ability to chew, and it may create sore spots in the mouth that make eating painful. A bridge that becomes loose or breaks can also make eating difficult or painful.

SWALLOWING PROBLEMS

As a result of a stroke or other neurological disorder, some of your residents will have difficulty controlling the muscles of the mouth and throat that are used to swallow. When the person tries to eat or drink, she may cough, choke, or make a "gurgling" sound. Feeling like you are going to choke can be very scary. Like chewing problems, swallowing problems increase the energy it takes to eat and can cause a person to tire before the meal is over.

DEMENTIA

Over the course of this illness, there are different problems that can affect the person's ability to eat. During the middle stage of dementia, the

Caring For Those With Dementia

You might find that it is difficult to get a person with dementia to focus on eating at meal times. The person may forget why she is at the table, or become distracted by others at the table or by discomfort (such as that caused by the need to use the toilet). The person may not be able to recognize the plate of food, and she may forget how to use eating utensils. She may become overwhelmed by the choice of foods. Some people with dementia will tell you they cannot eat because they do not have money to pay for the food.

To help meal time go more smoothly for your residents with dementia:

- Help the person prepare for the meal. Before going to the dining room, assist the person with toileting and dressing for the meal. Make sure the person is seated comfortably at her place at the table.

- If the person is easily distracted by others at the table or the general activity in the dining room, consider serving the meal in a more quiet setting, such as the resident's room.

- In some facilities, areas used for dining may be used for other activities as well, such as crafts or games. When it is time for the meal, make sure the area where the meal will be served looks like it is set for dining. This helps the person with dementia recognize what activity is supposed to be taking place at that time.

- Learn about the person's familiar meal time routine (for example, wash hands, set a place at the table, say grace), and help the person to follow it.

- Limit food choices by providing only one or two items at a time.

- Use hand-over-hand cueing to help the person use eating utensils. Provide "finger foods" (such as small sandwiches or cut-up vegetables or fruit) if necessary.

- Use a tablecloth or a placemat that contrasts with the color of the plate to help the person identify the plate on the table.

- If the person has concerns about paying for the meal, give the person a "meal ticket" or voucher to use in the dining room.

person may not recognize the sensation of hunger or thirst and will not seek food or beverages. The person may not recognize food as food, and as a result, may not eat. Other people have difficulty because they cannot remember how to use a knife and fork, or how to get food from the plate to the mouth. During the late stage of dementia, the person will not remember how to swallow. Often, the person will hold the food in the mouth without swallowing. The food is "pocketed" in the person's cheeks as the person accepts more bites of food without swallowing previous bites.

SPECIAL DIETS

Meals prepared for residents of long-term care facilities are specific to each person's individual needs. Personal preferences are taken into account when planning meals. During the admissions process, the nurse gathers basic information about the resident's eating habits, food likes and dislikes, and foods that should be avoided. The nurse may get this information from the resident, or from the resident's family if the resident is unable to provide the information himself. The dietitian also interviews the resident (or the family) to obtain additional details about the resident's usual eating habits and nutritional intake (Fig. 25-3). The dietician then completes a dietary assessment, which is used to plan a diet for the person that he will enjoy eating and that will keep him healthy.

The type of diet that is ordered for a person in a health care setting is determined by many factors. People with illnesses such as diabetes, heart disease, or kidney disease require special diets. Just the normal changes in the digestive system that accompany aging may require foods that are

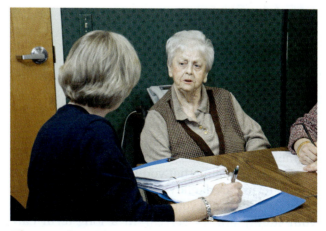

Figure 25-3

The dietitian interviews the resident (and possibly the resident's family members as well) to obtain information that will help her to plan the resident's diet.

easier to chew, easier to digest, and have added fiber to help prevent constipation. Specific diets are ordered by a doctor and an appropriate menu is prepared by a dietitian.

Brief descriptions of some of the special diets that you may see ordered in a long-term care facility are provided in Box 25-1. It is important for you to familiarize yourself with your facility's specific diets and the foods that they include. That way, if a mistake is made in the kitchen and the wrong meal is delivered for one of your residents, you will be able to recognize that an error has been made. Be aware that a resident can have an order for a combination of different diets. For example, a resident might have an order for a regular diet with mechanical chopped meats. Another resident might have an order for a carbohydrate-controlled diet with a sodium restriction.

Some of your residents will have **nutritional supplements** that are either offered with the meal or as an in-between meal snack. These nutritional supplements, which can be used to supply extra calories or protein, often take the form of a flavored shake or drink. These drinks are convenient and easy to serve. People with diabetes may require snacks in between meals to keep their blood glucose levels stable. The dietitian will plan for the nutritional supplements. It is usually the nursing assistant's responsibility to serve these nutritional supplements at specific times throughout the day and record that the supplements have been consumed. If your resident refuses an ordered supplement, please report this to the nurse right away.

MEAL TIME

A tasty meal, good company, and a relaxed dining atmosphere satisfy physical needs (hunger), as well as emotional ones (the need for love and belonging). In most cultures, eating is a social event. We eat at parties and celebrations, we eat on dates, we eat certain foods on certain holidays, and we look forward to catching up with family members and friends over the dinner table (Fig. 25-4). Now imagine that you have just moved into a long-term care facility. Who will you share your meals with? Would you miss one special dish that your family always serves? In a long-term care facility, you may have others to eat with, and the food can be quite good. However, the facility is still not the home you are used to. You might find yourself feeling a little lonely and homesick.

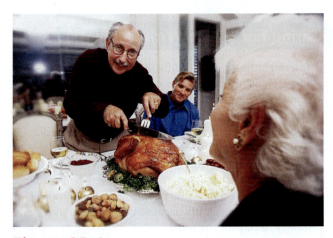

Figure 25-4
In most cultures, food plays a central role in many celebrations, and eating is a social experience.

Meal time for residents in a long-term care facility can be difficult for many reasons:

- The person may miss family members or familiar foods.
- Food choices may be limited due to a special diet, or the food may not be prepared the way the person likes it. For example, think about how many different ways there are to season and prepare a chicken! If chicken is on the menu at your facility, some residents may really like they way it has been prepared, but others may think that it isn't very good.
- Meals are usually served at specific times, not just when the person feels like eating. Most of us develop set routines for eating. For example, a resident might prefer a late breakfast and no lunch, but at the long-term care facility, breakfast is served at 8:00 AM and lunch is at 12 noon, and lunch is the big meal of the day. Imagine how hard it might be for the resident to adjust to this new schedule, after a lifetime of following a different schedule. Also, imagine what it would be like not to have the freedom to go to the kitchen and prepare yourself a snack when you are hungry. If a resident is hungry between meals, he must ask someone to bring a snack, and his choices will be limited to what is available at that time.
- Meal time can be lonely, especially if the person cannot take meals in the dining room. Some residents may eat in their rooms because they are simply too weak or too ill to take meals in the dining room. Residents

BOX 25-1 Special (Therapeutic) Diets

Regular ("house") diet. This is simply a well-balanced diet. There are no restrictions on foods or condiments (for example, salt, pepper, ketchup, salad dressing). There are many variations to the regular diet. For example, a high-calorie or low-calorie version may be ordered to promote weight gain or weight loss. A low-residue or high-fiber version may be ordered to either decrease or increase dietary fiber for people with certain digestive problems. A bland diet contains foods that are easy to digest and will not irritate the digestive tract.

Mechanical diet. A mechanical diet is a diet that has been changed slightly to remove foods that are hard to chew or digest. The texture of the foods is altered to make them easier to eat, and fried or high-fiber foods may be eliminated or very limited. A *mechanical chopped* diet provides foods cut in small pieces to make them easier to chew. Some people only need chopped meats. Others may also need vegetables chopped, depending on the vegetable. A *mechanical soft* diet includes foods that are ground up. For example, a sirloin steak would be put through a meat grinder and served as ground meat. Vegetables and other foods may also need to be altered to make them easier to chew.

Pureed diet. For a pureed diet, the food is blended to a smooth consistency, similar to that of pudding or very moist mashed potatoes. Some people may require a *drinkable puree.* To create a drinkable puree, the food is blended to a liquid, milkshake-like consistency. Pureed and drinkable puree diets are often prepared for those who have very poor dentition, are very frail, or who have end-stage disease. Pureed food may not be very appealing to you, but it is important not to voice or show that opinion while serving or feeding this diet to others!

Carbohydrate (CHO)–controlled diet. This diet, which contains limited amounts of carbohydrates, is ordered for people who have diabetes. The person's specific energy and nutritional requirements determine the amounts of fat, protein, and carbohydrates that are permitted. Because these amounts vary among individuals, this diet is different for each person. The amount of carbohydrates that should be eaten daily is calculated by the dietitian. This amount is then spaced out throughout the day between the three main meals and snacks. This helps to maintain steady blood glucose levels throughout the day. Carbohydrate intake needs to be balanced with any medications that the person may be taking to lower blood glucose levels. When caring for a person with diabetes, you must make special note of the amount of food the person eats at each meal.

Low-cholesterol, low-fat diet. Foods on this diet are low in saturated fat and cholesterol, and prepared in ways that do not add additional fats. The addition of butter, shortening, and margarine to foods is avoided, and foods such as fruits and vegetables, whole grains, and skim milk are encouraged. Those with heart disease usually have orders for a low-cholesterol, low-fat diet, but this diet is considered "heart healthy" for everyone!

Sodium-restricted diet. Sodium restriction is helpful for the treatment of certain types of heart disease, hypertension (high blood pressure), and kidney disease. A person on a sodium-restricted diet may be allowed to have a small amount of salt, or none at all. For example, some people may be able to eat foods that have some salt in them, but they will not be allowed to add extra salt at the table or eat very salty foods, such as pickles. Some people on sodium-restricted diets may use salt substitutes. If you have a resident who has been placed on a sodium-restricted diet, make sure you know whether he is allowed to use a little bit of salt or a salt substitute, or none at all. Other people may have severe restrictions placed on their salt intake. For these people, food will be prepared without any salt at all, and of course, the person will not be able to add salt to the food at the table. Because food can be very bland and unappetizing without salt, a packet of seasoning spices that can be sprinkled on the food to add flavor in the absence of salt may be provided. If these spices are provided, add them to the food as the person desires.

Clear liquid diet. Clear liquids are substances that can be poured at room or body temperature and that you can see through. Foods that are considered clear liquids include water, gelatin, fat-free broth or bouillon, popsicles, clear juices (for example, apple, cranberry, grape), clear carbonated sodas, and coffee and tea (without cream). Some medical tests require a person to be placed on a clear liquid diet for a short period of time before the test. A person who is nauseous, vomiting, or having diarrhea may be given a clear liquid diet until the symptoms have improved. Clear liquids do not contain enough nutrients to maintain health for very long, so the person will be progressed into a more nutritious diet as soon as the body can tolerate it.

BOX 25-2	Aspects of the Resident's Dining Experience Regulated by the Omnibus Budget Reconciliation Act

- Meals must meet the individual nutritional needs of each resident.
- Food must be served at the proper temperature.
- Food must be appealing to look at and seasoned to the individual resident's preference.
- Special diets, such as those followed for religious reasons, must be provided.

- Dining in the company of other residents is recommended.
- Residents in rehabilitation who are learning how to eat independently again must have a private area in which to eat.

with functional difficulties may choose to eat in their rooms because they are embarrassed to eat in front of others, either because of their "sloppiness" during meals or because of their need for staff assistance.

- Physical problems (such as pain or nausea) and emotional problems (such as anxiety or depression) can affect a person's appetite.

Long-term care facilities that receive government funding must follow Omnibus Budget Reconciliation Act (OBRA) regulations pertaining to meals (Box 25-2). These regulations ensure that each resident's rights are respected. They help to ensure that meal time is as enjoyable as possible for the resident. However, even if you work in a facility that is not required to follow OBRA regulations, you must make an effort to make meal time as pleasant as possible for your residents.

By providing companionship and assistance as needed, you can help to make sure that meal time remains a pleasant part of your resident's daily routine. Food should be presented in a way that will stimulate the appetite. Offering small portions of favorite foods frequently throughout the day can help increase a person's desire to eat. A clean, fresh mouth makes food taste better. A comfortable position, whether the person is seated at a regular table in the dining room or is using an over-bed table in bed, keeps the person focused on the food. If the person uses glasses or a hearing aid, make sure that these aids are in place. Provide pleasant conversation. All of these measures help to set a relaxed atmosphere and stimulate the appetite.

PREPARING FOR MEAL TIME

You will need to help your residents get ready for each meal. Be sure to give your residents enough time to prepare for meals. Allowing time to prepare

is especially important before breakfast, because early morning care must be completed before the meal. In a long-term care facility, residents are encouraged to eat in the dining room. Necessary care must be provided to help residents with grooming and dressing so that they are properly attired for the dining room. Residents may also need physical assistance to the dining room.

The assistance you provide will vary, depending on the person you are helping. Some people only need to be reminded that it is "almost time for lunch" and they will prepare themselves to eat. Others will need your help to get ready for the meal. The following actions are taken to help prepare a person for meal time:

- Assist the person with toileting. Help him to the bathroom, or offer the bedpan or urinal.
- Assist the person with basic hygiene and grooming. Help him to wash his hands and face and brush his teeth. If the person wears dentures, glasses, or a hearing aid, make sure these items are clean and in place.
- Position the person for eating. Residents in long-term care facilities are walked to the dining room, or taken in a wheelchair. In many facilities, the resident is helped from the wheelchair into a standard dining chair for the meal. If the person will be eating his meal in bed, smooth the bed linens and position the bed in a high Fowler's position, if permitted. Clear the over-bed table of clutter and wipe down the surface if necessary.
- Provide a pleasant environment. Remove any offensive or odorous items, such as bedpans or emesis basins, from the room. Adjust the lighting for comfort and turn on the radio or television if the person asks you to. Many people like to listen to music or watch a favorite program while they eat.

Helping Hands and a Caring Heart

FOCUS ON HUMANISTIC HEALTH CARE

Meal times can be difficult for residents of a long-term care facility. The person may miss his family members. Favorite foods that the person once enjoyed may not be prepared the same way at the facility, they may not be available at all, or they may no longer be allowed on the diet ordered by the doctor. Pain, anxiety, depression, illness, and medication side effects can cause the person to have little or no appetite. Part of providing humanistic care is assisting and encouraging your residents to eat adequate amounts of food, despite eating difficulties or loss of appetite. Actions such as making sure the food is served at the appropriate temperature, providing pleasant conversation, and assisting the person to be physically comfortable help the person to relax and enjoy the meal.

ASSISTING THE PERSON TO EAT

Once these preparations are completed, it is time to eat! Meals should be served as soon as they are delivered from the kitchen. This helps to ensure that hot foods are hot and cold foods are cold. Check that the name on the meal tray matches the name of the resident who will be receiving it (Fig. 25-5). Also, make sure that the diet noted on the tray matches the diet noted on the person's care plan or medical chart. If the meal is not as ordered, ask a nurse to confirm that a mistake has been made, and then call the kitchen for a replacement meal with the correct diet.

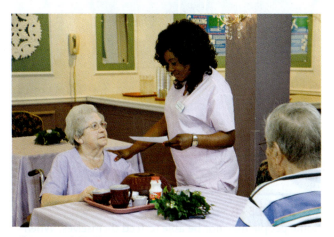

Figure 25-5
Always make sure that the right meal tray is being delivered to the right person.

In many long-term care facilities, a cloth or plastic clothing protector is used. This protector is placed over the person's chest to prevent the clothing from being soiled with food during the meal. Wearing a clothing protector is a matter of personal choice, so always ask the resident if it is all right for you to put the clothing protector on her before the meal. Please do not refer to the clothing protector as a "bib." An adult, especially one who is already feeling self-conscious because she needs help eating, will not appreciate being likened to a baby!

Help the person to eat as necessary. Encourage your residents to do as much for themselves as possible to help promote their independence. Assistive devices for eating (see Chapter 10) allow many residents with physical impairments to manage eating quite well on their own. The care plan will have basic information about the type of assistance the person needs, or you can ask the nurse.

Helping Hands and a Caring Heart

FOCUS ON HUMANISTIC HEALTH CARE

Think for a moment—when you are hungry, you sit down and eat. You cut your juicy steak, butter your hot rolls, and never give the act of eating a second thought. How would it feel to have to rely on another person to feed you, or cut up your food? Would you feel like a small child again, or like a burden? Be sensitive to your residents' feelings as you assist them with meals. Realize how very much they would like to be able to perform routine activities like eating without a second thought, just like you do.

To assist a person with eating, first remove the cover from the tray and tell the person what foods are on the tray. No one likes "mystery meat" for dinner! Depending on the person's abilities, you may also need to help the person with opening milk cartons or removing silverware from its wrapper, buttering bread, or cutting up meat (Fig. 25-6). If the person needs help seasoning the food, make sure that you add salt, pepper, and condiments according to the person's tastes, not your own. If the person has poor eyesight, you will need to tell her where items are on the tray. Describe the food and help the person to find it on the plate by referencing a clock face (Fig. 25-7).

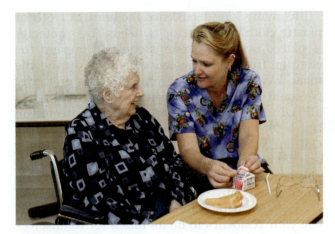

Figure 25-6
Some people will be able to eat on their own if you give them a little bit of assistance.

For example, you might say, "Okay, Mrs. Diaz—your pork chop is at 12 o'clock. The potatoes are at 3 o'clock, the green beans are at 6 o'clock, and the corn is at 9 o'clock. Your milk is on the upper right corner of the tray and your roll is on a bread plate to the left of your dinner plate."

When assisting a person to eat, be observant for signs that the person is having difficulty chewing or swallowing. Be descriptive about any problems that you observe. The information you provide will ensure that the person is appropriately assessed and modifications are made to make it easier for the person to eat. For example, after assessing the person, the dietitian may rec-

ommend a mechanical diet that is easier to chew, or the speech therapist may recommend eating (or feeding) techniques to improve the person's ability to swallow.

TELL THE NURSE

Signs that a person is having difficulty chewing or swallowing include the following and should be reported to the nurse right away:

- The person complains of tooth or mouth pain, or seems to favor one side of the mouth when chewing.
- The person complains of poorly fitting dentures.
- The person complains of sores in the mouth or on the tongue, or you notice sores when providing oral care.
- The person refuses to eat.
- The person coughs or gags frequently when eating or drinking.
- The person makes gurgling sounds.

FEEDING DEPENDENT RESIDENTS

Some residents may not be able to feed themselves at all (Fig. 25-8). Even though these residents will depend on you to do most of the work, it is very important that you involve them as

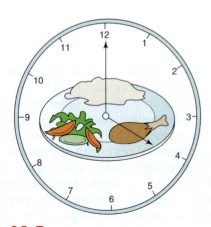

Figure 25-7
You can help a person with poor eyesight locate food on the plate by describing its location in terms of a clock face.

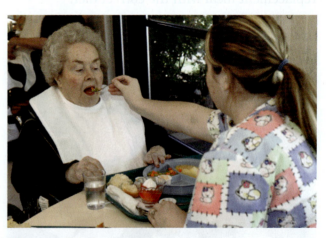

Figure 25-8
Some people may not be able to feed themselves. When you are feeding a resident, be sure to carry on a pleasant conversation, and engage the person in the process as much as possible.

much as possible in the process of eating. For example, you might ask the resident to help you by holding her own napkin. Remember that meal time is a very social time in a person's day. *Keep the person engaged with pleasant talk throughout the meal,* even if the person does not answer you. Hearing your voice and knowing that you care will increase the person's appetite and aid digestion. Remember, the resident being fed is a *person.* Do not approach feeding the person as just another task that you need to do.

When feeding another person, always use a spoon, not a fork, because the blunt edge of the spoon is safer than the sharp tines of the fork. Fill the spoon only about one-third full for each bite, and offer the bites slowly to prevent choking. Never rush the person through eating. Be sure to tell the person what foods you are offering her. If the person is alert and able to respond, ask her in what order she would like to try the food on the plate. Make sure you have seasoned the food according to the person's preference. If she is unable to tell you her preference, season the food mildly. Give the person enough time to chew and swallow each bite. You may need to gently remind the person to chew and swallow, especially if the person has dementia.

Offer liquids frequently between bites. People who have difficulty swallowing can choke easily on liquids, so always offer liquids slowly. Some people find drinking through a straw to be easiest. However, sometimes a resident is not allowed to use a straw because the amount of liquid taken up through a straw may be more than the resident can safely swallow at one time, leading to choking. Be sure to ask the nurse or follow the care plan.

For residents who have difficulty swallowing, the doctor may order the use of a thickener, an additive that thickens liquids and makes them easier to swallow. The doctor orders a specific consistency for thickened liquids. These consistencies are:

- **Nectar.** A nectar consistency can be poured very easily. When poured, the stream has a ribbon-like appearance. The consistency can be compared to fruit nectar, such as apricot or pear.
- **Honey.** A honey consistency is thicker than a nectar consistency and is not as easily poured. When poured, the stream looks like a solid column, or it drizzles.
- **Pudding.** A pudding consistency "plops" rather than pours from a cup. Although it is a thickened liquid, this consistency is eaten with a spoon.

The nurse or therapist will show you how to use a thickener to thicken liquids if this is necessary for one of your residents. Guidelines for providing thickened liquids are given in Guidelines Box 25-1. Procedure 25-1 gives the steps for feeding a resident who needs complete assistance with eating.

MEASURING AND RECORDING FOOD INTAKE

Most long-term care facilities will require you to record the amount of food that the person eats. In some facilities, you will just have to note the portion of the total meal that was consumed (for example, Mrs. Wells ate 60% of her breakfast, 80% of her lunch, and 30% of her dinner). Many facilities will want you to tell the nurse if one of your residents eats less than 70% of the meal.

As a nursing assistant, you will play a key role in the ongoing evaluation of your residents' nutritional status. Of all the nursing team members, you will have the most contact with your residents during meal times. You will see which foods are eaten readily and which are left on the tray. When you notice that a food has not been eaten, you might talk to the person about it. For example:

Nursing assistant: Hi, Mr. Wheeling! How was your lunch? (*Noticing that the dessert has not been eaten.*) Oh! I see you didn't eat your dessert. Are you full, or do you just not like vanilla tapioca?

Mr. Wheeling: Well, actually, I am pretty full, so I decided to skip the tapioca today. It's not my favorite anyway. (*Wrinkling nose*) I don't like the lumps.

Nursing assistant: Well, I'm glad you told me! We ought to be able to avoid "lumpy" desserts in the future . . . maybe vanilla pudding or ice cream would be better instead?

Mr. Wheeling (*smiling*): Thanks, Nancy. That would be great. I do look forward to dessert!

Talking with the person about why a food was not eaten serves two purposes. First, it allows you to give the nurse information that she and the dietitian can use to plan future meals for the person. Second, when you notice that a food has gone untouched and take the time to ask the person about it, you let the person know that you care about him as an individual (Fig. 25-9).

WHAT YOU DO	WHY YOU DO IT
If thickened liquids have been ordered for a resident, thicken all of the liquids on the resident's tray, including soup.	Thickened liquids have been ordered for the resident because the resident has difficulty swallowing. Providing any liquid without the thickener puts the resident at risk for choking.
Carefully read and follow the instructions on the thickener to prepare the desired consistency.	There are several thickeners available, and the product used in the facility can change based on pricing. There may be some variation in the amount of product needed to produce a particular consistency.
When adding a thickener to a liquid, use a "sprinkle and stir" technique, rather than a "plop and stir" technique.	It is better to add the thickener gradually. "Plopping" a spoonful of the thickener into the liquid makes it more difficult to dissolve the thickener in the liquid. You do not want the resident to taste gritty particles of thickener when drinking. Also, plopping the thickener into the liquid often results in the liquid becoming too thick. If the liquid becomes too thick, then the consistency will need to be adjusted by adding more liquid.
Allow the liquid to sit for a minute or two before serving to make sure it is the right consistency.	It takes a few minutes for the full effect of the thickener to take place. If you think the liquid is the right consistency and serve it right away, the liquid will continue to thicken and in a few minutes it will no longer be the consistency ordered for the resident. If the liquid becomes too thick, then the consistency will need to be adjusted by adding more liquid.
Add all condiments (for example, creamer, lemon juice) to the liquid before adding the thickening product.	Adding anything to a prepared thickened liquid can change the consistency.
Do not add ice to thickened liquids.	As the ice melts, it thins down the liquid.
Check the resident's hot beverages periodically for changes in consistency.	Hot beverages thicken as they cool. Some additional hot liquid may need to be added to return the beverage to the correct consistency.
Do not give the resident any food item that melts at room temperature (such as gelatin or ice cream).	These kinds of foods melt in the mouth and may become too thin for the resident to swallow without choking.
Do not provide the resident with a bedside water pitcher.	Water must be thickened before drinking. Leaving unthickened liquid at the bedside puts the resident at risk for choking. You cannot thicken the water ahead of time to leave at the bedside because the water continues to thicken as it sits.
Offer thickened beverages throughout the day.	Like all residents, residents on thickened liquids need to drink throughout the day to maintain adequate hydration. Because the resident must depend on the staff to prepare all liquids, she cannot drink whenever she wants to, so it is important to offer beverages frequently throughout the day.

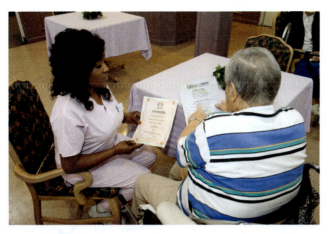

Figure 25-9
Respecting a person's preferences when it comes to food lets the person know that you care about him or her as an individual.

When there is concern about a resident's nutritional status, the dietitian may perform a **calorie count.** To perform a calorie count, the dietician reviews exactly what the resident has eaten over a certain number of days, and then calculates the average number of calories consumed each day. The dietitian also compares the resident's daily intake of specific nutrients to the recommended daily amounts of those nutrients. Although the exact procedure for doing a calorie count may vary, you will usually be responsible for assisting the dietician by keeping a record of the resident's intake for the required amount of time, usually 3 days. You will have to note what percentage of *each* food was eaten (for example, at dinner, Mr. Sommers ate 100% of his mashed potatoes, 50% of his salad, and 75% of his chicken breast). The dietitian then converts the percentages that

Be Smart About Surveys!

Good nutrition is essential for health. In addition, meal time is a very social time in the resident's day. Surveyors will monitor meal service in the facility to make sure that meal time is as pleasant as possible for the residents, and to ensure that every effort is being made to meet each resident's nutritional requirements. To help your facility remain without survey problems in this area:

- Ensure that the resident's toileting, hygiene, and grooming needs have been attended to in sufficient time so that he is ready to eat when the meal comes.
- Be attentive to the eating environment. Make sure it is clean, orderly, without unpleasant odors, and attractive and inviting for dining.
- Make sure the meal is attractive when served. For example, if a liquid has spilled on the tray, wipe up the spill and obtain a replacement if necessary. Do not serve the tray to the resident if it is delivered in unsatisfactory condition.
- Make sure that each resident gets the right tray, with the right diet.
- Ensure that foods are the appropriate temperature when served. Serve meals promptly, and avoid serving a resident his meal tray until you are available to sit down and assist him with the meal.
- Make sure that all of the residents seated at a table together are served their meals at the same time. Avoid having one resident at a table waiting on her meal while the others begin eating.

- Encourage socialization at meals.
- Help residents to be as self-sufficient as possible during meals. Prepare food items so that the resident can eat independently, if possible. However, if a resident appears to be struggling, step in to assist as needed.
- Follow any special feeding instructions as provided on the care plan.
- Follow any special orders for thickening fluids. Be sure that you know how to prepare thickened liquids to the ordered consistency.
- Continuously monitor how your residents are eating. If you see a resident who is not eating well, investigate why. Offer alternative food items as needed.
- Keep the nurse informed of any changes in a resident's appetite or insufficient intake.
- Accurately document the resident's intake after each meal, following facility policies and procedures.
- Provide for nutritious snacks throughout the day as the resident desires and is allowed to have. Be alert to any special orders or restrictions. Snacks should be offered to each resident at bedtime.
- If a resident is receiving enteral nutrition ("tube feedings"), be sure the head of the bed is raised during the feeding and for a period of time afterwards. Be alert to any problems with the enteral feeding and notify the nurse.

you provide into "total calories consumed." This number is used to help determine the resident's nutritional status.

OTHER WAYS OF PROVIDING FLUIDS AND NUTRITION

Drinking water and chewing, swallowing, and digesting food are the best ways to obtain fluids and nutrients. However, sometimes drinking and eating "the regular way" are simply not possible. For people who have problems chewing, swallowing, or digesting their food, fluids and nutrients must be provided another way. Three alternate methods of providing fluids and nutrition include intravenous (IV) therapy, enteral nutrition, and total parenteral nutrition (TPN, hyperalimentation).

INTRAVENOUS (IV) THERAPY

In **intravenous (IV) therapy,** fluids are given through a small catheter (tube) that is inserted into a vein (*intra* = in; *venous* = vein). The IV tubing (sometimes called an "IV line") is connected to a bag that contains the IV fluid (Fig. 25-10). The fluid slowly drips through the tubing and into the vein. Usually the IV line, which is thin, is inserted into one of the small veins in the arm or the back of the hand.

IV therapy is not a source of complete nutrition, but it is useful when a person needs fluids. In addition to water, the IV fluid usually contains glucose, vitamins, and minerals. Medications, such as pain medications or antibiotics, may also be added to the IV fluid. Sometimes, blood is given through an IV line.

You will not be responsible for managing IV therapy, but you may care for residents who have an IV line in place.

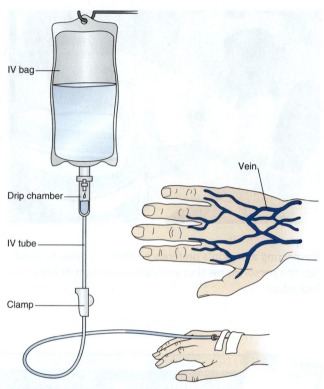

Figure 25-10

Intravenous (IV) therapy is used to give fluids. The IV fluid drips from the bag, into the tubing, and into the person's vein. The nurse uses the clamp to control the rate of flow.

ENTERAL NUTRITION

The word "enteral" comes from the Greek word for "intestines," *enteron*. **Enteral nutrition** involves placing food directly into the stomach or intestines, which eliminates the need for the person to chew or swallow. For example, a person who is unconscious is not able to chew and swallow, and will require enteral nutrition. Certain cancers, such as those that affect the mouth or throat, may also make enteral nutrition necessary. You may also see enteral nutrition used for a resident in end-stage disease (such as end-stage dementia) if the resident has specified in his advance directives that life-sustaining treatments, such as enteral nutrition, should be provided.

Enteral nutrition is sometimes called "tube feeding" because food, in the form of a formula-like fluid, is delivered through a tube that has been passed into the digestive tract. There are many ways to access the digestive tract with the feeding tube (Fig. 25-11):

- A **nasogastric tube** is inserted through the nose (*naso-*), down the throat, and into the stomach (*gastric*).

TELL THE NURSE !

When caring for a resident with an IV line, report any of the following observations to the nurse immediately:

- The tubing has become disconnected.
- The fluid bag is empty.
- The IV fluid is not dripping into the drip chamber.
- Blood has backed up into the IV tubing.
- The person complains of pain at the IV site.
- There is swelling or redness at the IV site.

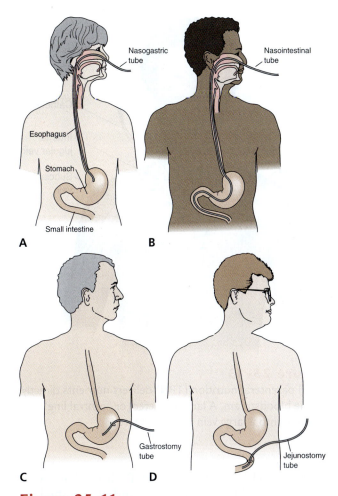

Figure 25-11

Enteral feeding tubes are inserted directly into the stomach or intestines. **(A)** A nasogastric tube is passed through the nose, down the throat, and into the stomach. **(B)** A nasointestinal tube is passed through the nose, down the throat, and into the small intestine. **(C)** A gastrostomy tube is inserted into the stomach through a surgical incision. **(D)** A jejunostomy tube is inserted into the small intestine through a surgical incision.

- A **nasointestinal tube** is inserted through the nose (*naso-*), down the throat, and into the small intestine (*intestinal*).
- A **gastrostomy tube** is inserted into the stomach (*gastro-*) through a surgical incision (*stoma*). The incision is made in the abdomen. A **percutaneous endoscopic gastrostomy (PEG) tube** is a special type of gastrostomy tube that is inserted into the stomach with the aid of an *endoscope*, a lighted, flexible tool that allows the doctor to see inside the body. Placement of a PEG tube is faster, cheaper, and less risky for the person than placement of a regular gastrostomy tube because open abdominal surgery is not needed.

- A **jejunostomy tube** is inserted into the jejunum (part of the small intestine) through a surgical incision (*stoma*). The incision is made in the abdomen.

When a person needs enteral nutrition for only a short time, a nasogastric or nasointestinal tube is usually used. These tubes do not require a surgical incision for placement. However, they can cause irritation of the nose and the back of the throat and may be difficult for the person to tolerate. The tube can be easily displaced, especially if the person vomits, coughs, or pulls on the tube. Because it is possible for the tube to become displaced during feeding, nurses are responsible for feeding people with nasogastric or nasointestinal tubes.

When a person needs enteral nutrition for more than a few days, a gastrostomy, jejunostomy, or PEG tube is used. These tubes are inserted through an incision in the abdomen, so irritation of the nose and throat is not a problem. Gastrostomy, jejunostomy, and PEG tubes are not as easily dislodged from their position as nasogastric or nasointestinal tubes are. However, they can come loose when a person moves, or during repositioning. People who are disoriented or confused may also pull them out.

Enteral feedings may be given at scheduled times, or continuously by an infusion pump. A person who is receiving nourishment through an enteral tube is at high risk for aspiration (inhalation of foreign material into the lungs). Aspiration can occur if the person regurgitates (vomits) the feeding formula and it goes down the windpipe and into the lungs. To help avoid regurgitation and aspiration, the head of the bed is raised during the feeding and for a period of time afterward (Fig. 25-12).

TELL THE NURSE

Notify the nurse if you suspect that a person who is receiving enteral nutrition has regurgitated or aspirated the formula or if you think that the feeding tube has become displaced. (Remember that only nurses can reconnect tubing that has been displaced.) Signs and symptoms of problems with enteral feeding devices include:

- Nausea, bloating, or pain during the feeding
- Coughing, gagging, or vomiting during the feeding
- Abdominal distention (a swollen abdomen)
- Diarrhea
- Drainage from around the tube insertion site
- Disconnected tubing

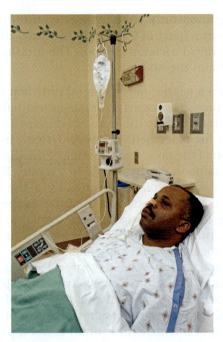

Figure 25-12
When a person is receiving enteral nutrition, the head of the bed must be raised during the feeding and for a period of time afterwards to help prevent regurgitation and aspiration.

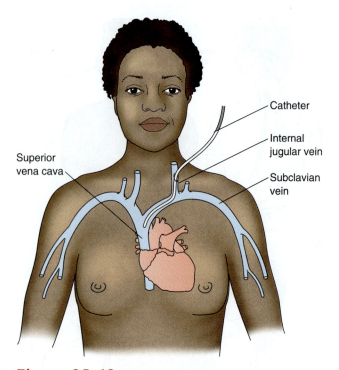

Figure 25-13
Total parenteral nutrition (TPN) delivers nutrients directly to the bloodstream. A large catheter (or "central line") is inserted into a large vein near the heart.

TOTAL PARENTERAL NUTRITION (TPN, HYPERALIMENTATION)

People who are very ill, injured, or recovering from surgery, especially gastrointestinal surgery, may not be able to tolerate food in the digestive tract. For these people, nourishment is delivered directly into the bloodstream through a large catheter (tube) inserted into a large vein near the heart (Fig. 25-13). This method of nutrient delivery is called **total parenteral nutrition (TPN)** or **hyperalimentation.** *Parenteral* means "by some way other than through the digestive tract." And *hyperalimentation* means "above (*hyper*) the alimentary (or digestive) tract." So you can see that both terms refer to a method of feeding that does not involve the digestive tract.

As you will recall from the beginning of the chapter, the digestive tract breaks food down into nutrients, and then these nutrients are absorbed into the bloodstream. If a person is receiving TPN, then the nutrients must be delivered to the bloodstream in their smallest form, because digestion does not occur. Water, glucose, vitamins, and minerals are small molecules, but proteins and fats are bigger. This is why a large catheter is

used for TPN, instead of an IV line. The large catheter used for TPN is wider and allows the bigger fat and protein molecules to pass through. An IV line is smaller and only allows smaller molecules, such as water, glucose, vitamins, minerals, and medications, to pass. The ability to administer fats and proteins, as well as the other four classes of nutrients, is where the "total" comes from in the term *total parenteral nutrition.*

As a nursing assistant, you will not be responsible for giving TPN feedings, but you may care for residents receiving them.

FLUIDS AND HYDRATION

FLUID BALANCE

As you learned earlier, water is just as necessary to life as food, if not more so. A healthy adult needs to drink between 1.5 to 3 quarts (48 to 96 ounces) of fluid each day just to keep up with the fluid that normally leaves the body in urine, feces, sweat, and the air we exhale. Most of these fluid needs are met by drinking water, juice, milk, and other beverages. However, certain foods, such as cucumbers, watermelon, grapes, and soup, have high water contents as well and provide for some of the fluid needed by the body. When the amount of fluid taken into the body equals the amount of fluid that leaves the body, a state of **fluid balance** occurs. Fluid balance is important for health.

Dehydration

Dehydration occurs when there is too little fluid in the tissues of the body. Causes of dehydration include diarrhea, vomiting, hemorrhage, severe burns, diaphoresis (excessive sweating), and simply not drinking enough fluids. In all of these situations, the amount of fluid that leaves the body is greater than the amount of fluid taken in.

Older people are at risk for dehydration because they do not feel thirsty as often as younger people do. In addition, some older people deliberately cut back on their fluid intake because problems with mobility make it difficult for them to get to the bathroom, or because they are afraid of having an incontinence accident. People with dementia are also at risk for dehydration because they may not recognize the sensation of thirst, or they may not be able to express the need for a drink. As a nursing assistant, you will play a very important role in ensuring that your residents' fluid intake is sufficient to meet their needs, and in preventing dehydration. Remember from Chapter 6 that dehydration is considered a "sentinel event," which means that the government considers dehydration to be a condition that should rarely, if ever, be seen in a resident of a nursing home.

Edema

The opposite of dehydration, **edema,** occurs when there is too much fluid in the tissues of the body. Kidney disease and certain types of heart disease can make it hard for the body to get rid of extra water, resulting in edema. In these situations, the amount of fluid that leaves the body is less than the amount of fluid taken in. For a person with edema, the doctor may restrict the person's fluid intake or order medications to help the body rid itself of the excess fluid.

OFFERING FLUIDS

Nursing assistants are responsible for providing fresh drinking water and other fluids to residents. Many of your residents will be allowed to have as much water as they like, and should be encouraged to drink (Fig. 25-14). If a person is allowed to have water, make sure that the water pitcher is

Be Smart About Surveys!

Many factors can place a resident of a nursing home at risk for dehydration. Dehydration can have many serious consequences, and may even lead to death or the need for hospitalization. Because dehydration is preventable with proper care, the government considers dehydration a "sentinel event." Surveyors will pay particular attention to the efforts made by the staff to ensure that each resident's fluid intake is adequate. To help your facility remain without survey problems in this area:

- Follow any special orders for increasing fluids or restricting fluids.
- If no fluid restrictions are in place, offer your residents a drink every time you interact with them, and make sure fresh water is always available and at the preferred temperature.
- If no fluid restrictions are in place, but the resident tends not to accept beverages when offered, try offering snacks that count as fluids such as popsicles, ice cream, or gelatin.
- If fluid restrictions are in place, know how much fluid the resident is allowed to have over the course of the day and spread the resident's total intake out over the course of the day.
- Serve beverages and foods that count toward the person's fluid requirements at the appropriate temperature to boost appeal and encourage intake.
- Keep the nurse informed of insufficient fluid intake.
- Accurately document the resident's fluid intake, following facility policies and procedures.

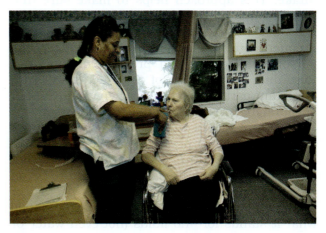

Figure 25-14
Water is essential to life. Residents should be assisted to drink throughout the day, including during evening and night hours.

filled with fresh, cold water. Add ice if the person prefers ice water. Replace the water in the pitcher when the pitcher is almost empty, or, if ice water is preferred, when the ice melts. People are more likely to drink fluids that taste good and are served at the appropriate temperature.

It is often a challenge to get some residents to drink a sufficient amount of fluid. If a resident has no restrictions on fluid intake, you should offer a drink every time you interact with the resident. This is especially important when the resident is confused or taking pain medications, because these residents might not remember to drink fluids often enough. Many residents will accept a drink if one is offered, even if they would not have asked for a drink on their own.

Sometimes, the doctor may either increase or restrict a person's fluid intake. An order to encourage fluids (sometimes called "force fluids") means that the person should increase her fluid intake. The nurse will give you information about the amount and type of fluids that should be offered. Most people do not like having to drink a large amount of liquid all at once. Frequently offering small amounts of a drink that the person likes throughout the day is a better approach. Make sure that the fluids you offer are cold or hot, and fresh. Not many people like room-temperature water, flat soda, or lukewarm tea. Also, remember that fluids do not necessarily have to take the form of a beverage. Foods such as gelatin, popsicles, ice cream, and broth can also count as fluids. Some residents may accept these items more easily than a beverage.

Offering small amounts of fluids at regular times throughout the day is also a good approach when the doctor has restricted a person's fluid intake. This approach helps to make sure that the person is never too thirsty, by spreading out his fluid intake over the course of the day. Frequent oral hygiene also helps to keep the person comfortable and prevent "dry mouth." Recording the amount of fluid taken in is an important part of your duties when you are either encouraging or restricting fluids for a person.

Some residents will not be allowed to have any fluids at all in preparation for a surgical or diagnostic procedure. A person who is not allowed to have any fluids at all is said to be on **"NPO status."** NPO stands for *nils per os*, or "nothing by mouth" in Latin. NPO means exactly what it stands for—no fluids (not even water or ice chips), no food, no hard candy, and no gum. If one of your residents has been placed on NPO status, empty his water pitcher and store it out of sight. You might also want to gently remind visitors that the person is not allowed to have anything to eat or drink, and suggest that they enjoy their own snacks and beverages in another room. Being on NPO status can be extremely uncomfortable. Being thirsty and not being able to drink is difficult. Frequent oral care helps to relieve some of the discomfort until the person is allowed to have fluids again.

MEASURING AND RECORDING INTAKE AND OUTPUT

Some residents may have an order to "maintain intake and output measurements." All of the fluids that enter and leave the body are measured and recorded on an **intake and output (I&O) flow sheet.** In health care facilities, fluids are measured and recorded in milliliters (mL) or cubic centimeters (cc). One mL is the same as one cc. One fluid ounce is equal to 30 mL or 30 cc.

Each time the person takes in fluids, or fluids leave the body, the amount is recorded. The amounts are totaled at the end of the shift and again at the end of the 24-hour reporting period. The amount of intake can then be compared with the amount of output to monitor the person's fluid balance.

Measuring Fluid Intake

Fluid intake includes all of the fluids that a person drinks, including those foods that are liquid at room or body temperature (such as gelatin, ice cream, pudding, and popsicles). Other fluids that are considered as part of a person's total intake include enteral or TPN feedings and IV fluids, but the nurse will be responsible for recording these amounts. Your facility will have a listing of the amount of fluid in common servings, and you will need to become familiar with the amount of fluid contained by the cups, glasses, and bowls used in your facility. Remember that 30 mL (30 cc) is equal to 1 fluid ounce, so an 8-ounce carton of milk would equal 240 mL ($8 \times 30 = 240$). But what if the person did not drink the entire carton of milk? In this case, you can estimate how much fluid was taken in. For example, if the person drank half of the carton of milk, then half of 8 ounces is 4, so 4×30 would be 120 mL. (Another way to arrive at this figure is to calculate what the total carton is worth in milliliters, and then divide by the amount consumed: $240/2 = 120$ mL.)

Sometimes it is necessary to calculate intake exactly. In this situation, you would calculate how

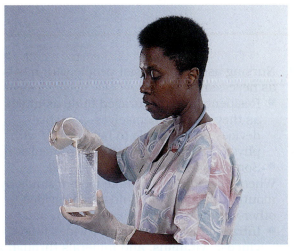

Figure 25-15
A graduate is a measuring device that is used to measure fluids. The graduate is marked with lines that indicate milliliters (mL) on the left and ounces (oz) on the right. (*Copyright B. Proud.*)

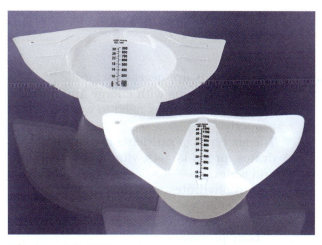

Figure 25-16
A collection device (sometimes called a "commode hat") is placed over the toilet seat before the person urinates, to contain and measure the amount of urine. (*Photograph courtesy of Medline Industries, Inc.*)

many fluids were offered to the person before he started to eat. For example, let's say a person's meal tray contained 150 mL of orange juice, 240 mL of milk, and 90 mL of water at the beginning of the meal. This would mean that 480 mL of fluid were offered (150 + 240 + 90 = 480). After the person has finished with the meal, you would take all of the fluids left in the glasses and pour them into a **graduate** (a measuring device) to measure the amount left (Fig. 25-15). Let's say that 40 mL of fluid are left. You would subtract the amount left (40 mL) from the total amount offered (480 mL) and record the total consumed as 440 mL.

Measuring Fluid Output

Fluids that are considered output are urine, vomit, blood, wound drainage, and diarrhea. Output is measured and recorded the same way that intake is. A person who is on I&O status will need to be reminded to urinate into a collection device, and instructed not to put toilet paper into the collection device. The urine cannot be discarded until you have measured and recorded the amount. Urine collection devices are available that can be used on a regular toilet, or with a bedside commode (Fig. 25-16). Urinals have measurements marked on the side so that you can easily see the amount that they contain. Urine from a bedpan or a urinary catheter drainage bag is poured into a graduate for measurement. (Urinary catheters are discussed in detail in Chapter 26.)

If a person vomits, the amount can be measured using the markings on the emesis basin. If the person vomited somewhere other than in the emesis basin (for example, on the floor or bed linens), then the nurse will estimate the amount of vomit. Blood and wound drainage is either estimated by the nurse or measured in a graduate if it is collected into a drainage device. Diarrhea is estimated for amount also.

Always remember to wear gloves when measuring output.

SUMMARY

- Food and fluids are necessary for life.
  - Food provides us with energy and nutrients that our bodies need to work properly.
  - The six types of nutrients are carbohydrates, proteins, fats, vitamins, minerals, and water.
    - Carbohydrates, proteins, and fat provide energy.
    - Vitamins, minerals, and water regulate body processes.
- To be healthy, we need to eat a variety of nutritious foods every day.
  - Not all foods are equally nutritious.
  - Nutrients work best in combination with other nutrients.
  - MyPyramid and nutrition labels on packaged foods can be used to plan a healthy diet.
  - People in the long-term care setting often have special needs as far as nutrition is concerned.
- Factors that influence a person's food preferences and eating habits include religion, culture, geography, finances, kitchen skills, and individual taste.
- Factors that affect an older person's food intake include loss of appetite (anorexia), functional problems, chewing problems, swallowing problems, and dementia. Factors that contribute to anorexia in older people include chronic health conditions, medications, decreased senses of taste and smell, and emotional difficulties, such as depression.
- Eating helps us to meet both physical and emotional needs.
  - Helping a person to prepare for meal time and serving meals promptly contributes to comfort and a relaxed atmosphere.
  - Respecting the individual's preferences is important when it comes to food.
  - Talking with the person as you assist with the meal is important, even if the person cannot answer you.
  - When our emotional needs are met, it is easier for us to meet our physical needs. Ensuring that meal time is pleasant can help improve a person's appetite.

- Nursing assistants assist people with meals, as necessary.
  - Residents are encouraged to do as much as they can for themselves. Assistive devices are available to help people with physical impairments to eat on their own.
  - Some residents will need to be fed.
- When a person cannot take food or fluids by mouth, nutrition and fluids are provided in other ways.
  - Intravenous (IV) therapy provides fluids, glucose, vitamins, and minerals through a small catheter inserted into one of the small veins of the arm or hand. IV therapy does not provide complete nutrition.
  - Enteral nutrition is provided by a tube that is placed directly into the stomach or intestines.
    - Nasogastric tubes, nasointestinal tubes, gastrostomy tubes, jejunostomy tubes, and percutaneous endoscopic gastrostomy (PEG) tubes are used for enteral feeding.
    - Formula-like food is usually delivered through an infusion device, either continuously or at specified times.
  - Total parenteral nutrition (TPN, hyperalimentation) involves the delivery of all six classes of nutrients through a catheter inserted into a large vein near the heart.
- Maintaining proper fluid balance is important for health.
  - The amount of fluids taken into the body should equal the amount of fluids that leave the body.
    - If the amount of fluid leaving the body is greater than the amount taken in, dehydration can occur.
    - If the amount of fluid leaving the body is less than the amount taken in, edema can occur.
  - The doctor may order a resident's fluid intake to be increased or restricted. Residents who have no fluid restrictions should be encouraged to drink frequently.
  - A person's fluid balance is monitored by measuring and recording fluid intake and output. One fluid ounce = 30 milliliters (mL) = 30 cubic centimeters (cc).

PROCEDURE 25-1

Feeding a Dependent Person

WHY YOU DO IT   A person who cannot feed herself will need to be fed to ensure that she receives proper nutrition. Providing companionship during the meal is just as important as providing assistance with the actual task of eating.

Getting Ready WORKSTEPS

1. Complete the "Getting Ready" steps.

Supplies

- gloves
- paper towels
- clothing protector
- oral hygiene supplies
- wash basin
- bedpan or urinal
- towel
- washcloth

Procedure

2. Help the person prepare for the meal. If the person is able to get out of bed, assist the person to the bathroom for oral hygiene, toileting, and washing of the hands and face. Otherwise:

   a. Cover the over-bed table with paper towels. Place the oral hygiene supplies on the over-bed table. Fill the wash basin with warm water (110°F [37.7°C] to 115°F [46.1°C] on the bath thermometer). Place the basin on the over-bed table.

   b. If the side rails are in use, lower the side rail on the working side of the bed. The side rail on the opposite side of the bed should remain up. Raise the head of the bed. Make sure that the bed is positioned at a comfortable working height (to promote good body mechanics) and that the wheels are locked.

   c. Put on the gloves.

   d. Assist the person with oral hygiene.

   e. Offer the bedpan or urinal. If the person uses the bedpan or urinal, empty and clean it before proceeding with the meal. Remove your gloves and dispose of them in a facility-approved waste container. Wash your hands.

   f. Assist the person with washing her hands and face.

3. If the person will be eating in the dining room, make sure she is properly dressed for the dining room. Assist the person to the dining room and make sure she is comfortably seated. If the person will be eating in her room, clear the over-bed table and position it over the bed at the proper height for the person.

4. Ask the person if she would like to use a clothing protector. Put the clothing protector on the person, if desired.

5. Get the meal tray from the dietary cart. (If the side rails are in use, raise the side rails before leaving the bedside.) Check the meal tray to make sure that it has the person's name on it and that it contains the correct diet for the person. Place the meal tray on the dining table or over-bed table.

6. Uncover the meal tray, and prepare the food for eating (for example, cut the meat, butter the bread, open any containers). Tell the person what is on the tray.

7. Take a seat close to the person.

8. Allow the person to choose what she would like to taste first. Using a spoon, offer a small bite to the person (fill the spoon no more than one-third full). Allow the person enough time to swallow the food.

(continued)

499

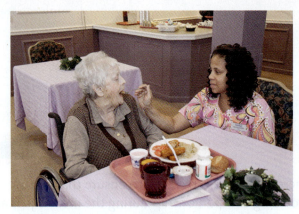

Step 8 Using a spoon, offer a small bite to the person.

9. Offer the person something to drink every few bites. Use the napkin to wipe the person's mouth and chin as often as necessary. Allow the person to assist with the eating process to the best of her ability.

10. Continue in this manner until the person is finished. Encourage the person to finish the food on the tray, but do not force the person to eat.

11. Remove the tray and the clothing protector when the person has finished eating. If the person has eaten in the dining room, assist her back to her room.

12. Assist the person with oral hygiene. If the person's clothes became soiled during the meal, assist the person to change the necessary items.

13. If the resident ate in bed and side rails are in use, return the side rails to the raised position. Lower the head of the bed as the person requests. Make sure that the bed is lowered to its lowest position and that the wheels are locked.

14. Gather the soiled linens and place them in the linen hamper or linen bag. Dispose of disposable items in a facility-approved waste container. Clean equipment and return it to the storage area.

15. Record the percentage of food eaten and the amount of fluid intake in the person's medical record, per your facility's policy. Report an abnormal appetite to the nurse (for example, less than 70% of the total meal consumed).

Finishing Up CLSOWR

16. Complete the "Finishing Up" steps.

WHAT DID YOU LEARN?

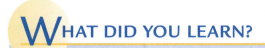

Multiple Choice

Select the single best answer for each of the following questions.

1. When assisting a person with eating, one of the first things you should do is
   a. Provide the person with privacy
   b. Butter the person's bread
   c. Wash your hands and the person's hands
   d. Cut the food into large pieces

2. Mrs. Wellington is blind. Which one of the following should she have during meal time?
   a. A mechanical soft diet
   b. Help identifying the location of the food on the plate
   c. A large spoon
   d. A cup holder

3. Mr. Jones is 98 years old and has no food restrictions on his diet. However, he is missing several teeth. Which type of special diet will most likely be ordered for Mr. Jones?
   a. Regular ("house")
   b. Carbohydrate (CHO)–controlled diet
   c. Mechanical soft diet
   d. Clear liquid diet

4. Which one of the following lists only items that would be included in fluid intake?
   a. Orange juice, soft-boiled egg, toast
   b. Milk, soup, gelatin
   c. Water, mashed potatoes, egg custard
   d. Milk, ham sandwich, ice cream bar

5. Miss Lee drank one third of an 8-ounce glass of iced tea. How many milliliters of fluid did Miss Lee drink?
   a. 60 mL
   b. 80 mL
   c. 100 mL
   d. 240 mL

6. Which one of the following lists foods that are good sources of protein?
   a. Steak, chicken, fish
   b. Spinach, carrots, beets
   c. Bread, cereal, rice
   d. Apples, oranges, bananas

7. Which one of the following nutrients accounts for 50% to 60% of our total body weight?
   a. Vitamin A
   b. Glucose
   c. Water
   d. Calcium

8. At the beginning of your shift, you give Mr. Gibson a water pitcher containing 270 mL of water. At the end of your shift, you note that 35 mL of water are left in the pitcher. How much water did Mr. Gibson drink?
   a. 35 mL
   b. 175 mL
   c. 235 mL
   d. 140 mL

9. Which of the following lists foods that are good sources of carbohydrates?
   a. Liver, fish, chicken
   b. Cereal, fruit, bread
   c. Milk, beans, cheese
   d. Water, soda, butter

10. Which one of the following can be harmful if too much is consumed?
    a. Folic acid
    b. Water-soluble vitamins (for example, vitamins C and B_{12})
    c. Fat-soluble vitamins (for example, vitamins A, D, E, and K)
    d. None of the above

11. Which health care professional is responsible for performing a calorie count to assess a resident's nutritional status?
    a. The nurse
    b. The dietitian
    c. The nursing assistant
    d. The doctor

12. Which one of the following can affect a person's food likes and dislikes?
    a. The person's religious beliefs
    b. The person's culture
    c. Where the person lives
    d. All of the above

Matching

Match the amount of fluid in milliliters (mL) with the same amount in ounces (oz).

_____ **1.** 240 mL

_____ **2.** 180 mL

_____ **3.** 300 mL

_____ **4.** 30 mL

_____ **5.** 120 mL

_____ **6.** 150 mL

a. 10 oz
b. 5 oz
c. 8 oz
d. 4 oz
e. 1 oz
f. 6 oz

STOP and Think!

- Mrs. Giovanni was recently admitted to your long-term care facility. She is a bit under-weight and her doctor wants her to consume more calories each day. The problem is Mrs. Giovanni will only eat about half of her meal at meal time. She says, "I just get full quickly." What are some ways you may be able to help Mrs. Giovanni improve her nutritional intake?

- Mrs. Wessel, a new resident in your long-term care facility, was living with her husband prior to her admission a week ago. She had been cared for at home by her husband, but he has been hospitalized with a stroke. Mrs. Wessel's daughter arranged for Mrs. Wessel's admission so that she would have help with her care during Mr. Wessel's hospitalization. Mrs. Wessel had a stroke 2 years ago, and since then has been paralyzed on her right side. She needs assistance with all of her care and has some difficulty swallowing. You have encouraged Mrs. Wessel to come out of her room to meet other residents, but she refuses. She also refuses to eat her meals in the dining room. She usually eats about 50% of her meal, and when she is offered alternatives, she always declines them. Her daughter commented that this is unusual because her mother has always had a healthy appetite. She loved her husband's cooking! Mrs. Wessel's daughter has not been able to visit much because she has been staying at the hospital with her father. Mrs. Wessel repeatedly asks about her husband and expresses worry about when she can return home with him. What do you think are some of the factors that are affecting Mrs. Wessel's food intake? Is there anything that you can do to help Mrs. Wessel maintain sufficient nutrition?

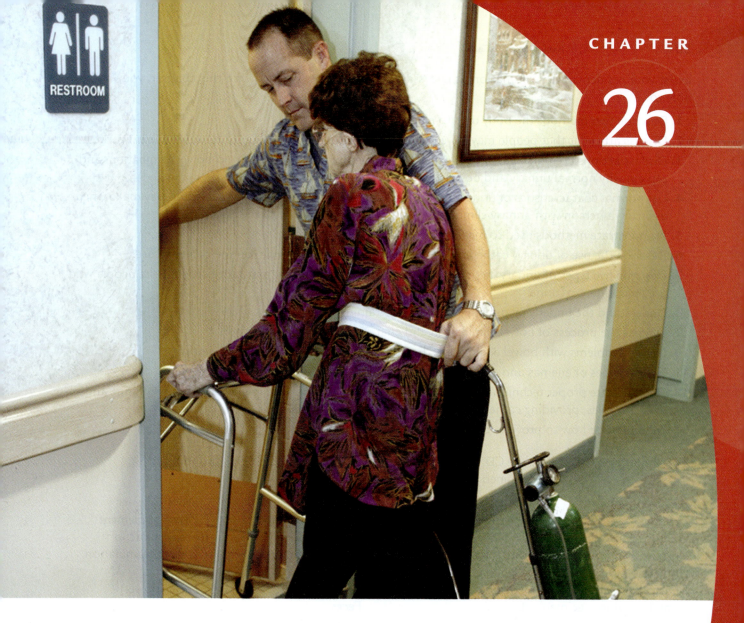

RESTROOM

Urinary and Bowel Elimination

WHAT WILL YOU LEARN?

In Chapter 25, you learned about how we take in food and convert it to energy in a process called *metabolism*. During this conversion process, waste materials (or by-products) are created. These waste products must be removed from our bodies, or we will become sick. Wastes are eliminated from the body in various forms. The urinary system rids the body of waste products that have been filtered from the bloodstream, along with excess fluid, in the form of urine. The digestive system rids the body of the solid waste that is left over from the foods that we eat, in the form of feces, or bowel movements. Although there are other ways the body rids itself of waste, urinary and bowel elimination is the subject of this chapter.

Your residents may have physical or mental difficulties that affect their ability to manage urinary or bowel elimination, or both. As a nursing assistant, you will need to

Photo: Nursing assistants help their patients or residents to meet their elimination needs by providing assistance as necessary.

assist your residents with elimination as necessary. When you are finished with this chapter, you will be able to:

1. Describe two methods the body uses to eliminate waste products.
2. Discuss attitudes that people may have regarding the processes of urinary or bowel elimination.
3. Discuss actions the nursing assistant can take to promote normal urinary and bowel elimination, and explain why normal urinary and bowel elimination is essential to health.
4. List normal characteristics of urine and describe observations that a nursing assistant may make when assisting a person with urinary elimination that should be reported to the nurse.
5. Demonstrate methods used to measure and record urinary output.
6. Describe the use of urinary catheters and demonstrate how to provide routine catheter care.
7. Describe five types of urinary incontinence and methods the nursing assistant uses to assist people who are incontinent of urine.
8. Understand the underlying principles of bladder training.
9. Discuss the process of bowel elimination and characteristics of normal stool.
10. Define problems with bowel elimination that are often seen in the health care setting.
11. List the types of enemas and discuss reasons why a person may require an enema.
12. Demonstrate proper technique for assisting with urinary and bowel elimination, obtaining urine and stool samples, providing catheter care, and administering enemas.
13. Demonstrate how to provide routine stoma care.

Vocabulary Use the CD in the front of your book to hear these terms pronounced and defined:

Bedside commode	Diuretic	Catheter care	Stool softener
Bedpan	Frequency	Urinary incontinence	Fiber supplement
Fracture pan	Urgency	Urinary retention	Fecal impaction
Urinal	Nocturia	Condom catheter	Digital examination
Urinalysis	Oliguria	Chyme	Flatulence
Midstream ("clean	Polyuria	Peristalsis	Fecal (bowel)
catch") urine specimen	Diuresis	Feces	incontinence
Urination	Anuria	Defecate	Enema
Voiding	Catheter	Stool	Stoma
Micturition	Straight catheter	Flatus	Ostomy
Dysuria	Indwelling catheter	Diarrhea	appliance
Hematuria	Suprapubic	Constipation	Ileostomy
Occult	catheter	Laxative	Colostomy

ASSISTING WITH ELIMINATION

ELIMINATION EQUIPMENT

Many of your residents will need no more assistance with elimination than a steady arm to lean on during the trip to the bathroom. The bathrooms in many long-term care facilities have special features that make them easier for people with physical disabilities to use (Fig. 26-1A). For example, handrails attached to the walls alongside the toilet or onto the toilet itself make it easier for the person to sit down and get back up. Some toilets have higher seats, so the person does not have to bend her knees as much to sit down and get back up. Modifications like these allow many residents to use the toilet in the bathroom with very little assistance from you. However, some of your residents may not be able to get out of bed at all, or they may be too weak or ill to walk to the bathroom. These people will need more help with elimination, and special equipment.

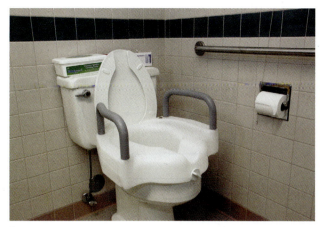
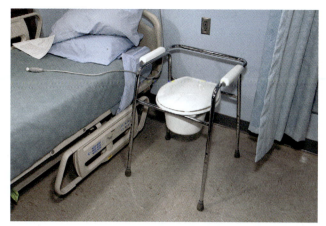

A   B

Figure 26-1

(A) Many toilets in health care facilities have special modifications that make them easier to use.
(B) A bedside commode can be used if a person can get out of bed but is not capable of walking the distance to the bathroom.

Bedside Commodes

For a person who is able to get out of bed, but who is not able to walk to the bathroom, a bedside commode can make toileting easier (Fig. 26-1B). The **bedside commode** is a chair frame with a toilet seat and a removable collection bucket. If the person is weak or unsteady, you will need to help her get out of bed and over to the bedside commode.

Bedpans

A **bedpan** is used for elimination when a person is unable to get out of bed at all (Fig. 26-2A). A woman who cannot get out of bed uses a bedpan to urinate, and for bowel movements. A man who cannot get out of bed uses a bedpan for bowel movements, and a urinal to urinate (see next section).

Bedpans, while sometimes necessary, must be used with extreme care. It is very easy to bruise or tear the fragile skin of an elderly or disabled person. In addition to causing immediate pain to the person, an injury like this can also lead to the formation of a pressure ulcer later on. Arthritis can make using a bedpan very painful, as can fractures of the back or legs. If a person has an injury or disability that makes it too uncomfortable or dangerous to use a regular bedpan, a special bedpan called a fracture pan is used. The **fracture pan,** which is wedge-shaped, is placed underneath the person's buttocks with the thin edge toward the person's back (Fig. 26-2B).

Using a bedpan is uncomfortable, and the discomfort alone can cause the person to have difficulty using it. Many facilities use disposable bedpans that are made from molded plastic. However, some facilities still use bedpans made from stainless steel. If the facility where you work uses metal bedpans, be sure to warm the bedpan before offering it to the resident. You can do this by wrapping the bedpan in a warm towel, or running warm water over the seat area and then drying it before use. Rubbing a small amount of powder on the rim of the bedpan can make it easier to slide under the person. If the person's condition allows, raise the head of the bed to promote a more natural elimination position. Provide as much privacy as safely possible. Procedure 26-1 describes how to help a person to use a bedpan.

Urinals

A man uses a **urinal** to urinate when he cannot get out of bed (Fig. 26-3). The urinal is designed to fit between the man's legs. To urinate, the man puts his penis in the opening of the urinal. If the man is very weak or disabled, you may need to place his penis inside the opening of the urinal for him. Procedure 26-2 describes how to help a man to use a urinal.

PROMOTING NORMAL ELIMINATION

Being in a health care facility can change a person's normal elimination patterns, which can cause health problems. The most effective method of treating urinary and bowel problems is to

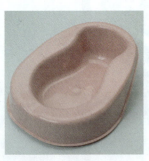

A. Regular bedpan

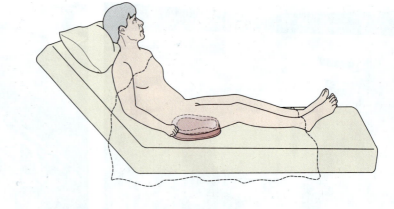

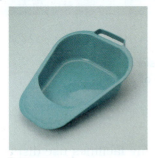

B. Fracture pan

Figure 26-2
Bedpans are used for women who cannot get out of bed to urinate. A bedridden man also uses a bedpan for bowel movements. **(A)** A standard bedpan. Position a standard bedpan like a regular toilet seat—the buttocks are placed on the wide, rounded shelf, with the open end pointed toward the foot of the bed. **(B)** A fracture pan. Position a fracture pan with the thin edge toward the head of the bed.

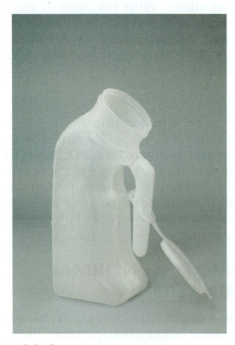

Figure 26-3
Men who cannot get out of bed to urinate can use a urinal.

prevent them from happening in the first place. As a nursing assistant, you can help promote normal urinary and bowel function for your residents. The following tips are simple, but effective.

- Encourage plenty of fluids, unless a resident has a medical condition that requires fluid restriction. Drinking plenty of fluids helps the kidneys to work properly, and regular urination flushes harmful bacteria from the bladder, helping to prevent urinary tract infections. In addition, drinking enough fluids helps to keep the feces soft, making bowel movements easier.
- Answer call lights promptly and take residents to the bathroom or provide them with a bedpan or urinal as soon as they ask you to. Many residents do not want to "bother" the nursing staff and will wait until the last minute to call for assistance with the bedpan or for help getting to the bathroom. If the person must wait too long for help to arrive, he or she may have an accident.

- Encourage your residents to call when they first feel the urge to void. This can help to prevent accidents. In addition, "holding" urine or feces is uncomfortable, and can lead to problems such as constipation.
- Offer residents the chance to eliminate frequently, especially if they are bed-bound or require assistance. Some residents may find it easier to accept an offer of assistance than to ask for help.
- Provide for privacy and comfort. A person is able to urinate or have a bowel movement much more easily if she is warm enough, in a comfortable position, and ensured of as much privacy as possible. Most women urinate and have bowel movements in a sitting or squatting position. Help a woman to sit upright by elevating the head of the bed (if she is using a bedpan), or have her lean forward a bit while seated on the toilet or bedside commode. Most men stand up to urinate and sit down to have a bowel movement. Some men have no difficulty using a urinal while lying down, but others will need to sit up or even to stand. In this case,

you may need to help the man to sit or stand up.

If a person is having difficulty urinating, there are some things you can do to help. For example, try turning on the faucet and allowing water to run into the sink. The sound of running water, which accompanied many of our early toilet training lessons, can help a person relax enough to start the urine stream. The sound of the running water also helps to cover up the sounds of urination, which may put some people more at ease. Putting the person's fingers in a basin of warm water can also help stimulate urination.

If a person is having difficulty moving his bowels, make sure that the person does not feel rushed. Many people like to read while having a bowel movement. Some people find that drinking warm fluids (such as coffee, tea, or warm water with lemon) helps stimulate the bowels to empty. Finally, regular exercise and foods that contain insoluble fiber help to promote regular bowel movements.

General guidelines for assisting a person with elimination are given in Guidelines Box 26-1.

Helping Hands and a Caring Heart

FOCUS ON HUMANISTIC HEALTH CARE

Everyone urinates and has bowel movements. However, most people consider elimination a private activity. Think about how it would affect you to be a resident of a long-term care facility. Nurses and nursing assistants ask you about your bathroom patterns. They want to know if you have had a bowel movement today, how big it was, and what it looked like. They want you to urinate into a container so that your urine can be observed and measured. You may have to share a bathroom, or worse yet, use a bedpan while being separated from other people in the room by only a curtain! Elimination, especially when it must take place in a fairly public way, is very embarrassing for many people.

A resident of a long-term care facility may have difficulty with elimination, especially if elimination must occur under conditions that are not as private as the person would like. Regardless of the amount of assistance that your residents need, privacy and consideration for individual preferences are essential. Provide privacy to the extent possible with regard to the safety of the person. Close the bathroom door, or close the privacy curtains

and the door to the room, if the person cannot use the regular toilet. Always make sure the call light is in reach so that the person can call you when he is ready for assistance. Some resident are too weak or unsteady to be left alone while they urinate or have a bowel movement. In fact, some residents will actually need for you to help hold them in the correct position during elimination. Being professional, kind, and straightforward will help to ease your resident's embarrassment.

Similarly, it is important to help your residents keep their sense of dignity. For many people, needing assistance with this most private of bodily functions is humiliating. Feelings of embarrassment and shame are made worse when residents accidentally soil themselves, their bed linens, or their clothing with urine or feces. This is a common occurrence in long-term care facilities. The effects of medications, being in a strange place, reluctance to ask for help, and physical or mental disabilities can all lead to accidents. Again, kindness, empathy, and a professional attitude can go a long way toward easing the resident's embarrassment.

Guidelines Box 26-1 Guidelines for Assisting with Elimination

WHAT YOU DO	WHY YOU DO IT
Always honor a person's request for assistance with elimination as quickly as possible.	Answering call lights quickly builds trust and prevents accidents. If a person who is bed-bound must wait too long for assistance, he could have an accident in the bed. A weak or unsteady person may try to walk to the bathroom on her own, rather than waiting for help to arrive. This puts the person at risk for a fall. Finally, it is very uncomfortable to "hold" urine or feces for a long time, and doing so can change the normal elimination patterns, causing health problems.
Always provide the person with as much privacy as safety considerations will allow.	Regular elimination is essential to health, so it is important to make this process as normal as possible for your residents. Many people have difficulty urinating or having a bowel movement if they think that someone else can hear them, or if someone else is in the bathroom with them.
If you leave the person alone, always make sure that the call light control is within easy reach of the person.	The person will need the call light control to let you know when she is finished, or if she needs help.
Make sure the toilet paper is within easy reach of the person. If the person is unable to wipe himself, assist with this task.	Wiping promotes comfort and helps to prevent irritation, odors, and infection.
Be sure to provide good perineal care as necessary, especially after bowel movements (see Chapter 23).	Good perineal care promotes comfort and helps to prevent irritation, odors, and infection.
Provide the person with the chance to wash his hands after elimination. This can be accomplished by stopping by the sink if the person is in the bathroom, or by providing a warm, wet washcloth after assisting the person from the bedside commode or removing the bedpan or urinal.	Most people prefer to wash their hands after using the toilet. Allowing people to follow their normal routines whenever possible is important, especially when other aspects of the routine need to be altered. In addition, handwashing is important for hygiene.
Always wear gloves when assisting a person with elimination, or when handling a bedpan, bedside commode bucket, or urinal that contains waste.	Urine and feces are considered body fluids and may contain pathogens.
Before disposing of waste, observe the feces or urine for amount and any unusual characteristics. Report and record your observations.	Abnormalities in the urine or feces could indicate a health problem.

WHAT YOU DO	*WHY YOU DO IT*
Never place a bedpan or urinal on an over-bed table or bedside table, even if the bedpan or urinal is clean. Dirty bedpans and urinals are taken to the bathroom immediately after use and cleaned and disinfected according to facility policy. Clean bedpans are either stored in a cabinet underneath the bedside table or returned to the equipment room. Clean urinals may be hung over the side rail, stored in a cabinet, or returned to the equipment room.	The over-bed table and bedside table are considered "clean" areas. Even if the bedpan or urinal is clean, most people do not want items associated with elimination placed on surfaces where they eat or have personal items displayed.
If there are odors in the room as a result of elimination, use an air freshener.	Most people will appreciate the use of an air freshener to make the air in the room smell fresher. Just be professional in any remarks you may make about the odor.
Disinfect equipment used for elimination carefully, according to facility policy.	Bedpans, urinals, and bedside commode buckets can act as fomites (that is, non-living objects that can transmit pathogens and cause infection) if they are not properly disinfected.

OBTAINING URINE AND STOOL SPECIMENS

Because the contents of a person's urine or feces can provide a doctor with clues about the person's overall health status, you may be asked to obtain a urine or stool specimen (sample) for laboratory study. When assisting with specimen collection, it is very important to make sure that the specimen container is properly labeled with the resident's name and room number. Otherwise, specimens could get mixed up and a resident may be diagnosed with, and receive treatment for, a condition he or she does not have! It is also important to make sure that the specimen is handled correctly after you obtain it. For example, in certain situations, the specimen may need to be delivered to the laboratory while it is still warm, or placed in a special plastic transport bag. If a specimen is not being delivered to the laboratory right away, then it needs to be stored properly until the scheduled pick-up time. Before collecting *any* specimen—of urine, feces, or any other body fluid—always ask yourself the following questions:

- Do I have the right person?
- What method is to be used to collect the specimen?
- Do I have the right type of specimen container?
- Is the specimen container properly labeled?
- What is the correct date and time?
- What storage and delivery method must I use?

Finally, always remember to wear gloves when assisting with specimen collection and when handling the specimen containers.

Obtaining a Urine Specimen

Urinalysis, or examination of the urine under a microscope and by chemical means, is a commonly used diagnostic tool. Substances found in urine during urinalysis can help doctors diagnose kidney disease, certain metabolic diseases, and infections. The collection and analysis of urine over a 24-hour period allows for evaluation of kidney function. To perform urinalysis, a urine specimen must be obtained.

Depending on the situation, the method of collecting a urine specimen may vary. For routine urinalysis, no special collection procedures are necessary. The person is asked to urinate directly into the specimen container, if possible. If this is difficult for the person, he or she can urinate into a specimen collection device ("commode hat," see Chapter 25, Fig. 25-16), or into a bedpan or urinal. The person must not have a bowel movement or place toilet paper in the collection device, because these actions will change the urinalysis results. The urine is then poured from the collection device, bedpan, or urinal into the specimen container. The procedure for obtaining a routine urine sample is described in Procedure 26-3.

In some situations, it may be necessary to obtain a **midstream ("clean catch") urine specimen** using a sterile specimen container. This method of collecting urine prevents contamination of the urine by the bacteria that normally live in and around the urethra. A midstream ("clean catch") urine specimen is usually ordered when the doctor suspects a urinary tract infection. This way, if any bacteria are found in the urine sample, the doctor knows that they are the ones most likely responsible for the infection. When a midstream ("clean catch") urine specimen is requested, the person is asked to clean the area around the urethral opening with a special cleansing wipe. The urine flow is started, then stopped, then started again. The urine sample is collected from the restarted flow. Procedure 26-4 describes how to assist a person with obtaining a midstream ("clean catch") urine specimen.

Your facility may train you to do a type of routine urine testing that involves dipping chemically treated paper strips into a urine sample. Chemicals on the paper react with certain substances that may be found in the urine, causing the chemical blocks on the paper to change color if these substances are present in the urine. The paper is then compared with a color chart that comes with the strips, and the results are recorded in the resident's chart and reported to the nurse.

Obtaining a Stool Specimen

Stool can be analyzed for the presence of blood, pathogens (such as parasites or bacteria), fat, and other things that are not normally found in feces. Because people do not have bowel movements as often as they urinate, if a stool specimen is needed, the person should be notified well in advance so that the specimen can be collected when it becomes available. Ask the nurse if there are any particular collection methods that should be used. Stool can be collected in a bedpan, bedside commode, or in a collection device placed onto a regular toilet. The person must not urinate or place toilet paper in the collection device, because these actions will change the test results. The procedure for collecting a stool specimen is given in Procedure 26-5.

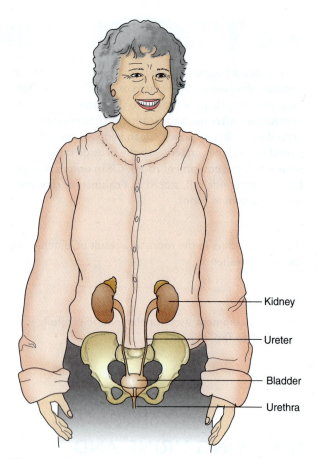

Figure 26-4
The urinary system.

URINARY ELIMINATION

NORMAL URINARY ELIMINATION

The urinary system, which is discussed in more detail in Chapter 39, is made up of the kidneys, ureters, urinary bladder, and urethra (Fig. 26-4). Blood passes through the kidneys, which remove waste products and excess fluid, forming urine. It takes the kidneys approximately 30 minutes to process the body's total blood volume. As it forms, the urine flows from the kidneys through the ureters and is stored in the urinary bladder. As the bladder fills, we begin to feel the urge to urinate. Urine leaves the body through the urethra.

The process of passing urine from the body is known by several terms, including **urination, voiding,** and **micturition.** Many of your residents will have their own terms for urinating, such as "peeing" or "passing water." When talking about urination with a resident, you should use words that the person is familiar with.

Urination should not cause discomfort. **Dysuria** is difficulty voiding that may or may not be associated with pain. Some people describe the discomfort they feel during urination as a "burning" or "cramping" sensation. Dysuria is often associatcd with bladder infections, prostate problems, and some sexually transmitted diseases (STDs).

Characteristics of Urine

In healthy people, urine is clear, without cloudiness or particles. Sometimes urine that has been in a container for a while will become cloudy as it cools. Healthy urine is pale yellow, straw-colored, or dark gold (amber) in color, with a slight odor. A slight red tinge to the urine may indicate **hematuria,** or the presence of blood in the urine. This is an abnormal finding. Sometimes hematuria is **occult** (that is, hidden) and must be detected using urinalysis. Some foods and medications can also affect the color and odor of urine. When you are helping a resident with urination, observe the urine and report any abnormalities to the nurse. Urine with an unusual odor or appearance could be a sign of illness or infection.

Urination Habits

The frequency of voiding, and the amount of urine voided each time, will differ from person to person. Many factors influence a person's urination habits, including the person's age, the amount of fluids the person drinks, and the types of medications the person takes. For example, many of your residents will be taking **diuretics** ("water pills" or "fluid pills"). These medications help the kidneys remove extra water from the body, and are often used in the treatment of kidney disease, certain types of heart disease (such as congestive heart failure), and hypertension. A resident who is taking a diuretic may have to urinate as frequently as every half hour!

You will soon become aware of the urination habits that are normal for each resident in your care. This knowledge will allow you to recognize any changes that may occur. For example, **frequency** is the term used to describe voiding that occurs more often than usual. Frequency is often accompanied by a feeling of **urgency,** or the need to urinate immediately. A person with a urinary tract infection may experience frequency and urgency. **Nocturia** is the need to get up more than once or twice during the night to urinate, to the point where sleep is disrupted. Nocturia can be a sign of pain or depression, a prostate or bladder disorder, or heart failure.

Urine Output

As you learned in Chapter 25, urine output is a key indicator of fluid balance. In a person who is maintaining a good fluid balance, urine output is neither too high nor too low.

- **Oliguria** is the state of voiding a very small amount of urine over a given period of time (for example, voiding only 100 to 400 mL of urine over 24 hours). *Olig-* means "few" and *-uria* means "urine." A person who is dehydrated might become oliguric (that is, have a urine output that is well below normal).
- **Polyuria** (*poly-* means "many") is excessive urine output. Polyuria, also known as **diuresis,** can be a sign of a health problem. For example, polyuria can be a symptom of poorly controlled diabetes. Or, polyuria may be the desired effect of a medication. For example, in a person who is taking a diuretic, polyuria is a sign that the medication is having the desired effect.

Evaluating a person's urine output is also a good way to determine how well a person's kidneys are working. **Anuria** (*an-* means "none") is defined as the state of voiding less than 100 mL of urine over a 24-hour period. Anuria usually indicates that a person is in kidney failure.

Not all of your residents will need to have their urine output measured and recorded, but residents who have illnesses or take medications that may alter the body's ability to maintain a healthy fluid balance will need to have their urine output measured and recorded each time they void. If a person uses a regular toilet, you will need to

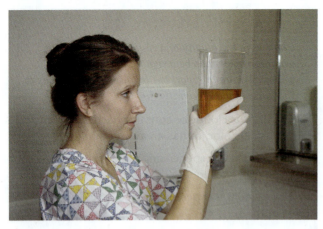

Figure 26-5
To measure urine output, the urine is poured into a measuring device, called a graduate. The graduate is held at eye level to properly determine the amount of fluid it contains.

remind the person to void into a specimen collection device ("commode hat") and to call you after he or she has finished voiding so that you can measure and record the amount of urine. Specimen collection devices, urinals, and the drainage bags used with urinary catheters often have markings that make measuring urine output easy. If they do not, then the urine output can be measured by pouring it into a graduate (Fig. 26-5). A graduate is also used to measure urine output if a person voids into a bedpan or bedside commode bucket.

If the urine output of one of your residents is being monitored, you will need to keep a record of the amount of urine passed at each voiding. Some intake and output (I&O) flow sheets will have spaces to record the amount of each individual voiding, while others may only have a space to record the end-of-shift amount. To obtain the end-of-shift amount, simply add the individual amounts together and record the total in the appropriate space.

URINARY CATHETERIZATION

Sometimes a person is unable to urinate using a toilet, bedpan, urinal, or bedside commode, due to disability or illness. In these situations, a urinary catheter is used. A **catheter** is a tube that is inserted into the body for the purpose of administering or removing fluids. A urinary catheter is inserted into the bladder through the urethra (or through an incision made in the abdominal wall) to allow the urine in the bladder to drain out. A urinary catheter is used in many different situations:

- A urinary catheter may be inserted to drain the bladder before or during a surgical

procedure, during recovery from a serious illness or injury, or to collect urine for testing.
- A urinary catheter may be used for a person who is incontinent of urine, if the person has wounds or pressure ulcers that would be made worse by contact with urine.
- A urinary catheter is necessary when a person is unable to urinate because of an obstruction in the urethra or an injury or illness that affects the spinal cord or the nerves that control bladder function.

Usually, inserting a urinary catheter is beyond the scope of practice for a nursing assistant, although in some facilities, nursing assistants are provided with additional training that allows them to insert urinary catheters. Inserting a catheter is a procedure that requires sterile technique because it involves putting a foreign object (that is, the catheter) into a person's body. If sterile technique is not used, the catheter can introduce infection-causing bacteria into the bladder. Even if you are not trained to actually insert urinary catheters, caring for people who have urinary catheters in place will certainly be a part of your daily duties.

Types of Urinary Catheters

You will see many different types of urinary catheters in use.

Straight catheters

A **straight catheter,** also known as a Robinson, Rob-Nel, or Red Rubber catheter, is used when the catheter is to be inserted and removed immediately. The catheter is introduced into the bladder, the urine is allowed to drain out, and the catheter is removed (Fig. 26-6A). The doctor may order catheterization with a straight catheter so that a sterile urine specimen can be obtained. A person with a spinal cord injury or an injury or illness that affects the nerves that control bladder function may also need to be catheterized with a straight catheter on a regular schedule to empty the bladder, because the person is not able to sense the need to urinate.

Indwelling catheters

An **indwelling catheter,** also known as a retention or Foley catheter, is left inside the bladder to provide continuous urine drainage. An indwelling catheter has a soft balloon that is inflated inside the bladder to keep the catheter from sliding out of the urethra (see Fig. 26-6B). Urine collects in a drainage bag, which is attached to the indwelling catheter by a length of tubing.

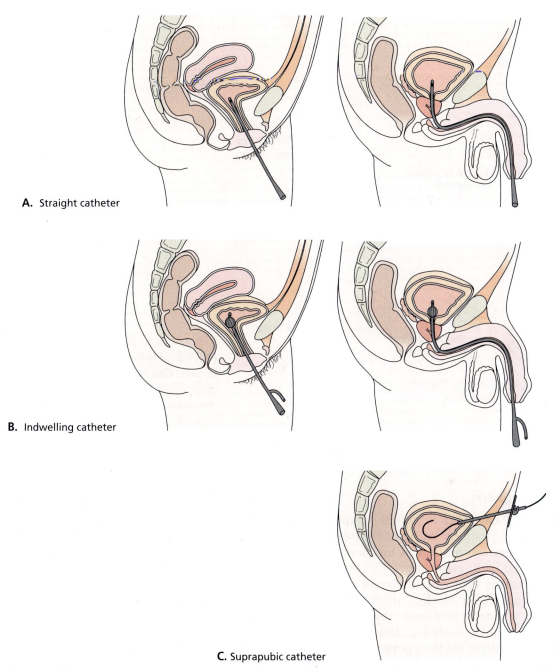

A. Straight catheter

B. Indwelling catheter

C. Suprapubic catheter

Figure 26-6

Types of catheters. **(A)** A straight catheter is inserted into the bladder, the urine is drained, and then the catheter is removed. **(B)** An indwelling catheter, also known as a Foley catheter or a retention catheter, remains in the body and urine drains continuously into a drainage bag. **(C)** A suprapubic catheter is inserted into the bladder through a surgical incision made above the pubic bone (*supra-* means "above"). A suprapubic catheter is a bit less likely to promote urinary infections because its location keeps the opening away from the contaminated perineal area.

An indwelling catheter may have two lumens or three lumens (Fig. 26-7). A double-lumen indwelling catheter has two lumens. One lumen, which connects to the catheter tubing, is for urine drainage. The other is used to inflate the balloon that holds the catheter in place. A triple-lumen indwelling catheter has three lumens. The extra lumen is used to flush the bladder with irrigation fluid. Regular flushing of the bladder with irrigation fluid helps to keep blood clots from forming inside the bladder. This is important in certain situations, such as when a man has just had prostate surgery.

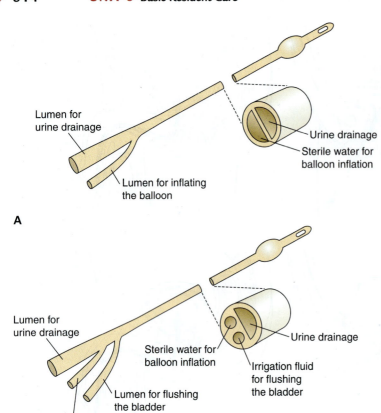

Lumen for
urine drainage

Urine drainage

Sterile water for
balloon inflation

Lumen for inflating
the balloon

A

Lumen for
urine drainage

Sterile water for
balloon inflation

Urine drainage

Irrigation fluid
for flushing
the bladder

Lumen for flushing
the bladder

Lumen for inflating
the balloon

B

Figure 26-7

(A) A double-lumen indwelling catheter has two lumens. One lumen is for urine drainage. The other is used to inflate the balloon that holds the catheter in place. **(B)** A triple-lumen indwelling catheter has three lumens. The additional lumen is used to flush the bladder with irrigation fluid.

Suprapubic catheters

A **suprapubic catheter** is a type of indwelling catheter. The suprapubic catheter is inserted into the bladder through a surgical incision made in the abdominal wall, right above the pubic bone (Fig. 26-6C). This type of catheter is most often used for people with blocked urethras, and for men. Men typically are not able to use an indwelling urinary catheter that is inserted through the urethra for long periods of time due to the anatomy of the male urethra. While a woman's urethra is straight and only about 2 inches long, a man's urethra is curved in an "S" shape and is about 6 inches long (Fig. 26-6B). In men, the pressure of the indwelling catheter on the curved areas of the urethra can cause erosion of the mucous membrane that lines the urethra.

Caring for a Person With an Indwelling Urinary Catheter

Indwelling urinary catheters are connected by a length of tubing to a urine drainage bag. Urine drains continuously from the bladder, through the catheter, down the tubing, and into the drainage bag (Fig. 26-8).

One type of urine drainage bag that is commonly used has a long length of tubing that allows the bag to be carried or secured to a bed frame or the back of a wheelchair. When a person has this type of urine drainage bag, using a cloth urine drainage bag cover can help minimize the embarrassment the person may feel about having a bag full of her own urine in plain view of others (Fig. 26-9). Another type of urine drainage bag, called a "leg bag," is connected to the catheter by a short length of tubing and secured to the person's thigh with straps. Leg bags are useful because they can be concealed underneath a person's clothing and they allow the person to move around freely. However, leg bags need to be emptied more frequently because they are smaller and hold less urine than a regular urine drainage bag.

When a regular urine drainage bag with a long length of tubing is being used, the tubing is secured loosely to the person's body near the insertion site using a catheter strap or adhesive tape. Securing the tubing to the person's body prevents the catheter from being accidentally pulled out during repositioning. In women, the tubing is attached to the thigh. In men, the tubing is attached to the thigh or lower abdomen

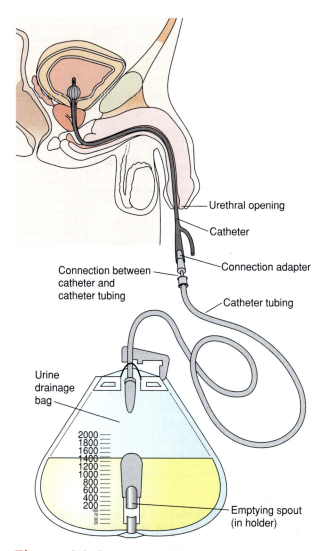

Figure 26-8

The indwelling urinary catheter drainage system consists of a catheter that is connected to a urine drainage bag by way of a length of tubing. The urine drainage bag has a connection adapter, where the tubing attaches, and an emptying spout, which is unclamped to allow the urine to drain from the bag. When not in use, the emptying spout is stored in a holder that is part of the bag.

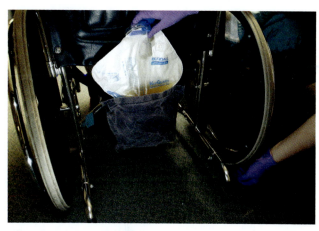

Figure 26-9

The urine drainage bag is placed inside a specially designed cloth cover to conceal it from view. Providing a resident with a urine drainage bag cover is a small gesture that can mean a lot to the resident.

(Fig. 26-10). A little bit of slack is left in the tubing to prevent the catheter from pulling against the bladder outlet and the urethral opening. The remaining length of tubing is then gently coiled and secured to the bed linens using a plastic clip (Fig. 26-10). Coiling the tubing prevents the tubing from becoming bent or kinked, which would stop the free flow of urine into the drainage bag. Coiling the tubing and securing it to the bed linens also keeps the weight of the tubing from pulling against the person's body. The drainage bag is then secured to the bed frame or the back

of the person's wheelchair, at a level lower than the person's bladder. If the drainage bag and tubing are higher than the person's bladder, then gravity could cause old, contaminated urine to run back down the tubing and into the person's bladder, causing an infection.

All urine drainage bags have a connection adapter (where the catheter tubing attaches) and an emptying spout that is opened to allow urine to drain from the bag. Because the inside of the catheter and tubing are sterile, it is safer for the person if the bag is not disconnected from the tubing once the catheter is in place. Disconnecting the bag from the tubing can allow harmful bacteria to enter the catheter. Occasionally, the tubing has to be disconnected from the bag (for example, to change the bag if it is leaking, to replace a regular drainage bag with a leg bag, or to perform certain procedures). If you must disconnect the tubing from the bag, be sure to prevent the end of the tubing from touching anything, and wipe the exposed tubing with an antibacterial wipe before reconnecting the drainage bag. General guidelines for caring for a person with an indwelling catheter are given in Guidelines Box 26-2.

Providing catheter care

As a nursing assistant, one of your responsibilities will be to provide catheter care for your residents with indwelling urinary catheters. **Catheter care** involves thorough cleaning of the perineal area (especially around the urethra) and the catheter tubing that extends outside of the body, to prevent infection. Providing good catheter care is important because the catheter provides a

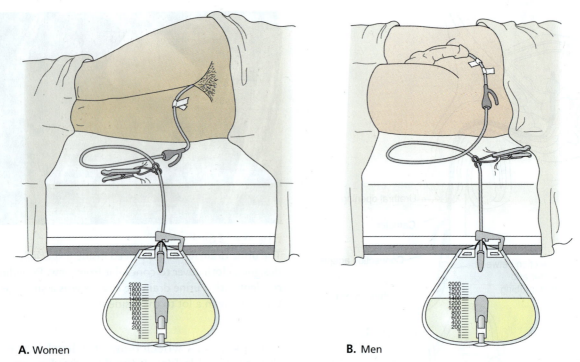

A. Women   **B.** Men

Figure 26-10

The catheter tubing is secured loosely to the person's body to prevent tension on the tubing and catheter, which could cause discomfort. Securing the tubing also prevents the catheter from accidentally being pulled out of the body during repositioning. **(A)** In women, the tubing is secured to the inner thigh. **(B)** In men, the tubing is connected either to the inner thigh or the lower abdomen.

pathway for bacteria to travel up from the perineum into the bladder, where they can cause infection. In addition, having a catheter in place eliminates the "flushing" action of normal urination, which helps to remove bacteria from the urinary tract naturally. Because bacteria can be introduced into the body both when a urinary catheter is inserted and after it is in place, urinary tract infections in catheterized people are among the most common health care–associated infections (HAIs). (Remember that HAIs are acquired in the health care setting.)

In an effort to reduce the risk of HAIs in people who are catheterized, many facilities require catheter care to be provided routinely (for example, once or twice daily), and again whenever the perineal area becomes soiled (such as when a person is incontinent of feces). Soap and water or a special antibacterial solution may be used when providing catheter care. The procedure for providing catheter care is given in Procedure 26-6.

Emptying urine drainage bags

Urine drainage bags are routinely emptied and the urine is measured at the end of each shift, unless ordered otherwise. Urine drainage bags should also be emptied if they become too full. The procedure for emptying a urine drainage bag is given in Procedure 26-7.

TELL THE NURSE

When caring for a resident with an indwelling urinary catheter, make sure you report any of the following observations to the nurse immediately:

- Changes in the color, clarity, or odor of the urine

- The urine is not flowing freely through the tubing (make sure that the tubing is not kinked or bent)

- The resident has pain or discomfort as a result of the catheter

- The catheter insertion site is red or swollen, or there is discharge from the catheter insertion site

- Urine is leaking around the catheter insertion site

Guidelines Box 26-2 Guidelines for Caring for People with Indwelling Catheters

WHAT YOU DO	WHY YOU DO IT
Loosely secure the catheter tubing to the person near the insertion site, using a catheter strap or adhesive tape.	Securing the catheter tubing helps to prevent the catheter from being pulled out during repositioning. Allowing a little bit of slack helps to prevent the catheter from pulling against the bladder outlet and the urethral opening.
Gently coil the remaining length of tubing and secure it to the bed linens using a plastic clip.	Coiling the tubing helps to prevent kinking, which could stop the free flow of urine into the drainage bag. It also keeps the weight of the tubing from pulling against the area where the tubing is secured to the person's body.
When repositioning a person who has an indwelling catheter, always make sure to unclip the coiled tubing from the linens before beginning the procedure. When you are finished with the procedure, secure the coiled tubing to the linens again.	The person needs to be able to move freely during procedures such as repositioning. If you try to move a person in the direction opposite from the length of tubing, and the length of tubing is still attached to the bed linens, then the catheter could be pulled out of the person's body.
Make sure that the person is not lying on the coiled tubing.	This would be uncomfortable for the person. In addition, the weight of the person's body on the tubing could stop the free flow of urine into the drainage bag.
Always make sure the urine drainage bag is placed at a level lower than that of the person's bladder.	Raising the urine drainage bag up higher than the bladder can cause old, contaminated urine to run back into the bladder, which can lead to infection.
Never attach a urine drainage bag to a side rail. Instead, attach the drainage bag to the bed frame.	Raising the side rail would raise the drainage bag to a level that is higher than the person's bladder. The bed frame does not move; therefore, the level of the drainage bag cannot change.
Keep the drainage bag off the floor. When emptying the drainage bag, be sure that the open emptying spout does not touch anything.	Bacteria can enter the closed drainage system in this manner. The presence of bacteria in the system can lead to health care-associated urinary tract infections in people with indwelling catheters.
Always wear gloves when emptying the urine drainage bag.	Urine is a body fluid and may contain pathogens.

Preparing for removal of an indwelling catheter

Use of an indwelling catheter can lead to temporary urinary incontinence when the catheter is removed, because the catheter allows the bladder to become "lazy." While the catheter was in place, urine drained out of the body continuously. The bladder did not have to fill up and then empty itself. This lack of activity can decrease the muscle tone of the bladder, leading to incontinence. To prepare the bladder for removal of the catheter and prevent temporary incontinence from developing, it is common to clamp the tubing of the catheter for a period of time to allow the urine to fill the bladder. The tubing is then unclamped and the urine is allowed to drain from the bladder. This procedure is repeated over a period of time, with the time between clamping and emptying becoming increasingly longer. Then the catheter is removed and the person is allowed to void normally. The nurse will let you know if you are to help prepare a person for removal of an indwelling catheter.

URINARY INCONTINENCE

Urinary incontinence is the inability to hold one's urine, or the involuntary loss of urine from the bladder. Urinary incontinence may be temporary or permanent. Temporary urinary incontinence can occur as a result of a bladder infection, or after an indwelling catheter that has been in place for a long time is removed. Permanent urinary incontinence can be caused by many things, including:

- Decreased muscle tone in the bladder or the muscles that support the bladder
- Injuries or illnesses that affect the spinal cord, the brain, or the nerves that control bladder function
- Dementia

Urinary incontinence can be emotionally devastating for both the incontinent person and the person's caregivers. For the person who is incontinent, having wet clothes or smelling like urine can be very embarrassing. Because the person may be self-conscious about odor or afraid of having an incontinence accident in public, he may start to avoid social situations. This can lead to feelings of anxiety, depression, and loneliness, and can have a very negative impact on the person's quality of life. Being incontinent of urine also places a person at risk for developing skin problems (such as rashes and pressure ulcers) and for falling (as the person rushes to the bathroom to avoid having an accident).

For the caregiver, caring for a person who is incontinent of urine can be frustrating and emotionally draining. It is common to change a person's clothes or bedding, only to have the person wet herself all over again. Because caring for an incontinent person can be so emotionally trying and time consuming, incontinence is the factor that most often leads family members to have a relative admitted to a long-term care facility.

Types of Urinary Incontinence

There are many types of urinary incontinence.

- **Urge incontinence** (overactive bladder, spastic bladder) is the involuntary release of urine right after feeling a strong urge to void. In urge incontinence, the person experiences bladder spasms (involuntary contractions of the smooth muscle in the walls of the bladder) that cause the bladder to release urine with little warning. This is the most common form of urinary incontinence among elderly people. Urge incontinence can be caused by neurological disorders that affect the nerves that control bladder function (such as multiple sclerosis or Parkinson's disease), pressure on the bladder (from tumors, an enlarged prostate, or fecal impaction), or irritation of the bladder (from infection or increased intake of caffeinated beverages or alcohol).
- **Stress incontinence** occurs when urine leaks from the bladder when the person coughs, sneezes, laughs, or exerts herself. Stress incontinence is most likely to occur when a person delays voiding and the bladder becomes too full. Stress incontinence is very common in older women. Childbirth, obesity, and loss of muscle tone as a result of aging are all factors that can contribute to stress incontinence. Stress incontinence can also occur in men after prostate surgery. Stress incontinence can often be corrected by following a regular schedule for toileting and by practicing exercises that strengthen the muscles that form the pelvic floor. Sometimes, medication or surgery is needed.
- **Overflow incontinence** occurs when the bladder is too full of urine. Overflow incontinence is associated with **urinary retention,** which is the inability of the bladder to empty completely during urination. Urinary retention can be caused by blockage of the bladder outlet (such as occurs with an enlarged prostate gland or the presence of a tumor). Urinary retention can also occur when the smooth muscle that forms the walls of the bladder loses its tone and cannot contract well enough to completely empty the bladder. Because the bladder does not empty completely when the person voids, urine is "retained" or kept in the bladder. The bladder refills with urine quickly (because it was never really empty), and the urine simply overflows. A person with overflow incontinence may "dribble" urine in between visits to the bathroom. If a person cannot empty

his bladder completely, it may be necessary to insert a catheter (either temporarily or permanently) to allow urine to drain from the bladder and prevent urinary retention and overflow incontinence from occurring. If the retention is caused by an obstruction, surgery may be necessary to remove the obstruction.

- **Reflex incontinence** occurs when there is damage to the nerves that enable the person to control urination. The bladder fills, but the person does not feel the urge to urinate. When the bladder is completely full, it empties reflexively (that is, automatically). Some people with certain disorders of the nervous system, such as paralysis from a spinal cord injury, will catheterize themselves with a straight catheter on a regular basis to prevent reflex urinary incontinence.

- **Functional incontinence** occurs as a result of confusion, disorientation, or problems with mobility that prevent the person from finding or reaching the bathroom in enough time (or waiting until a bedpan or urinal is provided). It is also thought that being in a strange environment (as a long-term care facility would be to someone who has just been admitted) can contribute to functional incontinence.

OBRA regulations require the health care team to evaluate a resident who is incontinent to determine the cause of the incontinence. In addition, the health care team is required to develop and follow a plan of care that seeks to reduce or eliminate incontinence accidents from occurring. The observations you make and the assistance you provide are critical for helping the health care team meet these requirements.

Managing Urinary Incontinence

Properly managing incontinence is a very important part of providing quality care for your residents. Managing incontinence reduces the resident's risk for physical complications (such as pressure ulcers and infections), and it helps the resident to maintain his dignity, which is important for the resident's quality of life. Residents should be checked at least every 2 hours (or more frequently, if needed) for incontinence. If a resident is found to be wet between routine checks, you need to provide incontinence care promptly. Keeping the skin clean and dry and using a barrier cream to protect the skin reduces the resident's risk for developing pressure ulcers and

other complications. (See Chapter 23 for a discussion of providing perineal care, which is especially important in people who are incontinent of urine, feces, or both.)

Many products are available to help manage urinary incontinence, including incontinence pads, incontinence briefs, and condom catheters. In addition, techniques such as bladder training may be used to help a person overcome certain types of incontinence. For some people, temporary or permanent catheterization may be necessary to manage the incontinence.

Incontinence pads and briefs

Products made for urinary incontinence are available to help prevent soiling of clothes and furniture (Fig. 26-11). Incontinence pads and briefs are specially made to absorb urine and hold it away from the person's skin. Keeping the skin dry helps to reduce the skin problems that can occur from prolonged contact with urine. Incontinence pads are placed inside the person's underpants to prevent wetting of the clothes and to draw the moisture away from the person's body. Incontinence briefs are worn instead of underpants. Incontinence pads and briefs are very useful for active people.

For a person who must stay in bed, bed protectors are used to help to keep the bed linens and mattress dry and to wick urine away from the person's skin. Many facilities have policies that specify that incontinence briefs are to be used only when the person is out of bed, and that bed protectors are to be used when the person is sleeping. Incontinence briefs tend to fit closely, which makes it difficult for air to reach the skin. Switching between briefs and bed protectors helps to prevent skin breakdown by allowing the

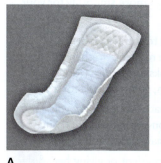 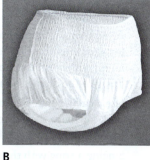

A   B

Figure 26-11

Incontinence pads and briefs are worn under clothing to absorb moisture and keep it away from the body. **(A)** DEPEND Guards for men. **(B)** DEPEND Extra Absorbency Underwear. (*Photographs courtesy of Kimberly-Clark Worldwide, Inc., Neenah, WI.*)

Caring For Those With Dementia

Elimination can present many problems for a person with dementia. The person may forget where the bathroom is, and she may not be may not be able to communicate to others that she needs to use the bathroom. Once in the bathroom, the person may not be able to recognize the toilet. She may also have difficulty moving the necessary clothing out of the way in order to use the toilet. All of these problems can cause the person to have incontinence accidents.

Assisting a person with dementia with elimination can be challenging for you as well. If the person has receptive aphasia, she may not be able to understand your questions or directions related to assisting her with elimination and incontinence care. The person may not recognize you, and she may not be able to understand why you are trying to remove her clothing or provide perineal care following an incontinence accident. As a result, the person may resist care.

To help your residents with dementia meet their elimination needs:

● Place a picture of a toilet on the bathroom door to help the resident identify the bathroom independently.

● Provide assistance with toileting on a regular schedule (for example, every 2 hours).

● Observe the resident's activity and body language, and provide assistance as needed. For example, a resident with dementia who needs to use the bathroom may become restless or demonstrate "searching" behavior as she wanders up and down the hall.

● Help the resident to select clothing with fasteners that are easy to manage (for example, pants with an elastic waist, instead of pants that zip).

To help incontinence care go more smoothly for your residents with dementia:

● Avoid bringing attention to the incontinence. Instead, offer to help the resident "freshen up" for an event the resident looks forward to (for example, going to the dining room, going outside for a walk).

● Use a calm, gentle approach. Your tone of voice and body language should convey that you are trying to be helpful, not that you have a dirty job to do!

● Singing a song with the resident or giving her something to hold (such as a stuffed animal or doll) while you are providing care may relax the resident and distract her from the task at hand.

● Keep your focus on the resident, not the task.

skin to be exposed to the air at night. As a nursing assistant, you must make sure that these incontinence products are changed frequently and that urine is cleaned from the skin whenever the change occurs.

Condom catheters

A **condom catheter** can be used to manage incontinence in men. A condom catheter is not a true catheter because it is not placed inside the body. It consists of a soft plastic or rubber sheath, tubing, and a collection bag for the urine (Fig. 26-12). The sheath is placed over the penis and the collection bag is attached to the leg. The urine flows through the tubing into the collection bag.

The condom must fit the penis. It should be fastened securely enough to prevent leaking, but not so snugly that it restricts circulation. Many condom catheters have adhesive material on the inside of the condom that allows for a good seal. Others must be secured with elastic tape. The tape strip is applied in a spiral fashion to allow for changes in the size of the penis (see Fig. 26-12).

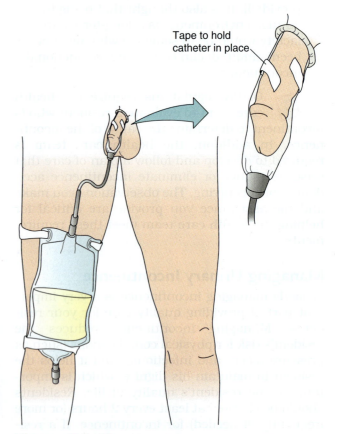

Tape to hold catheter in place

Figure 26-12

A condom catheter can be used to manage urinary incontinence in men. If tape is used to secure the condom catheter to the penis, it should be applied in a spiral fashion, not a circular fashion.

Tape that is applied incorrectly (that is, in an overlapping, circular fashion) puts the man at risk for developing a pressure ulcer on the penis and can compromise blood flow if the man has an erection, possibly causing permanent damage to the penis.

Use of a condom catheter requires good skin care. The penis must be cleaned, and the condom apparatus changed, daily.

Bladder training

Bladder training is commonly used to help people relearn how to control their urinary elimination. For example, a person may be encouraged to use the bedpan, urinal, or commode at scheduled times. Scheduling helps promote regular emptying of the bladder. The primary goal is for the person to be able to control involuntary urination. Even if this goal is not achieved, voiding at scheduled times can help to prevent some incontinence accidents from occurring. Reducing the number of incontinence accidents benefits the person both physically and emotionally.

The person's care plan will note any special bladder training techniques that are being used and the nurse will instruct you on any specific duties you will be assigned as part of that training.

BOWEL ELIMINATION

NORMAL BOWEL ELIMINATION

The digestive tract, which is discussed in more detail in Chapter 38, consists of the mouth, esophagus, stomach, small intestine, large intestine, rectum, and anus (Fig. 26-13). The rectum is actually part of the large intestine, and together, the large and small intestines are sometimes referred to as "bowels." Essentially, the digestive tract is a long, hollow tube. The food and fluids that we take in are broken down into smaller pieces and mixed together in the stomach, forming a partially digested food and fluid mixture known as **chyme.** From the stomach, the chyme passes slowly into the small intestine, where more digestion occurs and nutrients and fluid are absorbed, and then into the large intestine. Wave-like muscular movements, called **peristalsis,** move the chyme through the intestines. Finally, the chyme reaches the last part of the large intestine, called the rectum. At this point, all of the nutrients have been removed, and what remains is a semi-solid waste material, called **feces.** The presence of feces in the rectum stimulates the urge to **defecate**

(that is, have a bowel movement), and the feces leave the body through the anus, the very end of the digestive tract. Sometimes fecal material is referred to as **"stool"** after it leaves the body.

Flatus (or gas) is a natural byproduct of digestion, just as feces are. Eating certain foods, such as beans, broccoli, cabbage, cauliflower, and onions, can lead to the formation of flatus. The passing of flatus may be quite noisy and depending on what was eaten, the flatus may have a foul odor. For some people, passing flatus is very embarrassing.

Characteristics of Feces

In healthy people, feces are soft, brown, moist, and formed, with a distinct odor. Certain foods and medications can affect the color and odor of feces. When you are helping a resident with defecation, observe the feces and report any abnormalities to the nurse. Feces with an unusual odor or appearance could be a sign of illness or infection.

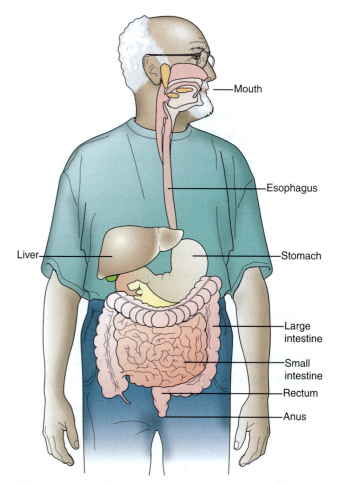

Figure 26-13

The digestive tract consists of the mouth, esophagus, stomach, small intestine, large intestine, rectum, and anus.

Bowel Habits

The frequency of a person's bowel movements, and the amount of feces passed each time, will differ from person to person. Many factors influence a person's bowel elimination pattern, including the amount of fluid the person drinks and the type of food he or she eats, the types of medications the person takes, the person's age, the person's level of activity, and the person's lifelong elimination habits. For example, some people have a bowel movement every morning. Other people are not so predictable. For some people, one or two bowel movements a day is normal. For others, one bowel movement every 2 or 3 days is normal. You will soon become aware of the bowel elimination pattern that is normal for each resident in your care. This knowledge will allow you to recognize any changes that may occur.

TELL THE NURSE

Changes in the quality of a person's feces or bowel elimination pattern can be a sign that something is wrong. Be sure to report the following observations to the nurse immediately:

- The person has diarrhea or is constipated
- There is blood or mucus in the stool
- The stool is black or dark green
- The stool is foul-smelling
- The person complains that the feces are painful or difficult to pass
- There is bleeding from the anus during or after a bowel movement
- The person has a swollen abdomen or complains of abdominal pain
- The person complains of liquid feces "seeping" from the anus
- The person has excessive flatus (gas)

PROBLEMS WITH BOWEL ELIMINATION

Problems with bowel elimination that are often seen in the health care setting include diarrhea, constipation, fecal impaction, flatulence, and fecal incontinence.

Diarrhea

Diarrhea is the passage of liquid, unformed stool. Diarrhea may occur frequently and can

be accompanied by abdominal cramping. If diarrhea is frequent or excessive, the loss of fluid from the body can quickly cause dehydration, especially in elderly people. When caring for a person with diarrhea:

- Practice good infection control techniques. A common cause of diarrhea is a bacterial or viral infection. Because the pathogen that caused the diarrhea will be present in the feces, it is important to use good infection control techniques when caring for a person with diarrhea.
- Answer the call light quickly to provide access to the toilet, commode, or bedpan. A normally continent person can have temporary fecal incontinence from diarrhea, which can be very humiliating. Being quick to respond, compassionate, and supportive can help the person to feel better.
- Provide gentle, thorough skin care after each bowel movement to prevent skin breakdown.
- Make sure to record and report the frequency and amount of each incident of diarrhea.

Constipation

The opposite of diarrhea is constipation. **Constipation** occurs when the feces remain in the intestines for too long. The delay allows too much fluid to be reabsorbed by the intestines, resulting in hard, dry feces that are difficult to pass. Constipation is fairly common among residents of long-term care facilities. Risk factors for developing constipation include:

- Taking medications that slow peristalsis (for example, pain medications)
- Not taking in enough dietary fiber or fluids
- Not getting enough exercise
- Delaying having a bowel movement after the urge occurs
- Lack of privacy

As you learned earlier in this chapter, there are many things a nursing assistant can do to help a resident maintain normal bowel function and prevent constipation. For example, encouraging residents to eat fiber-rich foods, drink plenty of fluids, and exercise regularly can help to keep bowel function regular. However, if a person is constipated and all other methods of promoting normal bowel function have failed, the doctor may order a laxative, stool softener, or fiber supplement.

- A **laxative** is a medication that chemically stimulates peristalsis so that material inside the intestines moves through at a faster pace. The resulting bowel movement is soft (or possibly liquid) and occurs within a few hours of taking the laxative, or overnight. Laxatives are acceptable for occasional use, but should not be used regularly. Regular laxative use causes the chyme to pass through the intestines too quickly for nutrients and fluids to be absorbed. This can result in poor nutrition and dehydration. The intestines also become used to being chemically stimulated to move and can become dependent on the laxative.

- **Stool softeners** help to keep fluid in the feces and are used to help prevent constipation for some people. Unlike laxatives, stool softeners do not chemically stimulate the intestines to cause a bowel movement.
- **Fiber supplements,** in the form of tablets or drink additives, can add bulk to the feces, causing the feces to hold fluid and preventing constipation.

Fecal Impaction

A **fecal impaction** occurs when constipation is not relieved. The feces build up in the rectum and become harder and harder as more and more fluid is absorbed. Eventually, it becomes almost impossible to pass the feces normally. The impaction blocks the passage of normal stool, but liquid stool may go around the impacted mass. A person with an impaction is usually very uncomfortable, and may complain of abdominal or rectal pain or of liquid feces "seeping" out of the anus. The person's abdomen may be swollen. The person may also have a decreased appetite, nausea, or vomiting.

If a person is thought to have a fecal impaction, the nurse will perform a **digital examination** (Fig. 26-14). *Digital* means "finger." During the digital examination, the nurse inserts a finger into the person's rectum to feel for the impacted mass. The impaction is removed by breaking the impacted feces apart and scooping it out of the rectum piece by piece. The doctor may also order the use of an oil retention enema or medication to help remove the impaction. Digital removal of a fecal impaction is very uncomfortable and embarrassing for most residents.

Many facilities require that a nurse remove an impaction. Nursing assistants are usually responsible for assisting the nurse during the procedure by supporting the person in the proper position, providing reassurance, and monitoring the person for signs of distress (because the nurse will not be

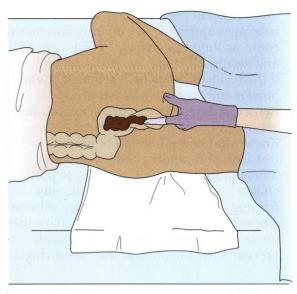

Figure 26-14
Digital examination. A finger is inserted into the person's rectum to check for a fecal impaction.

able to see the person's face). Rectal procedures can stimulate the vagus nerve, which can affect the person's heart rate and blood pressure. Be alert for a change in the person's color, shortness of breath, or loss of consciousness. If removing an impaction is within your scope of practice, make sure you have been adequately trained for the procedure and that it is part of your job description.

As you recall from Chapter 6, the government considers a fecal impaction a sentinel event (that is, a condition that should rarely, if ever, be seen in a resident of a nursing home). If a resident develops a fecal impaction, the survey team will be observing the care that is provided to all residents to maintain regular bowel elimination. The surveyors will also check documentation to make sure that proper care was provided to the resident who developed the fecal impaction. As a nursing assistant, you play a very important role in helping to prevent your residents from developing fecal impactions. To help prevent fecal impactions:

- Find out from the nurse how much fluid you need to provide to ensure that the resident takes in enough fluid to maintain effective bowel elimination and prevent dehydration. Be sure to tell the nurse immediately if you cannot get the resident to take the needed amount.
- Offer the resident fluids at every opportunity (unless the resident has orders for fluid restriction).

- If the resident does not find water or other beverages appealing, try offering snacks that count as fluids (such as ice cream, popsicles, and gelatin).
- If the resident needs help drinking or eating, provide the necessary assistance.
- Report to the nurse any problems you have getting the resident to take fluids.
- Know what bowel habits are normal for the resident, and report changes in bowel habits to the nurse immediately. Reporting changes, such as hard stool, difficulty passing stool, or more than 2 days without a bowel movement, promptly can allow the nurse to take quick action and possibly prevent a fecal impaction from occurring.

Flatulence

Flatulence is the presence of excessive amounts of flatus (gas) in the intestines, causing abdominal distension (swelling) and discomfort. Sometimes people have difficulty passing flatus because of a lack of activity or a recent surgical procedure. Getting out of bed and walking might be all that is needed to help the person to expel the gas. If walking is not allowed, positioning the person on her left side may help. If the flatulence cannot be relieved with these methods, a nurse may insert a rectal tube (a short piece of plastic tubing similar to the tubing used to administer an enema) to help the gas escape.

Fecal Incontinence

Fecal (bowel) incontinence is the inability to hold one's feces, or the involuntary loss of feces from the bowel. Like urinary incontinence, fecal incontinence can be temporary or permanent. Temporary fecal incontinence can occur with a severe case of diarrhea, simply because the person might not be able to get to the bathroom quickly enough. Some people experience temporary fecal incontinence if the call light is not answered soon enough. Diseases or injuries that affect the nervous system can also result in temporary or permanent fecal incontinence. A person who is unconscious will be incontinent of feces. A person who has dementia will develop fecal incontinence as the disease progresses.

Bowel training is very similar to bladder training and works to promote regular, controlled bowel movements. Offering the commode or bedpan at regular scheduled intervals is a common method of bowel training. Bowel training is often started by keeping track of when an incontinent person usually has a bowel movement, then making sure to provide the appropriate toilet facilities during that time period.

Be Smart About Surveys!

Assisting residents with urinary and bowel elimination is a very important part of providing quality care for your residents. Surveyors will want to see that staff members are taking the proper steps to promote normal urinary and bowel elimination and to manage incontinence. To help your facility remain without survey problems in this area:

- Make sure call light controls are within easy reach, and be sure to answer the call light promptly.
- Offer fluids each time you interact with a resident (unless the resident has orders for fluid restriction).
- Keep the nurse well informed of the resident's fluid intake and urinary and bowel habits.
- Be aware of, and maintain, toileting schedules, as specified on the resident's care plan.
- When a resident is incontinent, protect the resident's skin by providing good perineal care and applying a barrier ointment or cream after each episode of incontinence.
- For residents with indwelling urinary catheters, provide catheter care per your facility's policy.
- Take steps to promote quality of life. Provide residents who have indwelling urinary catheters with cloth covers for their urine drainage bags. For residents who are incontinent, maintain toileting schedules (to help prevent accidents) and assist with hygiene so that these residents can continue to enjoy social interactions without fear, worry, or self-consciousness.
- Document the care you provide per your facility's policy so that there is a record of the steps you have taken to promote normal urinary and bowel elimination and manage incontinence.

ENEMAS

An **enema** is the introduction of fluid into the large intestine by way of the anus for the purpose of removing stool from the rectum. There are several reasons a person would be given an enema.

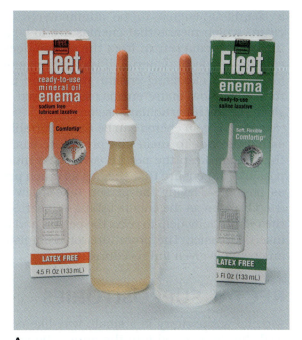
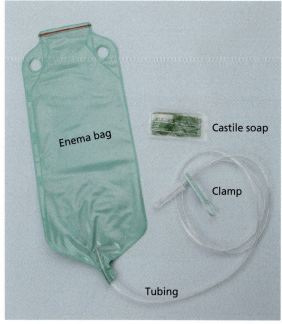

A   **B**

Figure 26-15
There are many different types of enema solutions. **(A)** Commercially prepared enema solutions. **(B)** A soapsuds enema is prepared using castile soap and water (not shown) and administered using an enema bag.

Enemas are used to relieve constipation and fecal impactions and to empty the intestine of fecal material before surgery or certain diagnostic tests. Sometimes enemas are used as part of a bowel-training program.

Types of Enemas

Several types of enemas are used in the health care setting (Fig. 26-15). Some are prepared by the nurse or nursing assistant, and others come prepackaged. The solution that is placed into the rectum varies according to the reason the enema was ordered.

- **Cleansing enemas.** Cleansing enemas are primarily used to remove feces from the lower large intestine. Tap water enemas and saline (salt water) enemas help soften the stool and stimulate peristalsis. Enemas containing these solutions should not be given repeatedly, because the intestine can absorb the solution, causing a fluid imbalance in the body. Soapsuds enemas consist of water and a small amount of a very gentle soap called *castile soap*. The soap solution irritates the lining of the

bowel, stimulating peristalsis. These, too, must be used with caution because too much soap can cause damage to the lining of the intestines.
- **Oil retention enemas.** An oil retention enema contains mineral, olive, or cottonseed oil. The oil lubricates the inside of the intestine and any stool that is present, making the stool easier to pass or remove. Oil retention enemas are useful for helping to remove fecal impactions.
- **Commercial enemas.** Commercially prepared and packaged enemas usually contain 120 mL of a solution that irritates the intestinal mucosa to promote peristalsis. Some commercial enemas contain a solution that is absorbed into the stool to make it softer and easier to pass.

Administering Enemas

Enemas are ordered by a doctor and usually given by a nurse. Some facilities allow nursing assistants to administer enemas after adequate training. Make sure you are familiar with your facility's policies on the administration of enemas. If you are permitted to give enemas, be sure to follow

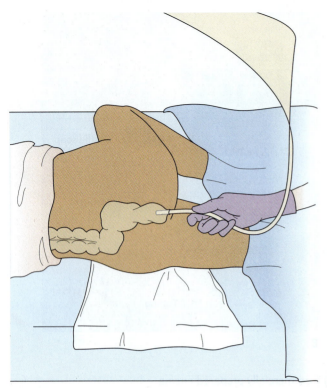

Figure 26-16
The left Sims' position is used when a person is to receive an enema. This position exposes the greatest amount of the bowel to the enema solution.

proper procedure and the doctor's orders closely. Make sure the solution is correct for the person, that you have the correct amount of solution, and that the solution is at the proper temperature. Enema solutions that are too cool can cause abdominal cramping and pain, while solutions that are too hot can cause serious injury and possibly even death. When you are assisting with the administration of an enema, make sure that a bed protector and bedpan are in place, or that the path to the bathroom is clear. When it comes time for the person to expel the enema, she will need immediate access to toilet facilities.

An enema is given with the person on her left side in Sims' position. When a person is lying on her left side in Sims' position, the intestine is positioned to take the best advantage of gravity. The solution will flow downward to clean a longer segment of bowel (Fig. 26-16). Having the person lie on her right side in Sims' position is not as effective, because the enema solution flows only as far as the rectum and does not clean as much of the bowel. After the enema has been administered, the person is asked to hold the solution in the bowel for the specified amount of time, and then to expel the solution. The doctor may order

a cleansing enema to be administered "until clear," which means that enemas are to be given until the enema return from the person does not contain any fecal material. If you are responsible for giving a cleansing enema, make sure to ask the nurse how many enemas are allowed to be given during a particular session.

Receiving an enema can be uncomfortable and embarrassing. To make the procedure easier for the person, keep the person covered as much as possible and ensure that she has as much privacy as possible. Having the person take a few slow, deep breaths as the enema tubing is inserted into the rectum may help to relax the person and make insertion easier. The procedure for administering an enema is given in Procedure 26-8.

RECTAL SUPPOSITORIES

A rectal suppository is a small, wax-like cone or oval that is inserted into the anus. The wax-like substance dissolves at body temperature, stimulating peristalsis or lubricating and softening the stool. Glycerin rectal suppositories are often used to help with bowel elimination, before resorting to an enema. Some rectal suppositories also contain medication. These should only be inserted by a nurse.

BOWEL DIVERSION

Some people may have some or all of their large intestine surgically removed as part of the treatment for illness or injury. Cancer, diverticulitis (an inflammatory disease of the bowel), and bowel trauma are reasons why surgical removal of all or part of the large intestine may be necessary. Depending on the location of the diseased part of the intestine and the length of the segment of the intestine that had to be removed, the person may need an alternate way of eliminating feces from the body following the surgery. In this case, the person will have a bowel diversion procedure. A **stoma** (a surgically created opening in the abdominal wall) is made and the remaining portion of the intestine is connected to it (Fig. 26-17). Feces pass through the stoma and into a pouch (called an **ostomy appliance**) that is worn over the stoma (Fig. 26-18).

- An **ileostomy** is created if the entire large intestine must be removed. The end of the small intestine (that is, the ileum) is attached to the abdominal wall. Because the chyme does not have the chance to travel through the large intestine (where water is

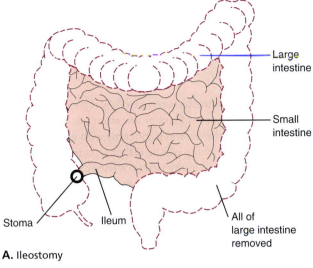

A. Ileostomy

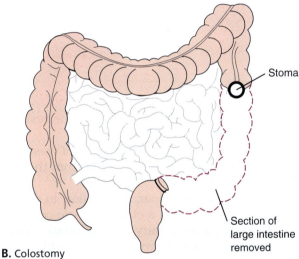

B. Colostomy

Figure 26-17

Some of the people you will care for may have had surgery to remove all or part of the large intestine. Such a surgery may be necessary because of cancer, a bowel obstruction, or trauma. **(A)** Ileostomy. The entire large intestine is removed. A stoma is made in the abdominal wall, and the end of the small intestine (the ileum) is sewn into place. **(B)** Colostomy. Part of the large intestine is removed. A colostomy can be done at any point along the large intestine; here, a section of the descending colon was removed. A stoma is made in the abdominal wall, and the healthy end of the remaining large intestine is sewn into place.

reabsorbed), the person's feces are very liquid and may flow fairly continuously. For this reason, a person with an ileostomy is quite prone to dehydration.

- A **colostomy** is created if part of the large intestine is still present. After the diseased part of the large intestine is removed, the healthy end is attached to the abdominal wall.

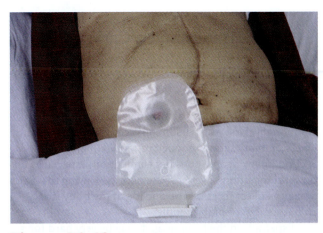

Figure 26-18

An ostomy appliance is worn over the stoma to collect the feces.

Sometimes, a temporary colostomy is done to allow a portion of the bowel to "rest." Later, the ends of the bowel are sewn back together and normal bowel elimination resumes. Among people with colostomies, the feces vary in consistency. If the portion of the intestine that was removed was near the beginning of the large intestine, then the feces will be more liquid because the chyme will spend less time in the large intestine. On the other hand, if the portion of the intestine that was removed was near the end of the large intestine, then the feces will be more solid and formed.

Ostomy appliances vary greatly. Some ostomy appliances consist of a bag with an adhesive opening that adheres to the skin around the stoma. Other ostomy appliances have two pieces—a ring of flexible rubber that is applied to the skin around the stoma, and a bag that is snapped on to the ring. Some appliances are used only once and then discarded, while others are emptied, cleaned, and used again.

Because the skin around the stoma comes into contact with feces, it must be kept clean to prevent irritation. If you are permitted to assist a resident who has had a bowel diversion procedure with ostomy care, make sure that you are familiar with the different types of ostomy appliances used in your facility and ask the nurse for help with any that are new to you. The ostomy appliance can be changed with the person sitting or standing in the bathroom, or while the person is in bed. If the ostomy appliance is being changed while the person is in bed, the person should either sit upright or lie flat. Procedure 26-9 describes how to assist a person who has had a bowel diversion procedure with routine ostomy care.

Helping Hands and a Caring Heart
FOCUS ON HUMANISTIC HEALTH CARE

For many people, having an ostomy is very difficult, emotionally. First, the person must cope with having an illness or injury serious enough to require major surgery. Second, many people consider elimination, especially bowel elimination, a very private activity. Having to wear a bag to collect feces on the outside of the body is very embarrassing for many people.

Especially in the beginning, it may be very hard for a person to accept the ostomy. If you are caring for someone who is getting used to the idea of having an ostomy, take the time to listen carefully if the person wants to talk about his fears or uncertainties. Be careful not to brush off the person's concerns with a comment such as "Oh, everything will be OK now; don't worry." Instead, put yourself in the person's shoes and think about how you would feel if you were in the same situation. Report the person's comments and questions to the nurse. Once the nurse knows that the person is having trouble adjusting to the ostomy, there are many things he or she can do to help the person adjust.

SUMMARY

- The elimination of waste products from the body is one of the most basic physical needs.
  - Although elimination is a natural function, many people are not comfortable discussing it or doing it in front of others. A person's culture and upbringing influence how comfortable he is with the body processes involved in elimination.
  - Normal urinary and bowel elimination can be promoted by encouraging fluids, answering the call light promptly, and providing for the person's privacy and comfort.
  - Incontinence is the inability to hold one's urine, feces, or both until a suitable receptacle (for example, a toilet, bedside commode, or bedpan) is made available. Incontinence has many causes and may be temporary or permanent.
    - Incontinence is difficult emotionally for both the person who is incontinent and that person's caregiver.
    - Being incontinent of urine or feces places a person at risk for skin breakdown. Providing good perineal care is essential when caring for a person who is incontinent of urine, feces, or both.
    - Fear of having an incontinence accident or self-consciousness about odor may cause a resident to avoid socializing with others. This can lead to feelings of isolation, depression, and anxiety, and

has a very negative effect on the resident's quality of life.
- The urinary system rids the body of waste products that have been filtered from the bloodstream.
  - Normal urine is clear, pale yellow to dark gold in color, with a characteristic odor. Urinary patterns vary among individuals. Any abnormal observations should be reported to the nurse.
  - A person who is having trouble urinating for physical or emotional reasons may need to have a urinary catheter placed to remove the urine from the bladder.
    - Urinary catheters may be left in place for an extended period of time, or inserted and then removed as soon as the bladder has been drained.
    - Providing good catheter care is essential to prevent health care-associated infections (HAIs). The use of urinary catheters is the leading cause of HAIs.
- The digestive system rids the body of waste products that are left over from digestion.
  - Normal stool is soft, brown, moist, formed, and has a distinct odor. Bowel elimination patterns vary among individuals. Any abnormal observations should be reported to the nurse.
    - Constipation occurs when feces remain in the intestine too long and excess fluid is absorbed, leaving the stool hard and

difficult to pass. Fecal impaction can result if constipation is not relieved.

- Diarrhea is the passage of liquid, unformed stool. Diarrhea can lead to dehydration.

- An enema is the introduction of solution into the large intestine. An enema is sometimes ordered by a doctor to treat or prevent bowel elimination problems.

  - The type of enema solution used is determined by the reason the enema has been ordered.

- Enemas are usually given by a nurse. However, in some facilities, enema administration is within the scope of practice of the nursing assistant. Enemas must be administered correctly, with special attention paid to the position of the person.

- You may care for a resident who has had a bowel diversion (for example, as a treatment for cancer). Assisting these residents with ostomy care helps to keep the stoma and surrounding skin clean and healthy.

PROCEDURE 26-1

Assisting a Person With Using a Bedpan

WHY YOU DO IT Bedpans are used for women who cannot get out of bed to urinate or have a bowel movement and for men who cannot get out of bed to have a bowel movement.

Getting Ready WGKIEPS
1. Complete the "Getting Ready" steps.

Supplies
- gloves
- bed protector
- toilet paper
- bedpan
- bedpan cover (or paper towels)
- perineal care supplies
- washcloth
- towel

Procedure
2. Make sure that the bed is positioned at a comfortable working height (to promote good body mechanics) and that the wheels are locked. If the side rails are in use, lower the side rail on the working side of the bed. The side rail on the opposite side of the bed should remain up. If necessary, lower the head of the bed so that the bed is flat (as tolerated).

3. Put on the gloves.

4. Fanfold the top linens to the foot of the bed. Place the bed protector on the bed. Adjust the person's hospital gown or pajama bottoms as necessary to expose the person's buttocks.

5. Place the bedpan underneath the person's buttocks. This can be accomplished by either helping the person to lie on her side, facing away from you, or by asking the person to bend her knees, press her heels into the mattress, and lift her buttocks. Slide the bedpan underneath the person (if the person is holding her buttocks away from the bed by bending her knees) or place the bedpan against her buttocks and help her to roll back onto it.

   a. A standard bedpan is positioned like a regular toilet seat.

b. A fracture pan is positioned with the narrow end pointed toward the head of the bed.

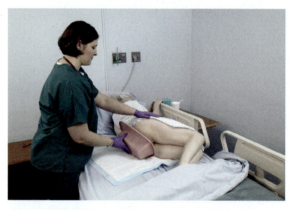

Step 5 Place the bedpan against the person's buttocks and help the person to roll back onto it.

6. Raise the head of the bed as tolerated. Draw the top linens over the person for modesty and warmth.

7. Make sure that the toilet paper and the call-light control are within reach. If the side rails are in use, return the side rails to the raised position.

8. Remove your gloves and wash your hands.

9. If safety permits, leave the room and ask the person to call you when she is finished. Remember to close the door on your way out.

10. Return when the person signals. Remember to knock before entering.

11. If the side rails are in use, lower the side rail on the working side of the bed. Lower the head of the bed so that the bed is flat (as tolerated).

12. Put on a clean pair of gloves.

13. Fanfold the top linens to the foot of the bed.

14. Ask the person to bend her knees, press her heels into the mattress, and lift her buttocks so that you can remove the bedpan and bed protector. (Or help the person to roll onto her side, facing away from you, while you hold the bedpan securely in place against the mattress to prevent the contents from spilling. Remove the bedpan and bed protector and then help the person to roll back.) If necessary, help the person to use the toilet paper.

15. Cover the bedpan with the bedpan cover or paper towels. Take the bedpan to the bathroom. (If the side rails are in use, raise them before leaving the bedside.)

16. Remove your gloves and dispose of them in a facility-approved waste container. Wash your hands.

17. Return to the bedside. Give the person a wet washcloth and help the person to wash her hands. Make sure the person's perineum is clean and dry. If necessary, provide perineal care.

18. Adjust the person's hospital gown or pajama bottoms as necessary to cover the buttocks. Help the person back into a comfortable

position, straighten the bottom linens, and draw the top linens over the person. Raise the head of the bed, as the person requests. Make sure that the bed is lowered to its lowest position and that the wheels are locked.

19. Return to the bathroom. Put on a clean pair of gloves. If the person is on intake and output (I&O) status, measure the urine. Note the color, amount, and quality of the urine or feces before emptying the contents of the bedpan into the toilet. (If anything unusual is observed, do not empty the bedpan until a nurse has had a chance to look at its contents.)

20. Gather the soiled linens and place them in the linen hamper or linen bag. Dispose of disposable items in a facility-approved waste container. Clean equipment and return it to the storage area.

21. Remove your gloves and dispose of them in a facility-approved waste container.

Finishing Up CLSOWR
22. Complete the "Finishing Up" steps.

PROCEDURE 26-2

Assisting a Man With Using a Urinal

WHY YOU DO IT   Urinals are used for men who cannot get out of bed to urinate.

Getting Ready WGKIEpS
1. Complete the "Getting Ready" steps.

Supplies
- gloves
- toilet paper
- urinal
- washcloth
- towel

Procedure
2. Ask the man what position he prefers—lying, sitting, or standing. If necessary, raise the head of the bed as tolerated. If the man would prefer to stand, help him to sit on the edge of the bed and then to stand up.

3. Put on the gloves.

4. Hand the man the urinal. If necessary, assist him in positioning it correctly.

5. Make sure that the toilet paper and the call-light control are within reach.

6. Remove your gloves and wash your hands.

7. If safety permits, leave the room and ask the man to call you when he is finished. Remember to close the door on your way out.

8. Return when the man signals. Remember to knock before entering.

9. Put on a clean pair of gloves. Have the man hand you the urinal, or remove it if he is unable to hand it to you. Put the lid on the urinal and hang it on the side rail while you

(continued)

assist the man with handwashing and perineal care as needed. Lower the head of the bed as the man requests.

10. Take the urinal to the bathroom. If the man is on intake and output (I&O) status, measure the urine. Note the color, amount, and quality of the urine before emptying the contents of the urinal into the toilet. (If anything unusual is observed, do not empty the urinal until a nurse has had a chance to look at its contents.)

11. Gather the soiled linens and place them in the linen hamper or linen bag. Dispose of disposable items in a facility-approved waste container. Clean equipment and return it to the storage area.

12. Remove your gloves and dispose of them in a facility-approved waste container.

Finishing Up CLSOWR

13. Complete the "Finishing Up" steps.

PROCEDURE 26-3

Collecting a Routine Urine Specimen

WHY YOU DO IT   A routine urine specimen is often requested for urinalysis. Proper collection and handling of the urine specimen helps to ensure that the urinalysis results are accurate.

Getting Ready WGKIEPS

1. Complete the "Getting Ready" steps.

Supplies

- gloves
- paper towel
- toilet paper
- specimen container and label
- plastic transport bag (if required at your facility)
- plastic bag or waste container
- specimen collection device ("commode hat"), bedpan, or urinal

Procedure

2. Complete the label with the person's name, room number, and other identifying information. Put the completed label on the specimen container. Take the specimen container to the bathroom. Place a paper towel on the counter. Open the specimen container and place the lid on the paper towel, with the inside of the lid facing up.

3. If the person will be using a regular toilet or bedside commode, fit the specimen collection device underneath the toilet or commode seat. Otherwise, provide the person with a bedpan or urinal, as applicable.

4. Assist the person with urination as necessary. Before leaving the room, remind the person not to have a bowel movement or place toilet paper into the specimen collection device, bedpan, or urinal. Provide a plastic bag or waste container for the used toilet paper.

5. Return when the person signals. Remember to knock before entering.

6. Put on the gloves.

7. If the person used a regular toilet or bedside commode, assist the person with handwashing and perineal care as necessary and then help the person to return to bed. If the person used a bedpan or urinal, cover and remove the bedpan or urinal and assist the person with handwashing and perineal care as necessary.

8. Take the covered bedpan, urinal, or specimen collection device (if the person used a bedside commode) to the bathroom. (If the side rails are in use, raise the side rails before leaving the bedside.)

9. If the person is on intake and output (I&O) status, measure the urine. Note the color, amount, and quality of the urine.

10. Raise the toilet seat. While holding the specimen container over the toilet, carefully fill it

about three-quarters full with urine from the specimen collection device, bedpan, or urinal. Discard the rest of the urine into the toilet.

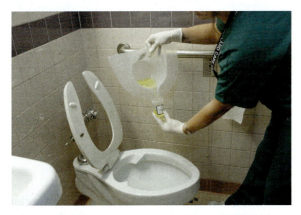

Step 10 Hold the specimen container over the toilet and fill it about three-quarters full with urine.

11. Put the lid on the specimen container. Make sure that the lid is tight. Put the specimen container on the paper towel on the counter.

12. Remove one glove and dispose of it in a facility-approved waste container. Holding the plastic transport bag in your ungloved hand, place the specimen container into the transport bag with your gloved hand. Avoid touching the outside of the transport bag with your glove.

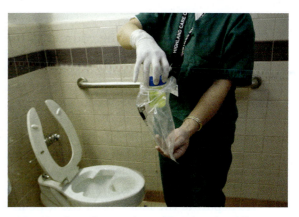

Step 12 Place the specimen container into the transport bag with your gloved hand.

13. Remove the other glove and dispose of it in a facility-approved waste container.

14. Gather the soiled linens and place them in the linen hamper or linen bag. Dispose of disposable items in a facility-approved waste container. Clean equipment and return it to the storage area.

15. Take the specimen container to the designated location.

Finishing Up   CLSOWR

16. Complete the "Finishing Up" steps.

PROCEDURE 26-4

Collecting a Midstream ("Clean Catch") Urine Specimen

WHY YOU DO IT   A midstream ("clean catch") urine specimen is often requested for urinalysis when the doctor suspects a urinary tract infection. Proper collection and handling of the urine specimen helps to ensure that the urinalysis results are accurate.

Getting Ready   WGKIEpS

1. Complete the "Getting Ready" steps.

Supplies

- gloves
- paper towel
- toilet paper
- specimen container and label
- "clean catch" kit
- plastic transport bag (if required at your facility)
- bedpan or urinal (if necessary)

Procedure

2. Complete the label with the person's name, room number, and other identifying information. Put the completed label on the specimen container.

3. If the person will be using a regular toilet or bedside commode, help the person to the bathroom or bedside commode. Otherwise, provide the person with a bedpan or urinal, as applicable.

(continued)

4. Put on the gloves.

5. Place a paper towel on the counter (if the person is in the bathroom) or on the over-bed table (if the person is using a bedside commode, bedpan, or urinal). Open the specimen container and place the lid on the paper towel, with the inside of the lid facing up.

6. Open the "clean catch" kit. Have the person clean his or her perineum using the wipes in the kit. Assist as necessary:

   a. **If the person is a woman:** Use one hand to separate the labia. Hold the wipe in the other hand. Place your wipe-covered hand at the top of the vulva and stroke downward to the anus.

   b. **If the person is a circumcised man:** Use one hand to hold the penis slightly away from the body. Hold the wipe in the other hand. Place your wipe-covered hand at the tip of the penis and wash in a circular motion, downward to the base of the penis.

   c. **If the person is an uncircumcised man:** Retract the foreskin by gently pushing the skin toward the base of the penis. Place your wipe-covered hand at the tip of the penis and wash in a circular motion, downward to the base of the penis.

7. Assist the person with urination as necessary. Before leaving the room:

   a. Make sure that the toilet paper, call light control, and specimen container are within reach.

   b. Remind the person that he or she must start the stream of urine, then stop it, then restart it. The urine sample is to be collected from the restarted flow. If the person is a woman, she must hold the labia open until the specimen is collected. If the person is an uncircumcised man, he must keep the foreskin pulled back until the specimen is collected.

8. Remove your gloves and dispose of them in a facility-approved waste container.

9. Return when the person signals. Remember to knock before entering.

10. Put on a clean pair of gloves.

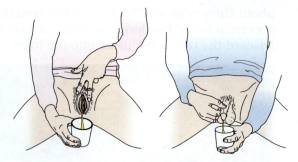

Step 7b Women must hold the labia open while voiding to prevent contamination of the urine sample. Uncircumcised men must keep the foreskin pulled back.

11. If the person used a regular toilet or bedside commode, assist the person with handwashing and perineal care as necessary and then help the person to return to bed. If the person used a bedpan or urinal, remove the bedpan or urinal and assist the person with handwashing and perineal care as necessary.

12. Put the lid on the specimen container, being careful not to touch the inside of the lid or container. Make sure that the lid is tight. Put the specimen container on the paper towel on the counter or over-bed table.

13. Remove one glove and dispose of it in a facility-approved waste container. Holding the plastic transport bag in your ungloved hand, place the specimen container into the transport bag with your gloved hand. Avoid touching the outside of the transport bag with your glove.

14. Remove the other glove and dispose of it in a facility-approved waste container.

15. Gather the soiled linens and place them in the linen hamper or linen bag. Dispose of disposable items in a facility-approved waste container. Clean equipment and return it to the storage area.

16. Take the specimen container to the designated location.

Finishing Up CLOSUR

17. Complete the "Finishing Up" steps.

PROCEDURE / **26-5**

Collecting a Stool Specimen

WHY YOU DO IT   A stool specimen is often requested for analysis. Proper collection and handling of the stool specimen helps to ensure that the test results are accurate.

Getting Ready WGKIEpS

1. Complete the "Getting Ready" steps.

Supplies

- gloves
- paper towel
- tongue depressor
- toilet paper
- specimen container and label
- plastic transport bag (if required at your facility)
- plastic bag or waste container
- specimen collection device ("commode hat") or bedpan

Procedure

2. Complete the label with the person's name, room number, and other identifying information. Put the completed label on the specimen container. Take the specimen container to the bathroom. Place a paper towel on the counter. Open the specimen container and place the lid on the paper towel with the inside of the lid facing up.

3. If the person will be using a regular toilet or bedside commode, fit the specimen collection device underneath the toilet or commode seat. Otherwise, provide the person with a bedpan.

4. Assist the person with defecation as necessary. Before leaving the room, remind the person not to urinate or place toilet paper into the specimen collection device or bedpan. Provide a plastic bag or waste container for the used toilet paper.

5. Return when the person signals. Remember to knock before entering.

6. Put on the gloves.

7. If the person used a regular toilet or bedside commode, assist the person with handwashing and then help the person to return to bed. Provide perineal care as necessary. If the person used a bedpan, cover and remove the bedpan and assist the person with hand-washing and perineal care as necessary.

8. Take the covered bedpan or specimen collection device (if the person used a bedside commode) to the bathroom. (If the side rails are in use, raise the side rails before leaving the bedside.)

9. Note the color, amount, and quality of the feces. Using the tongue depressor, take two tablespoons of feces from the bedpan or specimen collection device and put them into the specimen container. Dispose of the tongue depressor in a facility-approved waste container. Empty the remaining contents of the bedpan or specimen collection device into the toilet.

10. Put the lid on the specimen cup. Make sure that the lid is tight. Put the specimen container on the paper towel on the counter.

11. Remove one glove and dispose of it in a facility-approved waste container. Holding the plastic transport bag in your ungloved hand, place the specimen container into the transport bag with your gloved hand. Avoid touching the outside of the transport bag with your glove.

12. Remove the other glove and dispose of it in a facility-approved waste container.

13. Gather the soiled linens and place them in the linen hamper or linen bag. Dispose of disposable items in a facility-approved waste container. Clean equipment and return it to the storage area.

14. Take the specimen container to the designated location.

Finishing Up CLSOWR

15. Complete the "Finishing Up" steps.

PROCEDURE 26-6

Providing Catheter Care

WHY YOU DO IT   Providing proper catheter care helps to prevent the person from getting a urinary tract infection.

Getting Ready WORKERS

1. Complete the "Getting Ready" steps.

Supplies

- gloves
- paper towels
- bed protector
- bath thermometer
- wash basin
- soap or antiseptic solution
- bath blanket
- washcloths
- towels
- clean clothing

Procedure

2. Cover the over-bed table with paper towels.

3. Lower the head of the bed so that the bed is flat (as tolerated). Make sure that the bed is positioned at a comfortable working height (to promote good body mechanics) and that the wheels are locked.

4. Fill the wash basin with warm water (110°F [43.3°C] to 115°F [46.1°C] on the bath thermometer). Place the wash basin, soap, towels, and washcloths on the over-bed table.

5. If the side rails are in use, lower the side rail on the working side of the bed. The side rail on the opposite side of the bed should remain up.

6. Put on the gloves.

7. Spread the bath blanket over the top linens (and the person). If the person is able, have him or her hold the bath blanket. If not, tuck the corners under the person's shoulders. Fanfold the top linens to the foot of the bed.

8. Adjust the person's hospital gown or pajama bottoms as necessary to expose the person's perineum.

9. Ask the person to open his legs and bend his knees, if possible. If the person is not able to bend his knees, help the person to spread his legs as much as possible.

10. Position the bath blanket over the person so that one corner can be wrapped under and around each leg.

11. Position a bed protector under the person's buttocks to keep the bed linens dry.

12. Lift the corner of the bath blanket that is between the person's legs upward, exposing only the perineal area.

13. Form a mitt around your hand with one of the washcloths. Wet the mitt with warm, clean water and apply soap or antiseptic solution.

    a. **If the person is a woman:** Using the other hand, separate the labia. Place your washcloth-covered hand at the top of the vulva and stroke downward to the anus. Repeat, using a different part of the washcloth each time, until the area is clean. Rinse and dry the vulva and perineum thoroughly.

    b. **If the person is a circumcised man:** Place your washcloth-covered hand at the tip of the penis and wash in a circular motion, downward to the base of the penis. Repeat, using a different part of the washcloth each time, until the area is clean. Rinse and dry the tip and the shaft of the penis thoroughly.

    c. **If the person is an uncircumcised man:** Retract the foreskin by gently pushing the skin toward the base of the penis. Place your washcloth-covered hand at the tip of the penis and wash in a circular motion, downward to the base of the penis. Repeat, using a different part of the washcloth each time, until the area is clean. Rinse and dry the tip and the shaft of the penis thoroughly before gently pulling the foreskin back into its normal position.

14. Using a clean part of the washcloth, clean the catheter tubing, starting at the body and moving outward from the body about 4 inches.* Hold the catheter near the opening

---

*In some facilities, disposable antiseptic wipes may be used instead of a washcloth to clean the catheter tubing.

of the urethra. This will help to prevent tugging on the catheter as you clean it.

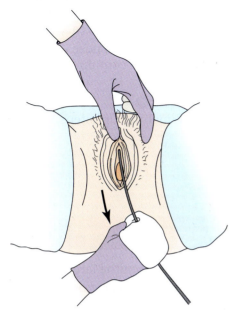

Step 14 Clean the catheter tubing, starting at the body and moving outward.

15. Dry the perineal area thoroughly using a towel.

16. Check that the catheter tubing is free from kinks. Make sure that it is securely taped to the person's leg.

17. Remove your gloves and dispose of them in a facility-approved waste container.

18. Assist the person into the supine position. Remove the bath blanket, and help the person into the clean clothing.

19. If the side rails are in use, return the side rails to the raised position. Raise the head of the bed as the person requests. Make sure that the bed is lowered to its lowest position and that the wheels are locked.

20. Gather the soiled linens and place them in the linen hamper or linen bag. Dispose of disposable items in a facility-approved waste container. Clean equipment and return it to the storage area.

Finishing Up CLSOWR

21. Complete the "Finishing Up" steps.

PROCEDURE 26-7

Emptying a Urine Drainage Bag

WHY YOU DO IT Urine drainage bags must be emptied whenever they are full and at the end of every shift (or as ordered).

Getting Ready WCKIEPS

1. Complete the "Getting Ready" steps.

Supplies

- gloves
- paper towels
- alcohol wipes (optional)
- graduate

Procedure

2. Put on the gloves.

3. Place a paper towel on the floor, underneath the urine drainage bag. Unhook the drainage bag emptying spout from its holder on the urine drainage bag. Position the graduate on the paper towel underneath the emptying spout.

4. Unclamp the emptying spout on the urine drainage bag and allow all of the urine to drain into the graduate. Avoid touching the

tip of the emptying spout with your hands or the side of the graduate.

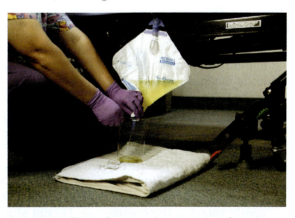

Step 4 Unclamp the emptying spout on the urine drainage bag and allow the urine to drain into the graduate.

(continued)

5. After the urine has drained into the graduate, wipe the emptying spout with an alcohol wipe (or follow facility policy). Reclamp the emptying spout and return it to its holder.

6. If the person is on intake and output (I&O) status, measure the urine. Note the color, amount, and quality of the urine before emptying the contents of the graduate into the toilet. (If anything unusual is observed, do not empty the graduate until a nurse has had a chance to look at its contents.)

7. Dispose of disposable items in a facility-approved waste container. Clean equipment and return it to the storage area.

8. Remove your gloves and dispose of them in a facility-approved waste container.

Finishing Up   CLSOWR

9. Complete the "Finishing Up" steps.

PROCEDURE 26-8

Administering a Soapsuds Enema

WHY YOU DO IT   A soapsuds enema may be ordered to remove feces from the large intestine prior to surgery or a diagnostic procedure. Proper administration of the enema is important to protect the person's safety and privacy during the procedure and to ensure that the enema is effective.

Getting Ready   WGKIEPS

1. Complete the "Getting Ready" steps.

Supplies

- gloves
- paper towel
- toilet paper
- bed protector
- lubricant jelly
- 5-mL packet of castile soap
- bedpan
- bedpan cover
- enema bag with tubing and clamp
- IV pole
- bath thermometer
- bath blanket
- perineal care supplies

Procedure

2. Make sure that the bed is positioned at a comfortable working height (to promote good body mechanics) and that the wheels are locked.

3. Prepare the enema solution in the bathroom or utility room. Clamp the tubing and then fill the enema bag with warm water (105°F [40.5°C] on the bath thermometer) in the specified amount (usually from 500 to 1500 mL). Add the castile soap packet and mix by gently rotating the enema bag. Do not shake the solution vigorously.

4. Release the clamp on the tubing and allow a little water to run through the tubing into the sink or bedpan. This will remove all of the air from the tubing. Reclamp the tubing.

5. Hang the enema bag on the IV pole and bring it to the person's bedside. Adjust the height of the IV pole so that the enema bag is hanging no more than 18 inches above the person's anus.

6. If the side rails are in use, lower the side rail on the working side of the bed. The side rail on the opposite side of the bed should remain up. Lower the head of the bed so that the bed is flat (as tolerated).

7. Spread the bath blanket over the top linens (and the person). If the person is able, have her hold the bath blanket. If not, tuck the corners under her shoulders. Fanfold the top linens to the foot of the bed.

8. Ask the person to lie on her left side, facing away from you, in Sims' position. Help her into this position, if necessary.

9. Put on the gloves.

10. Adjust the bath blanket and the person's hospital gown or pajama bottoms as necessary to expose the person's buttocks. Position the bed protector under the person's buttocks to keep the bed linens dry.

11. Open the lubricant package and squeeze a small amount of lubricant onto a paper

towel. Lubricate the tip of the enema tubing to ease insertion.

12. Suggest that the person take a deep breath and slowly exhale as the enema tubing is inserted. With one hand, raise the person's upper buttock to expose the anus. Using your other hand, gently and carefully insert the lubricated tip of the tubing into the person's rectum (not more than 3 to 4 inches for adults). Never force the tubing into the rectum. If you are unable to insert the tubing, stop and call the nurse.

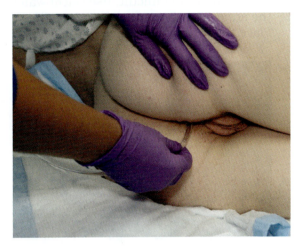

Step 12 Gently insert the top of the tubing into the person's rectum.

13. Unclamp the tubing and allow the solution to begin running. Hold the enema tubing firmly with one hand so that it does not slip out of the rectum. If the person complains of pain or cramping, slow down the rate of flow by tightening the clamp a bit. If the pain or cramping does not stop after slowing the rate of flow, stop the procedure and call the nurse.

14. When the fluid level reaches the bottom of the bag, clamp the tubing to avoid injecting air into the person's rectum.

15. Remove the tubing from the person's rectum and place it inside the enema bag. Gently

place several thicknesses of toilet paper against the person's anus to absorb any fluid.

16. Ask the person to retain the enema solution for the specific amount of time.

17. Assist the person with expelling the enema as necessary, using the bedpan, bedside commode, or toilet. If the person is using a regular toilet, ask her not to flush the toilet after expelling the enema.

18. If the person used a regular toilet or bedside commode, assist her with handwashing and then help her to return to bed. Provide perineal care as necessary. If the person used a bedpan, cover and remove the bedpan and assist her with handwashing and perineal care as necessary.

19. Raise the head of the bed as the person requests. Make sure that the bed is lowered to its lowest position and that the wheels are locked. (If the side rails are in use, raise the side rails before leaving the bedside.)

20. Take the covered bedpan or commode bucket (if the person used a bedside commode) to the bathroom.

21. Note the color, amount, and quality of feces before emptying the contents of the bedpan or commode bucket into the toilet. (If anything unusual is observed, do not empty the bedpan or commode bucket until a nurse has had a chance to look at its contents.)

22. Gather the soiled linens and place them in the linen hamper. Dispose of disposable items in a facility-approved waste container. Clean equipment and return it to the storage area.

23. Remove your gloves and dispose of them in a facility-approved waste container.

Finishing Up CLOSWR
24. Complete the "Finishing Up" steps.

PROCEDURE 26-9

Providing Routine Ostomy Care

WHY YOU DO IT   Because the skin around the stoma comes in contact with feces, it must be kept clean to prevent irritation.

Getting Ready WGKIEpS

1. Complete the "Getting Ready" steps.

Supplies

- gloves
- paper towels
- bed protector
- toilet paper
- 4 × 4 gauze pad
- clean ostomy appliance
- clean ostomy belt (if one is used)
- skin barrier
- bedpan
- bedpan cover (or paper towels)
- wash basin
- soap (or other cleansing agent, per facility policy)
- adhesive remover (optional)
- deodorant for ostomy appliance (optional)
- washcloths
- towel

Procedure

2. Cover the over-bed table with paper towels. Place the ostomy supplies and clean linens on the over-bed table.

3. Make sure that the bed is positioned at a comfortable working height (to promote good body mechanics) and that the wheels are locked.

4. If the side rails are in use, lower the side rail on the working side of the bed. The side rail on the opposite side of the bed should remain up. If necessary, lower the head of the bed so that the bed is flat (as tolerated).

5. Fanfold the top linens to below the person's waist.

6. Position the bed protector on the bed alongside the person to keep the bed linens dry. Adjust the person's clothing as necessary to expose the person's stoma.

7. Put on the gloves.

8. Disconnect the ostomy appliance from the ostomy belt if one is used. Remove the belt. If the ostomy belt is soiled, dispose of it in a facility-approved waste container (if it is disposable), or place it in the linen hamper or linen bag (if it is not disposable).

9. Remove the ostomy appliance by holding the skin taut and gently pulling the appliance away, starting at the top. If the adhesive is making removal difficult, use warm water or the adhesive solvent to soften the adhesive. Place the ostomy appliance in the bedpan.

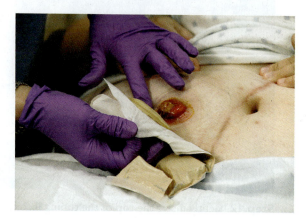

Step 9 Hold the skin taut and gently pull the ostomy appliance away.

10. Gently wipe the stoma with toilet paper to remove any feces or drainage. Place the toilet paper in the bedpan. Cover the stoma with the gauze pad to absorb any drainage that may occur until the new appliance is in place.

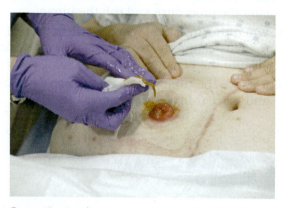

Step 10 Gently wipe the stoma with toilet tissue to remove drainage.

11. Cover the bedpan with the bedpan cover or paper towels. Take the bedpan to the

bathroom. (If the side rails are in use, raise them before leaving the bedside.)

12. Note the color, amount, and quality of the feces before emptying the contents of the ostomy appliance and the bedpan into the toilet. (If anything unusual is observed, do not empty the ostomy appliance until a nurse has had a chance to look at its contents.)

13. Dispose of the ostomy appliance in a facility-approved waste container.

14. Remove your gloves and dispose of them in a facility-approved waste container. Wash your hands.

15. Fill the wash basin with warm water (110°F [43.3°C] to 115°F [46.1°C] on the bath thermometer). Return to the bedside. Place the basin on the over-bed table. If the side rails are in use, lower the side rail on the working side of the bed.

16. Put on a clean pair of gloves.

17. Form a mitt around your hand with one of the washcloths. Wet the mitt with warm, clean water and apply soap (or other cleansing agent, per facility policy). Remove the gauze pad from the stoma and dispose of it in a facility-approved waste container. Clean the skin around the stoma. Rinse and dry the skin around the stoma thoroughly. Carefully observe the stoma and the surrounding skin. If you note any signs of irritation or inflammation, be sure to report these to the nurse.

18. Apply the skin barrier if needed, according to the manufacturer's directions.

19. Place the deodorant in the ostomy appliance if deodorant is used.

20. Put the clean ostomy belt on the person if an ostomy belt is used.

21. Make sure that the opening on the ostomy appliance is the correct size. Remove the adhesive backing on the ostomy appliance.

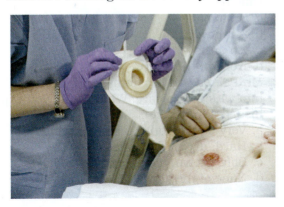

Step 21 Make sure the opening on the ostomy appliance is the correct size.

22. Center the appliance over the stoma, making sure that the drain or the end of the bag is pointed down. Gently press around the edges to seal the ostomy appliance to the skin.

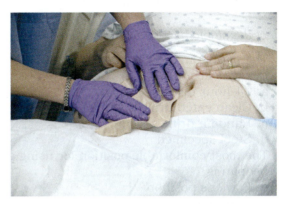

Step 22 Gently press the edges to seal the ostomy appliance to the skin.

23. Connect the ostomy appliance to the ostomy belt, if one is used.

24. Remove the bed protector.

25. Remove your gloves and dispose of them in a facility-approved waste container.

26. Adjust the person's clothing as necessary to cover the ostomy appliance. If the bedding is wet or soiled, change the bed linens. Help the person back into a comfortable position, straighten the bottom linens, and draw the top linens over the person. Raise the head of the bed, as the person requests.

27. If the side rails are in use, return the side rail to the raised position. Make sure that the bed is lowered to its lowest position and that the wheels are locked.

28. Gather the soiled linens and place them in the linen hamper or linen bag. Dispose of disposable items in a facility-approved waste container. Clean equipment and return it to the storage area.

Finishing Up CLOSWR

29. Complete the "Finishing Up" steps.

WHAT DID YOU LEARN?

Multiple Choice

Select the single best answer for each of the following questions.

1. The perineum (perineal area) is cleaned before collecting a
   a. 24-hour urine specimen
   b. Clean catch urine specimen
   c. Random urine specimen
   d. Stool specimen

2. The most comfortable position for using a bedpan is
   a. Fowler's position
   b. Sims' position
   c. Prone position
   d. Supine position

3. How far is an enema tube inserted into the rectum in an adult?
   a. 3 to 4 inches
   b. 5 to 6 inches
   c. 7 to 8 inches
   d. 12 to 16 inches

4. One of your residents needs to have an enema administered. How should you position the resident in preparation for the enema?
   a. Left Sims' position
   b. Fowler's position
   c. Supine position
   d. Right Sims' position

5. In a person with an indwelling urinary catheter, why must the urine drainage bag be kept lower than the person's bladder?
   a. Keeping the drainage bag below bladder level will prevent a bedridden person from seeing the bag, which he or she might find embarrassing
   b. Keeping the drainage bag below bladder level will keep the person comfortable in bed
   c. Keeping the drainage bag below bladder level will prevent urine from returning to the bladder, where it could cause infection
   d. Keeping the drainage bag below bladder level will prevent the urine from leaking out

6. Which one of the following describes normal urine?
   a. Cloudy with a strong odor
   b. Well-formed
   c. Red-tinged
   d. Clear, light yellow, or golden with a slight odor

7. A healthy person's feces will be:
   a. Black and tarry
   b. Soft, brown, formed, and moist with a distinct odor
   c. Hard and pellet-like
   d. Long and stringy

8. To help your residents or patients to maintain healthy bowel function, it is important to
   a. Answer call lights promptly
   b. Encourage them to eat a well-balanced diet and drink plenty of fluids
   c. Assist them with exercise
   d. All of the above

9. When caring for a person who is incontinent of urine or feces, it is important to:
   a. Provide good perineal care
   b. Let the person know that his or her behavior is inappropriate, so it will stop
   c. Take the person to the bathroom once daily
   d. Restrict fluids to reduce the chance of an accident

10. When caring for a person with an indwelling catheter, always remember to:
    a. Leave the drainage bag above the level of the bladder, while the person is in bed
    b. Tape any leaks at the connection site
    c. Wear gloves when providing catheter care
    d. Tape the drainage tube under the leg

11. What is the artificial opening for a colostomy called?
    a. A stoma
    b. A rectum
    c. An anus
    d. None of the above

12. Mr. Pak has an ileostomy, and you assist him with stoma care. What would you expect his feces to be like?
    a. Very liquid, continuously flowing
    b. Hard, dry, pellets
    c. Soft, brown, moist, and formed
    d. None of the above

Matching

Match each numbered item with its appropriate lettered description.

_____ **1.** Hematuria

_____ **2.** Peristalsis

_____ **3.** Micturition

_____ **4.** Defecation

_____ **5.** Nocturia

_____ **6.** Dysuria

_____ **7.** Urinalysis

_____ **8.** Anuria

_____ **9.** Oliguria

_____**10.** Polyuria

a. Excessive urine production
b. Excessive urination at night
c. Difficulty urinating
d. No urine production
e. Urination
f. Passing of feces
g. Routine urine test
h. Inadequate urine production
i. Blood in the urine
j. Wave-like muscular movement of the intestines

STOP and Think!

- You are a nursing assistant in a nursing home. Your new resident, Mrs. Walker, must use a bedpan because she is confined to bed. You notice that Mrs. Walker is finding it difficult to use the bedpan. What kinds of things could you do to help make using a bedpan easier for Mrs. Walker?

- You are caring for Miss Smiley, who has an indwelling catheter. When you are making your end-of-shift rounds, you note that Miss Smiley's urine drainage bag has very little urine in it. You know that the drainage bag was emptied right before you started your shift. That was almost 8 hours ago. Is this a cause for concern? Why or why not?

- Kelly has been assigned to care for Mrs. Ralph, who has a colostomy. She is unfamiliar with this term and doesn't know what to expect. If you were on Kelly's team, what would you tell Kelly to expect? What things would you tell Kelly to look for in caring for Mrs. Ralph?

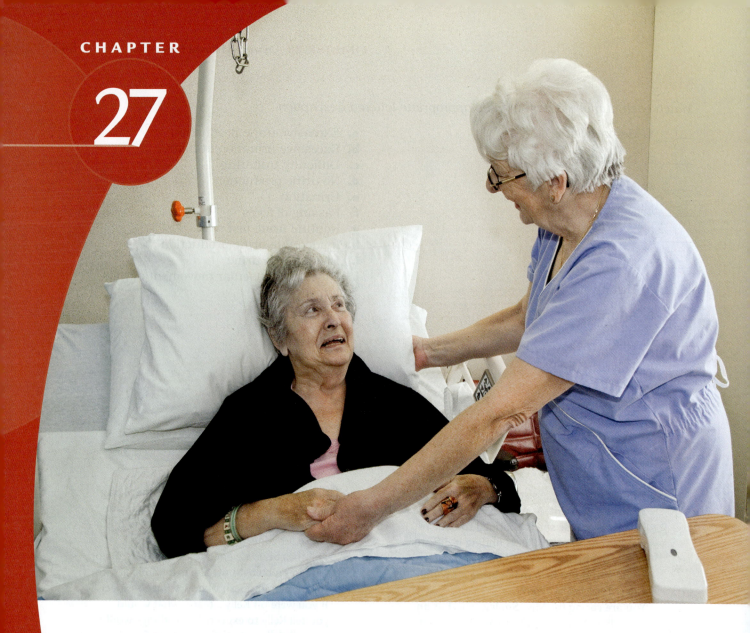

Comfort, Rest, and Sleep

WHAT WILL YOU LEARN?

When we are comfortable, we feel content, without pain or distress. We are able to rest, relax, and sleep. Helping residents to be as comfortable as possible and promoting rest and sleep are important parts of providing holistic care. In this chapter, you will learn about pain, which affects many residents' ability to be comfortable. You will also learn about rest and sleep, and why getting enough sleep is so important to a resident's well-being. When you are finished with this chapter, you will be able to:

1. Define pain and describe the difference between acute pain and chronic pain.
2. Discuss factors that can affect a person's response to pain.
3. List non-verbal signs of pain that a resident may show.

Photo: A nursing assistant helps to position a resident comfortably.

4. Describe methods a nursing assistant can use to gather more information about the nature of a resident's pain.

5. Explain the importance of promptly and accurately reporting a resident's pain.

6. Discuss the use of medications, physical therapy, and heat and cold applications to relieve pain and promote comfort.

7. Demonstrate how to safely use heat and cold applications in the long-term care setting.

8. Describe actions a nursing assistant can take to help a resident who is experiencing pain.

9. Explain the importance of rest and sleep to a person's overall well-being.

10. Describe the normal sleep cycle.

11. Describe factors that can affect a person's ability to obtain a good night's sleep.

12. Describe actions a nursing assistant can take to help residents get the rest and sleep that they need.

Vocabulary Use the CD in the front of your book to hear these terms pronounced and defined:

Pain	Pain threshold	Breakthrough	Continuous positive
Acute pain	Pain tolerance	pain	airway pressure
Chronic	Radiating pain	Insomnia	(CPAP) therapy
pain	Pain scale	Sleep apnea	

PAIN

Pain is an unpleasant sensation that can range from mild discomfort to intense suffering. Many of the residents in your care will have some type of pain. **Acute pain** is sharp, sudden pain, such as that which occurs with an injury. Acute pain lasts a short period of time and decreases as the body's tissues repair themselves and heal. **Chronic pain** is pain that lasts beyond the usual time that it would take for the tissues to heal. Pain may be caused by many conditions, such as

those listed in Table 27-1. Pain can make it difficult for a resident to rest, relax, and sleep.

HOW PEOPLE RESPOND TO PAIN

Pain is a totally subjective experience. Only the person who is experiencing the pain knows what it feels like. Different people do not experience pain in the same way due to differences in pain threshold and pain tolerance. A person's

Table 27-1   Examples of Conditions Associated With Pain

CONDITION	EXAMPLES	LOCATION OF PAIN
Circulatory conditions	Heart failure, peripheral vascular disease	Leg pain
Heart conditions	Coronary artery disease, myocardial infarction	Chest pain, angina
Inflammatory conditions	Arthritis, bursitis, tendonitis	Joint pain
Bone disorders	Fractures, osteoporosis, cancer	Bone pain
Gastrointestinal disorders	Heartburn, gastric ulcers, constipation	Abdominal pain, stomach ache
Skin disorders	Wounds, cellulitis	Varies
Neoplastic disorders	Cancer	Varies (for example, bone pain, abdominal pain, headache)
Neurologic disorders	Headache, sciatica, herniated disk, shingles	Varies (for example, head pain, back pain, skin pain)

pain threshold is the point at which the person becomes aware of pain. A person with a low pain threshold is very sensitive to pain, while a person with a high pain threshold is less sensitive to it. **Pain tolerance** is the level of pain that a person can endure before taking action to seek relief.

There are other factors that affect a person's response to pain as well. Culture and upbringing play a very large role in how people perceive and manage pain. For example, in some families, admitting to pain may be considered a sign of weakness. People who were raised in families that took a stoic approach to pain may feel that it is better to "grin and bear it" than to complain about the pain or ask for relief. Other people, however, may come from families where family members discussed every little ache and pain loudly and in great detail. People with a background like this might not hesitate to discuss or ask for relief from their own pain. A person's age and past experience with pain can also affect how the person responds to pain. For example, it is quite common for older people to think that pain is just a part of aging that needs to be tolerated. As a result, some residents may not mention their pain to caregivers, because they may feel that there is nothing to be done about it anyway. Some residents may not mention pain because they do not want to trouble caregivers for medication, or because they do not want to worry their loved ones.

It is very important to understand that each person experiences and expresses pain differently. As caregivers, we never want to assume that a person does not have pain, or that the person's pain is minimal, because the person does not complain. Nor should we ever assume that a person who complains about pain is exaggerating his pain, even if the person's pain seems out of proportion to the injury or condition causing the pain.

RECOGNIZING AND REPORTING PAIN

As a nursing assistant, you may be the first to notice that one of your residents is in pain. Sometimes the person will tell you about his discomfort. Other times, your observation skills will tip you off (Fig. 27-1). Non-verbal signs of pain may include:

- Facial expressions (such as grimacing or gritting the teeth)
- Moaning
- Crying
- Restlessness
- Calling out

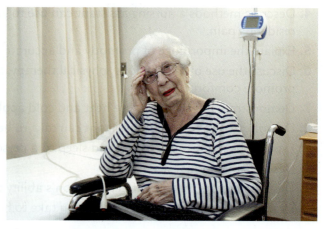

Figure 27-1

Paying close attention to non-verbal cues can help you to recognize when a resident is experiencing pain or discomfort.

- Rubbing the area of the body that is in pain
- Guarding (avoiding use of) the area of the body that is in pain
- Resisting care
- Redness or swelling in an area
- Profuse sweating
- Changes in the person's vital signs

When reporting a resident's pain to the nurse, it is helpful to provide additional details about the pain in your report, if possible. This additional information will help the nurse to assess what is happening and determine the appropriate action to take (Fig. 27-2). If the resident is able to

Caring For Those With Dementia

Residents with dementia often become resistant to care when they are experiencing pain or discomfort. The movement involved in routine care may cause pain or discomfort, which the person may not be able to verbalize because of the dementia. The only way the person with dementia may be able to express his discomfort is by resisting what you are trying to do. The person may grab or hit you, or push you away. If you see these behaviors in a resident with dementia, especially if the behaviors only occur during activities that require the resident to move, they may be an indication that the person is in pain. Report the behavior to the nurse, and describe exactly what you were doing when the behavior occurred. Tell the nurse how and where you were touching the resident, if contact with the resident was made. This information may help the nurse determine the source and the nature of the resident's pain.

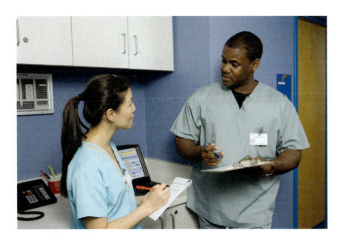

Figure 27-2

Finding out and reporting additional details about a resident's pain is a great help to the nurse.

understand and answer questions, try to obtain the following information:

- **Location of the pain.** Ask if the pain is localized (in one area), or if it travels anywhere else. Pain that travels from one area to another is called **radiating pain.**
- **Characteristics of the pain.** Not all pain or discomfort feels the same. Identifying the characteristics of the pain the resident is experiencing may help the nurse to identify the cause of the pain. Examples of words that can be used to describe pain include *aching, throbbing, stabbing, piercing, dull, sharp, cramping, burning, constant,* and *intermittent* (that is, the pain comes and goes).
- **Intensity of the pain.** The intensity of the pain is how much it hurts. As you have learned, pain is a subjective experience. Only the person experiencing the pain knows what the pain is like. A **pain scale** (a tool or guide that helps to translate a person's subjective rating of his or her pain into an objective measurement) can be helpful in understanding the extent of a person's pain (Table 27-2).
- **Circumstances surrounding the pain.** It will be useful for the nurse to know when the pain started, what the person was doing when the pain started, whether or not the person has ever experienced a similar pain before, and whether or not there is anything that makes the pain feel better or worse.

It is important for the nurse to know if a resident is in pain. If the pain is new, the nurse will need to take steps to find out what is causing the pain. Even if the pain is familiar and the cause of it is known, there may still be something the

nurse can do to help make the person more comfortable. Unrelieved pain and discomfort can lead to a significant decline in a resident's condition. Pain can negatively affect a resident's sleep, appetite, energy levels, and ability or desire to participate in self-care activities and to move. Pain also has an emotional impact, and can lead to depression. All of these factors affect the resident's general well-being and ability to attain or maintain her highest level of function.

TREATMENTS FOR PAIN

Treatments for pain include medication, physical therapy, and heat and cold applications.

Pain Medications

Over-the-counter pain medications—such as aspirin, acetaminophen (Tylenol), and ibuprofen (Advil)—can be very effective for relieving mild to moderate pain. Severe pain, such as that which often accompanies surgery, an acute illness, or some types of cancer, may only be controlled by the use of narcotics, such as morphine.

Residents with chronic pain need regular dosing of pain medication to keep the pain under control throughout the day and night (Fig. 27-3). The nurse and doctor will schedule the resident's doses of medication to stay ahead of the pain because if the pain is allowed to reoccur, a higher dose of medication may be necessary to relieve it. Some residents may experience **breakthrough pain** (pain that occurs before the next regularly scheduled dose of pain medication). It is important to recognize and report breakthrough pain so that the person does not have to be unnecessarily uncomfortable while waiting for the next scheduled dose of pain medication. By promptly

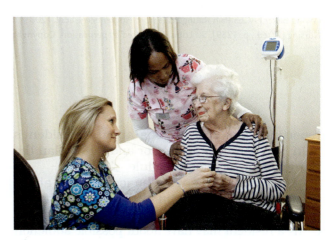

Figure 27-3

Many residents will take medication for pain.

Table 27-2   Pain Scales

TYPE OF SCALE	HOW IT IS USED
Verbal scale	The scale is made up of words such as "no pain," "mild," "moderate," "severe," "burning," "throbbing," and so on. The person chooses the words that best describe the pain.
Numeric scale	The scale is made up of a series of numbers (usually 0 to 10, or 0 to 5). The lowest number on the scale indicates "no pain" and the highest number on the scale indicates "the worst pain imaginable." The person chooses the number that best describes the pain.
Visual scales	The scale is a bar that includes words, color, numbers, or a combination of the three. The person is asked to place a mark on the bar to indicate the intensity of the pain.
Wong-Baker FACES Scale	The scale consists of six faces. The person is asked to choose the face that best describes how he or she is feeling.

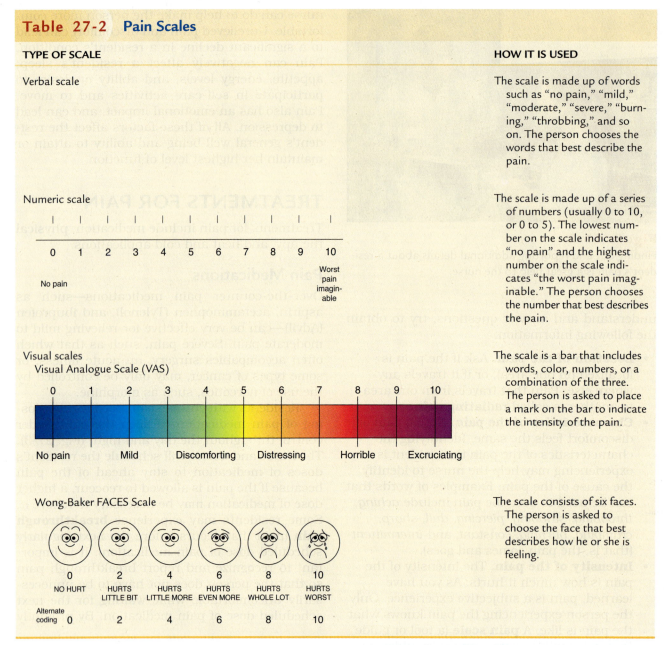

(Wong-Baker FACES Pain Rating Scale from Hockenberry, et al. [2005]. Wong's Essentials of Pediatric Nursing [7th ed., p. 1259]. St. Louis, MO. Used by permission. Copyright © Mosby.)

reporting your observations about a resident's pain, you can help the doctor and nurse plan the resident's medication schedule.

Some residents may be concerned about becoming addicted to pain medications. Although this can happen, it is rare. Promptly report any concerns a resident may have about possible addiction or side effects to the nurse. The nurse will work with the person to address those concerns.

Physical Therapy

Physical therapy can be useful for helping to relieve some types of pain. For example:

- **Exercise.** The physical therapist may assist the resident to perform exercises that stretch and strengthen the muscles, reducing the pain and stiffness that is often associated with musculoskeletal disorders.

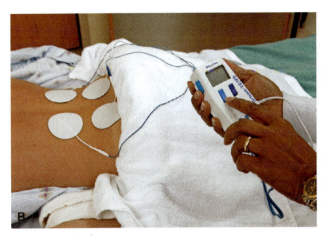

Figure 27-4
Transcutaneous electrical nerve stimulation (TENS) may be used to provide relief from some types of pain. Electrodes are attached to the skin over the painful area and a device is used to deliver electrical impulses through the electrodes. The electrical impulses help to block pain signals.

- **Ultrasound therapy.** The physical therapist uses an ultrasound device to transmit sound waves to muscle tissue and blood vessels in the painful area. The sound waves cause the tissue to relax and increase blood circulation in the area, reducing muscle tightness and spasms.
- **Transcutaneous electrical nerve stimulation (TENS).** The physical therapist uses a device to deliver electrical impulses through electrodes that are attached to the surface of the skin (Fig. 27-4). The electrical impulses help to block pain signals in the body.

Heat and Cold Applications

Many people with musculoskeletal pain can benefit from the application of heat or cold to an affected joint or muscle. The application of heat or cold can reduce or prevent tissue swelling, promote healing, ease pain, and promote comfort. Heat and cold have opposite effects on the body, which are summarized in Table 27-3. Because the application of heat or cold can be dangerous, these treatments require a doctor's order, and in some facilities, the application of heat or cold may be outside of the nursing assistant's scope of practice. However, even if you are not permitted to give these treatments, you will be involved with monitoring residents who are receiving them.

Older people are at very high risk for injury from the application of heat or cold, because their skin is very fragile and sensitive. Other factors

Table 27-3 Uses of Heat and Cold Applications

HEAT	COLD
Reduces pain and swelling and promotes circulation to speed healing	Reduces pain and swelling
Relieves muscle spasms	Numbs sensation and controls bleeding
Provides warmth	Reduces fevers

that can increase a person's risk for injury from the application of heat or cold include:

- **Fair skin.** Fair skin tends to be more sensitive to temperature changes than darker skin.
- **Impaired sensation.** People with impaired sensation, such as those who are paralyzed or who have diabetes, are at risk for injury because they are unable to detect whether an application is too hot or too cold.
- **Impaired consciousness.** People who are disoriented or taking pain medications may be unaware that an application is too hot or too cold, or unable to communicate to others the discomfort caused by the application.

People with these risk factors for injury must be monitored especially carefully during the application of heat or cold.

Heat applications

Heat relaxes the muscles, relieves pain, and promotes blood flow to the area. When heat is applied to the skin, the blood vessels dilate (widen), allowing more blood to flow to the tissues. Increased blood flow speeds healing by bringing more oxygen, nutrients, and infection-fighting white blood cells to the area. The increased blood flow helps to reduce swelling by removing excess fluid from the tissues. In addition, heat relaxes the muscles and helps loosen stiff joints.

Heat applications can be either moist or dry (Fig. 27-5). In moist applications, moisture comes in direct contact with the skin. Moist heat penetrates tissues more quickly and deeply than dry heat. For this reason, moist heat applications are used at a lower temperature to reduce the risk of burns. Examples of moist heat applications include warm compresses and hot water soaks (Fig. 27-5A).

Dry applications prevent moisture from coming in direct contact with the skin. Examples of dry heat applications include an electric heating pad or a hot water bottle wrapped in a towel. An Aquamatic pad (or K-pad) is a special type of

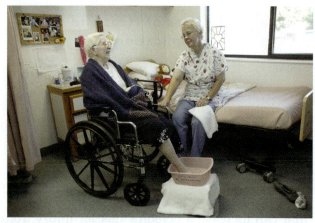

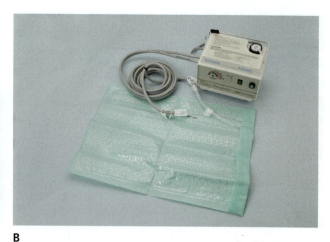

A   B

Figure 27-5

Heat applications are used to relax muscles, relieve pain, and promote blood flow to an area. Heat applications may be either moist or dry. **(A)** A warm soak is an example of a moist heat application. Soaks are done in either a wash basin (if the area to be soaked is small) or a tub (if the area to be soaked is large). **(B)** An Aquamatic pad is an example of a dry heat application. Water is heated in the heating unit. The heated water passes through the tubing and into a network of tubes inside the heating pad. The water never comes in contact with the person's skin.

electric heating pad (Fig. 27-5B). The pad is connected to a heating unit that heats water to a preset temperature. The water circulates through the pad and then back into the heating device so that a constant temperature is maintained. A key is used to set the temperature, and then the key is removed, preventing the heat from being turned up or down. Procedure 27-1 describes how to apply a dry heat application using an Aquamatic pad.

Burns are the most common complication of heat applications. Some burns, especially on thin, delicate skin, can be very severe, resulting in blistering, tissue loss, and the need for skin grafting. In addition to increasing the person's risk for burns, heat applications that are left in place for too long will eventually cause the blood vessels to constrict, putting the person at risk for tissue breakdown. For these reasons, heat applications should not be left in place for longer than 20 minutes. Make sure that you check the skin underneath the heat application every 5 minutes and stop the treatment immediately if you observe any evidence of burning. Warmth causes the skin to become pink or slightly reddened. Skin that is bright red or very pale could be burned. Report any observations that may indicate a burn to the nurse immediately, along with any complaints of pain, burning, or stinging.

Cold applications

Cold applications are often used for people who have musculoskeletal injuries resulting from trauma, such as sprains and fractures. Cold applications are also frequently used on incisions following surgical procedures. The application of cold reduces pain and swelling and decreases bleeding by cooling the skin and underlying tissues, causing the blood vessels to constrict (narrow). Because the blood vessels are constricted, less blood is carried to the tissues, resulting in less bleeding and decreased tissue swelling. The numbing effect of the cold helps to reduce pain.

Like heat applications, cold applications can be either moist or dry (Fig. 27-6). Moist applications allow the cold to penetrate the tissues more quickly and deeply. A cold compress, made by soaking a gauze pad, towel, or washcloth in cold water; wringing it out; and then applying it with pressure to the affected area, is an example of a moist cold application (Fig. 27-6A). Procedure 27-2 explains how to give a moist cold application.

Dry applications are usually colder than moist applications. An ice bag is an example of a dry cold application (Fig. 27-6B). Commercially prepared ice packs that are kept frozen until the time of use are available, or a dry cold application can be made by filling an ice bag with crushed ice and wrapping it in a towel or washcloth. Procedure 27-3 explains how to give a dry cold application.

When applied directly to a person's skin, cold can cause severe burns and blisters. Dry cold applications should be wrapped in a protective cloth to prevent the icy cold plastic from coming

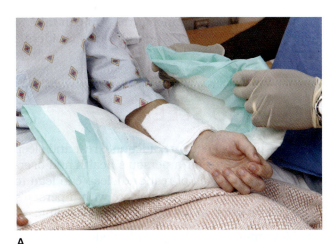

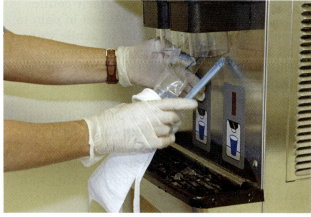

A   B

Figure 27-6
Cold applications are used to reduce pain and swelling. Cold applications may be either moist or
dry. **(A)** A cold compress is a moist cold application. **(B)** An ice bag is a dry cold application.

in direct contact with the person's skin. If a cold
application is left in place for too long, prolonged
constriction of the small blood vessels can keep
oxygen and nutrients from reaching the skin,
resulting in tissue death and skin breakdown.
For this reason, cold applications should not be
left in place for longer than 20 minutes. Make
sure that you check the skin underneath the cold
application every 10 minutes, and stop the treatment immediately if you observe any evidence of
a burn or blister. Pale skin, resulting from the
constriction of the blood vessels, should return to
its normal color quickly after the cold application
is removed. If it does not, or if you notice a burn
or blister starting to develop, inform the nurse
immediately. Also, if you have questions about
how to apply the cold application or for how long,
please ask the nurse for help.

THE NURSING ASSISTANT'S ROLE IN MANAGING PAIN

As a nursing assistant, there are many things
you can do to help a resident who is experiencing
pain and discomfort.

- Help the person to relax. Anxiety causes the
  body to become tense, which increases pain.
  Dim lights and a quiet environment can
  promote relaxation. Some people find that
  breathing slowly, regularly, and deeply in a
  calm, comfortable environment promotes
  relaxation and reduces pain.
- Provide distractions from the pain. Activities
  such as listening to music, watching television, reading, or sharing memories can help

to reduce pain and discomfort by giving the
person something to focus on, other than the
pain.
- Pay attention to positioning (Fig. 27-7).
  Positioning and supporting the body in
  proper alignment relieves strain on the muscles and joints and promotes comfort.
- Massage may help to relieve discomfort and
  can be very relaxing for the person. As with
  any personal care procedure, always check
  with the nurse or read the person's care plan
  before beginning to make sure that it is all
  right for the person to have a massage. In
  general, you should avoid massaging areas
  that are red, swollen, warm, and painful.

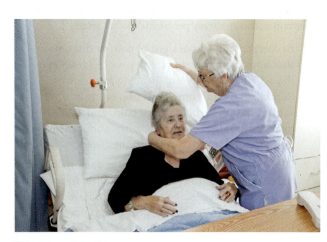

Figure 27-7
Positioning and supporting the body in proper alignment
promotes comfort. When the body is not in alignment,
unnecessary strain is put on the muscles and joints, which
increases pain and stiffness.

- Take things slow and be extremely gentle when you are assisting a resident in pain to move. Although you should be gentle with all of your residents, it is important to be especially gentle with residents who are in pain, because even the slightest movement may make the pain worse. In some cases, the nurse may administer pain medication before an activity to reduce the person's pain and make the activity more tolerable. When this is the case, wait until the pain medication takes effect before working with the resident.

Remember that each person's response to pain and the methods that he is most comfortable using to address it, will vary.

As the staff member who works most closely with the residents, you will play a vital role in helping to detect and manage pain. Being sensitive to what your resident is feeling and taking action to provide physical comfort and emotional support are important measures you can take to help promote comfort and relieve a resident's pain.

REST AND SLEEP

Just like physical comfort, adequate rest and sleep are very important for a person's health and overall well-being. A lack of rest and sleep can lead to many problems that can interfere with a person's ability to function at his or her best, including:

- **Worsened pain.** As a result of sleep loss, a person's ability to handle pain is often decreased. The person may experience a decrease in both pain threshold and pain tolerance.
- **Emotional and behavioral problems.** A lack of sleep can affect a person's ability to cope with everyday challenges. The person may become irritable, or cry easily. The person may even become depressed.
- **Decreased cognition.** A person who is not getting enough sleep may have difficulty concentrating, paying attention, remembering information, and making decisions. The person may even fall asleep during routine activities. This can make it difficult for the person to learn new information and skills, which can negatively affect the person's ability to reach his goals.
- **Fatigue and decreased physical ability.** Fatigue resulting from a lack of rest and sleep can affect the person's ability to participate in self-care or other activities. As a result, the person may experience a decrease in physical function, as well as emotional difficulties. Fatigue and decreased physical ability also increase the person's risk for falls and other injuries.
- **Increased risk for illness.** A lack of sleep and rest can decrease the immune system's effectiveness (putting the person at increased risk for infections) and affect heart function (resulting in high blood pressure and an irregular heartbeat).

NORMAL SLEEP

Sleep gives the body and the brain a chance to rest and recover from the activities and stresses of everyday life. During sleep, the eyes are closed and the muscles are completely relaxed. The person's respirations and heart rate slow down. The

Be Smart About Surveys!

As you have learned, OBRA requires us to help our residents achieve the goal of attaining or maintaining their highest level of function and well-being. When a resident is experiencing pain or discomfort, it is very difficult for the resident to work toward this goal. Surveyors will be looking to make sure that staff members recognize a resident's pain or discomfort, and take the appropriate measures (within their own scope of practice) to address it. To help your facility remain without survey problems in this area:

- Be alert to non-verbal signs of pain or discomfort that a resident may show. Ask your residents every day whether they are experiencing any pain. Report residents' complaints of pain, your observations of non-verbal signs of pain, and your residents' responses to your questions about the presence of pain to the nurse right away.
- When a resident is being treated for pain, help the nurse to monitor the resident's response to the treatment. If the resident continues to have pain, or you still see signs that the resident is not comfortable, keep the nurse informed.
- Provide for residents' physical comfort. Make sure that residents are positioned properly and supported in correct body alignment. Move residents gently.

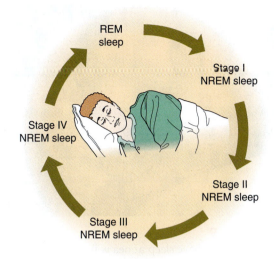

Figure 27-8

A complete sleep cycle includes four stages of non-rapid eye movement (NREM) sleep, followed by a period of rapid eye movement (REM) sleep. After REM sleep, the cycle begins again. On average, a person completes four or five sleep cycles during a night's sleep.

body works to heal and repair the tissues from the wear and tear of daily activity, strengthening the immune system and refreshing and re-energizing brain cells.

There are two different types of sleep: non-rapid eye movement (NREM) sleep and rapid eye movement (REM) sleep. A complete sleep cycle consists of four stages of NREM sleep, followed by a period of REM sleep (Fig. 27-8).

- **NREM sleep:** The four stages of NREM sleep progress from a light sleep to a very deep sleep. Each stage of NREM sleep lasts from 5 to 15 minutes.
- **REM sleep:** During REM sleep, there is increased activity in the brain. The heart and respiratory rates increase, and the eyes move back and forth rapidly. Dreaming occurs during REM sleep.

After completion of REM sleep, the cycle begins again. Through each cycle, REM sleep lasts a bit longer, eventually reaching approximately 1 hour. On average, a person completes four or five sleep cycles during a night's sleep.

Most adults need 7 to 8 hours of sleep per 24-hour period. Older people need this amount of sleep as well, but they often have a hard time getting this amount of uninterrupted sleep at night. Taking naps during the day may help an older person to meet the need for 7 to 8 hours of sleep per 24-hour period.

Caring For Those With Dementia

Many of your residents will take naps during the day. For residents with dementia who are confused as to the time of day, using a recliner for naps may be more appropriate than assisting the person to bed. Having the person nap in bed in the day time may confuse the person further, because the person may associate "going to bed" with night time.

FACTORS THAT CAN AFFECT SLEEP

A number of factors can affect a person's ability to obtain a good night's sleep.

Environment

Environmental conditions, such as noise, light, and room temperature, can affect a person's ability to sleep. For residents of long-term care facilities, environmental factors often cause problems sleeping. There may be more noise, or strange noises. The bed may feel different from the bed the person was used to at home. The person may have to adjust to having a roommate. The person (or the roommate) may require care during the night. Although the care is necessary, the person's sleep is disturbed when staff members enter the room.

Pain and Chronic Conditions

As you learned earlier, many residents experience some degree of pain or discomfort, and many have chronic health conditions. Pain and other symptoms of chronic health conditions (such as shortness of breath, coughing, or frequent urination) can make it hard for the resident to fall asleep, or to stay asleep. The medications a resident takes to manage chronic conditions may also disrupt sleep.

Sleep Disorders

Sleep disorders are medical conditions characterized by inadequate sleep, disturbed sleep, or sleep at inappropriate times. There are many different types of sleep disorders. Two of the most common sleep disorders are insomnia and sleep apnea.

Insomnia

Insomnia is a disorder characterized by an inability to fall asleep, or to stay asleep. The person may have trouble falling asleep, wake frequently during the night, or wake up too early in the morning and then be unable to fall back asleep. The person does not get an adequate amount of sleep, and the quality of the sleep that the person does get is poor.

Be sure to tell the nurse if a resident reports experiencing insomnia. The health care team will need to assess the resident to determine the cause of the insomnia, and to take actions to address it. Medications can aid in the treatment of insomnia, but these medications must be used with caution in older people. Some have side effects that cause the person to become groggy and less alert during the day, which can lead to falls and other accidents. Providing care and an environment that promotes sleep and rest without medication is preferred for older people with insomnia.

Sleep apnea

Sleep apnea is a disorder that causes the person to stop breathing for varying periods of time during sleep. There are several forms of sleep apnea, but the most common form is obstructive sleep apnea. In this condition, the soft tissue in the back of the throat collapses, blocking the airway and causing the person to stop breathing. When the person's blood oxygen level gets very low, the person wakes up and starts breathing again. Because the person's sleep is interrupted many times during the night, the quality of sleep is very poor. The person wakes up feeling tired, and may have difficulty staying awake during the day.

Sleep apnea is most common in men older than 40 years and people who are overweight. Symptoms include chronic, loud snoring; gasping and choking during sleep; and excessive sleepiness during the day. Mood changes (such as increased irritability) and cognitive changes can also occur.

There are several ways to manage sleep apnea. Lifestyle changes such as losing weight, avoiding alcohol and smoking, and avoiding certain positions while sleeping can help. Some people may have surgery to remove or reduce the tissue that causes the obstruction. However, one of the most common and effective ways of treating sleep apnea is with **continuous positive airway pressure (CPAP,** pronounced *see-pap*) **therapy.** In this treatment, the person wears a special CPAP mask while sleeping (Fig. 27-9). The CPAP mask forms a tight seal over the nose (and sometimes the mouth as well). The mask is attached to a machine that forces air into the airway, keeping it open during sleep. This keeps the person's blood oxygen level at an acceptable level, allowing the person to sleep through the night.

If you are caring for a resident who is receiving CPAP therapy, you may need to assist the resident

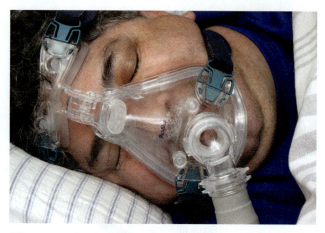

Figure 27-9
Many people who have sleep apnea will receive continuous positive airway pressure (CPAP) therapy. The special CPAP mask delivers air under pressure. The pressure keeps the airways open so that the person gets enough oxygen, allowing the person to sleep through the night. (© *Custom Medical Stock Photo.*)

with applying the mask and turning on the CPAP machine. The nurse will show you how the resident's mask should be applied and how the machine operates. You may also be responsible for helping the resident to keep the equipment clean.

TELL THE NURSE

When caring for a resident who is being treated with CPAP therapy for sleep apnea, be sure to report the following observations to the nurse:

- The person refuses to put on the mask, or takes it off
- There is a hissing noise coming from around the seal of the mask or the tubing
- The CPAP machine is not working properly

THE NURSING ASSISTANT'S ROLE IN PROMOTING REST AND SLEEP

As a nursing assistant, there are many things you can do to help your residents get the rest and sleep that they need.

Always respect each resident's preferences with regard to times for going to bed and waking up. Some people are "early to bed, early to rise." Other people are "night owls," meaning they like to go to bed late at night and sleep late in the morning. Disrupting these natural patterns can affect the person's quality of sleep.

Remember that a quiet, dark environment promotes rest and sleep. Sometimes the routines in long-term care facilities make it difficult for residents to sleep. When working during the evening and night hours, be especially mindful of things that you do that could affect a resident's ability to sleep. Take care to keep noise at a minimum, particularly at the change of shift when there is a lot of staff activity. Keep your voice low and encourage others to do the same. Avoid calling out to co-workers unless you need help in an emergency. Finally, be thoughtful about the use of lights. If you need to enter a resident's room to provide care, try to avoid turning on bright overhead lights. Use night-lights or other soft lighting, if possible. Gently awaken the resident who needs care, and be sure to explain to the resident who you are and what you are there to do. If more light is needed to safely complete the task, turn on only the lights you need. When you have finished providing care, make sure the resident is positioned comfortably, and turn out the lights as soon as you can.

Other actions you can take to promote rest and sleep are listed in Box 27-1. By being sensitive to the resident's needs, you can help to provide an atmosphere that promotes rest and sleep.

TELL THE NURSE ❗

As a nursing assistant, you may be the first to notice that a resident is having difficulty sleeping. Residents may also mention to you that they are having difficulties sleeping. Be sure to report any of the following observations about a resident's ability to sleep to the nurse right away:

- The resident is awake frequently during the night
- The resident lies awake for long periods before falling asleep
- The resident reports wakefulness or difficulty sleeping
- The resident seems sleepy during the day
- The resident gets up frequently during the night to urinate
- The resident tells you about, or shows signs of, pain or discomfort
- The resident reports an inability to get to sleep or stay asleep as a result of something in the environment (for example, the noise from another resident's television; being too hot or too cold)
- The resident expresses worry or anxiety about something

BOX 27-1 Actions to Promote Rest and Sleep for Your Residents

- Encourage increased physical activity during the day. Physical activity during the day promotes better sleep at night.
- Limit time for naps during the day. Although a short nap during the day can help an older person meet his sleep requirements, taking too many naps or naps that are too long can negatively affect the person's ability to sleep at night.
- Avoid giving the resident beverages with caffeine (such as regular coffee, tea, or cola) in the afternoon or evening. Many people are sensitive to caffeine and find that it keeps them up at night if they have it too late in the day.
- Promote relaxation by giving the resident a warm bath in the evening, or providing a massage. Finding out the resident's normal bed time routines, and following them as closely as possible, is also important for promoting relaxation and sleep.
- Offer the resident a snack at bed time.
- Assist the resident with elimination just before bed time.
- Create a comfortable environment for sleeping. Straighten the bed linens and fluff the pillows. Make sure items are put away and the room is neat and free of clutter. Close the blinds or draperies to darken the room, and turn off the overhead lights. (A night-light may be left on for safety.) Make sure the room temperature is not too hot or too cold.
- Turn off the television set or radio (unless the resident watches television or listens to the radio to relax before bed).
- Be observant. For example, if the resident seems upset or worried about something, you should report this to the nurse because stress or worry can impact the resident's ability to sleep. Similarly, if the resident seems to be in pain or have some other type of physical discomfort, report this to the nurse.

Caring For Those With Dementia

It is particularly important for residents with dementia to follow a consistent bed time routine. Remember that people with dementia have a great deal of difficulty adjusting to change. A change in the person's regular bed time routine may cause confusion and upset the person, affecting the person's ability to get the proper amount of rest.

Be Smart About Surveys!

Getting adequate rest and sleep are important to a resident's overall health and well-being. Surveyors will be very interested in the actions the health care team takes to ensure that residents get the sleep and rest that they need. To help your facility remain without survey problems in this area:

- Be aware of, and help residents to follow, their normal bed time routines. Make sure residents' basic needs (such as those related to toileting) are met as part of the bed time routine.

- Be attentive to the sleeping environment. Make sure it is dark, quiet, and comfortable.

- When a resident has an identified need to nap during the day, make sure the resident is positioned comfortably in either the bed or a recliner for the nap. Do not allow residents to nap sitting up in their chairs.

- Make an effort to limit noise on the unit, especially during the evening and night hours.

- Keep the nurse informed of any changes in a resident's ability to sleep or sleeping patterns.

- If a sleep medication has been ordered for a resident, take extra precautions to prevent falls and other accidents. Supervise or assist the resident with transfers, especially during the night.

SUMMARY

- Pain is an unpleasant sensation that can range from mild discomfort to intense suffering. Pain can be acute or chronic.
  - Each person experiences and expresses pain differently.
  - Nursing assistants play a very important role in recognizing and reporting pain. In this way, nursing assistants help other members of the health care team to determine the cause of the pain, and provide relief. Unrelieved pain decreases a resident's quality of life and can lead to a significant decline in a resident's condition.
  - Common treatments for pain include medication, physical therapy, and heat and cold applications. In addition, there are many things nursing assistants can do independently to help residents who are in pain.

- The body refreshes and repairs itself during sleep. Adequate rest and sleep are very important for a person's overall health and well-being.
  - Most adults, including older adults, need 7 to 8 hours of sleep per 24-hour period to function at their best.
  - Factors that can negatively affect a person's ability to sleep include environmental conditions (such as noise, light, or a room that is too hot or too cold), pain and other symptoms of chronic conditions, and sleep disorders (such as insomnia and sleep apnea).
  - Nursing assistants can help residents to get the rest and sleep they need by ensuring a restful environment, providing for physical comfort, and making an effort to minimize noise and other disruptions when providing care during the night.

Giving a Dry Heat Application With an Aquamatic Pad

WHY YOU DO IT   Heat applications relax the muscles, relieve pain, and promote blood flow to the area.

Getting Ready   WORKSTEPS

1. Complete the "Getting Ready" steps.

Supplies

- aquamatic pad
- cover
- heating unit
- ties or tape
- distilled water

Procedure

2. Check the pad for leaks. Make sure that the cord is not frayed and the plug is in good condition. Check the heating unit to be sure that it is filled with water. If you need to fill it, use distilled water. Tap water contains minerals that can corrode the unit.

3. Place the heating unit so that the tubing and pad are level with the heating unit at all times. Make sure that the tubing is free of kinks. Plug the cord into an outlet.

4. Allow the water to warm to the desired temperature, as specified by the nurse or the care plan. If the temperature is not preset, set the temperature with the key and then remove the key.

5. Place the pad in its cover.

6. Make sure that the bed is positioned at a comfortable working height (to promote good body mechanics) and that the wheels are locked.

7. Help the person to a comfortable position and expose only the area to be treated.

8. Apply the pad to the treatment site.

9. Leave the pad in place for the designated amount of time, usually 15 to 20 minutes. The pad may be secured in place with ties or tape, or the resident may assist by holding the pad in place. (Do not use pins to secure the pad. Pins can puncture the pad, causing it to leak.)

   a. Check the skin beneath the pad every 5 minutes. If the skin appears red, swollen, or blistered or if the person complains of pain, numbness, or discomfort, discontinue treatment immediately and notify the nurse.

   b. Refill the heating unit if the water level drops below the fill line.

   c. If you must leave the room, place the call light control within easy reach and ask the person to signal if he or she experiences numbness or burning.

10. When the treatment is complete, remove the pad.

11. Straighten the bed linens and make sure the person is comfortable and in good body alignment. Draw the top linens over the person.

12. Make sure that the bed is lowered to its lowest position and that the wheels are locked.

13. Gather the soiled linens and place them in the linen hamper. Dispose of disposable items in a facility-approved waste container. Clean equipment and return it to the storage area.

Finishing Up   CLOSURE

14. Complete the "Finishing Up" steps.

PROCEDURE 27-2

Giving a Moist Cold Application

WHY YOU DO IT   Cold applications reduce pain and swelling and decrease bleeding.

Getting Ready WGKIEPS

1. Complete the "Getting Ready" steps.

Supplies

- bed protector
- compress (for example, 4 × 4 gauze pad or washcloth)
- rolled gauze or ties (optional)
- bath basin
- ice
- bath towel

Procedure

2. Put the ice in the bath basin and fill the basin with cold water at the sink.

3. Make sure that the bed is positioned at a comfortable working height (to promote good body mechanics) and that the wheels are locked.

4. Help the person to a comfortable position and expose only the area to be treated.

5. Position the bed protector as necessary to keep the bed linens dry.

6. Moisten the compress with the ice water as ordered. Wring out the compress and apply it to the treatment site.

7. Leave the compress in place for the designated amount of time, usually 15 to 20 minutes. The compress may be secured in place with ties or rolled gauze, or the patient or resident may assist by holding the compress in place.

   a. Keep the compress moistened with ice water.

   b. Check the skin beneath the compress every 10 minutes. If the skin appears pale or blue or if the person complains of numbness or a burning sensation, discontinue treatment immediately and notify the nurse.

   c. If you must leave the room, place the call light control within easy reach and ask the person to signal if he or she experiences numbness or burning.

8. When the treatment is complete, remove the compress and carefully dry the skin.

9. Remove the bed protector. Straighten the bed linens and make sure the person is comfortable and in good body alignment. Draw the top linens over the person.

10. Make sure that the bed is lowered to its lowest position and that the wheels are locked.

11. Gather the soiled linens and place them in the linen hamper. Dispose of disposable items in a facility-approved waste container. Clean equipment and return it to the storage area.

Finishing Up CLSOWR

12. Complete the "Finishing Up" steps.

PROCEDURE 27-3

Giving a Dry Cold Application

WHY YOU DO IT   Cold applications reduce pain and swelling and decrease bleeding.

Getting Ready WGKIEpS

1. Complete the "Getting Ready" steps.

Supplies

- paper towels
- rolled gauze or ties (optional)
- crushed ice
- ice bag
- towel

Procedure

2. Fill the ice bag with water, close it, and turn it upside down to check for leaks. Empty the bag.

3. Fill the bag one-half to two-thirds full with crushed ice. Do not overfill the ice bag. Squeeze the bag to force out excess air, and close the bag.

4. Dry the outside of the bag with the paper towels and wrap it in the towel.

5. Make sure that the bed is positioned at a comfortable working height (to promote good body mechanics) and that the wheels are locked.

6. Help the person to a comfortable position and expose only the area to be treated.

7. Apply the ice bag to the treatment site.

8. Leave the compress in place for the designated amount of time, usually 15 to 20 minutes. The compress may be secured in place with ties or rolled gauze, or the resident may assist by holding the compress in place.

   a. Check the skin beneath the ice bag every 10 minutes. If the skin appears pale or blue or if the person complains of numbness or a burning sensation, discontinue treatment immediately and notify the nurse.

   b. Refill the bag with ice as necessary.

   c. If you must leave the room, place the call light control within easy reach and ask the person to signal if he or she experiences numbness or burning.

9. When the treatment is complete, remove the ice bag.

10. Straighten the bed linens and make sure the person is comfortable and in good body alignment. Draw the top linens over the person.

11. Make sure that the bed is lowered to its lowest position and that the wheels are locked.

12. Gather the soiled linens and place them in the linen hamper. Dispose of disposable items in a facility-approved waste container. Clean equipment and return it to the storage area.

Finishing Up CLSOWR

13. Complete the "Finishing Up" steps.

WHAT DID YOU LEARN?

Multiple Choice

Select the single best answer for each of the following questions.

1. Which one of the following can be used to treat and control pain?
   a. Medications, such as aspirin and morphine
   b. Back massage
   c. Heat and cold applications
   d. All of the above

2. The purpose of cold applications is usually to:
   a. Prevent heat exhaustion
   b. Speed the flow of blood to an injured area
   c. Prevent swelling
   d. Prevent the formation of scar tissue

3. What is a heat application used for?
   a. To relieve muscle spasms
   b. To reduce pain
   c. To promote circulation and speed healing
   d. All of the above

4. Dreaming occurs during which stage of sleep?
   a. Stage I non-rapid eye movement (NREM) sleep
   b. Stage IV NREM sleep
   c. Rapid eye movement (REM) sleep
   d. Stage II NREM sleep

5. Mrs. Moyer likes to go to bed at 11:00 p.m., and sleep in late the next morning. What could happen if Mrs. Moyer is required to go to bed earlier than her preferred bed time?
   a. Mrs. Moyer could experience a better quality of sleep
   b. Mrs. Moyer could have difficulty falling asleep, which could negatively affect her quality of sleep
   c. Mrs. Moyer could learn to become an "early bird"
   d. Mrs. Moyer could be at risk for having bad dreams

6. When might physical therapy be used for pain management?
   a. When a person is having musculoskeletal pain
   b. When a person is young
   c. When a person is in acute pain
   d. When pain medications are not effective

7. A resident who has difficulty sleeping may experience all of the following except:
   a. Difficulty remembering information
   b. Increased risk for falls
   c. Increased alertness
   d. Difficulty concentrating

8. Which of the following actions can disrupt a resident's sleep?
   a. Darkening the room and minimizing noise
   b. Performing routine incontinence care during the night
   c. Making sure the room temperature is comfortable
   d. Increasing the resident's level of activity during the day

9. Unrelieved pain can have which of the following effects?
   a. Increased sleep
   b. Depression
   c. Increased appetite
   d. Increased physical activity

10. You are assisting Mr. Levine to prepare for sleep. The nurse has informed you that Mr. Levine has sleep apnea and is receiving continuous positive airway pressure (CPAP) therapy. Which of the following should you do to ensure that Mr. Levine's treatment for this condition is being followed?
    a. Assist Mr. Levine to sleep on his back, supporting his neck in an extended position to open the airway
    b. Make sure that Mr. Levine's nasal cannula is secure and the oxygen is running at the right amount
    c. Make sure that Mr. Levine's mask is fit snugly over his nose, and that no hissing sound is heard when the continuous positive airway pressure (CPAP) machine is turned on
    d. None of the above

Matching

Match each numbered item with its appropriate lettered description.

_____ **1.** Pain tolerance

_____ **2.** Insomnia

_____ **3.** Radiating pain

_____ **4.** Pain threshold

_____ **5.** Transcutaneous electrical nerve stimulation (TENS)

_____ **6.** Pain scale

_____ **7.** Chronic pain

_____ **8.** Breakthrough pain

a. The point at which a person becomes aware of pain

b. A tool or guide that helps to translate a person's subjective rating of his or her pain into an objective measurement

c. Pain that lasts beyond the usual time that it would take for the tissues to heal

d. Pain that occurs before a person's next regularly scheduled dose of pain medication

e. A treatment for pain that uses electrical impulses to block pain signals

f. The level of pain that a person can endure before taking action to seek relief

g. Pain that travels from one area to another

h. A disorder characterized by an inability to fall asleep, or to stay asleep

STOP and Think!

● You are caring for Mrs. Lasorda, who has crippling rheumatoid arthritis. She has many "good" days when she is able to manage her personal care and get around pretty well. This week, however, she is having a severe flare-up of her illness. What are some measures that you may be asked to do to help Mrs. Lasorda be more comfortable?

● You are caring for Mrs. Benson during the night shift. She was just admitted to your facility from the hospital 2 weeks ago, following surgery for a broken hip. She goes to physical therapy daily. Lately, the therapy has not been going very well as she is having a hard time with the exercises. You enter the room for your first rounds around midnight and find Mrs. Benson awake. She tells you that she has not been able to fall asleep, and this is the third night this week that she has been like this. Mrs. Benson gets tearful as she talks to you, telling you that her inability to sleep makes her too tired to do what she needs to do in physical therapy. She is afraid that if she doesn't make progress, she won't be able to go back home. What can you do that may help Mrs. Benson?

Nursing Assistants Make a Difference!

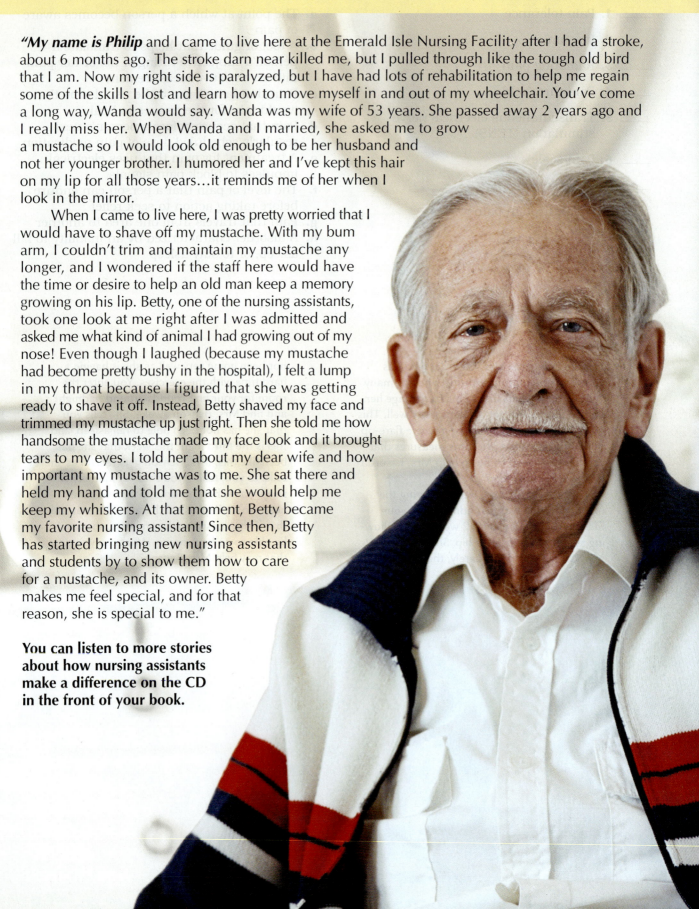

"My name is Philip and I came to live here at the Emerald Isle Nursing Facility after I had a stroke, about 6 months ago. The stroke darn near killed me, but I pulled through like the tough old bird that I am. Now my right side is paralyzed, but I have had lots of rehabilitation to help me regain some of the skills I lost and learn how to move myself in and out of my wheelchair. You've come a long way, Wanda would say. Wanda was my wife of 53 years. She passed away 2 years ago and I really miss her. When Wanda and I married, she asked me to grow a mustache so I would look old enough to be her husband and not her younger brother. I humored her and I've kept this hair on my lip for all those years…it reminds me of her when I look in the mirror.

When I came to live here, I was pretty worried that I would have to shave off my mustache. With my bum arm, I couldn't trim and maintain my mustache any longer, and I wondered if the staff here would have the time or desire to help an old man keep a memory growing on his lip. Betty, one of the nursing assistants, took one look at me right after I was admitted and asked me what kind of animal I had growing out of my nose! Even though I laughed (because my mustache had become pretty bushy in the hospital), I felt a lump in my throat because I figured that she was getting ready to shave it off. Instead, Betty shaved my face and trimmed my mustache up just right. Then she told me how handsome the mustache made my face look and it brought tears to my eyes. I told her about my dear wife and how important my mustache was to me. She sat there and held my hand and told me that she would help me keep my whiskers. At that moment, Betty became my favorite nursing assistant! Since then, Betty has started bringing new nursing assistants and students by to show them how to care for a mustache, and its owner. Betty makes me feel special, and for that reason, she is special to me."

You can listen to more stories about how nursing assistants make a difference on the CD in the front of your book.

DEATH AND DYING

Do not go gentle into that good night,
Old age should burn and rave at close of day
Rage, rage against the dying of the light.

—From *Do Not Go Gentle Into That Good Night*
by Dylan Thomas

In this poem by the Welsh poet Dylan Thomas
(1914–1953), the speaker begs his father to fight,
rather than accept, death. Although everyone who
lives must die, accepting the certainty of our own
death, or the death of someone we care about, is
rarely easy. In Unit 6, we will look at the final
stages of life and the role the nursing assistant
plays in providing compassionate care to those
who are dying, and their families.

Photo: Sunset off the coast of Layang
Layang Island, Malaysia.
(Scubazoo/Photo Researchers, Inc.)

DEATH AND DYING

who are dying, and their families.

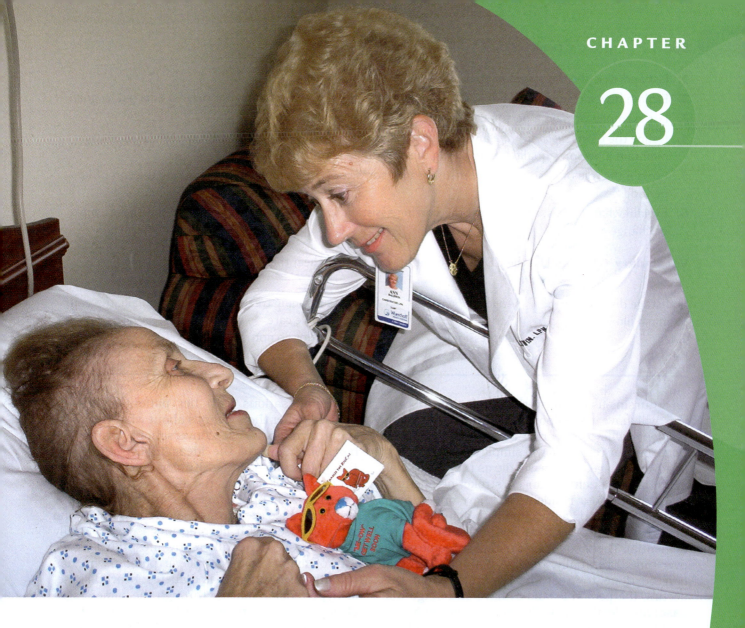

Caring for People During the End-of-Life Period

WHAT WILL YOU LEARN?

Many of your residents are entering the last phase of their lives when they come to live in a long-term care facility. In this chapter, you will learn about some of the emotions a resident and his family members may experience during the end-of-life period. You will also learn about some of the resources available to help ensure the resident's comfort, dignity, and best quality of life as death approaches. When you are finished with this chapter, you will be able to:

Photo: A hospice nurse cares for a terminally ill resident.
(Photograph courtesy of Wuesthoff Brevard Hospice & Palliative Care/Brenda Spakes.)

1. List and describe the stages of grief.

2. Explain how a resident, a resident's family members, and a resident's caregiver may be affected by grief.

3. List examples of ways a person can specify end-of-life care wishes.

4. Define the terms *supportive care* and *palliative care*, and explain how these types of care can be used to maintain a person's quality of life during the end-of-life period.

5. Explain the role of hospice care in ensuring a person's comfort and quality of life during the end-of-life period.

6. Explain what a will is, and describe the nursing assistant's role in assisting a person who wishes to make or change a will.

Vocabulary Use the CD in the front of your book to hear these terms pronounced and defined:

End-stage disease	Anger	Life-sustaining treatment	Palliative care
Terminal illness	Bargaining	Supportive care	Will
Grief	Depression	No code or do not	
Denial	Acceptance	resuscitate (DNR) order	

As a nursing assistant working in long-term care, you will have the opportunity to care for many residents who are nearing the end of their lives. Some of your residents will simply die as the result of advanced age. Others will die as the result of an acute illness such as cancer, stroke, or pneumonia. Many of your residents will have one or more chronic conditions associated with aging (such as heart conditions, chronic respiratory disorders, or dementia). These conditions usually become worse over time. Eventually, there is nothing more that can be done to treat the disorder. When this occurs, the person is said to have **end-stage disease,** and death is usually expected within a relatively short period of time. An illness or condition that has no cure and that will ultimately result in the person's death is referred to as a **terminal illness.**

GRIEF

Anyone experiencing any type of loss, be it the loss of health, loss of a marriage, loss of a loved one, or the impending loss of his own life will experience grief. **Grief** is defined as mental anguish, specifically associated with loss.

STAGES OF GRIEF

Dr. Elisabeth Kübler-Ross (1926–2004), a Swiss-born doctor who came to the United States in the 1950s, is the author of a famous book called *On Death and Dying.* Dr. Kübler-Ross, a psychiatrist, chose to work with terminally ill people. During her conversations with her patients, they expressed to her their feelings about what they were going through. These conversations formed the basis for many of the ideas in *On Death and Dying.* One key idea Dr. Kübler-Ross outlined in *On Death and Dying* is the idea that dying people experience distinct stages of grief. These same stages are also seen to some degree in people who are diagnosed with chronic illnesses, especially those illnesses that will greatly affect the person's way of living. For example, a person who has recently been told he has diabetes, heart disease, or hypertension may go through the same stages of grief that a person who has been told he is dying goes through. The stages of grief that Dr. Kübler-Ross identified are denial, anger, bargaining, depression, and acceptance:

- **Denial,** the first stage of grief, occurs when a person is told that he has a terminal illness. The person refuses to accept the diagnosis or feels that a mistake has been made (Fig. 28-1). He may ask for a second opinion, or act as if nothing is wrong and avoid returning to the doctor for a period of time. Denial helps to protect a person emotionally from overwhelming grief. This stage of grief can last only a few minutes, or it may last until the person actually dies. As a nursing assistant, it is not your place to convince the person that his illness exists, or to argue with the person about treatment or care issues. Instead, recognize that denial is a normal part of the grieving process, respond to the person in an honest yet neutral way, and communicate your observations to the nurse (Table 28-1).

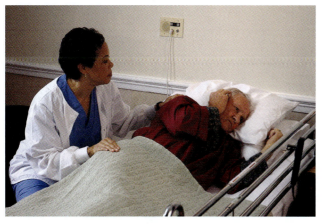

Figure 28-1
Denial helps to protect the person emotionally from overwhelming grief.

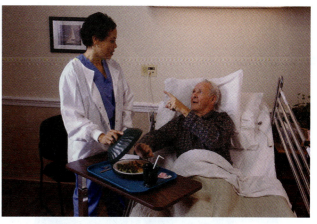

Figure 28-2
Many people who are grieving pass through a period of anger.

- **Anger** occurs when the person realizes that he is actually going to die (Fig. 28-2). People may feel angry for different reasons, and each person handles anger differently. Some people may be angry with themselves for not seeking help sooner, or for making a lifestyle choice that contributed to the illness, such as smoking. People express anger differently. Some people become moody and withdrawn, or uncooperative and hostile. Others may yell, or throw objects. If the person is religious, he may lose faith. Some people take their anger out on family members. Others may direct their anger toward health care

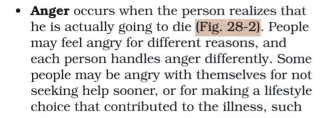

Table 28-1	Stages of Grief	
STAGE	**SAMPLE DIALOGUE**	**APPROPRIATE RESPONSE FROM NURSING ASSISTANT**
Denial	**Resident's daughter:** "They don't know what they're talking about. I know my mother is not dying. She has had pneumonia a number of times before, and she has always pulled through." **Nursing assistant:** "I'm sorry; it must be very hard for you to see your mother so sick."	Acknowledges what the person is saying by responding in an honest, yet neutral way
Anger	**Resident's husband:** "If the staff here wasn't so incompetent, my wife wouldn't be so sick!" **Nursing assistant:** "Mr. Smith, you seem so angry."	Acknowledges the person's anger and allows him to talk about it; by practicing empathy, you avoid feeling defensive or taking the person's anger personally
Bargaining	**Resident:** "I hope I can just hang on until my granddaughter has her baby. I would love to see my great-grandchild before I die." **Nursing assistant:** "We'll do all we can to help you do that. But until then, I'll be with you."	Offers support that she can realistically provide, and reassures the person that she will be cared for
Depression	**Resident:** "I don't want to die. . . . I'm so sad." **Nursing assistant** (sitting quietly and holding the resident's hand): "I'm here for you."	Offers comfort in the form of touch and silence; does not attempt to "cheer the person up"; if the person is refusing food or not sleeping, you could offer to obtain whatever foods appeal to the person's appetite or to talk to the nurse about arranging for medication to aid sleep
Acceptance	**Resident:** "I want to thank you for being so kind to me. It won't be long until I'm going on to my reward." **Nursing assistant:** "You're going on to your reward?"	Uses communication techniques that encourage the person to talk, such as rephrasing the person's statement as an open-ended question

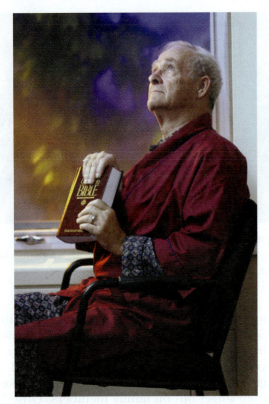

Figure 28-3
The bargaining stage is usually accompanied by a feeling of hope.

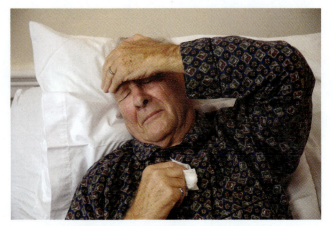

Figure 28-4
During the depression phase, the person realizes the full impact of his illness.

professionals. You must not take the anger personally—doing so can hurt your emotional well-being, as well as your ability to care for the person.

- **Bargaining** is typically done on a very private basis. The person wants to "make a deal" with someone he feels has control over his fate, such as God or a health care provider (Fig. 28-3). The person may want to live long enough to accomplish a goal, or to witness a specific event such as the birth of a child, a wedding, or an anniversary celebration. The will to live can be a very powerful force, and may, in fact, extend the person's life by a few months. As a nursing assistant, it is important for you to allow the person to experience the feeling of hope that accompanies this stage of grieving.
- **Depression** is the stage in which the person fully realizes that death will be the end result of the illness (Fig. 28-4). The person will be sad and may have regrets about things he was not able to accomplish during his lifetime. Some people are quite withdrawn and may say little, while others may want to openly mourn for their loss. Recognize that depression is a normal part of the grieving

process, and be supportive. Let the person know that it is all right for him to be feeling the way he is feeling. Tell the nurse if a grieving person's depression causes the person to cry constantly, refuse food, or fail to sleep. Some people will require medical intervention to treat their depression.

- **Acceptance** occurs when a person comes to terms with the reality of his own death, and is finally at peace with this knowledge (Fig. 28-5). Typically, people who have reached the acceptance stage will demonstrate their acceptance by completing unfinished business and saying their goodbyes. Many will plan their funeral service or write a poem or letter to be read after they are gone. Often, they will want to talk about their death, in an effort to help family members

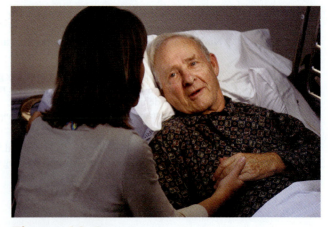

Figure 28-5
During the acceptance phase, the grieving person comes to terms with his death and begins to make plans for the future.

accept it also. The acceptance stage does not necessarily occur when death is near; some people gain acceptance months or even years prior to their eventual death from the illness.

It is important for you to recognize the stages of grief and understand that, although these stages have been identified, each person will experience them, and react to them, differently. Being able to recognize the stages of grief will enable you to provide better care to your residents and their families, because you will have a better understanding of what they are going through. This understanding will help you to be more effective in determining what your residents and their family members need from you.

A person who is grieving may not pass through all the stages of grief, and she may not pass through them in order. Many people work through the stages of grief, only to "relapse" and experience some of the earlier stages again. Throughout the grieving process, the one thing that usually persists is hope. Even the most realistic and accepting people hold onto the hope that a new drug will be developed, or that a new research project will yield a cure. Hope is what helps the person face another day or another painful treatment. It is what drives the person to keep up with normal activities, such as eating and praying, when she might otherwise feel like giving up entirely. As a nursing assistant, you must be responsive to, and nurture, a person's hope, without being unrealistic.

When you are caring for people who are grieving, be aware of the power of listening and touch. In many cases, it is not necessary to say anything at all. Listen to whatever the person needs to say, without imposing your own opinions or beliefs. Remember that this is the other person's grief, and he must work through it on his own terms.

GRIEF AND THE RESIDENT

Many of your residents will pass through the stages of grief over a period of many years. As a result, you may not actually see all of the stages of grief in a resident who is coming to terms with his own impending death. This is especially true of residents who have chronic conditions that they have struggled with for many years. These residents may have been hospitalized many times, when worsening symptoms put their overall health in danger. Each time such a health crisis occurred, the possibility of death loomed overhead. As a result, these residents may have worked through the various stages of grief over the course of many years as their condition worsened. Many live in a

state of acceptance, recognizing and accepting that death could come at any time.

One factor that influences how a person handles the grieving associated with the end of life is where the person is in his life in terms of responsibilities, commitments, accomplishments, hopes, and dreams. For example, an older person may feel more ready than a younger person may feel to die. The older person may feel more satisfied about what he has accomplished in life, which may make death easier to accept. On the other hand, an older person who is disappointed in how life turned out may feel bitter and angry about approaching death.

GRIEF AND THE FAMILY

The resident's family will also go through the stages of grief as they prepare for their loss. In fact, the stages of grief may be more apparent among the family members than in the resident who is approaching death. The resident may have already accepted the inevitability of illness and old age. However, for the resident's family, death may not seem like a reality until the person enters the active phase of dying.

Remembering that family members also experience the stages of grief will help you to understand behavior that may not seem fair or appropriate. For example, a family member may direct her anger at you, but the family member is not necessarily angry with you—she is angry that she is losing someone she loves. Like the dying person, the family members will each pass through the stages of grief individually and at their own order and pace. Sometimes there is emotional upset within a family when the members of the family (including the resident) are at different stages of the grieving process. Reporting your observations of this turmoil to the nurse will be helpful. Arranging for the assistance of clergy or other professionals experienced in grief counseling may be of great comfort to the person and the family.

TELL THE NURSE

When caring for a resident during the end-of-life period, pay attention to the person's emotional well-being, as well as her physical well-being. Report any of the following observations to the nurse immediately:

- The resident refuses treatment
- The resident cries constantly, refuses food, or cannot sleep

- There is tension and disagreement within the family
- The resident or a family member requests the assistance of clergy or a grief counselor
- The resident expresses interest in making or changing legal documents related to end-of-life care, such as advance directives or a will

GRIEF AND THE CAREGIVER

Caring for a resident during the end-of-life period will affect you. As we care for our residents, we become part of their lives and they become part of ours. When one of our residents is approaching death, we go through a grief process very similar to that experienced by the person and the family. Additionally, because members of the health care profession feel a great need to be able to help others, we often feel inadequate when we must watch others suffer and grieve, and there is little we can do to relieve their pain. We may even question our professional calling. Regardless of how long you work in the health care profession, a resident's declining health and death will impact you emotionally.

Taking time for yourself is very important. Doing this will help you to keep your feelings and emotions in perspective, and it will allow you to continue to give of yourself to others. Talking to your supervisor, a clergy member, or a mental health counselor about questions and fears you have about death can help you to clarify your feelings about death and dying (Fig. 28-6). In addition, you might find seeking advice from an "expert" helpful when you are trying to work through feelings concerning a specific situation with a resident.

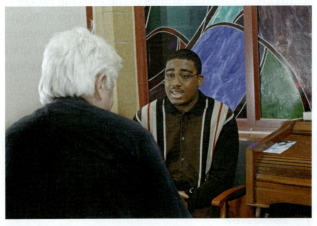

Figure 28-6
Clarifying your beliefs and confronting your fears about death and dying can help you to care for your residents more effectively.

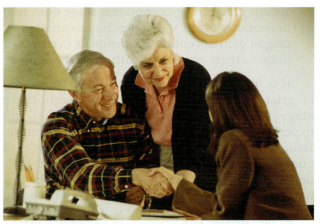

Figure 28-7
Having a living will, a durable power of attorney, or both helps to ensure that a person's wishes regarding his end-of-life care are known and honored in case the person is not able to make these wishes known himself. Many people seek a lawyer's assistance in completing these documents, just so they have them in case they ever need them. Long-term care facilities also have staff members who are able to assist residents with writing a living will or durable power of attorney. (© *Jupiter Images*)

DYING WITH DIGNITY

All people have the right to die in a way that is as peaceful and dignified as possible. Advance directives and hospice care can help to ensure a person's comfort and dignity during the end-of-life period.

ADVANCE DIRECTIVES

In Chapter 4, you learned that advance directives are documents that allow a person to make her wishes regarding health care known to family members and health care workers, in case the time comes when she is no longer able to make those wishes known herself. You will recall that a person's advance directive could include a living will, the naming of a durable power of attorney for health care (also known as a health care agent), or both.

Many people arrange for living wills, durable powers of attorney, or both as a way of ensuring that their wishes regarding their end-of-life care are known and honored (Fig. 28-7). Many people specify in their advance directives that they would like to avoid **life-sustaining treatments** (treatments that will prolong life) if by having these treatments, their quality of life will be compromised. Examples of life-sustaining treatments include respiratory ventilation, cardiopulmonary resuscitation (CPR), and the placement of a feeding tube or intravenous (IV) line for the provision of nutrition. Instead, the person may specify that only supportive care should be provided. **Supportive care** includes treatments that will not prolong life but will make the person more comfortable such as oxygen therapy, nutritional supplementation, pain medication, range-of-motion exercises, grooming and hygiene, and positioning assistance. A person who has made the decision to receive only supportive care at the end of her life will have a **no-code** or **do not resuscitate (DNR) order** written on her chart. This means that the usual efforts to save the person's life will not be made. The entire health care team should be aware of this order so that the person will be allowed to die with the compassion and dignity she has requested.

HOSPICE CARE

Hospice care is provided to ensure the person's comfort and dignity as death approaches, and to maintain the person's best quality of life until that time. There are Medicare benefits available for hospice care. A person becomes eligible for these benefits when the doctor documents in the person's medical record that the person's condition is end-stage or terminal, and that the person has approximately 6 months left to live.

Hospice care can be provided in a long-term care facility, in a hospital, in a facility that specializes in providing hospice care, or in the home. Hospice care is provided by a multidisciplinary team (made up of nurses, nursing assistants, clergy, social workers, doctors, mental health providers, and other professionals). The hospice team seeks to meet the physical, emotional, and spiritual needs of both the person and the person's family members. After the person's death, the hospice team provides grief counseling and other types of assistance for the family. Hospice care is available to residents and families 24 hours a day, 7 days a week.

The hospice team focuses on promoting the person's comfort. In addition to supportive care, the person usually also receives palliative care. **Palliative care** focuses on relieving uncomfortable symptoms, not on curing the problem that is causing the symptoms (Fig. 28-8). Examples of palliative treatments include the administration of medications to control pain, the administration of medications to prevent or treat constipation, and the use of oxygen to make it easier for the person to breathe. Treatments such as surgery, chemotherapy, and radiation may also be consid-

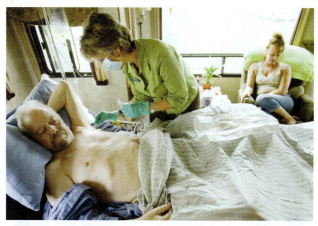

Figure 28-8

Hospice care seeks to promote comfort and quality of life for those who are dying. Here, a hospice worker checks a central line that is being used to administer pain medication. (*AP Photo/Coeur d'Alene Press, Jerome A. Pollos*)

ered palliative treatments when they are done primarily to increase the person's comfort, not to cure the person's disorder. For example, surgery may be performed to reduce the size of a tumor that is causing pain. Palliative care also involves eliminating certain routine procedures or treatments when they no longer offer any benefit to the person. For example:

- Medications that no longer serve a purpose may be discontinued.
- A therapeutic diet may be eliminated, and instead food and fluids are provided according to desire and tolerance.
- Routine weight measurements may be eliminated (unless they are needed for calculating medication dosages).
- Blood draws for laboratory tests may be eliminated (unless they are needed to monitor medication therapy).

Many people say that hospice is about living, not dying. Hospice helps people spend their remaining time in a way that is most meaningful to them. For some people, this may include enjoying simple pleasures, such as spending time in the courtyard so that they can enjoy the feeling of the sunshine and the smell of flowers (Fig. 28-9). Other people have a great need to reflect on, and talk about, their lives. This helps the person assign meaning to his life. Many people will find it important to spend time with loved ones to express feelings of love, appreciation, and hopes for the future. The opportunity to discuss regrets or make peace with those with whom they have had disagreements or misunderstandings may

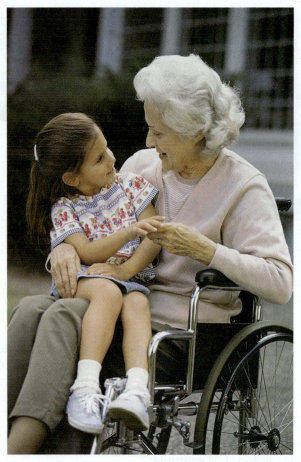

Figure 28-9
Care for a dying person includes helping the person to find pleasure and enjoyment during the time that is left.

also be important. The person can take much comfort in knowing that her wishes for living life and experiencing a dignified and peaceful death will be honored and that hospice is there to offer support and comfort to the family.

WILLS

A **will** is a legal statement that expresses a person's wishes for the management of her affairs after death. For a will to be valid, the person must be deemed competent, or "of sound mind," at the time the will is made or changed. If a resident expresses a desire to make or change a will, you should relay this information to the nurse. Many long-term care facilities have people on site who are able to provide assistance with wills, or the resident may wish to contact his own lawyer. As a nursing assistant, you may be asked to sign a will as a witness. If you sign as a witness, your signature means that you saw the person sign the document and that, to the best of your knowledge, the document accurately expresses that person's wishes. You should never sign a will as a witness if you have been named as a benefactor of the will. A benefactor is a person who will receive money or other items belonging to the person who has died when the will is read. You should also not sign a will as a witness if it is against your facility's policy for you to do so.

SUMMARY

- Applying the concept of holistic care—caring for the whole person by attending to the person's physical, emotional, and spiritual needs—is very important when you are caring for people at the end of life's journey.
- Caring for people during the end-of-life period requires an understanding of the ways in which people grieve.
  - Dr. Elisabeth Kübler-Ross, a noted authority on death and dying, identified five stages of grief: denial, anger, bargaining, depression, and acceptance.
  - Having an understanding of these stages and what the person is feeling during each one enables us to be more compassionate and understanding toward both the person and the family.
  - When caring for a person during the end-of-life period, recognize that you will also go through the grieving process as part of caring for the person, and make allowance for this.

- Advance directives and hospice care seek to preserve a person's right to die in as peaceful and dignified a manner as possible.
  - Many people arrange for living wills, durable powers of attorney, or both as a way of ensuring that their wishes regarding their end-of-life care are known and honored.
  - Hospice care seeks to preserve the person's comfort and dignity as death approaches, and to maintain the person's best quality of life until that time. A person becomes eligible for hospice care benefits through Medicare when the doctor documents in the person's record that the person's condition is terminal or end-stage, and the person has 6 months or less to live.
- A will is a legal document that expresses a person's wishes for the management of her affairs after death.

WHAT DID YOU LEARN?

Multiple Choice

Select the single best answer for each of the following questions.

1. Denial is:
   a. The stage of the grieving process in which the person becomes very depressed
   b. A form of bargaining with God for more time
   c. The final step of the grieving process
   d. The time during the grieving process when the person believes the diagnosis is incorrect

2. An organization that cares only for people who are dying is a:
   a. Skilled facility
   b. Sub-acute care unit
   c. Long-term care facility
   d. Hospice organization

3. The stage of grief when a person begins to say goodbye and make arrangements for his or her death is the:
   a. Bargaining stage
   b. Anger stage
   c. Denial stage
   d. Acceptance stage

4. Hospice care is designed to:
   a. Keep the person comfortable
   b. Prolong the person's life
   c. Treat the person aggressively
   d. All of the above

5. A resident with terminal cancer says he plans to live long enough to meet his first great-grandchild, who is due to be born in 2 months. This is an example of:
   a. Acceptance
   b. Depression
   c. Bargaining
   d. Denial

6. The legal document that expresses a person's wishes for the management of her affairs after death is a(n):
   a. Advance directive
   b. Durable power of attorney
   c. Living will
   d. Will

STOP and Think!

- Mrs. Brown, a resident in your long-term care facility, has a heart condition that is terminal. You have been caring for Mrs. Brown for a year or so now and have observed her working through the stages of grief as her condition has worsened. She seems to be in acceptance about her impending death and often talks about her funeral. The trouble is with Mrs. Brown's son. He used to visit quite often and was always friendly and courteous to the staff. Over the last few months, however, he has been visiting less often. When he has visited, he has been critical of you and the other caregivers, and once or twice he has even snapped at you. Just yesterday, you overheard him angrily telling his mother that he didn't want to hear anything else about a funeral! Why do you think Mrs. Brown's son is acting this way, and how can you help?

- You are caring for Mr. Lucas, an 82-year-old resident with chronic obstructive pulmonary disease (COPD) and heart failure. For the last 6 months, Mr. Lucas has needed to use oxygen periodically to help him breathe easier when he is feeling short of breath. Mr. Lucas has smoked for more than 50 years, and he continues to go to the smoking area at least once a day for a cigarette. He says that his cigarette is the highlight of his day. You have learned that Mr. Lucas has just been diagnosed with lung cancer. The doctor has talked to both Mr. Lucas and his family about his diagnosis. The doctor has told them that Mr. Lucas can undergo surgery, but that it would be very risky because of the COPD. Chemotherapy is not recommended due to the likelihood of serious damage to the heart. Without treatment, Mr. Lucas will most likely die within the year. Mr. Lucas does not want to do anything about his cancer. He wants to live out his days without feeling sick or exhausted by the cancer treatment. His family is very upset. They are angry about Mr. Lucas' smoking and they are demanding that the staff stop assisting him to the courtyard for his daily cigarette. Mr. Lucas asks you what you think he should do. What would you say to Mr. Lucas? Should you take him to the courtyard for a smoke? Can you do anything to help him in this situation?

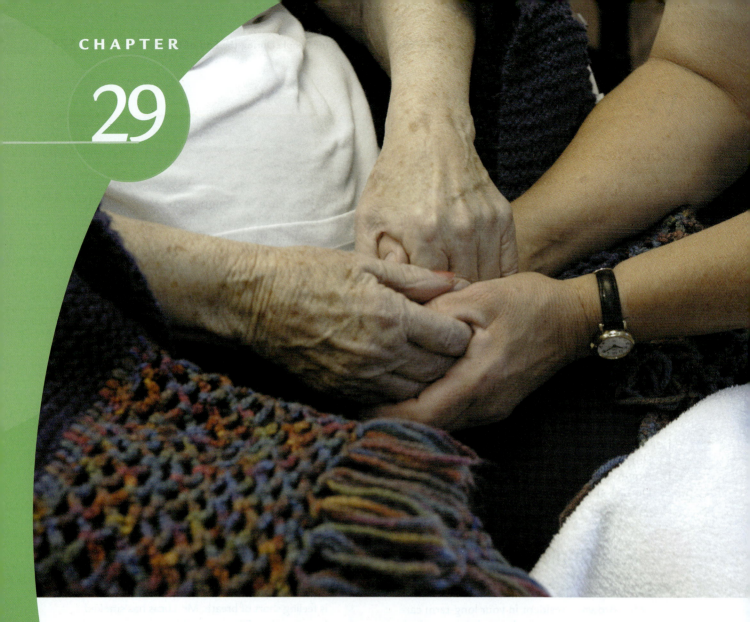

Caring for People Who Are Dying

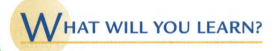HAT WILL YOU LEARN?

Each person is born to one possession which outvalues all the others—his last breath.
—Mark Twain

Most of us give little, if any, thought to what our "last breath" will be like. In the quote above, the American writer Mark Twain (1835–1910) suggests that the very end of life is an important life experience, just like all of the experiences leading up to that moment. As a nursing assistant, you will find yourself in the position of caring for residents who are dying. In this chapter, you will learn how you can help the dying person, and his or her family, in the time leading up to the person's "last breath," so that when the time comes, it is as peaceful as possible. You will also learn how to care for a person's body after death occurs. When you are finished with this chapter, you will be able to:

Photo: Sometimes, a simple gesture like holding someone's hand is the best thing you can do.

1. Describe the physical signs that frequently signal impending death.
2. Discuss how a nursing assistant's own feelings about death can affect the care given to a dying resident.
3. Describe ways in which the nursing assistant can provide comfort for the dying person.
4. Discuss how cultural and religious influences can affect how the dying person views death.
5. Describe the different ways in which family members may show grief.
6. Describe ways that a nursing assistant can help the family of a dying person.
7. Discuss the various responsibilities that a nursing assistant may have following the death of a resident.

Vocabulary Use the CD in the front of your book to hear these terms pronounced and defined:

Cyanotic	Afterlife	Postmortem care	Autopsy
Cheyne-Stokes respiration	Reincarnation	Rigor mortis	Shroud

SIGNS OF APPROACHING DEATH

Some people die suddenly, with little warning. Other people, however, may show certain characteristic physical signs in the time leading up to death, caused as the body begins to "shut down." These signs may appear over the course of a few hours or a few days, or in some cases, within the space of a few minutes. Some people may not show these signs. However, recognizing these physical signs and understanding why they occur will help you to know what type of care to give the dying person. Family members may also notice these signs, and become concerned. In this case, you will need to reassure them that these signs are normal signs of dying. (Any specific questions regarding the person's condition should be directed to the nurse.) Physical signs of impending death include the following:

- As circulation fails, the person's blood pressure drops and the pulse becomes rapid and weak. The person's skin feels cool and clammy, even though the person's body temperature is increasing. The person may perspire heavily and the skin may appear mottled (blotchy), very pale, **cyanotic** (blue-tinged), or grayish. Although you may be tempted to cover the person warmly, the person will need only light bed coverings.
- The respiratory pattern changes. The person may take very irregular, shallow breaths, in an alternating fast–slow pattern. This pattern of breathing is called **Cheyne-Stokes respiration.** As the person weakens, fluid or mucus may collect in the air passages, caus-

ing the noisy, rattling breathing that is often known as the "death rattle."
- The digestive system slows down. The person may experience nausea, vomiting, abdominal swelling, fecal impaction, or bowel incontinence. The person may not want food or water. Offering ice chips and providing frequent oral care helps to keep the mucous membranes of the mouth moist.
- Urine output decreases as the kidneys respond to the lack of blood flow. In addition, the person may become incontinent of urine.
- Nervous system changes result in decreased muscle tone and sensation. The muscles relax and the person may be too weak to reposition himself. Some people lose the ability to speak. The person may lose sensation in his arms or legs, and pain may decrease. Vision may become blurred. (You may notice that the person will turn toward a light in an effort to see better.) Hearing, however, usually remains normal until the moment of death.
- Consciousness may be altered. Some dying people lose consciousness and become comatose as death approaches. As consciousness decreases, pain usually does too. Some people remain conscious and oriented until the moment of death. It is common for a person who has drifted into and out of a semi-comatose state to become alert and oriented right before he or she dies.

When you are caring for a person who is dying, take note of any physical changes that you observe. Report these changes to the nurse and record them in the person's medical chart, per facility policy.

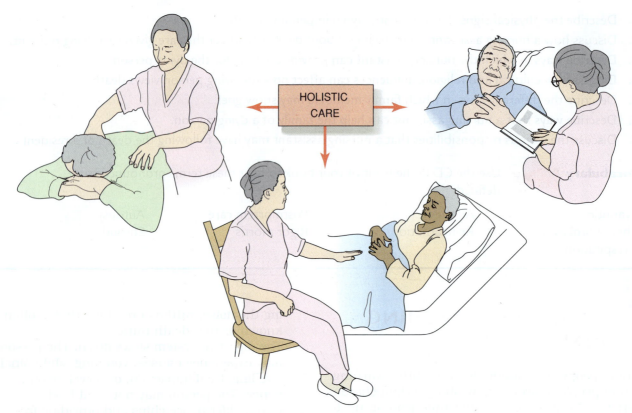

HOLISTIC
CARE

Figure 29-1

The nursing assistant provides for the dying person's physical and emotional comfort. Examples of physical comfort measures include providing frequent oral care and back massages. Examples of emotional comfort measures include caring for the family, helping the person to meet spiritual needs (for example, by reading aloud from a book that has special meaning for the person), and simply spending quiet time with the person.

CARING FOR A DYING PERSON

A holistic approach to care is taken with a person who is dying, just as with any other person (Fig. 29-1). Residents who are dying, like all residents, have physical and emotional needs. These needs may change dramatically as the time of death approaches, and will vary greatly depending on the person. Every person has the right to die peacefully and with dignity (Box 29-1). As a nursing assistant, it is your job to do everything you can to ensure that this right is honored.

Many nursing assistants (especially new nursing assistants) compromise the care they give to a dying resident, without being fully aware that they are doing so. For example, a nursing assistant might not check in on the dying person as often as she checks in on her other residents. She might provide only the necessary care and then leave the person's room quickly, because she might be afraid that if she stays, the person may actually die while she is in the room! Or, the nursing assistant may be overly cheerful around the person, hoping that this will keep the person from talking about death. These avoidance behaviors usually occur because the nursing assistant has not yet explored her own feelings about death. Many people who are new to the health care profession express concerns such as, "I'm afraid I'll cry if my resident dies," "I don't want to get too attached," or "I've never touched a dead person before and I'm scared." All of these are normal concerns. As noted in Chapter 28, talking to your supervisor, a clergy member, or a mental health counselor can help you to come to terms with your own feelings and beliefs about death. This knowledge of your own feelings will serve you well as you care for others who are dying.

Facing the death of a resident never gets any easier. You will become very attached to your residents. Although the relationship you have with the resident can make providing end-of-life care very emotionally difficult for you, it is this relationship that will allow you to provide the holistic care that the dying person needs so much.

BOX 29-1   The Dying Person's Bill of Rights

I have the right to be treated as a living human being until I die.

I have the right to maintain a sense of hopefulness, however changing its focus may be.

I have the right to be cared for by those who can maintain a sense of hopefulness, however changing this might be.

I have the right to express my feelings and emotions about my approaching death in my own way.

I have the right to participate in decisions concerning my care.

I have the right to expect continuing medical and nursing attention, even though "cure" goals must be changed to "comfort" goals.

I have the right not to die alone.

I have the right to be free from pain.

I have the right to have my questions answered honestly.

I have the right not to be deceived.

I have the right to have help from and for my family in accepting my death.

I have the right to die in peace and dignity.

I have the right to retain my individuality and not be judged for my decisions, which may be contrary to beliefs of others.

I have the right to discuss and enlarge my religious and/or spiritual experiences, whatever these may mean to others.

I have the right to expect that the sanctity of the human body will be respected after death.

I have the right to be cared for by caring, sensitive, knowledgeable people who will attempt to understand my needs and will be able to gain some satisfaction in helping me face my death.

_____

(Created at the workshop *The Terminally Ill Patient and the Helping Person,* in Lansing, Michigan, sponsored by the Southwestern Michigan Inservice Education Council and conducted by Amelia J. Barbus, Associate Professor of Nursing, Wayne State University, Detroit.)

MEETING THE DYING PERSON'S PHYSICAL NEEDS

A dying person becomes more and more dependent on others for basic physical care as the time of death approaches. As the focus of care becomes comfort, the nursing assistant has the opportunity to help the person feel that he is not alone in this last stage of life. Basic aspects of physical care for the dying person include the following:

- **Care of the skin.** More frequent skin care and linen changes are needed because of the urinary or bowel incontinence and the moist skin that often occur as the person nears death. The person will need to be checked regularly for incontinence of both urine and feces. His skin will need to be cleaned gently, and soiled clothing and linens must be changed.
- **Care of the mucous membranes.** Frequent oral care helps keep the mouth moist and more comfortable, especially if the person is comatose or not taking food or drink. Sometimes as death nears, the person does not blink as often, and a mucus crust may form around the eyelids. Gentle cleaning with a warm, wet washcloth helps to remove the dried mucus. The nurse may apply an ointment to keep the eyes moist. If the person is comatose, moist eye pads may be used for protection. Medical equipment, such as oxygen cannulas, may cause irritation and crusting of mucus around the nostrils. Gently removing the mucus crust with a warm, wet washcloth and applying a lubricant can help to keep the person comfortable.

- **Positioning.** As the person's condition worsens, the person may not be able to reposition herself without assistance. Frequent, regular position changes help to prevent pressure ulcers and promote comfort. The use of pillows or other positioning devices helps to maintain the body in proper alignment. If the person is in pain, you will need to be extra gentle and slow with position changes. Always tell the nurse if the person seems to be in pain so that necessary medications can be administered. A person who is having difficulty breathing will probably be more comfortable positioned with her head elevated.
- **Other comfort measures.** Receiving a back massage, listening to soft music, or being read to can help a person to rest and feel better. Enemas may be necessary to assist with bowel elimination. Secretions may collect in the person's airways, making breathing difficult. If you notice that a person is

having difficulty breathing, report this to the nurse. Suctioning and oxygen therapy can make breathing easier and more comfortable for the person. Keep the room well lit and ventilated. Remove soiled linens, bedpans, or emesis basins and use air freshener to help eliminate unpleasant odors.

As death nears, there may be changes in the dying person's ability to communicate with others. As the person's ability to communicate pain, thirst, or other physical needs decreases, he will rely more and more on the nursing team to notice those needs and take care of them. In addition, you must take measures to make communication easier:

- Remember that as death approaches, the person's vision may become blurry. Keep the room well lit to help the person to see better. Also, make sure you introduce yourself when entering the room and encourage family members to do the same. Imagine how you would feel if you could no longer see well, and you could not tell who was entering and leaving your room!
- Speaking may become difficult for the person. In this case, asking simple "yes or no" questions will make communication more effective.
- Hearing usually remains quite sharp up until the time of death, even if the person is comatose. Always talk to the person as if he is able to hear you, even if he cannot respond. Explain procedures to the person and offer reassurance that you are there and will return soon when you leave the room. Gently remind family members that the person may still be able to hear their conversations, and encourage them to talk to the person. Hearing the voices of family members can be comforting for the dying person. However, family members should be advised that potentially upsetting topics should be discussed elsewhere, out of earshot of the dying person.

A person's family members may wish to assist in providing physical care. If a family member says that she would like to be involved in caring for the dying person, encourage this by suggesting ways that the family member can help. For example, you might ask the family member if she would be willing to help you out by giving the person ice chips, and then show the family member how to do this (Fig. 29-2). Family members often feel useless or helpless when it becomes clear that there is nothing left to do except wait for death to arrive. Participating in the care of a dying loved one can help a family member to feel better about the situation.

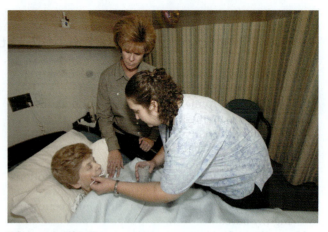

Figure 29-2
Sometimes, family members want to assist in meeting a dying person's physical needs. Here, a nursing assistant is showing a family member how to ease the person's thirst by giving ice chips.

MEETING THE DYING PERSON'S EMOTIONAL NEEDS

Emotionally, people prepare for death very individually. People may have many fears regarding death, such as a fear of the unknown or a fear of losing dignity and self-control. Some may fear that death will be painful, or worry about the effects of their death on the people left behind. Some people have concerns about unfinished business. Another concern that many dying people have is a fear of facing death alone (Fig. 29-3). Some people are able to talk about their fears, while others remain silent, unable to talk about what frightens them the most.

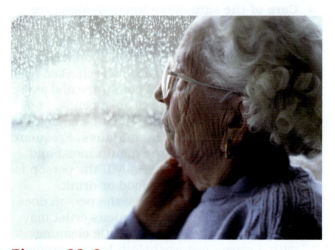

Figure 29-3
Many people have fears related to death, such as a fear of dying alone or of dying in pain. As a nursing assistant, you can help to relieve some of these fears.

Being a Good Listener

A nursing assistant can help meet a dying person's emotional needs by being a good listener (Fig. 29-4). A dying person may want to talk about her fears related to dying, or what she expects the afterlife to be like. Or, the person might just want to remember significant events in her life, and share those memories with you now. If you sense that a person wants to talk, use the communication techniques you learned in Chapter 5 to encourage her and let her know that you are there to listen. Even though you may be uncomfortable at first when a resident brings up the subject of death, do not change the subject, make yourself "busy," or simply pat the person on the hand and say, "Oh, don't worry, honey; you've got lots of time left." Many dying people are very aware of their situation and they may tell you that their time here is very short. Do not avoid spending time with a dying person because you are afraid that the person will bring up the subject of dying and you will not know what to say in response. You do not need to say anything—you just need to listen to what the person wants to tell you.

Other dying people do not want to talk and can become annoyed at your attempts to make small talk. Use your observation skills to note when a person would prefer not to talk. Although the person may not want to have a conversation, she will still want to know that you are nearby and watching out for her. Check on the person frequently and regularly and remind her that you are close by if she needs anything.

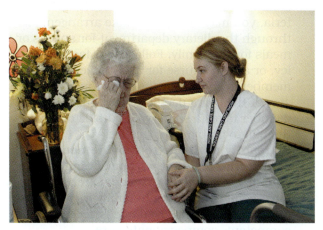

Figure 29-4

A nursing assistant helps to meet a dying person's emotional needs by being a good listener. Although you may think that the dying person is the one who benefits the most from these times spent together, quite frequently you will find that you benefit too. These moments spent listening can help you to understand yourself better, as well as your residents.

Helping Hands and a Caring Heart

FOCUS ON HUMANISTIC HEALTH CARE

Many dying people genuinely appreciate it when someone takes the time to sit near them quietly. Touch can convey so much more than words can in a situation like this. Gently hold the person's hand or touch her shoulder when you are speaking to her. Gently smooth the person's hair after you have finished straightening the bed linens or repositioning the pillow, or comfort the person with a back massage. All of these actions let a person know that she is cared for and not alone.

Culture, Religion, and Spirituality

Cultural and religious beliefs influence how a person feels about death and prepares for it. For example, some people may not feel comfortable talking about dying, because in their culture, death is considered a very private matter. Other people may seem very accepting of death, because their culture or religion has taught them that death is not to be feared.

Many dying people find peace and comfort in their religious faith. They may wish to visit with clergy members, surround themselves with religious items, or spend time alone in prayer, meditation, and reading of religious texts. Some people may ask you to read to them. Although you may not share the person's religious beliefs, you should honor this request. For the dying person, hearing familiar words that reflect the person's deepest beliefs can bring great comfort. You must respect the beliefs of other people, even if you do not share these beliefs.

A dying person may request that you call a clergy member to administer religious blessings or "last rites." If such a request is made, report it immediately to the nurse so that the necessary arrangements can be made. When the clergy member arrives, make sure that there is a place for the clergy member to sit, and ensure privacy. As part of preparing for death, people often want to confess to a clergy member, and they will want privacy to do this.

Religion is but one aspect of spirituality and many people are very spiritual without belonging to any particular religious group. Most people who are "spiritual" believe that a higher being or spirit offers hope and peace, although this higher being may not necessarily be one that is recognized by the world's various religions. Spirituality gives a person inner strength to face life's challenges. It gives meaning to a person's life. Many people exhibit their inner spirituality by listening to music, reading poetry, or just watching a sunset.

When cultural and religious or spiritual beliefs provide an explanation for what happens to a person after death, they can be a source of comfort for the dying person (as well as for the person's family members). For example, many people believe in an **afterlife,** a state of being where the dead meet again with loved ones who have passed on before them. Other people believe in **reincarnation,** the idea that a person's spirit or soul will live again on Earth in the form of an animal or human being, yet to be born.

CARE OF THE FAMILY

Knowing that a loved one will die soon can be difficult for family members. Family members must cope with their own grief, and possibly that of other family members as well. The stress and grief experienced by family members can cause them to act in ways that may seem strange to you. For example, some people may treat you rudely, or snap at you in anger. Be polite and do not take offensive actions or words personally. Usually, these offensive behaviors are just a result of the person's grief. If a family member seems to be getting overly agitated or angry, or if arguing or aggression between family members occurs, notify the nurse immediately.

As a nursing assistant, you may feel overwhelmed at the thought of caring for the family, as well as for the resident. However, there are many simple things you can do to comfort the family (Fig. 29-5).

- **Ensure good communication between the family members and the health care team.** Often, family members will have worries or fears related to the person's care or condition, and they may want to discuss these with you or another member of the health care team. If a family member asks you a question that you do not know the answer to or are not qualified to answer, make sure to relay this request for information to the nurse so that the family member's concerns can be addressed.
- **Allow family members to stay with the dying person, and to participate in the person's care if they want to.** When a person is dying, many families wish to remain close by. Visiting hours are usually relaxed, allowing family members to stay with the dying person for as long as they like.

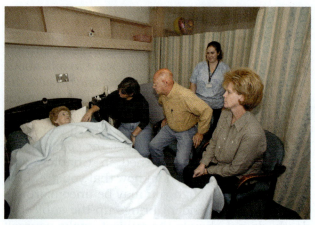

Figure 29-5
Family members will often seek reassurance and comfort from the nursing staff. As a nursing assistant, there are many simple kindnesses you can extend to the family that will help make this ordeal easier for them. Here, a nursing assistant has brought in an extra chair for a family member who has just arrived at the bedside.

Encourage family members to talk to the dying person and to help with the person's care. However, do not push family members to do this if they seem hesitant.

- **Ensure that the family members' basic needs are met.** Make sure that there are enough chairs in the room so that everyone can sit down. Encourage family members to rest and take meals as necessary. Show them how to find the restrooms, public telephones, vending machines, and cafeteria, if one is available. If your facility does not have a cafeteria, you may be able to make arrangements through the dietary department for snacks or meals for the family. Follow your facility policy, or ask the nurse for assistance. If a family member is showing signs of weariness, offer to stay at the dying person's side while the family member takes a short walk outside or down the hall to grab a cup of coffee.
- **Be readily available to provide needed care to the resident without being intrusive of the family's privacy.** Often, the most comforting thing to family members is knowing that their loved one is receiving competent, compassionate care.

Although you have responsibilities to the family, your first responsibility is to your resident. When providing physical care to the resident, be sure to ask the family members to step outside for a moment (unless they have chosen to help you) and close the curtains to help maintain the person's dignity. Also, too many visitors for too long a period of time can be tiring for some residents. If you suspect that the number of visitors or the length of time that they are staying is causing your resident to become overly tired, please report your observations to the nurse.

TELL THE NURSE !

When you are caring for a person who is dying, be sure to report the following to the nurse immediately:

- The person seems to be in pain

- The person is having trouble breathing

- The person asks to see a clergy member

- The person seems overwhelmed by the number of visitors or the length of time that they are staying

- A family member has a question about the person's care or condition that you are not qualified to answer

- The person has died

POSTMORTEM CARE

If you are present when one of your residents dies, you must notify the nurse that the person has died, and note the time. You may need to document the absence of vital signs. A doctor must be called to legally pronounce the person dead. The time of death is recorded on the person's death certificate. After the doctor has pronounced the person dead, you may be required to assist the nurse in giving postmortem care, depending on your facility's policy.

Postmortem care is the care of a person's body after the person's death. Cultural and religious beliefs often dictate how the body is to be cared for after death (and by whom). In some cultures, family members help to clean and prepare the body for whatever lies ahead, in accordance with cultural and religious traditions.

Postmortem care is necessary to keep the body in proper alignment and to prevent skin damage and discoloration. The skin is cleaned of any mucus, urine, feces, or other fluids. Standard precautions are followed when performing postmortem care, because bodily fluids are still potentially infectious, even after death. The body is placed in proper alignment before rigor mortis occurs. **Rigor mortis** is the stiffening of the muscles that usually develops 2 to 4 hours after death. Once rigor mortis occurs, it is difficult to reposition the body. It is common for air that has

been trapped in the lungs or the digestive tract to be released from the body when the body is repositioned as part of postmortem care. It may sound like the person has sighed or moaned. This natural occurrence may frighten you, unless you are aware of its cause.

In some cases, an autopsy may be required to confirm or identify the cause of the person's death. An **autopsy** is an examination of the person's organs and tissues after the person has died. In most cases, the doctor is responsible for obtaining a family member's permission to perform an autopsy. If an autopsy is to be performed, medical devices, such as tubes, drains, catheters, and intravenous (IV) lines, are not removed as part of postmortem care. If an autopsy is not necessary, the nurse will usually remove these medical devices as part of the postmortem care procedure.

Many facilities only prepare the person's body for the family to view before sending it to the morgue or funeral home, where the funeral director completes the postmortem care procedure. In this case, the bed linens are straightened (or changed, if they are soiled). The body is cleaned, dressed in a clean gown or pajamas, and positioned in a natural position on the bed (Fig. 29-6). Draw the top sheet up to the person's shoulders and cuff it neatly. (Do not cover the person's face with the sheet. This can be very disturbing for family members.) Make sure that the room is neat, and adjust the lights so that they are not too bright. As always, provide for privacy. You will need to help collect the person's personal belongings to be sent with the family. Dentures are either placed in the person's mouth, or labeled and sent with the body to the funeral home.

After the family has viewed the body and left, the body may be wrapped in a **shroud** (a covering used to wrap the body of a person who has died) for

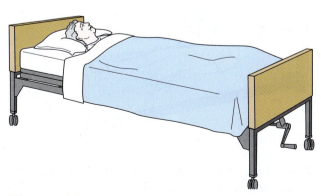

Figure 29-6

The body is placed in the supine position for viewing by the family. A pillow is placed under the person's head and shoulders.

transport to the morgue or funeral home. A shroud is contained in the preassembled postmortem kits used by many facilities (Fig. 29-7). The shroud may be a plastic sheet that is secured with pins, tapes, or ties (Fig. 29-8), or it may zip closed. The postmortem kit also usually contains safety pins or tape for securing the shroud, ties for holding the person's hands together, identification tags, a chin strap for securing the person's jaw, a plastic bag or envelope for the person's belongings, and 12″× 12″ gauze pads to absorb drainage. The procedure for postmortem care is given in Procedure 29-1. You show your respect for the person and the person's family by working quietly and preserving the person's privacy, even after death.

Providing postmortem care can be emotionally difficult. Health care workers often become very attached to their residents and grieve when they die. It is perfectly acceptable to feel sad and cry at the passing of a resident. You might be surprised to know that even the most experienced health care workers often seek a "shoulder to cry on." Talking about your feelings with a co-worker, supervisor, clergy member, or counselor can help you work through your own grief. Allow yourself to be a human being and to feel emotions. It might also help to think of providing postmortem care as a way of paying your last respects to the dead person. In this way, the ritual of providing this care becomes a way of coping with your grief.

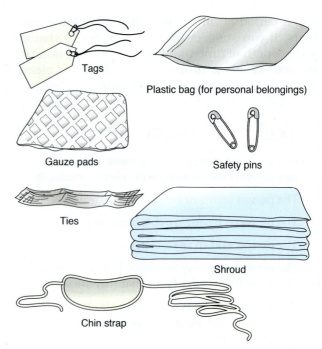

Figure 29-7

The contents of the postmortem kit vary, but most contain a shroud, something for securing the shroud, ties, gauze pads, a chinstrap, identification tags, and a plastic bag or envelope for the person's belongings.

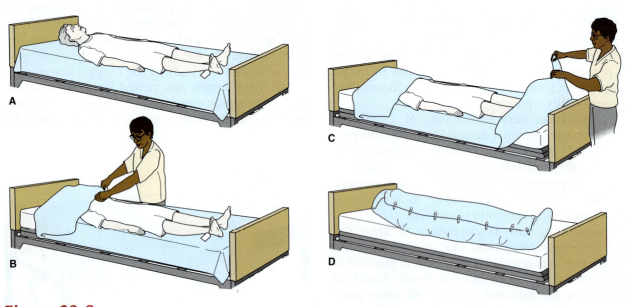

Figure 29-8

A shroud may be placed on the body after the family has left and before the body is taken to the morgue or funeral home. **(A)** The shroud is unfolded on the bed, and the body is placed on the shroud. **(B)** The top of the shroud is brought over the person's head. **(C)** The bottom of the shroud is brought over the person's feet. **(D)** The sides of the shroud are folded over the person's body and pinned, taped, or tied together. An identification tag is secured to the outside of the shroud.

SUMMARY

- Providing holistic care is as important at the end of life as it is at any other time. Nursing assistants must take steps to prevent their own discomfort with the subject of death from compromising their ability to care for people who are dying.
  - A dying person becomes very dependent on others for basic physical care. Recognizing the physical signs of impending death helps the nursing assistant to provide the necessary care.
  - A dying person will need assistance to meet emotional and spiritual needs as well.
    - Emotionally, people prepare for death in their own individual ways. Cultural and religious beliefs greatly influence a person's response to illness and death.
    - Often, the best thing a nursing assistant can do is listen if the person wants to talk, or spend quiet time with the person if he or she does not want to talk.
- Family members of a dying person require support as well.
  - Being respectful, thoughtful, and kind can do much to make family members feel better.
  - Some family members react poorly to grief and stress and may take out their frustrations on nursing assistants or other members of the health care team.
- Postmortem care is done to prepare the body for the morgue or funeral home. In some facilities, the body is prepared for the family's immediate viewing, and then postmortem care is done at the morgue or funeral home.

Providing Postmortem Care

WHY YOU DO IT   Postmortem care keeps the body in proper alignment and prevents skin damage and discoloration.

Getting Ready WCKIEPS

1. Complete the "Getting Ready" steps.

Supplies

- gloves
- paper towels
- cotton balls
- bed protector
- postmortem kit*
- wash basin
- soap
- comb
- bath blanket
- washcloth
- towel
- clean gown
- clean linens (if necessary)

Procedure

2. Cover the over-bed table with paper towels. Place your supplies on the over-bed table.

3. Make sure that the bed is positioned at a comfortable working height (to promote good body mechanics) and that the wheels are locked. Lower the head of the bed so that the bed is flat. Fanfold the top linens to the foot of the bed.

4. Put on the gloves.

5. If instructed to by the nurse, remove or turn off any medical equipment.

6. Place the body in the supine position. Position the pillow under the person's head and shoulders. Undress the body and cover it with the bath blanket.

7. Close the eyes. Put a moistened cotton ball on each eyelid if the eyes do not stay closed. If the person has an artificial eye, this should be in place, unless you are instructed otherwise.

8. Replace the person's dentures, unless you are instructed otherwise. Close the mouth and, if necessary, gently support the jaw with the chin strap, a light bandage, or a rolled hand towel.

9. Remove any jewelry and place it in a plastic bag or envelope for the family. List each piece of jewelry as you remove it. Do not remove engagement or wedding rings, unless it is your facility's policy to do so.

10. Fill the wash basin with warm water. Place the basin on the over-bed table. Wash the body and comb the hair.

11. If the family is to view the body, dress the body in a clean gown. If the bedding is wet or soiled, change the bed linens. Draw the top linens over the person, forming a cuff at the shoulders. (Do not cover the person's face.) Straighten the room, lower the lights, and provide for the family's privacy.

12. After the family leaves, collect all of the person's belongings, noting each item on your list.

13. Fill out three identification tags:
    a. Attach one to the right great toe or the right ankle.
    b. Attach one to the person's belongings.
    c. Save the last to be attached to the outside of the shroud (if used).

14. If a shroud is to be used, apply it now and attach the third identification tag to the outside of the shroud.

15. Gather the soiled linens and place them in the linen hamper. Dispose of disposable items in a facility-approved waste container. Clean equipment and return it to the storage area.

---

*The contents of the postmortem kit vary, but most contain a shroud, something for securing the shroud, ties, gauze pads, a chin strap, identification tags, and a plastic bag or envelope for the person's belongings.

16. Remove your gloves and dispose of them in a facility-approved waste container.

17. Transfer the body from the bed to a stretcher for transport to the morgue, if appropriate. If the family has made funeral arrangements, leave the body in the room with the door or curtain closed.

18. Report the time the body was transported and the location of the person's belongings to the nurse.

Finishing Up

19. Complete the "Finishing Up" steps.

WHAT DID YOU LEARN?

Multiple Choice

Select the single best answer for each of the following questions.

1. When caring for a person who is dying, you should:
   a. Keep family members away from the dying person
   b. Keep the room dark
   c. Provide for the person's physical and emotional needs
   d. Change the subject if the person starts to talk about death or dying

2. A common sign of approaching death is:
   a. Severe pain that gets worse
   b. Normal or increased vital signs
   c. Cool, moist skin
   d. Increased appetite

3. Postmortem care is done:
   a. Right before the person dies
   b. After the doctor pronounces the person dead
   c. After rigor mortis sets in
   d. If there is time

4. As death approaches, the last sense to be lost is:
   a. Sight
   b. Hearing
   c. Smell
   d. Taste

5. Which one of the following is a true statement about providing postmortem care?
   a. Standard precautions are used because the body may be infectious
   b. Dentures are removed from the mouth and given to the family to take home
   c. There is no need for privacy because the person is dead
   d. All of the above

6. In caring for the dying person, the nursing assistant also needs to care for the family. Which of the following can the nursing assistant do to support the family?
   a. Allow family members to stay with the dying person
   b. Be respectful of the family
   c. Provide the family with privacy
   d. All of the above

7. You are helping to care for Mrs. Winger, who has a terminal illness. One day when you are in Mrs. Winger's room, she tells you that during difficult times she has always found comfort in reading poems by her favorite poets. What is this an example of?
   a. Culture
   b. Spirituality
   c. Religion
   d. Reincarnation

8. Which of the following meets a dying person's physical needs?
   a. Providing frequent skin care
   b. Listening if the person wants to talk
   c. Preventing rigor mortis
   d. All of the above

Matching

Match each numbered item with its appropriate lettered description.

_____ 1. Reincarnation

_____ 2. Cheyne-Stokes respiration

_____ 3. Rigor mortis

_____ 4. Postmortem care

_____ 5. Autopsy

a. Examination of a person's tissues and organs after death
b. Stiffening of the muscles that occurs 2 to 4 hours after death
c. Care of a body after death
d. The belief that the soul of a dead person returns to Earth in the form of another human being or animal, yet to be born
e. Pattern of rapid–slow respirations

STOP and Think!

- You have been caring for Mr. Cole, who is dying. Now it appears that the time of death is rapidly approaching. Even though Mr. Cole is having trouble talking, he does manage to say to you, "I don't want to die alone." What can you do to help Mr. Cole?

Nursing Assistants Make a Difference!

"My mother recently passed away at Clayton County Nursing Home. Although Mom had been in poor health for some time, her death was hard on me. I must say, though, that the staff at Clayton County made this difficult time more bearable through their kindness and competence.

Last Monday, the phone rang and it was Elaine, one of the night nurses on duty. Elaine said that we needed to gather the family and come out, that Mom was dying. Soon, we had quite a crowd in Mom's room. I guess the staff was expecting us, because they had moved Mom's roommate to another room and brought in chairs so we would all have someplace to sit. One of the nursing assistants, Patty, was so great. She actually brought us a tray with a pot full of hot coffee, coffee cups, sugar, and creamer on it! We sat with Mom throughout the night and morning hours as she slowly weakened. Patty checked in with us often and would help turn Mom and change her when she soiled the bed. Sometimes she brought the nurse in to suction Mom when she started having trouble breathing. Although Mom could not talk to us, she regained consciousness about an hour before she died and looked us each in the eyes as we said our tearful good-byes.

When Mom took her last breath, we all knew what had happened. My sister went out into the hall to look for help. Luckily, Patty was nearby, and she quickly returned to the room to check Mom's vital signs. Then the doctor came in, and pronounced Mom dead. I asked Patty if I could help her wash Mom's body and get her into a clean gown, and Patty said that would be fine. Together, Patty and I prepared Mom for the funeral home. My family and I were allowed to stay in the room for a while after Mom died, just to reflect on things and finish making plans for the funeral.

Patty was really a godsend to me and my family during this difficult time. The excellent way Patty handled Mom's death spoke volumes about the care she gave to Mom while she was alive."

You can listen to more stories about how nursing assistants make a difference on the CD in the front of your book.

STRUCTURE AND FUNCTION OF THE HUMAN BODY

The human body is truly remarkable in its ability to maintain health and to heal from disease. In this unit, we will explore how each organ system functions normally, as well as how disease or injury affects the function of the organ system. We will also explore the measures that are taken to help the body return to its best level of functioning after injury or illness. Knowing how the body works when it is healthy helps us to understand how to help the body heal and function more effectively during illness.

Photo: The human body has amazing capabilities. This resident is celebrating her 107th birthday! (AP Photo/Argus Leader, Cory Myers).

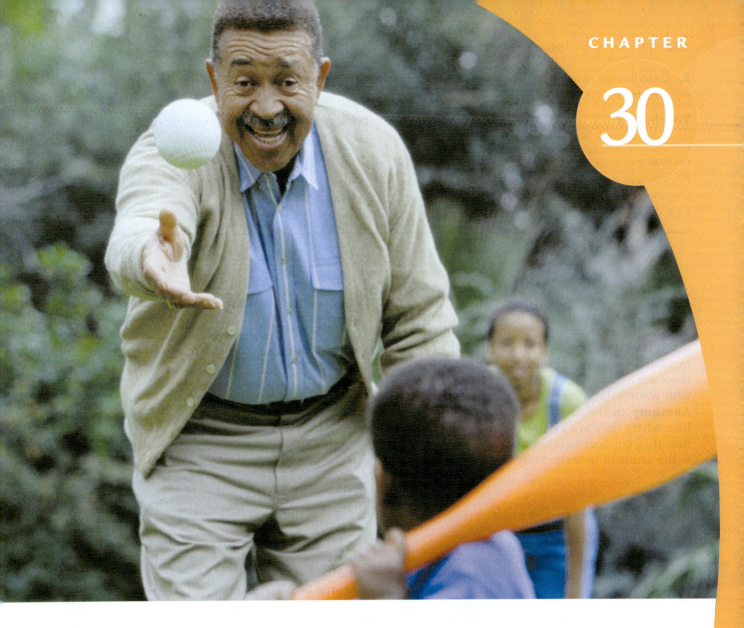

Basic Body Structure and Function

WHAT WILL YOU LEARN?

In this chapter, we will take a look at the body as a whole, functioning unit. You will learn about how changes in a person's normal anatomy or physiology can lead to disease or disabilities, and about the body's remarkable ability to correct small problems before they become large ones. When you are finished with this chapter, you will be able to:

1. Define the terms *anatomy* and *physiology*.
2. List and describe the basic levels of organization of the body.
3. Define the term *homeostasis* and give examples of how the body maintains the balance necessary for life.
4. Discuss how the body's inability to maintain homeostasis affects a person's health.

Photo: When we are healthy, our bodies allow us to do the things we like to do.

591

5. Describe the categories of disease and list some factors that may put a person at risk for developing a certain disease.

Vocabulary Use the CD in the front of your book to hear these terms pronounced and defined:

Anatomy	Organelles	Tissue	Homeostasis
Physiology	Cytoplasm	Organ	Disease
Organism	Nucleus	Organ system	
Cell	Cell membrane		

The human body is a wonder of design. In a healthy person, all of the body's parts work together effortlessly, like those of a highly efficient machine. To understand how a machine works, a mechanic studies the machine's parts and how they work together. The same is true of people who want to know how the human body works. **Anatomy** is the study of what body parts look like, where they are located, how big they are, and how they connect to other body parts. **Physiology** is the study of how the body parts work.

HOW IS THE BODY ORGANIZED?

All living things, from a jellyfish that washes up on the beach to the largest elephant roaming the plains of Africa, share the same general organization. The basic unit of life is the cell. Cells group together to form tissues. Tissues group together to form organs, and organs group together to form organ systems. Every living thing, or **organism**, shares these levels of organization, whether it is an animal or a plant (Fig. 30-1). The reason

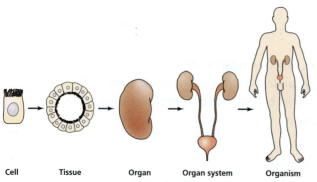

| Cell | Tissue | Organ | Organ system | Organism |

Figure 30-1
All living things (organisms) share the same basic levels of organization. Cells form tissues, tissues form organs, and organs form organ systems.

not all living things look alike or function alike is because at each level, there are variations specific to the type of organism. Let's take a closer look now at the levels of organization that make up each organism—cells, tissues, organs, and organ systems.

CELLS

A **cell** is the basic unit of life. A cell is so small that it can only be seen with a microscope. A single cell, as small as it is, has all of the characteristics of life. It is capable of organization, which means that it can join with other similar cells to perform a common function. It is capable of metabolism, which means that it takes in "raw materials" and converts them into the energy it needs to stay alive. It is capable of growth, which means that it changes in size over time. And finally, it is capable of reproduction, which means that it can make a copy of itself. Organization, metabolism, growth, and reproduction are basic qualities that make a living thing different from a non-living thing.

The human body is made up of millions of cells, of all different shapes, sizes, and functions. Each type of cell in the body has a specific duty. Our overall health depends on the ability of the cells of the body to do their jobs.

To function properly, cells require oxygen, water, nutrition, and the ability to eliminate waste products. Structures inside of the cell, called **organelles,** help the cell to make the energy it needs to stay alive and to rid itself of waste products (Fig. 30-2). The organelles float in a jelly-like substance called **cytoplasm.** In addition to organelles and cytoplasm, the cell contains a nucleus. The **nucleus** of the cell is like the cell's "brain." It contains all of the information the cell needs to do its job, grow, and reproduce. A **cell membrane** surrounds the cytoplasm and gives the cell its shape.

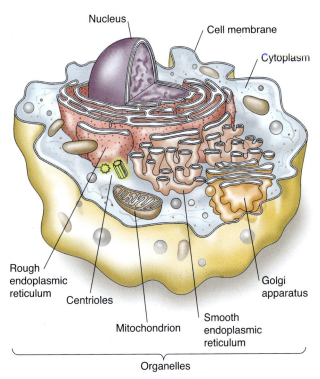

Figure 30-2
A cell contains organelles and a nucleus, which float in a jelly-like substance called cytoplasm. A cell membrane surrounds the cytoplasm and gives the cell its shape.

TISSUES

When cells that are similar in structure and specialized to perform a specific function join together, they form **tissue** (Fig. 30-3). There are four main types of tissue in the human body.

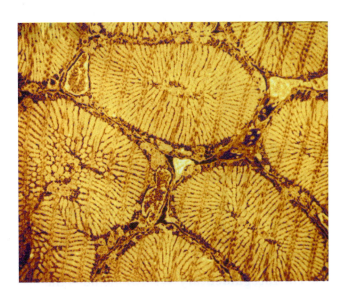

Figure 30-3
Cells join together to form tissues. (© *Scott Camazine/Photo Researchers, Inc.*)

Epithelial Tissue

Epithelial tissue covers the outside of the body, lines its internal structures, and forms glands. The purpose of epithelial tissue is protection. Epithelial tissue forms the outer part of the skin. It forms the mucous membranes that line our digestive, respiratory, urinary, and reproductive systems. It also covers organs, such as the lungs and heart, and lines the inside of the blood vessels, abdominal cavity, and chest cavity.

Connective Tissue

Connective tissue does what its name suggests—it connects other tissues together. Connective tissue supports and forms the framework for all of the parts of the body. Examples of connective tissue include bone, cartilage, ligaments, tendons, and fatty tissues. Blood is also considered a form of connective tissue.

Muscle Tissue

Muscle tissue produces movement. There are three types of muscle tissue found in the body (Table 30-1).

- *Skeletal muscle* allows you to move your arms, legs, and other parts of the body. Because you can decide when and how to move the parts of your body that contain skeletal muscle, skeletal muscle is said to be "voluntary," or under the control of the individual.
- *Smooth muscle* lines the walls of organs such as the intestines, the stomach, and the blood vessels. The movement provided by smooth muscle is involuntary, or out of your control. For example, it is the smooth muscle in the walls of the intestines that produces peristalsis (the wave-like movements that pass digested food through the intestines). You do not need to think about moving food through your intestines. Instead, this action occurs automatically.
- *Cardiac muscle* forms the heart. Contraction and relaxation of the cardiac muscle pumps blood throughout the body. Like smooth muscle, cardiac muscle is involuntary.

Nervous tissue

Nervous tissue conducts information. The brain, spinal cord, and nerves are made of nervous tissue. Nervous tissue allows one part of the body to "talk" to another part. For example, nerves carry information to the brain to be processed and

Table 30-1   Types of Muscle Tissue

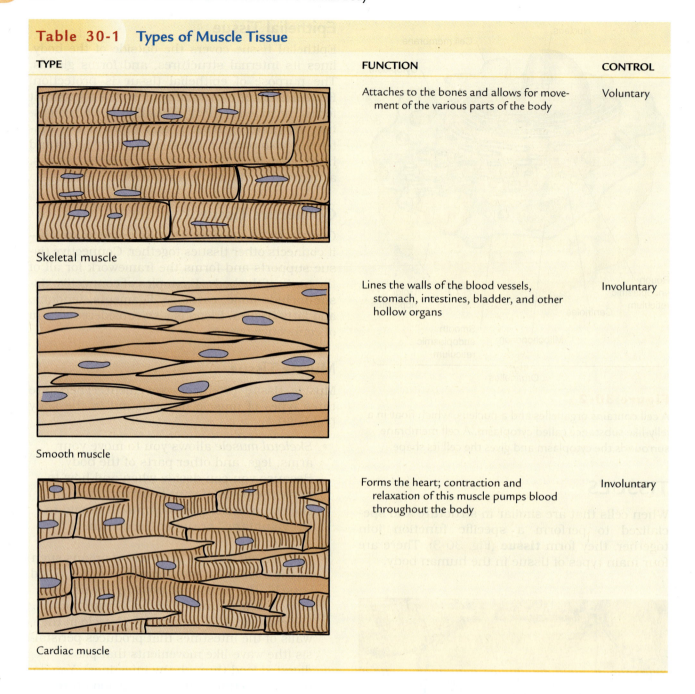

TYPE	FUNCTION	CONTROL
Skeletal muscle	Attaches to the bones and allows for movement of the various parts of the body	Voluntary
Smooth muscle	Lines the walls of the blood vessels, stomach, intestines, bladder, and other hollow organs	Involuntary
Cardiac muscle	Forms the heart; contraction and relaxation of this muscle pumps blood throughout the body	Involuntary

interpreted. In addition, the brain sends commands to other parts of the body through the nerves.

ORGANS

A group of tissues functioning together for a similar purpose form an **organ.** For example, the heart is made of all four tissue types, and its main function is to pump blood throughout the body. Other examples of organs include the stomach, liver, kidneys, and lungs. An organ may have one specific function, or it may have several.

ORGAN SYSTEMS

An **organ system** is a group of organs that work together to perform a specific function for the body. For the organ system to work properly, each organ within the system must function well. Human beings have 10 main organ systems (Fig. 30-4):

• The **integumentary system** includes the skin and its glands, the hair, and the nails. The function of the integumentary system is to protect the body.

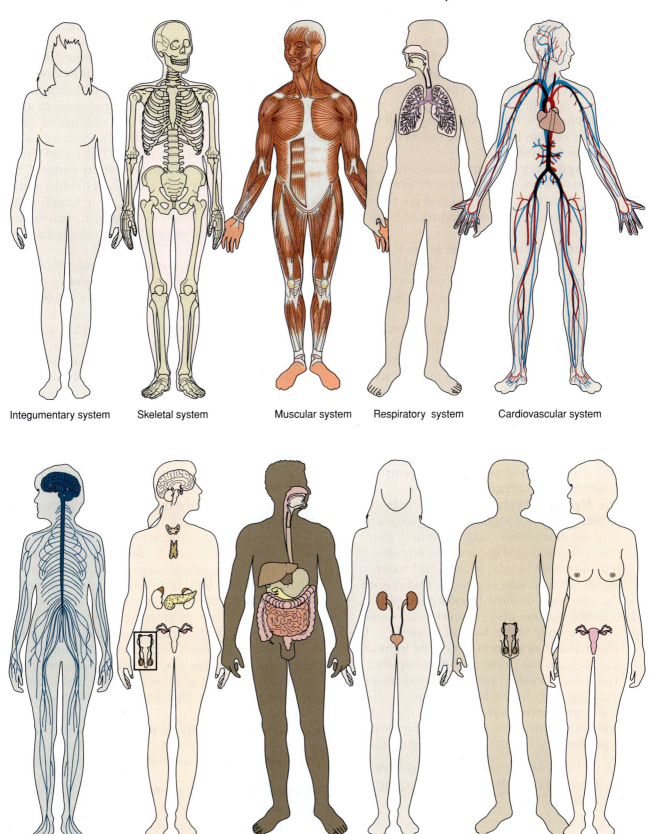

Integumentary system   Skeletal system   Muscular system   Respiratory system   Cardiovascular system

Nervous system   Endocrine system   Digestive system   Urinary system   Reproductive system

Figure 30-4
There are 10 organ systems in the human body.

- The **skeletal system** includes the bones. The function of the skeletal system is to provide a frame for the body and to give the body shape.
- The **muscular system** includes the muscles. The muscular system works along with the skeletal system to enable the body to move. Sometimes, the muscular system and the skeletal system together are called the musculoskeletal system.
- The **respiratory system** includes the lungs and the airways. The respiratory system allows us to take in oxygen and get rid of carbon dioxide, a waste product of cellular metabolism.
- The **cardiovascular system** is made up of the blood, the heart, and the blood vessels. The cardiovascular system transports nutrients and oxygen to the cells of the body, and carries waste products away.
- The **nervous system** includes the brain, spinal cord, and nerves. The nervous system controls the functioning of the other organ systems. It also allows us to interact with our environment through the **special senses** (sight, hearing, smell, taste, and touch).
- The **endocrine system** is made up of glands found in specific locations throughout the body. These glands secrete chemical substances called hormones, which control the function of certain organs.
- The **digestive system** includes the teeth, salivary glands, tongue, esophagus, stomach, small intestine, large intestine, liver, pancreas, and gallbladder. The digestive system allows us to take in food and water, digest the food into nutrients, and absorb the nutrients into the bloodstream. The digestive system also removes solid waste from the body in the form of feces.
- The **urinary system** includes the kidneys, the bladder, the ureters, and the urethra. The urinary system removes liquid waste from the body in the form of urine.
- The **reproductive system** allows the human body to produce new life. Without a means of reproduction, human life would cease to exist.

As you can see, organ systems do not work alone. They work together to maintain the life of the organism.

HEALTH AND DISEASE

All of the organ systems work together to maintain **homeostasis,** or balance. Homeostasis is a basic concept in physiology. The word comes

from the Greek words *homoios,* which means "same," and *stasis,* which means "standing." So, homeostasis means "staying the same." For an organism to stay alive, certain conditions within the body must remain the same, within a range of normal limits. You were introduced to this idea in Chapter 22, when we discussed vital signs. For example, the body temperature must remain within a certain range. The blood pressure must remain within a certain range. The fluids that keep our cells moist and healthy must not be too acidic or too basic. Our blood must contain the right amount of oxygen, nutrients, and other substances needed for metabolism at all times.

All of the organ systems are constantly working together to maintain a state of balance. When the external or internal environment changes, the organ systems must make adjustments to compensate for the change. For example, imagine that you are playing basketball at the park with your friends on a very hot day. You begin to sweat. This is your body working to cool you down. As you continue to play and sweat, you begin to get thirsty. This is your body telling you that it needs more water. As you run back and forth on the court, you breathe harder and your heart rate increases as your respiratory and circulatory systems work to send extra oxygen to your tissues. Your tissues need the extra oxygen because they use it to help produce the energy that allows you to keep playing.

Most of the time, you are not even aware of the adjustments your body is making to keep everything within the normal range. Even when you are sitting perfectly still, little adjustments are being made to keep the internal environment stable. Perhaps you are wondering how your body "knows" that an adjustment is needed. The answer is, through a feedback mechanism. Although all of the organ systems play a role in maintaining homeostasis, most of these feedback mechanisms are controlled by the nervous and endocrine systems.

The body's ability to maintain balance is an indicator of good health. There are times when the body's ability to maintain homeostasis is altered. This imbalance is usually the result of a disease. A **disease** (or a "disorder") occurs when the structure or function of an organ or an organ system is abnormal. Diseases can be acute (temporary) or chronic (long-term). Chronic diseases can have acute episodes (when the symptoms flare up and cause the person to feel ill, or more ill than usual). Diseases can be mild or severe. Sometimes, the same disease may be severe in one person but mild in another.

CATEGORIES OF DISEASE

There are several common categories of disease. A disease may belong to more than one of these categories. Common categories of disease include:

- **Infectious.** Infections are believed to play a role in approximately half of all illnesses.
- **Degenerative.** To degenerate means to "break down." Degenerative diseases occur when the tissues of the body wear out or break down. Arthritis, muscular dystrophy, osteoporosis, and Alzheimer's disease are examples of degenerative diseases. These diseases can be inherited, or they can be caused by infection, injury, or aging. Sometimes there is no known cause.
- **Nutritional.** These disorders occur when a person's diet lacks certain nutrients. Consuming too much of any one nutrient (for example, vitamins) or too many calories can also cause nutritional disorders. For example, obesity is a nutritional disorder.
- **Metabolic (endocrine).** Metabolic disorders, such as diabetes, occur when the body is unable to metabolize or absorb certain nutrients. Metabolic disorders often occur when the body secretes either too much of one type of hormone, or not enough. Because the hormone is responsible for controlling the function of a particular organ, the organ does not function properly and an imbalance in homeostasis occurs.
- **Immune.** These disorders change the way the immune system behaves. Sometimes, as in acquired immunodeficiency syndrome (AIDS), the disease reduces the immune system's ability to fight off infection. Other times, the disease causes the immune system to start attacking the body's own tissues.
- **Neoplastic.** The word neoplasm means "new growth." Many people use the word "cancer" or "tumor" when they are talking about neoplastic disease. Neoplasms cause problems by invading otherwise healthy tissues. The presence of the new growth prevents the tissues from functioning properly.
- **Psychiatric.** Mental disorders that affect a person's ability to function normally, such as depression, are also considered diseases.

RISK FACTORS FOR DISEASE

Why do some people get certain diseases and others do not? Why does a certain disease affect one person very mildly but totally destroy the health of another person? As a nursing assistant, one of your many responsibilities will be to help improve or maintain the health of your residents. To do that, you need to know about the factors that can put a person at risk for disease, or negatively affect his or her ability to recover from disease. Some of these factors include the following:

- **Age.** Some disorders are more likely to occur in certain age groups. For example, chickenpox, a viral infection, is more common in children. Age can also influence how a person reacts to disease. For example, when an adult gets the chickenpox, the infection is usually much more severe. In general, older people are more at risk for certain diseases because the process of aging causes a lot of wear and tear on the body's tissues and organs.
- **Gender.** A person's gender can put the person at risk for certain diseases. For instance, breast cancer is much more common in women than in men. Women are also more likely than men to develop diabetes. However, men are more likely to have heart disease.
- **Heredity.** The genes that we inherit from our parents may put us at risk for developing certain diseases. For example, scientists now know that some types of cancer, diabetes, and heart disease are inherited.
- **Lifestyle.** A person's living conditions and health habits play a major role in the person's overall health status. For example, a person who is homeless is more likely to get sick than a person who has shelter from the weather. A person who gets too little rest and has poor nutritional habits is more likely to become ill than a person who gets enough sleep and eats well. A person who smokes is more likely to develop cancer, lung disease, or heart disease than a person who does not. A person who likes a deep, dark tan in the summer is more at risk for developing skin cancer than a person who uses sunscreen. These are just examples of the many ways in which lifestyle influences health.
- **Occupation.** Many jobs put a person at risk for certain diseases. For example, constant exposure to coal dust puts coal miners at risk for developing "black lung disease." Health care workers who do not take care to protect themselves are at risk for certain infections, such as human immunodeficiency virus (HIV) or hepatitis.
- **Chronic disease.** A person who has a chronic disease, such as diabetes or high blood pressure, is at increased risk for

developing another disease. For example, a person who does not manage his diabetes well is likely to develop heart disease, blindness, or kidney failure. In addition, a person who has a chronic disease is often more likely to experience more severe problems from something that would not really affect a healthy person. For example, an ingrown toenail will cause discomfort and inconvenience in a healthy person. However, in a person with diabetes, the ingrown toenail could cause a severe infection, because diabetes changes the internal environment of the body, placing the person more at risk for infection.

- **Emotional health.** A person's emotional health can directly affect her physical health. Emotional stress can create physical problems such as headaches, digestive disorders, and muscle strain. In addition, stress places the body more at risk for infection. If you remember from Chapter 8, just becoming a resident of a health care facility can significantly increase a person's level of emotional stress and make coping with physical illness or disability more difficult.

Awareness of the factors that can put your residents at risk for disease will help you to better meet their individual needs. When you meet your resident's specific needs, or observe and report signs that indicate that the person's body is struggling to return to a balanced state, you are making a very important contribution to the person's health.

Helping Hands and a Caring Heart
FOCUS ON HUMANISTIC HEALTH CARE

There is a fine line between our physical health and our emotional health. When we feel good physically, it is easier to be in a good mood, and it is easier to handle the day's tasks and activities. Now, think about a person who is living with a chronic disease. The disease impacts the person's physical health every day. What if every day you did not feel 100% physically? Many of the residents you will be caring for are in this situation. Some people are able to adapt and will resolve themselves to "making the best of a bad situation." Others may have difficulty adjusting emotionally to the effects the illness has on their lives, and they may have problems with mood and behavior as a result. When you provide emotional support in addition to caring for your residents' physical needs, you play a very important role in helping your residents find a sense of "balance."

SUMMARY

- Understanding how the healthy body works helps us to understand and treat disease.
- All living things share the same levels of organization.
  - A cell is the basic unit of life.
  - A group of cells that is similar in structure and specialized for a specific function forms tissue.
  - A group of tissues functioning together for a similar purpose forms an organ.
  - A group of organs that function together for the same general purpose forms an organ system.
  - A group of organ systems working together for the purpose of maintaining life forms an organism.

- All of the organ systems work together to maintain a state of homeostasis, or balance.
  - When the body's ability to maintain homeostasis is altered, disease or illness can result.
    - There are several common categories of disease. These categories often overlap.
    - Certain factors put some people more at risk for disease than others.
  - A nursing assistant who is aware of the factors that put a person at risk for disease is able to provide better care for her residents, because she has a better understanding of each individual's needs.

WHAT DID YOU LEARN?

Multiple Choice

Select the single best answer for each of the following questions.

1. Which of the following is a factor that might put a person at risk for disease?
   a. Age
   b. Heredity
   c. Gender
   d. All of the above
2. What is the purpose of epithelial tissue?
   a. To provide a frame for, and give shape to, the body
   b. To connect other types of tissue together
   c. To cover the body and line its cavities
   d. To conduct nerve impulses
3. To function properly, cells need oxygen, water, nutrients, and the ability to eliminate:
   a. cytoplasm
   b. organelles

   c. disease
   d. waste
4. Which type of muscle tissue allows for movement of body parts?
   a. voluntary
   b. involuntary
   c. smooth
   d. cardiac
5. Glands are part of what body system?
   a. cardiovascular
   b. digestive
   c. endocrine
   d. nervous

Matching

Match each numbered item with its appropriate lettered description.

_____ **1.** Anatomy

_____ **2.** Organ

_____ **3.** Cell

_____ **4.** Tissue

_____ **5.** Physiology

_____ **6.** Homeostasis

_____ **7.** Organ system

_____ **8.** Organism

a. Basic unit of life
b. Study of how the body parts work
c. Study of what body parts look like, where they are located, how big they are, and how they connect to other body parts
d. A group of organs that work together to perform a specific function for the body
e. A state of balance
f. A living thing, formed by a group of organ systems working together for the purpose of maintaining life
g. A group of tissues functioning together for a similar purpose
h. Formed when cells that are similar in structure and specialized to perform a specific function join together

STOP and Think!

• Mrs. Hitchcock, one of your residents, has rheumatoid arthritis, a chronic and painful condition of the joints, in her hands and her hips. Some days are better than others are for Mrs. Hitchcock. Today, a local poet is coming to the facility to do a poetry reading for the residents, and you know that Mrs. Hitchcock has been looking forward to attending the reading all week. But when you go into Mrs. Hitchcock's room to help her get dressed, she says, "I just can't go . . . the pain is too bad . . ." and she starts to cry. As a nursing assistant, what concerns would you have for Mrs. Hitchcock? Is there anything you can do to help Mrs. Hitchcock?

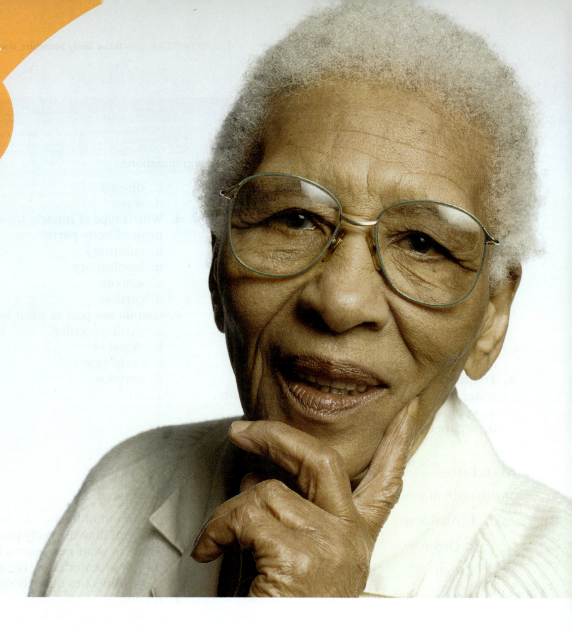

The Integumentary System

WHAT WILL YOU LEARN?

What is the largest organ in your body? Your skin! Just think—your body is covered in about 22 square feet of skin, and your skin alone weighs between 8 and 10 pounds. You already know that a major function of this very large organ is to cover and protect your body. But did you also know that the skin gives us clues about what is going on inside of a person's body? In this chapter, you will learn about the skin and the other organs that make up the integumentary system. You will learn about the importance of observing this organ system for changes that may indicate illness, and about actions you can take to help keep the skin (and its wearer!) healthy. When you are finished with this chapter, you will be able to:

1. List the layers of the skin.
2. Describe the accessory structures of the skin.

Photo: The integumentary system includes the skin, hair, and nails.

3. Discuss the major functions of the integumentary system.
4. Describe how normal aging processes affect the integumentary system.
5. Explain how pressure ulcers are formed and what conditions may increase a resident's risk of developing a pressure ulcer.
6. Describe how the nursing assistant helps to prevent residents from developing pressure ulcers.
7. Describe the different types of wounds that a resident might have.
8. Discuss the nursing assistant's duties regarding wound care.
9. Define terms used to describe skin lesions.

Vocabulary Use the CD in the front of your book to hear these terms pronounced and defined:

Jaundice	Subcutaneous tissue	Unintentional wound	Papule
Pallor	Sebum	Lesion	Vesicle
Flushing	Collagen	Rash	Pustule
Cyanosis	Bony prominences	Shingles (herpes zoster)	Excoriation
Epidermis	Necrosis	Dermatitis	Fissure
Keratin	Pressure points	Eczema	Ulcer
Melanin	Wound	Erythema	
Dermis	Intentional wound	Macule	

The integumentary system gets its name from the Latin word *integumentum,* which means "a covering." The integumentary system is made up of the skin, which covers the body, and the structures that develop from it, called *accessory structures* or *appendages.* The accessory structures of the skin are the nails, the hair, the sebaceous glands (which secrete oils to keep the skin moist), and the sweat glands.

Of all the body's organ systems, the integumentary system is the most easily observed. Healthy skin is glowing and vibrant, and may range in color from very light to very dark. A change in a person's normal skin color can indicate a serious health problem and should be reported to the nurse immediately. For example:

- **Jaundice** is a yellow discoloration of the skin and the whites of the eyes. Jaundice is usually associated with liver disorders.
- **Pallor** is paleness, and **flushing** is redness. Some people appear pale or flushed most of the time. In these people, pallor or flushing would be considered "normal." However, if you notice pallor or flushing in a person who is not normally pale or flushed, you should report this finding to the nurse.

- **Cyanosis** is a blue or gray discoloration of the skin, lips, and nail beds. Cyanosis develops when the skin does not receive enough oxygen. Cyanosis is a sign of a respiratory or circulatory disorder.

As you learned in Chapter 24, the condition of a person's hair and nails can also provide clues to the person's overall health. The hair should be shiny and soft, not brittle and dry, and the scalp should not be flaky or crusty. The nail beds of healthy nails are pink. The nails are flush with the nail bed and, when viewed from the side, the nails are slightly rounded.

TELL THE NURSE

The skin gives us many clues to a person's general health. Tell the nurse immediately if you observe any of the following:

- The person's skin looks abnormally pale or flushed, or has a bluish or yellowish hue
- The person has a new rash, or changes in an existing rash
- The person has a mole that has changed in appearance

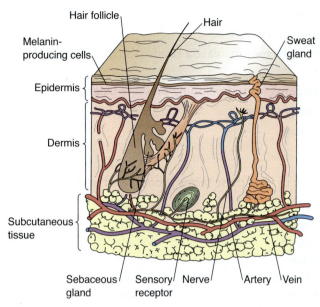

Figure 31-1

The skin has two layers, the dermis and epidermis. The skin rests on a layer of subcutaneous tissue.

STRUCTURE OF THE INTEGUMENTARY SYSTEM

SKIN

The skin is made up of two layers, the epidermis and the dermis (Fig. 31-1).

Epidermis

The **epidermis** is the outer layer of the skin. The epidermis is thickest on the soles of the feet and the palms of the hands, and very thin in areas such as the eyelids.

If you look at Figure 31-1, you will notice that the epidermis contains no blood vessels. You will also notice that it has two sub layers, a deep layer and a surface layer. New cells are produced in the deep layer of the epidermis. As the cells age, they work their way up, toward the surface of the body. As the maturing cells move toward the surface, they move further away from the blood vessels, which are located in the dermis. This means that as the cells age, they move further away from their supply of oxygen and nutrients. They also make **keratin,** a substance that causes them to thicken and become resistant to water. When the cells reach the surface of the body, they die and are shed away. This process takes approximately 28 days—so, each month, you get a "new skin!"

In addition to continually producing new cells, the deep layer of the epidermis produces a substance called melanin. **Melanin,** from the Greek word *melas* ("black"), is a dark pigment that gives our skin, hair, and eyes color. People with pale skin have less melanin than those with dark skin. Melanin helps to protect the skin from exposure to sunlight. In fact, continued exposure to sunlight causes the epidermis to produce more melanin, resulting in a tan. Sometimes, melanin is deposited throughout the epidermis in an uneven pattern, resulting in freckles.

Dermis

The **dermis** is the deepest layer of the skin (Fig. 31-1). The dermis consists of elastic connective tissue that allows it to stretch and move without damage. The dermis rests on a layer of fat called the **subcutaneous tissue.** Cutaneous is another word for "skin," and sub means "below," so *subcutaneous* means "below the skin." The blood vessels and nerves that supply the skin start in the subcutaneous tissue and send branches into the dermis. Looking at Figure 31-1, you can see that the sensory receptors that allow us to feel pressure, pain, and temperature are located in the dermis. (The sense of touch will be discussed in more detail in Chapter 36.) The sebaceous glands, the sweat glands, and the hair follicles are also found in the dermis.

ACCESSORY STRUCTURES (APPENDAGES)

The skin's accessory structures include the sebaceous glands, the sweat glands, the hair, and the nails.

Sebaceous (Oil) Glands

The sebaceous glands secrete **sebum,** an oily substance that lubricates the skin and helps to prevent it from drying out. The sebum is also slightly acidic. This acidity helps to protect the skin from harmful bacteria that may be present on its surface. The sebaceous glands open into the hair follicles, and the sebum passes along the hair and onto the surface of the skin (Fig. 31-1).

Sweat Glands

There are two types of sweat glands, eccrine glands and apocrine glands. Eccrine glands are found in the skin that covers most parts of our bodies. Eccrine glands produce a thin, watery liquid that contains salt and small amounts of other bodily wastes. The purpose of the eccrine glands is to help cool the body through the process of evaporation. As the watery sweat leaves the surface of the skin, it takes heat with it, cooling the body down. When you "work up a sweat," what you are experiencing is your eccrine glands at work! Another time you may have experienced your eccrine glands at work is when you have noticed your palms beginning to sweat as a result of being nervous. Many people sweat when they are nervous, and the palms of the hands contain a very large number of eccrine glands—hence, "sweaty palm syndrome."

The other type of sweat gland is the apocrine gland. Apocrine glands are found mostly in the skin of the armpits (axillae) and the perineum. The apocrine glands produce a thicker substance. When the bacteria that normally live on our skin mix with this substance, they produce what we know as "body odor." Apocrine glands become active when a person reaches puberty. As we age, the apocrine glands become less active.

Hair

Hair covers the entire body, except for the soles of the feet and the palms of the hands. Hair, especially that covering the scalp, helps to keep us warm. Most of the hair that covers the body is soft and fine, although in men, body hair tends to be thicker and more noticeable because of the action of certain hormones. In both men and women, the hair covering the scalp, armpits, and pubic area is thicker and coarser than the hair on the rest of the body.

Hair develops in the dermis of the skin from a sheath called a follicle (Fig. 31-1). The part of the hair that we can see consists of dead cells that have been hardened by keratin. The living cells that produce new hair cells, causing the hair to grow, are found at the bottom of the follicle or hair root. Melanin gives the hair its color. Blonde hair contains a small amount of melanin, while brunette hair contains much more.

Nails

Nails are made of special skin cells that have been hardened by the presence of keratin. Nail growth occurs from the nail root, the area where the nail emerges from the skin. Nails help to protect the ends of our fingers and toes.

FUNCTION OF THE INTEGUMENTARY SYSTEM

The integumentary system helps to maintain the body's homeostasis in three important ways. First, it offers a physical form of protection against microbes, chemicals, and other agents that could harm the body if they gained access to the delicate organs inside. Second, the skin, which is water resistant, helps to maintain the body's fluid balance by preventing excessive loss or absorption of water. Finally, the integumentary system helps to regulate the temperature of the body, ensuring that the temperature stays within a tolerable range.

PROTECTION

As you learned in Chapter 15, the body's first line of defense against the invasion of harmful microbes is intact skin. The skin is a physical barrier that prevents microbes from entering the body. The skin also offers us some protection against harmful substances, such as chemicals, that may be encountered in the environment.

MAINTENANCE OF FLUID BALANCE

Imagine what would happen if your skin were not resistant to water! Every time it rained or you took a shower, you would soak up the water like a sponge. And every time you went out in the sun, you would run the risk of having all of your internal organs dry out. Needless to say, without your water-resistant skin, maintaining the proper fluid balance would be a constant struggle. Fortunately, the keratin-rich cells of the epidermis, combined with the oils secreted by the sebaceous glands, work very well to form a water-resistant protective barrier between your internal organs and the outside world.

REGULATION OF BODY TEMPERATURE

The skin plays an important role in regulating the body temperature. When a person gets warm—for example, after working outside in the sun—the blood vessels in the dermis of the skin dilate (widen), allowing more blood to flow close to the surface of the skin. As the blood passes just beneath the surface of the skin, the heat the blood contains radiates out from the body, lowering the temperature of the blood. The cooled blood then travels, carrying its coolness, back to the central areas of the body, thus lowering the body temperature. The production of sweat on the skin enhances this process by cooling the skin even more so that the blood cools more effectively. In essence, this process is the body's way of "opening the windows" to allow a cool breeze to circulate through the house (Fig. 31-2A).

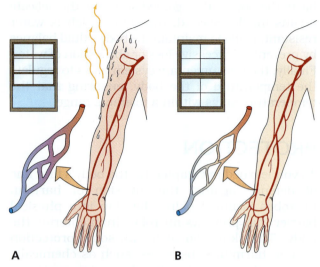

Figure 31-2

The skin plays an important role in maintaining the body's temperature within the proper range. **(A)** When the internal temperature is too high, the blood vessels in the skin dilate, causing more blood to pass near the surface of the skin and allowing heat to escape into the environment. Sweat evaporating from the surface of the skin also carries heat away from the body, contributing to the cooling process. **(B)** When the internal temperature is too low, the blood vessels in the skin constrict, causing less blood to pass near the surface of the skin and keeping the heat inside the body.

The reverse is true when a person gets cold, for example, following exposure to cold air. The blood vessels in the skin constrict (become narrower), limiting the amount of blood that passes close to the surface of the skin. By keeping the blood in the warmer, central areas of the body, the amount of heat that is lost to the outside environment is kept to a minimum. You have seen how your skin becomes pale or bluish when you have been outside in the cold air. Your body is essentially "closing the windows" to stop the breeze from cooling the house too much (Fig. 31-2B).

SENSATION

The skin contains millions of sensory receptors, special structures that allow us to detect pain, pressure, temperature, and touch. The sensory receptors and the role they play in sensation are discussed in detail in Chapter 36.

VITAMIN D PRODUCTION

Vitamin D is a nutrient that helps our bodies absorb and use calcium, a mineral that keeps our bones healthy. The skin produces vitamin D when it is exposed to the sun. In fact, sun exposure is our main source of this important vitamin! Vitamin D is also obtained by eating foods such as milk and fish.

ELIMINATION AND ABSORPTION

The skin is an active organ that is capable of both removing substances from the body and taking substances into it. For example, sweat contains small amounts of waste materials, which leave the body when the sweat evaporates. The skin can also absorb some substances, such as chemicals. We use the ability of the skin to absorb chemicals when we give medications using a "patch." An adhesive patch containing the medication is applied to the skin, and the medication is slowly absorbed through the skin and into the blood vessels. You may be familiar with patches that prevent motion sickness, provide birth control, or help a person to stop smoking. In all of these cases, the medication on the patch is absorbed through the skin.

THE EFFECTS OF AGING ON THE INTEGUMENTARY SYSTEM

As we age, changes occur in all of our organ systems. These changes are not related to illness. Rather, they are normal changes that occur in everyone who reaches a certain age. These changes may just affect the person's appearance, or they may actually affect the way the person's body functions. Because many of the people you will be caring for will be elderly, it is important for you to know about the changes that normally occur in each body system with aging. This knowledge will allow you to recognize age-related changes as normal. It will also allow you to provide better care for your elderly residents, because you will be aware of their special needs.

CHANGES IN PHYSICAL APPEARANCE

Perhaps because the integumentary system is the most visible organ system, we have come to associate "getting old" with many of the physical changes that occur in the integumentary system as we age. Wrinkles, gray hair, and "age spots" are all very visible signs of aging! Wrinkles form due to the loss of **collagen,** a protein that supports connective tissue, such as that found in the dermis. In addition, the adipose (fatty) tissue in the subcutaneous layer that supports the dermis thins with age, making the subcutaneous layer less supportive of the dermis. As a result, the skin loses elasticity, leading to the formation of wrinkles. Melanin also is responsible for many of the changes typically associated with aging. Gray hair is caused by the loss of melanin from the hair. "Age spots" (sometimes called "liver spots") are caused by deposits of melanin in certain areas, such as the backs of the hands or the face. Whether or not a person's skin "shows his age" depends on many factors, such as heredity; the amount of time the person spends in the sun; the person's use of tobacco, drugs, or alcohol; and the person's overall state of health. Think about all of the people you know. Do any look much younger than their actual age, or much older? What factors do you think might be responsible for the person's remarkably youthful appearance, or unusually old appearance?

FRAGILE, DRY SKIN

There are many changes that occur to the integumentary system with aging that affect more than just our appearance. As collagen is lost from the dermis and the subcutaneous layer thins, the skin becomes thinner, more fragile, and more prone to injury (Fig. 31-3). Blood flow to the dermis decreases, and the cells of the epidermis do not replace themselves as rapidly. The decrease in blood flow to the skin means that when an injury occurs, the skin takes longer to heal itself,

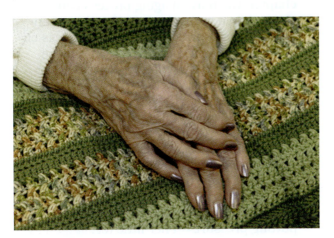

Figure 31-3
As skin ages, it becomes more delicate and prone to injury.

and the person is more at risk for developing an infection.

The number of sebaceous glands decreases, and as a result, so does the output of sebum. This leads to drying of the skin, which increases the risk for skin tears and injuries. In addition, with less sebum on the skin, the bacteria that normally live on the surface of our skin have more of a chance to cause trouble. (Recall that the acidity of sebum helps to keep these bacteria in check.)

When caring for an elderly person, keep the delicate nature of older skin in mind. Actions that would not cause harm in a younger person, such as gripping the person's arm to help her to stand or accidentally grazing her skin with your fingernails while helping her to put on her socks, can cause injury in an older person. It is very easy to tear an older person's skin, causing it to bleed. In addition, the skin of an older person is more sensitive to the drying effects of bathing than that of a younger person. In Chapter 23, you learned about some of the things that you can do to increase comfort and help to keep an older person's skin healthy, such as applying lotion after a bath to keep the skin soft and pliant.

THICKENING OF THE NAILS

As we age, our nails thicken and become yellow. This is especially true of the toenails. Because the nails are so tough, they are difficult to cut, and the person may be injured during the process. As you learned in Chapter 24, a nurse or a podiatrist is usually responsible for trimming an elderly person's toenails. The nurse or podiatrist may use a tool that looks like a sander to accomplish this task safely.

LESS-EFFICIENT TEMPERATURE REGULATION

Changes to the integumentary system that occur with aging also affect the older person's ability to adjust to changes in the environmental temperature. The sweat glands decrease in number and the production of sweat decreases, making an older person more vulnerable to overheating. In addition, the decreased blood flow to the skin interferes with the skin's ability to participate in temperature regulation. These changes must be considered when an older person is outside on a hot day, because they affect the ability of the body to cool itself and put the person at increased risk for heat-related problems, such as heat stroke.

DISORDERS OF THE INTEGUMENTARY SYSTEM

Many people in your care will have a disorder of the integumentary system. Sometimes, this disorder is the reason the person is in the health care facility. For example, this might be the case for a person who has a non-healing wound. Other times, the disorder develops after the person is already in the health care facility. For example, a person might develop a rash or a pressure ulcer, or have surgery that results in a surgical wound that must heal. As a nursing assistant, you will play an important role in observing signs and symptoms of skin disorders, preventing the development of skin disorders, and helping people with skin disorders to heal.

PRESSURE ULCERS

Pressure ulcers, also known as *decubitus ulcers* or *bedsores,* form when a part of the body presses against a surface such as a mattress or chair for a long period of time. Lying on wrinkled bed linens or an object in the bed, sitting on a bedpan for a long period of time, or wearing a splint or brace that presses against the skin can also start the process of skin breakdown that leads to the formation of pressure ulcers.

Pressure ulcers are particularly likely to form over **bony prominences,** or parts of the body where there is very little fat between the bone and the skin. The weight of the person's body squeezes the soft tissue between the bony prominence and the surface the person is resting on, disrupting the flow of blood to the tissue. Lack of blood flow to the tissue deprives the tissue of oxygen and nutrients, causing it to die. Tissue death as a result of a lack of oxygen is called **necrosis.** The necrotic (dead) skin and underlying tissues peel off or break open, creating an open sore (Fig. 31-4). The sore is very painful and creates an opening for microbes to enter the body. Pressure ulcers may be very deep, extending all the way down to the bone. They are very difficult to heal once they have occurred.

You will remember from Chapter 20 that many residents are not able to change position easily, due to weakness, disability, or illness. This inability to change position without help places the person at high risk for developing a pressure

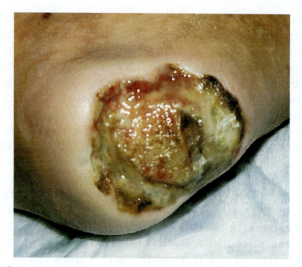

Figure 31-4
Pressure ulcers are painful, difficult to treat, and potentially fatal.

ulcer. The most common sites for pressure ulcers to form are on the heels, ankles, knees, hips, toes, elbows, shoulder blades, ears, the back of the head, and along the spine (Fig. 31-5). These particular areas are referred to as **pressure points.**

Risk Factors for Pressure Ulcers

The constant application of pressure on pressure points as a result of immobility is the basic cause of all pressure ulcers. Unfortunately, many people with limited mobility also have other risk factors for developing a pressure ulcer. The presence of any one of the following risk factors in a person with limited mobility makes it even more likely that the person will develop a pressure ulcer:

- **Advanced age.** As described earlier in this chapter, the normal aging process causes changes in a person's skin. The skin of an older person is fragile and thin, with less circulation. While a younger person may be able to tolerate staying in one position for 2 hours, an elderly person may need much more frequent position changes.
- **Decreased sensation.** Our sense of touch may decrease with age or certain diseases (such as diabetes). A person with decreased sensation may not feel the discomfort that unrelieved pressure can cause. She may not realize that she has been sitting in one position for too long, or that her shoe has been putting pressure on her little toe.
- **Poor nutrition and hydration.** For skin to remain healthy, good nutrition and proper

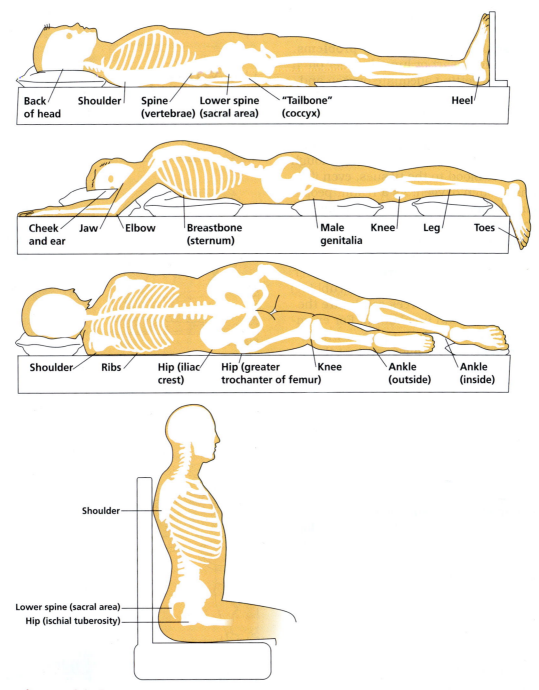

Back of head | **Shoulder** | **Spine (vertebrae)** | **Lower spine (sacral area)** | **"Tailbone" (coccyx)** | **Heel**

Cheek and ear | **Jaw** | **Elbow** | **Breastbone (sternum)** | **Male genitalia** | **Knee** | **Leg** | **Toes**

Shoulder | **Ribs** | **Hip (iliac crest)** | **Hip (greater trochanter of femur)** | **Knee** | **Ankle (outside)** | **Ankle (inside)**

Shoulder

Lower spine (sacral area)

Hip (ischial tuberosity)

Figure 31-5
Pressure points are areas where pressure ulcers are likely to form.

hydration are essential. People who are not receiving adequate nutrition or fluids, because of illness, depression, or other conditions are more likely to develop pressure ulcers. Poor nutrition will also delay the healing of any pressure ulcers that have already formed.

• **Moisture.** Prolonged contact with water, urine, feces, or sweat causes the epidermis

to soften and break down. Areas where skin touches skin (such as between the thighs, the folds of the abdomen, the armpits, and under the breasts) are places where sweat or bath water may become trapped on the skin, leading to skin breakdown. Bodily fluids like sweat, urine, and feces also contain irritants such as salt, ammonia, and bacteria, which further contribute to the breakdown of the skin. Once skin breakdown begins, the door is wide open for a pressure ulcer to form.

- **Cardiovascular and respiratory problems.** A person with a heart or lung disorder often has problems getting adequate oxygen and nutrients to the tissues. In a person with a respiratory disorder, the blood that is delivered to the tissues may not contain enough oxygen. The heart of a person with a cardiovascular disorder may not be strong enough to deliver the blood to the tissues, even if it contains enough oxygen. As a result, people with circulatory or respiratory problems are at even greater risk for developing pressure ulcers, because their tissues are already deprived of oxygen and nutrients.

- **Friction and shearing injuries.** In Chapter 20, you learned about how friction (rubbing) and shearing (pulling) forces can injure the skin and lead to skin breakdown. For example, shearing occurs when a person who is sitting up in bed slides down against the sheets. Shearing and friction injuries can also occur during repositioning.

Stages of Pressure Ulcers

Pressure ulcers develop in four stages (Fig. 31-6):

- **Stage 1.** A stage 1 pressure ulcer is characterized by a reddened area of skin that does not return to the normal color after the pressure is removed. The reddened area may then become very pale or white and develop a shiny appearance. Every time you reposition a resident, you should look carefully for reddened areas. If the person's circulation is normal, the skin will return to its normal color within a few minutes. If the skin stays red, feels hot to the touch, or is painful, you should report this finding to the nurse immediately. A reddened area that turns white means that blood flow has been compromised to the point that tissue damage has occurred.

- **Stage 2.** A stage 2 pressure ulcer looks like a blister, an abrasion, or a shallow crater. The epidermis peels away or cracks open, creating a portal of entry for microbes. The dermis may be partially worn away as well.

- **Stage 3.** In a stage 3 pressure ulcer, the epidermis and dermis are gone, and the subcutaneous fat may be visible in the crater. There may be drainage from the wound.

- **Stage 4.** The crater of damaged tissue extends all the way through the tissues to the muscle or bone.

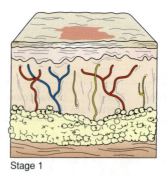 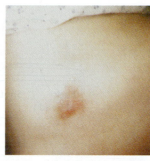
Stage 1

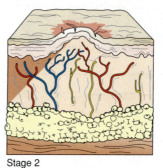 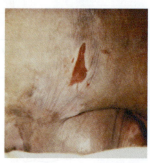
Stage 2

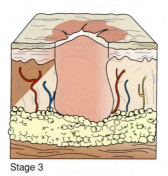 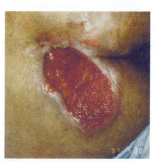
Stage 3

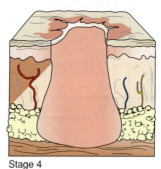 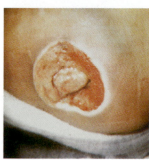 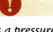
Stage 4

Figure 31-6
The four stages of pressure ulcer development.

TELL THE NURSE ❗

When caring for a person who has a pressure ulcer or is at risk for developing a pressure ulcer, report the following observations immediately:

- The person has redness over a pressure point that does not go away within 5 minutes.

- An area over a pressure point that was previously red has become pale, white, or shiny.

- An area over a pressure point that was previously red is hot to the touch or painful.

- A pressure ulcer has changed in size or depth.

The Nursing Assistant's Role in Preventing Pressure Ulcers

The prevention of pressure ulcers is a major concern of the nursing team. Pressure ulcers are very painful and difficult to treat, and they put the person at risk for infection. Ultimately, they can cause a person to die. For these reasons, every effort must be made to prevent a pressure ulcer from forming in the first place. As a nursing assistant, there are many things that you can do to help keep a person's skin healthy and prevent pressure ulcers from forming (Fig. 31-7).

- **Avoid allowing a person to remain in one position for a long period of time.** To prevent a pressure ulcer from forming, you must prevent any one part of a person's body from being under pressure for a long period of time. This means that you should not leave a resident sitting on a bedpan for a long period of time, because the bedpan places a lot of pressure on the lower spine,

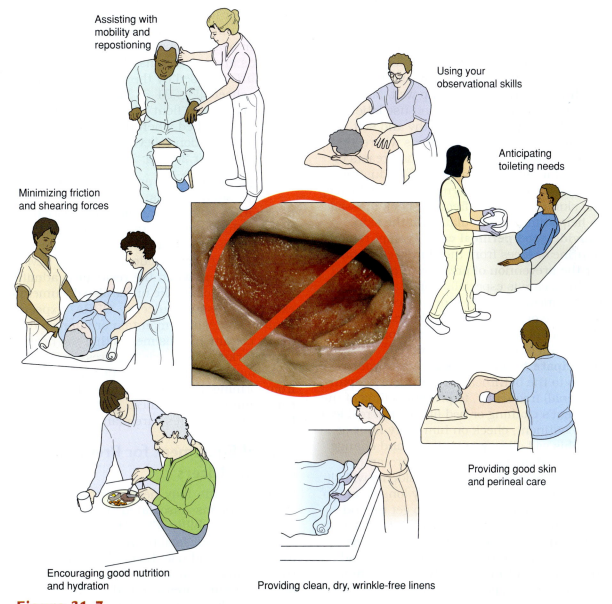

Assisting with mobility and repostioning

Using your observational skills

Anticipating toileting needs

Minimizing friction and shearing forces

Providing good skin and perineal care

Encouraging good nutrition and hydration

Providing clean, dry, wrinkle-free linens

Figure 31-7

There are many things you can do to help prevent a person from getting a pressure ulcer. (*Photograph © Garry Watson/Photo Researchers, Inc.*)

one of the pressure points. It also means that a resident who must stay in bed or in a wheelchair should be repositioned at least every 2 hours. A resident who has additional risk factors for developing a pressure ulcer, as described earlier, may need to be repositioned even more often. The care plan will specify how often the resident should be repositioned, and the sequence of positions.

- **Use your observation skills.** Look carefully at the skin of your residents each and every time you provide care. After repositioning a resident, move clothing and linens aside to check for reddened areas on the side of the body that had been bearing the resident's weight. When assisting a resident with bathing, changing wet or soiled linens, or giving a back massage, take that opportunity to look carefully at the resident's skin.

- **Provide good skin care.** When assisting with a bath, clean skin gently and thoroughly and rinse off the soap well. Make sure the skin is dried well and use lotion to keep the skin's surface healthy and soft. Thoroughly clean and dry areas where skin touches skin, such as under the breasts or other skin folds, and apply a light dusting of a powder containing corn starch to help keep the skin dry. Provide frequent back massage to help stimulate circulation in the skin.

- **Provide good perineal care.** Prompt removal of urine or feces from the skin is essential for the prevention of pressure ulcers. Good perineal care is especially important if a resident is incontinent of urine or feces. Clean any urine or feces from the skin each time the resident is incontinent, and apply a barrier cream or ointment, as ordered.

- **Anticipate toileting needs.** Assist your residents to the bathroom (or provide a bedpan or urinal) frequently, to prevent soiling of the resident's clothing or bed linens. If a resident is incontinent, check on him every hour or so. This will allow you to detect and change wet, soiled linens and clothing promptly.

- **Encourage mobility.** Some residents will sit in a chair or wheelchair all day long if you do not actively encourage them to get up and move around. Ask the resident to take a walk with you every 2 hours, if she is able. The exercise helps to stimulate circulation and keeps the resident from sitting in the same position for long periods of time. If a resident is paralyzed, assist her to change positions in her chair or have her move between the chair and the bed to prevent skin breakdown.

- **Minimize skin injury caused by friction or shearing.** Use lift devices and lift sheets when moving and repositioning residents to prevent injuries caused by friction and shearing. To help prevent shearing caused by the resident sliding down in bed, do not elevate the head of the bed more than 30 degrees.

- **Encourage good nutrition and hydration.** Offer refreshing drinks frequently. Encourage your residents to eat well. If a resident is not eating, report this observation to the nurse.

- **Take steps to relieve or reduce pressure.** Many devices are available to help reduce pressure and minimize the risk of skin breakdown. Special gel and foam pads that fit on beds or in chairs help to distribute body weight more evenly, preventing any one area from bearing most of the pressure. Elbow pads and booties may help prevent friction injuries caused by the skin rubbing against the sheets (Fig. 31-8). Placing a pillow under the calves to "float" the heels above the surface of the bed when the person is in the supine position relieves pressure on the heels (see Chapter 20, Fig. 20-5).

Because a pressure ulcer can have such serious consequences for a resident, OBRA expects that the health care team will do everything possible to prevent residents from getting pressure ulcers. The nurse is responsible for assessing each resident's risk for developing pressure ulcers when the resident is admitted to the nursing home. The nurse also documents any existing pressure ulcers. OBRA expects the health care team to maintain or improve the resident's condition. This means that the health care team works to heal existing pressure ulcers and takes measures to prevent new pressure ulcers from forming. Nursing assistants help the health care team to achieve these goals by carefully following the resident's care plan.

Special Equipment for Preventing Pressure Ulcers

Some residents may need a special bed to help avoid problems associated with prolonged bed rest and immobility (Fig. 31-9). If specialty beds are used in your facility, you will receive training in their care and use. Examples of specialty beds that you may see in use include air-fluidized beds and alternating pressure beds.

An air-fluidized bed supports the person on a fabric-covered layer of tiny ceramic beads (see Fig. 31-9A). The beads are kept in constant movement

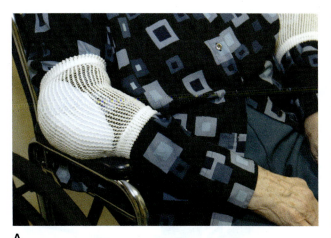

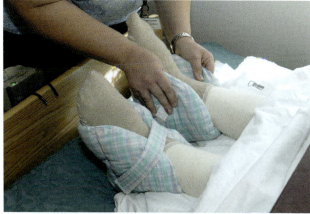

A   B

Figure 31-8

Pressure-reducing devices such as **(A)** elbow pads and **(B)** heel booties help to prevent the skin from rubbing against sheets and other surfaces.

by a current of air. The moving beads create a fluid-like effect, much like a waterbed but without the water, that helps to prevent pressure ulcers by relieving pressure on pressure points. In addition, the circulating air keeps the person's skin dry.

An alternating pressure bed supports the person on a series of compartments that fill with air and then deflate on a rotating basis (see Fig. 31-9B). The shifting areas of inflation shift the areas of pressure from place to place, helping to improve blood flow to the skin and underlying tissues and helping to prevent pressure ulcers. Alternating pressure can also be provided in the form of a mattress overlay that is placed on top of the person's regular mattress.

WOUNDS

A **wound** is an injury that results in a break in the skin (and often the underlying tissues, as well).

Be Smart About Surveys!

Pressure ulcers can be painful and difficult to heal, and they place the resident at risk for serious infection and death. Because the consequences of pressure ulcers are so serious, surveyors will pay special attention to how well staff members recognize a resident's risk for developing a pressure ulcer, and how well they take action to prevent a pressure ulcer from occurring. A pressure ulcer in a resident who is at low risk for developing a pressure ulcer is considered a sentinel event. To help your facility remain without survey problems in this area:

● Know which interventions listed in the care plan are for pressure ulcer prevention, and follow them.

● Be diligent about changing the resident's position at least every 2 hours, or according to the care plan.

● Use supportive devices to help maintain proper body alignment and relieve pressure on pressure points.

● Use pressure-reducing devices to reduce pressure on pressure points.

● Prevent friction and shearing injuries by using a lift sheet (draw sheet) when moving a resident up in the bed or chair.

● Take steps to make meal time as pleasant as possible for the resident. Ensuring that meal time is pleasant can help improve a person's appetite and food intake. Similarly, make an effort to offer appealing beverages throughout the day to encourage adequate hydration.

● Provide good skin and perineal care.

● Alert the nurse if a resident's food or fluid intake decreases, the resident experiences more frequent episodes of incontinence (or develops incontinence), the resident's function or mobility decreases, or the resident resists preventive care measures.

● Document the care you provide per your facility's policy so that there is a record of the preventive care that you have provided.

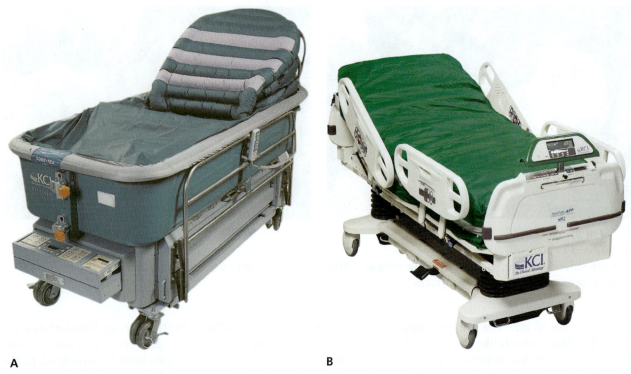

A   B

Figure 31-9

Specialty beds help to prevent problems related to prolonged bed rest and immobility. **(A)** The Fluidair Elite® airflow bed. **(B)** The TheraPulse®ATP™ alternating pressure bed. (*Photographs courtesy of Kinetic Concepts Inc. [KCI], San Antonio, Texas.*)

Although this discussion focuses on wounds that occur as a result of surgery or trauma, pressure ulcers and burns (also discussed in this chapter) are technically considered "wounds" too.

Type of Wounds

An **intentional wound** is a wound that is the result of a planned surgical or medical intervention (Fig. 31-10A). For example, a person who is recovering from surgery to repair a broken hip will have an intentional wound caused by the surgery. Intentional wounds also occur when intravenous (IV) lines, percutaneous endoscopic gastrostomy (PEG) tubes, or other medical devices are inserted into the body through a "man-made" opening. Intentional wounds are usually created under controlled conditions. Precautions are taken to minimize the risk of infection. The edges of the wound are usually clean and even, and held together with stitches (sutures) or staples.

An **unintentional wound** is an unexpected injury that usually results from some type of trauma. Wounds that occur from falls, accidents, and physical violence are examples of unintentional wounds (Fig. 31-10B). Unintentional wounds can be *open*, which means that the surface of the skin is broken. The risk of infection is high with open wounds, because the open skin creates a portal of entry for microbes. In addition, the uneven wound edges and amount of tissue damage may make closing the wound difficult. A *closed* wound is one where the skin is not broken, but there is damage to the underlying tissues. The deep tissue damage associated with a closed wound can be considerable, even though the only signs of injury may be redness, swelling, or bruising of the overlying skin.

Wound Healing

The human body is quite efficient at healing wounds, especially when it is otherwise healthy. Having multiple, severe injuries; a chronic illness; or an impaired immune system can limit a person's ability to heal on his own. A person who is very young or very old may heal more slowly, or have a limited ability to heal. The same is true of a person who is malnourished.

For a wound to heal properly, there must be adequate blood flow to the injured area. This blood flow is responsible for the inflammation that is usually seen around an injury. Inflammation is characterized by redness, swelling, heat, and pain.

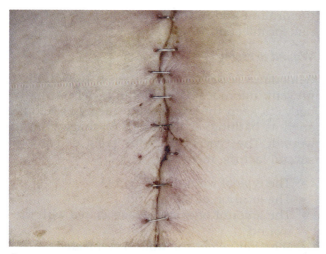

A. Intentional wound

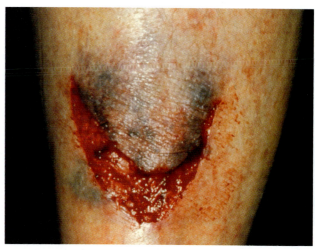

B. Unintentional wound

Figure 31-10

Wounds can be intentional or unintentional. **(A)** Intentional wounds, like this surgical incision, are created under controlled conditions, minimizing the risk of infection. The edges of the wound are usually brought together and secured with stitches or staples (shown here) to promote healing and minimize scarring. **(B)** Unintentional wounds are the result of an accident and carry a high risk of infection because they are often contaminated with dirt and microbes. The edges of the wound are often jagged, making it difficult to close the wound neatly. This unintentional wound on the leg of an 80-year-old woman was the result of a fall. (**B**, © *Dr. P. Marazzi/Photo Researchers, Inc.*)

It is a sign that the body is working to heal itself. Healing tissues also need good hydration and nutrition. Recall from Chapter 25 that adequate protein intake is especially important when the body is trying to rebuild injured tissues.

In the health care setting, we do many things to help support the wound healing process. Some of the measures taken by the health care team to support the wound healing process include closing the wound, inserting drains, and applying dressings. As a nursing assistant, your duties related to wound care will vary, depending on your employer and the state where you work. Usually, nursing assistants are asked to assist the nurse with wound care. However, some facilities may train you to perform specific duties related to wound care on your own. As always, if you are asked to perform a task that is new to you, make sure that the task is covered by your job description and that you have received the training you will need to perform the skill properly. No matter where you work, the most important role you will play with regard to wound care is that of "observer." As a nursing assistant, you will have the best opportunity to notice and report signs that might indicate that a wound is not healing properly or has become infected.

Wound closure

If a wound is kept clean but otherwise left alone, eventually the tissue will repair itself and the wound will close on its own. However, this can take a long time, it increases the risk of infection, and it often results in a scar. To speed this process up, minimize the risk of infection, and reduce the amount of scarring, the doctor may decide to close the wound. The timing for, and approach to, wound closure varies depending on the situation:

- In *first-intention wound healing*, the wound is closed surgically with sutures or staples. If the wound is minor (such as a cut from a fall), Steri-strips (small adhesive strips that are applied across the wound to hold the edges together) may be used. Pulling the edges of the skin and underlying tissues together and holding them closed helps speedup the healing process and minimize scarring.

- In *second-intention wound healing*, the wound is left open to heal from the inside out. Chronic wounds, such as late-stage pressure ulcers and venous (stasis) ulcers, often heal by second intention. Second-intention

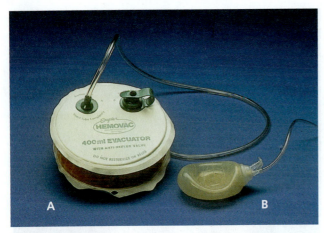

Figure 31-11
When drainage from a wound is significant, a drain may be placed. The drainage tube is placed in the wound and attached to a suction device, which draws the fluid out of the wound. Many types of drains are available. **(A)** A Hemovac drain. **(B)** A Jackson-Pratt or "grenade" drain.

wound healing results in a wider, more noticeable scar after the wound has healed.
* In *third-intention wound healing*, the wound is left open for a period of time to make sure that an infection is not going to occur. Then the wound edges are cleaned and closed to speed the healing process.

Wound drains

As part of the healing process, some wounds produce a lot of fluid, or drainage. A wound that is infected or bleeding also often produces a lot of drainage. Fluid that is allowed to collect in a wound can promote infection, delaying the healing process. Therefore, wound drains are often used to allow blood and other fluids to flow out of the wound (Fig. 31-11).

Some drains allow fluid to collect in the wound dressing (the material covering the wound). Others are connected to a collection device. If a resident you are caring for has a drain, take note of the characteristics of the drainage every time you check the dressing or the collection device. Is there more drainage than you expected? Does it have a foul odor that it did not have before? Has the appearance of the drainage changed? Report any unusual observations to the nurse.

When repositioning a resident with a drain, take care not to pull on the drain tubing. Pulling on the drain tubing could pull the drain out of the wound. The loss of the drain will allow fluid to collect in the wound until the doctor can replace the drain. Fluid in the wound puts the person at risk for infection.

Wound dressings

Sometimes, dressings are applied to wounds to prevent microbes from gaining access to the body, to keep the wound dry during procedures such as bathing, or to absorb drainage from the wound. The type of dressing used depends on several factors, including:

* The type of wound
* The location of the wound
* The amount of drainage associated with the wound
* Whether or not the wound is infected
* Whether or not the wound must be kept dry
* How often the dressing must be changed

The doctor writes the order for the type of dressing that is to be used.

Transparent dressings are thin, clear, single-layer dressings that are used on small wounds, drain sites, and IV insertion sites (Fig. 31-12A). Transparent dressings are not used on wounds that are draining. These dressings adhere directly to the skin. They protect the wound from moisture and microbes, but allow air to circulate freely. Because they are transparent, the health care team can inspect the wound without removing the dressing.

Some dressings have multiple layers. A contact layer is applied directly to the wound to pull excess drainage away from the wound and into the upper layers of the dressing. The contact layer is non-adherent, which means it will not stick to the surface of the healing wound when it is removed. A secondary layer, made of gauze or a similar material, is applied on top of the contact layer to absorb wound drainage. The layers of the dressing are held in place by a bandage (see Fig. 31-12B). Bandages can be made out of tape; an elastic material (such as an ACE bandage); or a soft, stretchy woven material (such as Kling gauze). In elderly people, tape is rarely used to secure bandages, because elderly skin is very fragile and can be damaged when the tape is removed.

When a wound is draining heavily and the dressing must be changed often, a Montgomery tie may be used. A Montgomery tie consists of a strip of adhesive that is attached to a cloth tie. The dressing is placed on the wound. Then, the adhesive strip of the Montgomery tie is applied to the person's skin alongside the dressing. Another Montgomery tie is placed in the same way on the other side of the dressing. Then, the ties are tied

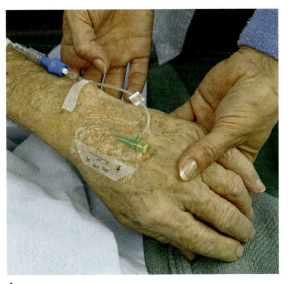
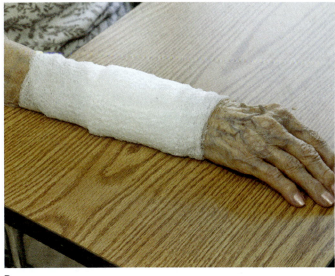

A   B

Figure 31-12
There are many different types of dressings. **(A)** A transparent dressing. **(B)** A dressing held in place with a bandage made of stretchy gauze.

together over the dressing to hold it in place (Fig. 31-13). When it is time to change the dressing, the ties are untied, the dressing is replaced, and then the ties are retied. Because there is no need to remove the adhesive tape to change the dressing, Montgomery ties help to protect the person's skin from damage caused by the frequent removal and reapplication of tape.

Procedure 31-1 explains how to help the nurse with a dressing change.

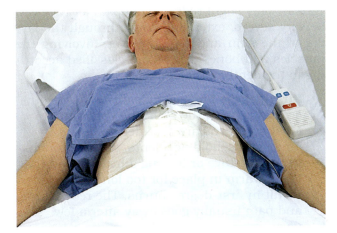

Figure 31-13
Montgomery ties can be used to secure a dressing that needs to be changed often. The adhesive is applied and then left in place. The ties secure the dressing and can be easily untied when a new dressing is needed. (© B. Proud.)

Vacuum-assisted closure (VAC) therapy

Vacuum-assisted closure (VAC) therapy may be used to help promote healing of complicated or chronic wounds. In VAC therapy, the wound is covered with a foam-like dressing. Tubing is embedded in the foam. Then, the foam, the tubing, and a margin of healthy skin are covered with transparent adhesive film, forming a seal. The end of the tubing is connected to a vacuum pump. When the pump is turned on, it creates suction. The suction removes wound drainage from the surface of the wound, stimulates blood flow to the wound, and stimulates the growth of new tissue (Fig. 31-14). When caring for a resident with a wound that is being treated with VAC therapy, it is important to make sure the system is functioning properly. Tell the nurse right away if the tubing is kinked, the vacuum pump is not functioning (there is no suction), or the dressing has become loose. An increase in bright red drainage in the collection device should also be reported right away.

TELL THE NURSE

When caring for a resident who has a wound, report the following observations immediately:

- The resident complains of increased pain or discomfort

- There is increased redness, swelling, or warmth around the wound

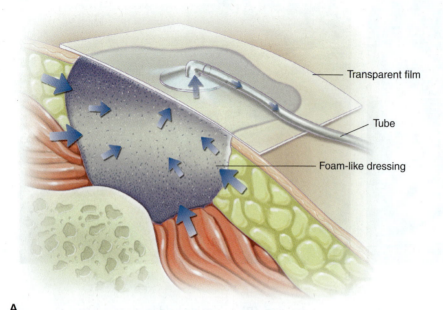

A

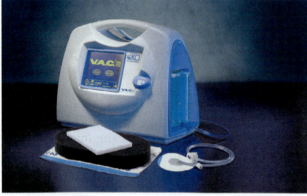

B

Figure 31-14
Vacuum-assisted closure (VAC) therapy is often used to promote healing of complicated or chronic wounds. **(A)** The wound is filled with a foam-like dressing. A tube is inserted into the foam, and then the area is sealed with a transparent film. When the pump is turned on, it creates suction, which draws fluid out of the wound and stimulates blood flow and the growth of new tissue. **(B)** The V.A.C.® ATS device. (*Courtesy of KCI Licensing, Inc. 2007.*)

- The resident has a fever

- Drainage from the wound has changed in amount or appearance, or has developed a foul odor

- The dressing is excessively wet or soiled, or has become loose

- The drain tubing has pulled out or has become disconnected

- The VAC therapy system is not functioning properly (for example, the tubing is kinked or there is no suction)

BURNS

Burns are injuries to the skin and underlying tissues caused by contact with extreme heat (thermal burns), chemicals (chemical burns), or electricity (electrical burns). Burns can be minor, causing only slight redness and pain, or they can be very severe, extending down through the layers of the skin and possibly even involving the muscles and bones. Burns are classified according to the depth of the damage:

- **First-degree burns** cause injury to the outermost layer of the skin, the epidermis. Most sunburns are first-degree burns. Minor household accidents, such as touching a hot stove or leaving a heating pad that is too warm in place for too long, can also result in first-degree burns. The redness and pain usually goes away after a few days.

- **Second-degree burns** penetrate into the dermis of the skin. Second-degree burns are often associated with blisters. These burns are very painful and the loss of the epidermis increases the risk of infection. Because an older person's skin is thin and fragile, injuries that would cause a first-degree burn in a younger person may cause a second-degree burn in an older person.

- **Third-degree burns** involve the epidermis and dermis, the subcutaneous layer, and often the underlying muscles and bones as well. People with third-degree burns need surgery, skin grafts, and extensive rehabilitation to heal. Third-degree burns are associated with very high infection rates, because the skin has been destroyed. In addition, the scarring that results from severe burns can cause severe disfigurement and contractures of the extremities. Because of the special care they require, people with third-degree burns are cared for in the acute care setting, often in specialized burn units.

LESIONS

Lesion is a general term used to describe any break in the skin. Often you will see the term *lesion* used when discussing rashes or other skin disorders. Lesions often occur in groups, forming a **rash.** Rashes can be *localized* (limited to one area) or *systemic* (occurring all over the body).

Rashes may be caused by a systemic infection. In this case, the skin itself is not infected, but it is showing signs of an infection inside of the body. The rash seen in shingles is a good example of a rash that is caused by a systemic infection. **Shingles (herpes zoster),** a disorder most commonly seen in people older than 65 years of age, is caused by the same virus that causes chickenpox. Following a case of the chickenpox, the virus remains in the person's body, but in an inactive state. The virus can become active again if the person's resistance to infection is lowered, which often happens with age. The virus causes a red rash of small, fluid-filled blisters (Fig. 31-15). Because the virus lives in the nerve cells, the rash usually follows the path of a nerve and is often accompanied by itching, stinging, or burning pain. For many people, the pain is severe, and it can last for weeks or months. Even the touch of clothing against the area may be very painful. Because shingles is most common in older people, you may care for a resident with this disorder. A resident with shingles should only be cared for by a person who has already been exposed to the chickenpox virus, because it is possible to get chickenpox from a person with shingles if you have not been exposed to the virus before. It is also very important to follow your facility's infection control procedures when giving care, to prevent others in the facility from being exposed to the virus.

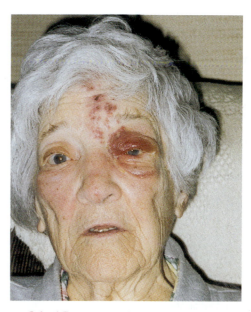

Figure 31-15
The shingles rash is a painful rash made up of fluid-filled blisters (vesicles). It is usually localized to one area or one side of the body, often in a stripe pattern.

Rashes may also be caused by contact with an irritant, such as poison ivy. In people with sensitive skin, contact with substances like bath soap or laundry detergent can cause a rash called *contact dermatitis.* **Dermatitis** is a general term for inflammation of the skin. **Eczema** is a type of chronic dermatitis that is usually accompanied by severe itching, scaling, and crusting of the surface of the skin.

Itching, burning, or redness of the skin accompanies many skin lesions. The redness of the skin that often accompanies these lesions is known as **erythema.** Dermatologists (doctors who specialize in knowledge of the skin) look at the characteristics of the lesions on the skin, as well as the location of the lesions and the person's other signs and symptoms, to find clues to their cause. There are many different types of skin lesions (Table 31-1):

- A **macule** is a small, flat, reddened lesion. Macules form the rash that is seen in measles.
- A **papule** is a small, raised, firm, lesion. Papules can be easily felt by passing your fingers lightly over the affected area.
- A **vesicle** is a small, blister-like lesion that contains watery, clear fluid. Vesicles form the rash that is seen in shingles.
- A **pustule** is a vesicle that contains pus, a thick, yellowish fluid that is a sign of infection. Pustules are seen in acne.

Table 31-1   Types of Skin Lesions

LESION	DESCRIPTION
Macule (© Custom Medical Stock Photo)	Small, flat, red lesions
Papule (© Custom Medical Stock Photo)	Small, raised, firm bumps
Vesicle	Small, fluid-filled, blister-like lesions
Pustule	Small, pus-filled, blister-like lesions
Excoriation (© Custom Medical Stock Photo)	Abrasion (wearing away of the surface of the skin)
Fissure	A crack in the skin
Ulcer	A crater-like open sore

- An **excoriation** is an abrasion, or a scraping away of the surface of the skin. Excoriations can be caused by trauma, chemicals, or burns (including friction burns from sliding a person across a sheet). Urine or feces, if left on the skin for too long, can cause a chemical excoriation.
- A **fissure** is a crack in the skin. Fissures can be caused by extreme dryness. Fungal infections, such as tinea pedis (athlete's foot), can also cause fissures.
- An **ulcer** is a shallow crater that is formed when the tissue dies. The dead tissue is shed, leaving a crater behind. Venous (stasis) ulcers, a common type of ulcer, develop as a result of poor blood flow through the veins in the legs.

Because skin lesions disrupt the skin's protective barrier, they place the person at increased risk for infection. Secondary bacterial infection of the skin is especially common when the lesion is itchy and the person scratches it excessively. *Secondary* means that the infection is occurring on top of the original problem. This is similar to what happens when you have a mosquito bite that you cannot stop scratching—eventually, you scratch it raw, it gets infected, and then it takes much longer for the bite to heal than it would have if you had just left it alone.

When you are caring for a person with skin lesions, there are several things that you can do to increase the person's comfort and promote healing of the skin:

- Make sure that you are aware of any adjustments to the normal bathing and skin care routine that may be necessary. For example, you may need to use a special soap or lotion as part of the person's skin care. The nurse will be able to tell you about any necessary changes to the routine, or you can check the care plan.
- Help the person to choose clothing that does not rub or irritate the skin lesion.
- Discourage the person from scratching itchy or irritated skin. Although scratching may bring temporary relief, it causes additional skin injury and puts the person at risk for infection. Soft mitt restraints or gloves may be necessary to prevent a confused resident from scratching the lesions.
- Observe the lesions for changes in color, or for bleeding or drainage. Report any changes to the nurse immediately. Also, note whether the lesions seem to be getting larger, or spreading to other parts of the body.

Summary

- The integumentary system consists of the skin and its accessory structures (hair, nails, sweat glands, and sebaceous glands).
- As the body's most visible organ system, the integumentary system can provide clues to a person's overall health. Changes in a person's skin tone or the development of a rash may signal an internal problem, such as liver disease, a heart or lung problem, or an infection.
- The integumentary system has three major functions that help maintain the body's homeostasis.
  - The skin protects us from microbes, chemicals, and other agents that could harm the body.
  - The skin helps us to maintain our internal fluid balance.
  - The integumentary system plays a major role in temperature regulation. Narrowing and widening of the blood vessels in the skin helps our bodies to maintain or release heat, respectively. The sweat glands help to cool our bodies through evaporation. Hair on our scalps and bodies helps to keep us warm.
- Like all organ systems, the integumentary system changes as we age.
  - Changes that affect our appearance include wrinkles, gray hair, and age spots.
  - The skin becomes more fragile and more prone to injury with age. The number and output of the sebaceous glands decrease, making the skin dry. Circulation to the skin decreases.
  - The number and output of the sweat glands decrease. This change, along with the changes in the skin, makes it harder for the older person to adjust to changes in the environmental temperature.
  - The nails become tough and yellow, making them difficult to trim.
- Pressure ulcers are a major concern in the health care setting.
  - Pressure ulcers develop when soft tissues are squeezed between bone and a surface, such as a mattress or chair. The weight of the body disrupts the flow of oxygen-rich blood to the tissues, causing the tissues to die and leading to the formation of a pressure ulcer.
  - Immobility is the underlying cause of all pressure ulcers. Several factors, including old age, poor nutrition, and moisture trapped in the folds of the skin, can increase an immobile person's risk of developing a pressure ulcer.
- Warning signs of pressure ulcers include:
  - A reddened area that does not return to its normal color after the pressure is relieved
  - A previously reddened area that is hot to the touch or painful
  - An area that is pale, white, or shiny
- Prevention of pressure ulcers is very important, because pressure ulcers are extremely painful, difficult to treat, and potentially fatal. The nursing assistant does many things to prevent residents from developing pressure ulcers, including repositioning, observing, providing good skin and perineal care, changing wet and soiled linens promptly, and encouraging exercise.
- A wound is a break in the skin. The underlying tissues are usually affected as well.
  - A wound can be intentional or unintentional.
  - A break in the skin puts the person at risk for infection. The health care team does many things to help wounds to heal quickly and with minimal complications.
  - Nursing assistants are in an excellent position to notice and report signs and symptoms that suggest that the wound has become infected or is not healing well, such as a foul-smelling discharge or excessive drainage or bleeding.
- Burns are injuries caused by heat, chemicals, or electricity.
- Lesions are breaks in the skin.
  - Many different types of skin lesions can form rashes.
    - The type of lesion is often a clue to the cause of the rash.
    - Rashes can be localized (limited to one area) or systemic (occurring all over the body).
  - Skin lesions can be caused by infections inside the body, infections of the skin itself, or irritation of the skin.
  - Nursing assistants are often the first to notice an unusual lesion on a resident.
  - Older people are at high risk for developing shingles (herpes zoster), a rash caused by the same virus that causes chickenpox.

Assisting the Nurse With a Dressing Change

WHY YOU DO IT   Helping the nurse with a dressing change minimizes the chance that the nurse's hands or other surfaces will become contaminated by the drainage on the soiled dressing. It also helps to ensure that the new dressing remains free of pathogens that could contaminate the wound.

Getting Ready   WGKIEpS

1. Complete the "Getting Ready" steps.

Supplies

- gloves
- gown (if necessary)
- mask (if necessary)
- paper towels or a bed protector
- plastic bag
- Bandaging material
- dressing
- scissors

Procedure

2. Cover the over-bed table with paper towels or the bed protector. Place the dressing supplies on the over-bed table. Fold the top edges of the plastic bag down to make a cuff. Place the cuffed bag on the over-bed table.

3. Make sure that the bed is positioned at a comfortable working height (to promote good body mechanics) and that the wheels are locked. If the side rails are in use, lower the side rail on the working side of the bed. The side rail on the opposite side of the bed should remain up.

4. Help the person to a comfortable position that allows access to the wound.

5. Fanfold the top linens to the foot of the bed. Adjust the person's clothing as necessary to expose the wound.

6. Put on the mask, gown, or both, if necessary. Put on the gloves.

7. The nurse will remove the old dressing. The nurse may ask you to take the old dressing and place it in the cuffed plastic bag. Be careful to keep the soiled side of the dressing out of the person's sight. Do not let the dressing touch the outside of the plastic bag.

8. Remove your gloves and dispose of them in a facility-approved waste container.

9. Wait while the nurse inspects the wound and measures it, if necessary.

10. Put on a clean pair of gloves.

11. Assist as the nurse applies a new dressing.

    a. Open the wrapper containing the dressing and hold it open so that the nurse can remove the dressing. Do not touch the dressing. Dispose of the wrapper in a facility-approved waste container.

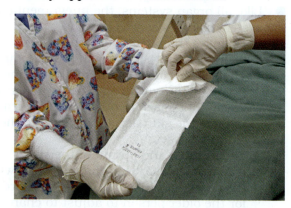

Step 11a Hold the wrapper open so that the nurse can remove the dressing.

    b. If the dressing will be secured with tape, cut four pieces of tape for securing the dressing. For a 4 × 4 dressing, each piece of tape should measure 8 inches long. Hang the tape from the edge of the over-bed table.

    c. If the nurse asks you to, use the tape strips to secure the dressing by placing one piece of tape along each side of the dressing. Center each piece of tape equally over the dressing and the person's skin.

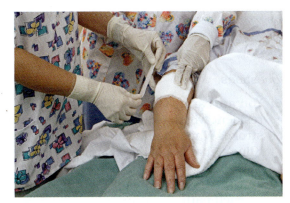

Step 11c If the dressing will be secured by tape, place one piece of tape along each side.

12. Remove your gloves (and gown and mask, if using) and dispose of them in a facility-approved waste container. Wash your hands.

13. Adjust the person's clothing as necessary to cover the dressing. Help the person back into a comfortable position, straighten the bottom linens, and draw the top linens over the person.

14. Make sure that the bed is lowered to its lowest position and that the wheels are locked. If the side rails are in use, return the side rail to the raised position on the working side of the bed.

15. Dispose of disposable items in a facility-approved waste container. Clean equipment and return it to the storage area.

Finishing Up CLOSUR

16. Complete the "Finishing Up" steps.

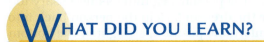WHAT DID YOU LEARN?

Multiple Choice

Select the single best answer for each of the following questions.

1. Where are pressure ulcers most likely to form?
    a. On the heels, ankles, and toes
    b. On the elbows and shoulder blades
    c. On the spine
    d. All of the above

2. Why is it important to prevent pressure ulcers from forming?
    a. Pressure ulcers are disgusting to see.
    b. People who have pressure ulcers require more care than people who do not, and this is expensive for the facility.
    c. Pressure ulcers are difficult to treat and can lead to a person's death.
    d. Pressure ulcers interfere with the skin's ability to make vitamin D.

3. What is the underlying cause of all pressure ulcers?
    a. Continuous pressure applied to one area
    b. Poor nutrition
    c. Incontinence
    d. All of the above

4. Which of the following factors can increase a person's risk of getting a pressure ulcer?
    a. Advanced age
    b. Incontinence
    c. Poor nutrition
    d. All of the above

5. Mr. Underwood has developed a white, shiny area on his left hip about the size of a quarter. Yesterday, this same area was red and hot to the touch. If you were Mr. Underwood's nursing assistant, what would be your biggest concern?
    a. That Mr. Underwood has shingles
    b. That Mr. Underwood has a stage 1 pressure ulcer
    c. That Mr. Underwood's wound is not healing properly
    d. That Mr. Underwood has jaundice

6. You are caring for Mrs. Kling, a 93-year-old resident who has limited mobility following a stroke. What should you do to minimize Mrs. Kling's chances of developing a pressure ulcer?
    a. Dry Mrs. Kling's skin thoroughly after each bath
    b. Reposition Mrs. Kling regularly, according to the care plan
    c. Encourage Mrs. Kling to eat well
    d. All of the above

7. Which one of the following is an example of an intentional wound?
    a. A wound that resulted from physical abuse
    b. A surgical incision
    c. A lesion
    d. A burn

8. Why is it important to keep the skin healthy?
    a. The skin protects the body from microbes and helps to maintain the body's fluid balance
    b. The skin protects the body from sunburn
    c. It is easier to detect signs of disease in a person with healthy skin
    d. Keeping the skin healthy helps to prevent wrinkles in old age

9. You are assigned to Mrs. Peebles, and you hear in report that she has shingles. You know that you must:
    a. Use a gown, gloves, and mask to keep from catching shingles yourself
    b. Tell the nurse that you have never had chickenpox
    c. Tell the nurse that you have never had measles
    d. Scrub the lesions vigorously to remove the dried scabs

Matching

Match each numbered item with its appropriate lettered description.

_____ **1.** Macules

_____ **2.** Melanin

_____ **3.** Dermatitis

_____ **4.** Vesicles

_____ **5.** Erythema

_____ **6.** Papules

_____ **7.** Pustules

_____ **8.** Excoriation

_____ **9.** Fissure

_____ **10.** Age spot

a. Redness of the skin that often accompanies rashes

b. Often seen on the backs of the hands; caused by melanin deposits

c. Cracks in the skin, such as those seen in athlete's foot

d. Abrasion or wearing away of the top layer of skin; caused by trauma, chemicals, or burns

e. Filled with pus, a thick yellow fluid associated with infection

f. Blister-like lesions that contain watery fluid, such as those seen in chickenpox and shingles

g. Flat, reddened lesions, such as those seen in measles

h. Firm, raised bumps

i. General term for inflammation of the skin

j. Gives the skin its color

STOP and Think!

- You have been assigned to help Mrs. Sills with her morning care. While you are helping Mrs. Sills to put on her socks, you accidentally scratch Mrs. Sills' ankle, causing her to bleed. What should you do? What are some steps you can take to avoid scratching a person's skin when you are providing care?

- Richard is providing care to Mr. O'Meara, who has just been transferred to Willow Wood Care Center. Mr. O'Meara is confined to a wheelchair. While giving Mr. O'Meara a back massage as part of evening care, Richard notices a reddened area at the base of Mr. O'Meara's spine. What are the possible explanations for this finding? What should Richard do?

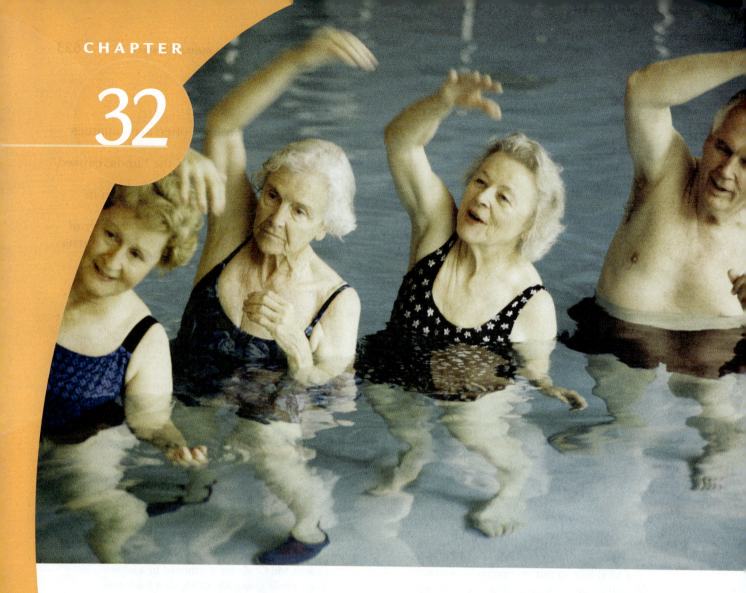

CHAPTER

32

The Musculoskeletal System

WHAT WILL YOU LEARN?

Think about everything you have done so far today. Before you even left the house this morning, you did a number of different tasks requiring the services of your musculoskeletal system—getting out of bed, brushing your teeth, eating breakfast, and taking the dog for a walk or feeding the cat, just to name a few. Think about all of the individual movements that each of these small tasks requires, and you will get a sense of how very important the musculoskeletal system is to our daily functioning.

The muscular system and the skeletal system work together to enable us to move. As you learned in Chapter 30, sometimes these two organ systems are referred to together as the *musculoskeletal system* because they work so closely together. In this chapter, you will learn about the structure and function of the musculoskeletal system, and about how it is affected by aging and illness. You will also learn about how nursing assistants help

624

Photo: Exercise helps to keep the bones, joints, and muscles healthy.

residents to maintain proper function of the musculoskeletal system. When you are finished with this chapter, you will be able to:

1. List the major parts of the musculoskeletal system.
2. List and describe the four types of bones found in the skeletal system.
3. Define terms used to describe joint movement.
4. List and describe the three types of muscles found in the muscular system.
5. Discuss the main functions of the musculoskeletal system.
6. Describe how normal aging processes affect the musculoskeletal system.
7. Describe some of the disorders that can affect the musculoskeletal system.
8. Define normal range of motion and describe methods used to maintain joint function in the health care setting.
9. Demonstrate how to help a person to perform range-of-motion exercises.

Vocabulary Use the CD in the front of your book to hear these terms pronounced and defined:

Skeleton	Muscle tone	Fracture	Hip fracture
Joints	Atrophy	Pathologic	Osteomyelitis
Range of motion	Muscular dystrophy	fracture	Amputation
Cartilage	Arthritis	Reduction	Stump
Ligaments	Osteoporosis	Fixation	Phantom pain
Tendons	Kyphosis	Traction	

STRUCTURE OF THE MUSCULOSKELETAL SYSTEM

The musculoskeletal system consists of the skeletal system and the muscular system.

THE SKELETAL SYSTEM

The skeletal system consists of the bones. The 206 bones in the human body form a framework called the **skeleton** (Fig. 32-1). The skeleton gives structure and shape to the body, and protects key vital organs (such as the heart and the brain) from injury.

The bones of the skeleton vary in size and shape. Bones are classified according to their shape (Fig. 32-2):

- **Long bones.** When we think of a "bone," what we often picture in our mind is an example of a long bone. The long bones are found in the arms and the legs. Long bones consist of a shaft and two rounded ends.
- **Short bones.** Short bones are round or cube-shaped. Short bones are found in the wrists and ankles.

- **Flat bones** are relatively thin and may be curved. Examples of flat bones include the ribs and the bones that form the skull.
- **Irregular bones** are oddly shaped bones that are not flat. Irregular bones are found in the spinal column and face.

Bones must be strong enough to support and protect the body, yet light enough to allow us to move. Can you imagine how heavy a large bone like the bone in your thigh would be, if it were solid? Instead, bones have two layers. The outside of the bone is hard and solid. The inside of the bone is sponge-like and airy. Thin strands of bone form a net-like structure, and the spaces in between the thin strands of bone are filled with bone marrow (Fig. 32-3). This combination of a solid, hard outside and a sponge-like inside results in bones that are very strong and able to resist a great amount of force, yet lightweight. The cells that form the bones are constantly broken down and replaced with new bone cells throughout a person's lifetime. A complex network of blood vessels supplies the bone cells with the oxygen and nutrients they need.

The areas where two bones join together are called **joints.** Joints allow us to move. The **range of motion** of a joint is the complete extent of

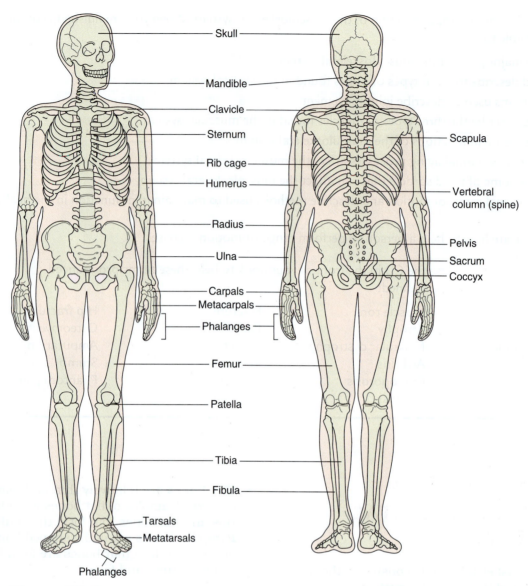

Figure 32-1
The human skeleton contains 206 bones. Some of the major bones are labeled here.

movement that the joint is normally capable of without causing pain. Joints can be classified according to the amount of movement they allow (Fig. 32-4):

- **Fixed joints** do not permit any movement at all. The joints between the bones of the skull are examples of fixed joints.
- **Slightly movable joints** allow for limited movement. Slightly movable joints are found between the vertebrae in the spine, and where the ribs attach to the sternum (breastbone). **Cartilage,** a tough, fibrous substance, fills in the space between the bones in the slightly movable joint. The cartilage permits limited movement and

acts as a "shock absorber" between the bones.
- **Freely movable joints** allow for a wide range of movement. Examples of freely movable joints include the knees, elbows, finger and toe joints, and hip joints. Some of the ways in which freely movable joints move are shown and defined in Table 32-1. The ends of the bones that form the freely movable joint are covered with cartilage, which provides a smooth surface for the other bones to move against. A capsule formed of connective tissue encloses the ends of the bones, forming a joint cavity. The lining of the capsule secretes a thick fluid called *synovial fluid* into the joint

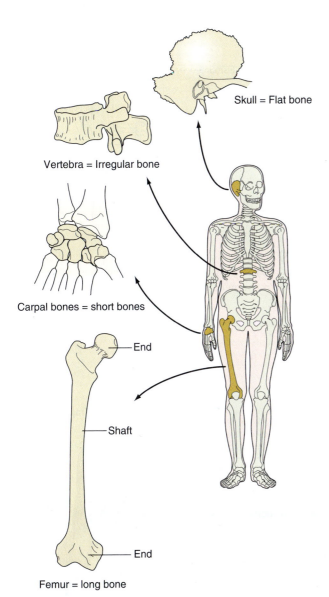

Skull = Flat bone

Vertebra = Irregular bone

Carpal bones = short bones

End

Shaft

End

Femur = long bone

Figure 32-2
Bones can be categorized by their shape. General types of bones include long bones, short bones, flat bones, and irregular bones.

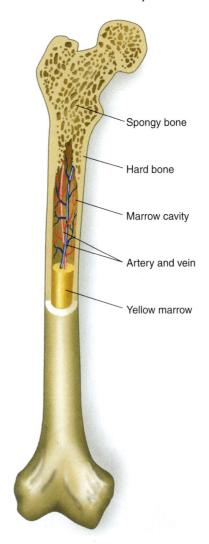

Spongy bone

Hard bone

Marrow cavity

Artery and vein

Yellow marrow

Figure 32-3
Bones have two layers, a solid outside and a net-like inside. As a result, bones are very strong, yet lightweight.

cavity. The synovial fluid lubricates the joint, which helps the joint to move smoothly. **Ligaments,** which are very strong bands of fibrous tissue, cross over the joint capsule, attaching one bone to another, and stabilizing the joint. If the ligament is torn or weak, the joint may be able to move too much in any one direction.

THE MUSCULAR SYSTEM

The muscular system consists of the muscles. As you learned in Chapter 30, there are three types of muscle tissue found in the body (see Chapter 30,

Table 30-1). Of the three types, skeletal muscle is the type of muscle tissue found in the musculoskeletal system. Skeletal muscle is said to be *striated*, because the muscle fibers make the muscles look like they have stripes. (*Striations* is another word for "stripes.")

There are almost 700 individual skeletal muscles in the body (Fig. 32-5). These muscles account for about 40% of a person's total body weight. Skeletal muscles vary in shape. Some are long, thick, and band-like. Others are flat or fanlike. Muscles are named according to their location, their shape, or their function.

The skeletal muscles are attached to the bones by bands of connective tissue called **tendons.** Occasionally, skeletal muscles are attached to

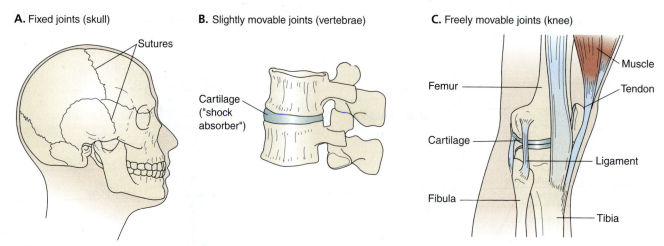

Figure 32-4

Joints are often categorized by the amount of motion they permit. **(A)** Fixed joints, such as the joints that join the bones of the skull, do not allow for any movement. **(B)** Slightly movable joints, such as those between the vertebrae in the spinal column, permit some movement. **(C)** Freely movable joints, such as the knee joints, allow for a wide range of movement.

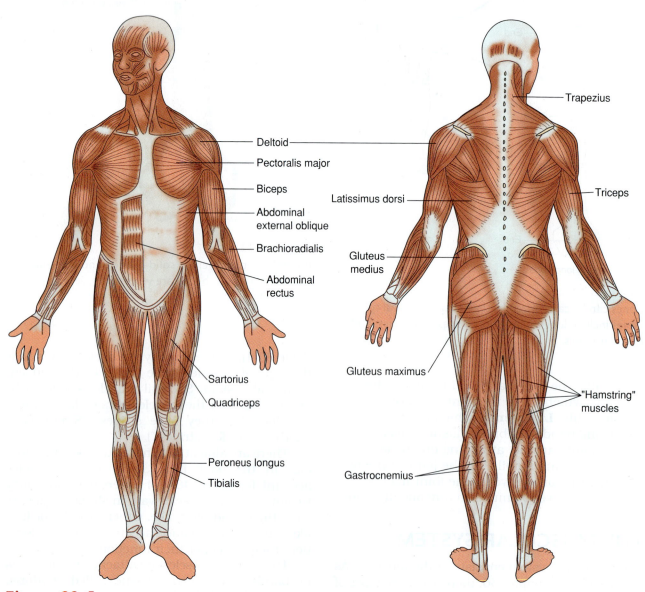

Figure 32-5

There are about 700 skeletal muscles in the body! Some of the more familiar ones are labeled here.

Table 32-1   Words Used to Describe Movement

	WORD	DEFINITION
Flexion / Extension	**Flexion** **Extension**	Bending of a joint Straightening of a joint
Abduction / Adduction	**Abduction** **Adduction**	Moving a body part away from the midline of the body Moving a body part toward the midline of the body
Rotation	**Rotation**	Twisting or turning of a joint
Supination / Pronation	**Supination** **Pronation**	Rotation of the palm so that it is facing up or forward Rotation of the palm so that it is facing down or backward
Eversion / Inversion	**Eversion** **Inversion**	Rotation of the sole of the foot outward Rotation of the sole of the foot inward
Dorsiflexion / Plantar flexion	**Dorsiflexion** **Plantar flexion**	Bending the foot upward at the ankle by pulling the toes toward the head Flexing the arch of the foot by pointing the toes downward

other muscles by a broad, flat sheet of tendon called an *aponeurosis*.

FUNCTION OF THE MUSCULOSKELETAL SYSTEM

The musculoskeletal system has several vital functions.

PROTECTION

The bones of the skeletal system protect delicate internal organs. For example, the skull bones surround and protect the brain, and the rib cage surrounds and protects the lungs and heart.

SUPPORT

The bones of the skeleton form a framework that supports and gives shape to the body. **Muscle tone,** or the steady contraction of the skeletal muscles, helps us to maintain an upright posture, such as sitting or standing. The muscles of the back, neck, shoulders, and abdomen are responsible for maintaining posture.

MOVEMENT

Voluntary movement occurs when a skeletal muscle contracts (shortens) or relaxes (lengthens) across a freely movable joint. In freely movable joints, each skeletal muscle attaches to the bone in two places, the origin and the insertion. The origin and the insertion points are on opposite sides of the joint. So, when the muscle contracts, the muscle shortens and the origin and insertion points are drawn closer to each other, causing the part of the body to move (Fig. 32-6).

Skeletal muscles usually work in groups to provide body movement. For example, your biceps muscle is located on the front of your upper arm. When you contract your biceps muscle, your lower arm is drawn toward your body. When you are lifting a heavy object, the brachioradialis muscle, which is also located in your upper arm, also contracts, helping to stabilize the elbow and assisting the biceps muscle with lifting. When it is time to straighten the arm again, the biceps muscle relaxes and the triceps muscle, located on the back of the upper arm, contracts, pulling the lower arm back into a straight position.

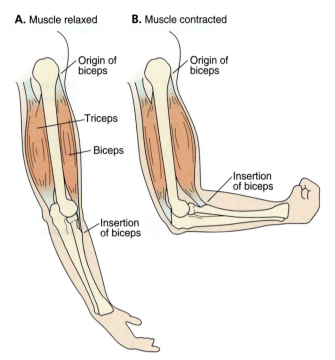

A. Muscle relaxed   **B.** Muscle contracted

Origin of biceps — Origin of biceps — Triceps — Biceps — Insertion of biceps — Insertion of biceps

Figure 32-6
The muscular and the skeletal systems work together to produce movement. The muscle attaches to the bone in two places, the origin and the insertion. **(A)** Shown here are the attachments of the biceps muscle, the muscle in your upper arm that bulges when you "make a muscle." **(B)** When you contract your biceps muscle, the origin and insertion points are drawn closer together. As the muscle shortens, it pulls on the bone, bringing your lower arm toward your body.

HEAT PRODUCTION

Contraction of the skeletal muscles produces heat and helps to maintain a constant body temperature. This is why we feel warmer when we move back and forth and stamp our feet while waiting outside on a cold day for a bus. The movement of the muscles produces heat, which makes us feel warmer. This is also why, when it is very cold, we may start to shiver. Shivering occurs when the skeletal muscles contract rapidly in unison. The involuntary contractions help to increase the heat output of the muscles, raising the body temperature and making us feel warmer.

CALCIUM STORAGE

Calcium is an important mineral that is necessary for the proper functioning of skeletal and cardiac muscle. Calcium is also what makes the bone tissue hard and strong. Most of the calcium we need to function on a daily basis is obtained from calcium-rich foods and beverages, such as milk, cheese, yogurt, broccoli, leafy greens, tofu, and calcium-fortified orange juice. However, if we do not take in enough calcium through our diets, then calcium is released from the bones as it is needed. Consuming enough calcium when we are young is essential for building up the calcium stores in our bones.

PRODUCTION OF BLOOD CELLS

In addition to storing calcium, the bones also function as a factory for the production of blood cells. There are many different types of blood cells, with many different functions. For example, some blood cells play a role in the immune response, and help us to fight off infection. Other blood cells carry oxygen to the tissues of the body. Blood cells form in red bone marrow, which is found in flat bones and the ends of the long bones. In young children, the shaft of the long bones also contains red bone marrow, but that red bone marrow is gradually replaced by yellow bone marrow as the person grows older. Yellow bone marrow is made up mostly of fatty tissue that can be used by the body for energy if necessary.

THE EFFECTS OF AGING ON THE MUSCULOSKELETAL SYSTEM

The normal processes of aging cause significant changes in the musculoskeletal system. It is the rare older person who does not have some degree of disability or discomfort related to the functioning of his or her musculoskeletal system! Aches, pains, and stiffness often accompany these changes. When it is difficult or painful to move, we tend to move less frequently. Decreased use of the musculoskeletal system leads to decreased strength and flexibility. Age-related changes in the musculoskeletal system are worsened when the person becomes less active and can be a major cause of disability in older people.

Exercising regularly and eating properly are measures that can delay or decrease the effects of aging on the musculoskeletal system. Engaging in some form of weight-bearing exercise, such as brisk walking, aerobics, or moderate weight training, has been shown to have many positive effects, even in older people (Fig. 32-7). Weight-

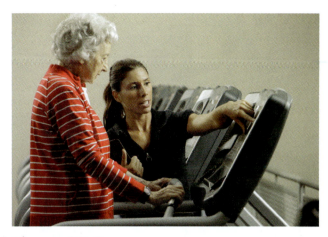

Figure 32-7
It is never too late to begin exercising! Regular exercise strengthens the muscles, helps to build bone mass, and lessens joint pain and stiffness.

bearing exercise helps to maintain bone strength by stimulating the body to store extra calcium in the bones. It improves blood flow, allowing more oxygen and nutrients to be carried to the tissues of the musculoskeletal system. Continued use of the muscles helps to retain strength. Flexibility of the joints is improved with regular exercise, which leads to fewer aches and pains.

People typically begin to experience age-related changes to the musculoskeletal system after the age of 40 years, although the onset of these changes may be significantly delayed in people who exercise regularly and are relatively healthy. The normal age-related changes that affect the musculoskeletal system include loss of bone tissue, loss of muscle mass, and wear and tear on the joints.

LOSS OF BONE TISSUE

Aging decreases the body's ability to absorb calcium, a critical nutrient. When the body cannot get the amount of calcium it needs from the diet alone, it begins to draw on the calcium stored in the bones. Some people begin drawing on their calcium stores at a relatively young age, for example, when they are in their 40s. The continuous, gradual loss of calcium causes the bones to lose their strength and hardness, making them more fragile and prone to breaking. If other conditions, such as poor nutrition, poor circulation, or a lack of physical activity are present, the loss of strong bone tissue occurs much more rapidly.

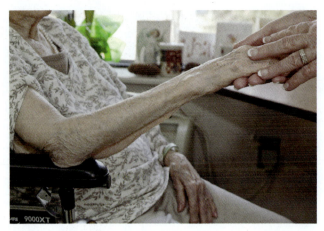

Figure 32-8
Muscle atrophy, or loss of muscle mass, is a normal age-related change. Immobility can make muscle atrophy much more severe.

LOSS OF MUSCLE MASS

The number of muscle cells also starts to gradually decrease when a person is in his or her 40s, resulting in a decrease in the size and strength of each individual muscle. The loss of muscle size and strength is called muscle **atrophy** (Fig. 32-8). If a person is poorly nourished, is not physically active, or has a chronic medical condition, muscle atrophy progresses at a much faster rate. If you have ever had a broken bone that required a cast, you probably noticed that after the cast was removed, the affected limb was smaller and weaker than the other one. What you noticed was muscle atrophy as a result of not being able to use the muscle during the time that the limb was in the cast!

Significant loss of muscle tissue can leave a person too weak to walk or carry out routine activities of daily living (ADLs). Loss of muscle tissue also affects the body's ability to produce heat. This is one reason why an elderly person might feel chilly in a room that a younger person would consider warm or even hot.

WEAR AND TEAR ON THE JOINTS

As we age, we lose the proteins that make the ligaments, tendons, and cartilage elastic and flexible, which can lead to stiffness and pain in the joints. The normal demands of daily life also cause a lot of wear and tear on the joints, which can, over time, lead to stiffness and pain. Overuse or injury of a joint, or being overweight, places extra strain on

certain joints and will make the normal changes associated with aging more severe. Joint pain and stiffness can make simple activities, such as walking or getting out of a chair, difficult. Joint stiffness can also make a person more likely to fall.

DISORDERS OF THE MUSCULOSKELETAL SYSTEM

It is likely that many of the people in your care will have some degree of musculoskeletal disability, simply as a result of their age. You may also care for people who have musculoskeletal disability as a result of disease or trauma.

MUSCULAR DYSTROPHY

Muscular dystrophy is a general term for a group of disorders that cause the skeletal muscles to become progressively weaker over time. These disorders are inherited. The types of muscular dystrophy vary according to the muscles that are affected, the age of the person typically affected, and the rate at which the disease progresses. Some people with muscular dystrophy experience only moderate disability, while others may die from the disease.

Muscular dystrophy is a common reason why a younger person may become a resident of a long-term care facility. Duchenne's muscular dystrophy, the most common form of muscular dystrophy, develops during childhood and usually causes death by the age of 20 years. As muscle weakness progresses and affects more of the person's body, the person becomes totally dependent on others for care. The person dies because the muscles that allow him to breathe eventually become too weak to perform this vital function.

The most common form of muscular dystrophy affecting adults is myotonic muscular dystrophy. A person with myotonic muscular dystrophy has difficulty relaxing the muscles after contracting them, and the muscles may spasm. In addition, the person experiences weakness and shrinking of the muscle tissue. People with myotonic muscular dystrophy also often have heart problems, endocrine disorders, and cataracts (yellowing and hardening of the lens of the eye).

A resident with muscular dystrophy will need your assistance with range-of-motion exercises, walking, positioning, and activities of daily living (ADLs).

ARTHRITIS

Arthritis is inflammation of the joints, usually associated with pain and stiffness. Arthritis is the most common disorder of the musculoskeletal system, affecting people of all ages. There are more than 20 different types of arthritis. Three of the most common types are osteoarthritis, rheumatoid arthritis, and gout.

Osteoarthritis

Osteoarthritis is the leading cause of physical disability among elderly people. In osteoarthritis, the cartilage that covers the ends of the bones wears away, making movement of the joint difficult and painful. Osteoarthritis appears to be the result of normal wear and tear on the joint, which is why it is seen most often in elderly people. However, obesity, previous joint injury, or a family history of the disease may increase a person's risk of developing osteoarthritis earlier in life and more severely.

Osteoarthritis usually affects weight-bearing joints, such as the knees, hips, and joints of the spinal column. Osteoarthritis begins when the smooth cartilage on the ends of the bones becomes rough, due to normal use of the joint. The rough area then becomes inflamed, and bony deposits build up. These bony deposits rub against the cartilage, causing even more damage. This cycle repeats until the cartilage has been worn down to the point where bone is actually rubbing against bone as the joint moves. The joint becomes swollen, stiff, and very painful.

A person with osteoarthritis may take medications to decrease both the pain and swelling. Heat and cold applications, which you learned about in Chapter 27, can also increase a person's level of comfort. Mild exercise that places the affected joints through their range of motion helps to diminish stiffness and maintain joint function. People who have very severe osteoarthritis may need surgery to replace the joint. Hips and knees are the joints most commonly replaced, but replacement of shoulder, elbow, wrist, and hand joints is also possible. Joint replacement surgery, also called total joint replacement, involves removing the ends of the bones in the affected joint and replacing them with parts made from metal and plastic (Fig. 32-9).

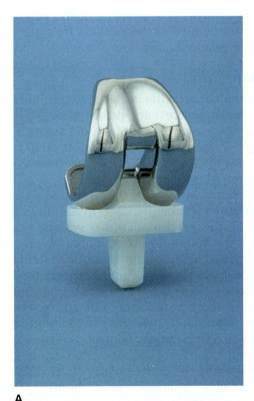

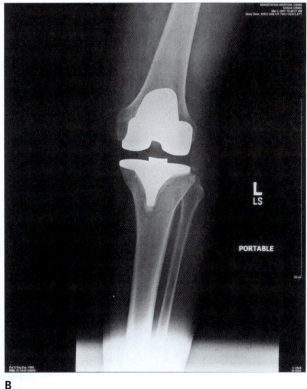

A   B

Figure 32-9

In joint replacement surgery, a damaged joint is replaced with an artificial (prosthetic) joint. **(A)** An artificial knee joint. **(B)** X-ray of an artificial knee joint in place. (*A, © SIU Bio Med/Custom Medical Stock Photo*)

As a nursing assistant, you may be responsible for caring for a resident who is recovering from joint replacement surgery. Residents who have had a joint replaced are not allowed to bear weight on the affected joint for a period of time after the surgery, so you will need to help them with transfers. In addition, residents who have had a hip joint replaced have several special care requirements during the recovery period:

- Following the surgery, the muscles and ligaments that normally hold the hip joint in place are weak, making it very easy for the head of the femur (the thigh bone) to dislocate, or pop out of joint. To prevent this from happening, the resident's legs must be spread apart (abducted) when the resident is in the supine or lateral position. Most residents who have had hip replacement surgery will have a special wedge-shaped pillow, called an *abduction pillow,* which goes between the legs and attaches to each leg with Velcro™ fasteners (Fig. 32-10). The abduction pillow helps to keep the legs spread. If an abduction pillow is not available, a regular pillow can be used instead.
- When sitting, a resident who has had hip replacement surgery must use a straight-backed chair. The resident's hips must be flexed no more than 90 degrees, and his feet must rest flat on the floor. This rule also applies when the resident is using the toilet or commode. A special device may be used to raise the height of the toilet seat to prevent flexion in excess of 90 degrees when the resident is using the toilet.

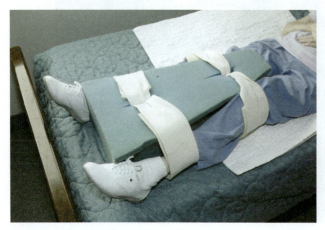

Figure 32-10
When a person is recovering from hip joint replacement surgery, an abduction pillow is used to help prevent the hip joint from becoming dislocated during the recovery period.

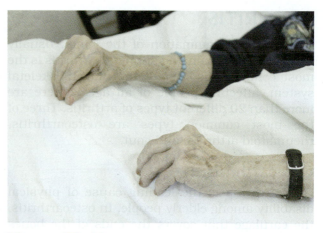

Figure 32-11
This woman has rheumatoid arthritis in the joints of her hands.

- A resident who has had hip replacement therapy will most likely be receiving physical therapy. Make sure that you learn about any specific ambulation and transfer techniques that the therapist prescribes for your resident.

As always, you should ask the nurse about any instructions or restrictions that are specific to your resident.

Rheumatoid Arthritis

Rheumatoid arthritis is a crippling condition that can cause severe joint deformities (Fig. 32-11). Unlike osteoarthritis, rheumatoid arthritis affects people much younger in life, most often between the ages of 20 and 40 years. This disease is more common in women than in men.

Researchers believe that rheumatoid arthritis is an autoimmune disorder. In autoimmune disorders, the body's immune system begins to attack the body's own tissues. So, for example, in rheumatoid arthritis, the immune system attacks and destroys the cartilage that covers the ends of the bones. Scar tissue develops within the joints, causing them to become stiff and useless. For many months, a person's rheumatoid arthritis may seem to be under control, but then the person will experience an acute flare-up of the disease. During the acute phases of the disease, the person may experience pain, swelling, redness, and heat in the joints, as well as fever and general weakness. Bed rest may be necessary, and splints can help decrease joint deformity. The gentle use of range-of-motion exercises helps to maintain joint mobility.

Gout

Gout is a type of arthritis that is caused by a disturbance in the body's metabolism. Uric acid is a waste product of metabolism that is usually eliminated from the body in the urine. If the body produces too much uric acid or the kidneys are unable to properly process the uric acid, the uric acid builds up in the body, forming crystals that are deposited within the joints. These uric acid crystals are extremely irritating to the tissues in the joint, and, as a result, the joint becomes inflamed and painful. While gout can affect any joint, the big toe is most commonly affected. Men past middle age are more commonly affected than women.

OSTEOPOROSIS

Osteoporosis is the excessive loss of bone tissue. Although everyone experiences some loss of bone tissue as a normal part of aging, people with osteoporosis lose excessive amounts of bone tissue, causing the bones to become crumbly and very fragile (Fig. 32-12). The bones most commonly affected by osteoporosis are the bones of the spine, the pelvis, and the long bones in the arms and legs.

Although osteoporosis can occur in older men, it is most common in older women who have gone through menopause. This is because estrogen, a hormone that is present in the bodies of women who are still having menstrual periods, helps to prevent bone loss. However, when a woman's periods stop, her body stops producing estrogen, and this puts her more at risk for bone loss. Other risk factors for the development of osteoporosis include:

- White race
- Petite body build ("small bones")
- Smoking
- Inactivity or immobility
- Diseases of the thyroid and adrenal glands
- A diet lacking in calcium, vitamin D (necessary for the absorption of calcium), and protein
- Therapy with certain medications, such as steroids

Osteoporosis causes bones to break more easily, and physical activity becomes very difficult.

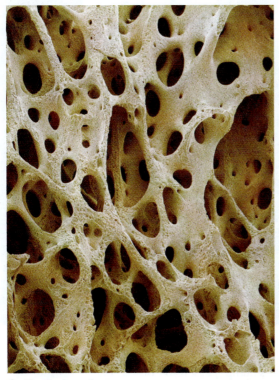

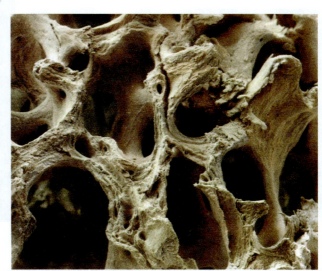

A. Healthy bone tissue

B. Osteoporotic bone tissue

Figure 32-12

Osteoporosis is a disease process that causes excessive loss of bone tissue, resulting in bones that are very brittle and prone to breaking. **(A)** Normal, healthy bone tissue. **(B)** Osteoporotic bone tissue. (*A,* © *Susumu Nishinaga/Photo Researchers, Inc.; B,* © *Dee Breger/Photo Researchers, Inc.*)

Sometimes bones are so brittle that a person can break them just by bumping into a piece of furniture. Bones that have been fractured are difficult to repair and heal slowly.

Osteoporosis can result in compression fractures of the vertebrae (the bones of the spine). Because of the osteoporosis, the vertebrae cannot support their load. Some of the vertebrae collapse, or become "compressed." Multiple compression fractures of the vertebral column result in **kyphosis** (an abnormal forward curvature of the upper spine) and are the cause of the "dowager's hump" that is commonly seen in elderly women with osteoporosis (Fig. 32-13). The spinal column fractures that occur as a result of osteoporosis are very debilitating. They cause stiffness, pain, and tenderness in the spine, which may lead to limited mobility. The person may also have trouble breathing, because the curvature of the spine allows less room for the lungs to expand. Taking in less oxygen when breathing can contribute to fatigue.

Medications that slow the rate of bone loss or help to build bone, calcium and vitamin D supplements, and resistance training (lifting weights) can all help to slow the progression of osteoporosis by helping to promote bone strength. However, as with most things, prevention is the best medicine! Osteoporosis can be prevented in many cases by exercising regularly and eating a diet rich in calcium, protein, and vitamin D, starting early in life.

When caring for a resident with osteoporosis, it is important to promote bone health and protect against injury. Carefully observe and document the types of foods and liquids the resident eats and drinks, and encourage snacks that are high in calcium, such as milk, yogurt, ice cream, and cheese. Encourage exercise by having the resident take frequent walks with you. Because a fall can have serious consequences for a person with osteoporosis, preventing falls is very important (see Chapter 18, Guidelines Box 18-2). When assisting the resident with transfers, be gentle.

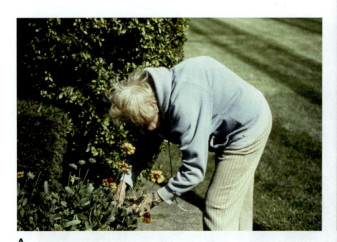

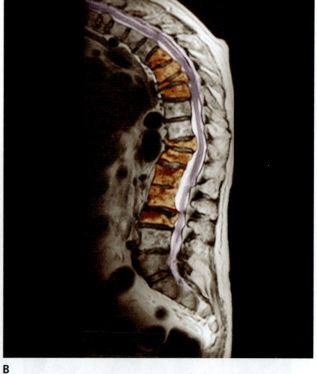

A   B

Figure 32-13
(A) Many people with osteoporosis develop kyphosis (a "dowager's hump") as a result of compression fractures of the spine. **(B)** A magnetic resonance imaging (MRI) scan of the spine of a person with osteoporosis. This is a side view (the person is standing, facing the left). The vertebrae (*brown*) enclose the spinal cord (*pink*). Some of the vertebrae have collapsed (*orange*) as a result of fractures, causing the spine to curve forward into kyphosis or a "dowager's hump." (*A, © Larry Mulvehill/Photo Researchers, Inc.; B, © Zephyr/Photo Researchers, Inc.*)

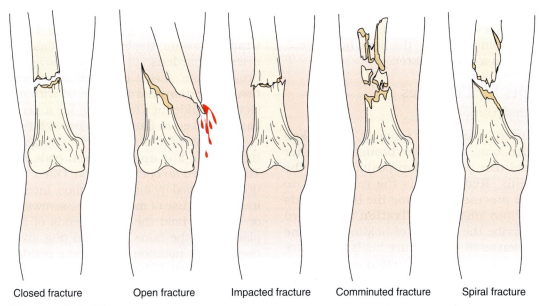

| Closed fracture | Open fracture | Impacted fracture | Comminuted fracture | Spiral fracture |

Figure 32-14
There are many different types of fractures.

Report any loss of function, swelling, or complaints of pain to the nurse immediately. These signs and symptoms may indicate a new fracture in a fragile bone.

FRACTURES

A **fracture** is a broken bone. Many fractures occur as a result of trauma, such as a fall. Some fractures, called stress fractures, occur when a bone is put under constant and repeated stress. Other fractures, called **pathologic fractures,** occur in bones that have been weakened by a disease process, such as osteoporosis or bone cancer.

Older people are especially at risk for fractures, because the bones become more fragile with age. Older people are also more likely to have diseases that put them at risk for pathologic fractures. Weak, brittle bones can fracture easily, often from a seemingly minor fall or stumble. For example, hip fractures are quite common in older women who have fallen just a short distance, such as from a standing position to the floor or sidewalk.

Not only do the bones of an older person fracture more easily, they also take longer to heal and they may heal improperly. Delayed or improper healing may cause prolonged difficulty with mobility, putting the person at risk for developing complications such as pressure ulcers, pneumonia, or blood clots. Other complications can develop as well, such as chronic pain, loss of

independence, loss of self-confidence, and fears related to falling and experiencing another fracture. These complications can have a serious impact on the person's overall quality of life. Your attention to safety and fall prevention for all residents is crucial in helping to avoid fractures and all of the problems associated with them.

Types of Fractures

Fractures can occur in almost any bone in the body and are classified in the following manner (Fig. 32-14):

- **Closed fracture.** The bone is broken, but the broken ends do not protrude through the overlying skin.
- **Open (compound) fracture.** The bone is broken, and the sharp ends of the broken bone have broken through the skin. Because the skin is broken, open fractures carry a very high risk of infection.
- **Impacted fracture.** The bone is broken all of the way through, and the broken ends of the bone are jammed into each other. These fractures are often seen in people who have jumped or fallen from a height, for example, off of a roof or ladder.
- **Comminuted fracture.** The bone is splintered into several little pieces. This type of fracture is common when a bone has been crushed under a great weight. The surrounding tissues, such as muscle and skin, may be seriously injured as well.

- **Spiral fracture.** The break circles around the bone in a winding fashion. Spiral fractures are common when the bone has been subjected to a twisting force.

Treatments for Fractures

Reduction and fixation

For a fractured bone to heal properly, the broken ends of the bone must be brought together (aligned) and then held in that position until the fracture heals. **Reduction** is the word used to describe the process of bringing the broken ends of the bone into alignment. **Fixation** is the word used to describe the process of holding the bone in one position until the fracture heals. There are many ways to accomplish reduction and fixation. The method used depends on the type and location of the fracture.

In a *closed reduction*, the doctor lines up the broken ends of the bone by simply pushing them back into place. In a closed reduction, it is not necessary to create a surgical incision to access the broken bone. Following a closed reduction, a cast (made of fiberglass or plaster of Paris) is applied to keep the bone in the proper alignment until healing occurs (Fig. 32-15A). First, a thin layer of cotton is placed on the skin to protect it. Then, the casting material is soaked in water and wrapped around the limb. As the casting material dries, it hardens, preventing movement of the broken bone. A cast is a method of *external fixation,* or fixation that is achieved without surgery. General guidelines for caring for a person with a cast are given in Guidelines Box 32-1.

Sometimes it is necessary to surgically expose the bone to line up the broken ends of the bone. This is called an *open reduction*. Often, open reduction is followed by *internal fixation*. Internal fixation involves the use of metal plates, screws, rods, pins, or wires to hold the broken ends of the bone in place until the bone is healed (Fig. 32-15B). You may see the notation "ORIF" on a resident's chart. This means that the resident has had surgery to achieve an "**O**pen **R**eduction, **I**nternal **F**ixation."

Traction

Some fractured bones cannot be repaired surgically for a period of time. In these cases, traction is used to keep the broken ends of the bone in alignment until the fracture can be permanently repaired by surgery or casting. In **traction,** the ends of the bones are placed in the

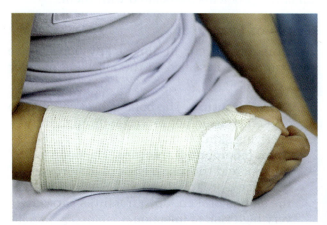

A. External fixation

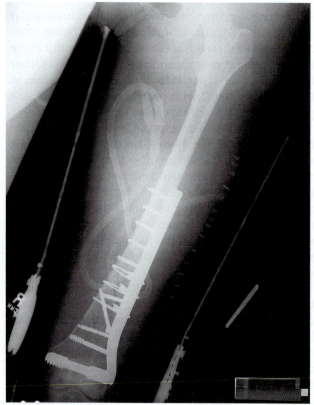

B. Internal fixation

Figure 32-15
With any fracture, the broken ends of the bone need to be brought back together (reduction) and held in place (fixation). **(A)** Fixation can be accomplished externally, with a cast, or **(B)** it can be accomplished internally, with devices such as plates, screws, pins, or wires. (**A,** © Lea Paterson/ Photo Researchers, Inc.)

Guidelines Box 32-1 — Guidelines for Caring for a Person With a Cast

WHAT YOU DO	WHY YOU DO IT
Do not cover the cast or place it on a plastic-covered pillow until it has dried completely.	The casting material produces heat as it dries. Covering the cast can cause the person's skin underneath the cast to burn.
Do not touch the cast with your fingertips until it is totally dry. If you must handle the cast, use the palms of your hands.	Touching the cast can cause it to dent, creating pressure spots against the person's skin.
Keep the casted body part elevated on a pillow for several days.	Elevating the casted body part helps prevent and reduce swelling around the fracture site.
Because the skin underneath the cast can start to itch, the person may try to slide an object between the cast and the skin to scratch the itchy area. Advise the person that placing objects inside of the cast should be avoided.	Sliding an object between the cast and the skin may injure the skin, which puts the person at risk for infection.
Make sure the person's toes (or fingers, if the cast is on the arm) are pink, warm, and moving. Report any complaints of increased pain, numbness, or tingling. Report any observations of cyanosis, increased swelling, cold toes or fingers, increased drainage on the cast, or a foul odor immediately.	Cyanosis; increased swelling; increased pain, numbness, or tingling; or cold fingers or toes may indicate that swelling inside the cast is interfering with blood flow. If the tissues do not receive enough oxygen and nutrients, tissue death and skin breakdown may occur. Increased drainage or a foul odor may indicate infection.
Keep the cast clean and dry.	Plaster cast material becomes soft again when it becomes wet.
Do not allow the person to place pressure or weight on the cast unless he has been specifically instructed to do so.	Placing too much pressure or weight on the cast can cause the cast to break.
Regularly inspect the condition of the cast and the skin around the edges of the cast.	A crack in the cast can cause the cast to become loose or break, which could delay healing of the broken bone. Rough edges on the cast can irritate or break the skin, putting the person at risk for infection and other problems.

proper alignment and then weight is applied to exert a constant pull and keep the bone in alignment. In skin traction, weight is suspended from a traction unit that is attached to the person's skin (Fig. 32-16A). In skeletal traction, weight is suspended from pins that are driven through the bone (Fig. 32-16B).

A resident in traction has several special care needs, many of which arise from the resident's limited ability to move or change position:

- You may be asked to assist the resident with range-of-motion exercises to work the unaffected joints and keep them limber.

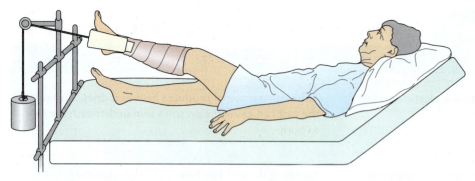

A. Skin traction

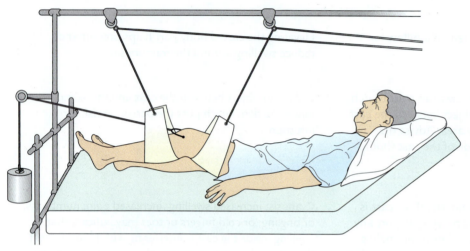

B. Skeletal traction

Figure 32-16
Traction is used to hold the broken ends of a bone in alignment until the fracture can be repaired permanently. **(A)** In skin traction, a device is attached to the person's skin, and weight is suspended from it. **(B)** In skeletal traction, pins are driven through the bone to support the weight.

- The resident will have to use a fracture bedpan (see Chapter 26, Fig. 26-2B), which is easier to slide under the buttocks.
- Pressure ulcers are always a concern, so it is important to keep the resident's skin clean and dry, and to monitor for signs of skin breakdown.
- Two staff members usually work together to change the bed linens, and the linens are changed from the top of the bed (working down), instead of from side to side. If you need to do this, the nurse will show you how.

When you are caring for a resident who is in traction, be very careful not to disturb or remove the weights attached to the traction unit. When you lower the bed height, check to make sure the weights are not resting on the floor. They must hang freely to apply the correct amount of tension to the affected limb.

Hip Fractures

As a nursing assistant working in long-term care, it is very likely that you will care for residents who are recovering from hip fractures. A **hip fracture** is a fracture that occurs at the top of the femur (thigh bone) (Fig. 32-17). The two factors that put a person at high risk for a hip fracture are a tendency to fall and fragile bones (as a result of the normal aging process or a disease process, such as osteoporosis). For these reasons, hip fractures are common in elderly people, especially elderly women.

A significant number of older people die within a year of experiencing a hip fracture. In addition, a person who has experienced one hip fracture is at increased risk for falling and experiencing another fracture in the future. Most of the time, a fractured hip requires surgery. However, surgery may not be an option for an older person who is frail, or has numerous medical problems. In this situation, traction may be used, but being in traction for an extended period of time puts the person at risk for serious complications from immobility, such as pressure ulcers and pneumonia. Even when surgical repair is possible, the person is still at risk for serious complications resulting from the immobility that occurs during

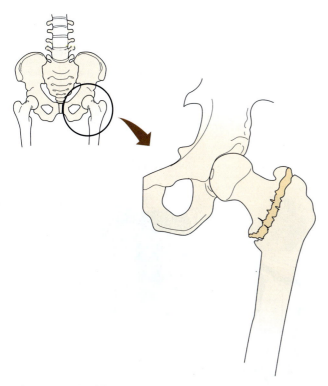

Figure 32-17
A hip fracture is a fracture that occurs at the top of the femur (thigh bone). Older people are at high risk for hip fractures, which can have devastating consequences.

and after treatment. Infection (either of the surgical wound, or a pressure ulcer, if one develops) is also a concern.

Most hip fractures are surgically reduced and stabilized with the use of plates, screws, or pins. Some people may also require joint replacement with an artificial (prosthetic) joint. During the recovery period, the person will need extensive rehabilitation to help regain strength and mobility. A resident who is recovering from a hip fracture will have very specific orders regarding mobility status. It is important for you to know what these orders are, and to follow them closely. The resident will most likely have limitations for positioning, mobility, and weight bearing. As the resident gains strength and mobility through rehabilitation, weight bearing and mobility will gradually be increased.

Recovering from a hip fracture can take 3 months, or longer. During this time, the resident may become very anxious and depressed. The resident may worry about falling again and experiencing another fracture. She may worry about her ability to continue to live on her own, or whether a change in living arrangements will be necessary in the future. She may be having a hard time adjusting to the loss of abilities, or the

need to use a walker or cane when she never needed to use one in the past. Your steady support and emotional encouragement will help the resident maintain a positive attitude, which is important for her recovery.

OSTEOMYELITIS

Osteomyelitis (infection of the bone tissue) is a serious and painful condition. Osteomyelitis is most often caused by bacteria. Bacteria from another site of infection in the body can reach the bone by traveling through the bloodstream. Trauma or surgery that exposes the bone also places a person at risk for osteomyelitis. A person with osteomyelitis experiences bone pain, fever, and swelling, redness, and warmth in the affected area.

When the bone tissue becomes infected, the bone marrow swells and presses against the hard outer layer of the bone. The swelling compresses the blood vessels that run through the bone marrow, preventing oxygen and nutrients from reaching the bone tissue. As a result, areas of the bone tissue die.

Osteomyelitis can be acute or chronic. Whether acute or chronic, osteomyelitis requires long-term antibiotic therapy. Because compression of the blood vessels makes it difficult for the antibiotics to reach the infected bone tissue, osteomyelitis can be difficult to treat, especially chronic osteomyelitis. Surgical removal of the affected area of the bone and surrounding tissue may be necessary. In severe cases, amputation may be necessary.

AMPUTATIONS

The removal of all or part of an arm or a leg is called an **amputation.** For example, a person may lose just a toe, or the leg from the knee down, or the entire leg. Trauma is a common cause of amputation. A body part may be severed from the body, or the body part may be so seriously damaged that the only treatment option is to surgically remove it. Disease may also make amputation necessary. For example, some types of cancer are treated by amputation of the affected limb.

Diseases that interfere with blood flow, such as diabetes, can also result in the need for amputation. As you learned in Chapter 24, people with diabetes tend to have circulatory problems, and often, blood flow to the feet is poor. The poor blood flow to the feet is usually associated with poor sensation as well as an increased risk for

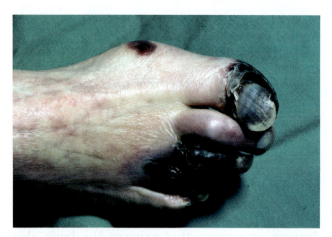

Figure 32-18
Impaired blood flow causes death of the tissues (gangrene). Once gangrene develops, the only treatment option may be amputation of the affected part. (© M. English/Custom Medical Stock Photo.)

infection. If a person with diabetes gets a foot infection, it may go unnoticed for a long time, and when it finally is noticed, it may be very difficult to treat. Eventually, death of the tissue (gangrene) occurs because the tissue is deprived of oxygen and nutrients (Fig. 32-18). Once gangrene develops, the only treatment option may be to remove the damaged part through amputation.

The loss of a body part, especially an arm or leg, can be very emotionally traumatic. It may take the person a long time to adapt to the changes in appearance, mobility, and functional ability caused by the amputation. These changes may significantly affect the person's daily routines and activities. Imagine what it would feel like to have to find new ways to do things that in the past you could do easily. For some people who have had a body part either partially or completely amputated, a prosthetic (false) part may allow the person to regain mobility, function, and a more normal appearance (Fig. 32-19).

The **stump,** or the end of the amputated limb that is left after surgery, must be cared for properly. Positioning is used to keep the muscles and tendons from shortening, and nearby joints are put through range-of-motion exercises to help maintain normal joint function and mobility. Wrapping the end of the stump with elastic bandages helps to shrink and shape the stump properly (Fig. 32-20). When assisting with caring for a person's stump, make sure to follow the nurse's or physical therapist's instructions exactly, as always. As you assist your resident with general care, you will have many opportunities to observe the stump for any drainage, bleeding, or pain. These findings could be signs of poor tissue heal-

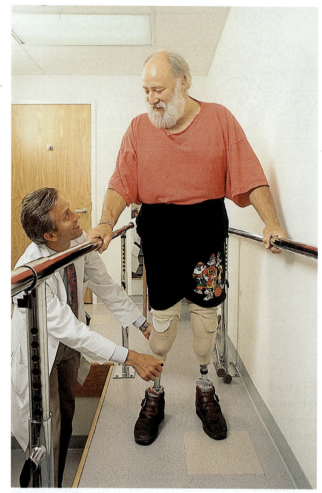

Figure 32-19
A prosthetic body part can help a person who has had an amputation regain function and mobility.

ing or infection, and must be reported to the nurse immediately.

Many people who have had an amputation experience what is known as **phantom pain,** or the feeling that the amputated body part is still

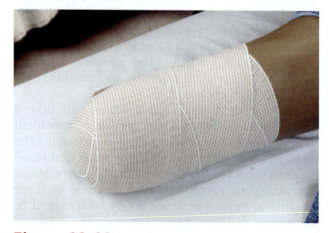

Figure 32-20
Wrapping the stump in bandages helps to shape it properly.

present. Aching, itching, and other sensations are all types of phantom pain. The sensations are caused by the healing of the nerves that were cut when the body part was removed. Phantom pain usually goes away a short while after surgery, but some people report having these episodes for years afterward. A resident who is confused (for example, as a result of the lingering effects of anesthesia following the surgery, or because of dementia) may forget that the amputated limb is no longer there. If the resident is experiencing phantom pain and does not remember that his leg has been amputated, he might get out of bed, attempt to walk to the bathroom, and fall. Be sure to take the necessary safety precautions to prevent incidents like this from occurring.

TELL THE NURSE

There are many signs and symptoms that may accompany disorders of the musculoskeletal system. As a nursing assistant, you have the opportunity to become very familiar with each of your residents' physical abilities and limitations. Report any of the following observations to the nurse immediately:

- The resident has fallen
- An area has become swollen, red, bruised, tender, or painful to the touch
- The resident complains of pain when moving a joint
- The resident's usual range of motion of a joint has decreased
- The resident limps or has pain while walking, or makes excuses to avoid walking
- The resident guards or rubs a joint, even when not moving
- The resident has decreased muscle strength

RANGE-OF-MOTION EXERCISES

Range-of-motion exercises—movements that put each joint through its complete range of motion—are done to prevent complications of immobility and maintain or restore musculoskeletal function. As you learned earlier, the range of motion of a joint is the complete extent of movement that the joint is normally capable of without causing pain. Normal activities—such as dressing, grooming, walking, and eating—usually put all of our joints through their complete range of motion several

times throughout the day. However, some of the people you will be caring for will have conditions that prevent them from doing the activities that would normally exercise their joints and muscles.

Immobility can have a serious impact on the musculoskeletal system. Muscle atrophy, loss of bone strength, and stiffness of the joints can quickly lead to permanent muscle weakness, brittle bones, and even contractures. As a nursing assistant, you will play a key role in preventing these complications by helping your residents with range-of-motion exercises as ordered.

Range-of-motion exercises are usually performed at least twice a day, often along with other personal care activities, such as bathing or dressing. The exercises can be done while the resident is in bed or sitting down. Depending on the situation, range-of-motion exercises may be performed for only one, some, or all of the joints. Sometimes, the resident will be able to perform the exercises on his own, and your role will be to provide guidance and encouragement. Other times, you will need to help the resident to perform the exercises.

- In **active range-of-motion exercises,** the resident performs the exercises independently, with verbal guidance from you.
- In **passive range-of-motion exercises,** you move the resident's joints through the exercises, without active involvement on the part of the resident. For example, you might perform passive range-of-motion exercises for a resident who is in a coma.
- In **active-assistive range-of-motion exercises,** the resident performs the exercises with some hands-on assistance from you. For example, the resident may be able to lift his arm out to the side, but will need your help to complete the movement of bringing the arm up near the head.

Procedure 32-1 explains how to assist a resident with passive range-of-motion exercises. Range-of-motion exercises can cause injury to the joints if they are not performed properly. Usually a physical therapist or nurse will evaluate the resident and determine which joints should be exercised. When assisting a resident with range-of-motion exercises, always follow the care plan (or the nurse's or physical therapist's instructions) exactly. This is important for two reasons:

1. There may be some exercises that the resident is not allowed to do.
2. The physical therapist or nurse will most likely change the care plan as the resident's condition either improves or worsens.

Guidelines Box 32-2 Guidelines for Assisting With Range-of-Motion Exercises

WHAT YOU DO	WHY YOU DO IT
Use good body mechanics.	Using good body mechanics saves energy and prevents muscle strain and injury.
Remove pillows and other positioning devices.	Pillows and positioning devices can prevent a person from achieving full range of motion of the joint.
Position the person so that each joint can be moved through all of the usual positions.	Positioning the person in a position that will allow each joint to be moved through all of its usual positions saves time (because the person will not have to be repositioned in between exercises) and helps to ensure that all of the exercises will be completed.
Move through the exercises in a systematic way (for example, from the head down).	Developing a routine helps to ensure that no exercise will be forgotten.
Unless instructed otherwise, perform the same exercise on each corresponding body part (for example, do the same thing for the right arm that you do for the left).	Exercising corresponding joints equally ensures that both sides of the body remain equally strong and flexible.
Support each joint as you exercise it.	Support reduces discomfort and strain on the joint.
Do not push a joint past its point of resistance.	Each joint has a limit to its range of motion. Attempting to exceed this limit can lead to joint pain and injury.
Watch the person's face for signs of pain or discomfort.	A person may not be able to tell you if what you are doing hurts. Therefore, it is important to watch the person's face for nonverbal cues, such as grimacing or wincing.
Avoid exercising a painful joint.	Exercising a painful joint can cause additional injury.
If you notice sudden, continuous contractions of the related muscles (spasticity), take a break or move the limb more slowly to allow the muscles to recover. Applying gentle pressure to the muscle can also relieve spasticity.	Spasticity is a sign that the muscles are working too hard. It may also indicate that the person is in pain, or that the joint's range of motion has been exceeded.
Expect the person's respiratory rate and heart rate to increase during the exercise. If these vital signs do not return to their normal resting rates after the activity ends, report this to the nurse immediately.	During activity, the tissues require more oxygen and nutrients, so the heart and lungs work harder to supply the tissues. However, once the activity ends, the heart rate and respiratory rate should return to normal because the tissues' demand for oxygen and nutrients will be less.
Encourage the person to help with the exercises as much as possible.	Active participation increases the person's sense of independence and improves function.

In addition to checking the care plan, you should make sure that helping the resident with the ordered exercises is within your scope of practice. For example, in some facilities, nursing assistants are not allowed to assist residents with range-of-motion exercises involving the neck. General guidelines for assisting a resident with range-of-motion exercises are given in Guidelines Box 32-2.

SUMMARY

- The musculoskeletal system consists of the bones, skeletal muscles, and joints.
  - The primary function of the musculoskeletal system is movement.
    - Joints are the areas where two bones meet. Most movement occurs at freely movable joints.
    - The skeletal muscles attach to the bones. When the muscle contracts (shortens), it pulls against the bone, causing the body part to move.
  - Other functions of the musculoskeletal system include protection, support, heat production, calcium storage, and blood cell production.
- As we age, we lose bone tissue and muscle mass, and our joints begin to show the effects of a lifetime of wear and tear. Consuming a diet rich in calcium, vitamin D, and protein and exercising regularly throughout life can help to delay or decrease the effects of aging on the musculoskeletal system.
- Disorders of the musculoskeletal system can make mobility very difficult.
  - Muscular dystrophy is a general term for a group of disorders that cause the skeletal muscles to become very weak over time. Muscular dystrophy is a genetic disorder, which means that it is inherited.
  - Arthritis is inflammation of the joints.
    - Osteoarthritis typically affects older people. In osteoarthritis, the cartilage that covers the ends of bones is worn away through normal use of the joint. Many people with osteoarthritis have joint replacement surgery to correct the condition.
    - Rheumatoid arthritis is a type of arthritis that develops at a younger age and can cause severe joint deformities. Rheumatoid arthritis is thought to be an autoimmune disorder, which means it is caused by a person's immune system attacking his or her own tissues.
    - Gout is a type of arthritis that results from the build-up of uric acid in the joints.
  - Osteoporosis is the excessive loss of bone tissue, resulting in bones that break very easily.
  - Fractures are broken bones.
    - Older people are especially at risk for fractures because of the normal loss of bone tissue that is a part of aging, and they are more likely to have diseases that put them at risk for fractures. Fractures may take longer to heal in an older person, and can significantly impact the person's quality of life.
    - Fractures may be treated by casting or by surgical placement of plates, screws, pins, or wires. Traction may be necessary to hold the ends of the broken bone in alignment until the fracture can be permanently repaired.
  - Osteomyelitis is infection of the bone tissue.
  - Amputation is the removal of a limb or part of a limb.
    - Amputation may be necessary because of trauma or complications related to a medical condition, such as osteomyelitis or diabetes.
    - Proper care of the stump promotes healing and increases the likelihood that a person can be fitted with a prosthetic limb.
- Range-of-motion exercises are used to preserve joint and muscle function in people who have conditions that limit their use of the musculoskeletal system. Range-of-motion exercises are usually performed at least twice a day.
  - Active range-of-motion exercises are performed by the resident.
  - Passive range-of-motion exercises are performed by the nursing assistant or nurse on behalf of the resident.
  - Active-assistive range-of-motion exercises are performed by the resident with some help from the nursing assistant or nurse.

Assisting a Person With Passive Range-of-Motion Exercises

WHY YOU DO IT   Range-of-motion exercises help to keep the joints and muscles healthy in people who have a limited ability to move.

Getting Ready WGKIEPS

1. Complete the "Getting Ready" steps.

Supplies
- bath blanket

Procedure

2. Make sure that the bed is positioned at a comfortable working height (to promote good body mechanics) and that the wheels are locked. If the side rails are in use, lower the side rail on the working side of the bed. The side rail on the opposite side of the bed should remain up. Raise or lower the head of the bed to a horizontal or semi-Fowler's position.

3. Assist the person into the supine position.

4. Spread the bath blanket over the top linens (and the person). If the person is able, have him hold the bath blanket. If not, tuck the corners under his shoulders. Fanfold the top linens to the foot of the bed.

5. Perform each range-of-motion exercise in steps 6 through 13 according to the person's care plan, being careful to expose only the part of the body that is being exercised. Repeat each exercise three to five times, as written in the care plan.

6. If your facility permits, exercise the person's neck:

a. Forward and backward flexion and extension (neck). Support the person's head by putting one hand under his chin and the other on the back of the head. Gently bring the head forward, as if to touch the chin to the chest, and then bring it backward, chin pointing to the sky.

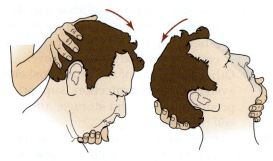

Step 6a Gently bring the head forward, then backward.

b. Side-to-side flexion (neck). Support the person's head by putting one hand under his chin and the other near the opposite temple. Gently tilt the head toward the right shoulder and then toward the left.

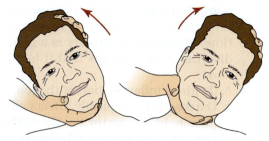

Step 6b Gently tilt the head toward the right shoulder, then the left.

c. Rotation (neck). Support the person's head by putting one hand under his chin and the other on the back of the head.

Gently move the head from side to side, as if the person were shaking his head "no."

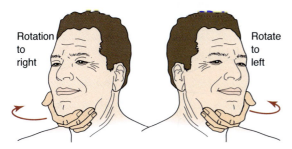

Step 6c Gently move the head from side to side.

7. Exercise the person's shoulder:

a. **Forward flexion and extension (shoulder).** Support the person's arm by putting one hand under his elbow and the other under his wrist. Keeping the person's arm straight with the palm facing down, lift the arm up so that it is alongside his ear and then return it to its original position.

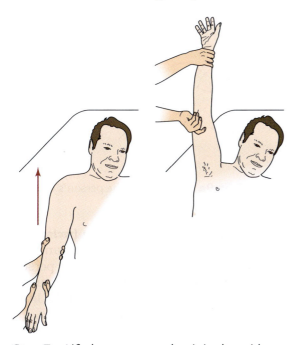

Step 7a Lift the arm up so that it is alongside the person's ear, then return it to its original position.

b. **Abduction and adduction (shoulder).** Support the person's arm by putting one hand under his elbow and the other under his wrist. Keeping the person's arm straight with the palm facing up,

move his arm away from the side of his body and then return it to its original position.

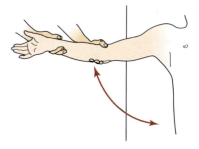

Step 7b Move the arm away from the person's side, then return it to its original position.

c. **Horizontal abduction and adduction (shoulder).** Support the person's arm by putting one hand under his elbow and the other under his wrist. Keeping the person's arm straight with the palm facing up, move his arm away from the side of his body. Gently bending the person's elbow, touch his hand to the opposite shoulder, then straighten the elbow and bring the arm back out to the side.

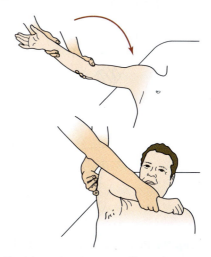

Step 7c Move the arm away from the person's side, then touch the person's hand to the opposite shoulder.

d. **Rotation (shoulder).** Support the person's arm by putting one hand under his elbow and the other under his wrist. Move the person's arm away from the side of his body and bend his arm at the elbow. Gently move the person's forearm up so that it

(continued)

forms a right angle with the mattress and then back down. This movement is similar to the motion a police officer makes when he or she is signaling someone to stop.

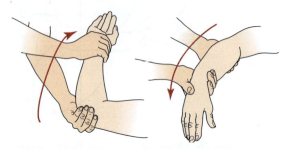

Step 7d Move the person's forearm up, then back down.

8. Exercise the person's elbow.
   a. **Flexion and extension (elbow).** Support the person's arm by putting one hand under his elbow and the other under his wrist. Starting with the person's arm straight and with the palm facing up, bend his elbow so that his hand moves toward his shoulder. Then, straighten out the elbow, returning the person's hand to its original position.

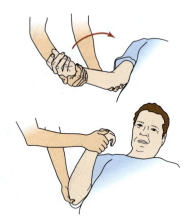

Step 8a Bend the arm so that the hand moves toward the shoulder, then return it to its original position.

   b. **Pronation and supination (elbow).** Support the person's arm by putting one hand under his elbow and the other under his wrist. Move the person's arm away from the side of his body and slightly bend his arm at the elbow. Gently move the person's forearm up so that it forms a right angle with the mattress. Gently turn the person's hand so that the palm is facing

the end of the bed. Then turn the hand the other way so that the palm is facing the head of the bed.

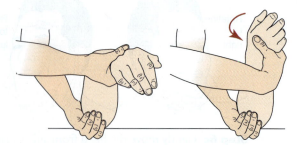

Step 8b Turn the hand so that the palm is facing the end of the bed, then turn the hand the other way so that the palm is facing the head of the bed.

9. Exercise the person's wrist.
   a. **Flexion and extension (wrist).** Support the person's wrist with one hand. Use the other hand to gently bend the person's hand down and then back.

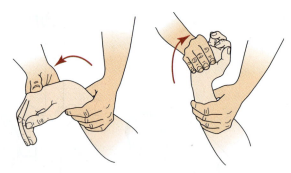

Step 9a Gently bend the person's hand down, then back.

   b. **Radial and ulnar flexion (wrist).** Support the person's wrist with one hand. Use the other hand to gently turn the person's hand toward his thumb. Then turn the hand the other way, toward the little finger.

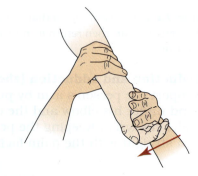

Step 9b Gently turn the person's hand one way, then the other.

10. Exercise the person's fingers and thumb.
   a. **Flexion and extension (fingers and thumb).** Support the person's wrist with one hand. Using your other hand, flex the person's fingers to make a fist, tucking his thumb under the fingers. Then straighten each finger and the thumb, one by one.

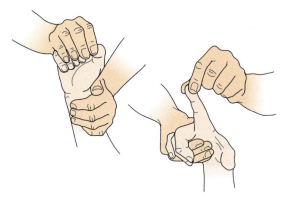

Step 10a Flex the person's fingers to make a fist, then straighten each finger and thumb, one by one.

   b. **Abduction and adduction (fingers and thumb).** With one hand, hold the person's thumb and index finger together. With the other hand, move the middle finger away from the index finger. Then move the middle finger back toward the index finger and hold the middle finger, index finger, and thumb together. Next, move the ring finger away from the other two fingers and thumb, then move it back toward the group. Do the same with the little finger. Finally, reverse the process. Hold the little finger and the ring finger together, and move the middle finger away and back. Complete with the index finger and thumb.

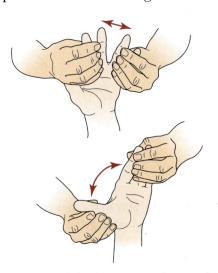

Step 10b Spread the fingers away from each other, then back together again.

   c. **Flexion and extension (thumb).** Bend the person's thumb into his palm, then return it to its original position.

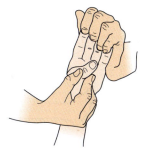

Step 10c Bend the thumb into the palm, then return it to its original position.

   d. **Opposition.** Touch each fingertip to the thumb.

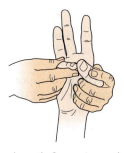

Step 10d Touch each fingertip to the thumb.

11. Exercise the person's hip and knee.
   a. **Forward flexion and extension (hip and knee).** Support the person's leg by putting one hand under his knee and the other under his ankle. Gently bend the person's knee, moving it toward his head. Then straighten the person's knee and gently lower the leg to the bed.

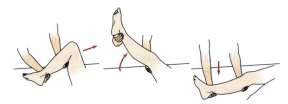

Step 11a Gently bend the knee, moving it toward the head. Then straighten the leg and lower it to the bed.

   b. **Abduction and adduction (hip).** Support the person's leg by putting one hand under his knee and the other under his ankle. Keeping the person's leg straight, move his

(continued)

leg away from the side of his body and then return it to its original position.

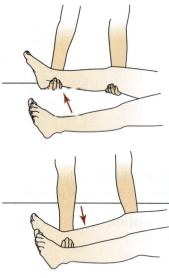

Step 11b Move the leg away from the person's side, then return it to its original position.

c. **Rotation (hip).** Support the person's leg by putting one hand under his knee and the other under his ankle. Keeping the person's leg straight, gently turn the leg inward and then outward.

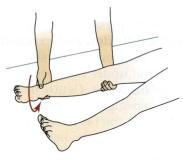

Step 11c Gently turn the leg inward, then outward.

12. Exercise the person's ankle and foot.
    a. **Dorsiflexion and plantar flexion (ankle and foot).** Support the person's ankle with one hand. Use the other hand to gently bend the person's foot up toward the head and then back.

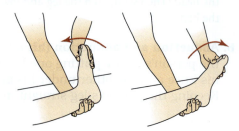

Step 12a Gently bend the foot toward the head, then back.

b. **Inversion and eversion (ankle and foot).** Support the person's ankle with one hand. Use the other hand to gently turn the inside of the foot inward and then outward.

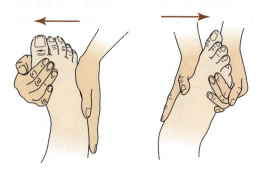

Step 12b Gently bend the foot inward, then outward.

13. Exercise the person's toes.
    a. **Flexion and extension (toes).** Put one hand under the person's foot. Put the other hand over the person's toes. Curl the toes downward and then straighten them.

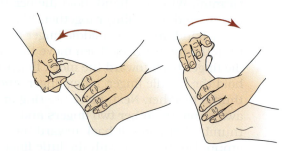

Step 13a Curl the toes downward, then straighten them.

b. **Abduction and adduction (toes).** Spread each toe the same way you spread each finger in step 10b.

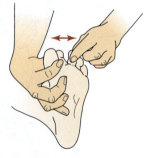

Step 13b Spread the toes away from each other, then back together again.

14. Straighten the bed linens and make sure the person is comfortable and in good body alignment. Draw the top linens over the person and remove the bath blanket.

15. If the side rails are in use, raise the side rail on the working side of the bed. Make sure that the bed is lowered to its lowest position and that the wheels are locked.

Finishing Up CLSOWR

16. Complete the "Finishing Up" steps.

WHAT DID YOU LEARN?

Multiple Choice

Select the single best answer for each of the following questions.

1. When a muscle atrophies, it:
   a. Becomes larger and stronger
   b. Becomes thinner and weaker
   c. Becomes stiffer
   d. Becomes more flexible

2. Which musculoskeletal disorder causes severe joint deformities and often affects people in their younger years?
   a. Osteoarthritis
   b. Rheumatoid arthritis
   c. Multiple sclerosis
   d. Muscular dystrophy

3. What is the term for a fracture where the broken ends of the bone do not penetrate the skin?
   a. Impacted fracture
   b. Comminuted fracture
   c. Spiral fracture
   d. Closed fracture

4. Excessive loss of bone tissue is:
   a. Osteoarthritis
   b. Osteoporosis
   c. Osteomyelitis
   d. Gout

5. What does the skeletal system do?
   a. It acts as a storage site for calcium
   b. It works with the muscles to produce movement
   c. It produces blood cells
   d. All of the above

6. Mrs. Vaughn broke her hip when she fell in the bathroom. Surgery is required to align the broken bone, and then the bone fragments are held together with metal plates and screws. What is the name of the procedure Mrs. Vaughn has had?
   a. Open fracture, internal fixation
   b. Open reduction, internal fixation
   c. Open reduction, external fixation
   d. Traction

7. What does the muscular system do?
   a. It produces heat
   b. It helps to maintain posture
   c. It works with bones to produce movement
   d. All of the above

8. Mr. Owen has severe osteoarthritis in his hips. You are caring for Mr. Owen following his hip replacement surgery. What do you need to remember?

   a. Mr. Owen's legs must always be kept together (adducted).
   b. When assisting Mr. Owen with range-of-motion exercises, make sure to flex the hips beyond 90 degrees to maintain flexibility in the joint.
   c. Mr. Owen should use an abduction pillow to keep his legs spread apart when he is in a supine or lateral position.
   d. Mr. Owen should be encouraged to get up and walk around within a day or two of the surgery.

9. Mrs. Curtis has just had a cast put on her right arm to treat a fracture resulting from a fall in the day room. What should you remember when you are helping Mrs. Curtis?
   a. Mrs. Curtis's arm should not be elevated.
   b. You should check Mrs. Curtis's fingers frequently to make sure that the cast is not too tight.
   c. Mrs. Curtis should be reminded that if the skin underneath the cast begins to itch, she can slide a tongue depressor inside the cast to scratch the itchy area.
   d. Mrs. Curtis should be encouraged to get out of bed and take a shower as soon as the cast dries.

10. Mr. Jefferson has poorly controlled diabetes. He injured his toe, resulting in a severe infection. Now, his toe is completely black as a result of gangrene. What is the most likely treatment for Mr. Jefferson's toe?
    a. Outside reduction, internal fixation (ORIF)
    b. Amputation of the toe
    c. Casting of the foot
    d. Range-of-motion exercises

11. Phantom pain refers to pain associated with:
    a. Amputation
    b. Bone infection
    c. Severe injury
    d. Swelling beneath a cast

12. The vertebrae are examples of which kind of bone?
    a. Long bones
    b. Flat bones
    c. Irregular bones
    d. Short bones

Matching

Match each numbered item with its appropriate lettered description.

_____ **1.** Flexion/extension

_____ **2.** Supination/pronation

_____ **3.** Dorsiflexion/plantar flexion

_____ **4.** Rotation

_____ **5.** Abduction/adduction

_____ **6.** Inversion/eversion

a.

b.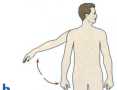

c.

d.

e.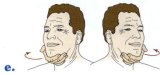

f.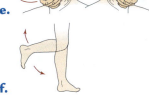

STOP and Think!

- You are assigned to care for Mr. Kuhlman. Mr. Kuhlman is 85 years old and fairly healthy, but he does have arthritis. One of your responsibilities is to assist Mr. Kuhlman to the dining room for meals. Today, while you are walking Mr. Kuhlman to breakfast, you notice that he is limping a bit and trying not to put weight on his left leg. You ask him if he is in pain, and he says, "I'm fine; it's just old age." What should you do?

- You have cared for Mrs. Green for several months. She has been able to walk independently with the aid of a walker. She has a stooped-over posture that you recognize as a "dowager's hump" due to her osteoporosis. A few weeks ago, Mrs. Green fell when she was walking to the dining room and suffered a broken hip. Mrs. Green is now back at your facility, after being discharged from the hospital following surgical repair of her broken hip. How should you change your usual approaches to meet Mrs. Green's current needs?

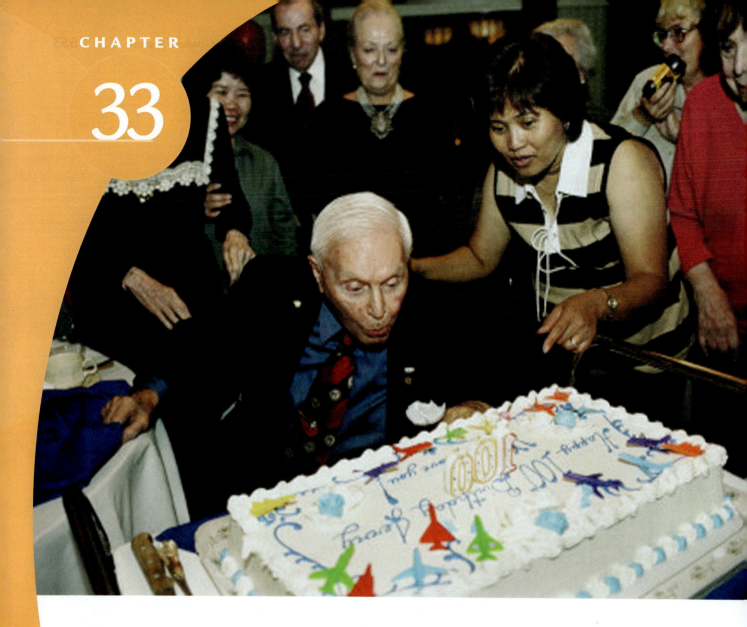

The Respiratory System

WHAT WILL YOU LEARN?

Have you ever heard the phrase, "It's as natural as breathing?" Breathing is certainly something that many of us take for granted, because we don't have to think about it. Air enters and leaves our lungs without any conscious effort on our part. With each breath, life-giving oxygen is delivered to the body, and carbon dioxide, a waste product of cellular metabolism, is removed from the body. Breathing is the function of the respiratory system, the subject of this chapter. When you are finished with this chapter, you will be able to:

1. List and describe the main parts of the respiratory system.

2. Discuss the main functions of the respiratory system.

Photo: A resident of a retirement community celebrates his 100th birthday by blowing out the candles on his cake. Regular physical exercise and avoidance of tobacco smoke and other pollutants help to keep the respiratory system functioning well into old age. (Zed Nelson/Getty Images).

3. Describe how normal aging processes affect the respiratory system.

4. Describe some of the disorders that can affect the respiratory system.

5. Describe how oxygen therapy is used to assist a person with respiration.

6. Describe the guidelines that a nursing assistant should follow when caring for residents receiving oxygen therapy.

7. Discuss other methods used to help a person who is having trouble with respiration.

Vocabulary Use the CD in the front of your book to hear these terms pronounced and defined:

Mucous membrane	Bronchioles	Influenza	Facemask
Mucus	Alveoli (alveolus)	Asthma	Suctioning
Nasal cavity	Gas exchange	Chronic obstructive	Hypoxic
Pharyngitis	Pleura	pulmonary disease	Nasopharyngeal airway
Pharynx	Diaphragm	(COPD)	Oropharyngeal airway
Larynx	Pneumonia	Emphysema	Mechanical ventilation
Laryngitis	Sputum	Chronic bronchitis	Endotracheal tube
Trachea	Hemoptysis	Respiratory therapy	Tracheostomy
Bronchi (bronchus)	Pleurisy	Flow meter	Pneumothorax
Lungs	Bronchitis	Nasal cannula	Hemothorax
Respiration			

STRUCTURE OF THE RESPIRATORY SYSTEM

The respiratory system consists of the lungs and a series of passages, collectively referred to as the *airway* (Fig. 33-1). You may hear people refer to the "upper respiratory tract" and the "lower respiratory tract." The upper respiratory tract consists of the structures located outside of the chest cavity (the nasal cavity, pharynx, and larynx). The lower respiratory tract consists of the structures located inside the chest cavity (the trachea, bronchi, bronchioles, and lungs).

AIRWAY

The purpose of the airway is to move air from the outside of the body to the lungs, and from the lungs to the outside of the body. The airway consists of a series of passages that become smaller in diameter as they approach the lungs. These passages are lined with a **mucous membrane,** a special type of epithelial tissue that lines many of the organ systems in the body. The surface of the membrane is kept moist by **mucus,** a slippery, sticky substance that is secreted by special cells.

Nasal Cavity

Air enters the body through the nostrils and passes into the **nasal cavity,** which is lined by a mucous membrane and coarse hairs. The coarse hairs and the mucous membrane help to trap dirt, dust, microbes, and other foreign particles, preventing these substances from entering the delicate lungs. The plentiful blood vessels in the mucous membrane transfer body heat to the air, warming it up to a comfortable temperature. In addition, the air picks up some of the moisture from the warm, moist nasal cavity. Warm, moist air is less likely than cold, dry air to damage the delicate lung tissue.

Pharynx

When you have a "sore throat," the part of your body that hurts is your pharynx. (You may have heard the term **pharyngitis,** which means inflammation of the pharynx, or a sore throat.) Both the nasal cavities and the oral cavity open into the **pharynx,** or throat region (Fig. 33-1). This means that air passes through the pharynx on its way to the lungs, and food and fluids pass through the pharynx on their way to the stomach. This sharing of space is convenient when you have a stuffy nose, because it means that you have another way to get air into your body (that

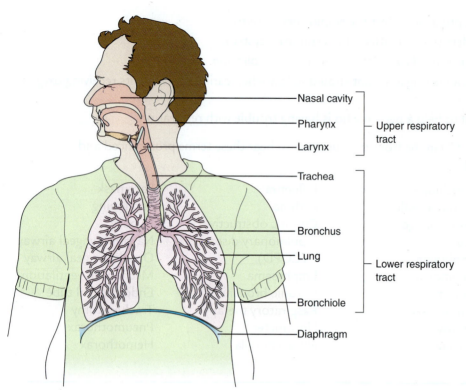

Nasal cavity
Pharynx — Upper respiratory tract
Larynx

Trachea
Bronchus
Lung — Lower respiratory tract
Bronchiole
Diaphragm

Figure 33-1

The respiratory system consists of the lungs and a series of passages collectively referred to as the "airway." The structures that form the airway include the nasal cavity, pharynx, larynx, trachea, bronchi, and bronchioles. The upper respiratory tract consists of those structures located outside the chest cavity, while the lower respiratory tract consists of those structures located inside the chest cavity.

is, through your mouth). However, this sharing of space can also lead to complications, such as choking, which occurs when you try to breathe and swallow at the same time. The pharynx is divided into three sections: the nasopharynx (located right behind the nasal cavities), the oropharynx (located behind the mouth), and the laryngeal pharynx (located above the larynx).

Larynx

From the pharynx, air passes into the **larynx.** The opening of the larynx is covered by a flap of cartilage called the epiglottis, which snaps shut when you swallow, closing off the opening and preventing food from passing into the lower respiratory tract.

In addition to serving as part of the airway, the larynx is the organ responsible for speech. The larynx, often referred to as the "voice box," contains the vocal cords. When air flows over the vocal cords, it causes them to vibrate, producing sound. Humans and other animals make recognizable sounds by controlling the flow of air over the vocal cords. An inflammation of the larynx, or **laryngitis,** usually affects a person's ability to talk.

Trachea and Bronchi

The **trachea,** also called the "windpipe," is the passage that carries air from the larynx down into

the chest toward the lungs. "C"-shaped rings of cartilage give the trachea its characteristic ridged appearance (Fig. 33-1). These cartilage rings support the trachea and keep it open. At its lower end, the trachea divides into two separate passages called the **bronchi** (singular, **bronchus**). One bronchus goes to the right lung and the other goes to the left lung.

The mucous membrane lining of the trachea and bronchi contains millions of tiny hair-like structures called *cilia*. The cilia constantly move in a waving or beating fashion, moving mucus upward toward the pharynx so that it can be coughed up and removed from the respiratory tract along with any trapped particles or microbes.

LUNGS

The **lungs** are the main organs of **respiration,** the process the body uses to obtain oxygen from the environment and remove carbon dioxide (a waste gas) from the body. Once inside the lungs, the bronchi divide into smaller and smaller branches called **bronchioles** (Fig. 33-2). There are more than a million bronchioles in each lung! At the end of each bronchiole, there is a grape-like cluster of tiny air sacs called **alveoli** (singular, **alveolus**). Each alveolus is surrounded by a network of tiny blood vessels (Fig. 33-3). The transfer of oxygen into the

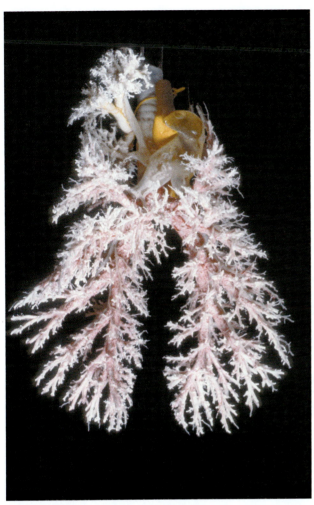

Figure 33-2
A resin cast of human lungs clearly shows the trachea, bronchi, and bronchioles. (© A. Siegel/Custom Medical Stock Photo.)

blood, and carbon dioxide out of it, occurs in the alveoli. This process is called **gas exchange,** and it is described in more detail later in this chapter. The tissue of healthy lungs is elastic (stretchy) and sponge-like, because of all of the air-filled alveoli. The many blood vessels that surround the alveoli give healthy lung tissue its brilliant pink color.

The lungs are divided into sections called lobes. The right lung has three lobes and the left lung has only two. The left lung is slightly smaller than the right lung because of the position of the heart in the chest cavity.

The lungs are located in the chest cavity. The inside of the chest cavity is lined with a membrane called the **pleura,** which also covers the outside of the lungs. Because the lungs almost fill the chest cavity, the pleura on the outside of the lungs almost touches the pleura on the inside of the chest cavity. The pleura secretes a thin fluid that allows the lungs to slide easily against the chest cavity walls during the process of breathing.

FUNCTION OF THE RESPIRATORY SYSTEM

The main purpose of the respiratory system is respiration. Respiration is accomplished through the processes of ventilation and gas exchange.

VENTILATION

Ventilation is the mechanical process of moving air in and out of the lungs (breathing). Ventilation has two phases: inhalation and exhalation. The **diaphragm** is a strong, dome-shaped muscle that separates the chest cavity from the abdominal cavity (Fig. 33-1). When we inhale, the diaphragm contracts, moving downward and making the chest cavity bigger. Air flows into the lungs, filling the alveoli and causing them to expand. When we exhale, the diaphragm relaxes, moving upward and pushing the air in the alveoli out of the lungs. Another group of muscles, called the intercostal muscles, helps with the respiratory effort as well. The intercostal muscles are located between the ribs.

The rate and depth of breathing is controlled mainly by the central nervous system, in the part of the brain called the medulla. Special cells, called chemoreceptors, are located in the medulla and in some of the major arteries. The chemoreceptors monitor the amount of carbon dioxide and oxygen in the blood and adjust the rate and depth of breathing as necessary. For example, if you are resting quietly, your body does not need as much oxygen, and the amount of air inhaled and exhaled is minimal. But, if you are exercising, your body's need for oxygen is greatly increased, and ventilation increases as well. Although the brain ensures that breathing occurs automatically, you also have some voluntary control over breathing (for example, when you hold your breath while swimming).

GAS EXCHANGE

So, we now know how air moves in and out of the lungs. But, just moving air in and out of the lungs is not enough. How does oxygen get from the air into the blood? How does the carbon dioxide in the blood get into the air we exhale? This is where the second phase of respiration, gas exchange, comes into play.

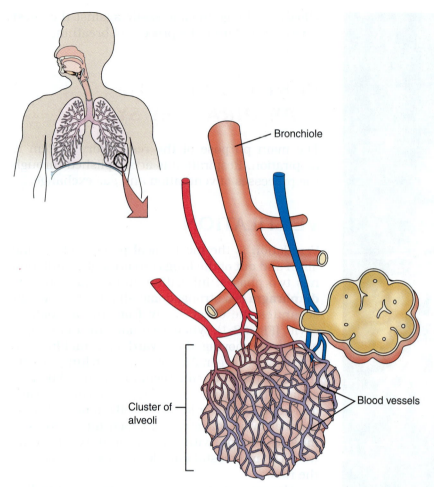

Bronchiole

Cluster of alveoli

Blood vessels

Figure 33-3

A cluster of air sacs, called alveoli, is found at the end of each bronchiole. The alveoli are surrounded by tiny blood vessels, which make gas exchange between the blood and the lungs possible.

Gas exchange occurs in the alveoli (Fig. 33-4). The walls of the alveoli are very thin—just one cell thick. Each alveolus is surrounded by a network of tiny blood vessels. The walls of the blood vessels are very thin too. As the blood passes through the blood vessels, it is brought very close to the air in the alveolus. Because the concentration of oxygen is greater in the air than it is in the blood, the oxygen in the air moves (diffuses) across the wall of the alveolus into the blood vessel, oxygenating the blood. At the same time, carbon dioxide moves from the blood (where it is more concentrated) into the alveolus, and is removed from the body when we exhale.

THE EFFECTS OF AGING ON THE RESPIRATORY SYSTEM

There is a good chance that many of the older people you will care for will have some type of respira-

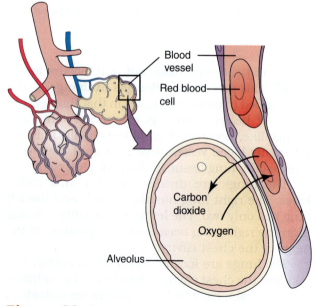

Blood vessel

Red blood cell

Carbon dioxide

Oxygen

Alveolus

Figure 33-4

Gas exchange occurs in the alveoli. Oxygen moves from the alveolus into the blood vessel, and carbon dioxide moves from the blood vessel into the alveolus.

tory problem. When the processes of aging are combined with chronic illness, immobility, or a lifetime of exposure to toxic chemicals (such as those in pollution and tobacco smoke), the respiratory system's ability to function properly is significantly reduced. For example, many people who are in their 60s, 70s, and 80s today began to smoke before anyone really knew about the harmful effects of tobacco smoke. In addition, many older people worked before regulations such as those resulting from the Occupational Safety and Health Act (OSHA) were in place to keep them safe on the job. As a result, many were exposed to substances in the workplace that we now know are very harmful to the lungs, such as asbestos and coal dust.

When we inhale toxic substances (such as those in tobacco smoke and polluted air) day after day, the delicate membranes inside the lungs and airways become inflamed and stay that way. The chronic inflammation leads to scarring and may even cause changes that lead to cancer. In addition, chemicals in tobacco smoke paralyze the tiny cilia that line the trachea and bronchi. The purpose of the cilia is to sweep mucus upward, toward the pharynx, so that it can be eliminated from the respiratory tract. When the cilia are no longer able to perform this function because they have been paralyzed by tobacco smoke, the person must work harder to keep the airway and lungs clear of mucus. These attempts to keep the airway clear are what many of us know as a "smoker's cough." Fortunately, if a person is able to stop smoking, the cilia do regain their function and the tissues of the lungs will heal if the damage is not too severe.

Our respiratory health in our older years is influenced by what we do when we are young. Regular physical exercise and avoidance of tobacco smoke and other pollutants help to keep the respiratory system functioning properly (Fig. 33-5). However, as a person ages, changes occur to the respiratory system, even if the person is otherwise healthy. These changes include less efficient ventilation and a decreased cough reflex.

LESS-EFFICIENT VENTILATION

As you have learned in other chapters, loss of tissue elasticity and loss of muscle mass occur as a person ages. In the respiratory system, these changes result in less-efficient ventilation. The very elastic lung tissue loses some of its ability to expand and bounce back as a person breathes, which reduces the amount of air that is taken in and let out with each breath. The diaphragm and intercostal muscles become weaker, which means that the chest cavity may not expand as much

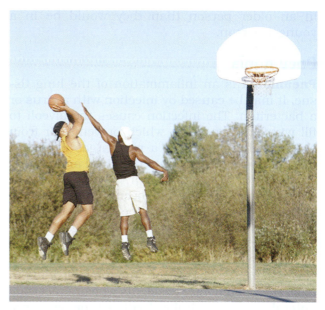

Figure 33-5
Exercise, especially when combined with avoidance of smoking and exposure to pollution, is an effective way of keeping your respiratory system healthy throughout your lifetime.

with each breath, so the amount of air taken in will be smaller. In healthy older people who do not smoke, these changes do not usually cause any problems. Often, the person will not be aware of any change, except possibly during exercise, when oxygen demands are significantly increased.

DECREASED COUGH REFLEX

The cough reflex helps us to keep the airway clear of secretions. With age, the cough reflex decreases, affecting the older person's ability to keep the airway clear. As a result, the person may have a harder time eliminating microbes and secretions from the respiratory tract. This puts the person at increased risk for respiratory tract infections. The decreased cough reflex also puts the person at risk for choking on food or saliva.

DISORDERS OF THE RESPIRATORY SYSTEM

INFECTIONS

A decreased cough reflex, the less efficient functioning of the immune system that occurs with age and immobility put older people at high risk for respiratory tract infections. In general, respiratory tract infections are likely to be more severe in an older person than they would be in a younger person.

Pneumonia

Pneumonia is an inflammation of the lung tissue. It may be caused by infection with a virus or a bacterium. The infection causes the alveoli to fill with fluid and pus, which prevents air from entering the alveoli. As a result, gas exchange (the transfer of oxygen into the blood and carbon dioxide out of it) cannot occur.

Aspiration pneumonia occurs when foreign material (such as food, tube-feeding formula, saliva, or vomit) is inhaled into the lungs. The foreign material can damage the lung tissue, causing the alveoli to fill with fluid. The foreign material can also carry bacteria into the lungs, leading to bacterial pneumonia. Residents who are receiving enteral nutrition (tube feedings) or who are unconscious are at increased risk for developing aspiration pneumonia because they are unable to protect their airway (by coughing or gagging).

Signs and symptoms of pneumonia include fever, pain when breathing, cyanosis (bluish skin as a result of decreased oxygen levels in the blood), and a productive cough. A productive cough is one in which a person coughs up **sputum** or "phlegm" (mucus and other respiratory secretions that are coughed up from the lungs, bronchi, and trachea). **Hemoptysis** is the coughing up of blood or blood-stained sputum (*heme* means "blood," and *–ptysis* means "to spit"). Hemoptysis may be seen in pneumonia, and can also occur with other respiratory disorders. In an older person, pneumonia may cause a fairly sudden change in mental status or delirium (see Chapter 9). The decreased oxygen levels in the blood impact the brain's ability to function and may result in increased confusion, behavioral changes, or both.

Pneumonia is usually diagnosed with a chest x-ray and treated with antibiotics. Knowledge about which microbe is causing the pneumonia will allow the doctor to prescribe the most effective antibiotic therapy. You may be asked to assist by collecting a sputum specimen for analysis. Guidelines for collecting sputum specimens are given in Guidelines Box 33-1.

Pleurisy is an inflammation of the pleura, the membrane that lines the chest cavity and covers the lungs. Pleurisy often accompanies lower respiratory tract infections, such as pneumonia. The inflammation of the pleura causes pain during breathing as the layers of membrane rub against each other when the lungs expand and relax. Fluid may also collect in the space between the chest cavity and the lung. This build-up of fluid prevents the lungs from expanding fully. The doctor may need to insert a needle into the chest cavity to drain the fluid.

Bronchitis

Bronchitis is an inflammation of the bronchi. Like pneumonia, bronchitis can be caused by a viral or bacterial infection. Bronchitis may cause a dry, non-productive cough that sounds like a "bark." Bacterial bronchitis is usually treated with antibiotics. Both bacterial and viral bronchitis can turn into pneumonia if the bronchial infection is not treated promptly.

Influenza

Influenza, commonly referred to as "the flu," is an acute respiratory infection caused by the influenza virus. You are probably already familiar with symptoms of the flu: sore throat, dry cough, stuffy nose, headache, body aches, weakness, and fever. Influenza is different from the "common cold," which can be caused by many different types of viruses and usually only affects the upper respiratory tract.

Influenza season runs from November through April. The influenza virus is very contagious. Most people who get the flu will recover in about a week. However, elderly people, very young children, and people with chronic health conditions who get the flu are at risk for developing serious complications, such as an extremely severe form of pneumonia. Because an outbreak of influenza in a long-term care facility can have such serious consequences for the residents, flu shots are usually given to residents and staff members each fall, before the start of flu season (Fig. 33-6).

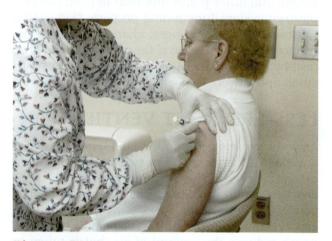

Figure 33-6

A resident receives a "flu shot." Vaccinating both residents and staff against the influenza virus is an effective way of preventing outbreaks of influenza in long-term care facilities.

Guidelines Box   33-1   Guidelines for Collecting a Sputum Specimen

WHAT YOU DO	WHY YOU DO IT
Explain to the person that the sputum for the specimen should be coughed up from deep down in the respiratory tract.	The sputum for analysis must come from the lungs, because that is where most of the infection-causing microbes are located. Explaining this to the person helps to ensure that he produces a specimen that will result in an accurate diagnosis. If you do not explain this to the person, he may just cough up saliva, which will not result in an accurate diagnosis.
Provide privacy.	Having to spit mucus into a cup can be embarrassing and unpleasant for some people.
Have the person rinse her mouth with water before coughing up the specimen.	Rinsing with plain water helps to remove microbes that are normally present in the mouth, resulting in a "cleaner" specimen.
Do not have the person rinse with mouthwash before coughing up the specimen.	The antiseptic effects of the mouthwash might actually kill the microbes in the sputum specimen that are responsible for the infection, which will result in inaccurate test results.
Have the person spit the specimen directly into a sterile specimen container and close the lid.	Having the person spit directly into the sterile specimen container reduces the risk of contaminating the specimen and results in more accurate test results.
Make sure that the specimen container is labeled properly and that the information is correct.	Labeling errors can result in misdiagnosis or the need to repeat the test.
Take the specimen container to the laboratory immediately after collecting the specimen or ask the nurse how to store it.	Allowing a specimen to sit around or storing it the incorrect way can result in the need to repeat the test.

ASTHMA

Asthma is a condition that affects the bronchi and bronchioles. In people with asthma, triggers (such as cold weather, allergies, respiratory infections, stress, smoke, and exercise) cause the bronchi and bronchioles to constrict (become narrower). This makes breathing difficult, because air does not flow freely through the airways. An asthma attack can be very frightening for the person experiencing it, because the airways can narrow to the point that breathing becomes almost impossible. If one of your residents is having trouble breathing or is making wheezing sounds, you should call the nurse immediately.

An acute asthma attack is usually treated with inhaled medications called bronchodilators (Fig. 33-7). Bronchodilators stop the muscle spasms responsible for the constriction of the airways. People with chronic asthma may need to take medication on a regular basis to prevent attacks from occurring. These medications may be given orally, or they may be inhaled.

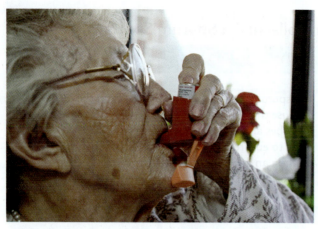

Figure 33-7
Asthma medications are often delivered through inhalers.

CHRONIC OBSTRUCTIVE PULMONARY DISEASE (COPD)

Chronic obstructive pulmonary disease (COPD) is a general term used to describe two related lung disorders, emphysema and chronic bronchitis. These disorders often occur together in the same person, which is why some health care professionals prefer the more general term, COPD. The leading cause of COPD is smoking.

Emphysema

Emphysema is a form of COPD that involves damage to the alveoli. As you learned earlier, the walls of the alveoli are very thin and delicate. When a toxin, such as tobacco smoke, is inhaled, it damages the thin walls of the alveoli. Over time, the damage causes the fragile walls of the alveoli to break. Eventually, instead of having millions of tiny alveoli where gas exchange can take place, the person has fewer, large "merged" alveoli that are no longer effective for gas exchange (Fig. 33-8). Because the lung tissue is damaged, it is no longer "springy," and the air gets trapped in the large, damaged alveoli. The trapped air cannot be exhaled and exchanged for new oxygen-rich air, which limits the amount of oxygen the lungs are able to supply to the body. In addition, excess fluid can collect in the damaged alveoli, creating an excellent place for infection-causing microbes to collect and multiply.

A person with emphysema has trouble getting a "proper breath." The person's breathing is shallow and rapid, and he may have to stop to catch his breath quite frequently when talking or engaging in any type of physical activity. As the person's emphysema gets worse, he will need

supplemental oxygen just to carry out even the simplest activities of daily living (ADLs). If you are caring for a person with emphysema, you may notice that his chest is enlarged and rounded. This finding is referred to as "barrel chest" and is caused by years of having extra air trapped in the lung tissue, which causes the chest cavity to enlarge over time.

Chronic Bronchitis

The other form of COPD is chronic bronchitis. **Chronic bronchitis** is caused by long-term irritation of the bronchi and bronchioles, such as that caused by inhaling tobacco smoke. The irritation leads to the production of thick mucus, which blocks the airways. Because the air cannot pass freely through the bronchi and bronchioles, breathing is impaired. In addition, infection-causing microbes can collect in the mucus and multiply, leading to infection.

A person with chronic bronchitis has a nagging, productive cough. She may complain of a "tightness" in her chest, or difficulty breathing. She is likely to have frequent respiratory tract infections. Like a person with emphysema, a person

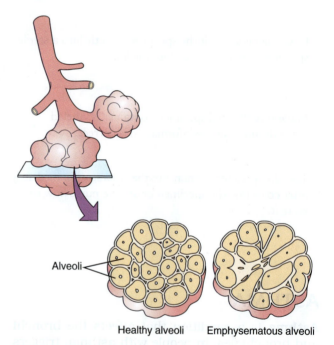

Alveoli

Healthy alveoli   Emphysematous alveoli

Figure 33-8
Emphysema occurs as a result of damage to the alveoli. The damage to the alveoli makes it difficult for the body to obtain oxygen and get rid of carbon dioxide. A healthy lung contains millions of tiny alveoli, where gas exchange takes place. In a person with emphysema, the walls of the alveoli break down, forming large areas where air can get trapped.

with chronic bronchitis will eventually need oxygen therapy.

Helping Hands and a Caring Heart

FOCUS ON HUMANISTIC HEALTH CARE

Residents who have chronic conditions of the respiratory system, such as asthma or COPD, may be quite "needy." You may become frustrated with their frequent use of the call light control to ask for seemingly trivial things. Please stop for a moment and try to understand how frightening it would be to suddenly feel that you could not breathe! A resident who is having an asthma attack or experiencing a flare-up of COPD feels that each breath might be his last. He might be afraid that in the event of another flare-up or attack, help will not arrive soon enough. Using the call light control frequently is the resident's way of making sure that someone will actually come quickly if he calls. Instead of giving in to the desire to avoid a needy resident, be patient and understanding of the underlying fears the resident may have. Spend more time with the resident, and get into the habit of stopping by to check on him, even when he has not called you. By addressing the resident's underlying need for safety and security, you will be providing truly humanistic care.

CANCER

In the United States, cancers involving the lungs and airway are the most common cause of cancer-related death in both men and women. The types of cancers that affect the upper respiratory tract include tumors of the mouth, tongue, and vocal cords. Cancers of the lower respiratory tract can involve the lungs or the lining of the bronchi. People who smoke cigarettes are 10 times more likely to develop lung cancer than non-smokers are. In addition, some cancers that begin in other body parts, such as the breast or intestines, commonly spread to the lungs.

There are many different ways of diagnosing and treating cancer, which are discussed in detail in Chapter 43. Treatment of lung cancer may involve surgical removal of all or part of the lung. Treatment of cancer of the mouth, tongue, or vocal cords may involve surgery to remove the cancer and possibly some of the surrounding tissues as well. This type of surgery often changes the person's appearance, in very noticeable ways.

For many people, coping with the change in their appearance as well as the diagnosis of cancer is very difficult.

Helping Hands and a Caring Heart

FOCUS ON HUMANISTIC HEALTH CARE

When a resident has a smoking-related illness, be careful not to be judgmental about the role the person's actions may have had in causing her disease. A resident with a smoking-related illness, such as cancer or COPD, may choose to continue smoking, even though she knows doing so may significantly shorten her life. Smoking is very physically addictive and quitting can be extremely difficult, especially when the person is trying to cope with the stress of having a chronic or terminal condition. Each of your residents must be allowed to make decisions concerning her own quality of life. For some people, this may mean not giving up smoking, even when it would seem to be the best thing to do.

RESPIRATORY THERAPY

Respiratory therapy is any treatment that is used to help a person achieve satisfactory respiration. Some of these treatments are relatively simple. For example, a humidifier may be used to add moisture to the air, helping to loosen secretions during a bout of bronchitis or pneumonia. Other treatments may be quite complex and involve the use of medications, such as oxygen, or mechanical ventilation.

Many of the therapies that are used to help people with respiratory disorders can be carried out only by people who have received advanced training, such as nurses and respiratory therapists. However, many facilities offer additional training that will allow you to be more active in caring for people with special respiratory needs. Make sure that you have been adequately instructed in any special procedures that are required of you, and always be aware of what is and is not within your scope of practice, per your state's or facility's policy.

If you are caring for a resident with a respiratory disorder, watch the nurse or respiratory therapist and ask questions about the types of treatments the person is receiving. This knowledge will help you to better understand the resident's specific needs. The nurse or respiratory therapist can also alert you to signs or symptoms that you should watch for and report to the nurse immediately.

GENERAL CARE MEASURES

As a nursing assistant, you will play a very important role in observing your residents for signs of respiratory distress, and promoting comfort.

Observation

A nursing assistant's main responsibility in caring for any resident with a respiratory problem is that of observation. Because you are the one who will spend the most time with your residents, you will be the one who has the best opportunity to observe signs that a person may be having problems with ventilation or gas exchange. Some of your residents who have chronic respiratory problems will always have difficulty breathing when they exert themselves. It is important for you to be able to recognize what is normal for each of your residents, so that you can recognize changes if they occur. You should also be aware of a person's normal skin color, so that you are able to recognize changes that may indicate that the tissues are not receiving enough oxygen.

TELL THE NURSE ❗

Not receiving adequate oxygen, even for a very short time, places a person at risk for developing severe complications, or even dying. Tell the nurse immediately if you observe any of the following:

- A resident experiences the sudden onset of chest pain or difficulty breathing
- A resident develops noisy breathing (for example, wheezing, "barking," or "crowing")
- A resident begins to make fluid-like, gurgling sounds (this is especially important to report if the resident is very weak or unconscious)
- A resident's skin has a blue or gray tinge, either at rest or while exercising
- A resident coughs up sputum that is discolored (green, frothy, brown, or red-streaked)
- A resident becomes short of breath during a physical activity that he has performed without effort in the past

---

- A resident's respirations become very slow and shallow, or they stop
- A resident's respiratory rate increases
- A resident shows increased confusion or restlessness
- A resident's level of consciousness is decreased

Promoting Comfort

There are many things that a nursing assistant can do to help a resident with respiratory problems feel more comfortable. Positioning the resident in the Fowler's or semi-Fowler's position is often helpful. Some residents are more comfortable when they assume a forward-leaning position using pillows on the over-bed table (Fig. 33-9). If the doctor has not placed any restrictions on the resident's fluid intake, encourage the resident to drink plenty of fluids. Fluids help to thin respiratory secretions so that they are easier to cough up. Providing frequent oral care will also help keep the resident comfortable and will reduce the number of microbes that are present in the mouth.

OXYGEN THERAPY

The air we breathe contains only about 20% oxygen. The rest is nitrogen. People with reduced lung function (for example, people with emphysema) may have trouble getting the oxygen their bodies need from inhaled air alone. For these people, the doctor might prescribe supplemental (extra) oxygen to increase the amount of oxygen that they take in with each breath. The supplemental oxygen is pure, 100% oxygen.

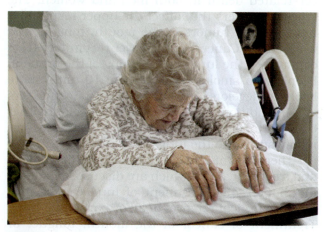

Figure 33-9

Certain positions make breathing easier for people with respiratory disorders. Many people find that leaning forward helps to make breathing easier.

Some people who are receiving supplemental oxygen will only need it for a short time. Others will need it for the rest of their lives. Oxygen can be given continuously, or it can be given on an as-needed basis. Some people only need supplemental oxygen when they are physically active.

Oxygen is considered a medication and requires a doctor's order to be used. The doctor determines the rate or concentration at which the oxygen should be delivered, and how it should be given. A nurse or respiratory therapist is responsible for setting up and adjusting the oxygen therapy. Many of the residents you will care for will be receiving oxygen therapy. Therefore, you need to understand how oxygen is given and what precautions are necessary while oxygen is being used. Some states and facilities do not allow nursing assistants to adjust or assist with the administration of oxygen, but others do. Always make sure that you are familiar with your specific job responsibilities with regard to oxygen therapy. General guidelines for oxygen therapy are given in Guidelines Box 33-2. You should also review Chapter 17 for safety considerations related to oxygen therapy.

Oxygen is usually delivered at a rate of 2 to 15 liters of oxygen per minute. The flow rate is set using a device called a **flow meter** (Fig. 33-10). Although you will not usually be responsible for adjusting the flow rate of oxygen, it is important for you to know what flow rate was ordered. You should check the flow meter frequently when you are caring for a resident who is receiving oxygen therapy to make sure that the flow rate is set

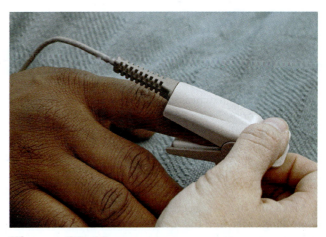

Figure 33-11
The pulse oximeter sensor is clipped to the person's fingertip. Pulse oximetry is used to monitor the amount of oxygen that is reaching a person's tissues.

properly. A resident (or a visitor) might change the setting on the flow meter. If you notice that the setting on the flow meter does not match the amount of oxygen that has been ordered, notify the nurse immediately. Receiving too much oxygen is just as dangerous as receiving too little oxygen.

Residents who are receiving oxygen therapy may need to be monitored to make sure that enough oxygen is reaching the tissues. Monitoring of the oxygen content of the blood is done using a device called a *pulse oximeter*. The pulse oximeter is clipped to the person's fingertip or earlobe (Fig. 33-11). Infrared light is passed through the tissue to a sensor on the other side of the device. The amount of light that reaches the sensor is translated into a measurement of how much oxygen the blood is actually carrying. A normal reading is between 95% and 100%. Readings below 85% indicate that the tissues are not receiving enough oxygen, and should be reported to the nurse immediately. An alarm will usually sound if the person's blood oxygen level is too low.

Because oxygen therapy can be very drying to the mouth or nose, moisture is often added to the supplemental oxygen using a humidity bottle. The humidity bottle is filled with distilled water. The oxygen passes through the water before it is delivered to the person. This increases the water content of the oxygen, making it less drying to the nose and mouth. As the oxygen flows through the water in the humidity bottle, it creates bubbles. You should check the humidity bottle frequently for bubbles, which indicate that the oxygen is flowing freely. You should also check the water level often, to make sure that it does not drop too

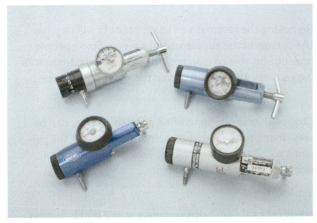

Figure 33-10
A flow meter controls the rate of oxygen flow. Flow meters come in a variety of styles. You should learn how the flow meters used by your residents work. This will allow you to check the flow meter to make sure that the person is receiving the ordered amount of oxygen.

Guidelines Box 33-2 Guidelines for Oxygen Therapy

WHAT YOU DO	WHY YOU DO IT
Avoid lighting matches or cigarette lighters in the person's room. Post a "No Smoking" sign, and remind the resident and any visitors not to smoke when oxygen is in use.	Use of oxygen therapy can increase the oxygen content of linens and clothing in the immediate area. If burning ashes from a cigarette should happen to drop on the bed, a fire would be more likely to start and would burn much faster as a result of the added oxygen.
Make sure that any electrical equipment is in good working order, and that cords are not frayed. Use a battery-operated razor or a blade razor when shaving a person who is receiving supplemental oxygen.	Electrical equipment that is not properly maintained can be the source of a spark, which could start a fire.
Make sure that the tubing through which the oxygen is delivered is free of kinks, and that the person is not lying on it.	If the tubing is obstructed in any way, oxygen flow will be impaired and the person will not receive the correct amount.
Do not adjust the flow rate of oxygen.	Adjusting the flow rate of oxygen is out of the nursing assistant's scope of practice. Receiving too much oxygen can be as harmful to the resident as receiving too little oxygen. The doctor decides how much oxygen the resident should receive.
When you are caring for a person who is receiving supplemental oxygen, be aware of the ordered flow rate, and tell the nurse if the flow rate on the flow meter does not match the ordered flow rate.	The setting on the flow meter may get changed accidentally. Checking frequently to make sure that the ordered flow rate matches the flow rate on the person's medical chart helps to keep your resident safe. Receiving too much oxygen can be as harmful to the resident as receiving too little oxygen.
When providing personal care, do not remove a person's facemask or nasal cannula, unless you are specifically told to do so by the nurse.	Removing the facemask or nasal cannula will deprive the person of the supplemental oxygen. Some people may not be able to tolerate a decrease in the amount of oxygen they are receiving, even for just a few minutes.
Make sure that the water level in the humidity bottle does not get too low. Tell the nurse if the water level is low and refilling or replacing the humidity bottle is not within your scope of practice.	Oxygen that is not humidified prior to delivery can be very drying to the mucous membrane lining of the person's nasal cavity and mouth. This dryness can be uncomfortable for the resident.
Provide oral care frequently, as directed by the nurse.	Frequent oral care helps to relieve some of the dryness of the nose and mouth that occurs with supplemental oxygen therapy.

(continued)

WHAT YOU DO	WHY YOU DO IT
Watch for signs of skin irritation behind the person's ears, over his or her cheeks, or under his or her nose.	The pressure and friction from the tubing that holds the facemask or nasal cannula in place can cause skin breakdown.
Follow your facility's policies and procedures for caring for the equipment used in oxygen therapy, such as nasal cannulas, tubing, and humidity bottles.	These policies and procedures are in place to prevent contamination of the equipment. Contaminated equipment can be a source of infection.

low. Your facility policy will specify how often the humidity bottle should be changed, and who is allowed to change it.

Sources of Supplemental Oxygen

Supplemental oxygen can be supplied through a wall-mounted delivery system, in a pressurized tank, or through an oxygen concentrator (Fig. 33-12).

Wall-mounted delivery systems

With a wall-mounted delivery system, the oxygen is piped into the resident's room from a central location. A special valve and flow meter device is inserted into the wall to access the oxygen (Fig. 33-12A). The nurse or respiratory therapist sets the flow meter so that the oxygen is administered at the correct rate.

Pressurized tank

These tanks, which are placed in the resident's room, contain oxygen under pressure. Some of these tanks are small enough for the resident to carry or wheel around (Fig. 33-12B). Always transport oxygen tanks in a "cage" or carrier made for that purpose. The cage helps to prevent the oxygen tank from being knocked over. Knocking over an unprotected oxygen tank could cause an explosion, because the oxygen is under pressure.

The nurse or respiratory therapist sets the flow meter on the tank so that the oxygen is administered at the correct rate. A gauge tracks the amount of oxygen remaining in the tank. You should note when the dial shows that the supply of oxygen is getting low. If you notice that the tank is nearly empty, tell the nurse or respiratory therapist so that she can exchange the nearly empty tank for a full one.

Oxygen concentrators

Oxygen concentrators are devices that take in air and filter out the nitrogen, leaving behind pure oxygen (Fig. 33-12C). The oxygen is then delivered to the person at the rate that has been programmed into the unit. Because the delivery amount is pre-set, the person (or caregiver) only has to turn the switch to "ON" when oxygen is needed. These units run on electricity and are often used in long-term care settings, especially if the person needs supplemental oxygen only once in a while.

Delivery of Supplemental Oxygen

A number of different devices are used to deliver oxygen to residents. The type of delivery device used depends on several factors, including the amount of oxygen ordered, the condition being treated, and the overall physical condition of the resident.

Nasal cannulas

A nasal cannula is the most common method of administering oxygen. A **nasal cannula** is two prongs of soft plastic tubing, which are inserted into the nostrils (Fig. 33-13A). The tubing to the cannula is connected to an oxygen source with a humidifier bottle and a flow meter. A nasal cannula is easy to apply, it does not interfere with eating or talking, and it is less likely to create a feeling of suffocation. However, the nasal cannula can dry out the mucous membranes in the nasal cavity if the oxygen is delivered at a high flow rate. The tubing can irritate the skin around the nostrils, on the cheeks, and behind the ears. Finally, a nasal cannula may not be suitable for use in a person who breathes through the mouth, because the concentration of oxygen delivered may not be high enough.

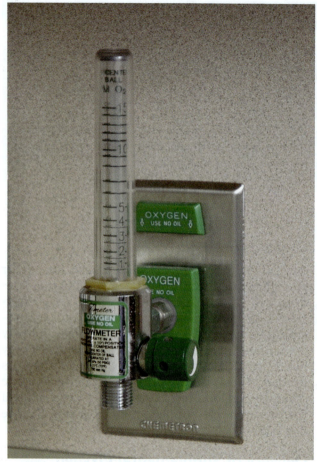

A. Wall-mounted delivery system

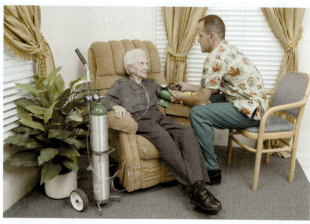

B. Pressurized tank

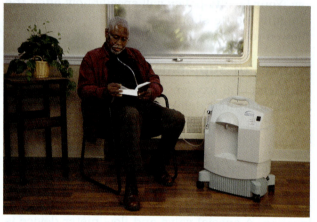

C. Oxygen concentrator

Figure 33-12

Supplemental oxygen can be supplied in various ways. **(A)** With a wall-mounted delivery system, the oxygen is piped into the person's room from a central location. A valve and flow meter device is inserted into the wall outlet to access the oxygen. **(B)** A pressurized tank of oxygen can go where the person goes. **(C)** An oxygen concentrator is often used in the long-term care setting, especially when the person only needs to use oxygen on an as-needed basis. Oxygen concentrators produce 100% oxygen by filtering the nitrogen out of room air.

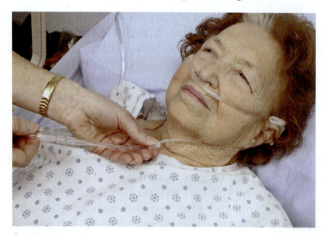

A. Nasal cannula

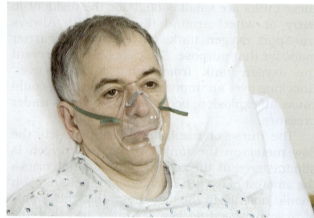

B. Facemask

Figure 33-13

Devices used for oxygen delivery. **(A)** A nasal cannula is a two-pronged device that is inserted into the nostrils to deliver oxygen to the person. A person who has a nasal cannula in place is able to eat, drink, and speak normally. **(B)** A facemask fits over the person's nose and mouth. A facemask may be used when a person requires a high level of supplemental oxygen. Facemasks come in a variety of styles.

Facemasks

Oxygen can also be delivered through a **facemask.** A facemask is made of soft, molded plastic material that fits over the nose and mouth (Fig. 33-13B). A facemask may be a simple device that just delivers the oxygen to the mouth and nose, or it may be quite complex, with attachments (such as bags that act as a holding place for extra oxygen). A facemask can deliver oxygen at a higher concentration than a nasal cannula can. In addition, a facemask is useful for a person who breathes through the mouth, instead of the nose. However, facemasks can make a person feel like he is suffocating (because they cover the person's nose and mouth), and they can interfere with the person's ability to eat, drink, and speak clearly. Sometimes a person is allowed to switch to a nasal cannula when it is time to eat or be shaved. Never remove a resident's facemask without first asking the nurse. Removing the facemask, even briefly, can have serious consequences.

TELL THE NURSE

When caring for a resident who is receiving oxygen therapy, be sure to report the following observations to the nurse right away:

- The oxygen flow rate on the oxygen flow meter does not match the ordered amount of oxygen

- The gauge on a pressurized oxygen tank indicates that the oxygen level is low

- The water level in the humidity bottle is low

- The screen on a pulse oximeter shows a reading of less than 85%

- The resident repeatedly tries to remove the nasal cannula or facemask

- The skin under the resident's nose, over the resident's cheeks, or behind the resident's ears is red or irritated, or the resident has developed a sore in any of these areas (if a nasal cannula is in use)

- There is a change in the rate or depth of respirations

MAINTAINING AN OPEN AIRWAY

If the airway is not clear, the person will not be able to meet the need for oxygen. Measures to maintain an open airway include suctioning and the use of airway devices.

Suctioning

People with respiratory disorders often need help removing secretions from the airway. Conditions such as pneumonia or chronic bronchitis can cause the production of large amounts of sputum, which builds up in the lungs and bronchi and makes it difficult to breathe. Other conditions interfere with a person's ability to cough up secretions. For example, a person who is unconscious or heavily sedated may not have an intact cough reflex. As a result, the person does not cough and the secretions continue to build up. **Suctioning** is the process of removing fluid and mucus from a person's airway.

Suctioning is done using various types of suction catheters. The suction catheter is attached to tubing and a suction source, which works like a vacuum cleaner to remove the secretions from the airway (Fig. 33-14). A Yankauer suction tip is used to remove secretions that collect in the back of the throat. A long, thin, flexible catheter is used when it is necessary to suction the airways in the lower respiratory system. This soft catheter can be passed through the nose or mouth, or down an endotracheal or tracheostomy tube.

Nursing assistants are not responsible for suctioning residents, but you will be responsible for letting the nurse know that suctioning may be needed, and for assisting during the procedure. Because suctioning removes air along with the bothersome secretions, a person can easily become **hypoxic** (that is, deficient of oxygen) during the suctioning procedure. During the suctioning procedure, the person may feel as if he is not getting enough air, which can be very frightening.

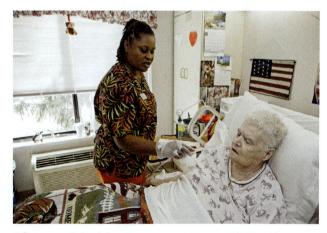

Figure 33-14
Suctioning is used to remove secretions from the airway. The nurse is responsible for performing this procedure, but you will play an important role in reporting a resident's need to be suctioned to the nurse.

Your calming and reassuring presence during the procedure can help keep the person calm and reduce discomfort.

Airway Devices

Sometimes a person is unconscious or has been sedated to the point that the muscles that keep the upper airway open relax. The lower jaw falls open and the tongue falls backwards into the throat, blocking the passage of air into the body. In this case, a nasopharyngeal airway or an oropharyngeal airway may be used.

A **nasopharyngeal airway** is a soft rubber tube that is inserted into the person's nose (Fig. 33-15A). It extends back toward the throat, providing an opening that air can flow through. An **oropharyngeal airway** is a hard plastic device that is

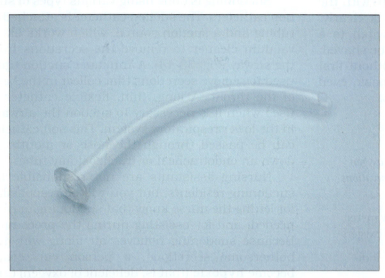
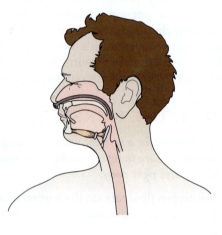

A. Nasopharyngeal airway

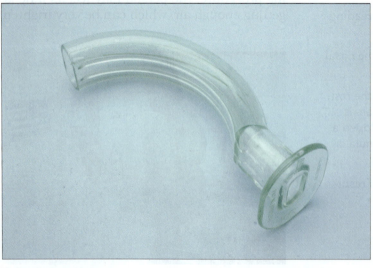
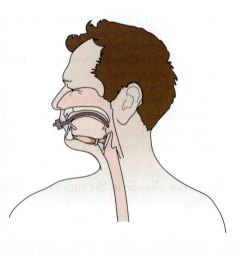

B. Oropharyngeal airway

Figure 33-15
An airway device may be used in a person who is unconscious or heavily sedated. The airway device keeps the airway open when the person cannot do this on his or her own. **(A)** A nasopharyngeal airway is inserted into the person's nose. **(B)** An oropharyngeal airway is inserted into the person's mouth.

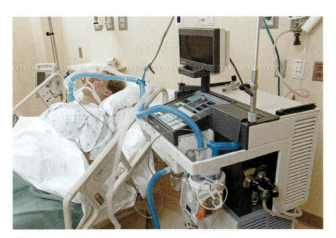

Figure 33-16

A mechanical ventilator performs the function of breathing for a person who cannot breathe on his own.

inserted into the person's mouth (Fig. 33-15B). The oropharyngeal airway stops the tongue from falling back into the throat, keeping the airway open. The oropharyngeal airway is used only for a person who is either heavily sedated or unconscious, because it can cause gagging and choking in a conscious person. You would be most likely to see these devices in use if you work in a subacute care unit or facility.

MECHANICAL VENTILATION

In **mechanical ventilation,** a machine called a *ventilator* breathes for a person who cannot breathe on his own (Fig. 33-16). Some people only need the ventilator for a short period of time, while others may need to be placed on a ventilator for the rest of their lives. Not all people who require mechanical ventilation are confined to bed. Some ventilators are portable (Fig. 33-17).

There are many reasons why a person might need to be put on a ventilator. For example, a serious head injury, stroke, or drug overdose can affect the breathing control centers in the brain, which means that regular breathing will no longer occur automatically. In these situations, mechanical ventilation is needed. A spinal cord injury or a neurologic disorder can interfere with the nerve impulses that cause the diaphragm to contract and relax automatically, resulting in the need for mechanical ventilation. Other conditions that may result in a person needing mechanical ventilation include acute respiratory infections and heart attacks. Mechanical ventilation is also often used both during and after surgery. In the long-term care setting, you would be most likely

to see mechanical ventilators in use in a subacute unit or other specialty unit.

A ventilator works by forcing air into the person's lungs. The air is delivered through a tube that is inserted into the airway. Depending on the situation, an endotracheal tube or a tracheostomy tube may be used (Fig. 33-18).

Endotracheal Intubation

Many people who require mechanical ventilation for only a short time will have an endotracheal tube. The **endotracheal tube** is inserted into the person's nose or mouth. It extends to the trachea, where a balloon cuff on the end holds it in place and prevents secretions that drain from the mouth from entering the respiratory tract (Fig. 33-18A). Being intubated with an endotracheal tube can be very uncomfortable and frightening.

- Because the endotracheal tube travels through the larynx (voice box), a person who

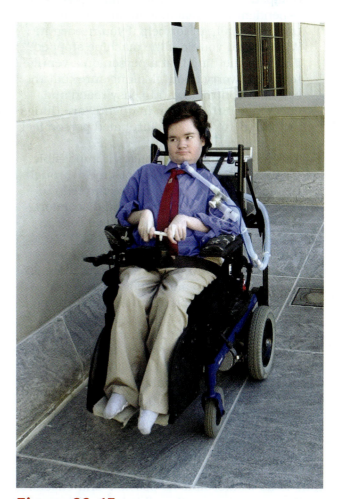

Figure 33-17

Portable ventilators allow some people with quadriplegia or other conditions that affect the muscles used for breathing to lead active lives. (*AP Photo/Jamie Martin.*)

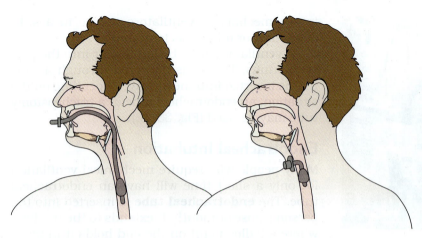

A. Endotracheal tube

B. Tracheostomy tube

Figure 33-18
Mechanical ventilation requires the use of an endotracheal tube or a tracheostomy tube. **(A)** An endotracheal tube is inserted into the person's nose or mouth and passed through the pharynx and larynx to the trachea. An inflatable balloon cuff at the end of the endotracheal tube holds it in place and helps to prevent secretions from passing into the lungs. **(B)** A tracheostomy tube is inserted into a surgically created opening in the neck called a tracheostomy.

has an endotracheal tube in place is unable to talk, and will need to communicate using some other method, such as writing on a notepad. Imagine what it would be like to be dependent on a machine to breathe and unable to call out for help if you needed it. What would you do if the machine stopped? This is something that a person on a ventilator might worry about. Making sure that the call light control is within easy reach and checking on the person frequently are things you can do to make an intubated person feel more secure.

- The endotracheal tube makes it impossible for the person to take food or fluids through the mouth. Frequent oral care can help to relieve some of the dryness and discomfort caused by having an endotracheal tube in place.

- Wrist restraints might be necessary for a person who is intubated, to keep the person from reaching up and removing the endotracheal tube from the airway. The tube is uncomfortable, and it is natural for a person to try and remove it. Although the wrist restraints may be necessary, they can add to the person's anxiety. As always, alternatives to restraints should be tried first. If restraints are applied, you will need to check on the person very frequently, and the restraints will need to be removed and reapplied at regular intervals.

Ensuring that a person with an endotracheal tube is as comfortable as possible and checking on the person frequently will help to relieve some of the person's worries and help her to feel safe. Always check to make sure that the endotracheal tube is still in place. Extubation (removal of the

tube) can have serious consequences for the person, including death.

Tracheostomy

If a person will need to be on a mechanical ventilator for more than a week or so, a tracheostomy is usually performed. A **tracheostomy** (often referred to as "a trach") is a surgically created opening in the neck that opens into the trachea. A short tube, called a tracheostomy or "trach" tube, is inserted into the opening and attached to the ventilator tubing (Fig. 33-18B). The tracheostomy tube is usually secured around the person's neck with ties or a special collar device (Fig. 33-19). If the tube is not secured, it could be

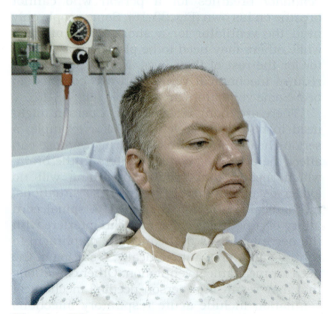

Figure 33-19
The tracheostomy tube is held in place with special ties or a collar.

coughed out very easily. As with an endotracheal tube, tell the nurse immediately if the person's tracheostomy tube has become dislodged!

A tracheostomy tube is much more comfortable for the person than an endotracheal tube. The person is able to eat and drink normally. The tracheostomy and tubing require special care, which is performed by the nurse. You are responsible for making sure that the tubing stays connected at all times and for observing the person for any signs that she is having trouble breathing.

Depending on the situation, a tracheostomy may be permanent or temporary. For example, a person who requires mechanical ventilation for several weeks will have a temporary tracheostomy that will be allowed to heal once the person no longer needs to be on the mechanical ventilator. However, a person who is paralyzed and will need to be on a ventilator for the rest of his life will have a permanent tracheostomy. A person who has had his larynx removed as a result of cancer will also have a permanent tracheostomy. The person breathes, talks, sneezes, and coughs through the tracheostomy because the airway between the pharynx and the trachea is no longer complete.

CHEST TUBES

Chest tubes are used to drain air or fluid (such as blood) that may build up in the chest cavity as a result of disease, trauma, or surgery. The build-up of air in the space between the lungs and the chest wall is called **pneumothorax.** The build-up of blood in the space between the lungs and the chest wall is called **hemothorax.** Pneumothorax and hemothorax are often complications of chest trauma. A severe lung infection can also cause the build-up of pus and fluid around the lung, making insertion of a chest tube necessary.

Fluid or air that builds up in the space between the lungs and the chest wall prevents the lungs from expanding fully. As a result, ventilation and gas exchange are affected, and the person is not able to meet the need for oxygen. In

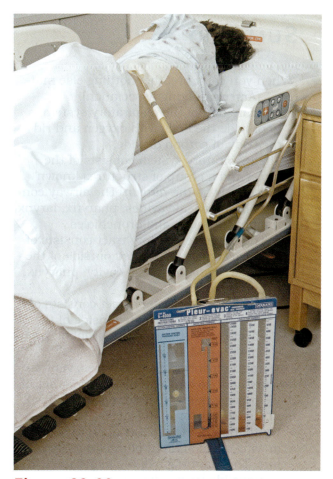

Figure 33-20

A chest tube drainage system is used to remove fluid (such as blood) or air that may build up in the chest cavity as a result of disease, injury, or surgery.

this situation, the doctor will insert a chest tube and connect it to a chest tube drainage system to remove the fluid or air that is preventing the lungs from expanding fully (Fig. 33-20). The nurse or respiratory therapist will tell you about the special care measures a person with a chest tube requires if you are responsible for caring for a resident who has a chest tube.

SUMMARY

- "When you can't breathe, nothing else matters." (American Lung Association)
  - The function of the respiratory system is to provide the body with oxygen and rid the body of carbon dioxide.
  - The respiratory system consists of the lungs and a group of structures known collectively as the *airway*. The airway consists of the nasal cavities, pharynx, larynx, trachea, bronchi, and bronchioles.
    - The upper respiratory tract consists of those structures located outside of the chest cavity (the nasal cavity, pharynx, and larynx).
    - The lower respiratory tract consists of those structures located inside of the chest cavity (the trachea, bronchi, bronchioles, and lungs).
- Respiration involves two processes, ventilation and gas exchange. If one or the other of these processes is impaired, respiration will not be effective.
  - Ventilation is the process of physically moving air in and out of the lungs (breathing). The diaphragm is the major muscle responsible for ventilation.
  - Gas exchange is the process of transferring oxygen from the air into the blood, and transferring carbon dioxide from the blood into the air. Gas exchange occurs in the alveoli.
- Like all organ systems, the respiratory system is affected by aging.
  - Loss of elasticity in the lung tissue and weakening of the muscles of respiration make breathing less efficient, because an older person is able to take in less air with each breath.
  - With aging, the cough reflex decreases.
  - Chronic health conditions, immobility, or a lifetime of exposure to pollution, chemicals, or tobacco smoke can make the effects of aging on the respiratory system much more noticeable. Regular physical exercise combined with healthy habits, such as the avoidance of smoking, help to keep the respiratory system healthy throughout a person's lifetime.
- Disorders of the respiratory system can make breathing very difficult.
  - Infections can be caused by bacteria or viruses and include pneumonia, bronchitis, and influenza. Respiratory tract infections can be very serious in older people.
- Asthma is a narrowing of the bronchioles in response to certain triggers such as allergies, cold air, exercise, smoke, or stress. An asthma attack can be very frightening for the person experiencing it.
- Chronic obstructive pulmonary disease (COPD) is a general term for two smoking-related disorders.
  - In emphysema, the alveoli are destroyed, and trapping of air in the lungs results. Breathing is difficult and gas exchange is impaired.
  - Chronic bronchitis affects the bronchi and bronchioles. Chronic bronchitis is associated with the production of excessive amounts of secretions.
- Cancers of the lungs and airway are the most common cause of cancer-related deaths in both men and women in the United States. People who smoke are 10 times more likely to develop lung cancer than non-smokers are.
- Respiratory therapy is used to help improve a person's processes of ventilation, gas exchange, or both.
  - A nursing assistant's responsibilities when caring for a resident with a respiratory disorder are mainly observation and the promotion of comfort. A nursing assistant also provides holistic care by helping the resident to feel safe and secure. Not being able to breathe easily can be very frightening for the resident.
- Oxygen therapy is the administration of supplemental oxygen.
  - Oxygen is a medication and requires a doctor's order to be used.
  - Oxygen may be supplied by way of a wall-mounted system, an individual pressurized tank, or an oxygen concentrator.
  - Oxygen can be administered through a nasal cannula or facemask.
- Suctioning is used to remove excessive secretions from a person's respiratory tract.
- Mechanical ventilation is used for a person who cannot inhale and exhale on his own. A person who needs the assistance of a mechanical ventilator must be intubated with an endotracheal tube or a tracheostomy tube.

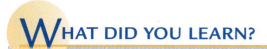

WHAT DID YOU LEARN?

Multiple Choice

Select the single best answer for each of the following questions.

1. Who has to write the order for oxygen to be used?
   a. The nurse
   b. The respiratory therapist
   c. The doctor
   d. No order is necessary

2. The nurse asks you to obtain a sputum specimen from Mrs. Long, who has pneumonia. Which one of the following is correct to do when obtaining a sputum specimen?
   a. Have Mrs. Long rinse her mouth with mouthwash before coughing up the specimen.
   b. Have Mrs. Long cough the specimen into an emesis basin, and then transfer the specimen to the specimen container.
   c. Explain to Mrs. Long that the specimen must come from deep within her chest.
   d. Put the specimen container in the refrigerator after you have collected the sputum specimen and labeled the container with Mrs. Long's name and room number.

3. What color is a healthy lung?
   a. Blue
   b. Gray
   c. White
   d. Pink

4. Where does gas exchange take place?
   a. In the alveoli
   b. In the bronchioles
   c. In the pleura
   d. In the nasal cavity

5. Which of the following is true about a person who has an endotracheal tube in place?
   a. The person is able to eat and drink normally.
   b. The person is able to talk normally.
   c. The person will need frequent oral care.
   d. The person is unconscious.

6. You have been assigned to care for Mr. Fenley, who has chronic obstructive pulmonary disease (COPD). He is on continuous oxygen by a nasal cannula at a rate of 4 liters per minute. One morning, you enter Mr. Fenley's room to do your morning checks, and you notice that the flow rate on the flow meter is set at 8 liters per minute. What should you do?
   a. Call the nurse immediately.
   b. Decrease the flow rate back to the prescribed 4 liters per minute.
   c. Tell Mr. Fenley that it is very dangerous for him to make adjustments to the flow meter on his own.
   d. Nothing. A resident can adjust the flow rate of oxygen to meet his own needs.

7. One of your responsibilities is to assist Mr. Tang with shaving. Mr. Tang is receiving continuous oxygen via a nasal cannula. What should you do when helping Mr. Tang to shave?
   a. Remove the nasal cannula before you begin the procedure.
   b. Use a battery-operated razor or a blade razor instead of an electrical razor.
   c. Increase the flow of oxygen during the procedure.
   d. Decrease the flow of oxygen during the procedure.

8. One of your newly admitted residents, Mr. Petersen, has emphysema. You are going to meet Mr. Petersen for the first time. Thinking back on what you learned during your nurse assistant training course about people with emphysema, which one of the following would you expect to be true of Mr. Petersen?
   a. His breathing will probably be shallow and rapid.
   b. He might need supplemental oxygen.
   c. He may have to catch his breath frequently while talking.
   d. All of the above

Matching

Match each numbered item with its appropriate lettered description.

_____ **1.** Respiration

_____ **2.** Lungs

_____ **3.** Nasopharyngeal airway

_____ **4.** Hemothorax

_____ **5.** Pharynx

_____ **6.** Trachea

_____ **7.** Pneumothorax

_____ **8.** Pleura

_____ **9.** Hypoxic

_____ **10.** Nasal cavity

a. Blood in the chest cavity

b. Also known as the "windpipe"; conducts air from the larynx to the bronchi

c. Membrane that covers the inside of the chest cavity and the outside of the lungs

d. Also known as the throat

e. A rubber tube that is inserted in a person's nose to keep the airway open

f. The process the body uses to obtain oxygen from the environment and remove carbon dioxide from the body

g. Primary organs of respiration

h. Space where air from the outside of the body is first warmed, humidified, and filtered

i. Air in the chest cavity

j. Deficient of oxygen

STOP and Think!

- You have been assigned to care for Mrs. Nielsen, who has severe respiratory problems resulting from a long history of asthma. The light above Mrs. Nielsen's door is on, and you go to find out what she needs. When you enter the room, Mrs. Nielsen asks you if it is almost time for dinner and whether or not you think she will need to wear a sweater. You answer Mrs. Nielsen's questions, and then ask her if there is anything else she needs, because surely there must be! She says, "no," she just wanted to ask you those questions. Do you think that Mrs. Nielsen has needs she may not be telling you about? What might you do for Mrs. Nielsen?

- Matthew is providing care for Mr. Thompson, who has smoked for more than 50 years. Mr. Thompson has advanced COPD, and requires a lot of assistance with nearly everything (including smoking, which he continues to do). One day, you and Matthew are leaving work together and you see all of the "smokers" outside having their cigarettes, shivering because it is the middle of winter. Matthew tells you that he thinks people who smoke are weak and lack willpower. How might Matthew's feelings about people who smoke affect his relationship with Mr. Thompson and other residents with smoking-related conditions?

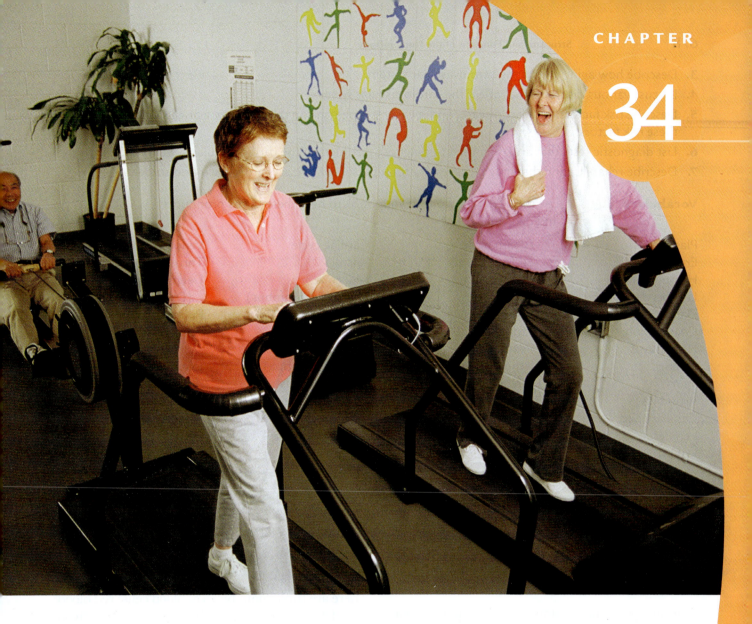

The Cardiovascular System

WHAT WILL YOU LEARN?

The heart and the other organs that make up the cardiovascular system are the subject of this chapter. According to the Centers for Disease Control and Prevention (CDC), about 61 million Americans live with the effects of either heart disease or stroke (a neurologic problem caused by cardiovascular disease). That is nearly 25% of the population! It is likely that some of the people you will care for daily will have some sort of a cardiovascular problem. Not only will an understanding of how the cardiovascular system works help you to better serve your residents, but it will also help you to keep your own cardiovascular system healthy. When you are finished with this chapter, you will be able to:

1. List and describe the major parts of the cardiovascular system.
2. Discuss the major functions of the cardiovascular system.

Photo: Residents of a continuing care retirement community (CCRC) use the equipment at an on-site fitness center. Exercising regularly is one way to keep the cardiovascular system healthy.

3. Describe how aging affects the cardiovascular system.

4. Discuss various disorders that affect the cardiovascular system.

5. Describe risk factors for heart disease, and measures a person can take to reduce or eliminate some of these risk factors.

6. List diagnostic tests that are often used to diagnose disorders of the cardiovascular system.

7. Describe rehabilitation that may be necessary for a person who has a cardiovascular disorder.

Vocabulary Use the CD in the front of your book to hear these terms pronounced and defined:

Plasma	Lymph node	Cardiac cycle	Venous thrombosis
Erythrocytes	Endocardium	Anemia	Thrombophlebitis
Hemoglobin	Myocardium	Leukemia	Deep venous thrombosis
Leukocytes	Epicardium	Thrombi (thrombus)	(DVT)
Platelets (thrombocytes)	Pericardium	Anticoagulants	Pulmonary embolism
Coagulation	Atria	Atherosclerosis	Venous (stasis)
Hemostasis	Ventricles	Plaque	ulcers
Arteries	Ischemia	Embolus (emboli)	Coronary artery
Veins	Circulation	Arteriosclerosis	disease
Arterioles	Pulmonary circulation	Peripheral vascular	Angina pectoris
Capillary bed	Systemic circulation	disease	Myocardial infarction
Venules	Systole	Varicose veins	Heart failure
Lymph	Diastole	Phlebitis	Cardiac rehabilitation

STRUCTURE OF THE CARDIOVASCULAR SYSTEM

The cardiovascular system, also known as the *circulatory system*, is made up of the blood, the blood vessels, the lymphatic system, and the heart. *Cardio* means "heart," and *vascular* means "vessels."

BLOOD

Blood is the life-giving fluid of our bodies. The blood has two main components, the plasma and the blood cells (Fig. 34-1A).

Plasma

More than half of the total blood volume is plasma. **Plasma** is the liquid part of the blood (Fig. 34-1B). Plasma is about 90% water. The other 10% is made up of substances that are dissolved in the water (such as glucose, amino acids, fats, and salts) and proteins. Important plasma proteins include albumin, fibrinogen, and globulins. Albumin plays a role in moving fluid in and out of the bloodstream. Fibrinogen is used as part of the blood clotting process. Globulins help to fight infection.

Blood Cells

There are three main types of blood cells: red blood cells (erythrocytes), white blood cells (leukocytes), and platelets (thrombocytes).

Red blood cells (erythrocytes)

Red blood cells, or **erythrocytes,** carry oxygen. The name *erythrocyte* comes from *eryth-*, which means "red," and *cyt,* which means "cell." There are approximately 5 million red blood cells per cubic millimeter of blood. Red blood cells are made in the red bone marrow (see Chapter 32) and are continuously replaced as old ones wear out.

Red blood cells are tiny, disc-shaped cells that are thinner in the center than at the edges (Fig. 34-1A). The "dent" in the center of the red blood cell contains a protein called **hemoglobin.** Oxygen molecules attach to the hemoglobin for transport to the tissues. When combined with oxygen, hemoglobin is bright red. This is what gives red blood cells their color and name.

The hemoglobin on each red blood cell can carry many oxygen molecules. The hemoglobin

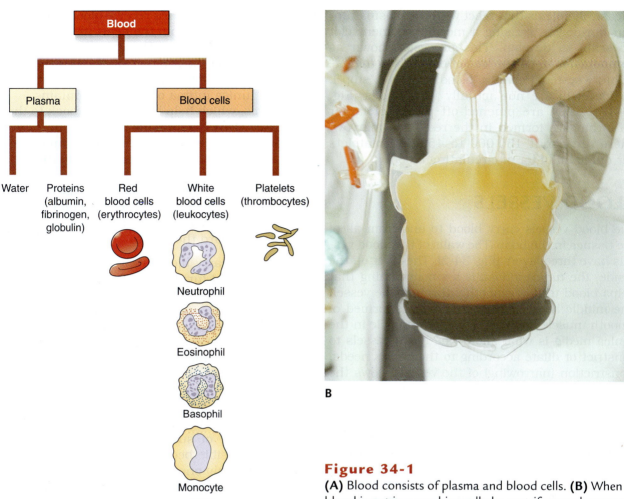

A

Blood
Plasma
Blood cells
Water | Proteins (albumin, fibrinogen, globulin) | Red blood cells (erythrocytes) | White blood cells (leukocytes) | Platelets (thrombocytes)

Neutrophil
Eosinophil
Basophil
Monocyte
Lymphocyte

B

Figure 34-1

(A) Blood consists of plasma and blood cells. **(B)** When blood is put in a machine called a centrifuge and spun at high speeds, the blood cells sink to the bottom while the plasma rises to the top. Human blood is about 55% plasma. (**B,** © *Antonia Reeve/Photo Researchers, Inc.*)

on red blood cells that have just received a full load of oxygen from the lungs is filled to capacity with oxygen, and therefore this blood is very bright red. As the blood circulates through the body, giving off oxygen and taking on carbon dioxide, the number of oxygen molecules on the hemoglobin decreases, and the blood becomes darker red in color.

White blood cells (leukocytes)

White blood cells, or **leukocytes,** fight infection. The name *leukocyte* comes from *leuk,* which means "white" and *cyt,* which means "cell."

The blood of a healthy person contains 5,000 to 10,000 white blood cells per cubic millimeter. There are five different types of white blood cells (Fig. 34-1A). Each type of white blood cell has a different function related to fighting infection.

Some destroy pathogens by surrounding them and "eating" them in a process called phagocytosis (see Chapter 15, Figure 15-2). Others secrete substances that cause the pathogen to die. Still others make proteins called antibodies, which prevent us from getting some diseases twice.

White blood cells are formed in the red bone marrow and the lymphatic system (discussed later in this chapter). An infection causes white blood cell production to increase, sending more "troops" into the bloodstream to battle the invading pathogen.

Platelets (thrombocytes)

Platelets (thrombocytes) are responsible for **coagulation** (clotting of the blood). When an injury occurs, the platelets stick together to form a temporary plug over the site of injury. They also release chemicals that react with the plasma protein fibrinogen, causing a more permanent clot (or scab) to develop. This process, known as **hemostasis,** stops the loss of blood from the circulatory system (*heme-* = "blood," *stasis* = "stop").

Platelets are not actually whole cells (Fig. 34-1A). They are pinched-off pieces of larger cells that are formed in the red bone marrow. There are about 150,000 to 450,000 platelets per cubic milliliter of circulating blood.

BLOOD VESSELS

The blood vessels carry blood to and from all of the tissues in the body. The walls of the blood vessels have three layers (Fig. 34-2). The layer on the inside, the *tunica intima,* is a smooth lining that helps blood to flow smoothly through the vessel. The middle layer, the *tunica media,* is formed of smooth muscle tissue. The smooth muscle in the tunica media is what allows the blood vessels to constrict or dilate according to the body's needs. Constriction (narrowing) of the vessels slows the flow of blood, while dilation (widening) of the vessels allows blood to flow more rapidly. The outer layer of the vessel wall, the *tunica externa,* is a tough protective layer of connective tissue.

Arteries carry blood away from the heart, and **veins** carry blood to the heart. Looking at Figure 34-2, you can see that there are two major differences between the walls of the arteries and the walls of the veins:

- The walls of the arteries contain more smooth muscle than those of the veins, because the arteries receive blood that is being pumped from the heart under great force and pressure. The smooth muscle in the walls of the arteries allows the arteries to handle the flow of blood from the heart.

- The tunica intima of the veins contains valves, which help blood to flow back to the heart. This is especially important in the arms and the legs, where blood would tend to flow away from the heart, due to the effects of gravity. The valves are assisted by contraction of nearby skeletal muscles. For example, when we walk, contraction of the leg muscles compresses the veins, pushing blood toward the heart.

Arteries carry blood away from the heart. As the arteries get further away from the heart, they branch into a network, becoming smaller and smaller in diameter (Fig. 34-3A). The smallest arteries are called **arterioles.** Arterioles send off branches called capillaries, which form a network in the tissues called the **capillary bed** (Fig. 34-4). As blood passes through the capillary bed, the oxygen and nutrients in the blood pass into the tissues, and carbon dioxide and other waste materials from the tissues pass into the blood. This transfer of substances in and out of the blood is possible because the walls of the capillaries have only one thin layer, as opposed to the three layers in the walls of the arteries and veins. After the blood passes through the capillary bed, it starts its journey back to the heart by way of very tiny veins called **venules** (Fig. 34-4). Venules drain into small veins, which become larger in diameter as they approach the heart (Fig. 34-3B).

LYMPHATIC SYSTEM

The pressure of the circulating blood through the tiny capillaries forces some of the blood plasma to leak out into the surrounding tissues. Approximately 10% of the circulating plasma leaks out of the capillaries in this manner. The lymphatic system helps to return the fluid that leaks into the tissues to the bloodstream. The lymphatic system also produces some of the white blood cells that fight invading pathogens.

The lymphatic system is actually a one-way, open-ended circulatory system (Fig. 34-5). Lymph capillaries absorb excess fluid from the surrounding tissues. (Once the fluid enters the lymph capillaries, it is called **lymph.**) The lymph capillaries join together to form larger vessels, called lymphatics. At certain points along the way, the lymph in the lymphatics passes through

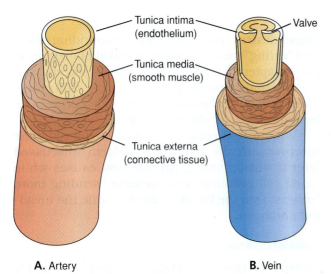

Tunica intima (endothelium)

Valve

Tunica media (smooth muscle)

Tunica externa (connective tissue)

A. Artery

B. Vein

Figure 34-2
The walls of the blood vessels have three layers. **(A)** An artery. **(B)** A vein.

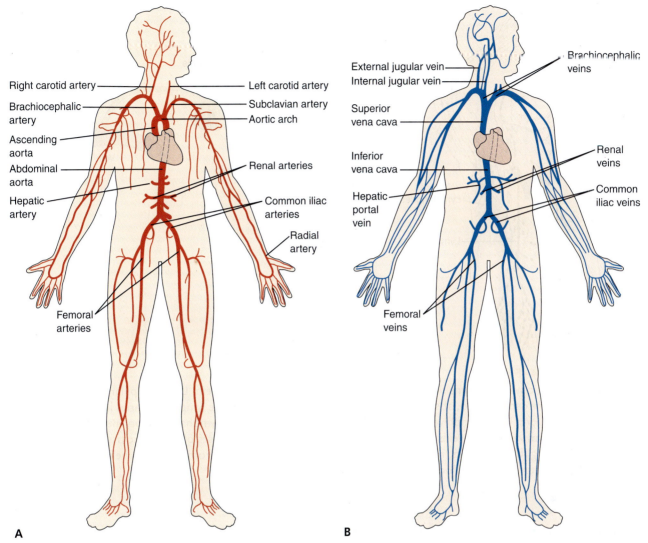

A

B

Figure 34-3

Blood vessels carry blood to every part of the body. **(A)** The major arteries of the body. Arteries carry blood away from the heart. Note how the arteries get smaller in diameter the further away they get from the heart. **(B)** The major veins of the body. Veins carry blood back to the heart. Note how the veins get larger in diameter the closer they get to the heart.

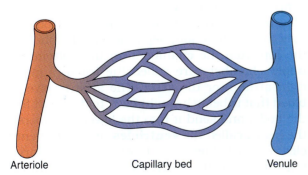

Figure 34-4

The capillary bed is where the transfer of substances between the blood and the tissues occurs.

lymph nodes, masses of lymphatic tissue that "clean" the lymph by removing bacteria and other large particles. Eventually, all of the lymphatics empty into the large veins in the shoulder region, returning the fluid to the general circulation.

Other parts of the lymphatic system include the thymus gland and the spleen. The thymus gland, which is located in the chest, secretes a chemical that stimulates the production of certain white blood cells (T cells) in the event of an infection. (Recall from Chapter 16 that T cells are the cells that the human immunodeficiency virus [HIV] virus attacks.) The spleen, located in the

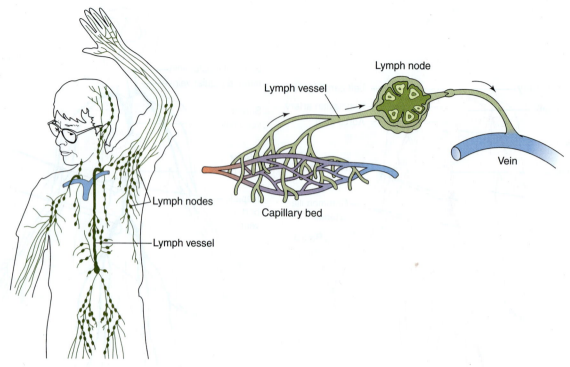

Figure 34-5

The lymphatic system returns fluid to the bloodstream. It is a one-way system. Lymph capillaries, located in the capillary bed, absorb fluid from the surrounding tissues. The lymph capillaries join together to form larger lymph vessels (called lymphatics). Eventually, the lymphatics empty into the subclavian veins, large veins in the shoulder region. Lymph nodes, masses of lymphatic tissue located along the lymphatics, remove bacteria and other foreign particles from the lymph before the fluid is returned to the bloodstream.

abdomen, helps to filter blood and break down worn-out red blood cells. The spleen also acts as a reservoir where extra blood is stored. The body draws on this "extra" blood supply during times of massive blood loss, for example, following a major injury.

HEART

The heart is a hollow, muscular organ about the size of a fist that lies in the center of the chest, tilted a bit toward the left, behind the sternum (breastbone). Like the walls of the arteries and veins, the walls of the heart are made of three layers of tissue. The **endocardium** is the smooth inner layer of the heart. The **myocardium,** the middle layer, is formed of cardiac muscle. Coordinated contraction and relaxation of the myocardium is what causes the heart to pump. The **epicardium** is the smooth outermost layer of the heart. The epicardium forms part of the **pericardium,** a double-layered protective sac that surrounds the heart. A thin film of fluid between the epicardium and the outer layer of the pericardium allows the pericardial layers to slide smoothly against each other each time the heart pumps.

Atria and Ventricles

The hollow interior of the heart is divided into four chambers (Fig. 34-6). A thick wall of muscle, called the septum, separates the left side of the heart from the right side of the heart. Valves, flaps of tissue that help to ensure that blood flows only in one direction, separate the chambers on the top from the chambers on the bottom. The upper chambers are called the left atrium and right atrium, or the **atria.** The atria receive the blood that is being brought back to the heart from the body, and send it into the lower chambers of the heart, called the **ventricles.** When the ventricles contract, they send blood from the heart to other parts of the body. Because the ventricles must send the blood much further with each contraction, they are larger than the atria, and have thicker, more muscular walls.

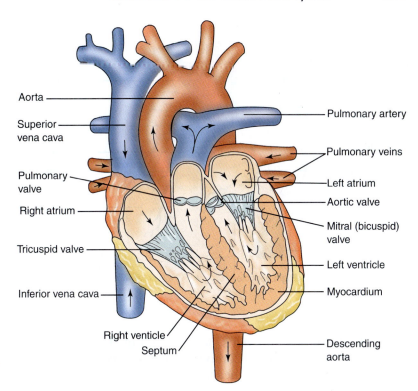

Aorta

Superior vena cava

Pulmonary valve

Right atrium

Tricuspid valve

Inferior vena cava

Right venticle

Septum

Pulmonary artery

Pulmonary veins

Left atrium

Aortic valve

Mitral (bicuspid) valve

Left ventricle

Myocardium

Descending aorta

Figure 34-6

The heart has four chambers. The atria receive blood that is being returned to the heart from the veins. Blood leaves the heart after passing through the ventricles.

Heart Valves

Blood can only flow through the heart in one direction. To keep blood flowing in the proper direction, the heart has four valves. Valves are flaps of tissue that snap shut after the blood passes through to prevent backflow.

- The tricuspid valve separates the right atrium from the right ventricle.
- The mitral (bicuspid) valve separates the left atrium from the left ventricle.
- The pulmonary valve is located where the pulmonary artery leaves the right ventricle.
- The aortic valve is located where the aorta leaves the left ventricle.

The four valves can be seen in Figure 34-6.

The valves that separate the upper and lower chambers of the heart may become diseased. For example, a type of infection called rheumatic fever can cause the valves to become thickened and scarred. Damaged valves are unable to create a seal when they close, which allows blood to backflow into the atria when the ventricles pump. This condition is called *valvular insufficiency*. A person with valvular insufficiency may need surgery to replace the defective valve.

Conduction System

The muscle cells that make up the myocardium are very specialized, so that they contract as a unit. This unified contraction is what allows the heart to work efficiently as a pump, moving blood continuously through the body. A small mass of special tissue in the heart, called the sinoatrial node (pacemaker), sets the pace for contraction by generating an electrical impulse. The electrical impulse travels through the myocardium via a special pathway called the conduction system. As it passes through, the electrical energy causes the cardiac muscle cells in the myocardium to contract. First the atria contract, there is a pause, and then the ventricles contract.

Coronary Circulation

Like all organs, the heart needs oxygen and nutrients. In fact, the heart's demand for oxygen and nutrients is very high because it works continuously, without rest. The normal resting heart rate of an adult is 70 beats/min, or about 100,800 beats in a 24-hour period! The heart cannot stop to rest when it is tired; it has to continue pumping blood through the body. All of this hard work adds up to a very high, and constant, demand for oxygen and nutrients.

The coronary circulation meets this demand (Fig. 34-7). (*Coronary* is another word for "heart.") Many people think that the cells of the heart just absorb oxygen from the blood that is passing through the chambers, but this is not the case. The tissues of the heart have their own special

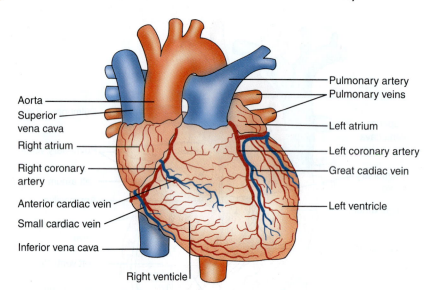

Aorta
Superior vena cava
Right atrium
Right coronary artery
Anterior cardiac vein
Small cardiac vein
Inferior vena cava
Right venticle

Pulmonary artery
Pulmonary veins
Left atrium
Left coronary artery
Great cadiac vein
Left ventricle

Figure 34-7

The heart has its own blood supply, called the coronary circulation.

network of arteries and veins, just like all of the other organs in the body. Coronary arteries carry oxygen-rich blood into the heart tissue. Coronary veins remove carbon dioxide and other waste products. Any disruption in the flow of oxygen-rich blood to the tissues of the heart can cause **ischemia** (lack of oxygen to the tissues). Prolonged ischemia causes the tissue to die, resulting in permanent damage to the heart muscle.

FUNCTION OF THE CARDIOVASCULAR SYSTEM

The main function of the cardiovascular system is that of transport. However, the cardiovascular system also plays a role in regulating temperature and protecting the body from disease.

TRANSPORT

Bringing oxygen, nutrients, and other necessary substances (for example, hormones) to the cells and taking waste materials away from them is one of the most important functions of the cardiovascular system. Oxygen, nutrients, wastes, and other substances are carried throughout the body by the blood. The heart powers the continuous movement of the blood (known as the **circulation**).

Pulmonary and Systemic Circulation

The pattern of circulation actually involves two circuits, the pulmonary circulation and the sys-

temic circulation (Fig. 34-8). The right side of the heart pumps blood to the lungs, where it picks up oxygen and releases carbon dioxide. This is the **pulmonary circulation** (*pulmonary* is another word for "lungs.") The left side of the heart pumps the newly oxygenated blood to the body. This is the **systemic circulation.**

The pattern of circulation goes like this (follow along on Figure 34-8):

Pulmonary circulation

- The largest veins in the body, the superior vena cava and the inferior vena cava, empty into the right atrium of the heart. The blood in these veins is returning from its journey to the tissues, so it has given up most of its oxygen and taken on a load of carbon dioxide.
- The right atrium pumps the oxygen-poor blood into the right ventricle.
- The right ventricle pumps the oxygen-poor blood into the pulmonary artery. The pulmonary artery branches into the right pulmonary artery, which goes to the right lung, and the left pulmonary artery, which goes to the left lung.
- Once in the lungs, the pulmonary arteries quickly branch into smaller arteries and arterioles to carry the oxygen-poor blood to the capillary beds surrounding the alveoli. As you remember from Chapter 33, gas exchange takes place in the alveoli. The oxygen in the alveoli moves into the blood, and the carbon dioxide in the blood moves into the alveoli, to be exhaled from the body.
- The blood, which now contains fresh oxygen, is carried by the network of venules, then

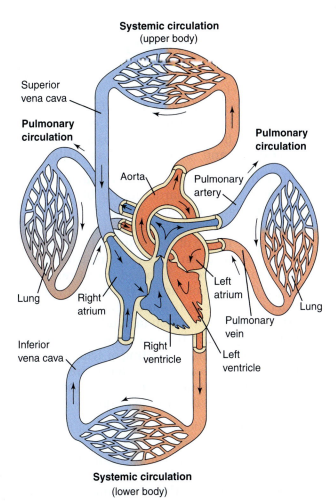

Systemic circulation
(upper body)

Superior
vena cava

**Pulmonary
circulation**

**Pulmonary
circulation**

Aorta

Pulmonary
artery

Lung

Right
atrium

Left
atrium

Lung

Pulmonary
vein

Inferior
vena cava

Right
ventricle

Left
ventricle

Systemic circulation
(lower body)

Figure 34-8

The pattern of circulation involves two circuits, the pulmonary circulation and the systemic circulation. In this diagram, *red* stands for oxygen-rich blood, and *blue* stands for oxygen-poor blood. Blood passes from the right ventricle into the pulmonary circulation. Once it is loaded up with oxygen, the blood returns to the left atrium, passes into the left ventricle, and is sent out to the rest of the body. This is the systemic circulation.

veins, to the pulmonary veins (right and left), which empty into the left atrium of the heart.

Systemic circulation

- The left atrium pumps the oxygen-rich blood into the left ventricle.
- The left ventricle pumps the oxygen-rich blood into the largest artery of the body, the aorta.
- The aorta branches very quickly into the coronary arteries to carry oxygen-rich blood to the heart muscle, and then into large branches of arteries that carry oxygen-rich blood to the rest of the body.

- The arteries branch into arterioles and then into capillaries, which join together to form a capillary bed. In the capillary bed, oxygen and nutrients move out of the blood and into the tissues, and carbon dioxide moves out of the tissues and into the blood.
- The blood, which now contains less oxygen, is carried by the network of venules, then veins, back to the right atrium, where the process begins again.

Cardiac Cycle

You may recall from Chapter 22 that the heart muscle contracts in two phases. During **systole,** or the active phase, the myocardium contracts, sending blood out of the heart. During **diastole,** or the resting phase, the myocardium relaxes, allowing the chambers to fill with blood. The atria are in systole when the ventricles are in diastole, and vice versa. The atria contract (atrial systole), sending the blood into the relaxed ventricles (ventricular diastole). Next, the atria relax (atrial diastole) while the ventricles contract (ventricular systole), sending the blood out to the body. This sequence is called the **cardiac cycle.**

The orderly sequence of systole and diastole is crucial for maximizing the amount of blood that is pumped throughout the body each time the heart contracts. During ventricular diastole, the ventricles are relaxed, which allows them to fill to capacity with blood. Without this rest period, the ventricles would never fill to capacity. Think about a plastic squirt bottle (the kind used at picnics to hold ketchup or mustard). If you fill the squirt bottle only partially with water, when you squeeze it, there is not enough force to push a large amount of water out of it. But, if you put as much water in the squirt bottle as it will hold and then squeeze, a small squeeze will cause a larger amount of water to squirt out with a lot more force. In other words, the heart is able to perform more efficiently when the ventricles are filled, because less force is required to send the maximum amount of blood out to the body.

As you may recall from Chapter 22, there are two distinct sounds that you will hear with your stethoscope when you are taking an apical pulse. The first sound, "lubb," is the sound of the tricuspid and mitral valves (the valves that separate the atria from the ventricles) snapping shut during ventricular systole. The second sound, "dupp," is the sound of the pulmonary and aortic valves closing during ventricular diastole. The two sounds heard together ("lubb–dupp") is what we know as a heartbeat.

REGULATION

Although transport is the cardiovascular system's major function, this system also plays a role in temperature regulation, as discussed in Chapter 31.

PROTECTION

The cardiovascular system helps to protect the body in two major ways. First, white blood cells, which play an important role in helping us to fight off disease, are circulated throughout the body in the blood. Second, when injury to the skin occurs, the blood has the ability to form a clot. The clot helps to protect us against excessive blood loss. It also helps to prevent microbes from gaining access to the body.

THE EFFECTS OF AGING ON THE CARDIOVASCULAR SYSTEM

As we age, some changes to the cardiovascular system take place. In a healthy older person, these changes do not have a major impact on day-to-day life. However, when the processes of aging are combined with a chronic health condition or a lifetime of unhealthy habits, the effect on cardiovascular function can be major. Age-related changes that occur include less efficient contraction of the heart, a loss of elasticity in the arteries and veins, and decreased numbers of blood cells.

LESS EFFICIENT CONTRACTION

Changes in the tissues of the heart, such as a loss of muscle tone and a loss of elasticity, affect the ability of the heart to contract forcefully, and it takes longer for the heart to complete the cycle of filling and emptying. A healthy older person might find that she tires faster while exercising, because the heart is not able to deliver oxygen and nutrients to the body as efficiently as it once was in times of increased demand. Medical conditions, such as obesity or hypertension, place additional strain on the heart muscle and make the effects of normal aging on the heart worse. The heart of an older person who is ill may barely be able to meet the body's needs for oxygen and nutrients when the person is at rest.

DECREASED ELASTICITY OF THE ARTERIES AND VEINS

As we age, the walls of the arteries and veins lose some of their elasticity.

The loss of elasticity in the walls of the arteries decreases the body's ability to control blood pressure and flow, because the arteries are not able to expand and "bounce back" as easily:

- When the walls of the arteries cannot expand easily, it becomes harder for the blood to flow through them. As a result, resistance increases. Remember from Chapter 22 that resistance is one of the factors that affect blood pressure. An increase in resistance leads to an increase in blood pressure.
- When the walls of the arteries cannot contract easily, the person may experience orthostatic hypotension (a sudden decrease in blood pressure that occurs when the person stands up from a sitting or lying position). This is because the arteries are not able to constrict quickly enough to maintain adequate blood flow to the brain.

The loss of elasticity in the walls of the veins causes them to "stretch out," slowing the flow of blood back to the heart. The valves in the walls of the veins become less effective, which also slows the return of blood to the heart. Immobility and bed rest can make the effects of aging on the veins worse, because the large muscles of the legs are not working to help move the blood back toward the heart.

DECREASED NUMBERS OF BLOOD CELLS

The production of blood cells slows as a person ages. A decreased number of red blood cells affects the blood's ability to deliver oxygen to the tissues. A decreased number of white blood cells puts the older person at higher risk for developing infections, because the body's ability to fight them off is reduced.

DISORDERS OF THE CARDIOVASCULAR SYSTEM

Disorders of the cardiovascular system can involve the blood, the blood vessels, or the heart.

DISORDERS OF THE BLOOD

Blood disorders are often detected through laboratory analysis of the blood. Common blood disorders include anemia, leukemia, and clotting disorders.

Anemia

Anemia is a condition that exists when the ability of the red blood cells to carry oxygen to the tissues is decreased. There are many different types of anemia, but only three major underlying causes:

- **Impaired red blood cell production.** Anemia can result when the body's ability to produce red blood cells is impaired. For example, a disorder that affects the bone marrow, where blood cells are made, can cause a decrease in the number of circulating red blood cells, leading to anemia. Or, the person's diet may not supply the vitamins and minerals that are needed to make red blood cells, or parts of red blood cells. For example, the body needs iron to make hemoglobin, the part of the red blood cell that binds with oxygen. If a person has a diet that is low in iron, the production of hemoglobin will be decreased, leading to anemia.
- **Increased red blood cell destruction.** Red blood cells can be destroyed as the result of an infection or poisoning. Inherited conditions, such as sickle cell anemia, can also result in the destruction of red blood cells. Normally, red blood cells last about 120 days, and then they are broken down and replaced with new red blood cells. In sickle cell anemia, the red blood cells are abnormally shaped and very fragile, and they break down faster than normal. The body cannot make new red blood cells fast enough to replace the ones that are broken down, leading to anemia.
- **Blood loss.** Slow chronic blood loss (such as that resulting from a stomach ulcer, a chronic health condition, or the use of certain medications) can also cause anemia, just by decreasing the amount of circulating blood.

Anemia is a very common disorder among older people. In fact, it is estimated that almost half of the residents in nursing homes have anemia. A person with anemia may experience fatigue, shortness of breath with exertion, a rapid heart rate (tachycardia), heart palpitations (an awareness that the heart is beating), and headaches. The person may feel cold all of the time. These symptoms can significantly impact the health and function of an older person. Older people with anemia have been found to have:

- Decreased mobility
- Increased dependence
- Repeated falls
- Worsening of other medical conditions
- Depression
- Impaired cognitive function
- Decreased life expectancy

As a nursing assistant, you will play an important role in supporting your residents with anemia, and minimizing complications related to the disorder. Guidelines for caring for a person with anemia are given in Guidelines Box 34-1.

Leukemia

Leukemia is the excessive production of white blood cells. The white blood cells are abnormal in structure and they cannot perform their job of protecting the body from infection. Leukemia can be caused by cancer of the bone marrow or by cancer of the lymphatic tissue. Leukemia occurs in people of all ages, and can cause death if treatment is started too late or is not effective. People who have leukemia are at higher risk for developing infections. They may also have bleeding disorders, which can cause them to bruise very easily or bleed from their gums during oral care.

Bleeding Disorders

There are two types of bleeding disorders. Either the blood clots too much, or not enough.

In some people, the blood clots too easily. Clots can form in the blood vessels, blocking the flow of blood and depriving the tissues of oxygen and nutrients. The blood clots are called **thrombi** (singular, **thrombus**). People who have blood that clots too easily may need to take medications called **anticoagulants** or "blood thinners" to help keep clots from forming where they are not needed.

Other people have the opposite problem—their blood does not form clots when it is supposed to (for example, after an injury). These people may lack fibrinogen, the protein in the blood plasma that assists with clotting. Or, they may have a low platelet count. (Recall that platelets are the blood cells that participate in

Guidelines Box 34-1   Guidelines for Caring For A Person With Anemia

WHAT YOU DO	WHY YOU DO IT
Provide for frequent rest periods, especially after activities that require exertion.	Anemia decreases the blood's ability to transport oxygen to the cells. As a result, a person with anemia will become tired very easily, and will need frequent rest periods.
Keep frequently used personal items within easy reach of the resident.	Keeping personal items handy reduces the amount of energy the person needs to use while carrying out daily activities.
Watch for signs of discomfort or distress during periods of activity.	To try to meet the body's demand for oxygen, the heart pumps faster, and the respiratory rate increases. As a result, the resident may experience chest pain, dizziness, and shortness of breath.
Take necessary safety precautions and provide appropriate support when assisting the resident with transferring or walking.	Older people who have anemia often experience dizziness when they stand up from a sitting or lying position. In addition, they may experience muscle fatigue. Both of these factors increase the person's risk for falls.
Provide the resident with warm clothing, or an extra blanket.	A person with anemia may become chilled very easily.
Encourage good nutrition, and report poor intake to the nurse.	Proper nutrition is necessary to provide the body with the vitamins and minerals necessary to make red blood cells and hemoglobin.

clot formation.) For these people, even a small bump can cause a large bruise, while a more severe injury can result in a fatal hemorrhage.

TELL THE NURSE

People who are taking anticoagulant medications and those with disorders that affect the ability of the blood to form clots are at risk for bleeding, which can have serious consequences. Be sure to report any of the following observations to the nurse immediately:

- Any signs of bruising or bleeding under the skin
- Bleeding from any area of the body (such as the gums or nose)
- Blood in the urine or stool

DISORDERS OF THE BLOOD VESSELS

Atherosclerosis

Atherosclerosis is blocking of the arteries. Blood is unable to flow freely through the arteries because **plaque** (a fatty deposit) builds up on the inside of the vessel wall (Fig. 34-9). The plaque impairs the flow of blood through the arteries, which means that less oxygen and nutrients are delivered to the tissues of the body. Plaque also makes the normally smooth inner lining of the artery rough, which can cause blood clots (thrombi) to form. Sometimes a blood clot breaks off and becomes an embolus. An **embolus** (plural, **emboli**) is a blood clot that breaks loose and moves through the bloodstream. An embolus can become stuck, blocking the circulation. If the

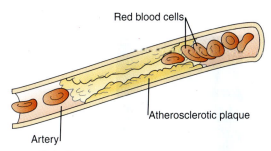

Figure 34-9

In atherosclerosis, fatty plaque builds up on the inside of the arteries, blocking the free flow of blood. This is particularly dangerous when the artery supplies a vital organ such as the heart, brain, or kidneys.

embolus blocks one of the important arteries of the brain, lungs, or heart, it can be life threatening. The plaque also interferes with the elasticity of the arterial walls, making them brittle and prone to breaking (a condition called **arteriosclerosis**). This "hardening of the arteries" can lead to hemorrhages (bleeding) in the small vessels.

Depending on which arteries are affected, atherosclerosis can have serious consequences. The arteries that supply the brain, heart, kidneys, and legs are affected most often.

- Atherosclerosis of the arteries that supply the brain can cause a stroke. Strokes are discussed in detail in Chapter 35.
- Atherosclerosis of the arteries that supply the heart can cause myocardial infarction ("heart attack"). Myocardial infarction is discussed later in this chapter.
- Atherosclerosis of the arteries that supply the kidneys can cause renal failure, discussed in Chapter 39.
- Atherosclerosis of the arteries that supply the legs can cause **peripheral vascular disease.** In peripheral vascular disease, decreased blood flow to the leg muscles causes pain and cramping when the person walks. The pain and cramping, called *claudication,* occurs because the muscles are not receiving enough oxygen. In severe cases, the tissues in the leg die from lack of oxygen, and amputation may be necessary.

Although the exact cause of atherosclerosis is unknown, we do know that several factors contribute to the development of atherosclerosis. Diabetes, hypertension, and obesity are all medical conditions that have been associated with atherosclerosis. Heredity and stress may also play a role. Smoking, eating a diet high in choles-

terol and saturated (unhealthy) fat, and a lack of physical activity can also increase a person's chances of developing atherosclerosis.

Venous Disorders

Loss of elasticity and decreased efficiency of the valves in the walls of the veins causes blood to "pool" in the legs, which can put the person at risk for several disorders:

- **Varicose veins.** In this condition, pooling of blood in the superficial veins (that is, the veins just underneath the skin) causes the veins to become swollen and "knotty" in appearance (Fig. 34-10). A person with varicose veins may experience pain, aching, swelling, or a feeling of heaviness in the legs. Varicose veins also put the person at risk for developing other venous disorders, such as phlebitis or venous (stasis) ulcers.
- **Phlebitis.** In this condition, pooling of blood in the vein causes the lining of the vein to become inflamed. The skin over the affected vein is reddened, and the area feels hard and hot to the touch. Phlebitis is often very painful.
- **Venous thrombosis.** In this disorder, blood clots (thrombi) form in the veins where the blood pools, because the blood is moving so slowly. When the blood clots cause inflammation of the lining of the vein, you may hear this condition referred to as **thrombophlebitis.** Blood clots can form in the superficial veins or the deep veins. When the blood clots occur in the deep veins, the condition is called **deep venous thrombosis (DVT).** Pain, redness, swelling, and warmth in the lower leg are all possible signs of DVT and should be reported to the nurse immediately. People with DVT are at high risk for **pulmonary embolism,** a life-threatening condition that occurs when an embolus becomes stuck in the pulmonary artery, the artery that carries unoxygenated blood from the heart to the lungs. If blood cannot reach the lungs, then it cannot pick up the oxygen it needs for the rest of the body.
- **Venous (stasis) ulcers.** These ulcers are seen on the lower legs, usually in the ankle area. The pressure of the pooled blood in the veins forces plasma out of the blood vessels and into the surrounding tissues. Swelling occurs, and the skin becomes fragile and inflamed. Eventually, the skin breaks down, resulting in an open sore.

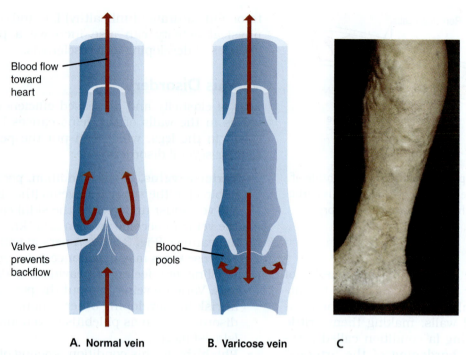

Blood flow toward heart

Valve prevents backflow

Blood pools

A. Normal vein   **B. Varicose vein**   **C**

Figure 34-10

Many older people, particularly women, have varicose veins. **(A)** In a healthy vein, the valves help blood to flow back toward the heart and prevent it from pooling. **(B)** In varicose veins, the valves no longer function properly, allowing the blood to pool. **(C)** The pooling of blood in the veins causes them to become swollen and "knotty" in appearance.

Generally, people with venous disorders experience pain and have difficulty with mobility. The doctor may order the use of leg exercises, anti-embolism (TED) stockings, or both to treat or prevent venous disorders.

Leg exercises

Leg exercises help to move blood back to the heart and prevent the formation of clots. The doctor or physical therapist may order the leg exercises you learned as part of the range-of-motion exercises described in Chapter 32 (Procedure 32-1) to be carried out at routine times. Or, a specific exercise routine may be ordered. Always check with the nurse to see if there are any specific instructions or precautions for your resident.

Anti-embolism (TED) stockings

Anti-embolism (TED) stockings are made of a tight-fitting elastic fabric. The stockings, which may be knee-high or thigh-high, are specially fitted for the person by the nurse or the physical therapist. The elastic fabric applies pressure, compressing the veins and helping to return blood to the heart. This helps to prevent pooling of blood in the legs.

Anti-embolism (TED) stockings are usually ordered to be applied before the person gets out of bed. Once the person stands up, gravity increases blood flow to the veins in the lower legs, causing the veins to widen and the blood to pool. The anti-embolism (TED) stockings are usually removed at bed time. Procedure 34-1 describes how to apply anti-embolism (TED) stockings.

DISORDERS OF THE HEART

Heart disorders are very common in the United States, especially among older people. Perhaps more than any other organ, the heart is affected by the choices we make in life (Box 34-1). Common heart disorders in adults include coronary artery disease, heart failure, and dysrhythmias.

Coronary Artery Disease

Coronary artery disease occurs when the coronary arteries narrow as a result of atherosclerosis. Recall that the coronary arteries supply the heart muscle with blood containing oxygen and nutrients. Initially, the heart muscle may receive enough oxygen to work properly when the body is at rest, but it may be unable to meet the increased needs brought on by activity. Eventually, one or

BOX 34-1 Risk Factors for Heart Disease

Conditions that are known to increase a person's risk of developing heart disease are called *cardiac risk factors.* We can control some of our risk factors for heart disease. Others are out of our control.

Risk factors for heart disease that we cannot change include the following:

- **Age.** The risk of developing heart disease increases with age.
- **Gender.** Men are at greater risk of developing heart disease at an earlier age than women are. However, after a woman goes through menopause, her risk of developing heart disease is the same as a man's.
- **Heredity.** People who have parents or siblings with heart disease are more likely to develop heart disease themselves.
- **Body build.** Some people tend to put on weight in the abdomen or chest ("apples"), while others tend to carry it in the buttocks or thighs ("pears"). "Apple"-shaped people are more likely to develop heart disease than "pear"-shaped people.

The following risk factors for heart disease can be controlled by making lifestyle changes:

- **Smoking**
- **Being physically inactive**
- **Being overweight or obese**
- **Consuming a diet high in saturated fat, cholesterol, and sodium**
- **Having poorly controlled hypertension**
- **Having poorly controlled diabetes**

Many national organizations, such as the American Heart Association, provide information and education about "healthy heart living." By following the advice of these organizations, many people are able to maintain good cardiovascular function well into old age. The keys to cardiovascular health are exercise; a diet that emphasizes fruits, vegetables, whole grains, and healthy fats and that is low in saturated (unhealthy) fats; and avoidance of smoking.

- **Exercise** helps to keep the heart muscle strong and working efficiently. Exercise also helps us to maintain a healthy body weight, and is an important measure for preventing or controlling conditions that can contribute to heart disease, such as diabetes and hypertension.
- **Eating a heart-healthy diet** helps to keep the heart muscle and blood vessels healthy. Like exercise, a heart-healthy diet also helps to prevent or control conditions that can contribute to heart disease such as excess weight, diabetes, and hypertension.
- **Avoiding smoking** is important because chemicals in tobacco smoke cause the blood vessels to constrict, depriving the heart of the oxygen and nutrients it needs to function properly.

more of the coronary arteries may become so narrow that no blood gets through, causing areas of the heart muscle to die.

Coronary artery disease is treated in a number of ways. Medications are available that help to keep the arteries open, permitting maximum blood flow. Balloon angioplasty is a technique that involves inserting a catheter with a small balloon on the tip into the narrow part of the affected artery. The balloon is inflated, pressing the plaque against the arterial wall to create a larger opening for the blood to flow through. Then the balloon is deflated and the catheter is removed (Fig. 34-11A). Sometimes, balloon angioplasty is done along with placement of a small coiled wire called a *stent.* The stent supports the artery walls, helping to keep the artery open (Fig. 34-11B). When the blockage is severe, surgery may be performed to bypass the blocked arteries and reestablish blood flow. The medical term for this type of surgery is coronary artery bypass graft (CABG) surgery. The acronym CABG is pronounced like "cabbage."

Conditions that are closely related to coronary artery disease include angina pectoris and myocardial infarction.

Angina pectoris

Angina pectoris is the classic chest pain that is felt as a result of the heart muscle being deprived of oxygen. Anginal pain varies among individuals. Some people describe it as a pain in the center of the chest. Others experience pain that starts in the chest and extends to the arm or neck. A person who is experiencing angina may feel as though he is suffocating, and he may become very anxious.

Many residents experience angina quite frequently and know what it is. These residents often keep nitroglycerin pills on hand to relieve the pain when it occurs. Nitroglycerin relaxes the arteries, increasing the flow of blood. If you have been trained to help a resident with her nitroglycerin, avoid handling the pills with your bare hands. The medication can be absorbed through the skin, which can cause a decrease in your blood pressure and a pounding headache.

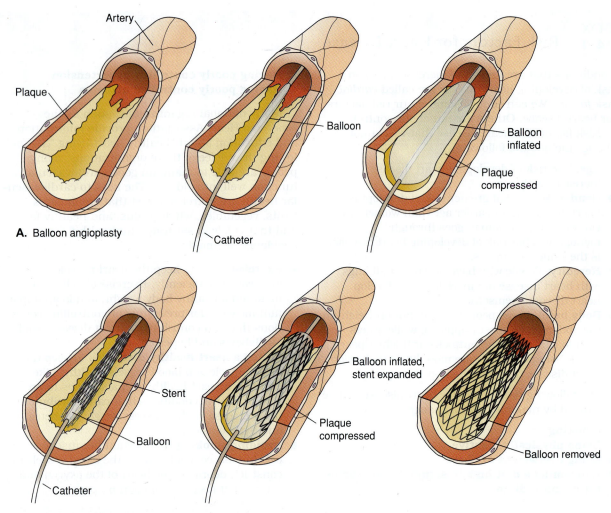

A. Balloon angioplasty

B. Balloon angioplasty with stent placement

Figure 34-11

(A) In balloon angioplasty, a catheter with a balloon on the tip is passed into the narrowed part of the artery. The balloon is expanded, pushing the plaque to the sides of the arterial wall and widening the artery. **(B)** Sometimes balloon angioplasty is done along with stent placement. The stent, a small wire cage, provides additional support to keep the artery open.

Myocardial infarction

A **myocardial infarction** is a "heart attack." A myocardial infarction occurs when one or more of the coronary arteries becomes completely blocked, preventing blood from reaching the parts of the heart that are fed by the affected arteries (Fig. 34-12). The lack of blood (and vital oxygen) causes the tissue to die. The dead tissue is called an *infarct*.

The severity of the myocardial infarction depends on the extent of the tissue damaged and the part of the heart affected. Although a myocardial infarction that affects the atria may not be life threatening, one that severely damages the ventricles can reduce the heart's ability to pump

blood to vital organs and cause death. Early recognition of the symptoms of a myocardial infarction (see Chapter 19) and early treatment can greatly increase a person's chances of surviving. Medications that help to maintain a normal heartbeat and restore blood flow to the affected area can greatly improve the person's outcome.

Heart Failure

Heart failure occurs when the heart is unable to pump enough blood to meet the body's needs. Heart failure has many causes. For example, disorders that cause the ventricles to lose muscle tone and become large and flabby can cause heart failure. Heart failure can also occur as a

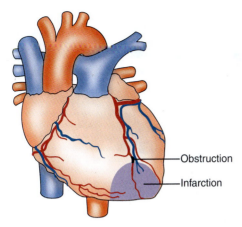

Figure 34-12

A heart attack occurs when one or more of the coronary arteries becomes blocked, preventing blood from reaching the myocardium. The lack of oxygen and nutrients causes the tissue that is supplied by the affected artery to die.

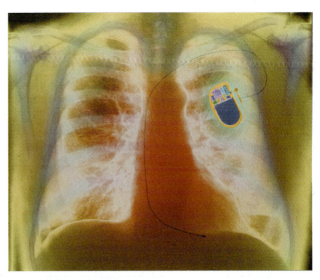

Figure 34-13

An electronic pacemaker is a battery-operated device used to treat heart block. The pacemaker sends out an electrical signal that stimulates the heart to contract when the person's heart rate drops below a pre-programmed rate. In this photograph, you can see the pacemaker above the person's ribcage. A dark blue lead connects the pacemaker to the person's heart, which is the red area in the lower right of the photograph. (© *Salisbury District Hospital/Photo Researchers, Inc.*)

result of a myocardial infarction that leaves the ventricles unable to function properly.

Heart failure can be either "right-sided" or "left-sided." Right-sided heart failure causes blood to back up in the venous system because the right ventricle's ability to pump the blood into the pulmonary circulation is impaired. In a person with right-sided heart failure, the veins in the legs and abdomen become swollen, and fluid may leak into the tissues, causing significant edema and skin breakdown. Left-sided heart failure (sometimes called *congestive heart failure*) causes the blood to back up in the lungs because the left ventricle's ability to pump the blood into the systemic circulation is impaired. The excess blood in the vessels of the lungs causes fluid to leak into the lung tissues, which causes congestion and makes breathing difficult.

For people with heart failure, medications may be used to help increase the heart's ability to pump more effectively and to pull excess fluid from the tissues. Many people with severe heart failure have their fluids restricted and their intake and output very carefully measured and monitored.

Dysrhythmias

A dysrhythmia is an irregular heart rate, rhythm, or both. There are many different types of dysrhythmias. Dysrhythmias can occur when the conduction system of the heart is not working properly. Dysrhythmias can cause a person to experience heart palpitations, fatigue, dizziness,

or fainting. Dysrhythmias can also increase the person's risk for a heart attack or stroke. Many of your residents will take medications to control a dysrhythmia.

Heart block is a common type of dysrhythmia. Heart block can result from a myocardial infarction that damages the conduction pathway, or it may occur as part of the normal aging process. A heart block causes the heart to slow down significantly, leading to dizziness or fainting episodes. Heart block is usually treated with an electronic pacemaker, a device that stimulates the heart to contract. The electronic pacemaker consists of a small, battery-operated device implanted under the skin below the collarbone and two wires that connect to the right side of the heart (Fig. 34-13). When the person's heart rate drops below a programmed rate, the battery-operated device sends a small electrical impulse through the wires that stimulates the heart muscle to contract. The electronic pacemaker must be checked routinely to make sure that it is functioning properly. A trained technician can perform these checks over the telephone using a special device. You may be responsible for escorting a resident to the telephone at the nurses' station for one of these appointments.

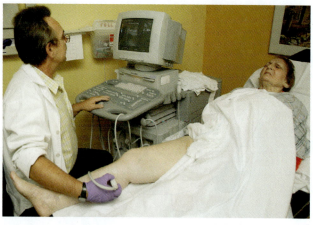

Figure 34-14
Doppler ultrasound is used to check the blood flow in the large vessels of the arms and legs. Here, the technician is using ultrasound to evaluate the blood flow through a resident's legs to make sure that deep venous thrombosis (DVT) or other problems do not develop. (© *Keith/Custom Medical Stock Photo*)

DIAGNOSIS OF CARDIOVASCULAR DISORDERS

Tests used to diagnose and monitor cardiovascular problems include the following:

- **Electrocardiography.** In electrocardiography, sensors are attached to the person's chest. These sensors pick up the electrical activity of the heart and record it on a piece of paper. The tracing is called an *electrocardiogram* (EKG, ECG). An EKG shows abnormalities in the conduction system of the heart.
- **Echocardiography.** In echocardiography, sound waves are bounced against the body to produce an image. A computer translates the sound waves into an image. Echocardiography can provide the doctor with much helpful information, including the size and shape of the heart, its pumping strength, and the location and extent of any damage to its tissues.
- **Doppler ultrasound.** In Doppler ultrasound, sound waves are used to check the blood flow in the large arteries and veins of the arms and legs (Fig. 34-14).
- **Radiography.** Radiographs, commonly known as "x-rays," are often used in the diagnosis of cardiovascular disease. A chest x-ray can show enlargement of the ventricles. Sometimes, a special dye is injected into the veins and then an x-ray is taken. The dye allows the doctor to see any abnormalities in the vessels of the heart or other parts of the body.

CARDIAC REHABILITATION

Cardiac rehabilitation focuses on helping a person with cardiovascular disease regain strength and adopt habits that will help the cardiovascular system become healthier. For example, a person who has had a heart attack or who is recovering from heart surgery may receive cardiac rehabilitation. Many people with cardiovascular disease benefit greatly from cardiac rehabilitation, especially if rehabilitation is started early. Cardiac rehabilitation gives people the energy and ability to pursue things that they enjoy doing, which improves quality of life.

A person who is in cardiac rehabilitation will begin an exercise program under the guidance of a therapist who specializes in cardiac disorders, or a nurse. The exercise program is designed to strengthen the heart muscle and make it a more effective pump. As the person grows stronger, the therapist or nurse will work with the person to develop an exercise plan that will become a part of the person's daily routine. A dietitian will work with the person to teach him about dietary changes that are needed to help control obesity and blood cholesterol levels. Avoidance of unhealthy habits, such as smoking, may require the use of medications and supportive emotional therapy.

Helping Hands and a Caring Heart
FOCUS ON HUMANISTIC HEALTH CARE

A person who has had a heart attack or heart surgery may not want to participate in cardiac rehabilitation. The person may be afraid that any type of activity will put too much stress on the heart. Or, the person may be depressed or in denial. When you are caring for a resident who needs cardiac rehabilitation, use empathy and good communication skills to help reassure and comfort the person. Report your observations of any emotional difficulties to the nurse immediately.

SUMMARY

- The cardiovascular system, also known as the circulatory system, is made up of the blood, the blood vessels, the lymphatic system, and the heart.
  - Blood consists of plasma and blood cells (red blood cells, white blood cells, and platelets).
  - Arteries carry blood away from the heart, and veins carry blood to the heart. The transfer of substances into and out of the blood occurs in the capillary bed.
  - The lymphatic system is a one-way system that returns fluid that leaks into the tissues to the bloodstream.
  - The heart is the muscular organ that powers circulation.
    - The heart has four chambers. The atria receive blood from the body, and the ventricles send blood to the body.
    - The heart valves make sure that blood flows through the heart in the proper direction.
    - The heart's conduction system makes and conducts the electrical impulses that cause the heart to contract regularly.
    - The coronary circulation supplies the heart with oxygen and nutrients.
- The main function of the cardiovascular system is to transport oxygen, nutrients, and other substances *to* the tissues, and remove carbon dioxide and other wastes *from* the tissues.
  - The pattern of circulation involves two parallel circuits. The right side of the heart

pumps blood into the lungs, where it picks up oxygen. The left side of the heart pumps the oxygenated blood to the rest of the body.
  - During systole, the heart contracts, sending blood out of the heart. During diastole, the heart relaxes, allowing the chambers to fill. The atria are in systole when the ventricles are in diastole, and vice versa.
- As we age, the heart contracts less efficiently, there is a loss of elasticity in the arteries and veins, and the number of blood cells decreases.
  - Less efficient contraction of the heart can cause an older person to tire more easily with exertion.
  - Loss of elasticity in the arteries decreases the body's ability to control blood pressure and flow, which can lead to hypertension and orthostatic hypotension. Loss of elasticity in the veins slows the return of blood to the heart and increases the person's risk for venous disorders that develop when blood pools in the legs.
  - A decrease in the number of blood cells puts the older person at risk for anemia and infections.
- Disorders of the cardiovascular system can affect the blood, the blood vessels, or the heart.
  - Disorders of the blood include anemia, leukemia, and bleeding disorders.

- Disorders of the blood vessels include atherosclerosis, varicose veins, phlebitis, venous thrombosis, and venous (stasis) ulcers.
  - Atherosclerosis is blocking of the arteries. Depending on which arteries are affected, atherosclerosis can lead to strokes, heart attacks, kidney failure, or peripheral vascular disease.
  - Disorders that affect the veins are usually caused by widening of the veins, which allows blood to pool in the legs. Venous disorders often cause pain and swelling, and contribute to mobility problems.
- Disorders of the heart include coronary artery disease, heart failure, and dysrhythmias.
  - Coronary artery disease is caused by a narrowing of the arteries that supply the heart muscle with oxygen and nutrients.
    - Angina pectoris is chest pain that results from the heart muscle being deprived of oxygen.
    - A myocardial infarction occurs when the blood supply to the heart muscle is completely obstructed.
  - Heart failure results from the heart's inability to pump blood in sufficient amounts to supply the body.
  - Dysrhythmias can occur when the conduction system of the heart is not working properly. A person with heart block, a type of dysrhythmia, may have an electronic pacemaker implanted to stimulate regular contraction of the heart.
- Tests used to diagnose and monitor cardiac problems include electrocardiography, echocardiography, Doppler ultrasound, and radiography.
- The goal of cardiac rehabilitation is to help a person with cardiovascular disease to regain strength and adopt habits that will improve the health of the cardiovascular system. An exercise plan and dietary and other lifestyle changes are part of cardiac rehabilitation.

Applying Anti-embolism (TED) Stockings

WHY YOU DO IT   Use of anti-embolism (TED) stockings as ordered helps to prevent the formation of blood clots in the lower legs.

Getting Ready WGKIEPS

1. Complete the "Getting Ready" steps.

Supplies

- anti-embolism (TED) stockings in the correct size

Procedure

2. Make sure that the bed is positioned at a comfortable working height (to promote good body mechanics) and that the wheels are locked. If the side rails are in use, lower the side rail on the working side of the bed. The side rail on the opposite side of the bed should remain up.

3. Help the person into the supine position.

4. Fanfold the top linens to the foot of the bed. Adjust the person's clothing as necessary to expose one leg at a time.

5. Turn the stocking inside out down to the heel.

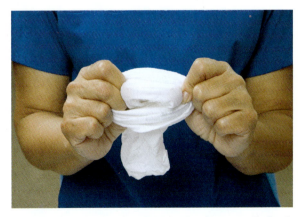

Step 5 Turn the stocking inside out down to the heel.

6. Slip the foot of the stocking over the person's toes, foot, and heel. The stocking has an opening in the toe area, which allows the health care team to assess the person's toes to make sure they are receiving enough blood. Depending on the manufacturer, this opening may be on the top or on the bottom of the stocking.

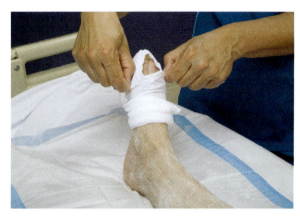

Step 6 Slip the foot of the stocking over the person's toes, foot, and heel.

7. Grasp the top of the stocking and pull it up the person's leg. The stocking will turn itself right-side out as you pull it up the person's leg.

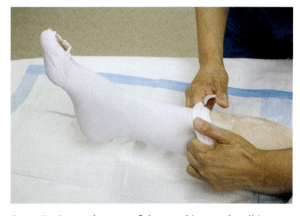

Step 7 Grasp the top of the stocking and pull it up the person's leg.

(continued)

8. Check to make sure that the stocking is not twisted and that it fits snugly against the person's leg, with no wrinkles. Also make sure that the stocking fits smoothly over the heel and that the opening in the toe area is correctly located in the toe region.

9. Cover that leg, expose the other leg, and repeat steps 5 through 8.

10. Prepare the person for transferring out of bed. If the person will be staying in bed, help the person back into a comfortable position, straighten the bottom linens, draw the top linens over the person, and raise the head of the bed as the person requests. Make sure that the bed is lowered to its lowest position and that the wheels are locked.

Finishing Up CLOSWR

11. Complete the "Finishing Up" steps.

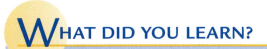

WHAT DID YOU LEARN?

Multiple Choice

Select the single best answer for each of the following questions.

1. The formation of artery-clogging plaque on the inside of the arteries is called:
   a. Atherosclerosis
   b. Arterioles
   c. Anemia
   d. Myocardial infarction

2. What is the function of the cardiovascular system?
   a. Transport of substances throughout the body
   b. Regulation of body temperature
   c. Protection of the body from blood loss and infection
   d. All of the above

3. Which circulation supplies the tissues of the heart with oxygen and nutrients?
   a. Pulmonary circulation
   b. Systemic circulation
   c. Coronary circulation
   d. Pericardial circulation

4. Which of the following is a risk factor for cardiovascular disease?
   a. Poorly controlled hypertension
   b. A diet high in cholesterol and saturated fats
   c. Lack of physical activity
   d. All of the above

5. Mrs. Briggs is on your regular assignment. She is 93 years old. The nurse tells you that Mrs. Briggs' blood work results show that she has anemia. Because of this condition, you know that you will need to take which of the following measures when caring for Mrs. Briggs?
   a. Elevate her lower limbs to control edema
   b. Provide rest periods in between care activities
   c. Apply anti-embolism stockings before she gets out of bed
   d. Examine her calves carefully for excessive redness and warmth

6. You are told that Mr. Deering is now taking an anticoagulant. Which of the following observations would be important to report to the nurse right away?
   a. His gums bleed when you provide oral care

   b. You notice that his urine is tinged with a pink color
   c. He has several new bruises that were not there yesterday
   d. All of the above

7. Mrs. Getz has orders to use anti-embolism (TED) stockings. Which of the following care measures is correct? Anti-embolism (TED) stockings must be:
   a. Applied before getting out of bed in the morning and removed at bed time
   b. Applied at bed time and removed before getting out of bed in the morning
   c. Applied like regular stockings
   d. Removed every 2 hours to check for reddened areas underneath

8. The purpose of cardiac rehabilitation is to:
   a. Strengthen the leg muscles to improve the resident's ability to perform a regular exercise routine
   b. Measure the electrical activity of the heart
   c. Provide emotional support to a resident who has had a heart attack
   d. Strengthen the heart muscle to improve its ability to pump blood to the body

9. Angina pectoris is a classic pain that is felt when the heart muscle is deprived of oxygen. This pain can be experienced in all of the following areas, except the:
   a. arm
   b. calf
   c. chest
   d. jaw

10. Deep vein thrombosis (DVT) is a serious condition that can occur in a person who has limited mobility. Which of the following statements is true about this condition?
   a. It is treated by a surgical procedure to implant a stent to keep the artery wall open.
   b. It occurs when the heart cannot pump effectively to meet the body's needs, causing the blood to back up in the body.
   c. It will cause a heart block that will disrupt the heart's normal rhythm.
   d. It usually causes pain and redness in the calf.

Matching

Match each numbered item with its appropriate lettered description.

Set 1

_____ **1.** Red blood cells (erythrocytes)

_____ **2.** White blood cells (leukocytes)

_____ **3.** Ventricles

_____ **4.** Veins

_____ **5.** Atria

_____ **6.** Arteries

_____ **7.** Systole

_____ **8.** Pulmonary circulation

_____ **9.** Systemic circulation

_____ **10.** Diastole

a. Upper chambers of the heart, which receive blood from the body

b. Vessels that carry blood away from the heart

c. Active phase of the cardiac cycle

d. Blood cells that help the body to fight infection

e. Circuit that sends newly oxygenated blood to the body

f. Resting phase of the cardiac cycle

g. Blood cells that contain hemoglobin and carry oxygen

h. Lower chambers of the heart, which pump blood to the body

i. Circuit that sends oxygen-poor blood to the lungs to pick up oxygen

j. Vessels that return blood to the heart

Set 2

_____ **1.** Atherosclerosis

_____ **2.** Embolus

_____ **3.** Varicose veins

_____ **4.** Phlebitis

_____ **5.** Dysrhythmia

_____ **6.** Electrocardiography

_____ **7.** Myocardial infarction

a. A blood clot that breaks off and moves through the bloodstream

b. The medical term for a "heart attack"

c. An irregular heart rate, rhythm, or both

d. A method of recording the electrical activity of the heart, used for diagnostic and monitoring purposes

e. Blocking of arteries caused by the build-up of plaque on the inside of the vessel wall

f. A condition that results from pooling of blood in the veins just underneath the skin, causing them to become swollen and "knotty" in appearance

g. Inflammation of a vein

STOP and Think!

You are caring for Mr. Becker, a 74-year-old man with a history of heart disease. Mr. Becker keeps nitroglycerin in his bedside table to use when he has an angina attack. As you are assisting Mr. Becker back into his room from the dining room, he starts to complain of a tightness in his chest and seems to be having difficulty breathing. His lips also look a little blue. He asks you to help him with his nitro-glycerin pill. What safety precaution needs to be taken while handling nitroglycerin? What else should you do?

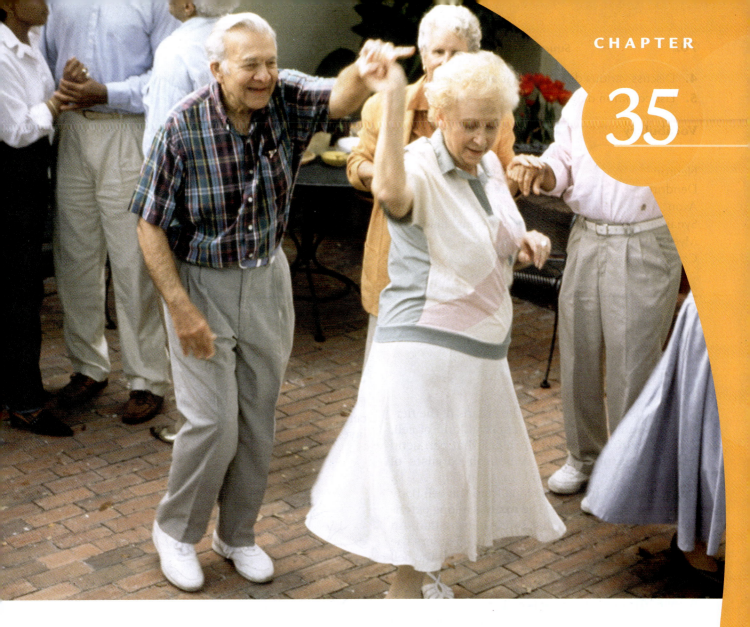

The Nervous System

WHAT WILL YOU LEARN?

The nervous system consists of the brain, the spinal cord, and the nerves. The nervous system receives information at a great rate, from both inside the body and outside of it. It then processes this information and issues instructions to other organ systems to carry out. "Command central" of the human body, the nervous system, is the subject of this chapter. When you are finished with this chapter, you will be able to:

1. List and describe the structures that make up the two main divisions of the nervous system.
2. Discuss the main functions of the nervous system.
3. Describe how aging affects the nervous system.

Photo: The nervous system helps us to move with grace and coordination by directing the activity of the muscles. (© Tom & Dee Ann McCarthy/CORBIS)

4. Discuss various disorders that affect the nervous system.

5. List common diagnostic procedures that are used to help detect nervous system disorders.

Vocabulary Use the CD in the front of your book to hear these terms pronounced and defined:

Neuron	Peripheral nervous	Transient ischemic	Coma
Dendrites	system (PNS)	attack (TIA)	Comatose
Axon	Meninges	Stroke	Persistent vegetative
Synapse	Cerebrospinal fluid	Hemiplegia	state
Myelin	(CSF)	Parkinson's disease	Quadriplegia
Central nervous system	Sensory nerves	Epilepsy	Paraplegia
(CNS)	Motor nerves	Multiple sclerosis (MS)	

STRUCTURE OF THE NERVOUS SYSTEM

Nervous tissue, which forms the organs of the nervous system, is made up of a special kind of cell, called a neuron. A **neuron** is a cell that can send and receive information. A neuron consists of dendrites, a cell body, and an axon (Fig. 35-1). **Dendrites** are short extensions from the cell body that *receive* information. The **axon** is a long extension from the cell body that *sends* information. An electrical signal, called a nerve impulse, enters the neuron at the dendrites. It passes through the cell body and travels down the axon, and then on to the dendrites of the next neuron in line. The movement of the nerve impulse is called *conduction*. The axon of one neuron does not actually connect with the dendrites of the next (Fig. 35-1). Instead, chemicals called neurotransmitters carry the nerve impulse across the gap between the axon of one neuron and the dendrites of the next. This gap is called a **synapse.** The axons of some neurons are wrapped in **myelin,** a fatty, white substance that protects the axon. Myelin also helps to speed the conduction of nerve impulses along the axon.

The nervous system has two main divisions, the central nervous system and the peripheral nervous system (Fig. 35-2). The **central nervous system (CNS)** consists of the brain and spinal cord. The central nervous system receives information, processes it, and issues instructions. The **peripheral nervous system (PNS)** consists of the nerves outside of the brain and spinal cord. A nerve is simply a bundle of axons, wrapped in a connective tissue sheath. The peripheral nervous system receives information from the environment, and carries commands from the brain and spinal cord to the other organs of the body, such as the muscles.

THE CENTRAL NERVOUS SYSTEM

Because it is so vital to the body's functioning, the central nervous system is well protected by three layers of connective tissue, called **meninges,** the

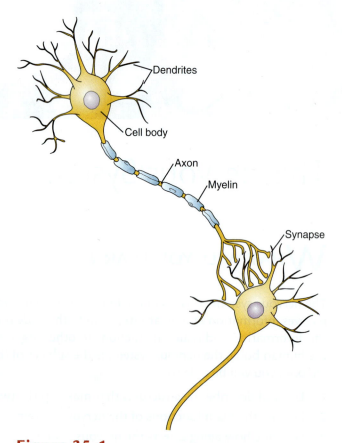

Figure 35-1
Neurons are special cells that have the ability to send and receive information.

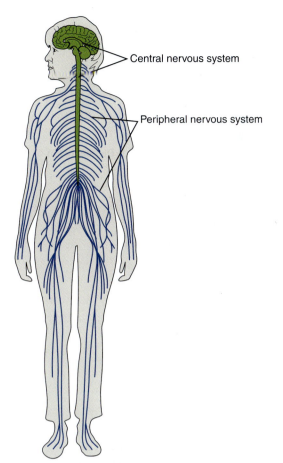

Figure 35-2
The nervous system has two main divisions, the central nervous system and the peripheral nervous system. "Peripheral" means "along the edge" or "away from the center."

Central nervous system

Peripheral nervous system

bony skull, and vertebrae (Fig. 35-3). The three meninges are, from the inside out:

- The *pia mater*, a thin delicate layer of tissue rich in blood vessels that is attached to the surface of the brain and spinal cord
- The *arachnoid mater*, the web-like middle layer
- The *dura mater*, a thick, tough outer layer that is attached to the inside of the skull and the vertebrae

The space between the pia mater and the arachnoid mater contains **cerebrospinal fluid (CSF),** a clear fluid that circulates around the brain and spinal cord and acts as an additional "shock absorber" to protect these structures.

The Brain

The brain, a large, soft mass of nervous tissue, is where information is processed and instructions are issued. The brain has four parts: the cere-

brum, the diencephalon, the brain stem, and the cerebellum (Fig. 35-3).

The cerebrum

The cerebrum is the largest part of the brain, with the characteristic "folds" that we always picture when we think of a brain (Fig. 35-3). The cerebrum:

- Controls the voluntary movement of muscles
- Gives meaning to information received from the eyes, ears, nose, taste buds, and sensory receptors in the skin
- Allows us to speak, remember, think, and feel emotions

A deep groove divides the cerebrum into two hemispheres, the left hemisphere (or "left brain") and the right hemisphere (or "right brain"). The right and left hemispheres communicate with each other and are connected by a structure called the *corpus callosum*. The right side of the brain controls the left side of the body, and vice versa. So, an injury to the tissues in the left side of the brain may result in loss of function on the right side of the body.

The diencephalon

The diencephalon contains the thalamus and the hypothalamus (Fig. 35-3). The thalamus sorts out the impulses that arrive via the spinal cord from other parts of the body and sends them to the correct part of the cerebrum. The hypothalamus controls body temperature, fluid balance, appetite, sleep cycles, and some of the emotions, and regulates the pituitary gland, a gland you will learn more about in Chapter 37.

The brain stem

The brain stem connects the spinal cord to the brain. It has three parts: the midbrain, the pons, and the medulla (Fig. 35-3). The medulla contains the centers that control respiration, heartbeat, and blood pressure.

The cerebellum

The cerebellum helps to coordinate the brain's commands to the muscles so that the muscles move smoothly and in an orderly fashion. It also plays a role in balance.

The Spinal cord

The spinal cord is a "cord" of nervous tissue that extends from the base of the brain downward, to a point approximately even with your

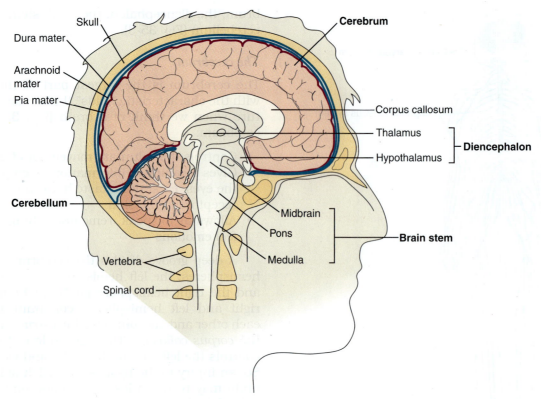

Figure 35-3

The brain and the spinal cord make up the central nervous system (CNS). The brain has four parts: the cerebrum, the diencephalon, the brain stem, and the cerebellum. Three layers of connective tissue, called the dura mater, the arachnoid mater, and the pia mater, help to cushion and protect the brain and spinal cord. Additional protection is provided by the bony skull and vertebrae.

bellybutton. The vertebrae (the bones that make up your spine) surround and protect the spinal cord.

The spinal cord is the main connection between the brain and the rest of the body. Pathways of nerve tissue in the spinal cord, called *tracts*, carry messages to and from the brain. Ascending tracts carry information from the peripheral nervous system to the brain. Descending tracts carry information from the brain to the peripheral nervous system.

THE PERIPHERAL NERVOUS SYSTEM

The peripheral nervous system consists of the nerves, or the lines of communication between the central nervous system and the rest of the body. Every part of the body is innervated, or supplied, by nerves, which form a vast network throughout the body.

The nerves that form the peripheral nervous system are either sensory nerves or motor nerves. **Sensory nerves** carry information from the "outside in." In other words, the sensory nerves carry information from the internal organs and the outside world to the spinal cord and up into the brain so that the brain can analyze the information. **Motor nerves** carry information from the "inside out." In other words, the motor nerves carry commands from the brain down the spinal cord and out to the muscles and organs of the body. Motor nerves allow the brain to control voluntary muscle movement and the involuntary functions of the internal organs.

Thirty-one pairs of nerves, called spinal nerves, connect to the spinal cord. Each spinal nerve consists of one sensory nerve and one motor nerve. The spinal nerves that innervate the arms and the upper part of the body are located in the neck region, while the spinal nerves that innervate the legs and the lower part of the body are located in the back.

Some nerves are connected directly to the brain. These nerves are called cranial nerves. There are 12 pairs of cranial nerves.

FUNCTION OF THE NERVOUS SYSTEM

The nervous system receives, processes, and responds to information.

REGULATION OF THE INTERNAL ENVIRONMENT

By now, you are familiar with the concept of homeostasis, or balance. For the body to function well, a state of homeostasis must be maintained. The nervous system regulates what is going on within the body and makes adjustments, as necessary, to keep things within the range of normal. For example, control centers in the hypothalamus monitor the body temperature, and control centers in the medulla monitor heart beat and respirations.

When the central nervous system detects an imbalance, a special part of the peripheral nervous system, called the autonomic system, is activated. The autonomic system has two divisions, the sympathetic nervous system and the parasympathetic nervous system. Generally speaking, the sympathetic nervous system speeds things up, and the parasympathetic nervous system slows them back down. Perhaps you have heard of the "fight-or-flight" response. When we are put in a dangerous situation, our heart rate and breathing increase, and the adrenal glands release adrenaline, a chemical that helps us to cope with stress. These changes allow us to run faster or be stronger in a fight, and they are caused by activation of the sympathetic nervous system. Once the danger has passed, the parasympathetic nervous system slows things back down.

INTERACTION WITH THE EXTERNAL ENVIRONMENT

The nervous system allows us to interact with the world around us. The special senses—touch, taste, smell, sight, and hearing—provide the brain with information about the outside world. The brain responds to this information. The ability to receive information about the outside world and respond to it makes life more pleasurable, and it helps to protect us from harm. (The special senses are discussed in detail in Chapter 36.)

THE EFFECTS OF AGING ON THE NERVOUS SYSTEM

Neurons cannot divide and reproduce as other body cells do. That means that we keep the same 100 billion neurons our whole lives, give or take a few! Despite the fact that neurons are not replaced, they experience relatively little wear and tear over the course of a lifetime. Still, some structural changes occur as a result of aging, which can result in slowed conduction times and slight memory changes.

SLOWED CONDUCTION TIMES

You may notice that some of your elderly residents are not as quick to react to things as they used to be. This is a normal age-related change that is caused by changes in the myelin sheath and the amount of neurotransmitters. As we age, the amount of myelin surrounding the axons decreases, reducing the speed of nerve conduction by approximately 10%. In addition, neurotransmitter imbalances can interfere with the ability of a nerve impulse to travel across a synapse, slowing conduction. These changes are a normal part of the aging process, and they occur gradually over time.

Slowed conduction times can increase an elderly person's risk for falling and other accidents. It will take an older person longer to regain his balance if he starts to fall, or to avoid an obstacle (such as a pet or small child) that suddenly darts into his path. For this reason, it is especially important to remember the general safety guidelines from Chapter 18 when caring for an older person. For example, when helping an older person to walk, you will want to make sure that the pathway is well-lit and clear, that the person's clothes and shoes fit properly, and, if the person wears glasses, that she is wearing them.

MEMORY CHANGES

Memory and thought processes usually remain intact with normal aging. It may take an older person slightly longer to remember names, dates, or other information from the past, but given

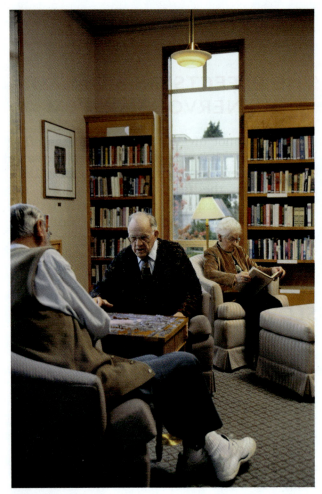

Figure 35-4
Use it or lose it! Studies have shown that actively exercising your mind throughout life helps to preserve mental function.

enough time, the person will eventually remember. Many older people experience a mild loss of memory for recent events, while still having excellent long-term memory. Engaging in activities that stimulate the mind (such as reading, traveling, working crossword puzzles, and doing crafts and other handiwork) throughout life helps to keep thought processes sharp and active well into old age (Fig. 35-4).

DISORDERS OF THE NERVOUS SYSTEM

There are many types of nervous system disorders. Some disorders affect a person's ability to control movement, or experience sensation. Other disorders may affect a person's ability to speak. Still other disorders affect a person's memory or

behavior. Disorders can be the result of a disease process, such as Parkinson's disease, or the result of an injury that damages the brain, spinal cord, or peripheral nerve pathways. Disorders of the nervous system are one of the most common causes of disability among elderly people. Approximately 50% of the disabilities seen in people older than 65 years are caused by a disorder of the nervous system.

TRANSIENT ISCHEMIC ATTACKS (TIAS)

Ischemia is decreased blood flow to the tissues. The tissue that is not getting enough blood is said to be *ischemic.* **Transient ischemic attacks (TIAs)** are temporary (transient) episodes of dysfunction that are caused by decreased blood flow (ischemia) to the brain. Any condition or situation that decreases blood flow to the brain can cause a TIA. For example, small blood clots can form in the heart or the arteries that supply the brain. These clots can break off and travel into the narrow arterioles of the brain, where they temporarily block the blood flow. Low blood pressure, certain medications, cigarette smoking, or standing up suddenly after lying down can also lead to a TIA.

Symptoms of a TIA vary according to the part of the brain affected by the decreased blood supply. Common symptoms may include dizziness, nausea, blurring or loss of vision, double vision, paralysis on one side of the body or face (with or without loss of sensation), or the inability to speak or swallow. The symptoms of a TIA may only last a few minutes, or they may last for several hours. The person usually recovers completely within 24 hours.

If you suspect that one of your residents is having (or has just had) a TIA, please report this to the nurse immediately. TIAs are usually a warning that the person could have a stroke in the near future. A TIA may also be a sign of an underlying medical condition that needs to be addressed.

STROKE

As you remember from Chapter 19, a **stroke** occurs when blood flow to a part of the brain is completely blocked, causing the tissue to die.

Causes of Stroke

The most common cause of a stroke is a blood clot that blocks the flow of blood to a part of the brain. As a result, people who smoke, have atherosclerosis, or have poorly controlled hypertension or diabetes are at high risk for having a stroke. Another, less common, cause of a stroke is cerebral hemorrhage. A cerebral hemorrhage occurs when a small artery in the brain bursts. The bleeding into the surrounding brain tissue puts pressure on the delicate tissue, damaging it. A cerebral hemorrhage is more likely in people with chronic hypertension, arteriosclerosis ("hardening of the arteries"), or certain deformities of the blood vessels in the brain.

Effects of Stroke

The lasting effects of a stroke depend on the area of the brain that is affected and the amount of tissue that is damaged. For example, a stroke that affects the vital control centers of the brain stem will result in death, while a stroke that affects part of the cerebrum may result only in disability. The most common disabilities resulting from a stroke are hemiplegia and aphasia.

Hemiplegia is paralysis on one side of the body. (Remember that the right side of the brain controls the left side of the body, and the left side of the brain controls the right side of the body—so a stroke that damages the right side of the brain will affect the left side of the body, and vice versa.) Depending on the amount of tissue damage, the hemiplegia may be mild or severe. A person with mild hemiplegia may have slight muscle weakness or shaking on the affected side, while a person with severe hemiplegia may not be able to move or feel any type of sensation at all on that side of the body. A person with severe hemiplegia who has lost sensation on one side of the body will need frequent repositioning to maintain proper body alignment and prevent pressure ulcers from forming. Care must also be taken to prevent other injuries, such as burns, because the person will not have the ability to detect heat, cold, or pain on the affected side.

Another common disability caused by a stroke is aphasia. Aphasia, as you learned in Chapter 9, affects the ability of the person to communicate with others. A person who has had a stroke may have expressive aphasia, receptive aphasia, or both.

- *Expressive aphasia* is caused by damage to the motor centers of the brain that control the ability to speak or form sounds into meaningful words. A person with expressive aphasia may also have trouble swallowing, increasing her risk of choking.
- *Receptive aphasia* is caused by damage to the area of the brain that allows the person

to understand words. The person can speak clearly, but he no longer knows the meaning of the words. As a result, a person with receptive aphasia may not be able to follow your verbal instructions.

Treatment of Stroke

In the past, the treatment of stroke focused on stabilizing the person's medical condition and then using aggressive physical therapy to help retrain disabled muscles to perform simple tasks. However, now treatments are available that can help to minimize the permanent damage caused by the stroke. For example, medications that dissolve blood clots are sometimes used to reestablish blood flow to the brain before permanent damage can occur. To work, these medications must be given very soon after the onset of the stroke. The signs and symptoms of a stroke are described in Chapter 19. As a nursing assistant, your ability to recognize that a resident may be having a stroke could enable the resident to receive treatment faster and experience less disability following the stroke.

Treatment immediately following a stroke depends on the severity of the damage to the brain, and on whether the person or the person's health care agent wants life-support measures to be taken. A person who has had a stroke may be very critically ill initially and need intensive care nursing. During this crisis period, the person's family members face uncertainty and difficult decisions may have to be made. The person's health care agent may need to decide whether or not to prolong life-support measures. Or, if the person survives the stroke, decisions may need to be made about where the person will live in the future. In many cases, a stroke is the event that makes a move to long-term care facility necessary.

A person who suddenly experiences a stroke and regains consciousness only to find that she is paralyzed or unable to communicate can be totally devastated. Rehabilitation, which is started as soon as the person's medical condition stabilizes, can be physically and emotionally difficult (Fig. 35-5). Depression, frustration, anger, and behavioral and personality changes can be expected. As a nursing assistant, you will be responsible for supporting the person both physically and emotionally during this difficult phase of his or her life.

PARKINSON'S DISEASE

As you learned earlier, neurotransmitters are chemicals that carry nerve impulses across the gap between the axon of one neuron and the dendrites

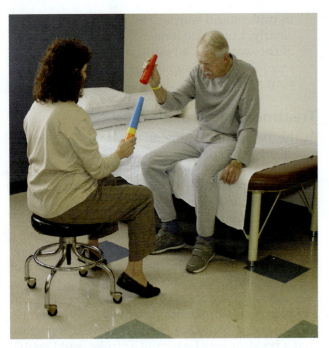

Figure 35-5
For a person who has experienced a stroke, rehabilitation can be a long and frustrating experience. Learning about the rehabilitation techniques that are being used with your resident and providing emotional support is important.

of the next. There are many different types of neurotransmitters. In **Parkinson's disease,** one of these neurotransmitters, called *dopamine,* is not produced in sufficient amounts. Dopamine is necessary for proper functioning of the motor neurons. In a person with Parkinson's disease, the brain's instructions regarding muscle movement never reach the muscle, because of the lack of dopamine. Without enough dopamine, the impulse cannot be passed on to the next neuron in line. Because of this nervous system "short circuit," the brain loses its ability to properly control body movement. We do not know exactly what causes the neurons to stop producing dopamine.

Parkinson's disease is a progressive disease, which means that it gets worse with time. The average age for the onset of Parkinson's disease is 55 years. Men are affected more often than women.

Effects of Parkinson's Disease

The effects of Parkinson's disease can be easily remembered by thinking of the word "TRAP:"

T stands for *tremor.* Parkinson's disease usually starts with a faint tremor that gets worse over a long period of time. The tremor is most apparent when the person is resting and decreases when the person attempts purposeful movement.

R stands for *rigidity.* The muscles become increasingly stiff. When rigidity is combined with the tremor, there is a cogwheeling effect. Cogwheeling is the term used to describe the jerky, ratcheting feel to the movement.

A stands for *akinesia* (lack of movement). *Bradykinesia,* or slowed movement, is also noted in Parkinson's disease.

P stands for *postural instability.* The person's ability to maintain his balance becomes increasingly worse, increasing the person's risk for falls.

As a result of these changes, the person has an abnormal gait. The person's steps are "shuffling," which means that they are short, there is a slight hesitation as the person tries to move the foot forward, and the foot barely comes off the floor. The person's posture is stooped forward, and he loses the natural arm swing that helps us to maintain balance (Fig. 35-6). The person has difficulty initiating movement, but once the person gets going, the short, shuffling steps and forward posture make it difficult for him to control his speed and maintain balance. In addition, the person has difficulty turning. Instead of twisting the body and pivoting on the toes, a person with Parkinson's disease turns his whole body as one unit, taking many small steps to complete the turn. Because of these abnormal movements, the person with Parkinson's disease is at very high risk for falling and incurring significant injuries.

Difficulty controlling the muscles around the face and throat cause other symptoms that are characteristic of Parkinson's disease. The person loses the ability to move the small muscles of the face that are responsible for facial expression, giving the face a "mask-like" appearance. Because the muscles used for swallowing are also affected, the person has trouble eating, and is at high risk for choking and aspiration. Drooling is common.

The muscles used for speech are also affected. The person is unable to project his voice, so the volume is low and the speech pattern is monotone (that is, without variation). Sometimes the person's words come out very rapidly, and are difficult to understand. Picture boards and asking simple questions that can be answered with a

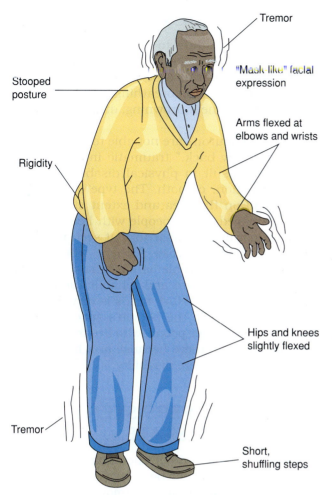

Tremor

"Mask-like" facial expression

Stooped posture

Arms flexed at elbows and wrists

Rigidity

Hips and knees slightly flexed

Tremor

Short, shuffling steps

Figure 35-6
People with Parkinson's disease often develop a characteristic shuffling gait with a forward lean.

nod or shake of the head can help improve the person's ability to express himself.

Other problems that are common with Parkinson's disease include skin disorders, sleep disturbances, constipation, and as the disease progresses, incontinence. In the later stages of the disease, the person may develop dementia. In the end stage of Parkinson's disease, the person becomes totally dependent on others for care, and will be at risk for all of the complications of immobility.

Treatment of Parkinson's Disease

Medications used in the treatment of Parkinson's disease support dopamine activity in the brain. They are given on a set schedule to help maintain muscle control and coordination throughout the day. A person who is taking medications for Parkinson's disease may seem to have "on" times and "off" times throughout the day. When the person is "on," the person's symptoms are well controlled by the medication and the person may be able to perform his daily activities with minimal problems. During the "off" times, however, the medication dose is beginning to wear off, and the person's symptoms may reappear. You should report your observations about the person's "on" and "off" times to the nurse. This information can help the nurse and the doctor schedule the person's doses of medication to achieve the best control of the person's symptoms. In addition, scheduling personal care and activities during the person's "on" times can help promote independence, because the person functions better during these times.

Other treatments for Parkinson's disease may include speech therapy to help with swallowing problems and physical therapy to help with movement difficulties. Some people with Parkinson's disease may be candidates for surgical treatment. Surgical treatment involves implanting an electrode in the brain to stimulate the part of the brain that is responsible for muscle coordination and movement.

EPILEPSY

Epilepsy is a disorder characterized by chronic seizure activity. Seizures are caused by interruptions of the normal electrical activity in the brain. A person with epilepsy experiences seizures periodically. The seizures may be grand mal seizures, which are characterized by generalized and violent contraction and relaxation of the body's muscles, or they may be petit mal (absence) seizures, which can be very mild and hardly noticeable. Care for a person who is having a grand mal seizure is described in Chapter 19.

There are many possible causes of epilepsy. For example, a person may develop epilepsy following a head injury, brain infection, or stroke. Many times, the exact cause of a person's epilepsy is never determined.

Medications are available that help to reduce the frequency of seizures. For some people with epilepsy, these medications do not work, but for others, they are very successful.

MULTIPLE SCLEROSIS (MS)

It is thought that **multiple sclerosis (MS)** is an autoimmune disorder—the immune system attacks and destroys the myelin sheaths that protect the nerves, resulting in faulty transmission of nerve impulses. MS usually affects the nerves in the hands, feet, and eyes first, and then moves inward toward the central nervous system. Muscle weakness, tingling sensations, twitching of the eyes, and visual disturbances may be early signs of MS.

MS usually strikes people early in life, between the ages of 20 and 40 years. The disorder progresses at different rates, depending on the individual. Some people may have a period of remission (mild or no symptoms) followed by a relapse (the symptoms return and are much worse). In the late stages of the disease, the person may become totally paralyzed. At this time, there is no cure for MS, although some medications have been shown to slow the progression of the disease.

MS is a reason why a younger person may become a resident of a long-term care facility. Because a person with MS has difficulty controlling muscle movement, he is at increased risk for injury. It may be necessary to pad hard surfaces in the environment that could cause injury if the person accidentally bumps into them. Be aware of, and follow, any specific instructions for seating and positioning that are included on the person's care plan. Range-of-motion exercises may be ordered to help maintain muscle tone and prevent contractures. A person with MS often has difficulty with bowel and bladder elimination as a result of nerve damage. For example, the person may experience urinary retention, constipation, or incontinence. Be sure to communicate with the nurse about your resident's specific needs. Your attention to these needs is important to help minimize problems, promote comfort, and maintain the person's sense of dignity.

AMYOTROPHIC LATERAL SCLEROSIS (ALS, LOU GEHRIG'S DISEASE)

Amyotrophic lateral sclerosis (ALS), like MS, is a nervous system disorder that causes progressive muscle weakness. In ALS, the nerves that transmit impulses between the spinal cord and the muscles are totally destroyed. People in the late stages of the disease are totally paralyzed, yet their minds remain sharp. Death occurs when a person loses the ability to breathe and swallow.

ALS usually affects people later in life, between the ages of 40 and 60 years. Men are affected more often than women. Most people who have ALS die within 10 years of the diagnosis.

HEAD INJURIES

Head injuries leading to brain damage can be caused by falls, accidents, and physical violence. Brain damage can also occur from events that cause a person to stop breathing for a long period of time, such as near drowning, drug overdose, or choking.

Because neurons are not able to repair themselves or "grow back," traumatic injuries to the brain often result in physical disability, loss of mental function, or both. The type of disability will depend on the area and extent of the brain tissue damaged. Some people with head injuries will have paralysis similar to that seen in people who have had a stroke. Others will develop epilepsy, memory problems, or behavioral problems. The type of care and rehabilitation that a person with a head injury needs is very individualized, according to the person's specific needs. Many of the younger people who live in long-term care facilities are there because of a head injury that resulted in severe disability.

COMA AND PERSISTENT VEGETATIVE STATE

A **coma** is a deep state of unconsciousness from which a person cannot be aroused. A coma can be caused by head injury, a tumor, a lack of oxygen, exposure to toxins, or illness. A person who is in a coma (that is, a person who is **comatose**) is unaware of his environment and cannot deliberately respond to people or things in it. The person cannot move on his own, and he cannot talk or respond to commands. A coma generally lasts only 2 to 4 weeks.

Some people will come out of the coma and make a full recovery, or they will experience only some disability. Others will come out of the coma, but still lack the ability to respond to their environment. When this occurs, the person is said to be in a **persistent vegetative state.** A person in a persistent vegetative state has sleep–wake cycles, and is able to breathe on his own. In addition, it may seem like the person in a persistent vegetative state is responding to his environment. For example, the person may open his eyes when someone is talking to him, and his eyes may even move toward the person who is speaking. The person may even laugh, smile, or grimace. However, these are involuntary responses. The person is not actually deliberately responding to his environment. A person can live in a persistent vegetative state for years.

It is generally believed that if a person remains in a persistent vegetative state for longer than 1 year, the condition is permanent.

A person who is comatose or in a persistent vegetative state is totally dependent on others for care. Care measures are aimed at keeping the person physically healthy. For example, preventing infection and pressure ulcers is a primary concern. Nutritional support is provided by enteral nutrition.

SPINAL CORD INJURIES

Injuries to the spinal cord are usually caused by trauma, but they can also be caused by birth defects or tumors of the spine. Trauma can cause the vertebrae to break, and the sharp fragments of bone can cut the soft tissue of the spinal cord, causing damage. Permanent damage can also result when the soft tissue of the spinal cord swells following an injury. The bones that surround the spinal cord do not "give." As a result, the spinal cord is squeezed, cutting off blood flow and resulting in tissue death from lack of oxygen.

The disability that results from a spinal cord injury depends on the severity of the injury and the level of the spine where the injury occurred. Remember that the spinal cord is the line of communication between the brain and the rest of the body. If this line is broken at any point, then nerve impulses cannot travel beyond the break in the line. So, an injury to the spinal cord in the neck area can result in **quadriplegia** (paralysis from the neck down), because nerve impulses are not able to travel past the neck. An injury further down the spinal cord may result in **paraplegia** (paralysis from the waist down). The paralysis may be partial or complete, depending on the severity of the injury.

As with other types of disorders of the nervous system, the care and rehabilitation needed by a person with a spinal cord injury will depend on the severity and extent of the injury. A person with quadriplegia will usually need total assistance with his activities of daily living (ADLs), while a person with paraplegia may require little or no assistance following rehabilitation. For some people, the emotional effects of a spinal cord injury are very hard to overcome. Loss of control over one's body, and the accompanying loss of independence, can be devastating.

DIAGNOSIS OF NEUROLOGIC DISORDERS

When a person is showing signs or symptoms that suggest a neurologic disorder, the doctor may order one of several diagnostic tests to help determine the exact cause of the person's signs and symptoms. Improved diagnostic tools have led to the earlier detection of many neurologic disorders. Diagnostic tests that are often ordered for people with signs and symptoms of a neurologic disorder include the following:

- **Imaging studies.** Tumors of the nervous system can occur in the brain, the spinal cord, or along the peripheral nerve tracts. Many of these tumors are not cancerous, but they may cause problems as they grow and press on healthy brain tissue or nerves. Imaging studies, such as radiography ("x-rays"), computed tomography (CT), and magnetic resonance imaging (MRI), are used to help locate tumors of the brain, spinal cord, or surrounding bony structures. Imaging studies are also useful for detecting fractures of the skull or vertebrae. When used with special dyes (injected into a vein), imaging studies can help to reveal abnormalities in the blood vessels that supply the brain.
- **Electroencephalography.** An electroencephalogram (EEG) records the electrical activity of the brain. EEGs are used to pinpoint seizure activity within the brain. Also, when there is a possibility that someone is "brain dead" (for example, following a severe head injury), electroencephalography is used to monitor the person's brain activity. If there is no electrical activity for the period of time specified by the law (usually 24 hours or more), the person may be declared dead.

SUMMARY

- Neurons are the basic cell of the nervous system.
  - A neuron can send and receive information.
  - Information, in the form of a nerve impulse, enters the neuron at the dendrites, travels through the cell body and down the axon, and then across the synapse and onto the dendrites of the next neuron in line.
- The nervous system consists of the central nervous system (CNS) and the peripheral nervous system (PNS).
  - The central nervous system consists of the brain and the spinal cord. The central nervous system receives information, processes it, and issues commands. These delicate organs are protected by three layers of tissue (called meninges), the cerebrospinal fluid (CSF), and the bony skull and vertebrae.
    - The brain processes information and issues commands. The brain has four parts: the cerebrum, the diencephalon, the brain stem, and the cerebellum.
    - The spinal cord carries information to and from the brain.
  - The peripheral nervous system consists of the nerves. The nerves carry information to and from the central nervous system.
    - Sensory nerves carry information from the "outside in." Sensory nerves give the brain information about other organ systems or the outside world.
    - Motor nerves carry information from the "inside out." Motor nerves allow the brain to control the movement of muscles.
- The nervous system receives, processes, and responds to information.
  - The nervous system receives information from other organ systems and reacts to it, helping the body to maintain a state of homeostasis.
  - The nervous system allows us to experience the world around us. Without our nervous systems, we would not be able to enjoy the taste and smell of a ripe peach, a beautiful piece of music, the sight of a loved one, or the soft fur of a favorite pet. We would not be able to move, think, or create.
- The changes in the nervous system that result from normal aging are relatively few.

- Older people are not as quick to react to things as younger people, which increases the older person's risk for falling and other accidents.
- Memory and thought processes usually remain intact with normal aging, although it may take an older person a little bit longer to recall information.
- Disorders of the nervous system can affect the brain, spinal cord, or nerves.
  - Transient ischemic attacks (TIAs) are caused by decreased blood flow to the brain. Once blood flow returns, the person's symptoms go away. Although the effects of a TIA are not lasting, a person who has had or is having a TIA needs medical attention, because TIAs are often warnings that the person could have a stroke in the near future.
  - A stroke can be caused by a blood clot or hemorrhage that disrupts blood flow to the brain. The part of the brain that does not receive enough blood dies, due to lack of oxygen and nutrients. The effects of a stroke are permanent and can be mild or severe.
  - Parkinson's disease affects the brain's ability to conduct motor impulses to the muscles because of a lack of the neurotransmitter dopamine. A resident with Parkinson's disease is at high risk for falls, choking accidents, and, as the disease progresses, complications of immobility.
  - Epilepsy is a seizure disorder caused by abnormal electrical activity in the brain.
  - Multiple sclerosis (MS) is a nervous system disorder that affects the motor neurons, resulting in muscle weakness that gets worse over time.
  - Head injuries that result in brain damage and spinal cord injuries are a major reason why many younger people come to live in long-term care facilities.
  - A person who is in a coma or a persistent vegetative state requires total care to maintain physical health.
- Diagnostic procedures used to detect disorders of the nervous system include imaging studies—such as x-rays, computed tomography (CT) scans, and magnetic resonance imaging (MRI) scans—and electroencephalograms (EEGs).

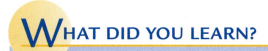

WHAT DID YOU LEARN?

Multiple Choice

Select the single best answer for each of the following questions.

1. Any condition that temporarily decreases blood flow to the brain can cause what to occur?
  a. A "senior moment"
  b. A transient ischemic attack (TIA)
  c. A heart attack
  d. A cerebral hemorrhage

2. Mrs. Romanelli has had a stroke and has a lot of trouble forming words. What term is used to describe Mrs. Romanelli's difficulty with language?
  a. Aphasia
  b. Dysphasia
  c. Paraplegia
  d. Hemiplegia

3. Mr. Owens had a stroke that left him paralyzed on the left side of his body. Which one of the following statements is true?
  a. The stroke occurred in the left side of Mr. Owens' brain.
  b. The stroke occurred in the right side of Mr. Owens' brain.
  c. The stroke affected Mr. Owens' brain stem.
  d. Mr. Owens has paraplegia.

4. Which of the following can increase a person's risk for a transient ischemic attack (TIA)?
  a. Low blood pressure
  b. Certain drugs
  c. Smoking
  d. All of the above

5. Which nervous system disorder is characterized by a lack of the neurotransmitter dopamine?
  a. Multiple sclerosis (MS)
  b. Epilepsy
  c. Parkinson's disease
  d. Dementia

6. What neurologic disorder is characterized by chronic seizure activity?
  a. Multiple sclerosis (MS)
  b. Epilepsy
  c. Parkinson's disease
  d. Stroke

7. What diagnostic test is used to monitor electrical activity of the brain?
  a. Electrocardiogram (EKG)
  b. Imaging studies, such as computed tomography (CT)
  c. Electroencephalogram (EEG)
  d. There is no test available to monitor the electrical activity of the brain

8. How does aging affect the nervous system?
  a. Older people usually become "senile" and forgetful.
  b. Older people lose the ability to form or understand words.
  c. Older people may take slightly longer to react to things.
  d. Aging does not affect the nervous system because old neurons are constantly replaced.

9. Mrs. Page has Parkinson's disease. Sometimes she is able to walk to the bathroom independently with her walker, and other times she calls for help as her steps become "frozen," and she is not able to get moving again. What is the best explanation for this behavior?
  a. Mrs. Page's medication dose is wearing off when she has increased difficulty with movement.
  b. Mrs. Page cannot move well when her feet are cold.
  c. Mrs. Page is having emotional difficulties accepting her condition and as a result has become very needy for attention.
  d. Mrs. Page has dementia from the Parkinson's disease and no longer remembers how to walk.

10. Mr. Luking has been admitted to your long-term care facility, because he is in a persistent vegetative state. Which of the following statements about persistent vegetative state is true?
  a. Mr. Luking will have normal sleep–wake cycles.
  b. Mr. Luking will be able to respond in a meaningful way to visitors.
  c. The persistent vegetative state could turn into a coma.
  d. Care measures will focus on meeting Mr. Luking's emotional needs.

Matching

Match each numbered item with its appropriate lettered description.

_____ **1.** Meninges

_____ **2.** Cerebrospinal fluid (CSF)

_____ **3.** Central nervous system

_____ **4.** Peripheral nervous system

_____ **5.** Axon

_____ **6.** Myelin

_____ **7.** Dendrite

_____ **8.** Neuron

_____ **9.** Synapse

a. Sends a nervous impulse
b. Consists of the brain and spinal cord
c. Fatty white substance that speeds the conduction of nerve impulses
d. A cell that can send and receive information
e. Receives a nervous impulse
f. The gap between the axon of one neuron and the dendrites of the next
g. Three layers of connective tissue that protect the brain and spinal cord
h. Consists of the nerves
i. Clear fluid that cushions the brain and spinal cord

STOP and Think!

Cordella is a new nursing assistant at your facility. She has been assigned to take care of Mr. Vittorio, who has Parkinson's disease. When you are talking with Cordella in the break room, she mentions to you that she is finding it very difficult to care for Mr. Vittorio. She tells you that sometimes he functions very well and needs little assistance from her. Other times, especially first thing in the morning, it is like she is dealing with a completely different resident! During these times, Mr. Vittorio seems very uncooperative. He resists her efforts to get him to move, and when she tries to communicate with him, he stares at her blankly and mumbles in such a low voice that she cannot understand what he is saying. Cordella said that the nurse told her that Mr. Vittorio is at risk for falls; however, Cordella can't get him to follow her safety instructions. When he does walk, he doesn't pick his feet up, and he won't stand up straight. Cordella is also finding it difficult to assist Mr. Vittorio during meals. He cannot keep the food on his fork long enough to get it to his mouth, and as a result he makes a huge mess at the table. He frequently coughs when he is trying to swallow, and Cordella reports that she constantly has to wipe drool from his chin. Can you help Cordella to better understand Mr. Vittorio's problems? Can you make any suggestions to her that might help with his care?

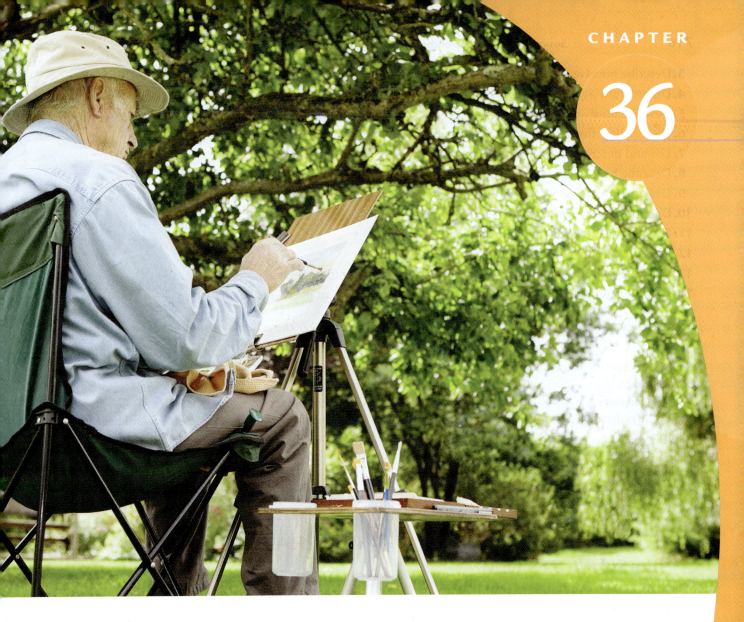

The Sensory System

WHAT WILL YOU LEARN?

We rely on our special senses—sight, hearing, taste, smell, and touch—to understand and interact with the world around us. Our sensory system allows us to experience the beauty and joy of the world we live in. It also helps to protect us from harm. Many of the people you will care for will have disorders or disabilities involving the sensory system. In this chapter, you will learn about how the sensory system works and about some of the disorders that can affect the sensory system. You will also learn how you can help to meet the needs of people who cannot see or hear well. When you are finished with this chapter, you will be able to:

1. Describe the main function of the sensory system.
2. List and define the two main divisions of the sensory system.

Photo: Our sensory system allows us to experience and enjoy the world around us.

3. Describe how we experience taste and smell.

4. Discuss how aging affects a person's senses of taste and smell.

5. Describe how we experience sight.

6. Discuss the effects of aging on the eye.

7. List and describe disorders that can affect the eye.

8. Describe how to care for eyeglasses, contact lenses, and prosthetic (artificial) eyes.

9. Describe special considerations that are taken when caring for a blind person.

10. Describe how we experience sound.

11. Discuss the effects of aging on the ear.

12. List and describe disorders that can affect the ear.

13. Describe techniques for communicating with a hearing-impaired person.

14. Demonstrate proper technique for inserting and removing an in-the-ear hearing aid.

Vocabulary Use the CD in the front of your book to hear these terms pronounced and defined:

Sensory receptors	Presbyopia	Cerumen	Conductive hearing
Sense organs	Conjunctivitis	Presbycusis	loss
Tactile receptors	Cataract	Cerumen impaction	Otosclerosis
Referred (radiating) pain	Glaucoma	Otitis media	Sensorineural hearing
Myopia	Diabetic retinopathy	Otitis externa	loss
Hyperopia	Macular degeneration	Vertigo	
Astigmatism	Braille	Tinnitus	

STRUCTURE OF THE SENSORY SYSTEM

The sensory system is part of the nervous system. The sensory system consists of **sensory receptors,** specialized cells or groups of cells associated with a sensory nerve. The sensory receptor picks up information, called a *stimulus,* and translates it into a nerve impulse, which is then sent to the brain for interpretation, via the sensory nerve. Sensory receptors are found throughout the body. Some are found in the **sense organs,** which you probably can name already—the eyes, the ears, the nose, and the taste buds. Other sensory receptors are found throughout the skin, and even in the tissues of internal organs.

The sensory system is sometimes divided into two major parts. This division is based on the location of the sensory receptors. The first part is called general sense. The sensory receptors that are responsible for general sense are found everywhere throughout the body. The second part is called *special sense.* The sensory receptors that are responsible for special sense are located in the specific sense organs (the eyes, the ears, the nose, and the taste buds).

GENERAL SENSE

General sense is responsible for our sense of touch, position, and pain.

TOUCH

Our sense of touch allows us to feel textures (such as the plush velvet of a party dress or the hot sand between our toes at the beach) and the shapes of objects. The sense of touch is made possible by tactile receptors found in the skin (Fig. 36-1). (*Tactile* is another word for "touch.") The **tactile receptors** are stimulated when something comes in contact with the surface of the body and presses on them, causing them to change shape. Some areas of the skin have more tactile receptors than others, and are therefore more sensitive to touch. For example, the tips of the fingers and toes and the lips contain many tactile receptors and are more sensitive to touch than other parts of the body.

Some of the tactile receptors in the skin allow us to sense pressure, also known as *deep touch.* Intolerance to prolonged pressure is what makes us shift our position when we have been sitting in

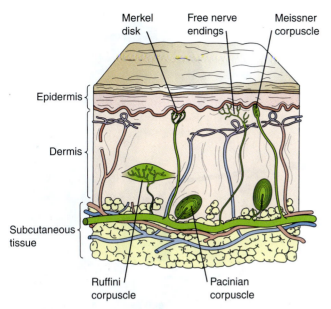

Figure 36-1

Tactile receptors and free nerve endings in the dermis of the skin allow us to feel things that come in contact with our bodies. There are four main types of tactile receptors: Ruffini corpuscles, Meissner corpuscles, Pacinian corpuscles, and Merkel disks.

one position for a long time. A person who is unable to sense pressure (for example, a person who is paralyzed) does not become uncomfortable from being in one position for a long time. Therefore, the person is not motivated to change positions. What effect do you think this has on the person's risk for developing skin breakdown and pressure ulcers?

POSITION

Position receptors, found in the muscles, tendons, and joints, keep the brain informed about the position of various body parts in relation to each other. For example, you can tell if your leg is bent or straight without actually looking down to check its position. These same receptors also relay information to the brain about the degree of muscle contraction, especially when the muscle is contracting against resistance (for example, when you are lifting weights). Position sense provides us with muscle tone and the ability to move our muscles in a smooth, coordinated way.

PAIN

Pain is the body's distress signal. Pain tells us that we have been injured, that we have overworked a muscle group, that an organ is not

working properly, or that we are ill. Pain can be acute (sharp, sudden pain that occurs with an injury and goes away after the tissues have healed) or chronic (pain that lasts beyond the usual time that it would take the tissues to heal).

Free nerve endings (dendrites) in the skin and the tissues of our internal organs allow us to detect pain. Your brain is usually pretty good at identifying what hurts when the cause of the pain is on the surface of your body (for example, when you burn your finger while removing a hot dish from the oven). But your brain may have more trouble pinpointing the exact location of pain that is coming from an internal organ. This results in the phenomenon known as **referred (radiating) pain.** For example, a person who is having a heart attack may complain of pain in the shoulder, neck, arm, or jaw. Gallbladder disease may cause pain in the back and shoulder on the person's right side. A back injury may cause pain to radiate down the leg and into a person's foot. Figure 36-2 shows how pain from certain internal organs can be referred to other areas of the body.

Many of the people you will care for will have some type of pain. The nursing assistant's role in

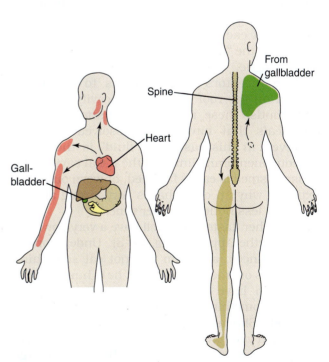

Figure 36-2

Pain may not always be felt at its exact source. Pain from the heart may be felt in the arm, shoulder, neck, or jaw (*red shading*). Pain from the gallbladder may be felt in the back and shoulder on the person's right side (*green shading*). A back injury can cause pain to radiate down the leg and into the foot (*yellow shading*).

caring for a person who experiences pain is described in Chapter 27.

TASTE AND SMELL

The sense organs of taste and smell are the taste buds and the roof of the nasal cavity, respectively. Special cells in these areas, called chemoreceptors, detect chemicals in the food we eat, the beverages we drink, and the air we breathe. The chemical signal is changed to an electric one and carried by sensory neurons to the brain, which tells us what we are tasting or smelling.

Taste buds cover the surface of the tongue. We have thousands of taste buds, and each taste bud consists of about 100 chemoreceptors, plus some supporting cells. The taste buds are bathed in fluid (either saliva or the liquids that we drink). The fluid contains dissolved chemicals, which stimulate the taste buds.

There are four basic tastes: sweet, salty, sour, and bitter. The taste buds that detect these four basic tastes are arranged in a particular pattern on the tongue. The "sweets" are found on the tip of the tongue. The "salties" are found on each side of the tongue, toward the front. The "sours" are located on each side of the tongue, toward the back. And the "bitters" are located across the back of the tongue.

The receptors that allow us to smell are located on the roof of the nasal cavity. Like the taste buds, these receptors are stimulated by chemicals that have been dissolved in fluid. However, in this case, the "fluid" is the moist mucous membrane lining of the nasal cavity. The sense of smell is easily fatigued, or worn out. This explains why an odor that is very strong at first becomes less noticeable over time.

Together, taste and smell have a very powerful effect on the appetite (Fig. 36-3). Under normal circumstances, a person will not eat something that tastes or smells bad, even if he is hungry. But, how often have you found yourself eating too much of something just because it tastes or smells so good? Similarly, how often have you noticed that when you have a head cold and a stuffy nose, food seems to lose appeal? This happens in large part because you can't smell the food!

As we get older, the number of chemoreceptors on the tongue and on the roof of the nasal cavity decreases. In addition, we produce less saliva, which makes it harder to dissolve the chemicals that stimulate the taste buds. As a result of these changes, the senses of taste and smell become less intense, leading to an overall

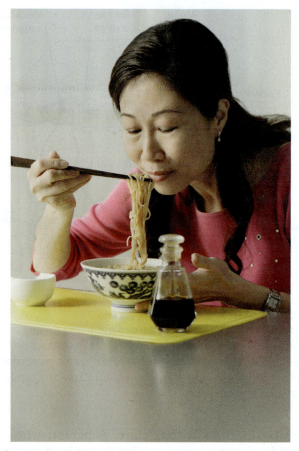

Figure 36-3
The senses of taste and smell are closely related. Fragrant soup is a treat for the tongue and the nose!

decrease in appetite. To make up for a diminished sense of taste and smell, older people often season their food more heavily than younger people.

There are many dangers associated with a diminished ability to taste or smell. For example, an older person may not be able to tell that food has spoiled, and become ill from eating it. Or, he may not be able to detect the smell of smoke or a gas leak. It is surprising how much we rely on our senses of taste and smell to keep us safe.

SIGHT

Our sense of sight allows us to detect light, color, and shape.

STRUCTURE OF THE EYE

The sense organ of sight is the eye. Each eye is protected by the bones of the skull, which form a protective cavity ("orbit," "eye socket") around the eye. Only the very front of the eyeball lacks the bony protection of the skull. To protect the front

A. External structure of the eye

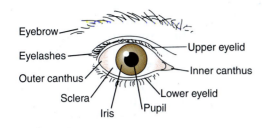

B. Internal structure of the eye

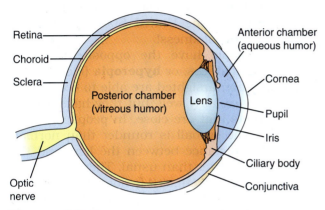

Figure 36-4
The eye. **(A)** External view of the eye. **(B)** Internal structures of the eye.

of the eye, we have eyelids that close and eyelashes and eyebrows that serve as "dust catchers" (Fig. 36-4A). Lacrimal glands, located above the eye in the orbit, form tears that help to keep the eye moist and free of dust and bacteria. Skeletal muscles located around the eyeball allow us to move our eyes.

It may be helpful to look at Figure 36-4B as we go through the internal structure of the eyeball. The eyeball itself is made up of three layers of tissue—the sclera, the choroid, and the retina:

- The *sclera* is the tough outer layer. The sclera is made of connective tissue. Although most of the sclera is white (hence the term, "white of the eye"), the front of the sclera, which is called the *cornea*, is clear. Light passes through the cornea to the inside of the eye.
- The *choroid* is the middle layer. This layer contains the blood vessels that supply the retina and other parts of the eye. At the front of the eye, the *choroid* also forms the ciliary body and the iris. The *ciliary body* is a muscular structure that attaches to the *lens*, a flexible, transparent, curved structure that adjusts to focus light rays onto the retina. The ciliary body changes the shape of the lens, allowing the eye to focus. The other

structure formed by the choroid, the *iris*, is the colored part of the eye. The iris is actually a round muscle with an opening in the center (the *pupil*). The iris controls the amount of light that enters the eye through the pupil.

- The *retina* is the innermost layer. The retina contains receptors, called *rods* and *cones*, which turn light into nerve impulses. The nerve impulses travel through the *optic nerve* to the brain for interpretation.

The eyeball also has two fluid-filled chambers (Fig. 36-4B):

- The *anterior chamber* is located between the cornea and the lens. Special cells in the ciliary body secrete *aqueous humor*, a watery fluid that fills the anterior chamber. The aqueous humor passes through the anterior chamber and is reabsorbed back into the bloodstream.
- The posterior chamber is located between the lens and the retina. The posterior chamber is filled with *vitreous humor*, a jelly-like substance that gives the eyeball its shape.

FUNCTION OF THE EYE

Think about how a camera works. To take a picture, you need light and film. You also need a way of controlling the amount of light that enters the camera, and adjusting the distance between the camera lens and the film. If the amount of light entering the camera is not sufficient, or if the distance between the lens and the film is not correct, the resulting photograph will be out of focus.

The human eye works much like a camera:

- The retina is the "film."
- The iris and pupil control the amount of light that enters the eye. In bright sunlight, the iris constricts, making the pupil smaller so that less light is allowed into the inner part of the eye. In low light, the iris dilates, making the pupil bigger so that more light can enter the eye.
- The cornea and lens work to focus light rays onto the retina, resulting in a clear image. First, the curve of the cornea focuses the light rays as they enter the eye. Next, the light rays pass through the lens, where the focus is refined (Fig. 36-5A). If the object the person is looking at is close, then the ciliary body contracts, causing the lens to become shorter and rounder. If the object is far away, then the ciliary body relaxes, causing the lens to become longer and flatter. The curved lens bends the light rays and brings them into focus on the retina, forming an image.

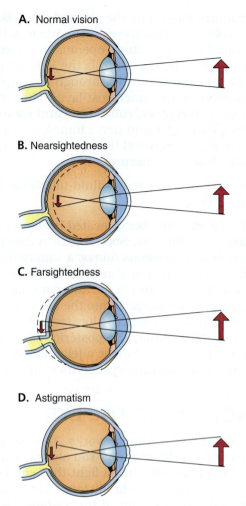

A. Normal vision

B. Nearsightedness

C. Farsightedness

D. Astigmatism

Figure 36-5
Many people need corrective lenses, such as glasses or contact lenses, to achieve clear vision. Three common problems that require the use of corrective lenses are nearsightedness (myopia), farsightedness (hyperopia), and astigmatism. **(A)** Normal vision. Light rays pass through the cornea and the lens and are focused on the retina. **(B)** Nearsightedness (myopia). The eyeball of a person who is nearsighted is more oval in shape than normal, which increases the distance between the lens and the retina. As a result, the image comes into focus before the retina. **(C)** Farsightedness (hyperopia). The eyeball of a person who is farsighted is more round in shape than normal, which decreases the distance between the lens and the retina. As a result, the image is not yet focused when it hits the retina. **(D)** Astigmatism. In astigmatism, the cornea is not perfectly curved. Some of the light rays that pass through the cornea are focused on the retina, but others are not, resulting in blurred vision.

Clear, sharp vision is indeed a true gift. Many people need some help (in the form of corrective lenses, such as glasses or contact lenses) to see clearly. People who wear corrective lenses need help focusing the image properly on the retina.

Some people need help focusing because of the shape of their eyeball. For example, the eyeball may be a little more oval than normal, causing the distance between the lens and the retina to be greater than usual. This results in nearsightedness, or **myopia** (Fig. 36-5B). People who are nearsighted are able to see fairly well close up, but they have trouble seeing images that are far away. This is because the distance between the person's lens and retina is longer than usual, which means that the image actually comes into focus before it hits the retina. This is a very common problem—20% of the people in the United States have some degree of nearsightedness!

Some people have the opposite problem, called farsightedness, or **hyperopia** (Fig. 36-5C). People who are farsighted are able to see objects in the distance fairly well, but they have trouble seeing objects that are close. In people who are farsighted, the eyeball is rounder than normal, causing the distance between the lens and the retina to be shorter than usual. Therefore, when the image hits the retina, it is not yet in focus.

Other people have trouble focusing images properly because the cornea is not perfectly curved. This condition is called **astigmatism** (Fig. 36-5D). The irregular curve of the cornea bends the light rays in funny ways, which results in a blurred, distorted image.

THE EFFECTS OF AGING ON THE EYE

As we age, many changes occur in the eye that can affect vision:

- The number of receptors in the retina decreases, and the lens becomes more opaque (cloudy). As a result, images are not focused as sharply as in younger days, and colors may not be as bright.
- The iris becomes more rigid, which means that it takes longer for an older person's eyes to adjust when she moves from a bright area to a dim one, or vice versa.
- The lens becomes less flexible, which affects the older person's ability to focus on objects that are close, a condition known as **presbyopia.** Presbyopia is why many people start using reading glasses in their 40s (Fig. 36-6).
- There is a decrease in tear production, which leads to dryness and irritation of the eyes. Many older people use lubricating eye drops to help keep the eyes moist and comfortable.

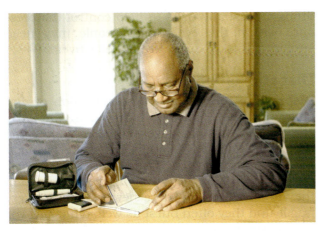

Figure 36-6
Presbyopia, which occurs when the lens becomes less elastic with age, is a common age-related change. People with presbyopia often need to use reading glasses to help them focus on things that are close.

DISORDERS OF THE EYE

Conjunctivitis ("Pink Eye")

Conjunctivitis is infection and inflammation of the conjunctiva, a clear membrane that lines the inside of the eyelids and covers most of the surface of the eye (Fig. 36-4B). In conjunctivitis, the white of the eye appears red. The eye may itch or burn, and it tears excessively (Fig. 36-7). There may be a sticky white or yellow discharge.

There are many different causes of conjunctivitis. Microbes that cause colds and sinus infec-

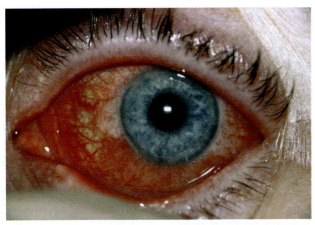

Figure 36-7
Conjunctivitis, or "pink eye," is a very contagious infection of the conjunctiva, the clear membrane that covers most of the surface of the eye and lines the inside of the eyelids. The affected eye is red, itchy, and teary, and there may be a sticky white or yellow discharge. (© *Science Photo Library/Photo Researchers, Inc.*)

tions can travel through the tear ducts and onto the surface of the eye, causing an infection. Or, microbes from an infection somewhere else in the body can be transferred into the eye when the person touches the infected area and then rubs his eyes. For example, methicillin-resistant *Staphylococcus aureus* (MRSA) and herpes virus can cause conjunctivitis in this way.

Conjunctivitis is highly contagious. Rubbing the eyes and then touching something transfers the microbes to that surface, where someone else can easily pick them up. All that person has to do is touch her own eyes, and she could find herself with her own case of conjunctivitis! Conjunctivitis is usually treated with eye drops or an eye ointment prescribed by a doctor.

Cataracts

Cataracts are very common in older people, but they can occur in younger people as well. It is thought that excessive exposure to sunlight increases a person's chances of developing cataracts. A **cataract** is the gradual yellowing and hardening of the lens of the eye. The lens becomes opaque and eventually prevents light from passing through to the retina. The person's vision becomes more and more cloudy as the cataract worsens (Fig. 36-8). It is like looking through a sheer curtain panel. When you look through one thickness of the sheer panel, your vision is only slightly cloudy. If you fold the panel to make a double thickness, your vision gets cloudier. And, if you fold the panel again to make a triple thickness, your vision becomes cloudier still. This is what a person with a cataract experiences. Total blindness can result as a cataract becomes more opaque.

Many people with cataracts have surgery to remove the opaque lens and replace it with an artificial one. Improvements in equipment and surgical techniques have made this procedure simple and routine. Surgery is often performed on an outpatient basis, using only a local anesthetic. The person usually can return home a few hours after the procedure. Cataract surgery enables people with cataracts to once again enjoy activities such as needlework and reading that would have been nearly impossible before.

Glaucoma

Glaucoma is a disorder of the eye that occurs when the pressure within the eye is increased to dangerous levels. This occurs when the aqueous humor in the anterior chamber is not reabsorbed into the bloodstream. As more and more aqueous humor is formed, it creates pressure, which builds up in the eye. The pressure squeezes the nerves

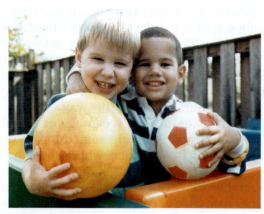

A. Normal vision

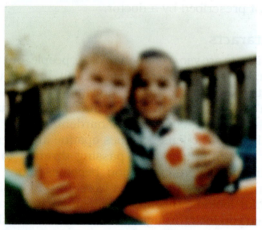

B. Cataract

Figure 36-8

Cataracts occur when the lens of the eye becomes yellow and hard over time, resulting in cloudy vision. This is what the world looks like to **(A)** a person with normal vision and **(B)** a person with cataracts. (*Courtesy of the National Eye Institute, National Institutes of Health.*)

and the blood vessels in the retina. Eventually, the nerves are destroyed and vision is lost.

People who are older than 40 years and have a family history of glaucoma are at high risk for developing glaucoma themselves. Glaucoma also seems to be more common in people with dark irises (brown eyes), as opposed to light ones (blue or green eyes). The most common type of glaucoma occurs gradually, over a long period of time. However, in some people, the onset of glaucoma happens suddenly, and is accompanied by a great deal of pain. Both chronic and acute glaucoma can lead to blindness if left untreated.

Early detection and treatment of glaucoma can help to save the person's vision. This is why routine eye examinations are essential. If a person is found to have glaucoma, medicated eye

drops are usually used to help control the pressure within the eye. Some people may need surgery if the eye drops are not effective.

Diabetic Retinopathy

Diabetic retinopathy is a complication of diabetes that can lead to blindness. In the early stages, the tiny blood vessels that supply the retina burst, leading to hemorrhages and damaging the retina. As the retina tries to heal, new blood vessels start to grow along the retina and in the vitreous humor. These new vessels are very fragile and they often burst as well, damaging the retina even more.

The number of cases of blindness caused by diabetic retinopathy in the United States is rapidly increasing. Early detection during an eye examination is essential for preserving the person's vision. Laser treatment is often necessary to help seal off hemorrhages in the retina.

Macular Degeneration

The macula is the small area in the middle of the retina where images are sharpest. In **macular degeneration,** deposits build up in the macula. The receptors in the area become damaged. The person's vision becomes increasingly blurry, with a blind spot in the middle of the visual field. Factors that can increase a person's risk for developing macular degeneration are smoking, excessive exposure to sunlight, a diet high in cholesterol, and an inherited tendency for the disorder.

Blindness

Blindness has many different causes and takes many different forms. Some people may have low vision (that is, partial sight), and others may be totally blind. Some people see nothing but darkness, but many others can see light, movement, shapes, and even colors, just not clearly enough to distinguish between them. Some people have been blind since birth and have never seen anything, while others may have lost their sight later in life. Most people who are blind adapt well and are very independent. People who have recently lost their sight, however, may be very frightened, especially of walking or moving around on their own.

Rehabilitation for a person who has recently lost his sight focuses on safety and the person's return to independence. Navigation skills are taught so that the blind person can be independent again. During rehabilitation, a blind person may learn to work with a companion animal that

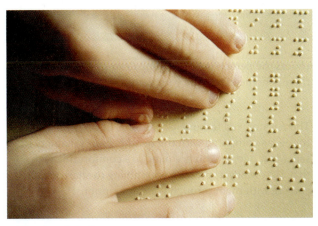

Figure 36-9
Braille uses a system of letters formed from raised dots to enable a blind person to read. (*Will & Deni McIntyre/Photo Researchers, Inc.*)

has been specially trained to guide the person as she walks. The person may learn **Braille**, a system that uses letters made from combinations of raised dots (Fig. 36-9). The person runs her fingers over words written in Braille to read them. In addition, many books are available on compact disc (CD) for the person to listen to.

As a nursing assistant, treating a person who is blind with respect and allowing the person to be as independent as possible are the best things you can do to help the rehabilitation effort. Learn the techniques that your resident is being taught and reinforce them by helping the person to practice them continuously. Guidelines for caring for a person who is blind are given in Guidelines Box 36-1.

CARING FOR EYEGLASSES, CONTACT LENSES, AND PROSTHETIC EYES

Many of your residents will wear glasses or contact lenses. Some may even have a prosthetic (artificial) eye. Many people are able to care for their own vision accessories, but others may need your help.

Eyeglasses

Eyeglasses are commonly used to correct vision. Some people wear eyeglasses only for reading or close work, while others may need to wear them all the time when they are awake. Always make sure that your residents who need glasses wear them, especially if the resident is confused or disoriented. Being unable to see clearly can make

confusion and disorientation worse and adversely affect the person's quality of life.

Eyeglasses are very expensive to replace if broken or lost. As with all of your residents' personal belongings, you should be careful when handling a person's eyeglasses. Clean eyeglasses with cloths or a special solution made specifically for that purpose, or with warm water (Fig. 36-10). If water or a special cleaning solution is used to clean the lenses, finish by drying them with a soft cloth or tissue. Paper towels or napkins may scratch the lenses and should not be used. When not in use, the person's eyeglasses should be stored in their case within easy reach.

Contact Lenses

Contact lenses are also commonly worn to help make vision sharp. Contact lenses are made of molded plastic and fit directly on the eyeball. Contacts may be soft or hard. How long they can be worn before taking them out depends on the type of lens. Some lenses are removed and cleaned daily, while others can be left in for several days at a time.

Contact lenses must be cared for carefully to prevent infection and irritation of the eyes (Fig. 36-11). Special cleaning and soaking solutions are used to clean and store the lenses. The types of solutions that are used vary according to the type of lens. Each lens is kept in its own case ("left" and "right") because the correction and size for the left and right eyes may be different. If one of your residents wears contact lenses, make sure you are familiar with the proper technique for helping the person to care for them. Report any complaints of eye irritation or discharge to the nurse immediately.

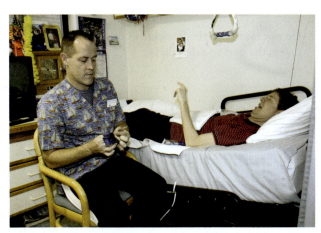

Figure 36-10
Take special care when handling a person's eyeglasses. They are expensive to replace.

WHAT YOU DO	WHY YOU DO IT
Speak in a normal tone of voice.	Unless the person is hearing impaired as well as blind, there is no need to raise your voice.
It is fine to use words such as "see," "look," and "watch." Be descriptive in the things you see around you. For example, tell the person that the sky is a beautiful shade of blue or that there are lovely yellow flowers blooming right outside the window.	There is no need to be self-conscious about your ability to see, as compared with the blind person's inability to see. Most people who are blind are comfortable with that fact. Many appreciate your ability to share what you see with them through your descriptions.
Ask the person about the extent of her blindness, and do not hesitate to ask the person what type of help she needs from you.	Asking the person about her blindness will help you to better care for the person. You might be surprised at what the person is able to do for herself, with little or no assistance from you!
When you enter the person's room, knock and tell the person who you are and why you are there. Similarly, when you leave, tell the person that you are leaving.	If you do not announce yourself when you enter the room, you could startle the person. Imagine how frightening it would be to hear someone walking around in your room and not know who they are or what they are doing! Similarly, if you do not tell the person that you are leaving, he may not be aware that you have left. How would you feel if you started talking to someone who was no longer in the room and were left to figure it out on your own that the other person had left?
Make sure you explain procedures completely and descriptively. Throughout the procedure, tell the person what type of equipment you are using, what you are doing, and what you are going to do next.	With all residents, you should take care to explain procedures thoroughly. However, with a blind person, you may have to modify your approach a bit. For example, instead of just showing the person a piece of equipment, you will need to describe it to him, or let him touch it. Also, you should tell the person what is happening as it happens so that the person is not left wondering where you are in the procedure, or what is coming next.
Do not rearrange the furniture in the person's room, unless the person asks you to.	The person is used to moving around the room on her own. If you move the furniture, the person could injure herself by running into something that has been moved and is now in an unfamiliar location.
Leave the door either completely open or completely closed.	If the door is partially open, the person may feel for the door, think that it is all the way open, and walk into the edge of the door.
When helping a blind person to walk, do not propel the person in front of you. Instead, let the person walk beside you and slightly behind you as she rests a hand on your elbow. Walk at a normal pace. Let the person know when you are about to turn a corner, or when a curb or step is approaching (and whether or not you will be stepping up or down).	In this way, you guide the person and reduce the risk of stumbles over unforeseen obstacles.

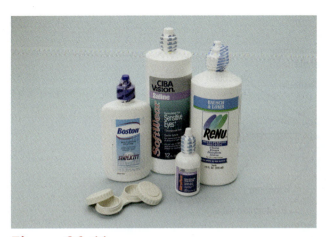

Figure 36-11
Contact lenses must be cleaned and stored properly to prevent infection and irritation of the eyes.

Prosthetic Eyes

Sometimes a person's eye must be surgically removed, because of either injury or disease. A person who has had an eye removed may choose to wear a patch to cover the missing eye, or he may wear a prosthetic (artificial) eye. Prosthetic eyes are made of ceramic or plastic and are usually designed to be very close in appearance to the person's own eye, in terms of color and shape (Fig. 36-12). When the person's natural eye is removed, a supporting structure is often inserted into the empty socket and the tissues inside the eyelids (the conjunctiva) are closed over it. Many times, the muscles that move the eyeball are attached to the supporting structure. This allows

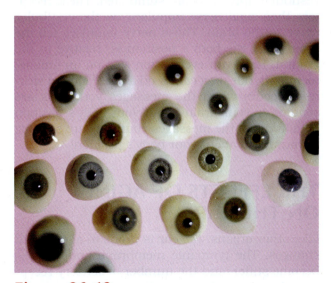

Figure 36-12
Artificial eyes are custom-made to look very similar to the person's other eye. (© *Lawrence Lawry/National Artificial Eye Service/Photo Researchers, Inc.*)

the prosthetic eye, if the person chooses to wear one, to move with the other eye.

A prosthetic eye is usually a curved disc (not a ball) that fits underneath the person's eyelids. Some prosthetic eyes are removable and others are permanent. If your resident's prosthetic eye is removable, you may need to help him with cleaning and storing it. Like eyeglasses, a prosthetic eye is very expensive to replace and should be cared for carefully. Improper handling can cause scratches or nicks on the prosthetic eye that can injure or irritate the person's eyelids. Handling the prosthetic eye with dirty hands or not cleaning it properly can result in an infection. If one of your residents wears a prosthetic eye, make sure you have been instructed in the proper way to care for it.

HEARING AND BALANCE

The sense organ of hearing and balance is the ear.

STRUCTURE OF THE EAR

The ear has three main sections: the outer ear, the middle ear, and the inner ear (Fig. 36-13).

The Outer Ear

The outer ear consists of the part of the ear that you can see (called the *pinna* or the *auricle*), plus a short canal called the *external auditory canal* (Fig. 36-13). The shape of the pinna allows it to collect sound waves and direct them down the external auditory canal toward the *tympanic membrane* (also called the eardrum). The external auditory canal is lined with small hairs and special glands that secrete **cerumen** (ear wax). Cerumen helps to protect the ear canal by trapping dirt and other particles.

The Middle Ear

The middle ear consists of an air space containing three very small bones (called *ossicles*) and the opening of the *eustachian tube*. The eustachian tube connects the middle ear to the pharynx (throat) and serves to equalize the pressure in the middle ear. If you have ever gone up or down a mountain or flown in an airplane, then you have probably felt your eustachian tube at work. As you change altitudes, your ears feel funny and you yawn to open them. The yawn allows air to travel through the eustachian tube, making the air pressure in the middle ear equal to the air pressure outside of your body. Equalizing the air

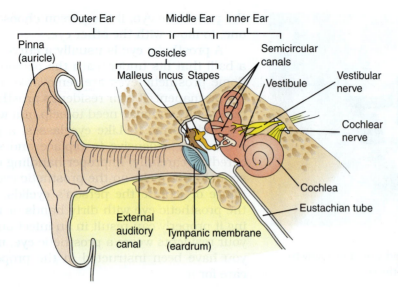

Figure 36-13
The ear.

pressures prevents the tympanic membrane from rupturing.

The three small bones (ossicles) in the middle ear are connected to the tympanic membrane. These bones, individually called the *malleus,* the *incus,* and the *stapes,* form a tiny bridge between the tympanic membrane and the inner ear (Fig. 36-13).

The Inner Ear

The most complex part of the ear is the inner ear, which contains the receptors that make hearing and balance possible. The part of the inner ear that is responsible for hearing is called the *cochlea.* The cochlea looks like a snail's shell and is filled with fluid (Fig. 36-13). Receptors for hearing are found within the cochlea.

The other part of the inner ear consists of two sac-like structures, called the *vestibule,* and three *semicircular canals* (Fig. 36-13). Like the cochlea, the semicircular canals are filled with fluid. The vestibule and the semicircular canals, which are referred to together as the *vestibular apparatus,* help us to keep our balance.

FUNCTION OF THE EAR

Hearing

Sounds travel in the form of sound waves. Sound waves are captured by the pinna and sent down the external auditory canal. As the sound waves travel down the external auditory canal, they come in contact with the tympanic membrane, causing it to vibrate. The tympanic membrane vibrations are then passed to the first bone of the

middle ear, the malleus; which sends the vibrations to the second bone, the incus; and then to the last bone, the stapes. The stapes rests against the oval window, a membrane at the opening of the cochlea. When the stapes vibrates, it causes the oval window to vibrate, sending the vibrations through the fluid inside the cochlea. The moving fluid stimulates the receptors inside the cochlea, which then send nerve impulses via the cochlear nerve to the brain. The brain interprets these nerve impulses as sound.

Balance

When your body position changes, receptors in the vestibular apparatus are stimulated. These receptors then send nerve impulses via the vestibular nerve to the brain. These nerve impulses tell the brain what the body's position is, relative to the ground. Have you ever gotten sick on an amusement park ride, in a car, or on a boat? Motion sickness occurs when the messages your ears are sending to your brain about your body's position do not match the messages your eyes are sending to your brain about your body's position!

THE EFFECTS OF AGING ON THE EAR

Like other organs, the ear is prone to age-related changes. The tympanic membrane and ossicles become stiffer, and the number of sensory receptors decreases. As a result, many older people gradually lose the ability to hear high-pitched sounds. This type of hearing loss is called **presbycusis.**

A person with presbycusis has trouble telling the difference between similar-sounding high-pitched sounds like *th* and *s,* which can lead to frequent misunderstandings. Conversations can be difficult to follow, especially when many people are talking at once or there is a lot of background noise. As a result, an older person with presbycusis may start to avoid social situations, because she cannot hear well and is embarrassed to have to keep asking others to repeat themselves. Avoiding social gatherings can lead to a feeling of isolation and a decreased quality of life for the older person.

Many older people with presbycusis are mistakenly labeled "confused" or "disoriented" by family members, friends, or health care professionals. But think about it, how can a person answer a question correctly if she cannot hear it clearly in the first place? When speaking with an elderly person with presbycusis, it is helpful to speak slowly using a lower tone of voice. This may make it easier for the person to understand what you are saying.

DISORDERS OF THE EAR

Cerumen Impaction

Cerumen impaction is a condition that occurs when ear wax (cerumen) builds up and becomes packed in the external auditory canal. In addition to decreased hearing, the person may experience a sense of fullness in the ear, ringing, itching, or pain. Routinely placing an object in the ear (such as a hearing aid or cotton swab) can cause cerumen impaction, because the object pushes the cerumen deep into the external auditory canal. Treatment usually involves irrigating (flushing) the ear with a special solution to remove the wax. Some residents have to use special ear drops on a routine basis to prevent this condition from occurring.

Ear Infections

Otitis media is an infection of the middle ear that occurs when fluid builds up in the middle ear. Bacteria from the throat find their way into the middle ear through the eustachian tube. Once there, they start to grow and multiply in the trapped fluid. Otitis media is usually accompanied by ear pain, fever, and difficulty hearing. If untreated, otitis media can cause scarring of the tympanic membrane and a permanent loss of hearing. If the infection is bacterial, antibiotics are usually given to treat it.

Another infection commonly seen in the ear involves the external auditory canal. **Otitis externa,** commonly referred to as "swimmer's ear," is an infection of the lining of the external auditory canal. Otitis externa is common in people who swim frequently or get the insides of their ears wet during showering or bathing. The ear becomes very painful to the touch. Antibiotic ear drops are usually needed to treat the infection.

Ménière's Disease

Ménière's disease, named after the French doctor who first described it, is a disease of the inner ear. Doctors do not know exactly what causes Ménière's disease. People with this disorder periodically experience episodes of dizziness (**vertigo**), ringing in the ear (**tinnitus**), temporary hearing loss, and a feeling of pressure or fullness in the ear. One or both ears may be affected, and with time, many people begin to experience permanent hearing loss in the affected ear or ears. There is usually no cure for this disorder.

Although Ménière's disease is not fatal, it can be very difficult to live with. Each attack can last between 2 and 4 hours, and is often accompanied by nausea, vomiting, or both. A person who is having an attack should lie down and keep his eyes fixed on an object that is not moving. This helps to reduce the nausea and lowers the risk of falling as a result of the dizziness. After a severe attack, the person may be very tired. A person with Ménière's disease may need to take more time when getting up from a sitting or lying position to prevent an attack from occurring.

Deafness

Like blindness, deafness has many different causes and takes many different forms. Some people have been deaf since birth, while others may have lost their hearing gradually later in life. Deafness can be partial or complete. The two main types of deafness are conductive hearing loss and sensorineural hearing loss:

- **Conductive hearing loss** occurs when something prevents sound waves from reaching the receptors in the cochlea. For example, the external auditory canal may be blocked by built-up cerumen, or by a tumor. The tympanic membrane may be damaged and not vibrate well, or the ossicles might not move freely. **Otosclerosis** is a disorder that causes a change in the stapes, preventing it from moving properly. Often, surgical removal and replacement of the stapes with a wire prosthesis can help to restore some hearing in people with otosclerosis.
- **Sensorineural hearing loss** occurs when the receptors are unable to receive stimuli

or transmit nerve impulses. Presbycusis, or age-related hearing loss, is sensorineural. However, there are many other causes of sensorineural hearing loss that are not necessarily the result of aging. For example, prolonged exposure to loud noise (especially industrial noise), recurrent ear infections, trauma to the ear, and some types of medications can all cause sensorineural hearing loss.

A person with hearing loss may work with a speech therapist to learn how to speak more clearly. In addition, many adaptive devices are available to help a person with hearing loss maintain his independence. For example, telephone devices for the deaf (TDD systems) can be used in combination with a standard phone to allow a hearing-impaired person to communicate using the telephone. Television shows are available with "closed captioning," a system that prints the words that are being spoken at the bottom of the screen so that the person can read them.

Communicating with a person who is hearing-impaired

When caring for a person with hearing loss, there are a few easy things you can do to ensure good communication:

- **Minimize background noise.** Background noise, such as a television set, other people talking, or the clank of silverware and dishes in the dining room, can make it difficult for the person to hear you. If a television set or radio is contributing to background noise, ask the person if you might temporarily turn it down (or off) so that you can talk to her. If the person is in an area where there are several other people or lots of activity, you may need to move with the person to a quieter location.
- **Face the person when you are speaking to him.** Many people who lose their hearing gradually develop the ability to partially lip-read what people are saying to them. You should always face the person as you speak so that the person has a clear view of your mouth (Fig. 36-14). Make sure that you are not standing in front of a window, or other bright light. The glare from the light will prevent the person from seeing your face clearly, and he will not be able to read your lips. Also, avoid chewing gum or speaking fast. These actions can also make it difficult for the person to lip-read.
- **Use a notepad to write down important questions or directions so that the person**

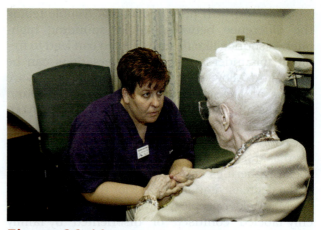

Figure 36-14
Always give a person who is hearing impaired an unobstructed view of your mouth. This will help the person to lip-read.

can read them. This helps to eliminate misunderstandings. If the person cannot read or reads in a language that is unfamiliar to you, a picture board (see Chapter 5, Fig. 5-4) may be helpful.
- **Make sure that the person fully understands what you said.** Some people, especially if the hearing loss is recent, hesitate to ask other people to repeat themselves. They may feel embarrassed by their hearing loss. When you are the "sender," you need to make sure that the person has gotten the message you were trying to send. If you are not sure that a person has understood what you have said to her, simply ask the person to repeat what you said back to you. For example, say, "If you could please repeat back to me what I said, I can make sure I told you everything I needed to." When the request is phrased in this way, the person feels as though she is helping you to do your job by repeating back the information. This helps to preserve the person's self-esteem and is a much better approach than just saying, "Now, what did I say?"
- **Let the person know if you cannot understand what he is saying to you.** Many people with hearing impairments have difficulty speaking clearly. If you cannot understand what the person is saying to you, let the person know this. The person may be trying to tell you something that is vitally important to his care or health. Tell the person that you did not understand and look for another way for him to get his message across. For example, you might offer him a notepad so that he can write down what he needs to tell you.

- **Consider learning sign language.** Residents who have significant hearing loss may use sign language to communicate (Fig. 36-15). Knowing how to communicate in this manner can be a very useful skill for a nursing assistant to have.

Hearing aids

Many people who are hearing-impaired use a hearing aid. A hearing aid is a battery-powered device that amplifies sound (makes it louder) before it enters the external auditory canal. There are many different styles of hearing aids (Fig. 36-16). Some styles fit entirely within the external auditory canal. Others attach behind the ear or to the person's eyeglasses. Others take the form of a small box that the person carries in his pocket.

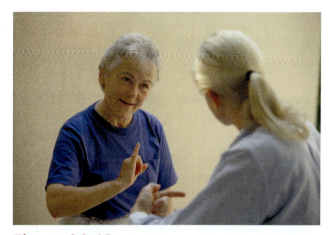

Figure 36-15
Some people who are deaf use sign language to communicate. (© Will & Deni McIntyre/Photo Researchers, Inc.)

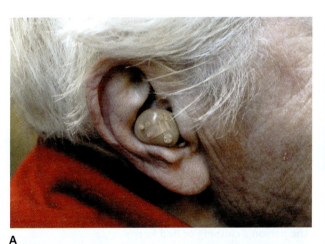

A

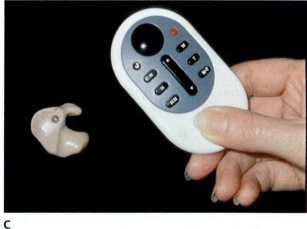

C

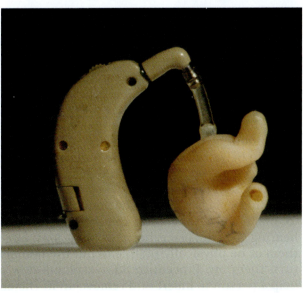

B

Figure 36-16
Hearing aids come in a variety of styles. **(A)** This type of hearing aid fits entirely inside the external auditory canal. **(B)** This type of hearing aid fits behind the person's ear. **(C)** This type of hearing aid is carried in a pocket. (B, © Bishop/Custom Medical Stock Photo; C, © SPL/Custom Medical Stock Photo.)

Guidelines Box 36-2   Guidelines for Caring for Hearing Aids

WHAT YOU DO	WHY YOU DO IT
Clean the hearing aid daily, according to the manufacturer's instructions.	If the hearing aid is not cleaned daily, the sound passages can become blocked with cerumen. The cerumen build-up can cause the hearing aid to stop working properly.
Make sure that the person has a spare set of batteries on hand at all times, and replace dead batteries immediately.	The hearing aid is battery-operated and will not work if the batteries are dead. It is very inconvenient for a person who uses a hearing aid to be without it for any length of time.
Keep hearing aids away from heat and moisture.	Heat and moisture can damage the plastic ear mold.
Do not use hairspray or other hair care products on a person who wears a hearing aid while the hearing aid is in place.	The chemicals in many hair care products can damage the plastic ear mold.
Store hearing aids at room temperature when they are not being worn.	Hearing aids are delicate instruments. Exposure to very hot or very cold temperatures is not good for them.
Keep the hearing aid in a designated place (for example, in its case in the bedside table drawer) when it is not in use.	Hearing aids are small and can be easily lost. Getting into the habit of always storing the hearing aid in the same place when it is not in use can prevent it from getting lost.
Check clothing and bed linens for the hearing aid before placing these items in the laundry.	The resident may remove the hearing aid and place it in his pocket or on the bed beside him. The hearing aid will be damaged if it goes through the laundry with the person's clothing or bed linens.

Not all people with hearing loss can benefit from the use of a hearing aid. It depends on the type of hearing loss the person has. An otologist (ear specialist) evaluates the person's hearing deficit to determine whether a hearing aid will be useful, and to determine what type of hearing aid should be used.

Hearing aids amplify all sounds, not just the voice of the person who is speaking. Noises from the environment, such as other people talking, the handling of dishes, or background music in the dining room, are also amplified. This can be distracting to a person wearing a hearing aid, and as a result, the person may choose to keep his hearing aid turned off most of the time.

Hearing aids are expensive and must be cared for carefully. General guidelines for caring for hearing aids are given in Guidelines Box 36-2. If one of your residents uses a hearing aid, make sure that you know how to care for it and operate it. If a person who uses a hearing aid seems unable to hear you, make sure the hearing aid is turned on, and that the volume is turned up high enough. If the hearing aid still does not seem to be working, check the batteries to see if they need to be replaced and make sure the sound passageway is not blocked with cerumen. As with eyeglasses, it may be your responsibility to make sure that your residents have their hearing aids in place because they may forget them or be physically unable to put them in and turn them on. Procedure 36-1 explains how to help a person to insert and remove an in-the-ear hearing aid.

SUMMARY

- The sensory system protects us from harm and lets us experience the world that we live in. The sensory system has two main divisions: general sense and special sense.
  - The receptors for general sense are spread throughout the body.
  - The receptors for special sense are located in special sense organs (the eyes, the ears, the nose, and the taste buds).
- General sense is responsible for our sense of touch, position, and pain.
  - Tactile receptors in our skin allow us to feel textures and the shapes of objects.
  - Position receptors in our muscles, tendons, and joints let us know where our body parts are in relation to each other.
  - Pain receptors (free nerve endings) in our skin and internal organs let us know when we are injured or ill.
- Chemoreceptors in the taste buds and the roof of the nasal cavity give us our senses of taste and smell. Together, taste and smell play a very large role in stimulating the appetite. These senses also help to keep us safe by alerting us to signs of danger (such as spoiled food, a gas leak, or smoke from a fire).
- The eye is a complex organ that gives us our sense of sight.
  - Many people need corrective lenses (eyeglasses or contact lenses) to see clearly. Common problems with focusing include myopia (nearsightedness), hyperopia (farsightedness), and astigmatism.
  - Changes in the eye as a result of aging can lead to presbyopia (an inability to focus on objects that are close), cataracts, and dry eyes. In addition, older people need more time to adjust when moving from a brightly lit area to a dim one, or vice versa.
- Some eye disorders, such as glaucoma and diabetic retinopathy, can lead to permanent vision loss if they are not treated.
- There are many different degrees of blindness.
  - Most people who are blind manage quite well on their own.
  - When caring for a person who is blind, you may have to make a few changes in the way you normally do things, to make up for the person's inability to see.
- Always handle your residents' eyeglasses, contact lenses, and prosthetic (artificial) eyes with care. These items are expensive and difficult to replace. In addition, improper handling of contact lenses or prosthetic eyes can lead to infection of the eye.
- The ear is responsible for our senses of hearing and balance.
  - Sensory receptors for sound are located in the cochlea.
    - Presbycusis is age-related hearing loss caused by a gradual decrease in the number of sensory receptors for sound.
    - There are many different degrees of hearing loss. Hearing loss may be conductive or sensorineural in origin.
    - When talking to a person with hearing loss, minimize background noise when possible, be sure that the person can see your face, take care to speak clearly, and clarify information as necessary. Sometimes, it may be necessary to write information down or use a picture board to ensure complete understanding.
  - Sensory receptors for balance are located in the vestibular apparatus, which consists of the vestibule and the semicircular canals. These receptors tell the brain where the body is in relation to the ground.

36

PROCEDURES

PROCEDURE 36-1

Assisting a Person With an In-the-Ear Hearing Aid

WHY YOU DO IT   Being able to hear clearly makes communication easier and enhances the person's quality of life.

Inserting an In-the-Ear Hearing Aid

1. Complete the "Getting Ready" steps.
   WGKIEPS

2. Check the hearing aid to make sure the volume is down and the hearing aid is turned off.

3. Help the person to a comfortable position, with his head turned so that the ear needing the hearing aid is closest to you.

4. Inspect the ear canal for excessive cerumen (ear wax). If you see excessive wax build-up in the ear canal, gently wipe the ear canal with a warm, moist washcloth.

5. Gently insert the tapered end of the hearing aid into the external auditory canal. Gently rotate the hearing aid so that it fits into the curve of the ear. With one hand, push up and in. Use your other hand to pull gently down on the person's earlobe. The hearing aid should fit snugly but comfortably, flush with the ear.

6. Turn on the control switch. Adjust the volume by talking to the person as you increase the volume. Stop increasing the volume when the person can hear you.

7. Complete the "Finishing Up" steps.
   CLSOWR

Removing an In-the-Ear Hearing Aid

1. Complete the "Getting Ready" steps.
   WGKIEPS

2. Turn off the hearing aid.

3. Gently pull up on the person's ear. This will allow you to lift the hearing aid up and out of the person's ear.

4. Remove the batteries before storing the hearing aid in its case. Make sure the case is labeled with the person's name.

5. Complete the "Finishing Up" steps.
   CLSOWR

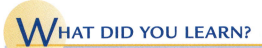

WHAT DID YOU LEARN?

Multiple Choice

Select the single best answer for each of the following questions.

1. Where are sensory receptors that are responsible for "special sense" located?
   a. In the muscles, tendons, and joints
   b. In the eyes, ears, nose, and taste buds
   c. In the brain and spinal cord
   d. In all of the organs of the body

2. Mrs. Knight is having a heart attack. She complains to the nurse of pain in her arm and jaw. What type of pain is Mrs. Knight experiencing?
   a. Chronic pain
   b. Referred (radiating) pain
   c. Imagined pain
   d. Musculoskeletal pain

3. One of the residents in the facility where you work, Mr. Hepberg, is 85 years old and in fairly good overall health. Mr. Hepberg always says to you, "Don't ever get old, honey! When you get old, even the food doesn't taste good anymore." Why might Mr. Hepberg feel this way?
   a. The meals at the facility are very bland for dietetic reasons.
   b. Mr. Hepberg is depressed.
   c. As we get older, our sense of taste and smell decreases, making food less appealing.
   d. Mr. Hepberg has a head cold.

4. Which one of the following symptoms of conjunctivitis should be reported to the nurse?
   a. Itching and burning of the eye
   b. Redness of the eye
   c. A sticky white or yellow discharge from the eye
   d. All of the above

5. Jessica is assigned to take care of Mr. Golden, who has recently become blind. What should Jessica remember when caring for Mr. Golden?
   a. Jessica should greet Mr. Golden and state her name when she enters his room.
   b. Jessica can help Mr. Golden to feel more secure when walking by walking a step or two ahead of Mr. Golden and letting Mr. Golden rest his hand lightly on her elbow.

   c. During procedures, Jessica should explain each step of the procedure to Mr. Golden as she does it so that he knows what is happening.
   d. All of the above

6. Which one of the following is true about cataracts?
   a. Many elderly people develop cataracts, but young people can develop them too.
   b. Cataracts are very painful.
   c. There is no cure for cataracts.
   d. Cataracts are a complication of diabetes.

7. Michael is taking care of Miss Jordan, who has a hearing loss. Miss Jordan is wearing her hearing aid, but it does not seem to be working. What should Michael do first?
   a. He should raise his voice.
   b. He should make sure that the hearing aid is turned on, and that the volume is high enough.
   c. He should remove the hearing aid and replace its batteries.
   d. He should report the problem to the nurse immediately.

8. Mr. Campi, one of your elderly residents, is very hard of hearing. What should you remember when you are talking to Mr. Campi?
   a. You should sit or stand so that Mr. Campi has a clear view of your face, and you should avoid chewing gum or speaking quickly.
   b. If you think that Mr. Campi has not completely understood what you are saying, you should demand that he repeat it back to you so that you can correct his mistakes.
   c. If you do not understand what Mr. Campi has said, you should just let it pass. Letting him know that you did not understand might embarrass or frustrate him.
   d. There is no point in talking to Mr. Campi. He cannot hear you anyway. It is better to just write everything down.

Matching

Match each numbered item with its appropriate lettered description.

_____ **1.** Iris

_____ **2.** Cornea

_____ **3.** Lens

_____ **4.** Myopia

_____ **5.** Astigmatism

_____ **6.** Retina

_____ **7.** Hyperopia

_____ **8.** Pupil

_____ **9.** Vitreous humor

_____ **10.** Ciliary body

a. Nearsightedness

b. Clear portion of the sclera, through which light passes to the inside of the eye

c. A round muscle; the colored portion of the eye

d. Farsightedness

e. A disorder of the cornea that results in blurred vision

f. The hole in the center of the iris

g. A flexible, transparent, curved structure that helps to focus images on the retina

h. Contains rods and cones, the sensory receptors responsible for vision

i. The jelly-like substance contained in the posterior chamber that helps to give the eyeball its shape

j. The muscle that allows the lens to either become shorter and rounder or longer and flatter

STOP and Think!

- You work in an assisted-living facility and have known one of the residents, Mrs. Zinner, for almost 6 years now. Mrs. Zinner is in her 70s and enjoys very good health. In fact, her only disability seems to be related to glaucoma, which is causing her to go blind. Mrs. Zinner's ability to see is now limited to being able to tell the difference between light and dark and make out the outlines of very large objects. What are some ways that you can help Mrs. Zinner adjust to her blindness physically? What are some things you can do that will help Mrs. Zinner adjust emotionally?

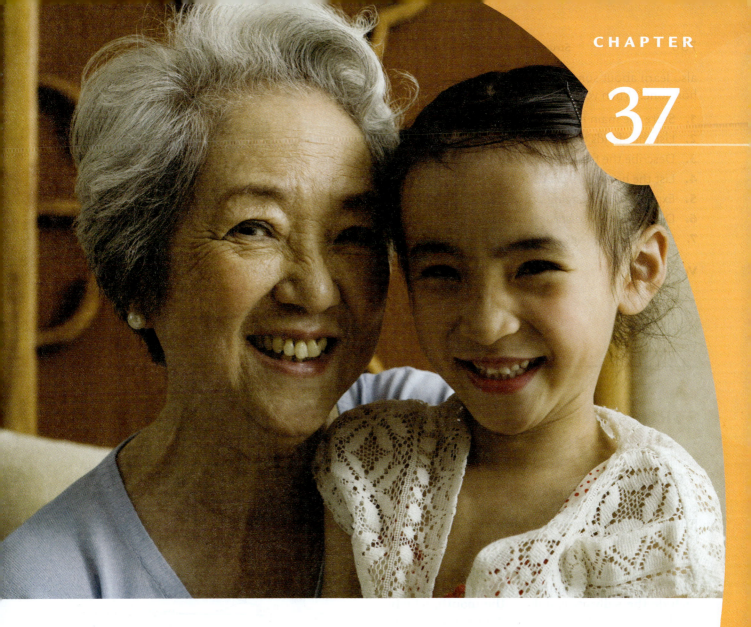

The Endocrine System

WHAT WILL YOU LEARN?

The endocrine system produces hormones, chemicals that act on cells to produce a response. The word "hormone" comes from the Greek word *hormaein*, "to set in motion." This is, in fact, exactly what hormones do—set things in motion. Sometimes, the effects of the hormone occur over a long period of time. For example, hormones allow us to grow to our adult height, and they cause the physical changes that turn boys and girls into men and women. Other times, the effects of hormones are more immediate. Hormones with short-term effects help the body to maintain homeostasis. For example, insulin is a hormone that regulates blood sugar levels.

The hormones produced by the endocrine system control many of the body's functions. In this chapter, you will learn about the glands of the endocrine system, some of the hormones they produce, and how these hormones act to "set things in motion." You will

Photo: The hormones produced by the endocrine system set processes in motion. For example, hormones are what cause us to grow!

also learn about some of the disorders that occur when the body produces too much or too little of a certain hormone. When you are finished with this chapter, you will be able to:

1. State the main function of the endocrine system.
2. List the glands that make up the endocrine system.
3. Describe the feedback mechanism that controls the endocrine system.
4. List the hormones produced by the different glands of the endocrine system.
5. Explain how the aging process affects the endocrine system.
6. Discuss various disorders that affect the endocrine system.
7. Discuss the special care needs of people who have endocrine system disorders.

Vocabulary Use the CD in the front of your book to hear these terms pronounced and defined:

Hormones	Hyperthyroidism	Diabetes mellitus	Hypoglycemia
Goiter	(Graves' disease)	Type 1 diabetes mellitus	Hyperglycemia
Tetany	Hypothyroidism	Type 2 diabetes mellitus	Glucometer

STRUCTURE OF THE ENDOCRINE SYSTEM

A group of glands, called the endocrine glands, make up the endocrine system. Be careful not to confuse endocrine glands and exocrine glands! Endocrine glands produce hormones and release them directly into the bloodstream. Exocrine glands produce substances that are not hormones and release them into a hollow organ or onto a surface. Examples of exocrine glands include the salivary glands in the mouth, which produce saliva, and the sweat glands in the skin, which produce sweat. Exocrine glands are not part of the endocrine system.

The endocrine glands are located in specific places throughout the body (Fig. 37-1):

- The *pituitary gland* is about the size of a cherry and lies underneath the brain. It is connected by a stalk to the hypothalamus.
- The *pineal gland* is also located underneath the brain.
- The *thyroid gland* is located in the neck. It is butterfly-shaped, with two oval lobes located on either side of the larynx. The lobes are connected by a narrow band of tissue called the isthmus.
- The *parathyroid glands* are four tiny glands that are embedded in the back of the thyroid gland.
- The *thymus gland* is located in the upper part of the chest above the heart.

- The *adrenal glands* are located on top of the kidneys.
- The *pancreas* is located in the abdomen.
- The *sex glands (gonads)* are the ovaries in women and the testes in men. These glands

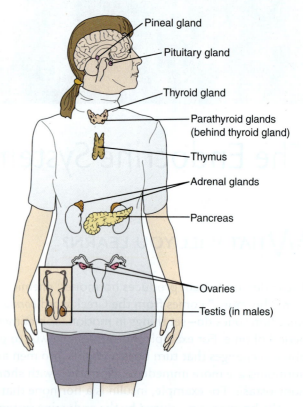

Figure 37-1
The endocrine system is made up of the endocrine glands, which are located throughout the body.

are also considered part of the reproductive system and are discussed in detail in Chapter 40.

FUNCTION OF THE ENDOCRINE SYSTEM

The endocrine system controls many of the body's processes such as growth and development, reproduction, and metabolism. It does this by producing **hormones,** chemicals that act on cells to produce a response. The hormones are released into the bloodstream, which means that they can affect cells far from the gland that produced them. The hormone travels in the blood until it reaches its target cell. Once there, it attaches to a special receptor in the cell wall. Just as turning a key in a lock causes a door to open, attaching a hormone to a receptor causes a specific reaction in the cell. Some hormones have receptors in all of the body's cells, while other hormones have receptors in only certain types of cells.

The release (secretion) of many hormones is regulated by a feedback system. In a feedback system, some change in the internal environment causes the gland to begin producing its hormone. The gland continues to produce the hormone until the amount of hormone (or some other related substance) reaches a certain level in the body. At that point, the gland stops producing the hormone. The feedback system works very much like a central heating unit in a house. The thermostat is pre-set to keep the temperature inside the house within a certain range. When the thermostat detects that the temperature has dropped below this pre-set range, the thermostat signals the furnace to turn on to heat the air. After the furnace creates heat and the temperature in the house rises to the desired range, the thermostat turns the furnace off.

In the rest of this section, we will explore the individual glands of the endocrine system, the hormones they secrete, and the effects of these hormones on the body.

PITUITARY GLAND

The pituitary gland, which is controlled by the hypothalamus, releases hormones that affect the function of other glands in the endocrine system. In this sense, the pituitary gland is like the "master gland." The pituitary gland has two parts, the posterior lobe and the anterior lobe.

Posterior Lobe Hormones

The posterior lobe of the pituitary gland stores and releases hormones that are produced by the hypothalamus. Two hormones are released by the posterior lobe (Fig. 37-2).

- *Antidiuretic hormone (ADH)* acts on the kidneys. ADH limits the amount of water that is lost from the body in the form of urine. When a person does not take in enough fluid or loses too much fluid through sweating, vomiting, or diarrhea, the hypothalamus detects a lower fluid level in the blood and signals the pituitary gland to release more ADH. The ADH causes the kidneys to save body fluid by decreasing the amount of urine produced. Similarly, when the hypothalamus detects that fluid levels are too high, it signals the pituitary gland to secrete less ADH. The lack of ADH causes the kidneys to produce more urine, eliminating the excess fluid from the body.
- *Oxytocin* is the hormone that causes labor to begin and is responsible for the let-down of milk in the breasts of a nursing mother.

Anterior Lobe Hormones

The anterior lobe of the pituitary gland makes and releases several different hormones (Fig. 37-2).

- *Growth hormone* is what causes our bodies to get bigger and taller as we move from infancy into adulthood. Growth hormone is usually released in greater amounts during short periods of time, resulting in a child's "growth spurts." Although the output of growth hormone is highest during childhood, the anterior lobe continues to release growth hormone long after the growing phase of development is finished. Cells need to be replaced throughout a person's lifetime, and growth hormone is necessary for that to occur.
- *Thyroid-stimulating hormone (TSH)* stimulates the thyroid gland to produce thyroid hormones, which affect the rate of metabolism in the body's tissues.
- *Adrenocorticotropic hormone (ACTH)* stimulates the adrenal glands to produce their hormones, which help the body to deal with stress.
- *Prolactin* stimulates the milk glands of the breast to produce milk when a baby is born.
- *Gonadotropins* regulate the functioning of the sex glands (gonads) in both males and females. There are two gonadotropins, *follicle-stimulating hormone (FSH)* and *luteinizing hormone (LH)*. The action of the gonadotropins is discussed in more detail in Chapter 40.

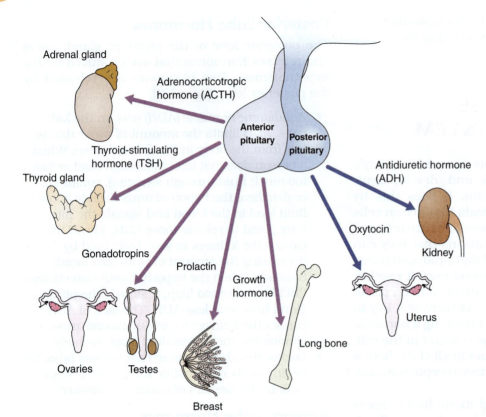

Figure 37-2
The pituitary gland, or "master gland," releases hormones that affect other glands in the endocrine system.

PINEAL GLAND

The pineal gland secretes *melatonin*, which helps to regulate the body's sleep–awake cycles. The pineal gland is stimulated by light and darkness and secretes melatonin during the dark part of the day.

THYROID GLAND

The thyroid gland produces two hormones that help to regulate the body's metabolism, the main one being *thyroxine*. In addition, the thyroid gland produces *calcitonin,* a hormone that helps to regulate the amount of calcium in the bloodstream.

Thyroxine

The hormone thyroxine sets the rate of metabolism for the cells of the body. How quickly body cells and tissues use nutrients (especially protein) and produce energy is determined by the amount of thyroxine present in the bloodstream. If the thyroid gland releases more thyroxine, the metabolic rate of the cells increases, and if the thyroid gland releases less thyroxine, the metabolic rate of the cells decreases.

The thyroid gland needs iodine to produce thyroxine. Iodine is found naturally in fish and shellfish and is added to salt and other commercial products. When a person does not get enough iodine in her diet, the thyroid gland is not able to produce adequate amounts of thyroxine. The sensors in the hypothalamus and pituitary gland detect a decrease in the level of thyroxine in the bloodstream and release TSH to stimulate the thyroid gland to produce more. However, because the thyroid gland has no iodine, it cannot respond to the request for more thyroxine, and the cycle repeats itself. The constant stimulation of the thyroid gland causes it to enlarge. An enlargement of the thyroid gland is called a **goiter** (Fig. 37-3). Iodine deficiency is just one cause of a goiter. A goiter can also occur when the thyroid gland does not produce enough hormone because of disease or tumors.

Calcitonin

Another important hormone produced by the thyroid gland is calcitonin. Calcitonin is one of the hormones that helps to maintain calcium levels in the bloodstream. As you learned in Chapter 32, calcium is important for proper functioning of the skeletal and cardiac muscle. Calcium helps transmit nerve impulses into and out of the

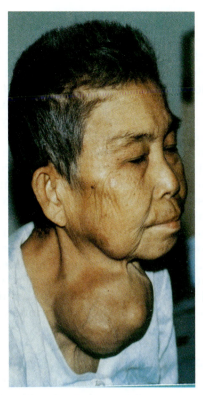

Figure 37-3
The swelling in this woman's neck is a goiter, or an enlarged thyroid gland. Goiter can be caused by a lack of iodine in the diet or by a tumor or disease that affects the thyroid gland's ability to produce thyroid hormone. (*From Rubin, R. & Strayer, D.S. [2008]. Rubin's Pathology: Clinicopathologic foundations of medicine [5th ed., p. 942]. Philadelphia: Lippincott Williams & Wilkins.*)

muscle fibers, allowing for the smooth contraction and relaxation of the muscles. Too little calcium makes the muscle fibers irritable and unable to relax after they contract, causing cramping. **Tetany** (cramping of the skeletal muscles and an irregular heartbeat) can occur if the calcium level drops too low. Too much calcium in the bloodstream causes muscles to become weak and slow to respond.

Calcitonin lowers the amount of calcium in the bloodstream by allowing the calcium to be deposited in the bones and eliminated by the kidneys. For example, if a person drinks a lot of milk or takes calcium supplements, the level of calcium in the bloodstream increases as the calcium is absorbed from the intestines. The high calcium level in the blood stimulates the thyroid gland to produce calcitonin. Calcitonin transports the extra calcium to the bones. Any calcium that cannot be stored in the bones is excreted by the kidneys, in the form of urine.

PARATHYROID GLANDS

The parathyroid glands produce *parathyroid hormone (PTH)*, which has the opposite effect of calcitonin. PTH causes calcium to be released from the bones into the bloodstream, increasing the amount of calcium in the bloodstream. In addition, PTH helps the kidneys to keep calcium, instead of excrete it in the urine. As you learned in Chapter 32, a calcium-rich diet is important to build up stores of calcium in the bones. PTH is what allows us to draw on these stores later in life, when our bodies become less efficient at absorbing the calcium that we eat. The actions of calcitonin and PTH balance each other and help to keep the levels of calcium in the bloodstream constant.

If the parathyroid glands are surgically removed or become damaged by disease, PTH is not produced in adequate amounts and the calcium levels may drop, causing tetany. Some tumors of the parathyroid gland can cause an overproduction of PTH that results in too much calcium being removed from the bones. The bones then become very fragile and fracture easily. Because the kidneys are responsible for excreting the excess calcium, kidney stones are likely to form.

THYMUS GLAND

The thymus gland secretes *thymosin*, a hormone that helps infection-fighting T cells to mature. An increase in the secretion of thymosin stimulates the body to produce more T cells during an infection or illness.

ADRENAL GLANDS

Each adrenal gland has two separate parts: the *medulla*, or inner portion, and the *cortex*, or outer portion (Fig. 37-4). Each part secretes distinct hormones.

Medullary Hormones

The medulla of the adrenal glands secretes two hormones that are responsible for the "fight-or-flight" response of the body in emergency situations. Those hormones are *epinephrine* (also known as adrenaline) and *norepinephrine*. Epinephrine and norepinephrine help the heart and lungs deliver more oxygen and nutrients to the muscles, preparing the body to "stand up and fight or turn tail and run." A "side effect" of these hormones is the dry-mouthed, heart-pounding reaction that occurs when you are frightened!

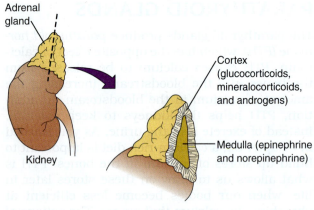

Figure 37-4

The adrenal gland consists of an inner part (the adrenal medulla) and an outer part (the adrenal cortex). Each part produces and secretes different hormones. Many of these hormones help us to deal with stressful situations.

Cortical Hormones

The outer portion of the adrenal glands secretes three main groups of hormones:

- *Glucocorticoids* play a role in the metabolism of fats and proteins, and help the body to maintain a reserve of glucose (sugar) that can be used in times of stress. They are also able to suppress the body's inflammatory response. For this reason, glucocorticoids are often given in the form of medications for severe inflammatory disorders, such as asthma, rheumatoid arthritis, or severe allergic reactions. Hydrocortisone is a common medication that is a glucocorticoid.
- *Mineralocorticoids* help to regulate the level of certain minerals in the body, particularly sodium and potassium. *Aldosterone* is the primary hormone in this group. Aldosterone helps the kidneys to reabsorb sodium and secrete potassium.
- *Androgens* are secreted in small amounts by the adrenal cortex. Androgens are converted by the body into the sex hormones *testosterone* (in men) and *estradiol* (in women).

PANCREAS

The pancreas is both an exocrine gland and an endocrine gland. It functions as an exocrine gland by producing and secreting enzymes into the small intestine that help to digest food. It functions as an endocrine gland by producing two hormones, *insulin* and *glucagon*.

Insulin

Special cells within the pancreas, called the *islets of Langerhans,* produce and secrete the hormone insulin. Insulin, which affects all of the body's cells, allows glucose (sugar) to be transported from the bloodstream into the individual cells, where it is used for energy. In this way, insulin lowers the blood glucose level.

When a person eats, food is digested and absorbed by the bloodstream in the form of glucose. The blood glucose levels determine how much insulin the pancreas releases. After eating, a person's blood glucose is elevated, and the pancreas releases insulin. The insulin causes the glucose to move from the bloodstream into the cells, where it can be used for energy. Any extra glucose is converted to glycogen. Glycogen is stored in the liver for later use, or it is converted to fat and deposited in various places on the body.

Glucagon

Glucagon has the opposite effect of insulin. While insulin is responsible for lowering blood glucose levels, glucagon is responsible for raising them. When the glucose levels in the bloodstream drop, as they normally do when a person has not eaten for some time, the pancreas secretes glucagon. The glucagon stimulates the liver to release the glucose that has been stored as glycogen into the bloodstream, to supply the cells of the body with fuel for energy. Insulin and glucagon work together to keep the body's blood glucose levels stable.

SEX GLANDS

The sex glands (or gonads) secrete the hormones that result in the onset of puberty and that regulate reproduction. Because the ovaries and testes are also considered a part of the reproductive system, these glands are discussed in greater detail in Chapter 40.

THE EFFECTS OF AGING ON THE ENDOCRINE SYSTEM

The normal processes of aging decrease the amount of hormones produced and slow their secretion by the glands of the endocrine system. Many of the physical changes that are part of aging are directly related to the smaller amounts of hormone released. For example, decreases in growth hormone levels slow the rate at which the body's cells and tissues divide and replace themselves, and decreases in thyroid hormone levels slow the body's metabolism.

In women, menopause (the end of menstruation, which signals the end of a woman's ability to bear children) occurs as a result of decreased hormone production by the ovaries. In men, secretion of hormones by the testes decreases, affecting sexual drive and function.

DISORDERS OF THE ENDOCRINE SYSTEM

Disorders of the endocrine system occur when the body produces too much or too little of a certain hormone. Imbalances in hormone secretion can be caused by disorders of the hypothalamus, the pituitary gland, the specific endocrine gland responsible for the hormone, or as a result of poor nutrition. Corrective measures may be needed to restore the body's homeostasis and prevent the imbalances from causing health problems. There are many different types of endocrine disorders. Some of the ones you will be most likely to encounter in the long-term care setting are described here.

ACROMEGALY

The secretion of too much growth hormone after a person has reached adulthood causes excessive growth of the bones of the hands, feet, and face. This condition is called acromegaly (Fig. 37-5). The person does not grow taller, but he does have a disproportioned appearance, especially in the face and hands.

THYROID GLAND DISORDERS

Remember that the secretion of the thyroid hormones is controlled by the pituitary gland. Therefore, thyroid disorders can be caused by abnormalities of the pituitary gland or by abnormalities of the thyroid gland itself. Thyroid disorders can also result from nutrient deficiencies, such as a lack of iodine. A simple blood test can be used to detect imbalances in thyroid hormones. Once detected, these imbalances can usually be treated.

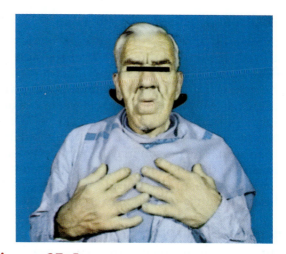

Figure 37-5
Secretion of too much growth hormone in an adult causes acromegaly, excessive growth of the bones of the hands, feet, and face.

Hyperthyroidism

Hyperthyroidism (sometimes called **Graves' disease**) is caused by the excessive secretion of thyroxine (*hyper* = "above"). In a person with hyperthyroidism, the metabolic rate of the body's cells is increased. Signs and symptoms of hyperthyroidism include increased hunger accompanied by weight loss, an irregular heartbeat, an inability to sleep, irritability, confusion, increased perspiration, and intolerance to heat. Hyperthyroidism may be treated by surgically removing part of the thyroid gland, or by destroying part of the gland with radiation.

Hypothyroidism

Hypothyroidism results when thyroxine secretion is too low (*hypo* = "below"). Hypothyroidism is more common among women and the elderly. Hypothyroidism causes signs and symptoms that are opposite those of hyperthyroidism. Signs and symptoms of hypothyroidism include fatigue, weakness, depression, anorexia, weight gain, constipation, and intolerance to cold. Hypothyroidism is treated by administering thyroxine in the form of a pill.

ADRENAL GLAND DISORDERS

Two of the most common adrenal gland disorders, Addison's disease and Cushing's syndrome, result from imbalances of the adrenal cortical hormones.

Addison's Disease

In Addison's disease, the adrenal cortex is destroyed, resulting in low levels of the adrenal cortical hormones. Because the glucocorticoids play a role in protein metabolism, a person with Addison's disease develops muscle weakness and atrophy. Dark discoloration of the skin and disturbances in the body's salt and water balance are also seen. The person may have hypertension as a result of the Addison's disease. A person with Addison's disease may need assistance with walking and range-of-motion exercises.

Cushing's Syndrome

Cushing's syndrome results from excessive secretion of glucocorticoids. Cushing's syndrome can be caused by disorders of the pituitary gland that affect ACTH secretion or by disorders of the adrenal gland itself. Some people develop Cushing's syndrome after taking high doses of steroid medications, such as hydrocortisone, for a long period of time. Because glucocorticoids help us to metabolize fat, people with Cushing's syndrome tend to develop pockets of fat in the abdomen, on the back, and in the face. Increased facial hair is also common (Fig. 37-6). A person with Cushing's syndrome will have high blood glucose levels, because one of the effects of glucocorticoids is to decrease the use of glucose by the tissues. Easy bruising of the skin and muscle weakness are also seen.

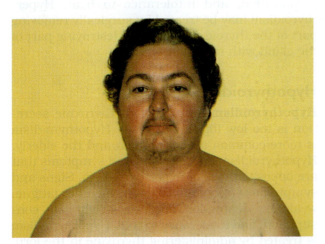

Figure 37-6
Cushing's syndrome results from excessive amounts of the adrenal cortical hormones. The excessive secretion of androgens, which are converted into sex hormones, is what caused this woman to develop facial hair. The accumulation of fat on the woman's back and face is the result of excess glucocorticoids. (*Reprinted with permission from Rubin, E., & Farber, J.L. [2005]. Pathology [4th ed., p. 1162]. Philadelphia: Lippincott Williams & Wilkins.*)

DIABETES MELLITUS

Diabetes mellitus results when the pancreas is unable to produce enough insulin, the body's cells are unable to properly use the insulin that is produced, or both. When there is not enough insulin in the body, or if the body's cells do not respond to the insulin that is produced, the body cannot use the glucose that enters the bloodstream. As a result, the amount of glucose in the bloodstream becomes very high. The high blood glucose levels may cause the person to experience symptoms such as fatigue, weakness, excessive thirst, excessive urination, blurry vision, and an increased number of infections. In an elderly person, high blood glucose levels also increase the person's risk for dehydration and falling. Over time, if the blood glucose levels are not controlled, the person can develop serious complications, such as blindness, kidney failure, nerve damage, and cardiovascular disease.

Diabetes mellitus can occur in people of all ages and races, but people between the ages of 65 and 74 years and people of Native American or African descent are affected most often. Diabetes mellitus is the most common of all endocrine gland disorders and is a leading cause of death among the elderly.

Types of Diabetes Mellitus

There are two types of diabetes mellitus, type 1 and type 2.

Type 1 diabetes mellitus

Type 1 diabetes mellitus, which accounts for 5% to 10% of all cases of diabetes, is caused by destruction of the insulin-producing cells of the pancreas. As a result, the body cannot produce its own insulin. A person with type 1 diabetes must receive regular injections of insulin in order to keep his blood glucose level within a normal range. Most people who have type 1 diabetes are diagnosed while they are children or young adults, which is why you may hear this type of diabetes referred to as "juvenile diabetes."

Type 2 diabetes

Type 2 diabetes, which accounts for 90% to 95% of all cases of diabetes, occurs when the pancreas still produces some insulin, but the cells of the body are unable to respond to the insulin. This results in higher blood glucose levels, because the body is unable to move the glucose out of the blood and into the cells. Risk factors for developing type 2 diabetes include being overweight or obese and increasing age. Because the number of people who are overweight or obese is increasing in the United States, we are seeing more and more cases of type 2 diabetes each year. And, while in the past, type 2 diabetes was mostly considered a disease of "old age," now more people are developing type 2 diabetes at a younger age, possibly even during childhood.

Some people, especially those who are overweight, develop a condition known as "pre-diabetes." This means that their blood glucose level is higher than it should be, but not as high as it would be in diabetes. Research has shown that people with "pre-diabetes" who make lifestyle changes (such as eating a healthy diet and exercising regularly) can often delay or prevent the onset of type 2 diabetes.

Management of Diabetes Mellitus

To keep blood glucose levels within the range of normal, three factors must be balanced: diet, exercise, and medication (Fig. 37-7). A change in any one of these factors can affect blood sugar control, resulting in **hypoglycemia** (a blood glucose level that is too low) or **hyperglycemia** (a blood glucose level that is too high). Box 37-1 reviews some of the causes and effects of hypoglycemia and hyperglycemia.

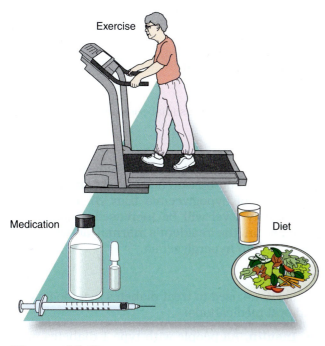

Figure 37-7
Diabetes mellitus is managed with diet, exercise, and medication. A change in any one of these three factors can affect the blood glucose level.

Diet

A person with diabetes needs to eat a well-balanced, nutritious diet, with limited sweets and fats. Following a proper diet helps to keep blood glucose levels within the normal range. A proper diet also helps the person achieve or maintain a healthy body weight, and reduces the person's risk for cardiovascular disease, which often accompanies diabetes.

Meals and snacks should be eaten at regular times throughout the day to help keep blood glucose levels steady. This is why, when you are caring for a person with diabetes, it is important to serve meals and snacks at the scheduled time (Fig. 38-8). You will also need to pay attention to how much the person eats, and what the person eats. Specific amounts of carbohydrates, sugars, fats, and proteins are needed to react with the medication the person takes for his diabetes. If the person refuses the meal or snack, or only partially finishes it, his blood glucose level may become too low. Similarly, if the person eats more food than usual, or food with higher sugar content than usual, the amount of medication will not be sufficient and his blood glucose level may become too high.

Following a diabetic diet may be quite difficult, especially for a person who enjoys sweets. Life-long eating habits can be hard to change. Sometimes special treats can be worked into the person's diet plan. However, some of your residents may keep stashes of candy or other sweets in their rooms. If you notice that a resident with diabetes is hoarding sweets, you should report this to the nurse.

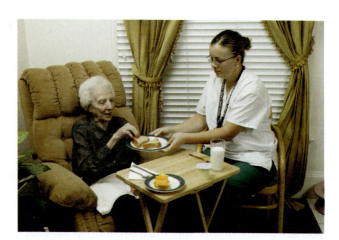

Figure 37-8
It is very important for a person with diabetes to eat regular, nutritionally sound meals and snacks. If one of your residents with diabetes refuses to eat or only eats part of a meal or snack, report this to a nurse immediately.

BOX 37-1 Hypoglycemia and Hyperglycemia

Hypoglycemia or hyperglycemia can result when diet, exercise, and medication are not in balance. A person's medication dose is planned to balance the person's usual food intake and amount of activity. A change in food intake or level of activity can lead to hypoglycemia or hyperglycemia if the person's medication dose is not adjusted accordingly. Both hypoglycemia and hyperglycemia can have serious consequences, including death, if they are not treated.

Hypoglycemia (low blood glucose levels)

Causes
- Missing a meal or a snack
- A delayed meal or snack
- Eating too little food
- Vomiting
- NPO status
- Increased level of activity
- Too much medication

Effects
- Cool, clammy skin
- Sweating
- Feeling "shaky"
- Confusion or difficulty concentrating
- Rapid heart rate and rapid breathing
- Headache
- Blurry or "double" vision
- Restlessness and irritability
- Trembling
- A tingling sensation in the mouth or tongue
- Hunger
- Loss of consciousness (insulin shock)

Hyperglycemia (high blood glucose levels)

Causes
- Eating too much food
- Decreased level of activity
- Too little medication
- Physical stress (illness or injury)
- Emotional stress
- Undiagnosed diabetes

Effects
- Excessive urination
- Excessive thirst
- Extreme hunger
- Unplanned weight loss
- Fatigue
- Blurry or "double" vision
- Headache
- Irritability
- Dry, flushed skin
- Sweet-smelling breath
- Dehydration
- Seizures
- Loss of consciousness (diabetic coma)

Exercise

When we exercise, our muscles use glucose for energy. This helps to lower blood glucose levels. In addition, exercise plays an important role in achieving or maintaining a healthy body weight. An older person's ability to exercise may be limited by a chronic health condition or disability. You should encourage the person to participate in whatever level of exercise he can tolerate. Be sure you are aware of any specific instructions for exercise that are included in the person's care plan.

When you are caring for a person with diabetes, be aware that changes in the person's normal activity level could result in hypoglycemia or hyperglycemia. For example, a resident with diabetes who is beginning a new physical therapy program should be watched closely for signs and symptoms of hypoglycemia (Box 37-1), because her activity level will be increased. Similarly, a decrease in the resident's normal activity level could lead to hyperglycemia.

Medication

Medications used to treat diabetes include insulin and oral medications:

- **Insulin.** All people with type 1 diabetes mellitus, and some people with type 2 diabetes mellitus, require insulin. Insulin can be administered using a needle and syringe, a special insulin "pen," or a pump (Fig. 37-9).

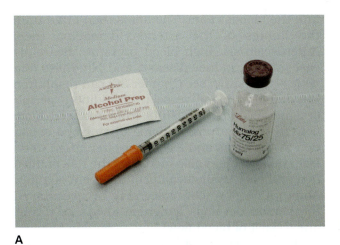

A

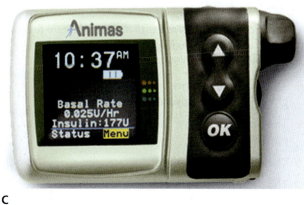

C

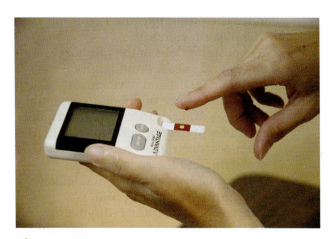

B

Figure 37-9

Insulin can be administered using **(A)** a needle and syringe, **(B)** an insulin pen, or **(C)** an insulin pump. (*B, Courtesy of sanofi-aventis, U.S. C, courtesy of Animas Corporation, West Chester, PA.*)

Several types of insulin are available. The types of insulin differ in the speed at which they start working and how long they last in the body. Most of your residents who take insulin for the treatment of diabetes will receive multiple insulin injections each day.

- **Oral medications.** Many people with type 2 diabetes mellitus take oral medications to help control their blood glucose levels. The different types of oral medications used to treat diabetes work in slightly different ways. Some stimulate the pancreas to produce more insulin, some act on the cells in the body to help them use the insulin that the body produces, and some decrease the amount of glucose that enters the bloodstream after eating.

Monitoring Blood Glucose Levels

As you have learned, diabetes control involves balancing diet, exercise, and medication. A person with diabetes needs to monitor her blood glucose levels regularly to make sure that her prescribed treatment is keeping her blood glucose level within the desired range. A **glucometer** is used to monitor blood glucose levels. Most glucometers use a drop of blood, obtained from the person's finger (Fig. 37-10). The "finger stick" method of monitoring blood glucose levels can be painful for the person and can also expose the health care worker to bloodborne diseases. If you

are allowed to assist a resident with blood glucose monitoring using this method, make sure to wear gloves.

Many people with diabetes monitor their own glucose levels, but some residents may need help with this. Different facilities will have different policies about who is responsible for blood glucose monitoring. You may work in a facility that allows nursing assistants to perform blood glucose monitoring. Make sure that you have been adequately trained in how to use the equipment and record your findings. Be aware of which glucose levels need to be reported to the nurse immediately.

Figure 37-10

A glucometer is used to monitor blood glucose levels.

TELL THE NURSE ❗

When caring for a person with diabetes, be sure to report any of the following observations to the nurse right away:

- The person has signs or symptoms of hypoglycemia or hyperglycemia (Box 37-1)
- The person refuses a meal or snack, or only eats part of it
- The person has vomited
- The person has received gifts of food from visitors
- The person is taking food from others
- The person's activity level has changed significantly (either more active or less active than usual)

Complications of Diabetes Mellitus

Many organ systems can be affected by uncontrolled diabetes mellitus of either type. Low insulin levels increase the release of lipids (fats) into the bloodstream. The lipids then build up in the linings of the arteries, damaging them. Atherosclerosis, high blood pressure, heart disease, stroke, kidney disease, and blindness (diabetic retinopathy; see Chapter 36) can result from the damaged blood vessels. In addition, peripheral nerve damage results from reduced blood flow to the neurons, causing diminished sensation in the arms and legs. Poor circulation to the feet and lower legs also increases the risk of infection and poor tissue healing in the event of injury. Amputation of a foot or leg may be necessary if the person develops gangrene (death of tissues due to lack of blood flow).

Early detection of diabetes mellitus is essential for preventing complications. Once diabetes mellitus is diagnosed, the person needs to take steps to keep his blood glucose level within the normal range. Following the recommended diet closely, exercising regularly, and taking prescribed medications correctly is very important. These actions help to keep the disease under control and minimize the person's risk of developing complications.

SUMMARY

- The endocrine system is made up of glands located in specific places throughout the body that produce hormones. Hormones are chemical messengers that allow the body to reproduce, grow, develop, metabolize energy, respond to stress and injury, and maintain homeostasis.
  - The pituitary gland is considered the master gland of the endocrine system, because it secretes hormones that affect other glands. The pituitary gland is controlled by the hypothalamus.
    - The posterior lobe of the pituitary gland stores and releases antidiuretic hormone (ADH) and oxytocin.
    - The anterior lobe of the pituitary gland produces and releases growth hormone, thyroid-stimulating hormone (TSH), adrenocorticotropic hormone (ACTH), prolactin, and the gonadotropins (luteinizing hormone [LH] and follicle-stimulating hormone [FSH]).
  - The thyroid gland produces thyroxine, which helps to regulate metabolism, and calcitonin, which helps to maintain calcium levels in the bloodstream.
- The parathyroid glands secrete parathyroid hormone (PTH), which helps to move calcium from the bones into the bloodstream.
- The adrenal glands produce hormones that help us to deal with stress.
  - The adrenal medulla secretes epinephrine and norepinephrine, which play a role in the "fight-or-flight" response.
  - The adrenal cortex secretes glucocorticoids, mineralocorticoids, and androgens.
- The pancreas secretes insulin and glucagon, which play a role in regulating blood glucose (sugar) levels.
- Disorders of the endocrine system result from either too much hormone or too little hormone.
  - Hypothyroidism (secretion of too little thyroid hormone) and hyperthyroidism (secretion of too much thyroid hormone) are common endocrine disorders. Thyroid hormone imbalances change the body's metabolic rate, causing many uncomfortable symptoms. Fortunately, hypothyroidism and hyperthyroidism can usually be treated.

- The most common of all endocrine disorders is diabetes mellitus.
  - There are two forms of diabetes mellitus.
    - Type 1 diabetes mellitus occurs when the insulin-producing cells of the pancreas are destroyed.
    - Type 2 diabetes mellitus occurs when the pancreas produces some insulin, but the cells of the body are unable to respond to the insulin that is produced.
    - Both types of diabetes mellitus are managed with diet, exercise, and medication.
  - A person with diabetes mellitus is prone to hyperglycemia (blood glucose levels that are too high) and hypoglycemia (blood glucose levels that are too low). Both hyperglycemia and hypoglycemia can cause complications, some of which are life threatening.
  - Keeping blood glucose levels within the range of normal is very important to prevent long-term complications of diabetes from developing such as cardiovascular disease, stroke, nerve damage, kidney failure, blindness, and amputation.

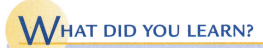

WHAT DID YOU LEARN?

Multiple Choice

Select the single best answer for each of the following questions.

1. Hormones are chemical messengers that allow the body to:
   a. Metabolize energy
   b. Grow
   c. Reproduce
   d. All of the above
2. Which endocrine disorder causes an increased metabolic rate, increased hunger, weight loss, an irregular heartbeat, an inability to sleep, irritability, and intolerance to heat?
   a. Hyperthyroidism
   b. Diabetes
   c. Acromegaly
   d. Pituitary gigantism
3. Mrs. Snow has diabetes mellitus. What special care considerations might a nursing assistant who is caring for Mrs. Snow need to keep in mind?
   a. Mrs. Snow will be unable to tolerate cold, and therefore, will often need a sweater.
   b. Mrs. Snow will need to eat meals and snacks on a regular schedule.
   c. Mrs. Snow may grow tired very easily.
   d. Mrs. Snow is likely to be irritable.
4. Why must a person with type 1 diabetes mellitus receive regular doses of insulin?
   a. The cells of the body do not respond to the insulin produced by the pancreas.
   b. The person's pancreas does not produce insulin on its own.

   c. The person's pancreas produces too much glucagon.
   d. People with type 1 diabetes do not need to take insulin; their disease can be controlled through diet, exercise, and oral medications.
5. Mr. Byron has type 2 diabetes mellitus. Although he knows that he should limit the amount of sweets that he eats, he has a real "sweet tooth" and often eats candy. In addition, he only monitors his blood glucose on days when he does not feel well. What complications is Mr. Byron at risk for developing if he does not make more of an effort to control his blood glucose levels?
   a. Kidney failure
   b. Blindness
   c. Heart disease
   d. All of the above
6. Mrs. Barney takes oral thyroxine to control her hypothyroidism. Without this medication, what sort of signs and symptoms do you think Mrs. Barney would have?
   a. Loss of appetite, weight gain, and constipation
   b. Frequent urination and excessive thirst
   c. Fat deposits on her back, abdomen, and face
   d. Excessive growth of the bones of the hands, feet, and face

Matching

Match each numbered item with its appropriate lettered description.

_____ **1.** Parathyroid hormone (PTH)

_____ **2.** Antidiuretic hormone (ADH)

_____ **3.** Growth hormone

_____ **4.** Thyroid-stimulating hormone (TSH)

_____ **5.** Calcitonin

_____ **6.** Adrenocorticotropic hormone (ACTH)

_____ **7.** Thyroxine

_____ **8.** Norepinephrine and epinephrine

_____ **9.** Glucocorticoids

_____**10.** Insulin

a. Secreted by the adrenal cortex; helps the body to deal with stress

b. Secreted by the posterior pituitary gland; acts on the kidneys to limit the amount of water lost in the urine

c. Secreted by the anterior pituitary gland; causes our bodies to get bigger and taller

d. Secreted by the pancreas; helps the body to manage blood glucose levels

e. Secreted by the thyroid gland; lowers the amount of calcium in the bloodstream

f. Secreted by the anterior pituitary gland; stimulates the adrenal glands to produce their hormones

g. Secreted by the thyroid gland; sets the metabolic rate for the cells of the body

h. Secreted by the parathyroid glands; stimulates the release of calcium from the bones into the bloodstream

i. Secreted by the anterior pituitary gland; stimulates the thyroid glands to produce their hormones

j. Secreted by the adrenal medulla; participates in the "fight-or-flight" response

STOP and Think!

- One of your residents, Mr. Singer, receives insulin injections for his diabetes. This morning, Mr. Singer had his injection and then ate most of his breakfast. About 30 minutes later, he vomited. Now, Mr. Singer tells you that he feels shaky, and you can see that he is sweating. Why is it important for you to report these observations to the nurse immediately?

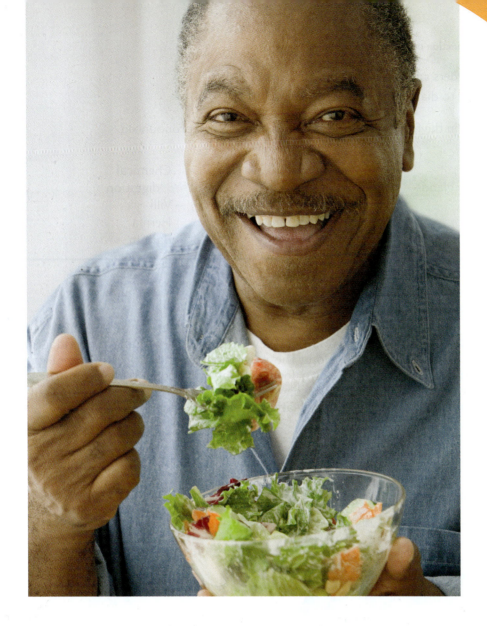

The Digestive System

WHAT WILL YOU LEARN?

Did you know that over the course of a lifetime, you will eat about 50 *tons* (100,000 pounds) of food? As you already know from Chapters 25 and 26, it is your digestive system's job to process that food so that your body can use it, and to rid the body of the solid waste that is created as part of the food processing process. In this chapter, you will learn more about the individual organs of the digestive system and how they work. You will also learn about some common disorders of the digestive system. When you are finished with this chapter, you will be able to:

1. List the organs that are part of the digestive system.
2. Describe the function of the organs of the digestive system.
3. Discuss the effects of aging on the digestive system.

Photo: The digestive system processes the food that we eat.

749

4. Discuss common digestive disorders and their symptoms.

5. Describe some of the tools used to diagnose digestive disorders.

Vocabulary Listen & Learn Use the CD in the front of your book to hear these terms pronounced and defined:

Esophagus	Rugae	Pancreas	Chemical
Stomach	Salivary glands	Mastication	digestion
Esophageal (cardiac)	Liver	Mechanical	Villi
sphincter	Bile	digestion	Hernia
Pyloric sphincter	Gallbladder	Enzymes	Barium

STRUCTURE OF THE DIGESTIVE SYSTEM

The digestive system, also known as the gastrointestinal system, is a long tube, or *tract*, consisting of the mouth, pharynx, esophagus, stomach, small intestine, and large intestine (Fig. 38-1). In addition, several accessory organs (appendages) along the way assist in the process of breaking down food so that our bodies can use it. These accessory organs include the teeth, tongue, salivary glands, liver, gallbladder, and pancreas.

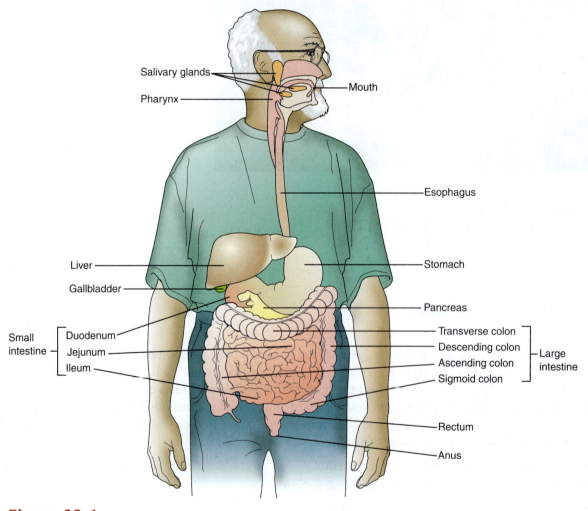

Figure 38-1

The digestive system breaks down food, absorbs nutrients, and gets rid of waste.

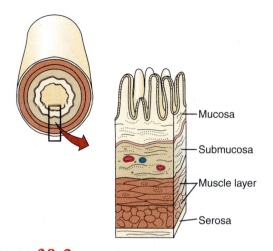

Figure 38-2
The walls of the digestive tract consist of four basic layers.

THE DIGESTIVE TRACT

The walls of the "tube" that forms the digestive tract are made up of four layers of tissue (Fig. 38-2). The layers are basically the same throughout the digestive tract, although there is some variation from region to region. The four basic layers are the mucosa, the submucosa, the muscle layer, and the serosa:

- The *mucosa*, a mucous membrane, lines the digestive tract. The mucosa helps to trap disease-causing microbes. This is important because the digestive tract is open to the outside world at both ends (that is, the mouth and the anus). In addition to trapping microbes, the mucosa helps to protect the delicate tissues of the digestive tract from stomach acid, a very harsh fluid produced by the stomach to help digest food.
- The *submucosa* contains blood vessels and nerves.
- The *muscle layer* contains smooth muscle. Recall from Chapter 30 that smooth muscle is not under voluntary control—it contracts and relaxes automatically. Peristalsis (contraction of the smooth muscle in the walls of the digestive tract) moves food through the system.
- The *serosa* is a tough outer layer of connective tissue.

Let's take a look now at the individual organs that form the digestive tract.

The Mouth, Pharynx, and Esophagus

Food begins its journey through the digestive tract at the mouth, or oral cavity. The mouth is lined with a mucous membrane and contains the teeth and tongue, accessory organs that assist with chewing and swallowing food. When you swallow, the epiglottis (a flap of cartilage that covers the opening to the larynx) snaps shut to prevent food from passing into the trachea. Instead, food moves into the pharynx (throat) and then into the esophagus.

The **esophagus,** a long narrow tube, serves mainly as a passageway for food to get from the pharynx to the stomach. The esophagus passes through the chest cavity, behind the heart (Fig. 38-1). It enters the abdominal cavity at the *hiatus,* an opening in the diaphragm (the large, flat muscle that separates the abdominal and chest cavities). After entering the abdominal cavity, the esophagus connects with the upper part of the stomach. The mucus secreted by the esophageal mucosa, as well as the action of the muscle layer, helps to move food downward and into the stomach.

The Stomach

The **stomach** is a hollow, muscular holding pouch for food. The stomach has three main regions (Fig. 38-3):

- The *fundus* is the upper region.
- The *body* is the main region. The esophagus enters the stomach here. The **esophageal (cardiac) sphincter,** a circle of muscular tissue, surrounds the place where the

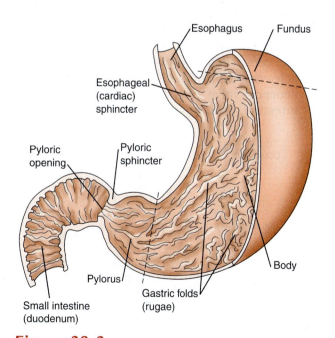

Figure 38-3
The stomach is a hollow holding pouch for food.

esophagus enters the stomach and keeps food from going back up the esophagus after it has entered the stomach.

- The *pylorus* is the bottom region. Food leaves the stomach through the **pyloric sphincter,** a circle of muscular tissue that surrounds the place where the stomach empties into the small intestine. The pyloric sphincter helps to prevent food from returning to the stomach once it enters the small intestine.

As most of us have experienced after eating a large holiday dinner, the stomach is capable of stretching and holding a large amount of food. Folds of the mucosa, called **rugae,** flatten out as food enters the stomach, almost doubling the stomach's holding capacity.

The Small Intestine

The small intestine, which is about 20 feet long, is so named because its diameter is much smaller than that of the large intestine. The small intestine has three regions, called the *duodenum*, the *jejunum*, and the *ileum* (Fig. 38-4).

The Large Intestine

The large intestine (also called the *colon*) is 4½ feet long and is much larger in diameter than the small intestine. Like the small intestine, the large intestine has several distinct regions (Fig. 38-5):

- The *appendix* is a tiny, closed pouch that dangles from the cecum. Inflammation or infection of the appendix causes *appendicitis*, a painful condition that is life threatening if not treated. Treatment is surgical removal of the appendix.
- The *cecum* is like a waiting room for food that is leaving the small intestine through the ileocecal valve and entering the large intestine. Food moves through the large

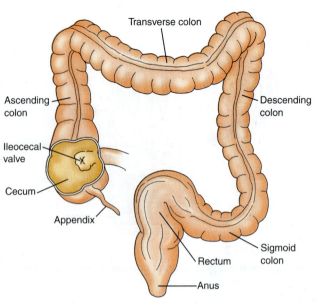

Figure 38-5
The large intestine has several regions: the cecum, the ascending colon, the transverse colon, the descending colon, the sigmoid colon, and the rectum. The appendix is a small pouch attached to the end of the cecum.

intestine much more slowly than it moves through the small intestine. Incoming deliveries from the small intestine need a place to wait until the next segment of the large intestine, the ascending colon, is able to accept more food for processing.
- The *ascending colon* travels upward from the cecum.
- The *transverse colon* travels across.
- The *descending colon* travels down.
- The *sigmoid colon* is an S-shaped curve at the end of the descending colon.
- The *rectum* is the last segment of the colon. The place where the rectum opens to the outside of the body is the *anus*.

THE ACCESSORY ORGANS

Several organs—the salivary glands, liver, gallbladder, and pancreas—play a role in digestion, but are not actually part of the digestive tract (Fig. 38-1).

- The **salivary glands** are located near the mouth. They produce and secrete saliva, a substance that helps with chewing and swallowing by moistening the food.
- The **liver** is a large organ located just underneath the diaphragm (Fig. 38-1). The liver produces and secretes bile into the

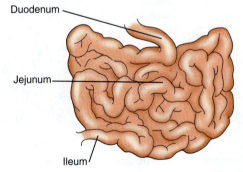

Figure 38-4
The small intestine has three regions: the duodenum, the jejunum, and the ileum.

duodenum. **Bile** is a substance that helps with the digestion of fats. The liver also has several other important functions that are not related to digestion. For example, it produces clotting factors (chemicals that help our blood to clot) and it helps to clear our blood of toxins, such as alcohol and drugs.

- The **gallbladder,** a small pouch that is attached to the liver, stores bile produced by the liver that is not secreted directly into the duodenum.
- The **pancreas** is located behind the stomach, in the curve of the duodenum (Fig. 38-1). The pancreas produces substances that aid in digestion and secretes them into the duodenum. The pancreas also produces insulin and glucagon, hormones that are secreted directly into the bloodstream. (Recall from Chapter 37 that insulin and glucagon regulate glucose levels in the blood.)

FUNCTION OF THE DIGESTIVE SYSTEM

The digestive system breaks down the food we eat into nutrients, which are then absorbed into the bloodstream for use by the body's cells. In addition, the digestive system removes unusable digested food from the body, in the form of feces.

DIGESTION

Digestion, or the breaking down of food into simple elements (nutrients), begins in the mouth. First, we physically break the food into smaller pieces by chewing it. Another word for chewing is **mastication.** This physical breaking up of the food, such as occurs when we chew, is called **mechanical digestion.** Next, chemical substances in our saliva start to work on the smaller pieces of food, breaking them down even more by breaking the bonds that hold the food molecules together. Substances that have the ability to break chemical bonds are called **enzymes.** The human body produces many different types of enzymes, each with a specific function. The process of breaking down food through the use of chemical substances, such as enzymes, is called **chemical digestion.**

After passing through the esophagus, the food we eat stays in the stomach for 3 to 4 hours, where digestion continues to take place. Special glands in the stomach lining produce hydrochloric acid (sometimes called "stomach acid") and

enzymes. The stomach acid and enzymes act on the pieces of food to break them down even further. The peristaltic action of the stomach helps to mix the food with the acid and enzymes, creating a liquid substance called *chyme.*

The chyme passes into the duodenum, the first segment of the small intestine. Once in the duodenum, the chyme mixes with bile (secreted by the liver) and digestive enzymes secreted by the pancreas. These substances cause further breakdown of the food. From the duodenum, the chyme passes into the jejunum.

ABSORPTION

Once the chyme reaches the jejunum, absorption of nutrients begins. At this point, the food is fairly well digested. Now, it is time to start moving the nutrients from the digestive tract into the bloodstream. To reach the bloodstream, the nutrients pass through the mucosa and into the blood vessels in the next layer, the submucosa. The mucosa of the small intestine has millions of tiny finger-like structures called **villi** (Fig. 38-6). The villi increase the small intestine's ability to absorb nutrients by increasing the surface area of the mucosa.

Although most of the absorption of nutrients takes place in the small intestine, the large intestine also plays a role in absorption. Bacteria that live in the large intestine act on the chyme to produce vitamin K and some B vitamins, which are absorbed by the body. The action of these bacteria on the chyme can also produce gas as a

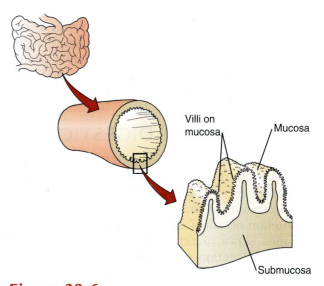

Figure 38-6
Villi are finger-like projections that increase the small intestine's ability to absorb nutrients.

by-product, especially when high-fiber foods, such as beans, onions, and broccoli, are part of the diet. As the chyme passes slowly through the large intestine, water is absorbed into the bloodstream. By the time the chyme reaches the end of the long intestine, all nutrients and most of the water have been removed, and the chyme has taken on the soft, moist, semi-solid consistency of normal feces.

EXCRETION

The feces (waste products of digestion) collect in the rectum, the last segment of the large intestine. The walls of the rectum gradually expand as the feces build up. At a certain point, the brain senses that the rectum is "full" and the urge to defecate (have a bowel movement) occurs.

EFFECTS OF AGING ON THE DIGESTIVE SYSTEM

Like all of the body's organ systems, the digestive system is affected by the process of aging.

LESS EFFICIENT CHEWING AND SWALLOWING

In older people, the production of saliva decreases, which may make chewing and swallowing more difficult. In addition, many older people have dental problems, such as missing or painful teeth. An older person may choke as a result of trying to swallow food that has not been chewed properly. Remember this when you are helping an older person to eat. Create a relaxed, social environment for eating and help the person to cut food up into small, easy-to-chew pieces.

LESS EFFICIENT DIGESTION

Food is most easily digested when it has been thoroughly chewed. Mechanical digestion increases the effectiveness of chemical digestion by making the pieces of food smaller. In an older person, the production of saliva, stomach acid, and digestive enzymes slows, making chemical digestion less efficient. Digestion is less efficient, because not only are fewer chemicals available for chemical digestion, but also the pieces of food that the chemicals must work on may be larger, due to inefficient chewing.

INCREASED RISK FOR CONSTIPATION

In an older person, the movement of food through the digestive tract may be slower. This can put the older person at risk for constipation. The chyme spends more time in the large intestine, which allows more water to be reabsorbed into the bloodstream. As a result, by the time the chyme reaches the end of the large intestine, almost all of the water has been removed and the resulting feces are hard, dry, and difficult to pass. Certain medications (such as prescription pain relievers) and immobility can also increase a person's risk for constipation. Measures that you can take to help your residents avoid constipation are described in Chapter 26.

DISORDERS OF THE DIGESTIVE SYSTEM

Because the digestive system contains so many different organs, there are many different disorders that can occur. Four of the most common digestive disorders that you are likely to see in the health care setting are ulcers, hernias, gallbladder disorders, and cancer.

ULCERS

Ulcers (sores caused by wearing away of the protective mucosa that lines the digestive tract) can occur anywhere along the digestive tract. The most common sites are the stomach (*gastric ulcer*) and the duodenum (*duodenal ulcer*). Ulcers occur when the stomach produces too much hydrochloric acid. Factors such as smoking, frequent use of over-the-counter pain medications, and infection with a bacterium called *Helicobacter pylori* can increase a person's risk for developing ulcers. In severe cases, the ulcer may affect all of the layers of the stomach or duodenum wall, not just the mucosa. This condition, called a *penetrating ulcer*, is life threatening.

A person with an ulcer may feel uncomfortably full or nauseous after eating. Stomach pain is common, especially within 3 hours of eating (or when the person does not eat). Most ulcers are chronic. The person will have periods of feeling well, interrupted by flare-ups of symptoms.

Most ulcers can be treated with medication. People with severe ulcers may need surgery.

HERNIAS

The abdominal cavity (the space in the body where most of the digestive organs are found) is bounded by muscular walls. The muscular walls of the abdominal cavity give structure to the body and help to keep the internal organs in the proper place. A **hernia** occurs when an internal organ bulges through a weakness in the muscular wall of the abdominal cavity (Fig. 38-7). Sometimes the weakness occurs at the site of an old surgical incision. Other times, the muscle is just weak in certain areas. If there is a weak area in the muscular wall, and the person does something that requires a lot of physical effort (such as lifting a heavy object), a hernia may occur. Hernias can occur in a number of different places:

- *Inguinal hernias* and *femoral hernias* occur when a loop of intestine bulges through the abdominal wall in the groin area. Inguinal hernias are more common in men, and femoral hernias are more common in women. These types of hernias are repaired surgically.
- *Umbilical hernias* occur around the navel (belly button). If the umbilical hernia is very small, no treatment may be needed. However, surgery may be required to repair a larger umbilical hernia.
- *Hiatal hernias* occur when part of the stomach passes through the hiatus, the opening in the diaphragm that allows the esophagus to pass into the abdominal cavity. People with hiatal hernias often have heartburn because the stomach acid moves back up into the esophagus. A person with a hiatal hernia may find that eating small, frequent meals and sitting up for at least 2 hours after every meal helps to relieve the heartburn. Medication can also provide relief of symptoms. People with severe symptoms may need surgery to repair the hernia.

Complications occur if the muscle tightens around the trapped tissue, cutting off its blood supply. This situation, called a *strangulated hernia*, is a surgical emergency.

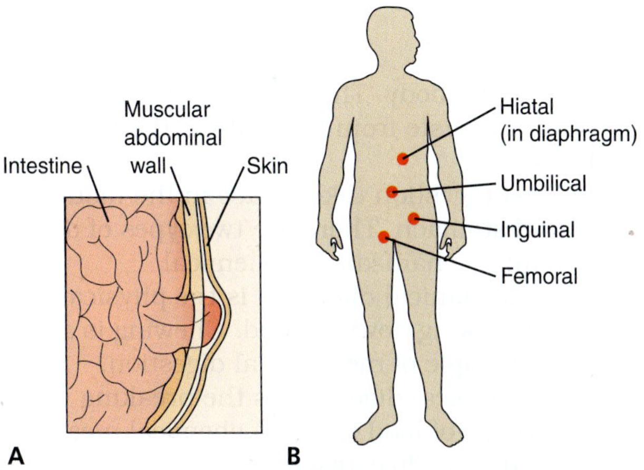

GALLBLADDER DISORDERS

Gallstones can form and block the flow of bile from the gallbladder into the duodenum (Fig. 38-8). This can lead to inflammation and infection of the gallbladder. A person with a gallbladder disorder has episodes of severe pain. The pain may stay in the upper abdominal region, or it may radiate to the back and shoulder on the person's right side. The person may also have indigestion, especially after eating foods that are high in fat. Because bile gives feces their characteristic brown color, in a person with a gallbladder disorder, the feces

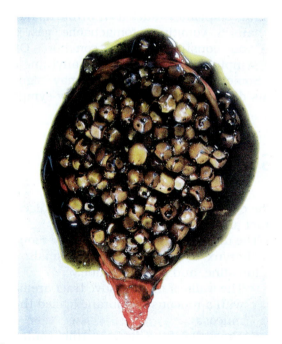

Figure 38-8
A gallbladder that has been removed and cut open to reveal the many gallstones inside. Gallstones can block the flow of bile into the duodenum, causing indigestion and severe pain. (*Rubin, R., & Stayer, D.S. [2008].* Rubin's Pathology: Clinicopathologic Foundations of Medicine *[5th ed., p. 668]. Philadelphia: Lippincott Williams & Wilkins.*)

Figure 38-7
(A) A hernia occurs when an internal organ bulges through a weakness in the abdominal wall. **(B)** Hernias can occur in a number of different places.

may be pale and "clay-colored" due to their low bile content. Remember also that bile helps the body to digest fat. In a person with gallbladder disease, the feces may float because they contain a great deal of undigested fat.

Medication or laser treatment may be used to dissolve the gallstones. In some cases, surgical removal of the gallbladder is needed.

CANCER

Any of the organs in the digestive system can be affected by cancer. The person's signs and symptoms will vary, depending on the location of the tumor. A person with cancer involving the digestive system may have one or more of the following signs and symptoms: loss of appetite, indigestion, pain, vomiting, constipation, changes in bowel movements, or blood in the stool. Depending on the location and type of cancer, it may be treated with surgery, radiation, chemotherapy, or a combination of these.

DIAGNOSIS OF DIGESTIVE DISORDERS

Digestive complaints—such as heartburn, indigestion, nausea, vomiting, stomachache, gas, diarrhea, and constipation—are common. Often, these symptoms are not a sign of anything serious. Sometimes, however, they may signal a serious disorder. Always report a new symptom, or a change in the person's symptoms, to the nurse immediately.

Sometimes, the doctor will order one or more tests to evaluate a person's symptoms. Some of these tests are simple, such as laboratory analysis of a stool sample. Others are more involved. Tests you may hear mentioned include the following:

- **Endoscopy** involves using a special instrument to look inside the digestive tract and obtain tissue or fluids for analysis. Endoscopy allows the doctor to look inside the digestive tract for tumors or other abnormal growths. The endoscope may be passed through the person's mouth (to view the upper digestive tract) or anus (to view the lower digestive tract).
- **Imaging studies,** such as x-rays, computed tomography (CT) scans, and magnetic resonance imaging (MRI) scans, allow the doctor to view the organs of the digestive system without actually entering the body. Sometimes, the person is asked to swallow barium or have a barium enema prior to the procedure. **Barium** is a liquid substance that coats the mucosa of the digestive tract and makes the organs appear on an x-ray.

A person who needs one of these diagnostic procedures may have a special diet in the days leading up to the procedure, or be placed on NPO status. Sometimes, an enema is ordered to clean out the large intestine prior to the procedure. The nurse will let you know of any special care needs for a person who is having one of these procedures.

SUMMARY

- The digestive system consists of the digestive tract and several accessory organs.
  - The digestive tract consists of the mouth, pharynx, esophagus, stomach, small intestine, and large intestine.
    - The walls of the digestive tract are lined with a mucous membrane (called the mucosa).
    - The walls of the digestive tract contain smooth muscle, which contracts to help move food through the tube (peristalsis).
  - Accessory organs include the teeth, tongue, salivary glands, liver, gallbladder, and pancreas.
- The digestive system breaks down the food we eat into nutrients that can be used by the

cells of the body. The digestive system also removes waste from the body in the form of feces.
  - Most digestion takes place in the mouth and stomach. There are two types of digestion: mechanical and chemical.
    - Mechanical digestion is the physical breaking down of food. Chewing is an example of mechanical digestion.
    - Chemical digestion is the breaking down of food through chemical means, such as digestive enzymes.
  - Most absorption takes place in the small and large intestines.

- Most absorption of nutrients takes place in the jejunum and ileum, the last two segments of the small intestine.
  - Water is reabsorbed into the bloodstream as the chyme passes through the large intestine.
- Feces are what are left after all of the nutrients and most of the water are removed from the chyme, during its passage through the small and large intestines. Feces collect in the rectum, the last segment of the large intestine, until the urge to defecate occurs.
- As a person gets older, he may have more trouble chewing and swallowing food.

Digestion is less efficient. In addition, the older person may be at higher risk for becoming constipated.
- Common disorders of the digestive system include ulcers, hernias, gallbladder disorders, and cancer. Always report a new gastrointestinal complaint, or a change in a person's usual symptoms, to the nurse immediately.
- A person who is having a diagnostic procedure to evaluate her digestive system may have special care needs prior to the test. The nurse will let you know of any special instructions, which should be followed carefully.

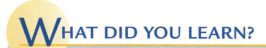

WHAT DID YOU LEARN?

Multiple Choice

Select the single best answer for each of the following questions.

1. Where does the process of digestion begin?
   a. In the stomach
   b. In the large intestine
   c. In the mouth
   d. In the esophagus
2. What is a hollow, muscular pouch for holding food?
   a. The appendix
   b. The gallbladder
   c. The duodenum
   d. The stomach
3. What is another term for the large intestine?
   a. Stomach
   b. Duodenum
   c. Colon
   d. Appendix
4. Where does most absorption of nutrients take place?
   a. In the jejunum and ileum of the small intestine
   b. In the rectum of the large intestine
   c. In the stomach
   d. In the liver
5. Where is most of the water absorbed from the chyme, resulting in the formation of formed, semi-moist feces?
   a. In the large intestine
   b. In the small intestine

c. In the stomach
   d. In the gallbladder
6. Normal changes in the digestive system related to aging include:
   a. Less efficient chewing and swallowing
   b. Less efficient digestion
   c. Increased risk for constipation
   d. All of the above
7. You have been caring for Mrs. Zimmerman for several months. Mrs. Zimmerman has always had a "sensitive stomach." She often tells you that she is "queasy" or that something she ate "didn't agree with her." Although she always complains about the food at the facility, she usually cleans her plate. Today, however, you noticed that not only did Mrs. Zimmerman not eat her lunch, but she also has seemed particularly listless all afternoon. What should you do?
   a. Nothing; Mrs. Zimmerman always has "stomach issues"
   b. Record Mrs. Zimmerman's lack of appetite in her chart; the nurse will follow up later
   c. Report this change in Mrs. Zimmerman's behavior to the nurse immediately
   d. Wait and see if Mrs. Zimmerman has any appetite for dinner

STOP and Think!

Mr. Scott is a resident on your routine assignment. He is 82 years old, and a retired police officer. You have gotten to know him quite well in the weeks that you have taken care of him. He always says he loves a good steak, a good cup of coffee, and a cigarette! Today, when you are helping him with mouth care, you notice a dark, reddened area inside of his mouth that you never noticed before. When you mention it to Mr. Scott, he brushes it off as nothing important, but you notice that is he is also refusing to put his partial denture in his mouth. Mr. Scott usually eats 100% of his meal, but today at lunch, you see that he barely ate 50% of the food that was on the meal tray. When you ask him about it, he just tells you that he isn't hungry. He also turns down the cup of coffee he usually has after his meal. What do you think might be going on with Mr. Scott? What should you do?

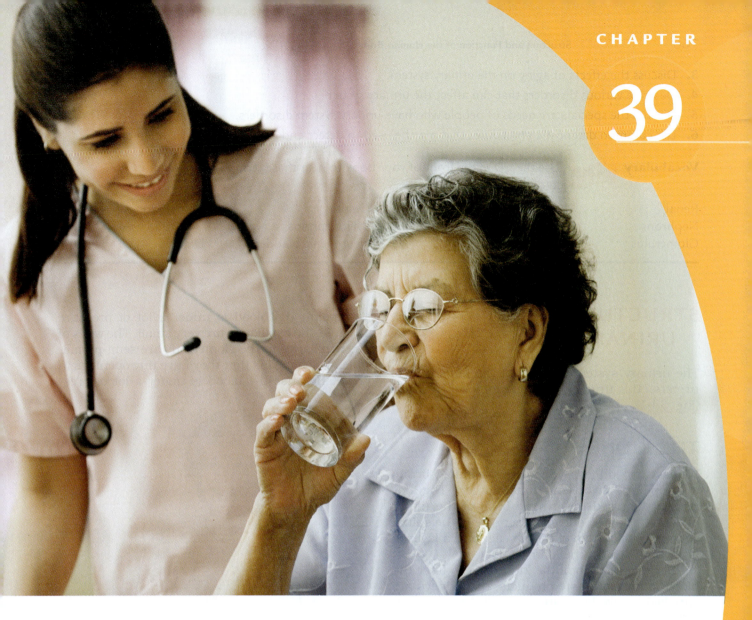

The Urinary System

WHAT WILL YOU LEARN?

As you learned in Chapter 26, the urinary system rids the body of waste products that have been filtered from the bloodstream, along with excess fluid, in the form of urine. In Chapter 26, you also learned how to assist residents with urinary elimination. In this chapter, you will learn a little bit more about the organs that make up the urinary system and how they work. As a nursing assistant, many of your daily responsibilities will allow you to observe changes in the functioning of a resident's urinary system that could indicate a serious problem. This is why it is important for you to know about the effects of aging on the urinary system, and about some of the disorders that can affect this very important organ system. When you are finished with this chapter, you will be able to:

1. List the organs that make up the urinary system.
2. Describe the primary function of each organ of the urinary system.

Photo: Drinking plenty of fluids helps to keep the urinary system healthy.

3. Discuss the effects of aging on the urinary system.

4. Describe various disorders that can affect the urinary system.

5. Discuss the special care needs of people who have urinary system disorders.

6. List common diagnostic procedures that may be used to detect and diagnose urinary system disorders.

Vocabulary Use the CD in the front of your book to hear these terms pronounced and defined:

Renal	Filtrate	Cystitis	Kidney stones (renal
Nephrons	Urine	Pyelonephritis	calculi)
Glomerulus	Urethritis	Neurogenic bladder	Dialysis

STRUCTURE OF THE URINARY SYSTEM

The urinary system consists of the kidneys, the ureters, the urinary bladder, and the urethra (Fig. 39-1).

THE KIDNEYS

We have two kidneys, which are like kidney beans in shape and color (only much larger). The kidneys are located toward the back of the upper abdominal cavity, one on either side of the spinal column. The bottom of the rib cage and a layer of fat help to protect the kidneys.

Because the job of the kidneys is to filter the blood to remove waste products, the kidneys are supplied by two large arteries, called the left and right renal arteries. (**Renal** is a word meaning "related to, involving, or located in the region of the kidneys.") The renal arteries are branches of the aorta, the largest artery in the body. The blood flow through the renal arteries is so efficient that the kidneys are able to filter all of the body's blood every half-hour.

Inside each kidney are approximately 1 million tiny **nephrons,** the basic functional units of the kidney (Fig. 39-2). The nephrons are responsible for actually filtering the blood that passes through the kidney. Each nephron consists of a glomerulus and a series of tubules (Fig. 39-2). The **glomerulus** is a capillary bed, enclosed within a structure called *Bowman's capsule.* The blood entering the kidneys through the renal arteries is under great pressure. Once inside the kidneys, the blood passes through a series of arteries that get smaller and smaller, until it reaches the capillary bed of the glomerulus. The blood enters the glomerulus through a vessel called the afferent arteriole (*afferent* means "enter") (Fig. 39-2). At

this point, the blood is under a lot of pressure because the capillaries are very small. The walls of the capillaries in the glomerulus are semi-permeable, which means that they have tiny openings in them. Because the blood is under a lot of pres-

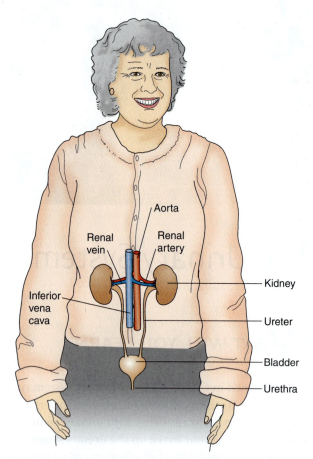

Figure 39-1

The urinary system consists of the kidneys, ureters, bladder, and urethra. Each kidney is supplied by a renal artery, which branches off of the aorta. After the kidneys filter the blood, the filtrate (urine) passes into the ureters and the blood passes into the renal veins, which empty into the inferior vena cava.

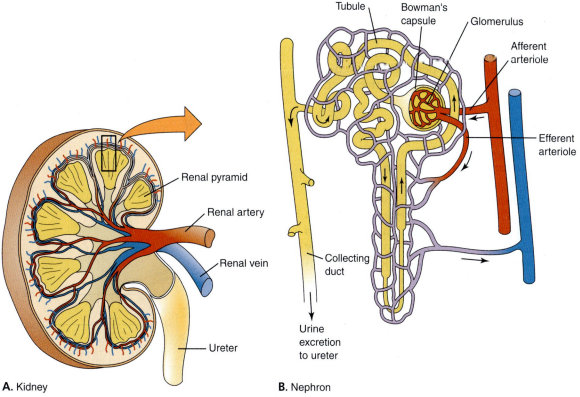

A. Kidney   **B.** Nephron

Figure 39-2

The kidney. **(A)** If you were to cut open the kidney and look at the tissue through a microscope, you would see nephrons, the functional units where filtration actually takes place. Each kidney contains about 1 million nephrons, arranged in a radiating pattern. **(B)** Each nephron consists of a glomerulus and a series of tubules. Blood (*red*) is filtered in the glomerulus, producing filtrate, the basis of urine (*yellow*). Filtered blood (*purple*) leaves the glomerulus through the efferent arteriole and is returned to the circulation through the renal veins.

sure, a lot of the liquid in the blood squeezes through the walls, taking the wastes and nutrients that are dissolved in it with it. This liquid, known as the **filtrate,** forms the basis of the urine. Next, two things happen (Fig. 39-2B):

- The filtered blood leaves the glomerulus through the efferent arteriole (*efferent* means "exit"). It is returned to circulation through the renal veins, which empty into the inferior vena cava (the largest vein in the body).
- Meanwhile, the filtrate enters Bowman's capsule, and from there, flows into the tubules that make up the rest of the nephron. Small capillaries surround the tubules of the nephron. As the filtrate passes slowly through the tubules, these small capillaries reabsorb useful substances, such as water, nutrients, and minerals, from the filtrate. By the time the filtrate reaches the end of the tubules, only excess fluid and waste substances remain. This is **urine.** The kidneys

produce 160 to 180 liters of filtrate each day, but only about 1 to 1.5 liters are excreted from the body in the form of urine. (One liter is equal to about one quart.)

Urine from each nephron is emptied into a collecting area, called the *renal pelvis.* From the renal pelvis, the urine flows into the ureters.

THE URETERS

Two ureters, slender, muscular tubes approximately 10 to 13 inches (25 to 32 cm) long, carry urine from the kidneys to the bladder (Fig. 39-1). The ureters are wider at the top where they connect to the renal pelvis, but they quickly become very narrow. Where the two ureters enter the bladder, a small triangular fold of tissue called the *trigone* keeps urine from flowing back into the ureters after it has emptied into the bladder.

The ureters are lined with a mucous membrane, which helps to protect against infection.

Smooth muscle in the walls of the ureters contracts rhythmically, moving urine away from the kidney and toward the urinary bladder. The peristaltic movements that help move urine through the ureters are similar to the peristaltic movements that help move food through the digestive tract.

THE BLADDER

The bladder is a hollow sac that is a holding place (reservoir) for urine. Urine is constantly produced by the kidneys and transported through the ureters to the bladder, where it is stored until urination occurs. The bladder is very small when empty, but can become quite large as it fills with urine. The *internal sphincter* (a ring of involuntary muscle), located where the bladder joins the urethra, keeps the bladder closed while it fills.

Like the ureters, the inside of the bladder is lined with a mucous membrane. The walls of the bladder contain three layers of smooth muscle. When the walls of the bladder contract, urination occurs.

THE URETHRA

The urethra is a tube that carries urine from the bladder to the outside of the body. The urethra begins at the *bladder outlet* (the place where the bladder and the urethra join, just below the internal sphincter) and ends at the external urinary opening (called the *urinary meatus* or *urethral orifice*). Below the internal sphincter, the *external urethral sphincter*, a ring of voluntary muscle, relaxes to allow urine to pass during urination.

Male and female urethras are very different in size and function (Fig. 39-3). In women, the urethra measures about 1½ to 2½ inches and is used only as a passageway for urine to leave the body. In men, the urethra measures about 6 to 8 inches and serves as a passageway for both urine and semen. In men, the urethra passes through the prostate gland soon after leaving the bladder outlet. The prostate gland produces seminal fluid, the fluid that, along with sperm cells, makes up semen.

FUNCTION OF THE URINARY SYSTEM

REMOVAL OF LIQUID WASTES

The main function of the urinary system is to filter the blood and remove waste products and excess fluid from the body. A moderately full bladder usually contains about 1 pint (470 mL) of

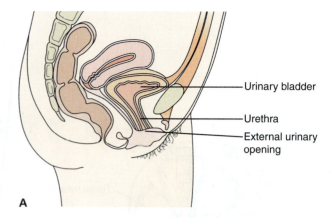

A

Urinary bladder
Urethra
External urinary opening

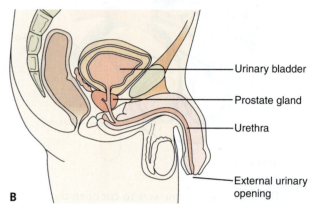

B

Urinary bladder
Prostate gland
Urethra
External urinary opening

Figure 39-3

While a woman's urethra **(A)** is straight and only about 2 inches long, a man's urethra **(B)** is curved in an "S" shape and is about 6 inches long. Because of the differences in anatomy, women are more prone to urinary tract infections than men are, but men are harder to catheterize than women are.

urine. When about 200 to 300 mL of urine collects in the bladder, the internal sphincter opens and allows urine to flood the upper segment of the urethra. At this point, the urge to urinate occurs. The person voluntarily relaxes the external urethral sphincter and the muscles of the bladder contract, allowing urine to pass out of the body through the urethra. Although it is possible to delay urination for some time, the bladder continues to fill with urine and eventually, the bladder will empty itself automatically.

MAINTENANCE OF HOMEOSTASIS

The urinary system plays several important roles in maintaining the body's homeostasis:

- The urinary system helps to keep fluid levels within the body constant. As the filtrate passes through the tubules in the nephrons, water is reabsorbed, as necessary, to maintain the body's fluid balance. Too much fluid in the blood can lead to fluid overload, causing swelling in parts of the body. Too little fluid can lead to dehydration.

- The urinary system regulates the levels of essential minerals—such as potassium, calcium, and sodium—by either saving them or releasing them through urine.
- The urinary system regulates the acidity of the blood. The pH scale, which you might remember from chemistry class, is used to rate the degree of acidity of a substance. Human blood is slightly above a 7 on the scale, which ranges from 1 to 14. Anything above 7 is basic, or alkaline. Anything below 7 is acidic. Our blood cannot be either too acidic or too basic. When there is even a slight change in the blood's pH, damage to the cells can occur. Acid is a normal by-product of cellular metabolism. So, to maintain the blood at a constant pH level, the kidneys excrete the excess acids produced by cellular metabolism.

THE EFFECTS OF AGING ON THE URINARY SYSTEM

The normal processes of aging affect the urinary system:

- **Less efficient filtration.** After a person reaches 40 years of age or so, the number of functioning nephrons in the kidneys starts to decrease, decreasing the kidneys' ability to filter waste products from the bloodstream.
- **Decreased muscle tone.** Loss of muscle tone as a result of aging can reduce bladder capacity and may contribute to stress incontinence (leaking of urine from the bladder when the person exerts herself).
- **Enlargement of the prostate gland (in men).** In older men, enlargement of the prostate gland is common. The enlargement may be benign (a normal effect of aging) or it may be due to cancer of the gland. As the prostate gland enlarges, it pushes against the urethra, causing it to narrow. Total emptying of the bladder of urine becomes difficult, and the man may experience episodes of overflow incontinence. As you recall from Chapter 26, overflow incontinence can occur when urine is retained in the bladder. Because the bladder does not empty completely when the man voids, it refills with

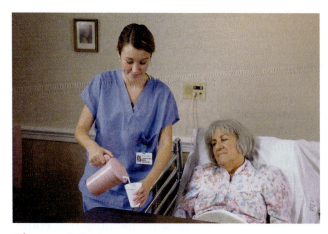

Figure 39-4
Encourage your residents to drink plenty of fluids, unless the resident has a medical condition that requires fluid restriction.

urine quickly, and the urine simply overflows. As a result, the man may "dribble" urine in between visits to the bathroom. An enlarged prostate is treated with medications, surgery, or both.

- **Increased risk for urinary tract infections.** Older people are also more likely to get urinary tract infections. Incomplete emptying of the bladder can contribute to the development of infections, as can a decrease in immune system functioning.

Although it is important for everyone to drink plenty of water and other fluids, it is especially important for older people. Drinking plenty of fluids helps the kidneys to work properly, and regular urination flushes harmful bacteria from the bladder, helping to prevent urinary tract infections (Fig. 39-4).

DISORDERS OF THE URINARY SYSTEM

Illness or injury to any part of the urinary system affects the whole system, and, eventually, the whole body. Common disorders of the urinary system include infections, neurogenic bladder, kidney stones, renal failure, and tumors.

INFECTIONS

Infections can affect any part of the urinary system:

- **Infection of the urethra (urethritis).** **Urethritis** is especially common in men, because the urethra is longer and curved. Microbes responsible for sexually transmitted infections (STIs), such as gonorrhea, herpes, and chlamydia, are common causes of urethritis in men. STIs are discussed in more detail in Chapter 40.

- **Infection of the bladder (cystitis).** Bladder infections **(cystitis)** are more common among women than men for two reasons. First, the urethral opening in women is located close to the anus. Because feces, which contain bacteria from the digestive tract, exit the body at the anus, this area is often contaminated with microbes that could cause a bladder infection. (This is why it is important to wipe from the front to the back when providing perineal care for a woman.) Second, a woman's urethra is short and straight, which means that once microbes gain access to the urinary tract, they do not have far to travel to infect the bladder.
- **Kidney infections (pyelonephritis).** If a bladder infection is not treated promptly with appropriate medications, the pathogens can travel up the ureters and infect the kidneys. A kidney infection **(pyelonephritis)** can cause severe illness. If untreated, the infection might result in permanent damage to the nephrons.

A change in the appearance or odor of a resident's urine or a change in a resident's voiding habits may be a sign of a urinary tract infection (Fig. 39-5). In younger people, symptoms of urinary tract infections include urinary frequency, burning, and cramping. However, many older people with urinary tract infections do not have these symptoms. Instead, an older person might show behavioral changes, such as increased confusion, decreased alertness, or unusual behaviors. As a nursing assistant, you may be the first to notice a change in a resident's urine, voiding pattern, or behavior that could indicate that a urinary tract infection is present.

NEUROGENIC BLADDER

Neurogenic bladder is a condition caused by problems with the nerves that control the bladder. Neurogenic bladder can be caused by a spinal cord injury, a stroke, a tumor, or complications from diabetes. The bladder is either overactive, or underactive:

- An overactive bladder is spastic, or highly sensitive to stimulation. The person experiences bladder spasms (involuntary contractions of the smooth muscle in the walls of the bladder) that result in the frequent, uncontrolled release of small amounts of urine from the bladder (urge incontinence). In this condition, the amount of urine the bladder is able to hold (that is, the bladder's capacity) is reduced. There are medications that can be used to treat overactive bladder, but these medications are not often recommended for older people, because of their side effects. Treatment measures include carefully controlling fluid intake and emptying the bladder completely at regular intervals (for example, by applying pressure over the bladder to stimulate voiding). Sometimes, catheterization with a straight catheter is ordered immediately following each attempt at voiding to check for residual urine (urine left in the bladder after voiding).
- An underactive bladder is flaccid, or unable to contract forcefully. The smooth muscle that forms the walls of the bladder loses its tone, causing the bladder to "stretch out." As a result, the bladder's capacity is increased. Because of nerve damage, the person may not be able to sense that the bladder is full, resulting in reflex incontinence (the bladder empties itself automatically when it becomes too full). Or, the muscular walls of the bladder may not be able to contract strongly enough to empty the bladder of all urine, leading to urinary retention and overflow incontinence. (You recall from Chapter 26 that overflow incontinence is characterized

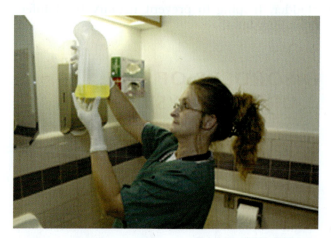

Figure 39-5

Urine that is cloudy or dark or that has an abnormal odor may be a sign of a urinary tract infection. Always look at the urine before discarding it. If you notice anything unusual, get the nurse before discarding the urine.

by dribbling of urine as the bladder overfills.) Treatment for an underactive bladder may include intermittent catheterization with a straight catheter or continuous catheterization with an indwelling urinary catheter to empty the bladder and prevent it from stretching, and careful monitoring of fluid intake and output.

Residents with neurogenic bladder may be very self-conscious about the leakage of urine, and the smell. Your actions to help them with hygiene to feel clean and fresh are very important.

KIDNEY STONES (RENAL CALCULI)

As you have learned, the main function of the kidney is to filter and remove waste products from the bloodstream. Many of these waste products are in the form of mineral salts, such as calcium salts and uric acid. If waste products become very concentrated, they can start to group together, forming tiny crystals that continue to grow in size as more of the mineral is deposited around them. These clumps of minerals are called **kidney stones,** or renal calculi (Fig. 39-6). Kidney stones are most common in middle-aged adults. Factors that may increase an older person's risk of developing kidney stones include immobility, not drinking enough fluids (which causes urine to be more concentrated with the waste salts), and infections of the urinary system.

Stones most often form in the collecting area (renal pelvis) of the kidney, but they can also form in the bladder. Kidney stones usually cause severe pain as they move downward through the ureter, and then through the urethra. The rough edges of the stone can damage the mucosal lining of the ureter or urethra, causing it to bleed, resulting in hematuria (blood in the urine). The person may complain of a cramping pain in the back or side in the area of the kidney or in the lower abdomen.

A person with a kidney stone usually needs to drink plenty of fluids to help flush the stone through the urinary tract. Medication may be necessary to help control the pain. You may be asked to collect all of the person's urine after each voiding and strain it to retrieve the stone. To strain the urine, place a piece of filter paper or a 4 × 4 gauze pad in a graduate, and then pour the urine into the graduate (Fig. 39-7). The urine will pass through the filter paper or gauze pad, leaving any stones behind. It is important to retrieve the kidney stones so that they can be sent to the laboratory

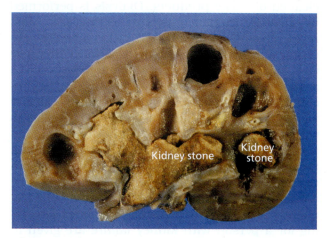

Figure 39-6
This is a kidney, cut open to reveal the kidney stones inside. Kidney stones can grow to be quite large, with sharp edges. They may cause obstruction of the ureters or urethra. Once the stone is passed, it is usually sent to the laboratory for analysis to determine which waste salt is causing the stones to form. (© Dr. E. Walker/Photo Researchers, Inc.)

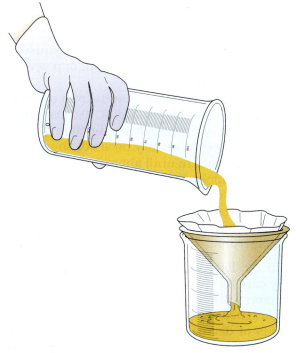

Figure 39-7
You may be asked to strain a person's urine to retrieve kidney stones. To strain urine, put a piece of filter paper or a 4″ × 4″ gauze pad in a graduate, and then pour the urine into the graduate. The urine will pass through the paper or gauze pad, leaving any stones behind. The stones are then transferred to a specimen container and sent to the laboratory for analysis.

for chemical analysis. Once the doctor knows which waste salt is causing the stones to form, he may be able to prevent future stones from developing.

If a stone becomes lodged in the narrow ureter, it can block the flow of urine to the bladder. The urine builds up, placing pressure on the delicate nephrons of the kidney. In this case, the person will need to have the stone removed surgically. Often, the stones are removed using a procedure called *lithotripsy.* In lithotripsy, high-frequency sound waves are directed at the stone, causing it to break into smaller pieces that can then be passed through the urinary tract. Sometimes, a surgical incision needs to be made for stone removal.

KIDNEY (RENAL) FAILURE

Kidney (renal) failure is the inability of the kidneys to filter blood effectively. As a result of kidney failure, waste products and fluid build up in the body, straining the heart and other organs. The person becomes very ill and can die if treatment is delayed.

Kidney failure can be either acute or chronic:

- Acute kidney failure can result from a medical or surgical emergency that causes a decrease in the amount of blood flow through the kidneys. It can also be caused by poisoning, a severe infection, or a severe allergic reaction.
- Chronic kidney failure results from a gradual loss of functioning nephrons. Because the kidneys lose their ability to function gradually, the person usually does not show signs of kidney failure until approximately 80% to 90% of kidney function is lost. The most common causes of chronic kidney failure are hypertension and diabetes, chronic conditions that damage the blood vessels in the glomerulus.

In the long-term care setting, you will most likely care for people with chronic kidney failure. A person with chronic kidney failure may feel ill and fatigued all of the time, and he may have periods of decreased mental alertness or agitation. Because the build-up of wastes in the bloodstream causes an unpleasant taste in the mouth, the person may have a loss of appetite (leading to unintentional weight loss) and the person's breath may have a distinct odor. The person's skin may itch all over and it may be discolored. The person may bruise or bleed easily. Late in the disease process, the person develops oliguria (a urine output of less than 400 mL in 24 hours), followed by anuria (the absence of urine output).

People with kidney failure often need to have dialysis. **Dialysis** does the job of the kidneys by removing waste products and fluids from the body. There are two types of dialysis:

- In *hemodialysis,* the person's blood is drawn intravenously, passed through a machine with filters and solutions that clean the blood of waste, and then returned to the person's body through another vessel (Fig. 39-8A). A person who is receiving regular hemodialysis treatments will have surgery to create a *fistula* or *graft.* The fistula or graft provides access for the needles and tubing used during the dialysis treatment. Sometimes, this access is provided through a temporary device called a *shunt.*
- In *peritoneal dialysis,* solutions that absorb waste products are instilled (placed) into a person's abdominal cavity through a tube that has been surgically inserted for this purpose (Fig. 39-8B). The solution remains in the abdominal cavity for a specified period of time so that waste products can be absorbed into the solution through the membrane lining the abdominal cavity. The used solution is then drained into a collecting bag and is discarded according to facility policy.

Dialysis takes several hours and must be performed several times a week to keep the blood cleaned of waste products. Dialysis is performed by specially trained nurses or technicians. Most residents who need dialysis travel to a health care center specifically designed to perform this service. Sometimes, a resident is too ill to be taken to a dialysis center, so the dialysis nurse or technician may bring portable equipment to the facility where you work. Many of your older residents with chronic kidney failure will not receive dialysis because they are too frail or weak to tolerate the procedure. However, if you are caring for a resident who receives dialysis, you may be asked to monitor the person's vital signs quite frequently after each treatment. Guidelines for caring for a person with kidney failure are given in Guidelines Box 39-1.

TUMORS

Tumors, which may or may not be malignant (cancerous), can affect all of the organs of the

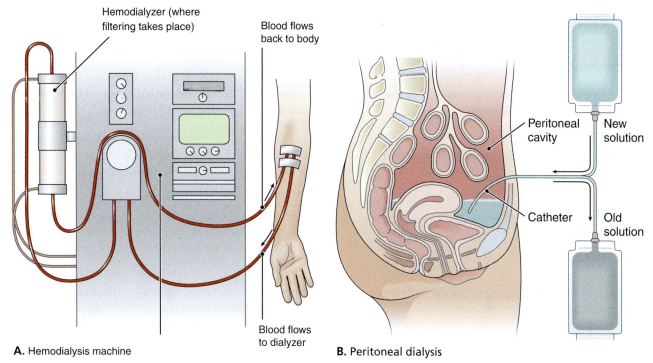

Hemodialyzer (where filtering takes place)

Blood flows back to body

Blood flows to dialyzer

A. Hemodialysis machine

Peritoneal cavity

New solution

Catheter

Old solution

B. Peritoneal dialysis

Figure 39-8

Dialysis machines perform the job of the kidneys for people who have kidney failure. **(A)** Hemodialysis. The dialysis machine receives blood drawn from an artery in the person's arm. The blood is filtered and then returned to the body. **(B)** Peritoneal dialysis. A special solution is placed in the person's abdominal cavity to absorb wastes, and then the solution is drained.

urinary system. Tumors can block the flow of urine through the urinary system, resulting in kidney damage. Kidney damage may also result from tumors of the kidney that invade the healthy tissue, damaging the nephrons. Surgical removal of the affected kidney is usually necessary, but as long as the remaining kidney is functioning properly, it should be able to handle removal of waste and fluid.

Tumors of the bladder are common among people who have smoked cigarettes. The risk for bladder cancer increases with age, and older men are twice as likely to develop bladder cancer as older women are. Bladder tumors are usually malignant and may spread to other organs. Tumors may be treated with medication, radiation, or surgery, depending on the type of tumor and whether or not it has spread to other parts of the body. In some cases, it is necessary to remove the bladder. Because the urine is no longer able to flow from the ureters into the bladder and then into the urethra to leave the body, a *urinary diversion* is created. The urine leaves the body through a stoma and drains freely into an ostomy appliance that is worn on the outside of the body.

- In a *ureterostomy*, one or both of the ureters are brought through the abdominal wall by way of small incisions, and sutured in place (Fig. 39-9A).
- In a *urostomy*, the ureters are attached to a small portion of the small intestine (Fig. 39-9B). One end of the segment of intestine is sealed off, and the other end is brought through the abdominal wall and sutured into place.

If one of your residents has had a urinary diversion procedure and you are permitted to assist the person with ostomy care, the nurse will show you how. The ostomy appliance needs to be emptied regularly, and good skin care around the stoma is essential. If urine leaks around the appliance, skin irritation and breakdown can occur. As always, the urine should be observed for any changes that might indicate infection or other urinary disorders. It may also be necessary to measure and record the amount of urine before discarding it.

Guidelines Box 39-1   Guidelines for Caring for a Person With Kidney Failure

WHAT YOU DO	WHY YOU DO IT
Carefully measure the person's urine output and document the amounts accurately.	The doctor will use this information to monitor how well the person's kidneys are functioning.
Assist with obtaining urine samples as requested.	Testing the urine for waste products is another way of monitoring how well the person's kidneys are functioning.
Follow the person's care plan carefully with regard to food and fluid intake.	To reduce the amount of work the kidneys have to do, the person's fluid intake may be restricted and a special diet that is low in salt and protein may be ordered.
Monitor vital signs according to the person's care plan, and report any changes to the nurse immediately.	Changes in fluid balance, especially after dialysis, can significantly raise or lower a person's blood pressure.
When measuring the blood pressure of a person who receives hemodialysis treatments, avoid measuring the blood pressure in the arm in which the person's fistula, graft, or shunt is located.	Pressure can decrease blood flow through the fistula, graft, or shunt, which can lead to clots. Clots can make the fistula, graft, or shunt unusable for dialysis.
Provide frequent skin care.	Skin care helps prevent the skin irritation and itching that can be caused by kidney failure.
When assisting a person who receives peritoneal dialysis treatments with bathing or dressing, take care not to accidentally dislodge the tube used for peritoneal dialysis.	If the tube becomes dislodged, it will be necessary to reinsert it.
Provide care measures, such as frequent repositioning and range-of-motion exercises, to help prevent the complications of immobility.	People in kidney failure may be on bed rest, which can put them at risk for complications from immobility.

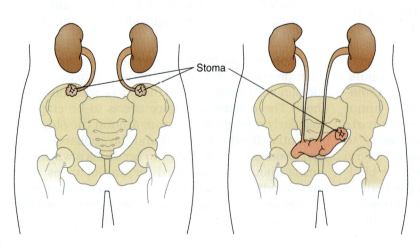

A. Ureterostomy   **B.** Urostomy

Figure 39-9
Urinary diversion procedures are necessary when part of the urinary system must be removed. **(A)** In a ureterostomy, one or both ureters are brought through the abdominal wall and sutured into place. **(B)** In a urostomy, the ureters are joined to a small segment of the small intestine, and then the intestine is brought to the surface of the body and sutured into place.

Observations that may be a sign of a urinary system disorder and should be reported to the nurse immediately include:

- Complaints of sharp, sudden pain in the abdomen, side, or back
- Blood in the urine (hematuria)
- A significant increase or decrease in the amount of urine voided in a period of time
- Changes in a person's voiding habits, especially increased or decreased frequency, or a new onset of incontinence
- Pain or burning when urinating
- Urine that appears dark or cloudy, or that has a strong ammonia smell
- Increased confusion, decreased alertness, or unusual behavior

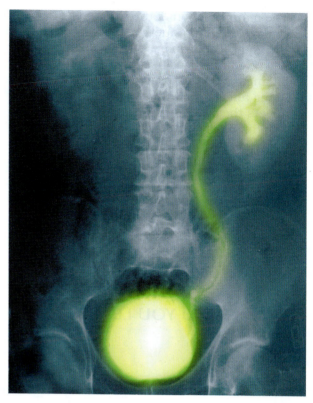

Figure 39-10
In intravenous pyelography (IVP), a type of radiographic (x-ray) procedure, a special dye is injected intravenously to allow visualization of the kidneys, ureter, and bladder. (© *Scott Camazine/Photo Researchers, Inc.*)

DIAGNOSIS OF URINARY DISORDERS

Observations that indicate problems affecting the urinary system are often non-specific. For example, kidney stones or urinary tract infections can cause abdominal pain, a common symptom of many digestive disorders as well. Usually, additional testing is needed to find out what the real problem is. Many types of tests are used to diagnose disorders of the urinary system:

- **Urinalysis.** In urinalysis, the urine is examined under a microscope and by chemical means.
- **Imaging studies.** Computed tomography (CT) scans, magnetic resonance imaging (MRI) scans, and radiographs (x-rays) can allow a doctor to see tumors and other abnormalities of the urinary system. With x-rays, a special dye may be injected into the veins before the x-ray is taken to high-light the kidneys, ureters, and bladder (Fig. 39-10).
- **Ultrasound.** Ultrasound may be used to detect tumors of the urinary system.
- **Cystoscopy and ureteroscopy.** A small, lighted scope is inserted through the urethra and used to view the inside of the bladder (cystoscopy) or ureters (ureteroscopy).

You may be asked to collect and measure urine for testing or to help prepare a resident for other diagnostic tests or procedures. Make sure that you are informed about any specific procedures that you will be responsible for, such as keeping the person on NPO status, restricting or encouraging fluids, or straining urine.

SUMMARY

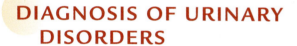

- The organs of the urinary system are the kidneys, the ureters, the urinary bladder, and the urethra.
  - The two kidneys filter the blood to remove waste products and excess fluid.
- The ureters carry urine from the kidneys to the bladder.
- The bladder is a holding place for urine.
- The urethra carries urine from the bladder to the outside of the body.

- The main function of the urinary system is to remove waste products and excess fluid from the body. The urinary system also plays a key role in homeostasis by maintaining fluid balance and regulating the pH of the blood.
- Aging affects the urinary system just as it affects the other organ systems.
    - In an older person, loss of muscle tone affects the bladder's ability to hold urine and empty properly.
    - Older men may experience difficulty voiding as a result of an enlarged prostate gland.
    - An older person is more likely to develop urinary tract infections, because of decreased immune function and incomplete emptying of the bladder.
    - As we age, the number of nephrons decreases, reducing the kidney's efficiency at filtering blood.
- Disorders of the urinary system include infections, neurogenic bladder, kidney stones (renal calculi), kidney (renal) failure, and tumors.
    - As a nursing assistant, you may be the first to notice signs and symptoms of a urinary problem that a resident is having.
    - You may also be involved in helping a resident to prepare for a diagnostic test used to evaluate the urinary system, or in assisting with treatment.

WHAT DID YOU LEARN?

Multiple Choice

Select the single best answer for each of the following questions.

1. Urine leaves the body through the:
   a. Nephrons
   b. Urethra
   c. Ureters
   d. Bladder
2. How does aging affect the urinary system?
   a. The number of nephrons is decreased, reducing the kidney's ability to filter blood efficiently
   b. The ability to empty the bladder completely is decreased
   c. Bladder capacity is decreased
   d. All of the above
3. How much urine does an average adult pass each day?
   a. 200 mL of urine per day
   b. 500 mL of urine per day
   c. 1 to 1.5 liters of urine per day
   d. 160 to 180 liters of urine per day
4. Why are urinary tract infections more common in women than in men?
   a. A woman's urethra is short, and the opening of the urethra is located close to the anus
   b. A woman's urethra is long and curved
   c. Women tend to be more careless with perineal care
   d. Women do not drink as much water as men
5. Which of the following might be a sign of a urinary tract infection?
   a. Pain or burning while urinating
   b. Extreme thirst
   c. Anuria (absence of urine)
   d. Kidney failure
6. Which procedure uses high-frequency sound waves to break up kidney stones?
   a. Lithotripsy
   b. Dialysis
   c. Filtration
   d. Urostomy
7. Mr. Loyd has a urostomy, which was done to treat his bladder cancer. What do you need to remember when caring for Mr. Loyd?
   a. He may develop kidney failure at any time
   b. He will require good skin care around the stoma to prevent skin irritation and breakdown
   c. He is more at risk for kidney stones
   d. He will not require any special care
8. How is the male urethra different from the female urethra?
   a. It is longer
   b. It serves as a passageway for urine and for semen
   c. The opening is further away from the anus
   d. All of the above
9. Sally is caring for Mrs. Brady, who has been going to the bathroom more frequently than usual. Now, Mrs. Brady is complaining of a burning sensation when she urinates. Why

is it important for Sally to report what she has observed to the nurse?

a. Mrs. Brady may be in kidney failure

b. Mrs. Brady may have a urinary tract infection

c. The nurse will assign another nursing assistant to help with Mrs. Brady's care

d. It is not necessary for Sally to report these observations to the nurse

10. Mrs. Offenheimer is very self-conscious about her frequent dribbling of urine. You know that this is a symptom of:

a. Attention-seeking behavior

b. An underactive bladder

c. An overactive bladder

d. Kidney failure

Matching

Match each numbered item with its appropriate lettered description.

_____ **1.** Cystitis

_____ **2.** Renal calculi

_____ **3.** Pyelonephritis

_____ **4.** Glomerulus

_____ **5.** Urethritis

a. Infection of the kidneys

b. Capillary bed in the nephron; surrounded by Bowman's capsule

c. Infection of the urethra

d. Kidney stones

e. Infection of the bladder

STOP and Think!

● Janice is assigned to care for Mr. Roberts, who has been having a cramping pain in his left side near his waist. The nurse told Janice that the doctor believes that Mr. Roberts is passing a kidney stone. This morning, while helping Mr. Roberts with his A.M. care, Janice noticed that the urinal hanging on Mr. Roberts' side rail was full. Because Janice knows that Mr. Roberts is being evaluated for kidney stones, what extra steps will she take when she empties his urinal?

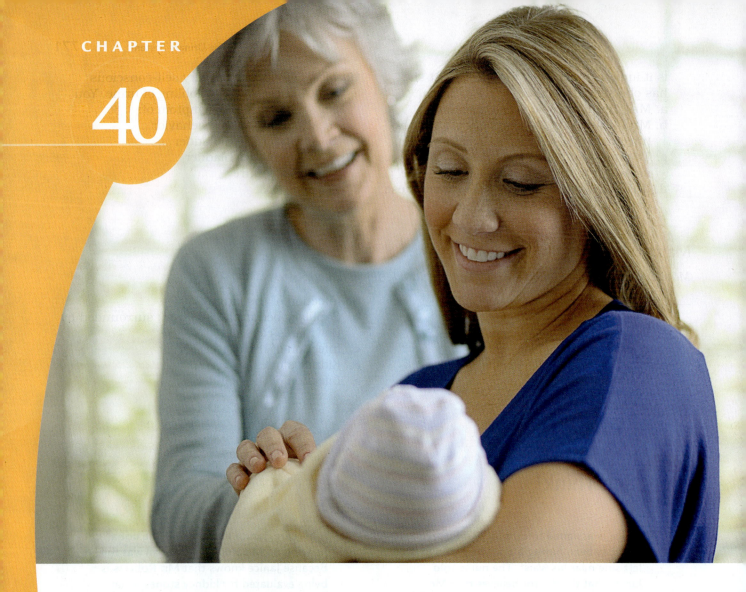

The Reproductive System

WHAT WILL YOU LEARN?

Of all of the systems that make up the human body, perhaps none is as fascinating and miraculous as the reproductive system. **Reproduction** is the process by which a living thing makes more living things like itself. Because all living things eventually die, the ability to reproduce is essential for the survival of any species. Without the ability to reproduce, the species would slowly die off and cease to exist.

In this chapter, you will learn about the male and female reproductive systems, which are very different from each other. You will learn about their structure and function, the effects of aging on each, and common disorders that can affect each. In addition, you will learn about sexually transmitted infections (STIs), which can affect both men and women. When you are finished with this chapter, you will be able to:

1. Describe the main function of the reproductive system.
2. List the organs that make up the female reproductive system.
3. Discuss the normal function of the female reproductive system.

Photo: A grandmother welcomes a new grandchild to the family.

4. Explain the effects of aging on the female reproductive system.

5. Describe the disorders that may affect the female reproductive system.

6. List the organs that make up the male reproductive system.

7. Discuss the normal function of the male reproductive system.

8. Explain the effects of aging on the male reproductive system.

9. Describe the disorders that may affect the male reproductive system.

10. Discuss sexually transmitted infections (STIs) that may affect the male or female reproductive systems.

Vocabulary 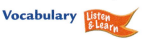 Use the CD in the front of your book to hear these terms pronounced and defined:

Reproduction	Ovulation	Uterine prolapse	Impotence (erectile
Sex cell (gamete)	Menstrual period	(prolapsed uterus)	dysfunction)
Sperm cell	Vaginitis	Pessary	Sexually transmitted
Egg (ovum, ova)	Pelvic organ prolapse	Gynecologist	infection (STI)
Conception	Cystocele	Postmenopausal bleeding	Pelvic inflammatory
(fertilization)	Rectocele	Ejaculation	disease (PID)

Has anyone ever told you that you have "your mother's eyes" or "the family nose?" Do you look very much like your brothers or sisters, or not much like them at all? Each of us receives our genes, the bundles of DNA that determine how we develop and what we look like physically, from our parents. Your mother gave you half of your genes and your father gave you the other half, to make a full set. This is why you may look a lot like either one of your parents, or like a blend of the two. Or, why you may look very much like one of your siblings, and not much like another one. It all depends on the combination of genes that you received.

Each species has a set number of genes, or chromosomes. For example, human beings have 46 chromosomes. This means that to keep the number of chromosomes the same from generation to generation, the father contributes 23 chromosomes and the mother contributes 23 chromosomes. The special cells contributed by each parent that contain half of the normal number of chromosomes are called **sex cells,** or **gametes.** The male sex cell is called a **sperm cell.** The female sex cell is called an **egg,** or **ovum** (*ova,* plural). When the sperm joins the egg, forming a cell that contains the complete number of chromosomes, **conception (fertilization)** occurs. During the 9 months leading up to the birth of a baby, the single original cell that formed at conception copies itself over and over again, forming all of the baby's tissues and organs.

One of the main functions of the reproductive system in both males and females is to produce and transport sex cells. However, unlike other organ systems in the body, the organs that make up the reproductive system are very different in men and women. The male reproductive system is designed to produce sperm and deposit it inside the female's body. The female reproductive system is designed to produce eggs, receive sperm cells, contain and nourish a developing baby, give birth, and provide nourishment after the baby's birth by producing breast milk. Because of the physical and functional differences between the male and female reproductive systems, we will look at each system separately in the sections that follow.

THE FEMALE REPRODUCTIVE SYSTEM

STRUCTURE OF THE FEMALE REPRODUCTIVE SYSTEM

The organs and structures of the female reproductive system are located both inside and outside of the body. The internal organs are the ovaries, fallopian tubes, uterus, and vagina (Fig. 40-1A). The outer structures are the labia, the clitoris, and the vaginal opening (Fig. 40-1B). These outer structures are sometimes referred to collectively as the *vulva.* In addition, the breasts (mammary glands) are considered accessory organs of the female reproductive system, because they play a role in nourishing a newborn baby.

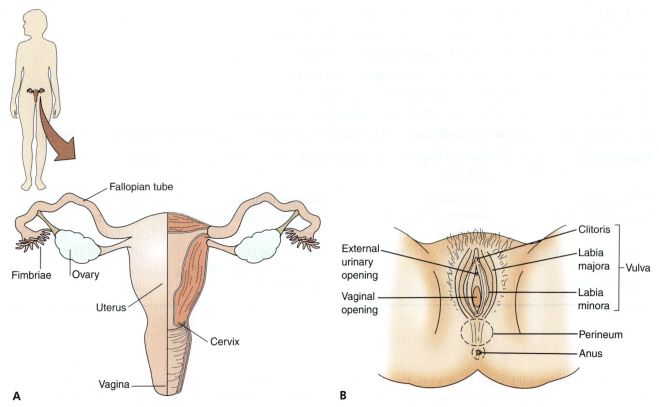

Figure 40-1
The female reproductive system. **(A)** Internal structures include the ovaries, fallopian tubes, uterus, and vagina. **(B)** External structures, collectively known as "the vulva," include the vaginal opening, labia, and clitoris.

The Ovaries

The ovaries are two small, almond-shaped organs located deep inside the abdomen on either side of the uterus (Fig. 40-1A). The ovaries store the ova, or eggs. When a baby girl is born, her ovaries contain all of the eggs that she will ever have. The stored eggs are kept in a "holding pattern" until they are needed. Once a girl passes through puberty and reaches reproductive age, she begins to ovulate. **Ovulation** is the release of a ripe, mature egg from the ovaries each month.

The Fallopian Tubes

The fallopian tubes, also called *uterine tubes* or *oviducts*, are slender tubes about 4 to 5 inches long that transport the egg from the ovary to the uterus. After leaving the ovary, the egg moves through the fluid in the abdomen to the entrance of the nearest fallopian tube. The open ends of the fallopian tubes nearest the ovaries have small, fringe-like projections called *fimbriae* (Fig. 40-1A). The fimbriae beat in a wave-like motion, helping to move the egg into the tube. Once in the fallopian tube, the egg moves

toward the uterus, helped along by the peristaltic contractions of the smooth muscle layer in the walls of the fallopian tube and the tiny, hair-like cilia on the lining of the fallopian tube. Like the cilia in the airways of the lungs, the cilia in the fallopian tubes move gently back and forth, creating a sweeping motion that helps to move the egg along the length of the tube. Conception, if it occurs, occurs in the fallopian tubes.

The Uterus

The uterus, sometimes referred to as the *womb*, is a hollow, pear-shaped organ (Fig. 40-1). The uterus has three sections:

- The *fundus* is the upper, rounded portion of the uterus.
- The *body* is the mid-portion of the uterus.
- The *cervix* is the lower, narrow portion of the uterus. Normally, the cervix is closed, except for a very tiny opening. This opening, which is no larger than a pinpoint, allows sperm to enter the uterus, and menstrual blood to pass out of it. When a woman is about to

give birth, the cervix dilates (opens), becoming as large as 10 centimeters in diameter. Dilation of the cervix creates an opening wide enough for the baby to pass through into the vagina.

The walls of the uterus are made of thick, smooth muscle tissue. The muscular walls of the uterus expand to accommodate a growing baby and then contract during labor to push the baby out. The inner cavity of the uterus is shaped like a capital "T" and is lined with tissue called *endometrium*.

The Vagina

The vagina is a muscular tube about 3 inches long that connects the uterus to the outside of the body (Fig. 40-1A). The vagina is the receiving organ for sperm. It also serves as the birth canal, through which a baby passes during birth. The mucous membrane lining of the vagina helps to lubricate the vagina during sexual intercourse and protect the body from infection. It contains many folds, which allow the vagina to expand enough to allow a baby to pass through.

The Vulva

The vulva consists of the vaginal opening, the labia, and the clitoris (Fig. 40-1B).

- The vaginal opening, also called the *vaginal orifice*, is where the vagina opens to the outside of the body. The vaginal opening is located between the external urinary opening (the urinary meatus or urethral orifice) and the anus. The area between the vaginal opening and the anus is often called the *perineum*. However, the term *perineum* can also be used to describe the entire external genital area of both men and women.
- The labia, or "lips," are folds of tissue that surround the vaginal opening. The many folds of the external female reproductive system can create difficulties with hygiene, especially if a woman is unable to provide for her own cleanliness needs. Perineal care and hygiene assistance is discussed in Chapter 23.
- The clitoris is located at the upper folds of the internal labia. This tissue, which is very sensitive to touch, helps to initiate a woman's sexual arousal.

The Breasts (Mammary Glands)

In women, the breasts are considered accessory organs of the reproductive system, because they

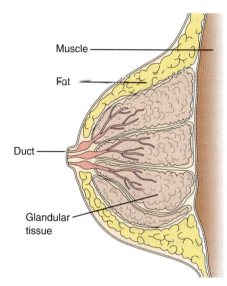

Figure 40-2
The breasts consist of glandular tissue and fat.

play a role in nourishing the newborn. Although the female breasts develop during puberty, they do not become functional until the end of pregnancy. The breasts are made up of lobes, or sections, that contain glandular tissue and fat (Fig. 40-2). When it is stimulated by the hormone prolactin (which is secreted by the pituitary gland at the end of pregnancy), the glandular tissue of the breasts produces milk, a process known as *lactation*. In response to an infant's suckling, the glandular tissue contracts, sending the milk through the ducts to the nipple.

FUNCTION OF THE FEMALE REPRODUCTIVE SYSTEM

Each month during a woman's reproductive years (from puberty to menopause), her body prepares itself to become pregnant. If pregnancy does not occur, the woman has a menstrual period and the cycle begins again.

The cycle begins when the pituitary gland releases follicle-stimulating hormone (FSH), a hormone that causes about 20 eggs in the ovaries to begin to grow and mature. Each egg grows within its own "shell," called a follicle. FSH also stimulates the follicles to produce estrogen, another hormone. As the estrogen level increases, it "turns off" FSH production. This feedback mechanism limits the number of follicles that mature each month. One egg-containing follicle continues to grow and mature, and the others die off.

When the egg has matured, luteinizing hormone (LH), another hormone released by the pituitary gland, causes the follicle to burst, releasing the egg from the ovary (ovulation). Following ovulation, the empty follicle continues to produce estrogen, and it also begins to produce progesterone. Estrogen and progesterone cause the uterus to begin to prepare itself to receive a fertilized egg.

In response to estrogen and progesterone, the lining of the uterus (the endometrium) thickens, creating a soft, nourishing environment for a fertilized egg, should one arrive. Estrogen and progesterone allow the fertilized egg to attach itself to the endometrium (a process called *implantation*). Once the fertilized egg implants, it begins to divide, forming the cells and tissues that will eventually become a new human being. If fertilization does not occur, the egg passes into the uterus, where it usually dissolves. The levels of hormones decrease, causing the endometrial lining to break down and pass through the vagina as the **menstrual period.**

This cycle of hormone secretion and egg development occurs in a regular pattern throughout a woman's reproductive years. The average cycle from the first day of one menstrual period until the start of another one is 28 days, but the cycle can be as short as 22 days or as long as 45 days.

THE EFFECTS OF AGING ON THE FEMALE REPRODUCTIVE SYSTEM

Unlike the age-related changes that affect other organ systems, the age-related changes that affect the female reproductive system are usually very noticeable.

Increased Difficulty Becoming Pregnant

Many women in their late 30s and early 40s have difficulty becoming pregnant. This is because each month, the number of healthy eggs remaining in a woman's ovaries decreases. Becoming pregnant is often still possible at this age, just more difficult. Fertility treatments, such as the use of drugs to cause more eggs to ripen each month or in-vitro fertilization (IVF), are often very helpful for women in this age group who wish to become pregnant.

Decreased Sex Hormone Production

As a woman ages, her body produces lower amounts of sex hormones, especially estrogen and progesterone. Eventually, this decreased hormone production results in menopause, the complete ending of a woman's menstrual cycles. Menopause occurs in most women sometime between the ages of 45 and 55 years and is caused by the loss of ovary function due to age. Menopause can cause many bothersome symptoms, including "hot flashes," irritability, a loss of energy, and an inability to sleep. Decreased production of estrogen and progesterone, which are "feminizing" hormones, may also cause some women to develop facial hair and a coarse ("scratchy") voice. Some women experience vaginal dryness and irritation that can make sexual intercourse uncomfortable. When this is the case, use of a lubricant during sexual intercourse can be helpful. Vaginal dryness and irritation can also lead to **vaginitis** (inflammation of the vaginal tissues). Vaginitis can cause itching, burning, and a vaginal discharge, and it increases the woman's risk for vaginal infections.

Many women who have gone through menopause choose to replace the hormones their bodies no longer produce by taking estrogen and progesterone orally. This is called hormone replacement therapy (HRT). HRT helps to minimize some of the more annoying "side effects" of menopause, such as hot flashes. In addition, research shows that taking estrogen and progesterone after menopause can help keep bones strong. However, research has also shown that HRT may increase a woman's risk for breast cancer, heart disease, and some types of dementia. Each woman must work with her health care provider to determine whether HRT is right for her, given her unique situation and health history.

DISORDERS OF THE FEMALE REPRODUCTIVE SYSTEM

Many types of disorders can affect the female reproductive system.

Cysts and Non-cancerous Growths

Many organs in the female reproductive system can be affected by cysts or other noncancerous growths. Although these cysts and growths are not cancerous, they can still cause problems.

- **Cysts** can form on the ovaries after ovulation, causing intense pain. Although not malignant, ovarian cysts may need to be surgically removed if they occur frequently and are painful. Cysts may also form in the lubricating glands located inside the vagina, creating a painful, infected lump that may have to be surgically drained.
- **Fibroids (myomas)** sometimes form in the muscle wall of the uterus.

Pelvic Organ Prolapse

The female reproductive organs, the urinary bladder, and the rectum are supported in the pelvic cavity by connective tissue and muscles. Childbirth and the loss of estrogen that occurs with menopause can cause these supportive structures to weaken. As a result, an older woman may experience **pelvic organ prolapse.** In pelvic organ prolapse, the affected organ shifts downward from its normal position (Fig. 40-3):

- **Cystocele** occurs when the bladder shifts downward, pressing into the front (anterior) vaginal wall. Cystocele can contribute to incomplete emptying of the bladder and stress incontinence (see Chapter 26).

- **Rectocele** occurs when the front wall of the rectum shifts downward, pushing into the back (posterior) vaginal wall. Women with this condition may feel pressure in the rectal area, have difficulties having a bowel movement, or feel as if the rectum is not empty following a bowel movement.

- **Uterine prolapse (prolapsed uterus)** occurs when the uterus shifts downward, into the vaginal canal. The uterus may slip only part way into the vagina, or it may pass all of the way through the vagina, so that it is visible on the outside of the body. Symptoms of uterine prolapse can include a feeling of pelvic pressure or fullness, low back pain, trouble having a bowel movement, leaking

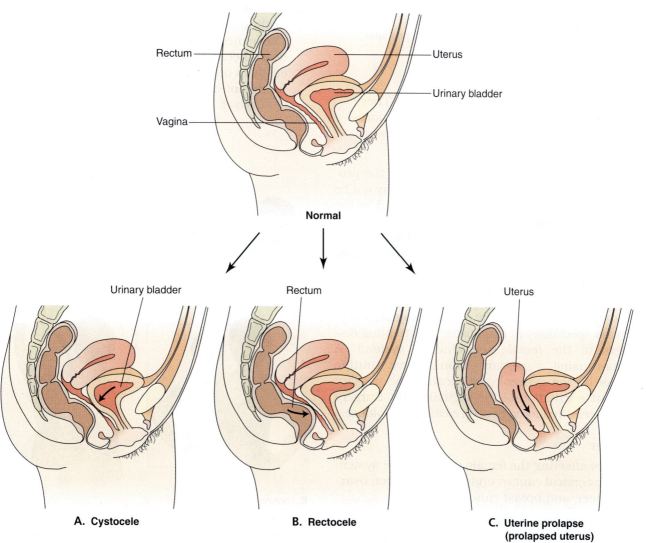

A. Cystocele   **B. Rectocele**   **C. Uterine prolapse (prolapsed uterus)**

Figure 40-3

Pelvic organ prolapse is common in older women. **(A)** In cystocele, the bladder shifts downward, pressing into the front (anterior) wall of the vagina. **(B)** In rectocele, the front wall of the rectum shifts downward, pressing into the back (posterior) wall of the vagina. **(C)** In uterine prolapse (prolapsed uterus), the uterus slips downward, into the vagina.

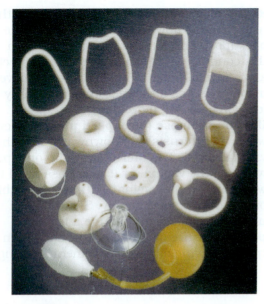

Figure 40-4
Pessaries, devices used to treat pelvic organ prolapse, come in a variety of styles.

of urine, and urinary incontinence. These symptoms are usually better in the morning, and become worse over the course of the day.

Treatment depends on the severity of the prolapse. If the prolapse is mild, treatment may not be necessary, or estrogen may be administered (in the form of a cream that is applied to the skin) to strengthen the supportive tissues and muscles. If the prolapse is more severe, a device called a **pessary** may be inserted into the vagina to support the prolapsed organ in the proper position. Pessaries come in a variety of styles (Fig. 40-4) and must be fitted by the doctor (usually a **gynecologist,** a doctor who specializes in diagnosing and treating disorders of the female reproductive system). A woman using a pessary should have routine checks by the gynecologist because the pessary can cause irritation of the vaginal walls. Surgery may be required for very severe cases of prolapse.

Cancer

Cancers affecting the female reproductive system include cervical cancer, endometrial cancer, ovarian cancer, and breast cancer.

- **Cervical cancer** (cancer of the cervix, the lower region of the uterus) is more common among women between the ages of 30 and 50 years and can be caused by a sexually transmitted viral infection. Other factors that can increase a woman's risk of developing

cervical cancer include having sexual intercourse at an early age and having multiple sexual partners. If diagnosed early enough, cervical cancer can be effectively treated without putting a woman's ability to have children at risk.
- **Endometrial cancer** (cancer of the lining of the uterus) is the most common type of cancer that affects the female reproductive tract. It is most common in women after menopause. The first sign of this type of cancer is **postmenopausal bleeding,** uterine bleeding that occurs after a woman has completed menopause. Postmenopausal bleeding can also result from hormone imbalances.
- **Ovarian cancer** (cancer of the ovary) most commonly occurs in women between the ages of 40 and 65 years. Ovarian cancer is a leading cause of cancer death for women. This cancer is associated with a high rate of death because it grows quickly and spreads easily to other organs. Early diagnosis and treatment can improve a woman's chances of survival.

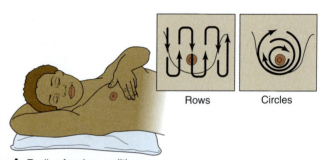

Rows   Circles

A. Feeling for abnormalities

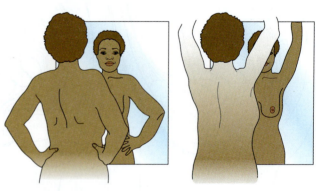

B. Looking for abnormalities

Figure 40-5
Women are encouraged to examine their breasts monthly, so that they become familiar with the way their breast tissue normally looks and feels. A breast self-exam (BSE) involves **(A)** feeling the breasts for abnormalities and then **(B)** looking at the breasts for abnormalities.

- **Breast cancer** is the most commonly occurring cancer in women. Early detection and new treatment methods for breast cancer allow many women to be completely cured of this disease. Breast cancer can develop in women with relatives with breast cancer, especially a mother or sister, but it can also develop in women who have no family history of the disease. Women of all ages are encouraged to examine their breasts regularly (Fig. 40-5). In addition, annual mammograms (x-rays of the breast tissue) are recommended for women 40 years of age and older to screen for breast cancer. Although there is no specific age at which a woman should stop getting mammograms, many of your elderly residents will not have routine mammograms, because their other health problems would not make them good candidates for treatment, even if the cancer was discovered.

TELL THE NURSE

Your duties will include assisting your female residents with their personal hygiene and toileting needs. Because of this, you may be the first to observe signs of a problem involving the reproductive organs. Or, a female resident may tell you about a problem that she is experiencing. Report any of the following observations or complaints to the nurse immediately:

- The woman has an unusual vaginal discharge
- The woman has vaginal bleeding, but she has already gone through menopause
- The woman has pain or cramping in her lower abdomen
- The woman complains of a feeling of pelvic pressure or fullness
- The woman complains of problems emptying her bowel or bladder
- There is a protrusion from the vaginal opening
- The woman reports itching or burning around the vulva
- The skin around the vulva is inflamed or irritated
- There are changes in skin coloring, sores that do not heal, lumps, unusual swelling, or thickened areas around the vulva
- There is a lump or thickened area in the breast
- There is a discharge from the nipples or puckering of the skin of the breasts

THE MALE REPRODUCTIVE SYSTEM

STRUCTURE OF THE MALE REPRODUCTIVE SYSTEM

The organs and structures of the male reproductive system include the testicles (testes), the epididymis, the vas deferens, and the penis (Fig. 40-6). Accessory organs include the seminal vesicles and prostate gland, which play a role in producing semen (the fluid that carries sperm cells out of the body).

The Testicles (Testes)

The testicles are two walnut-like organs located in the *scrotum*, a loose, bag-like sac of skin that is suspended outside of the body, between the thighs. The testicles have two important functions: they secrete testosterone, the hormone that is responsible for the development of male secondary sex characteristics and for the proper functioning of the male reproductive system and they produce sperm cells. The testicles are located outside of a man's body, because the temperature necessary for the proper development of sperm cells is lower than the temperature inside the body.

The Epididymis

After the sperm cells leave the testes, they move into the epididymis, a series of coiled tubes where the sperm cells mature and gain the ability to move. A sperm cell's ability to move comes from its whip-like "tail." The tail's whip-like motion moves the sperm cell forward, allowing it to move through the female reproductive tract in search of an egg to fertilize.

The Vas Deferens

From the epididymis, the sperm cells move into the vas deferens, a passageway that transports the sperm cells to the urethra (Fig. 40-6). While in the vas deferens, the sperm cells are mixed with the secretions from the seminal vesicles and the prostate gland. These secretions, which nourish and protect the sperm cells, form the fluid portion of semen. In the prostate gland, the vas deferens joins with the urethra, which is the final passageway through which the sperm cells leave the man's body.

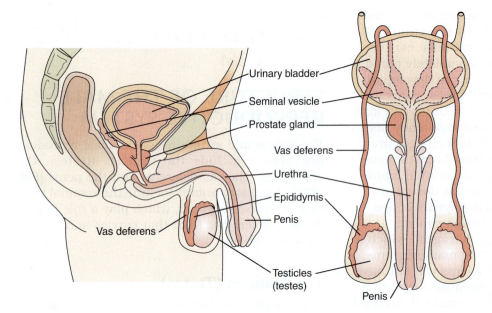

Figure 40-6
The male reproductive system consists of the testicles (testes), the epididymis, the vas deferens, and the penis. Accessory organs include the seminal vesicles and prostate gland.

The Penis

The male urethra, described in Chapter 39, is contained in the penis. Semen leaves the man's body through the external urinary opening, which is located at the tip of the *glans penis,* the enlarged end of the penis. If a male has not been circumcised, a loose fold of skin called the *foreskin* covers the glans penis.

The urethra is surrounded by "spongy" tissue. Stimulation by the nervous system causes this spongy tissue to fill with blood. This, in turn, causes the penis to become hard and erect. When erect, the penis can be inserted into a woman's vagina, allowing sperm cells to be deposited into the woman's reproductive tract.

FUNCTION OF THE MALE REPRODUCTIVE SYSTEM

The function of the male reproductive system is to produce and nourish male sex cells (sperm), and to deposit these cells inside the female's body so that fertilization can occur. The mature female reproductive system usually produces only one egg each month. In contrast, the mature male reproductive system produces sperm cells constantly. Many millions of sperm cells are needed to fertilize one egg because so many sperm cells die during their journey through the woman's reproductive tract. After puberty, sperm cells are produced in the testicles in response to the release of FSH by the pituitary gland. The pituitary gland also secretes interstitial cell-stimulating

hormone (ICSH), which stimulates the testicles to produce testosterone. Testosterone is needed for the continued development and growth of the sperm cells.

Sperm cells are deposited in the female reproductive tract through the process of **ejaculation.** During sexual intercourse, stimulation of the erect penis causes the forceful release of semen from the body. Ejaculation is how sperm cells leave the man's body and enter the woman's vagina so that the process of fertilization and reproduction can begin.

THE EFFECTS OF AGING ON THE MALE REPRODUCTIVE SYSTEM

As they get older, many men find that the frequency and duration of their erections decreases. Many men also develop enlargement of the prostate gland.

Decreased Frequency and Duration of Erections

Beginning at around the age of 20 years, production of testosterone and sperm begins to gradually decline. A man can remain fertile until late in life, even as late as 80 years of age, but most men find that as they get older, erections occur less frequently and last for shorter periods of time. This is a result of decreased production of testosterone. The ability to have and maintain an erection is also affected by the effects of aging on the cardiovascular system, which can result in decreased blood flow to the penis. Finally, medications taken for hypertension and other common disorders can also affect sexual abilities.

Enlargement of the Prostate Gland

As a man ages, the prostate gland tends to enlarge. Because the prostate gland surrounds the urethra, this enlargement can make urination difficult. Prostate problems associated with aging are discussed in Chapter 39.

DISORDERS OF THE MALE REPRODUCTIVE SYSTEM

Common disorders of the male reproductive system include impotence (erectile dysfunction) and cancer.

Impotence (Erectile Dysfunction)

Impotence (erectile dysfunction) is the inability to achieve or maintain an erection long enough to engage in sexual activity. A resident may experience erectile dysfunction for several reasons. Lowered levels of male hormones, circulatory problems that restrict blood flow to the penis, medications, or emotional disturbances can all affect a man's ability to have an erection, either temporarily or permanently. In many cultures, the

ability to have an erection and father children is often considered a mark of "manliness." Because of this, many men who have erectile dysfunction are embarrassed to tell a health care provider about this problem. However, once the cause has been discovered, many effective methods of treatment can allow a man to remain sexually active throughout his life span.

Cancer

Cancers affecting the male reproductive system include testicular cancer, prostate cancer, and penile cancer. In addition, men may get breast cancer, although this cancer is much less common in men than in women.

- **Testicular cancer** usually affects young to middle-aged adult men and can easily spread to other parts of the body through the lymphatic system before it is detected. Men of all ages are encouraged to examine their testicles regularly (Fig. 40-7). Testicular self-exams (TSEs) can help detect lumps and other abnormalities at an early stage. Early detection and treatment of cancer leads to a better survival outcome.
- **Prostate cancer.** Cancer of the prostate gland most commonly occurs in men older than 50 years of age. Rectal examination, during which a doctor inserts a finger into the man's rectum to feel for enlargement of

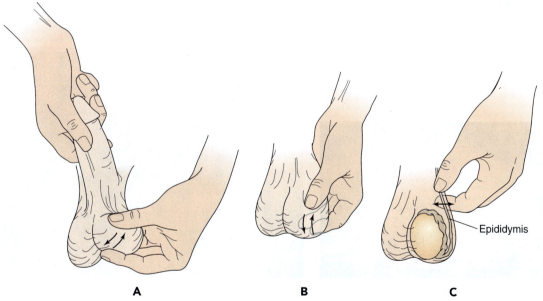

A   B   C

Figure 40-7

Men are encouraged to examine their testicles monthly. This is an effective and easy way to detect testicular cancer. A testicular self-exam (TSE) involves rolling each testicle between the fingers in a side-to-side motion **(A)** and then in an up-and-down motion **(B)**, and then feeling along the epididymis, the cord-like structure on the top and back of the testicle **(C)**.

the gland, can lead to early detection. A blood test can also be used to screen for prostate cancer. Prostate cancer typically grows slowly and has a good cure rate with early detection.

- **Penile cancer.** Occasionally, lesions that appear on the penis may be cancerous. As always, it is important for you to report any changes in the skin of residents, no matter what part of the body they appear on.

TELL THE NURSE

A conscientious nursing assistant always observes a resident for changes that indicate that something is "not quite right" and reports those observations to the nurse immediately. Listed below are some observations that may indicate disorders of the male reproductive system. Report any of the following observations or complaints to the nurse immediately:

- The man has an unusual discharge from the penis, especially if it contains blood or other discolored secretions
- The man has pain or burning when urinating
- There is a lump or thickened area in the testes
- There are changes in the skin surrounding the scrotum or penis
- There is reddened or irritated skin in the genital area
- The man complains of pain or aching in the scrotum or rectal area

SEXUALLY TRANSMITTED INFECTIONS

A **sexually transmitted infection (STI)** is an infection that is most often transmitted by sexual contact. These infections, also known as *sexually transmitted diseases (STDs)* or *venereal diseases*, can be caused by bacteria or viruses. The pathogens are transmitted through semen and vaginal secretions. Infection of the organs of the reproductive system is most common, although the mucous membranes of the eyes, mouth, or anus may also become infected following contact with infected semen or vaginal secretions. Some STIs, such as acquired immunodeficiency syndrome (AIDS), involve the entire body.

Some of the most common STIs include the following:

- **Herpes simplex** is a viral infection. There are two forms of herpes simplex. Herpes simplex type I causes the common "cold sore" or "fever blister" on the lip. Herpes simplex type II, or genital herpes, causes painful blisters to form around the vaginal opening and perineum (in women) or the external urinary opening (in men) (Fig. 40-8). There is no cure for genital herpes and the blisters may return over and over again throughout the lifetime of the person who is infected.

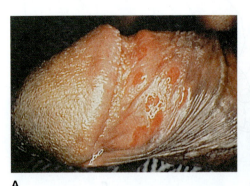
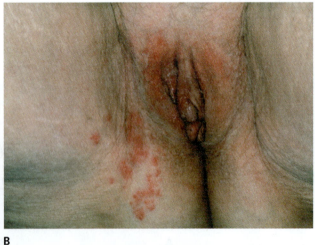

A   B

Figure 40-8
Genital herpes is a viral infection that causes blisters to form (**A**) on the penis (in men) and (**B**) on the vulva (in women). There is no cure for genital herpes. (**A**, *used with permission from Goodheart, H.P. [2003]: Goodheart's photoguide to common skin disorders. Diagnosis and management [2nd ed., p 284].* **B**, © Dr. P. Marrazi/Photo Researchers, Inc.)

- **Gonorrhea** is a bacterial infection. In men, the bacterium that causes gonorrhea infects the urethra. The man may experience a burning sensation during urination and notice a greenish discharge from the urethra, or he may have no symptoms at all. Women who are infected with the bacterium that causes gonorrhea may not have any symptoms. Because the infection may not be detected and treated for some time, the bacterium can travel to the fallopian tubes and into the abdominal cavity, resulting in a condition called **pelvic inflammatory disease (PID).** PID often results in severe pain and scar tissue. If detected, gonorrhea can be treated with antibiotics.
- **Chlamydia,** the most commonly occurring STI, is caused by a type of bacteria. Like gonorrhea, chlamydia often is not associated with any noticeable symptoms. Chlamydia can cause infertility in both men and women and is treated with an antibiotic.
- **Genital (venereal) warts** are caused by a virus. In men infected with the virus, small, wart-like growths may occur inside the urethra. In women, the warts may be seen around the vaginal opening, inside the vagina, or on the cervix. Infection with genital warts increases a woman's risk of developing cervical cancer. Treatment may involve removal of the growths with a laser.
- **Syphilis** is a bacterial infection. The signs and symptoms of syphilis occur in three stages. During the first stage, a painless lesion is seen on the genitals. This lesion

heals, and 2 to 4 weeks later, the person develops a skin rash and a fever. This is the second stage. If not detected and treated, the infection becomes latent. This means that the pathogen that is causing the infection is still in the person's body, but it is not active. As many as 20 or more years later, the pathogen can become active again, resulting in the third stage. The third stage usually involves damage to the cardiovascular and nervous systems, which can result in confusion, dementia, and paralysis.
- **AIDS** is caused by human immunodeficiency virus (HIV). The HIV virus can be transmitted in semen, vaginal secretions, or blood. To date, there is no cure for AIDS, and many people with AIDS die as a result of the disease. AIDS is discussed in detail in Chapters 16 and 44.

Although you may think that only young people are at risk for STIs, remember that many of your older residents continue to be sexually active and can still get an STI if they have sexual relations with an infected partner. Condoms, which help to prevent the transmission of infected secretions from one person to another, are very useful for preventing STIs, but many older people do not use condoms because they think of them primarily as a means of birth control, and pregnancy is not a concern after menopause. Avoiding sexual activity with infected partners is another important preventive measure. If one partner develops signs or symptoms of an STI, sexual relations should be avoided until both partners have been treated, or reinfection can occur.

SUMMARY

- Reproduction is the process by which a living thing makes more living things like itself. Although in both men and women, the reproductive system produces the cells and hormones that are necessary to create a new life, the organs that make up the reproductive system are very different in men and women.
- The female reproductive system consists of internal structures (the ovaries, the fallopian tubes, the uterus, and the vagina), external structures (the labia, the clitoris, and the

vaginal opening, referred to collectively as the vulva), and the accessory organs (the breasts).
  - The female reproductive system is designed to produce eggs, receive sperm cells, contain and nourish a developing baby, give birth, and provide nourishment after the baby's birth by producing breast milk.
  - Each month during a woman's reproductive years (from puberty to menopause), her body prepares itself to become

pregnant. If pregnancy does not occur, the woman has a menstrual period and the cycle begins again.

- A woman's ovaries stop functioning when the woman is between 45 and 55 years of age. This causes the onset of menopause. After a woman goes through menopause, she no longer menstruates and is not able to become pregnant.
- Disorders that can affect a woman's reproductive system include cysts and non-cancerous growths, pelvic organ prolapse, and cancer.

● The male reproductive system consists of the testicles (testes), the epididymis, the vas deferens, and the penis. Accessory organs include the seminal vesicles and prostate gland, which play a role in producing semen (the fluid that carries sperm cells out of the body). Sperm cells leave the body through the urethra.

- The male reproductive system is designed to produce sperm and deposit it inside the female's body.
- After puberty, the male reproductive system produces sperm cells continuously. Sperm cells are produced in the testes and mature in the epididymis. From the epididymis, they pass through the vas deferens and urethra to reach the outside of the body. Before leaving the body, the sperm cells are mixed with secretions from the seminal vesicles and the prostate gland, forming semen.

- As they get older, many men find that the frequency and duration of their erections decreases. Many men also develop enlargement of the prostate gland.
- Disorders of the male reproductive system include impotence (erectile dysfunction), cancer, and infection.

● Sexually transmitted infections (STIs) are infections of the reproductive system that are commonly transmitted by sexual contact.

- Common STIs include herpes simplex, gonorrhea, chlamydia, genital (venereal) warts, syphilis, and AIDS. Although some STIs can be treated, there is no known cure for herpes simplex or AIDS.
- Anyone who engages in sexual activity can get an STI. Using condoms and avoiding sexual activity with infected partners can lower a person's risk of getting an STI.

WHAT DID YOU LEARN?

Multiple Choice

Select the single best answer for each of the following questions.

1. What occurs when a male sex cell joins the female sex cell, forming a cell that contains the complete number of chromosomes?
   a. Ovulation
   b. Menstruation
   c. Menopause
   d. Conception (fertilization)

2. Which one of the following is a sexually transmitted infection (STI)?
   a. Breast cancer
   b. Herpes simplex
   c. Hepatitis A
   d. Tuberculosis (TB)

3. Which sexually transmitted disease (STI) is caused by a bacterium and may cause a man to have a burning sensation during urination and a greenish discharge from the urethra?

   a. Gonorrhea
   b. Syphilis
   c. Pelvic inflammatory disease (PID)
   d. Acquired immunodeficiency syndrome (AIDS)

4. As you are providing perineal care for Mrs. Baxter, an 82-year-old resident, you notice a slight bulge in the area of her vulva and pink, smooth tissue protruding from her vagina. You know that this must be reported to the nurse, and is most likely:
   a. A cancerous tumor
   b. An enlarged prostate gland
   c. A fibroid
   d. A prolapsed uterus

Matching

Match each numbered item with its appropriate lettered description.

_____ **1.** Sperm

_____ **2.** Estrogen

_____ **3.** Cystocele

_____ **4.** Egg (ovum)

_____ **5.** Vaginitis

_____ **6.** Menopause

_____ **7.** Testosterone

_____ **8.** Rectocele

_____ **9.** Impotence (erectile dysfunction)

a. Male sex hormone

b. Condition that occurs when the front wall of the rectum shifts downward, pressing into the back wall of the vagina

c. Male sex cell

d. Inflammation of the vaginal tissues

e. Female sex hormone

f. The complete ending of a woman's menstrual cycles

g. Female sex cell

h. Condition that occurs when the bladder shifts downward, pressing into the front wall of the vagina

i. Inability to achieve an erection

STOP and Think!

- Mrs. Janofsky is one of the residents in the long-term care facility where you work. She is 78 years old and has been widowed for a number of years. Mrs. Janofsky has talked to you a number of times about a gentleman friend who she looks forward to seeing. He comes to the facility frequently to visit Mrs. Janofsky, and she often asks for privacy when he visits. Mrs. Janofsky's friend visited last evening. Today as you are helping Mrs. Janofsky with her bath, she tells you that her vaginal area is very sore. When you tell her that you will report this to the nurse, she grabs your hand and seems embarrassed. She tells you that she is sore because she had sex with her friend. She mentions that as much as she likes the intimacy, it is uncomfortable for her because she is so dry. She tells you that she hopes that you do not think badly about her for having that kind of relationship with her friend. How should you respond to Mrs. Janofsky?

Nursing Assistants Make a Difference!

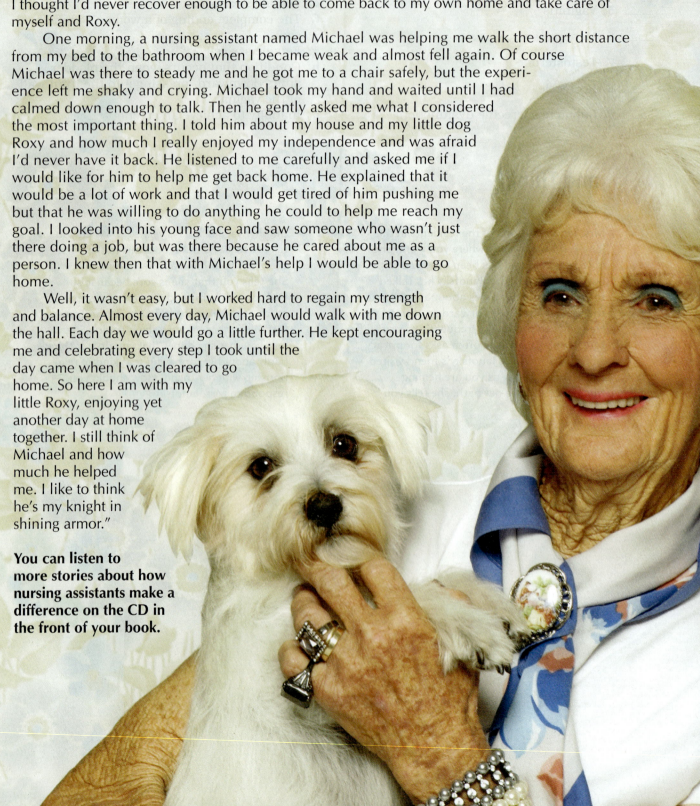

"Just look at me now, here with my little dog Roxy! A year ago, I would never have believed I'd be at home with Roxy again. You see it was about a year ago that I fell getting out of the bathtub and broke my right hip. I had surgery to repair the fracture, followed by several months of rehabilitation in a nursing facility. I'll tell you, my spirits were low the day they admitted me to the nursing facility. I thought I'd never recover enough to be able to come back to my own home and take care of myself and Roxy.

One morning, a nursing assistant named Michael was helping me walk the short distance from my bed to the bathroom when I became weak and almost fell again. Of course Michael was there to steady me and he got me to a chair safely, but the experience left me shaky and crying. Michael took my hand and waited until I had calmed down enough to talk. Then he gently asked me what I considered the most important thing. I told him about my house and my little dog Roxy and how much I really enjoyed my independence and was afraid I'd never have it back. He listened to me carefully and asked me if I would like for him to help me get back home. He explained that it would be a lot of work and that I would get tired of him pushing me but that he was willing to do anything he could to help me reach my goal. I looked into his young face and saw someone who wasn't just there doing a job, but was there because he cared about me as a person. I knew then that with Michael's help I would be able to go home.

Well, it wasn't easy, but I worked hard to regain my strength and balance. Almost every day, Michael would walk with me down the hall. Each day we would go a little further. He kept encouraging me and celebrating every step I took until the day came when I was cleared to go home. So here I am with my little Roxy, enjoying yet another day at home together. I still think of Michael and how much he helped me. I like to think he's my knight in shining armor."

You can listen to more stories about how nursing assistants make a difference on the CD in the front of your book.

SPECIAL CARE CONCERNS

As a nursing assistant working in long-term care, you may be involved with the care of residents who have developmental disabilities, mental illness, cancer, or HIV/AIDS. Along with the normal assistance needed for feeding, bathing, and toileting, these groups have other unique needs. The purpose of this unit is to introduce you to these groups and help you to recognize, and assist with meeting, their special needs.

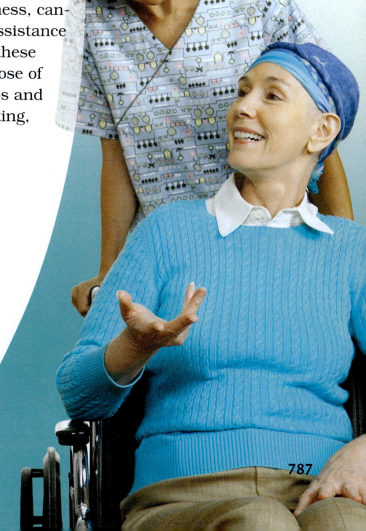

Photo: Some of your residents will have cancer.

As a nursing assistant working in long-term care, you may be involved with the care of residents who have developmental disabilities, mental illness, cancer, or HIV/AIDS. Along with the normal assistance needed for feeding, bathing, and toileting, these groups have other unique needs. The purpose of this unit is to introduce you to these groups and help you to recognize, and assist with meeting, their special needs.

Photo: Some of your residents will have special...

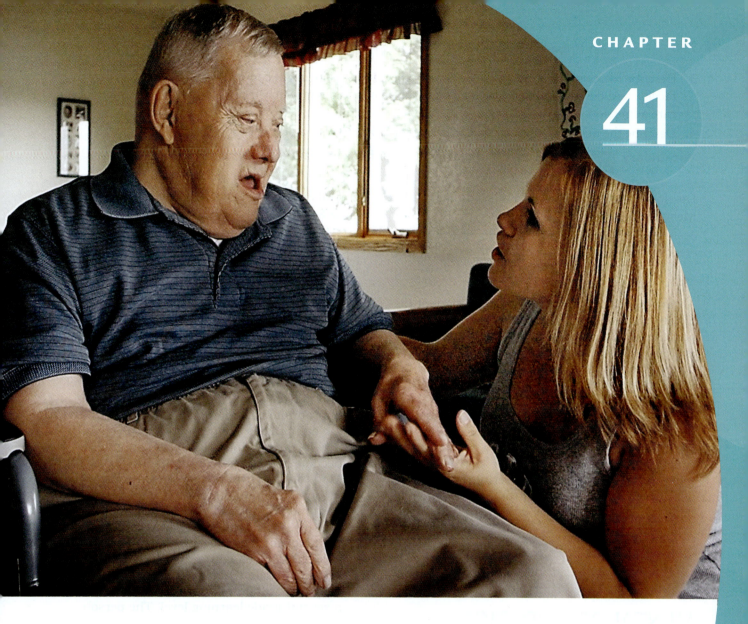

Caring for People With Developmental Disabilities

WHAT WILL YOU LEARN?

In this chapter, you will learn about caring for people with developmental disabilities. Permanent disabilities that affect a person before adulthood are called developmental disabilities because they interfere with normal physical or mental development. As a nursing assistant working in long-term care, you may have the opportunity to care for residents with developmental disabilities. When you are finished with this chapter, you will be able to:

1. Define the term *developmental disabilities* and discuss various causes.
2. List common developmental disabilities and describe characteristics of each one.

Photo: A resident with Down syndrome talks with a staff member. (AP Photo/Mankato Free Press, John Cross)

3. Describe reasons why a person with a developmental disability might come to live in a long-term care facility, and describe some of the challenges the person and family may face as a result of the long-term care admission.

4. Describe the nursing assistant's role in caring for a person with a developmental disability.

Vocabulary Use the CD in the front of your book to hear these terms pronounced and defined:

Developmental disability	Down syndrome	Cerebral palsy	Fetal alcohol syndrome
Mental retardation	Autism	Fragile X syndrome	Spina bifida

A **developmental disability** is a permanent disability that affects a person before he reaches adulthood (that is, before 19 to 22 years of age) and interferes with the person's ability to achieve developmental milestones. A developmental disability may be *congenital* (something a child is born with) or *acquired* (occurring after birth, as a result of trauma or illness). Common causes of developmental disabilities are shown in Box 41-1. A developmental disability may affect mental function, physical function, or both. Developmental disabilities vary in severity. Some people with developmental disabilities are very independent, while others require total care.

TYPES OF DEVELOPMENTAL DISABILITIES

MENTAL RETARDATION

A person with **mental retardation** has below-average intellectual functioning and problems with adaptive skills. *Intellectual functioning* is the ability to reason, think, and understand. One way intellectual functioning is measured is through an intelligence quotient (IQ) test. A person with mental retardation has an IQ score of less than 70 points (about 20 to 30 points below average). *Adaptive skills* are skills needed to live and work such as communication skills, social skills, and self-care skills. A person with mental retardation has limited adaptive skills in two or more areas.

Mental retardation can be caused by abnormalities in the brain that are present at birth. It can also be caused by problems that interfere with oxygen getting to the brain before, during, or after birth. The severity of mental retardation, like that of other disabilities, varies:

- **Mild mental retardation.** Most people with mental retardation fall into this category.

Mild mental retardation may go unnoticed until a child begins school and starts having trouble with reading or solving math problems. With special education, a person with mild mental retardation is usually able to achieve a third- to sixth-grade learning level and master the skills needed for socially appropriate behavior. Vocational (job) training can provide the person with the opportunity to earn an income, allowing him to become less dependent on others (Fig. 41-1).

- **Moderate mental retardation.** People with moderate mental retardation have delays in both motor (manual) skills and speech development. With special education, a person with moderate mental retardation is usually able to learn self-care skills, communication skills, and safety habits. However, academically, she will probably not progress beyond a second-grade learning level. The person

---

BOX 41-1 **Common Causes of Developmental Disabilities**

Congenital (present at birth)
Genetic (inherited) disorders
Consumption of alcohol, drugs, or other toxic substances during pregnancy
Infections during pregnancy, such as German measles (rubella) or human immunodeficiency virus (HIV)
Poor nutrition during pregnancy
Conditions that deprive the baby of oxygen

Acquired (occurring after birth)
Birth trauma
Head injury
Near drowning
Poisoning

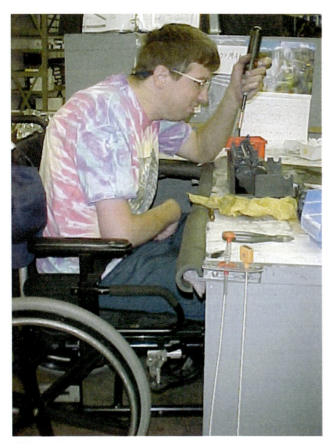

Figure 41-1
Vocational training helps to prepare people with disabilities for the work force. (*Courtesy of the Wood County Board of Mental Retardation and Developmental Disabilities, Bowling Green, OH.*)

may also have trouble learning socially appropriate behavior.

- **Severe mental retardation.** With special education, people with severe mental retardation are able to learn some communication and basic self-care skills. A person with severe mental retardation can usually learn to walk, if he does not have other physical disabilities.
- **Profound mental retardation**. *Profound* means "deep." People with profound mental retardation have minimal function in all developmental areas, physical and mental. These people need complete assistance with their activities of daily living (ADLs), and constant supervision to provide for their safety.

One of the great rewards that you will experience as a nursing assistant is the satisfaction of helping a person with mental retardation to feel loved, and allowing him to express love back to you (Fig. 41-2). Many people with mental retar-

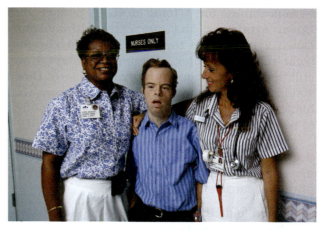

Figure 41-2
One of the great rewards that you will have as a nursing assistant is the satisfaction of helping a person with mental retardation to feel loved, and allowing him to express love back to you.

dation need guidance with "appropriate" methods of displaying their love and affection to other people. In the same manner that a child learns that hugging a kitty too hard may lead to being scratched, people with mental retardation may need gentle reminders that a hug may sometimes be too tight and that not everyone appreciates physical affection.

Adults with mental retardation may function mentally at the level of a 7- or 8-year-old, with child-like curiosity and innocence. However, they are adults and will experience the same hormonal changes and sexual drives as everyone else. Because the person may not understand what is happening, these physical drives may be very confusing. Education and guidance from caregivers is very important to help a person with mental retardation learn about appropriate touch and sexual behavior. In addition, caregivers must protect the person from sexual abuse. Because people with mental retardation tend to be very trusting, and because they are not able to understand what is happening to them, they are often targets of sexual abuse. As a nursing assistant, you must be especially observant for signs of sexual abuse when caring for a person with mental retardation. Any observations you make or suspicions that you have should be reported to the nurse immediately.

DOWN SYNDROME

Down syndrome is a developmental disability that is the result of a genetic disorder. Normally, each of our body's cells contains 23 pairs of chromosomes, for a total of 46. A person with Down syndrome has one extra chromosome. Down syndrome is the most common chromosome-related disorder, affecting 1 in every 1,000 children born. Although the exact cause of Down syndrome is unknown, studies have shown that babies with Down syndrome are born more often to women who have children later in life.

People with Down syndrome have some degree of mental retardation and muscle weakness. In addition, they have certain characteristic physical features (Fig. 41-3):

- Eyelid folds that give the eyes an almond-shaped appearance
- A large tongue in a small mouth
- Square hands with short fingers
- A small, wide nose and small ears
- Short stature and a wide, short neck

Many people with Down syndrome are also born with heart defects that require corrective surgery or medication. Frequent respiratory tract infections are also common among people with Down syndrome, due to muscle weakness (which affects the muscles used for breathing) and a compromised immune system. Adults with Down syndrome are at increased risk for thyroid disorders, heart valve disease, joint problems, pain, and seizures. They may experience age-related vision and hearing loss at an earlier age, and they are at very high risk for developing Alzheimer's disease.

More than 50% of people with Down syndrome who are older than 50 years have Alzheimer's disease. The onset of Alzheimer's disease occurs much earlier than usual in a person with Down syndrome, when the person is in her 40s or possibly even late 30s. In its early stages, Alzheimer's disease may be more difficult to recognize in a person with Down syndrome, because of limitations in mental functioning that the person may already have as a result of the Down syndrome. If you notice a change in the abilities of a resident with Down syndrome, even a slight change, it is important for you to report this change to the nurse.

AUTISM

A person with **autism** has extreme difficulty communicating and relating to other people and surroundings. Although the specific cause of autism is unknown, experts suspect a genetic link. Like Down syndrome, autism affects about 1 in every 1,000 children born. Boys are affected more often than girls are.

Autism affects a person's reasoning skills, language skills, ability to socialize, ability to perform self-care activities, and response to touch and pain. A person with autism may seem very withdrawn, like he is in his "own world" (*auto*- means "self"). The person may have lengthy or extreme tantrums, or show aggressive or violent behavior that can result in self-injury. Other disorders, such as mental retardation and seizure disorders, may accompany autism. However, many people with autism have average or above-average intelligence. Therapy focusing on communication and social skills can be very useful for a person with autism.

CEREBRAL PALSY

Cerebral palsy is caused by damage to the cerebrum, the part of the brain involved with motor control. Cerebral palsy has many possible causes, including physical brain deformity and conditions that interfere with the flow of oxygen to the baby's brain before, during, or shortly after birth. Babies who are born prematurely or have a low birth

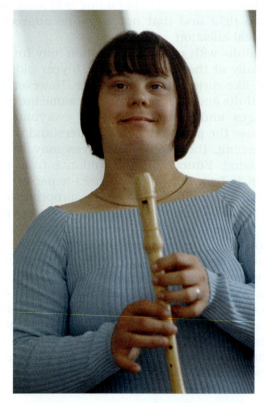

Figure 41-3
Certain physical characteristics are typical of Down syndrome, such as almond-shaped eyes; a wide, short neck; and square hands with short fingers. (© *Tim Garcha/ zefa/Corbis*)

weight are at higher risk for cerebral palsy. Accidents in early childhood can also cause cerebral palsy. For example, head trauma that causes swelling or bleeding in the brain and events that interfere with the flow of oxygen to the brain (such as choking, near drowning, or poisoning) can all cause this disability. The degree of disability depends on the extent of the damage to the brain.

The cerebrum plays a role in motor activity. This is why cerebral palsy typically affects the person's ability to voluntarily move parts of his body (Fig. 41-4). Body movements may be affected in different ways, leading to different types of cerebral palsy:

- **Spastic cerebral palsy**. The muscles are stiff and tight, and the reflexes are exaggerated.
- **Athetoid cerebral palsy.** The person experiences involuntary, slow, writhing movements of the affected parts of the body. The hands, arm, feet, and legs are affected most often. The muscles of the face and tongue may also be affected.
- **Ataxic cerebral palsy.** The person has difficulty coordinating movement. Some people experience problems because of decreased muscle tone, leading to muscle "floppiness."

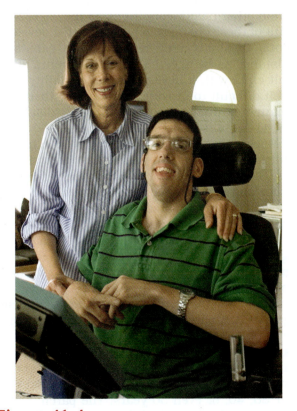

Figure 41-4
Cerebral palsy affects a person's motor function.
(*AP Photo/Steve Nesius*)

- **Mixed cerebral palsy.** A person may have more than one type of cerebral palsy. Most people with mixed cerebral palsy have both the spastic and the athetoid types.

If the muscles affected by the cerebral palsy are in the hands and arms, the person may be unable to perform self-care skills such as feeding, bathing, or dressing. If the muscles of the feet and legs are affected, the person may have difficulty walking, or be unable to walk. Varying degrees of mental retardation may also accompany the physical disabilities associated with cerebral palsy.

Cerebral palsy is not a progressive disorder (in other words, it does not get worse with time.) However, as a person with cerebral palsy ages, the effects of aging combined with the cerebral palsy can cause additional problems. For example, as the person ages, he may experience muscle and joint pain and problems with swallowing and bowel and bladder function. The person may have more difficulty breathing, and as a result, speaking may become more difficult as well.

FRAGILE X SYNDROME

Fragile X syndrome is an inherited type of mental retardation caused by a defect in the X chromosome. Fragile X syndrome is more common and usually more severe in boys, as compared with girls. People who have fragile X syndrome are usually moderately to severely mentally retarded and may have physical characteristics such as large, cupped ears; a slim build; wide-set, somewhat squinting eyes; and velvet-like skin. They usually have delayed speech and communication skills. They may be hyperactive, and prone to "mood swings." Autism may also accompany fragile X syndrome. As they age, people with fragile X syndrome are noted to have increased musculoskeletal problems, including an earlier onset of osteoporosis.

Treatments for this condition focus on minimizing symptoms and include physical therapy for motor control and speech therapy to improve language skills. Behavioral therapy and medication have been found to be helpful in managing mood, behavior, and sleep disturbances.

FETAL ALCOHOL SYNDROME

Fetal alcohol syndrome is a combination of physical and mental problems that affect a child whose mother consumed alcohol during pregnancy. The degree of disability seems to depend on the amount of alcohol the mother drank during her pregnancy, as well as on how frequently she drank. Babies born with fetal alcohol syndrome are usually smaller than normal and have mental retardation, behavioral problems, learning difficulties, and facial deformities. Although the disabilities caused by fetal alcohol syndrome are permanent, special education and therapy can help to maximize the person's abilities.

SPINA BIFIDA

Spina bifida is a congenital defect of the spinal column. Normally, the vertebrae enclose the spinal cord, protecting it from harm. In a person with spina bifida, the vertebrae do not close properly during development, leaving the spinal cord exposed. As with other developmental disabilities, spina bifida varies in severity. Some people with spina bifida have only a slight bone deformity that is not visible on the outside of the body, except for possibly a dimple or tuft of hair on the back. Other people have more severe deformities that result in the meninges, the spinal cord, or both bulging through a large opening on the back. The person may just have weakness in the legs, or she may be totally paralyzed below the waist. Problems with bowel and bladder control are common. Sometimes people with spina bifida also have mental retardation.

FACTORS LEADING TO LONG-TERM CARE ADMISSIONS

People with developmental disabilities become residents of long-term care facilities for many reasons. A person with a developmental disability may become a resident of a long-term care facility because her disabilities are simply too difficult or too numerous for the family to manage at home. Or, a move to a long-term care facility may become necessary because the person's parents or other caregivers die or become too frail to physically care for her.

Today, because of improvements in medical care and nutrition, people who have developmental disabilities are living much longer than they used to. People with developmental disabil-

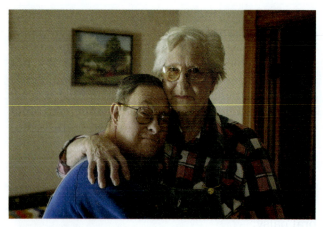

Figure 41-5
Parents of an adult child with a developmental disability face new challenges as they and their child age. Care becomes more difficult as the parents age, and many worry about how their child will be cared for after their own deaths. (*AP Photo/Lawrence Journal-World, Bill Snead.*)

ities experience the same changes that occur as a result of aging as everyone else. However, they usually experience these changes earlier, in middle age. In addition, many people with developmental disabilities are at risk for developing certain other health conditions as they age. As a result of these changes, a person with a developmental disability may require more care and assistance as he ages. The aging parents of an adult child with a developmental disability may find it difficult to provide that care for their son or daughter, due to their own frailty or disability (Fig. 41-5).

Moving to a long-term care facility can be difficult for the person, as well as his family members. Having to leave home—where the person felt comfortable and safe—and move into a long-term care facility can be incredibly traumatic for a person with a developmental disability, just as it can be for any other resident. The person may feel angry, deserted, or alone, and will need your compassion and understanding to help become comfortable in his new surroundings.

Family members may have difficulty adjusting as well. A parent may have difficulty trusting the care of his or her child to someone else. In many cases, the parent has been the child's primary caregiver for the child's entire life. You can imagine how hard it would be to give up that role after 30, 40, or even 50 years! The parents may worry about how to afford their own care, as well as that of their child. In addition, they may worry about paying for the continued care that their child will need after their death.

CARING FOR A PERSON WITH A DEVELOPMENTAL DISABILITY

The degree to which a person is disabled varies greatly from person to person. Some physical disabilities are very mild and may only cause minor muscle weakness and coordination problems. Others are more severe and may leave the person without any control over her muscles at all. The severity of mental disabilities also varies from person to person.

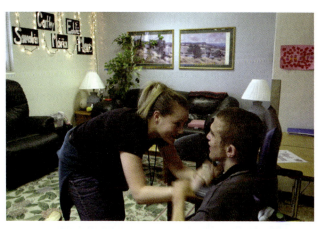

Figure 41-6
Good communication skills are especially important when working with people with developmental disabilities. (*Sacramento Bee/Jose Luis Villegas.*)

Helping Hands and a Caring Heart

FOCUS ON HUMANISTIC HEALTH CARE

When working with a person who has a developmental disability, the care that you provide must be specific to the person's abilities and disabilities. Learn as much as you can about each person in your care. Focusing on each person's abilities, whether developmentally disabled or not, will help you to provide the standard of care that each of your residents needs from you.

COMMUNICATING WITH A PERSON WITH A DEVELOPMENTAL DISABILITY

Many people with developmental disabilities have difficulty communicating with other people. Some are unable to speak or to learn language skills due to a lack of motor skills, mental capabilities, or both. Vision or hearing problems can also make communication difficult. However, many people with developmental disabilities find other ways of communicating. For example, they may rely heavily on non-verbal communication techniques, such as facial expressions, nods, and body language. When caring for a person with a developmental disability:

- Ask family members what communication techniques work best with the person.

Family members are often glad to share with you what they have learned about which communication methods work best.
- If the person has a mental disability, use simple words and short phrases. This allows the person to comprehend ideas or tasks, one at a time.
- Perhaps the most useful communication method is that of a touch, a smile, or a kind word, all of which transmit the message of your care and compassion for the person (Fig. 41-6).

Because many people with severe developmental disabilities have difficulty communicating, they may be unable to tell you if they are experiencing pain or discomfort. Learn to watch for small, subtle changes in your residents, such as changes in behavior, eating habits, or sleeping habits. Changes like these may be a sign that the person is ill. Because you will most likely be the member of the health care team who spends the most time with the person, you will likely be the first to notice that "something is not quite right." Always be sure to report your observations to the nurse.

TELL THE NURSE

A person with a developmental disability may not be able to tell you when something is wrong. Use your observation skills and be sure to report any of the following to the nurse immediately:

- There is a change in the person's vital signs, especially body temperature or pulse rhythm
- There is a change in the person's appetite

- There is a change in the person's level of activity
- There is a change in the person's physical abilities (for example, a person who usually has no trouble walking starts having falls)
- There is a change in the person's level of mental functioning (for example, the person seems confused or disoriented)
- There is a change in the person's behavior (for example, a normally gentle person becomes aggressive)
- The person complains of pain or discomfort
- The person's skin is red or swollen in areas
- The person shows signs of physical or mental abuse

MEETING THE PHYSICAL NEEDS OF A PERSON WITH A DEVELOPMENTAL DISABILITY

A person with a developmental disability has the same physical needs as everyone else. Because of the person's disability, however, he may need some help in meeting those needs. As always, you will need to consider the specific needs of each person. Nursing assistants often are involved with assisting people with disabilities with their ADLs, and with activities related to rehabilitation.

Assisting the Person With Activities of Daily Living (ADLs)

Depending on the severity and type of disability, the person may need varying levels of assistance with ADLs. Some types of disability, such as cerebral palsy, can cause muscle weakness on one or both sides of the body, making dressing and grooming difficult. The short fingers of a person with Down syndrome may make it hard for the person to manage buttons or zippers on clothing. Assistive devices, which you learned about in Chapter 10, allow many people with physical disabilities to manage their ADLs independently or with minimal assistance. A person with mental disabilities may simply need supervision and reminders (for example, about which step comes next) to complete his ADLs. As with all of your residents, helping the person achieve the greatest possible level of independence is the best type of assistance that you can give.

Assisting With Rehabilitation

A person with developmental disabilities may require rehabilitation to help maintain function and ensure the best quality of life. For example, a person who has physical limitations may need physical therapy to keep the affected parts of her body functional, or to reduce pain. A person who has difficulty swallowing may benefit from the services of a speech therapist. As a nursing assistant, you will play a very important role in supporting the rehabilitation effort, and helping the person to maintain or improve function.

MEETING THE EMOTIONAL AND SOCIAL NEEDS OF A PERSON WITH A DEVELOPMENTAL DISABILITY

Reassurance, love, and acceptance are vital for everyone's well-being, and especially for those with disabilities that can make them appear or feel "different." Similarly, all people have the need to interact with other people and participate in activities that they find enjoyable. When planning activities for a resident with developmental disabilities, it is important to take into consideration the person's skills, abilities, and interests.

SUMMARY

- Permanent disabilities that affect a person before she becomes an adult are called *developmental disabilities* because they interfere with that person's normal physical or mental development.
  - Developmental disabilities can be due to congenital abnormalities, traumatic injury, infection, disease, deprivation of oxygen or nutrition, or the result of poisoning or drug use.
  - Developmental disabilities can affect a person physically or mentally.
- There are many different types of developmental disabilities. The degree to which a

person's abilities are affected varies considerably, even among people who have the same type of disability.

- Mental retardation affects a person's general intellectual functioning. A person with mental retardation has an IQ score of less than 70 and limited adaptive skills in two or more areas.
- Down syndrome is a developmental disability that is the result of an extra chromosome. People with Down syndrome have some degree of mental retardation, as well as certain physical characteristics. A person with Down syndrome is at very high risk for developing Alzheimer's disease by middle age, as well as other health conditions.
- Autism is a congenital disorder. People with autism have extreme difficulty communicating with and relating to other people and their surroundings.
- Cerebral palsy affects the motor region of the brain (the cerebrum). A person with cerebral palsy has difficulty with movement. Some people with cerebral palsy also have some degree of mental retardation.
- Fragile X syndrome is an inherited type of mental retardation that is more common in boys.
- Fetal alcohol syndrome is a combination of physical and mental abnormalities that affect a child whose mother consumed alcohol during pregnancy.
  - Spina bifida is a defect of the spinal column that can cause paralysis of the lower extremities.
- New challenges for care arise as a person with a developmental disability grows into middle age. Admission to a long-term care facility may be necessary if the person's parents die, or become too frail themselves to provide care.
- Nursing assistants may care for people with developmental disabilities in the long-term care setting.
  - Because people with developmental disabilities may have trouble communicating with others, nursing assistants often must rely on their observation skills to tell when something is wrong.
  - Nursing assistants often must provide some or complete assistance with activities of daily living (ADLs). However, many people with developmental disabilities are able to manage their ADLs quite independently by using assistive devices.
  - Nursing assistants are often very involved in assisting people with developmental disabilities with tasks related to rehabilitation.
  - Nursing assistants play a very important role in helping people with developmental disabilities to meet their emotional and social needs.

WHAT DID YOU LEARN?

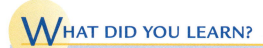

Multiple Choice

Select the single best answer for each of the following questions.

1. Which one of the following statements about mental retardation is correct?
   a. It affects the motor region of the brain
   b. It can occur before, during, or after birth
   c. It is always severe
   d. None of the above

2. What physical characteristics does a person with Down syndrome have?
   a. Large, cupped ears; a slim build; wide-set, somewhat squinting eyes; and velvet-like skin
   b. Almond-shaped eyes, square hands with short fingers, large tongue in a small mouth

   c. A large head
   d. Facial deformities and small stature

3. What do researchers think is a cause of autism?
   a. Genetics
   b. Oxygen deprivation at birth
   c. Drugs
   d. Trauma at birth

4. Cerebral palsy can be caused by:
   a. Infection during pregnancy
   b. A lack of oxygen to the brain
   c. An extra chromosome
   d. Alcohol intake during pregnancy

5. A person with autism may have:
   a. An extra chromosome
   b. Hearing and vision problems
   c. Problems relating to others socially
   d. Muscle weakness
6. A person with Down syndrome always has some degree of:
   a. Mental retardation
   b. Spastic movements
   c. Cerebral palsy
   d. Autism
7. Which one of the following statements about fetal alcohol syndrome is correct?
   a. It occurs when a woman smokes during pregnancy
   b. A newborn with fetal alcohol syndrome is larger than normal
   c. It occurs when a woman drinks alcohol during pregnancy
   d. It is caused by oxygen deprivation at birth

8. What is spina bifida?
   a. A seizure disorder
   b. A defect of the spinal column
   c. A shunt
   d. Another name for fragile X syndrome
9. What is common in a person with spina bifida?
   a. Autism
   b. Bowel and bladder incontinence
   c. Drooling
   d. Seizures
10. Which developmental disability is associated with a high risk for the development of Alzheimer's disease?
    a. Autism
    b. Cerebral palsy
    c. Down syndrome
    d. Fragile X

STOP and Think!

- Today a new resident has been admitted to the long-term care facility where you work. Mr. Theodore has severe cerebral palsy. He is an only child. His parents, who are in their 80s, are experiencing health problems of their own and are no longer able to provide the physical care that Mr. Theodore needs. Mr. Theodore is very upset. He is crying, and he keeps asking why his family doesn't want him anymore. What can you do in the coming days and weeks to help Mr. Theodore make the adjustment to his new home?

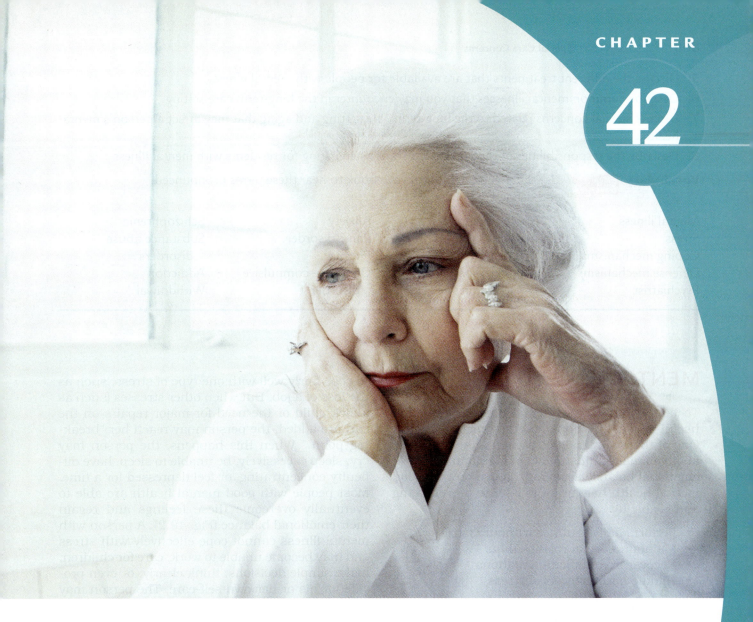

Caring for People With Mental Illness

WHAT WILL YOU LEARN?

A **mental illness** is a disorder that affects a person's mind, causing the person to experience emotional difficulties, to act in unusual ways, or both. (*Mental* means "mind.") A mental illness affects the way a person thinks. As a result, it changes the way the person sees herself, her relationships, and the world in general. As a nursing assistant, you will care for residents with mental illness. There are many different types of mental illness, and mental illness varies in severity from person to person. When you are finished with this chapter, you will be able to:

1. Define the term *mental illness*.
2. Describe some of the qualities that define good mental health.
3. Discuss methods that people use to cope with stress effectively.
4. List possible causes of mental illness.

Photo: Mental illnesses are disorders that affect the mind and emotions.

5. Discuss the different treatments that are available for people with mental illness.

6. Describe common mental illnesses that you may encounter in the long-term care setting.

7. Discuss special concerns related to the long-term care setting and aging that may affect a person's mental health.

8. Describe the responsibilities of the nursing assistant when caring for residents with mental illness.

Vocabulary Use the CD in the front of your book to hear these terms pronounced and defined:

Mental illness	Psychologist	Anxiety	Schizophrenia
Stress	Suicide	Panic disorder	Substance abuse
Coping mechanisms	Depression	Phobia	disorders
Defense mechanisms	Bipolar disorder (manic	Obsessive-compulsive	Addiction
Psychiatrist	depression)	disorder	Withdrawal

MENTAL HEALTH

To better understand mental illness, it is often useful to start by understanding mental health. One of the main qualities of mental health is the ability to make adjustments to maintain a state of emotional balance. Generally, a person with good mental health has an overall sense of well-being and is able to:

- Perform daily routines without distress
- Maintain normal relationships
- Recover from difficult situations
- Handle normal levels of stress

Stress, which results from any change in normal routine, affects a person's ability to maintain a state of balance. Changes that affect us physically, such as illness or disability, cause physical stress. Life events, such as getting married, getting divorced, starting a new job, having a baby, or losing a loved one, cause a great deal of mental stress. For most of us, stress is a constant in our lives. Even day-to-day activities, such as reading the newspaper, raising children, or performing our jobs, are sources of stress (Fig. 42-1). Stress that is not managed properly can affect a person's physical health, as well as his mental health. For example, not being able to manage stress can put a person at risk for cardiovascular problems, such as a heart attack, or digestive disorders, such as ulcers.

Each person has a limit to the amount of stress that she can effectively deal with at any given time. Fatigue, illness, and everyday stress sometimes affect our ability to cope well with change. Many times, stress does not come from a single source. For example, a person may be able to cope fairly well with one type of stress, such as the loss of a job. But when other stresses (such as a sick child or the need for major repairs on the car) are added, the person may reach her "breaking point." When this happens, the person may cry, sleep excessively, be unable to sleep, have difficulty concentrating, or feel depressed for a time. Most people with good mental health are able to eventually overcome these feelings and regain their emotional balance (Fig. 42-2). A person with mental illness cannot cope effectively with stress and may become unable to work, care for children, make simple decisions, think clearly, or even provide for his or her own self-care. The person may

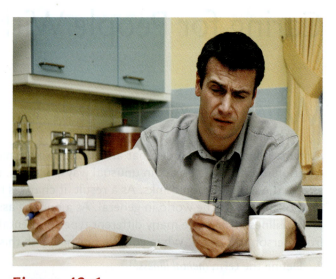

Figure 42-1

Stress is a constant in most people's lives. Money problems, work, family, and world events are common sources of stress.

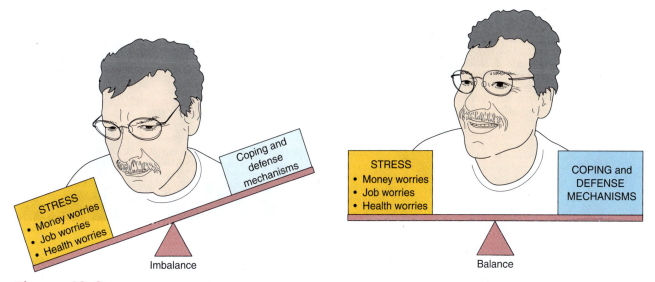

Figure 42-2
A person who is mentally healthy is able to maintain a state of emotional balance on most days. Stress can drag us down, causing the scale to tip out of balance, but a person who is mentally healthy is able to adjust to the stress and return to a state of emotional balance.

need medication, counseling, or support groups to help regain emotional balance.

COPING MECHANISMS

What do you do when you start to feel overwhelmed or "stressed out"? Maybe you exercise, practice a hobby, get together with friends, meditate or pray, or just find a quiet place to relax (Fig. 42-3). Over time, many people come to know what they can do to make themselves feel better when they start to feel overwhelmed by life's pressures. These conscious and deliberate ways of dealing with stress are called **coping mechanisms.**

Many people rely on positive coping mechanisms, such as exercise, prayer and meditation, getting together with friends, or engaging in a hobby. Other people rely on less effective coping mechanisms. These people seek short-term relief through behaviors such as nail biting, pacing, overeating or not eating enough, smoking, or abusing drugs or alcohol (Fig. 42-4). Initially, these behaviors may help the person to reduce stress. But over time, they place the person at risk for serious physical problems, mental problems, or both.

DEFENSE MECHANISMS

Defense mechanisms are methods of dealing with stress that "just happen." Usually the person is not even aware that he is using them. Defense mechanisms help to protect us from emotionally traumatic events. The behaviors associated with defense mechanisms occur when the mind attempts to restore or maintain emotional balance in response to stress. Common defense mechanisms include the following.

- **Compensation** means to make up for a loss by "filling in" or "substituting" something else. For example, a person who feels lonely may eat too much. This person is substituting food for affection.
- **Conversion** means "to change." For example, a person who is depressed (an emotional problem) may develop a stomach ache (a physical problem), and then use the physical problem as a reason to avoid participating in an activity.
- **Denial** is refusing to believe something that is true, especially if the truth is unpleasant. For example, a person who has been diagnosed with cancer may truly believe that the doctor has made the wrong diagnosis, and that she does not have cancer.
- **Displacement** is shifting an emotion from one person to another who is less threatening. For example, a resident who is angry with her daughter for moving her to a long-term care facility—and who is afraid of expressing this anger because she fears the daughter will abandon her—may take her anger out on the nursing assistant instead.
- **Projection** is blaming someone else for your own uncomfortable or unacceptable actions

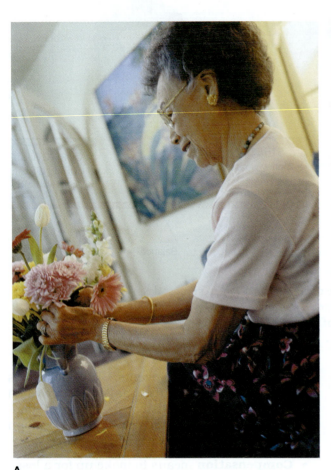

A

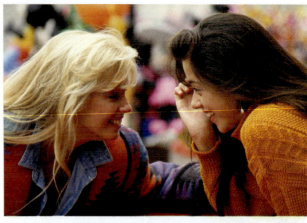

B

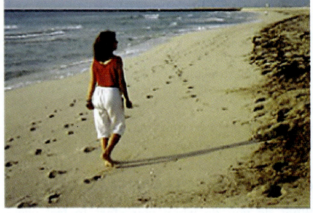

C

Figure 42-3
Our physical and mental health depends on our ability to manage everyday stress. Enjoying a hobby **(A),** laughing with friends **(B),** and taking a long walk **(C)** are just some of many positive approaches people take to relieve stress! (**B,** © *Christopher Briscoe/Photo Researchers, Inc.;* **C,** © *Jeff Greenberg/Photo Researchers, Inc.*)

or feelings. For example, a resident may accuse a nursing assistant of breaking a vase when in fact, the resident actually broke the treasured vase herself.

- **Rationalization** is making excuses or creating acceptable reasons for poor behaviors or actions. For instance, a student who does not study for a test and then fails it may tell herself that the reason she failed is because the teacher is "too hard."
- **Regression** means to turn back to a former or earlier state. For example, many older children who experience stress as a result of being hospitalized begin demonstrating behaviors from when they were younger, such as thumb-sucking or bedwetting.
- **Repression (suppression)** is the refusal to remember or think about a frightening or

painful memory. A person may repress memories of an automobile accident or childhood abuse.

CAUSES AND TREATMENT OF MENTAL ILLNESS

There are many different types of mental illness, and many different causes. Some types of mental illness run in families (that is, they are inherited). Others result from chemical imbalances in the brain. In Chapter 35, you learned about chemicals called *neurotransmitters.* An imbalance in these chemicals can lead to some forms of mental illness. Mental illness can also be caused by injury to the brain. Finally, some mental illnesses

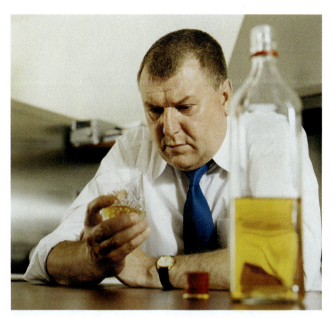

Figure 42-4
Many people drink alcohol excessively, use illegal ("street") drugs, or abuse legally prescribed drugs to deal with stress. This is called substance abuse. Although substance abuse may provide short-term relief from the pressures of daily life, in the long run it is not an effective coping mechanism.

may be caused by a person's environment. For example, a person who is abused by a family member may develop ineffective coping or defense mechanisms that lead to mental illness.

Fortunately, many mental illnesses, just like many physical illnesses, can be successfully managed with medications, psychiatric counseling, or both. The word *psychiatric* comes from the Greek words *psyche* (the soul) and *iatreia* (healing). A **psychiatrist** is a medical doctor trained in diagnosing and treating mental illness. A psychiatrist is allowed to prescribe medications. A **psychologist,** while not a medical doctor, has education and training that allows him to provide counseling services to help people with mental illness. A psychologist is not allowed to prescribe medications. Depending on the person's situation, he may need the services of a psychiatrist, a psychologist, or both. With treatment, many people with mental illnesses are able to lead happy, productive lives. Because many people with mental illnesses are at risk for committing **suicide** (taking their own lives, intentionally and voluntarily), diagnosis and treatment of mental illness is very important.

Treatment for mental illness has changed dramatically over the last 50 years. In the past, people with mental illnesses were usually sent to special hospitals ("mental institutions"), where

they were given large doses of medications to keep them quiet and sedated. Techniques such as electroconvulsive therapy (ECT) (the delivery of an electrical shock to the person's brain through electrodes applied to the scalp) and lobotomy (surgical removal of part of the brain) were used frequently, often with little success. Now, we know more about why mental illnesses occur and how they should be treated. For example, now that we know that moods and behaviors can be affected by chemical imbalances, we have developed new medications that help to restore the brain's chemical balance. Rather than simply sedating the person into submission, these new medications help the person to act and think more "normally." And, while ECT is still used in the treatment of certain mental disorders, improvements in technique have made the procedure much safer and much more effective.

TYPES OF MENTAL ILLNESS

In the sections that follow, we will review some of the more common mental illnesses, and special considerations you should be aware of when caring for residents with these disorders. When caring for residents with mental illnesses, be aware that two residents, both with the same diagnosis, may have very different symptoms and very different methods of coping with their illness. Do not make the mistake of assuming that every resident with the same diagnosis will behave in the same way. Also, as you care for residents with mental illnesses, make an effort to learn more about their conditions. The information in this book provides good basic information, but there is so much more to learn! Increasing your knowledge about your residents' specific conditions allows you to better understand and care for them.

MOOD DISORDERS

Mood disorders affect how a person feels emotionally. Depression and bipolar disorder (manic depression) are two very common types of mood disorders.

Depression

Depression is a disorder characterized by a persistent "low" mood and decreased pleasure. A person with depression may experience:

- Feelings of sadness, anxiety, or "emptiness" that do not go away

- Feelings of guilt, hopelessness, worthlessness, or helplessness
- A loss of interest in, or enjoyment of, usual activities
- Decreased motivation or energy and increased fatigue
- Difficulty concentrating or making decisions
- Difficulty remembering things
- Irritability, anger, or restlessness
- Changes in eating or sleeping habits
- Physical complaints, such as pain or digestive disorders

The incidence of depression increases with age (Fig. 42-5). Many medications, or combinations of medications, can cause depression as a side effect. Hormonal changes, such as menopause, can also be a contributing factor. Finally, some of the unique losses and challenges that an elderly person faces may overwhelm the person emotionally and promote depression (Fig. 42-6). For example:

- Elderly people face the loss of spouses, friends, and others close to them. Often, these losses occur within a short period of time, allowing no time for the person to complete the grieving process for one loss before experiencing another.
- Elderly people face the loss of physical abilities and independence, either as a result of illness or the normal processes of aging. As a result, many elderly people feel

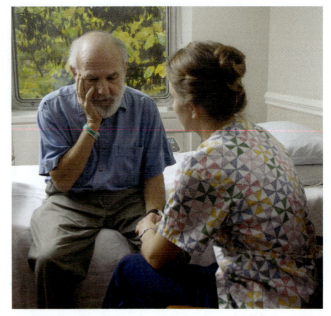

Figure 42-5
Depression is common among older people. If you think that one of your residents is depressed, you should report your suspicions to the nurse.

that they have become a burden to their families.
- Elderly people may have experiences that damage their self-confidence and self-esteem (such as falls, the onset of incontinence, or the need to give up a driver's license).

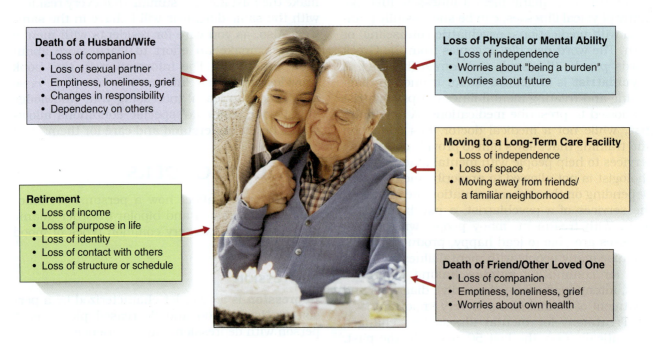

Death of a Husband/Wife
- Loss of companion
- Loss of sexual partner
- Emptiness, loneliness, grief
- Changes in responsibility
- Dependency on others

Loss of Physical or Mental Ability
- Loss of independence
- Worries about "being a burden"
- Worries about future

Moving to a Long-Term Care Facility
- Loss of independence
- Loss of space
- Moving away from friends/ a familiar neighborhood

Retirement
- Loss of income
- Loss of purpose in life
- Loss of identity
- Loss of contact with others
- Loss of structure or schedule

Death of Friend/Other Loved One
- Loss of companion
- Emptiness, loneliness, grief
- Worries about own health

Figure 42-6
As we age, we face very challenging life events. These additional stresses can put an elderly person at risk for clinical depression and other mental illnesses.

- Admission to a long-term care facility is associated with many losses and challenges. The person must give up his home, and possibly many treasured belongings as well. The person must adjust to having less privacy and less control over all aspects of her life. Separation from family and friends can be difficult.
- Retirement can also pose challenges. Although many people view retiring from a job as an event to be celebrated, some people miss the structure, routine, and sense of identity that their jobs gave them. Retirement also means that a person's income becomes fixed, which can lead to money worries.

These factors can easily lead to feelings of helplessness, worthlessness, and hopelessness. The person's self-esteem is lowered. As a nursing assistant working in a long-term care facility, you can play an important role in helping your residents to handle these life challenges and regain or maintain their sense of self-esteem. Being *present* for each resident you care for goes a long way in helping the person feel understood, valued, respected, and cared for. Meeting the person's love and belonging needs is critical for helping to maintain (or improve) the person's mental health.

Because depression is common among older people, many people assume that depression is "just a part of growing old." However, this is not the case. Depression is not a normal part of aging! When caring for your older residents, pay attention to changes in their behaviors or moods that may indicate depression. By reporting these observations to the nurse, you play a vital role in helping to ensure that the person receives treatment for the depression.

Treatment is extremely important, because untreated depression can lead to many serious problems. Loss of interest, lack of motivation, decreased enjoyment, and changes in eating and sleeping habits can cause the person to stop participating in usual routines and activities, which can lead to a decline in physical abilities, physical illness, or both. In addition, untreated depression can cause the person to have suicidal thoughts and wishes. Many people are surprised to learn that older people have a higher rate of suicide than any other age group. Older men, especially those who are widowed or divorced, are at the highest risk. Never assume that a resident living in a long-term care facility would not commit suicide. Although it is rare, it has happened.

Be alert to statements a resident may make that would indicate a wish to die or intent to commit suicide. For example, a resident might say something like, "I hope when I close my eyes tonight, I never wake up" or "There is no point in living like this! I will find a way out of here." It may make you feel uncomfortable to hear such statements, and you may be tempted to respond by saying something like, "Don't say things like that" or "Don't feel that way! I am sure you will have a better day tomorrow." However, responses like these "shut the door" on the resident's feelings, and his willingness to share them. Instead, it is better to respond with questions to explore exactly what the resident is feeling. For example:

Resident: "I'm tired of living. I don't want to be here anymore."
Nursing Assistant: "Is that how you really feel?"
Resident: "Yes, it is!"
Nursing Assistant: "Do you ever think about ending your own life?"
Resident: "Yes. I think about it all the time."
Nursing Assistant: "Do you have a plan? How would you do it?"
Resident: "I'm still thinking on that one! But when I figure it out . . . Just don't be surprised if I'm not here when you come to work one morning."

In this example, by asking just a few questions, the nursing assistant was able to find out exactly how the resident is feeling. Asking about a plan is important, because the resident's answer reflects the seriousness of his intent. Also, if the resident does respond with a specific plan, it will be important to check the resident's environment to determine whether or not he has what he needs to carry out his plan. All of the information that you learn from your questions should be reported to the nurse *immediately* so that the resident can get the help that he needs. Even if the resident says that he is not thinking about suicide, the fact that he is wishing for death is something that the health care team needs to know about and follow up on.

Communicating with a person who is depressed may be difficult. The person may not be fully alert and attentive to what you are saying. The person may find that it takes great effort to talk, and may choose to say little, or only speak when spoken to. Answers to your questions may be one or two syllables, if anything at all. Your efforts to engage the person in conversation may end up irritating the resident who would prefer to be left alone. When communicating with a person who is depressed, be patient, and make eye contact as much as possible. Making eye contact will help you to tell whether or not the person is paying attention to you, and you will also be able to see if the person is starting to get irritated. If you sense that the person is starting to get irritated or angry, do not take it personally and do not try to talk the person out of his feelings. Encouraging a person who is depressed to be more cheerful will only make the person feel more isolated and misunderstood. A more appropriate response would be to acknowledge what the person is experiencing and allow him some control. For example, you could say something like, "Mr. Joseph, I seem to be upsetting you with my questions. I apologize. I don't mean to upset you. I want to help you, but if you would rather I come back later, I can do that." or "Mr. Joseph, I understand that you are feeling very upset right now. Would you like to talk about what is bothering you?" These responses show the person that you are aware of his feelings, that you care, and that you are respecting him by allowing him some control.

Bipolar Disorder (Manic Depression)

Bipolar disorder (manic depression) is a mental health disorder that causes mood swings. The person experiences periods of depression, which can be severe, followed by periods of excessive excitement (mania). Between mood swings, a person with bipolar disorder may have periods of "normal" mood. A person with bipolar disorder may have mood swings several times a day, or less frequently, with days or even weeks passing between episodes. Experts believe that bipolar disorder is caused by chemical imbalances in the brain that affect a person's moods. People with bipolar disorder are often treated with medications that help to stabilize mood.

Most people with bipolar disorder are diagnosed with the disorder when they are young adults. However, it is possible that the condition could first be diagnosed when the person is older. If a resident seems to be experiencing mood swings, it will be important for you to report this to the nurse. If the person is known to have bipolar disorder and is receiving treatment for it, the treatment plan may need to be adjusted. Or, the mood swings may be the first sign of the disorder.

ANXIETY DISORDERS

Anxiety is a feeling of uneasiness, dread, apprehension, or worry. Anxiety is a normal feeling that we have in response to situations that are threatening to our body, lifestyle, values, or loved ones. A certain level of anxiety is normal and may actually lead us to do something positive about a bad or potentially dangerous situation. But too much anxiety or prolonged periods of anxiety can make it hard for us to function or cope with everyday situations. Feelings of anxiety can cause many physical signs and symptoms such as sleeplessness, restlessness, fatigue, changes in appetite, or an increased heart rate and blood pressure. It is also common for an anxious person to be irritable and to have difficulty thinking clearly.

Although we all have periods of increased anxiety, some people have periods of anxiety that continue to build until they can no longer function. Anxiety is a typical symptom in many common mental illnesses. However, in some mental illnesses, overwhelming anxiety is the key feature of the disorder. Some people experience generalized anxiety, and others experience particular anxiety disorders. Common anxiety disorders include panic disorder, phobias, and obsessive-compulsive disorder.

Specific Anxiety Disorders
Panic disorder

Panic is a sudden, overpowering fright. A person with a **panic disorder** has terrifying episodes or "panic attacks," during which she experiences sudden increases in anxiety and feelings of intense fear. A person who is having a "panic attack" usually also has physical signs and symptoms, such as chest or abdominal pain, a rapid heartbeat, shortness of breath, and dizziness (Fig. 42-7). These symptoms may be similar to those of a heart attack or other serious physical illness. Panic attacks can be brief, or they may last for some time. Some people will experience these attacks rarely while others will have them quite often. It is important to remember that even though the physical symptoms may not be a sign of a serious physical condition, they are no less real and frightening to the person who is experiencing them.

When speaking to a person who is having a panic attack, keep your voice low and calm. Ask the person to take a deep breath, and encourage her to focus on you. Reassure the person that she is safe and that you will help her. Remaining calm and speaking in a reassuring manner helps to lower the person's anxiety level.

Phobias

A **phobia** is an excessive, abnormal fear of an object or situation. For example, the person may

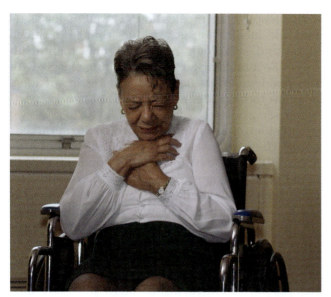

Figure 42-7
People with panic disorder suffer from "panic attacks," which are characterized by feelings of intense fear and anxiety, accompanied by physical signs and symptoms such as chest pain and a rapid heartbeat.

be abnormally afraid of a specific thing, such as dogs, birds, cats, or heights. Phobias can be incredibly disabling for the person affected by them. The person will do anything to avoid the thing she is afraid of, to the point where she may be unable to do something as simple as leaving her room.

It will be important for you to be aware of any phobias your residents may have so that you can avoid putting residents in situations that will cause them anxiety and distress. For example, a resident who is afraid of birds is likely to experience extreme anxiety if she is taken out to sit in the courtyard where there is a birdbath. Being unable to control the situation (for example, because she is in a wheelchair and must depend on you for help leaving the area) will further increase the resident's anxiety. This situation places the resident at risk for experiencing a panic attack, physical injury (for example, as she tries to get away from the area), or both. To prevent situations like this from occurring, ask the nurse or check the person's care plan for information about any phobias the resident may have.

Obsessive-compulsive disorder

Obsessive-compulsive disorder is an anxiety disorder that causes a person to suffer intensely from recurrent unwanted thoughts (*obsessions*). The obsessions are usually associated with rituals (repetitive behaviors) that the person feels obligated to complete constantly (*compulsions*). The person performs these rituals to try to reduce the anxiety associated with the obsession. Not performing the rituals increases the person's level of anxiety. When it is severe, obsessive-compulsive disorder takes over the person's life. The obsessions and rituals interfere with the person's ability to perform tasks that are associated with normal daily activities.

A resident who has obsessive-compulsive disorder may experience increased anxiety because disability or illness may prevent him from performing his ritual behaviors. As a result, the resident may ask you repeatedly to perform activities that he thinks will help him to feel better. For example, the resident may ask you over and over again to check his window to make sure it is locked, or to look for a certain object in his closet. This can affect your ability to complete your work in a timely way, and it can be extremely frustrating. It is important to recognize that the person cannot help these behaviors. Trying to convince the person to stop making these requests will only increase his anxiety. A planned, consistent approach to the resident is necessary. When a planned, consistent approach is taken, all members of the health care team follow the plan and respond to the person in the same way. For example, to help the resident with obsessive-compulsive disorder who is concerned about the window lock, staff members may be assigned to check the window lock on a regular schedule. This schedule is shared with the resident. In this way, the resident's needs are addressed, but limits are placed. The nurse will advise you about specific approaches that should be used with a resident who has obsessive-compulsive disorder. In addition, it will be important for you to communicate the resident's response to these approaches to the nurse.

Caring for a Person With an Anxiety Disorder

It may be difficult to get a resident with an anxiety disorder to do what you need her to do. The person may feel so overwhelmed by her worries that she does not really hear what you are asking her to do, or fully understand what you are trying to say. As a result, she may not follow your instructions, or she may deny ever getting instructions. When asking the resident to do something, make sure you have the person's full attention. You may need to ask the resident to turn off the television or radio temporarily to minimize distractions. Repeating instructions, writing reminders, and getting feedback from the resident may be helpful.

A resident who has an anxiety disorder may feel totally overwhelmed by making simple decisions. Limiting choices to only two or three options may help the resident cope with daily routines and activities. Avoid the temptation to make decisions for the resident. Doing this can cause the resident to feel a loss of control, which can be a contributing factor to both anxiety and depression.

SCHIZOPHRENIA

A person with **schizophrenia** has trouble determining what is real and what is imaginary. He may suffer from delusions, such as the belief that he is someone famous or that someone is spying on him or trying to take his belongings. He may also experience hallucinations, such as voices in his head telling him to perform a certain act. A person with schizophrenia often feels like others are controlling his thoughts. Conversations may be difficult to follow as the person switches from one topic to another, or makes up new words or patterns of speech. As a result of these symptoms, the person may say or do very strange things, making it hard for him to function normally in social situations. The person's behavior is often frightening and confusing to others.

Schizophrenia tends to run in families and may have a genetic basis. As with other mental illnesses, schizophrenia may be mild or severe. Schizophrenia is usually diagnosed in early adulthood. An older resident with schizophrenia has probably lived with, and been treated for, the disorder for many years.

Medications called *antipsychotics* are used for the treatment of schizophrenia. These medications may make the person dizzy or drowsy and lethargic, putting the person at increased risk for accidents. Prolonged use of some types of antipsychotics can cause problems with movement, such as muscle rigidity or tremors, muscle spasms, or restlessness that results in an inability to keep still. These movement problems also increase the person's risk for accidents. Other types of antipsychotics can increase the person's risk for developing diabetes and high cholesterol, which can lead to significant medical problems. If you are caring for a resident who is taking an antipsychotic, you will need to be observant for side effects of the medication, as well as for signs that the medication is working (that is, reduced signs and symptoms of the person's mental illness). As a nursing assistant working closely with the resident every day, you will be in an ideal position to help the nurse by making and reporting observations.

Residents who have mental disorders that cause them to lose touch with reality (such as schizophrenia) can present a real challenge when providing care. You must understand that what the person thinks he sees, hears, or feels *is* the person's reality. Listen very carefully to what the person is saying, and watch the person's facial expressions and other body language to try to understand what the person is experiencing. Then, respond to the mood or feeling that the person is conveying through his body language and tone of voice. As always, seek help from the nurse or your co-workers if you have difficulty understanding or caring for your resident.

SUBSTANCE ABUSE DISORDERS AND ADDICTION

Substance abuse disorders are disorders that involve the excessive or inappropriate use of drugs (legal or illegal), alcohol, or inhalants. Some people abuse more than one substance. A person with a substance abuse disorder can develop a physical and emotional dependence on the substance. When this occurs, the person must have the substance in order to function. If she cannot get the substance, she experiences physical symptoms (such as tremors and delirium) and emotional symptoms (such as anxiety). Addiction is a physical need for a substance that results in withdrawal signs and symptoms if the substance is withheld. Withdrawal is an emotional and physical reaction that occurs when use of the addictive substance is discontinued.

Alcohol is the substance most often abused by older people. Many older people are able to hide their substance abuse, particularly if they are living alone and do not socialize with others on a regular basis. However, admission to a long-term care facility may trigger withdrawal signs and symptoms when the person no longer has access to the substance that is being abused. Withdrawal signs and symptoms depend on the type of substance that was abused, how frequently, and how much the person was using.

TELL THE NURSE ❗

Withdrawal is a medical emergency. Any of the following signs and symptoms should be reported to the nurse immediately:

- Body tremors
- Mental status and mood changes
- Delirium
- Hallucinations (such as a feeling that something is crawling all over the skin)
- Restlessness
- Anxiety and fear
- Insomnia
- Nausea and vomiting
- Sweating
- Heart palpitations and rapid pulse
- Seizures

Residents with substance abuse disorders may still try to seek the substance they are abusing, even after admission to a long-term care facility. A visitor may bring the desired substance to the resident, or the resident may seek a staff member's help in obtaining the substance. You should never agree to these types of requests, and you must report them to the nurse immediately. You should also report any suspicions you may have about a visitor supplying the substance to the resident. Be alert for signs that suggest the resident is continuing to engage in substance abuse, such as changes in the resident's behavior or mental status, or the smell of alcohol. Reporting your observations is important to help protect the resident, as well as others in the facility.

CARING FOR A PERSON WITH MENTAL ILLNESS

It is likely that some of your residents will have or develop mental illnesses. Approximately 25% of elderly people in the United States have serious mental health problems. Of this 25%, approximately half are living in long-term care facilities.

ASSISTING WITH ACTIVITIES OF DAILY LIVING (ADLS)

Mental illness may affect a person's ability to eat, sleep, rest, or manage routine grooming and hygiene. People with mental illnesses will need different levels of assistance with their activities of daily living (ADLs), depending on the severity of their disorders. As always, help to promote the person's independence by allowing the person to provide as much of his self-care as possible. Because some mental illnesses affect a person's ability to think through the steps of routine care, you may need to gently remind the person of what step comes next. For instance, you may need to say, "OK, you're all dressed now...you just need to brush your teeth before we take our walk." Be sure to recognize the resident's efforts by praising accomplishments, no matter how small. For a person with mental illness, even routine tasks may seem very difficult. Your words of recognition and praise provide reassurance and help to motivate the person to continue working toward recovery.

LISTENING AND OBSERVING

Because nursing assistants are the "eyes and ears" of the health care team, good listening and observing skills are important to have with all residents. In some cases, your observations may lead to the diagnosis of a mental illness. As noted earlier, the diagnosis and treatment of mental illness is very important. In other cases, when a mental illness has already been diagnosed, your observations will help the health care team monitor the effectiveness of the treatment the person is receiving.

Sometimes another medical problem can cause a person to appear to be mentally ill. For example, the symptoms that accompany hypothyroidism and anemia are often mistaken for depression. Some of the behaviors seen in a person with dementia can be very similar to those seen in a person with some types of mental illness. Infections, dehydration, and the side effects of many medications can cause behavioral changes in elderly people that may be similar to behavioral changes seen in certain mental illnesses. When you notice a change in a resident's behavior or mental status, and report this change to the nurse, you are taking the first step toward making sure the person gets the help he needs. The health care team will work to determine the cause of the person's change in behavior, which will lead to prompt treatment.

When reporting and recording subjective information about residents, it is always important to use the resident's own words, and avoid adding your own opinions or judgments. This is especially important when caring for a person with mental illness, because certain phrases or words may have special meaning for the person. To accurately gauge the person's mental status, the health care team will need to know exactly what the person said.

TELL THE NURSE !

There are many signs and symptoms of mental illness. Sometimes another medical problem or a medication will make a person show signs of mental illness. As a nursing assistant, you must know what types of behaviors and moods are "normal" for each resident who is in your care. Watch for the subtle signs that something is not quite right and make sure to tell the nurse immediately if you notice any of the following in your residents:

- Changes in appetite, such as eating too much, or not eating enough
- Changes in sleep patterns, such as sleeping too much, or not being able to sleep
- Restlessness, pacing, or unusual "handling" of objects such as bed linens
- An inability to concentrate
- Crying for long periods of time or crying frequently
- Loss of interest in daily activities that were previously enjoyed
- Loss of interest in socializing with others
- An inability to focus during a conversation, or an unwillingness to make conversation
- Unusual mood or behavioral changes
- Fatigue or irritability
- Expressions of feelings of hopelessness or helplessness
- Expressions of a desire to die

SUMMARY

- One of the main qualities of mental health is a state of emotional balance.
  - Life causes stress, which can threaten our ability to maintain emotional balance.
  - People who are mentally healthy are able to manage stress effectively. People who are mentally ill have trouble effectively coping with stress.
  - Coping mechanisms and defense mechanisms help us to deal with stress.
    - Coping mechanisms are actions that a person does deliberately to manage stress, such as going to an exercise class or engaging in a hobby.
    - Defense mechanisms occur when the mind attempts to restore or maintain emotional balance in response to stress. Defense mechanisms often occur automatically, without conscious effort.
- A mental illness is a disorder that affects a person's mind, causing the person to experience emotional difficulties, act in unusual ways, or both.
  - Mental illnesses may be temporary or permanent, and of varying severity.
  - Mental illnesses may be caused by extremely stressful situations, genetics, chemical imbalances in the brain, brain damage or injury, or a person's environment.
  - Mental illnesses are typically treated using a combination of medication and psychiatric therapy.
  - Mental illness places a person at risk for committing suicide. Therefore, diagnosis and treatment of mental illness is extremely important.
- Common mental illnesses you may see among your residents include mood disorders (such as depression and bipolar disorder), anxiety disorders (such as panic disorder, phobias, and obsessive-compulsive disorder), schizophrenia, and substance abuse disorders and addiction.
  - Depression is characterized by feelings of excessive sadness and hopelessness that do not go away with time.
    - Depression is common among elderly people.
    - Detection and treatment of depression is very important.
  - Bipolar disorder (manic depression) is a mental illness that causes mood swings. The person's mood varies between periods of mania (extreme highs) and depression (extreme lows).

- Anxiety disorders are characterized by overwhelming feelings of uneasiness, dread, apprehension, or worry.
- Schizophrenia is a mental illness that causes a person to have trouble determining what is real and what is imaginary. The person may have delusions and hallucinations.

- Substance abuse disorders are disorders that involve the excessive or inappropriate use of drugs (legal or illegal), alcohol, or inhalants. Substance abuse can lead to addiction, a physical need for a substance that results in withdrawal signs and symptoms if the substance is withheld.

WHAT DID YOU LEARN?

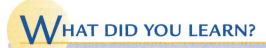

Multiple Choice

Select the single best answer for each of the following questions.

1. Which physical sign or symptom can be caused by anxiety?
   a. Sleeplessness
   b. Fatigue
   c. Increased heart rate and blood pressure
   d. All of the above
2. What is depression?
   a. An overwhelming feeling of uneasiness, dread, apprehension, or worry
   b. A persistent "low" mood and decreased pleasure
   c. A sudden, overpowering fright
   d. Recurrent, unwanted thoughts
3. You are caring for a resident who has schizophrenia. You know that when you are recording or reporting subjective information about this resident, you should:
   a. Report or record what the resident has said, using his own exact words
   b. Report or record your interpretation of what the resident has said, since the resident often says things that do not make much sense
   c. Report or record your own opinion about what the resident has said, in addition to reporting or recording the subjective information in the resident's own words
   d. Avoid reporting or recording any subjective information about this resident at all

4. One of your elderly residents, Mrs. Sigfried, has been acting strangely the last few days. She is refusing to eat, and she insists on sleeping all of the time. Why is it important for you to report your observations to the nurse immediately?
   a. Refusing to eat and extreme sleepiness are signs that death is approaching.
   b. Mrs. Sigfried's change in behavior could be caused by a physical or mental problem, and sharing your observations with the nurse will help Mrs. Sigfried to get the help she needs, sooner.
   c. Mrs. Sigfried is in violation of facility policy.
   d. Mrs. Siegfried is a danger to the other residents.
5. One of your residents tells you that he hears voices inside his head, telling him to contact aliens on another planet. What is this resident experiencing?
   a. The effects of doing too many drugs in the '70s
   b. Hallucinations
   c. Delusions
   d. Mania
6. Which one of the following is a negative way to manage stress?
   a. Smoking in moderation
   b. Taking an exercise class
   c. Taking a bubble bath
   d. Getting together with friends

Matching

Match each numbered item with its appropriate lettered description.

_____ **1.** Panic disorder

_____ **2.** Phobia

_____ **3.** Obsessive-compulsive disorder

_____ **4.** Schizophrenia

_____ **5.** Bipolar disorder (manic depression)

_____ **6.** Substance abuse disorder

_____ **7.** Withdrawal

a. An emotional and physical reaction that occurs when use of an addictive substance is discontinued

b. An anxiety disorder characterized by an extreme, abnormal fear of an object or situation

c. A mental illness characterized by an inability to tell what is real from what is imaginary

d. An anxiety disorder characterized by recurrent unwanted thoughts and rituals that the person cannot control

e. An anxiety disorder characterized by sudden increases in anxiety, often accompanied by physical signs and symptoms, such as a rapid heartbeat and chest pain

f. A disorder that involves the excessive or inappropriate use of drugs (legal or illegal), alcohol, or inhalants

g. A mental illness characterized by mood swings, from extreme highs to extreme lows

STOP and Think!

● Mrs. Gordon, one of your residents, is 83 years old. She has been confined to a wheelchair for the past 2 years due to circulatory problems and pain in her legs. She needs a great deal of help with most of her activities of daily living (ADLs). She tires very easily, and spends at least half of the day in bed. She used to enjoy reading, but she has very poor vision now, because of cataracts. Her husband, Leo, died 5 years ago. They had been married for 52 years. They never had children. She has a niece and nephew who visit occasionally. While you are caring for Mrs. Gordon, she says, "I don't know why the Lord is keeping me here. I lived out my purpose. I am no good to anyone anymore. I want to join Leo." How would you respond to Mrs. Gordon's statements? What would you report to the nurse, and why? What are some reasons that Mrs. Gordon might be feeling this way? What can you do to help her?

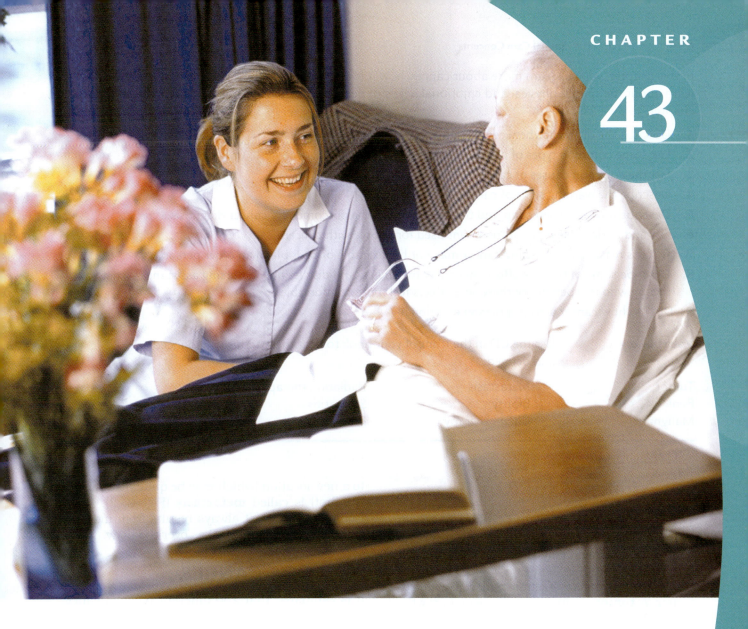

Caring for People With Cancer

WHAT WILL YOU LEARN?

Cancer is the second leading cause of death in the United States. Only heart disease kills more people in this country each year. However, it is important to remember that many people who are diagnosed with cancer survive it, especially when the cancer is diagnosed and treated early. As a nursing assistant, you will play an important role in making sure that changes in a resident that might be early signs of cancer are reported to the nurse promptly. In addition, you will care for people who have already been diagnosed with cancer and are receiving treatment for it, or who are waiting to find out if they have cancer.

Photo: A nursing assistant talks with a resident who is receiving chemotherapy to treat cancer. A common side effect of chemotherapy is hair loss. (© Colin Cuthbert/Photo Researchers, Inc.)

In this chapter, you will learn more about cancer, how it is diagnosed, and how it is treated. You will also learn about the special physical and emotional needs of people with cancer. When you are finished with this chapter, you will be able to:

1. Describe the difference between benign and malignant tumors.
2. List some common types of cancer.
3. List the common causes of cancer.
4. Describe the warning signs of cancer.
5. Describe how early detection and treatment affects the outcome of a cancer diagnosis.
6. List and explain the types of treatment used for people with cancer.
7. Discuss reasons why treating cancer may not be desirable or possible in an older person.
8. Describe some of the side effects of cancer treatment, and discuss how a nursing assistant can help a person who is experiencing these side effects feel more comfortable.
9. Discuss how cancer affects a person emotionally.

Vocabulary Use the CD in the front of your book to hear these terms pronounced and defined:

Tumor	Metastasis	Radiation therapy
Benign	Biopsy	Stomatitis
Malignant	Chemotherapy	Prognosis

WHAT IS CANCER?

The word *cancer* comes from the Greek word *karkinos,* or "crab." Indeed, cancers are "crab-like," with a central body and arms that reach out into the surrounding tissues (Fig. 43-1). The central body is a mass of abnormal cells, called a tumor. A **tumor** is simply an abnormal growth of tissue. Not all tumors are necessarily cancer.

Tumors that are not cancerous are called benign. (*Benign* means "kind.") A **benign** tumor is made of abnormal cells that tend to stay together, without spreading into surrounding tissues. In addition, benign tumors tend to grow slowly, because their cells do not divide rapidly. Many benign tumors are easily treated, because they are slow growing and their cells tend to stay together. However, an untreated benign tumor can enlarge and press on vital organs, which can cause serious problems (or even death), depending on the organs that are affected.

Cancerous tumors are called malignant. (*Malignant* means "evil.") A **malignant** tumor is made up of abnormal cells that do not function properly. Malignant cells divide rapidly and invade nearby healthy tissue. Malignant cells can also travel through the bloodstream to other parts of the body, where they "take root" and start a new cancerous tumor. The process by which cancer cells spread from their original location in the body

to a new location (which may be quite distant from the first) is called **metastasis** (Fig. 43-2). Death from cancer almost always results from metastasis. The cancer simply takes over the body.

TYPES OF CANCER

It is estimated that 200 different types of cancer can affect the human body. All organ systems can

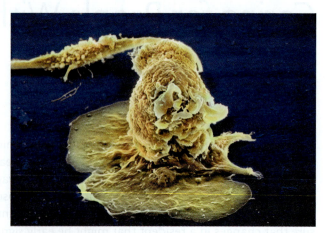

Figure 43-1

Cancerous tumors have the ability to send crab-like arms of cancerous cells into the surrounding tissue. This is a scanning electron micrograph (SEM) of a breast cancer cell. Color has been added to the photograph to make the cancer cell stand out. (© *Biophoto Associates/Photo Researchers, Inc.*)

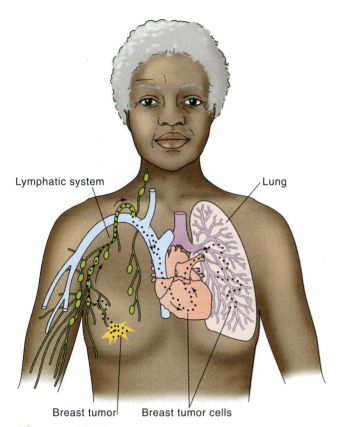

Figure 43-2

Metastasis is the process by which malignant cells spread to other parts of the body, or metastasize. A common example of metastasis is when a woman with breast cancer also develops lung cancer. First, the malignant cells of the breast tissue gain access to the lymphatic system, which empties into the bloodstream. The malignant cells are pumped, along with the blood, through the right side of the heart. Some of the malignant cells are deposited in the tiny blood vessels in the lungs, where they begin to multiply and grow, forming a new tumor.

be affected by cancer. Some cancers are very rare, while others are quite common. Common cancers that you may have heard of include skin cancer, lung cancer, breast cancer, brain cancer, colon cancer, ovarian cancer, prostate cancer, leukemia, and lymphoma. Cancer can occur at any age, but 67% of cancer deaths occur in people older than 65 years. The most common cancers seen in elderly people are breast, lung, prostate, and colon cancer.

CAUSES OF CANCER

There has been much research into what causes cancer and why some people get cancer and others do not. At present, the exact cause of cancer

is still unknown. Currently, researchers believe that whether or not a person develops cancer may be related to a combination of many factors, including:

- **Genetics.** Some cancers seem to "run in families." For example, a woman with a mother or sister who has breast cancer is more likely to develop breast cancer herself. This suggests that genetics may play a role in whether or not a person develops cancer.
- **Environmental factors.** What we are exposed to on a daily basis also seems to play a role in the development of cancer. For example, a person who smokes or spends a lot of time around people who smoke is more likely to develop lung cancer than a person who is not exposed to tobacco smoke. Some people work in jobs or live in places that expose them to cancer-causing agents (*carcinogens*), such as radiation, asbestos, chemicals, and pollution.
- **Lifestyle.** Factors such as a person's diet and the amount of time he spends exercising have been shown to play a role in the person's risk for developing cancer. For example, diets that contain lots of fruit and vegetables are known to lower a person's risk for many cancers, while diets that are high in fat increase a person's risk for some cancers. Similarly, exercising on a regular basis can lower a person's risk for developing cancer, while not exercising can increase the person's cancer risk.

The American Cancer Society (ACS) reports that approximately one third of the deaths caused by cancer in the United States are the result of smoking, and another third are related to dietary habits. Eating a healthy diet, exercising, and avoiding smoking and job-related carcinogens are important steps that people can take to lower their risk of developing cancer.

DETECTION OF CANCER

Early detection of cancer can lead to early treatment, which greatly improves a person's chances of surviving the disease. Many cancers are caught in their early stages when a person notices signs and symptoms and reports them to a health care provider. For example, a person may feel an odd lump, or notice blood in the stool. Other cancers are caught in their early stages through routine physical examinations and screening tests.

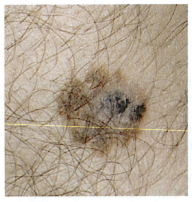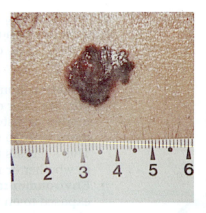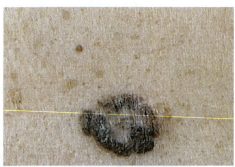

Figure 43-3

Moles that change in appearance or bleed, have jagged borders, display two or more colors (for example, brown, black, pink, gray, or white), or are larger than a pencil eraser may be malignant melanoma. Malignant melanoma is the most lethal type of skin cancer, accounting for 4% of deaths from cancer overall. (*Photographs courtesy of Goodheart, H.P. [2008]. Goodheart's photoguide to common skin disorders: Diagnosis and management, 3e [pp. 325, 354]. Philadelphia: Lippincott Williams & Wilkins.*)

WARNING SIGNS OF CANCER

Our bodies are good at letting us know when something is not quite right. A person who has cancer may experience one or more of the following early warning signs. These warning signs can be remembered by thinking of the word *CAUTIONS:*

Change in bowel or bladder habits. A person with colon cancer may have diarrhea or constipation, or he may notice that the stool has become smaller in diameter. A person with bladder or kidney cancer may have urinary frequency and urgency.

A sore that does not heal. Small, scaly patches on the skin that bleed or do not heal may be a sign of skin cancer. A sore in the mouth that does not heal can indicate oral cancer.

Unusual bleeding or discharge. Blood in the stool is often the first sign of colon cancer. Similarly, blood in the urine is usually the first sign of bladder or kidney cancer. Postmenopausal bleeding (bleeding after menopause) may be a sign of uterine cancer.

Thickenings or lumps. Enlargement of the lymph nodes or glands (such as the thyroid gland) can be an early sign of cancer. Breast and testicular cancers may also present as a lump.

Indigestion or difficulty in swallowing. Cancers of the digestive system, including those of the esophagus, stomach, pancreas, and biliary system, may cause indigestion, heartburn, or difficulty swallowing.

Obvious change in a wart or mole. Moles or other skin lesions that change in shape, size, or color should be reported (Fig. 43-3).

Nagging or persistent cough or hoarseness. Cancers of the respiratory tract, including lung cancer and laryngeal cancer, may cause a cough that does not go away or a hoarse (rough) voice.

Sudden, unexplained weight loss. Loss of a significant amount of weight (for example, about 10 pounds) without trying may be an early sign of cancer.

Some people recognize these early warning signs of cancer, but put off making an appointment with a health care provider because they are embarrassed or scared. Others, especially older people, may disregard a warning sign because they assume that it is just another problem caused by aging or an existing chronic health condition. Some older people may not notice the warning sign at all. As a nursing assistant, you may be the first to notice that a resident has an early warning sign of cancer. Reporting your concerns to the nurse immediately can lead to early detection and treatment. Early detection and treatment plays a very important role in preventing deaths due to cancer.

ROUTINE PHYSICAL EXAMINATIONS AND SCREENING TESTS

Many cancers are detected during routine physical examinations, or by screening tests that are done on a regular basis. Examples of screening tests include mammograms (used to detect breast cancer), Pap smears (used to detect cervical cancer), and fecal occult blood tests (used to detect colon cancer). These tests can help to detect cancer long before the person develops noticeable signs or symptoms of the disease. The early detection of cancer allows the cancer to be treated before it has time to spread (metastasize) to nearby tissues or other organs.

If physical examination or screening tests reveal that a person might have cancer, the doctor may order additional studies or exploratory surgery (surgery that is performed when a person is thought to have a significant medical problem, but the doctors do not know the extent of the problem or what is causing it). Examples of additional studies that may be ordered for a person who might have cancer include the following.

- **Imaging studies,** such as x-rays, computed tomography (CT) scans, and magnetic resonance imaging (MRI) scans, allow the doctor to see the tumor without actually entering the body.
- **Endoscopic studies** involve using a special lighted instrument to look inside the body and obtain tissue or fluids for analysis. Examples of endoscopic studies include *bronchoscopy* (when a scope is passed into the lungs through the mouth), *gastroscopy* (when a scope is passed into the stomach through the mouth), and *colonoscopy* (when a scope is passed into the large intestine through the anus).
- **Biopsy** is the surgical removal of cells or a small piece of tissue for microscopic examination. Biopsy is done to determine if cells are cancerous, and to determine exactly what type of cancer is present.

TREATMENT OF CANCER

There are three main approaches to treating cancer. The approach used depends on the type of cancer and the extent to which the cancer has spread to other tissues and organs. Treatment methods may be used alone or in combination with each other, depending on the type and extent of the cancer.

- Surgery involves cutting away the tumor and surrounding tissue to remove the cancer and stop the spread of the disease. Many cancer surgeries change the person's physical appearance significantly. For example, a woman with breast cancer may lose one or

both breasts. A person with bone cancer may lose all or part of an arm or leg. A person with colon cancer may need to use an ostomy appliance for the rest of his life. Although it is a relief to have the cancer gone, the person must still deal emotionally with the change in his or her appearance.

- **Chemotherapy** involves the use of medications (chemical agents) to destroy the cancer cells. There are many different chemotherapy drugs available now, each for specific types of cancer. Chemotherapy is often used in combination with surgery to help destroy any malignant cells that the surgery may not have removed completely. Chemotherapy works by killing cells that divide rapidly, such as cancer cells. Unfortunately, some types of normal cells in the body also divide rapidly, such as the cells in the hair follicles. This is why people who are receiving chemotherapy often experience hair loss (alopecia). Many people, especially women, may be very self-conscious about their hair loss. These people may find that wearing a wig, hat, or scarf helps them to feel more confident about their appearance (Fig. 43-4).
- **Radiation therapy** involves the use of powerful x-ray beams to destroy the cancer cells.

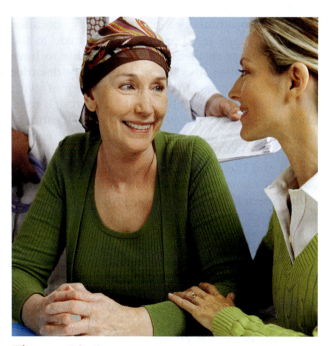

Figure 43-4

Hair loss (alopecia) is a common side effect of cancer chemotherapy. Many people who have lost their hair temporarily as a result of chemotherapy find that wearing a wig, hat, or scarf helps them to feel more confident about their appearance.

The beams are directed at the tumor to destroy the cells. Sometimes tiny pellets that contain radiation are placed inside the tumor so that the cells are destroyed from the inside. This is a common method of treating prostate cancer—radioactive pellets are placed inside the prostate gland with a needle-like instrument to destroy the cancer cells.

Surgery, chemotherapy, and radiation may be either *curative* or *palliative*. When a treatment is performed with the goal of curing the person of cancer by completely removing the cancerous cells from the body, the treatment is said to be *curative*. However, sometimes the cancer cannot be cured. When this is the case, the goal of treatment is to make the person as comfortable as possible until death occurs. This sort of treatment is referred to as *palliative* (see Chapter 28, Figure 28-9). Examples of palliative cancer treatments include surgery to bypass an obstruction caused by a tumor and chemotherapy or radiation to shrink a large tumor that is pressing on an organ and causing pain.

Many of your older residents with cancer will receive palliative treatment, or no treatment at all. Because of advanced age, a chronic health condition, or both, the person may be too frail to tolerate aggressive treatment of the cancer. For example, a resident with heart disease may not be able to tolerate the recommended chemotherapy, because the medications used are potentially toxic to the heart. Another resident may not be able to have surgery, because his chronic respiratory disorder makes anesthesia too risky. A resident with dementia may not be able to sit still through radiation treatments. In cases like this, the treatment may be harder on the person than the cancer itself! As a result, the person (or his health care agent) and the doctor may agree not to screen for common cancers (or not to do further testing for cancer even if the person has symptoms that suggest cancer). Instead, palliative care is provided to minimize symptoms and keep the person as comfortable as possible.

Helping Hands and a Caring Heart

FOCUS ON HUMANISTIC HEALTH CARE

A person who has cancer may need to decide among several different treatment options. Sometimes, the person will have to decide whether she even wants to go ahead with treatment. Some people may choose to have every type of treatment available. Others may choose to skip treatment, even if it means a chance for longer survival. You must always remember that each resident has the right to choose. The reasons behind treatment choices are unique and specific for each individual person. Although one choice may be right for one person, a different choice will be the right one for another. To truly provide humanistic care to a person with cancer, you must respect the person's decisions and choices concerning treatment. You do not have to necessarily agree with your residents' choices, but you must respect what they have decided to do. Use your listening skills to show the person that you care. Allow the person to verbalize his fears and feelings without adding your own opinion as to whether you think the person is doing the right thing or not. When you respect the decisions of the people you provide care for and support them emotionally, you demonstrate true compassion and caring.

CARING FOR A PERSON WITH CANCER

Many of us know someone who has had cancer. In fact, the experience of losing someone to cancer, or of witnessing someone's recovery from cancer, may be what inspired you to become a nursing assistant in the first place. Like all residents, those with cancer have special physical and emotional needs that must be met.

MEETING THE PHYSICAL NEEDS OF A PERSON WITH CANCER

People with cancer have special physical needs that are directly related to the cancer, the treatment, or both. Cancer can be very painful. The pain may be temporary, related to surgery or radiation treatment. Or, it may be chronic, related to the cancer itself. In addition, many of the treatments used for cancer have unpleasant side effects. As a nursing assistant, you will play an important role in helping your residents who have cancer to manage their pain and deal with the unpleasant side effects of treatment.

Managing Pain

Pain control is an essential part of the treatment for a person with cancer. Advanced cancerous tumors often cause severe pain that can only be relieved by the regular use of strong pain medications. Report any observations that suggest that a resident is in pain, or any complaints that the person may have of pain, to the nurse promptly. (See Chapter 27 for a complete discussion of pain, and the nursing assistant's role in detecting it and helping to control it.) As a nursing assistant, you will also need to be aware of and look for side effects of pain medication, such as constipation. The discomfort from the constipation alone may be as bad as the tumor pain. Recall what you learned in Chapter 26 about the measures you can take to help prevent your residents from becoming constipated. And if one of your residents does become constipated, please report this to the nurse immediately.

MANAGING SIDE EFFECTS OF TREATMENT

The treatments used for cancer, especially chemotherapy and radiation therapy, may have severe side effects:

- **Digestive problems.** Nausea, vomiting, anorexia (loss of appetite), and diarrhea are common with chemotherapy and radiation treatments. Residents who are having digestive problems as a result of cancer treatment will appreciate frequent mouth care. In addition, you can offer ice chips or popsicles to prevent the person from becoming dehydrated. Many people are able to tolerate ice chips or popsicles when nothing else will stay down. If the person is able to tolerate some foods or liquids and has an appetite for something special, try to accommodate the person's request.
- **Skin problems.** A person who is receiving radiation treatment will have tattoo marks on the skin that indicate where the radiation is to be directed. Be careful not to use lotions, perfumes, or other products that may contain alcohol in that area, because the alcohol may cause a burn during treatment. Even if products that contain alcohol are avoided, the radiation itself can cause irritation and burning of the skin. Gentle, thorough skin care can help to prevent skin breakdown.
- **Mouth problems.** People who are having chemotherapy may develop **stomatitis** (inflammation of the mouth). Sores in the mouth may be very painful and cause discomfort during eating. Drinks that are blended with ice, ice cream, yogurt, and fruit may be very soothing and can provide much-needed nutrition. Frequent, gentle oral care

is necessary to prevent infection. A special mouthwash or spray may be used to numb the inside of the person's mouth before providing oral care.
- **Fatigue.** People who are receiving cancer treatment may be very tired, all of the time. Rest periods should be scheduled between all of the resident's daily activities.
- **Increased risk for infection.** Some cancer treatments temporarily interfere with the body's ability to fight off infections. People who are having these treatments will be at high risk for getting contagious illnesses, such as colds or the flu. In addition, if they do get a cold or the flu, it could turn into something more serious, such as pneumonia. For this reason, you must be very careful to protect residents with lowered immunity from contact with other people who have a contagious illness.

TELL THE NURSE

When caring for a person who has cancer, be sure to report any of the following observations to the nurse immediately:

- The person has severe nausea, vomiting, or both
- The person has pain or sores in the mouth
- The person's skin is red or irritated in areas
- The person has an unusual discharge or bleeding from the vagina, urethra, or rectum
- The person complains of pain, or shows body language that suggests he is in pain
- The person has diarrhea or is constipated
- The person has redness, swelling, or pain around an intravenous (IV) or venous access site
- The person has a fever or other signs of infection

MEETING THE EMOTIONAL NEEDS OF A PERSON WITH CANCER

A person who is awaiting test results or who has just been diagnosed with cancer will have many emotional needs. The word *cancer* is very frightening to many people, because the disease is so often associated with death. However, a diagnosis of cancer is not necessarily a "death sentence." Many types of cancer can be successfully treated. Still, many people are very anxious about their prognosis, especially right after the cancer is diagnosed. A **prognosis** is the doctor's prediction of the course of a disease, and his estimation of the person's chances of recovering from it.

A person who has cancer may have many other fears as well. For example, the person may fear the side effects of treatment. Or, he may worry about how his body will look during treatment or following surgery. The person may be afraid of experiencing a great deal of pain as a result of the cancer or treatment. The person may worry that even if the cancer is treated successfully now, it may return later.

If one of your residents has been diagnosed with cancer, be sure to check in on the person as often as you check in on your other residents. Spend time with the person. Many nursing assistants are uncomfortable with the subject of cancer, and as a result may avoid a person with cancer without even being aware that they are doing so. You might be afraid that you won't know what to say if the person's cancer is not treatable. Remember, caring for a person with cancer does not require you to say anything—the person will be comforted just by the fact that you are there and willing to listen.

Often, people with cancer find comfort in their spiritual beliefs and practices. The person may request visits from clergy members. Time spent praying, reading religious texts, meditating, or listening to spiritual music may be comforting to the person. Provide privacy for the person during these times, and make sure you relay any requests for clergy visits to the nurse per facility policy so that the appropriate calls can be made.

SUMMARY

- A tumor, or mass of abnormal cells, may be *malignant* (cancerous) or *benign* (not cancerous). The cells that make up malignant tumors divide rapidly and spread into nearby tissues. They can also enter the bloodstream and spread to distant organs, a process called *metastasis.*
- Early detection of cancer can lead to early treatment, which greatly improves a person's chances of surviving the disease.
  - The nature of your duties as a nursing assistant will put you in an ideal position to observe changes in a resident that may be early warning signs of cancer.
  - Many cancers are detected at an early stage through routine physical examinations or screening tests. If cancer is suspected, the doctor might recommend follow-up tests (such as radiologic studies, endoscopic studies, or biopsy).
- The three main approaches to treating cancer are surgery, chemotherapy, and radiation therapy.
  - These approaches may be used alone or in combination, depending on the type of cancer and whether it has spread.
  - Treatment may be curative or palliative. The goal of curative treatment is to rid the body of the disease. The goal of palliative treatment is to keep the person comfortable when the disease cannot be cured.
  - Cancer treatment can be associated with unpleasant side effects, including hair loss (alopecia), nausea, vomiting, diarrhea, loss of appetite (anorexia), mouth sores (stomatitis), skin breakdown, lowered immunity, and fatigue.
- A person with cancer often faces many treatment choices, including the choice of not having treatment at all. It is important to respect the person's choice, even if you do not agree with it.
- An older person may not be a good candidate for cancer treatment, because of advanced age, the effects of chronic disease, or both.
- A resident with cancer requires humanistic care, just as any other resident does. Nursing assistants must take steps to prevent their own discomfort with the subject of cancer from compromising their ability to care for their residents with the disease.
  - A person with cancer has many physical needs that are directly related to the cancer, or to its treatment. Nursing assistants play an important role in helping the person with cancer to manage pain and deal with unpleasant side effects of cancer therapy.
  - A person with cancer will need assistance to meet emotional and spiritual needs as well. Often, the best thing a nursing assistant can do is listen if the person wants to talk, or spend quiet time with the person if he or she does not want to talk.

WHAT DID YOU LEARN?

Multiple Choice

Select the single best answer for each of the following questions.

1. Which one of the following statements best describes a malignant (cancerous) tumor?
   a. It consists of abnormal cells that divide rapidly and are capable of spreading to nearby tissues and distant organs.
   b. It consists of abnormal cells that divide slowly and tend to stay together.
   c. All tumors are malignant.
   d. All malignant tumors are fatal.

2. Which one of the following factors plays a role in whether or not a person develops cancer?
   a. Genetics
   b. Lifestyle choices, such as diet and exercise
   c. Environment
   d. All of the above

3. Mrs. Worthington is receiving chemotherapy following surgery to remove a malignant tumor. Following each treatment, she is nauseous, and often she vomits. What could you do to help Mrs. Worthington feel better?
   a. Offer her strong pain medications
   b. Offer her ice chips, and sit with her and hold her hand
   c. Enter her room only when necessary to avoid disturbing her
   d. Serve her meal tray as usual, in hopes that the smell of the food will increase her appetite

Matching

Match each numbered item with its appropriate lettered description.

_____ 1. Alopecia

_____ 2. Stomatitis

_____ 3. Biopsy

_____ 4. Metastasis

_____ 5. Palliative

_____ 6. Tumor

_____ 7. Prognosis

a. Surgical removal of cells or tissue for examination under a microscope
b. Treatment done with the goal of reducing pain and discomfort, not curing the disease
c. Loss of hair
d. The doctor's prediction of the course of a person's disease, and the person's chance of recovering from it
e. Inflammation of the mouth
f. The spread of malignant cells to other parts of the body
g. Abnormal growth of tissue

STOP and Think!

- You are caring for Mr. Lukens, a resident who was recently diagnosed with cancer. The doctors have presented Mr. Lukens and his family with a number of different treatment options, and for the last few days, Mr. Lukens has been weighing the pros and cons of each. In addition, he is still trying to adjust to the diagnosis he has just been given, and what it means for his future. One morning, while you are making Mr. Lukens' bed, he starts to talk to you about his father, who died of cancer after going through several months of agonizing treatments. He tells you that he is scared that he, too, will go through the treatments and in the end, all of his suffering might be for nothing. "Maybe it would just be easier to give up now and die peacefully," he says. How would you react to what Mr. Lukens is telling you? Is there anything you can do or say that might help Mr. Lukens with the difficult choices he needs to make?

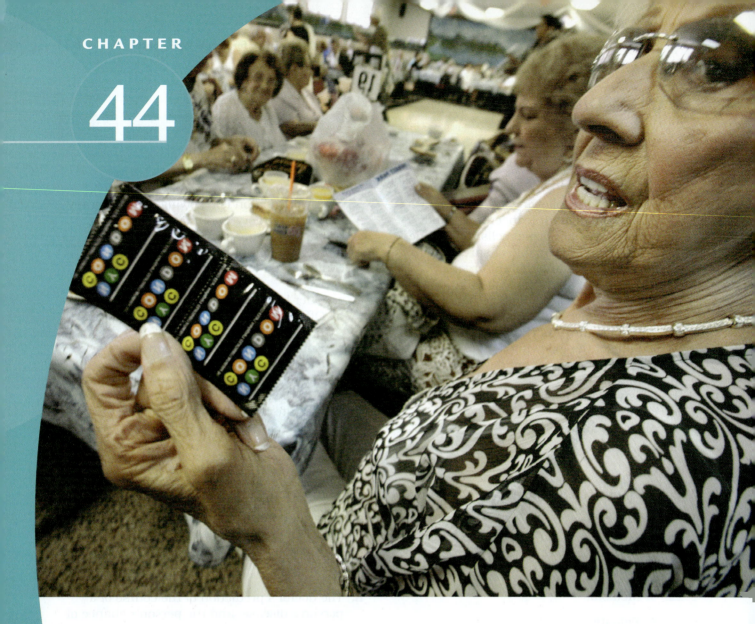

Caring for People With HIV/AIDS

WHAT WILL YOU LEARN?

In Chapter 16, you learned how human immunodeficiency virus (HIV), the virus that causes acquired immunodeficiency syndrome (AIDS), is transmitted. You also learned about measures you can take to protect yourself from HIV infection in the workplace, and about how HIV takes over the body's immune system, eventually leading to the condition known as AIDS. In this chapter, you will learn more about AIDS, and how it affects the people who have it, physically and emotionally. When you are finished with this chapter, you will be able to:

1. Describe the progression of HIV infection to AIDS.
2. Discuss who is at risk for HIV infection and AIDS.

Photo: Seniors attend an HIV/AIDS educational presentation and screening held by the New York City Department of Aging. Although many people think of HIV/AIDS as a disease that affects young people, older people are at risk too. (AP Photo/Bebeto Matthews)

3. Discuss legal concerns related to caring for people with HIV/AIDS.
4. Describe how HIV/AIDS affects a person physically.
5. Describe how HIV/AIDS affects a person emotionally.
6. Recognize the importance of the nursing assistant's responsibility to provide for the physical and emotional needs of the person with HIV/AIDS.

Vocabulary Use the CD in the front of your book to hear this term pronounced and defined:

HIV-positive

HOW DOES HIV INFECTION BECOME AIDS?

Currently, more than one million people in the United States are infected with HIV. A person who is infected with HIV is said to be **HIV-positive,** because he has tested positive on the blood test for HIV antibodies. HIV invades a person's white blood cells. In doing so, the virus destroys the cells that are responsible for protecting the body. As HIV takes over the body's immune system, the infected person begins to have more and more health problems, such as severe infections and aggressive cancers. Most HIV-positive people eventually develop AIDS, an advanced stage of HIV infection. AIDS is said to occur when the person's battered immune system is no longer able to fight off infections and malignancies. People with AIDS do not die from the virus that has infected their bodies. Rather, they die from infections and malignancies that the body is no longer able to fight.

Most people who become infected with HIV experience a brief, flu-like illness about 2 to 4 weeks after they are first exposed to the virus. During this brief illness, the person may have a fever, swollen lymph nodes, a sore throat, a rash, or any combination of these signs and symptoms. These signs and symptoms eventually go away, and may be forgotten. In many cases, if the person is tested for the virus within the next 3 to 6 months, the test will not be positive, even though the person is infected with the virus. A person can be infected with HIV for many years before developing AIDS, or he may never develop AIDS. The amount of time that it takes before AIDS develops and death occurs varies greatly from person to person. For example, in children and people in poor health, HIV infection is likely to progress to AIDS more quickly. As HIV infection progresses, the person is likely to experience:

- Loss of appetite, nausea, vomiting, or diarrhea
- Weight loss
- Fever (with or without night sweats)
- Pain or difficulty swallowing (dysphagia)
- Fatigue
- Swollen lymph nodes in the neck, armpits, and groin
- A cough or recurrent episodes of pneumonia
- Sores or white patches in the mouth
- Bruises or dark bumps on the skin that do not heal (Kaposi's sarcoma; Fig. 44-1)
- Forgetfulness and confusion
- Dementia

To date, there is no cure for HIV/AIDS, although medications have been developed that can delay the onset of AIDS in HIV-positive people. These medications can cost more than $10,000

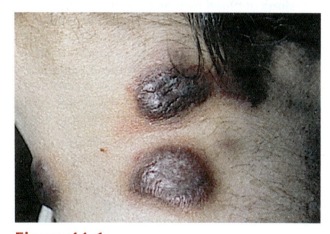

Figure 44-1
As a result of their weakened immune systems, people with AIDS often develop malignancies, such as Kaposi's sarcoma. The lesions of Kaposi's sarcoma are often seen on the skin and mucous membranes of people with advanced HIV infection (AIDS). (Photograph courtesy of Goodheart, H.P. [2003]. *Goodheart's photoguide of common skin disorders: Diagnosis and management* [p. 374]. Philadelphia: Lippincott Williams & Wilkins.)

per year and are not always successful. In addition, they often have severe and disabling side effects such as headache, dizziness, nausea, diarrhea, fever, skin rash, severe anemia, and extreme fatigue. Currently, no medication can kill HIV and offer a complete cure for AIDS.

WHO IS AT RISK FOR HIV/AIDS?

Although the first cases of HIV/AIDS were reported in homosexual men, we now know that *anyone* can get AIDS—young, old, homosexual, heterosexual, male, or female. In Chapter 16, you learned that HIV is transmitted from one person to another through body fluids such as blood, semen, and vaginal secretions. Exposure to HIV can also occur either before or during birth, or through breast milk. Behaviors and situations that increase a person's risk for becoming infected with HIV include the following:

- **Having unprotected sex.** Unprotected sexual intercourse, both homosexual and heterosexual, is the most common method of HIV transmission.
- **Sharing of needles.** Sharing of needles among people who abuse intravenous drugs is the second most common method of transmission.
- **Receiving tissue transplants or transfusions of blood or blood products.** Before 1985, people who received blood transfusions may have been exposed to HIV. This method of transmission is less common now in developed nations with more advanced health care systems, because donated blood is screened for the virus. However, some developing countries still do not screen their blood supplies.

In the United States, the highest rate of HIV infection is among adults between the ages of 30 and 39 years. However, this is not the only at-risk age group. Although many people do not consider the elderly population to be at risk for becoming infected with HIV, the Centers for Disease Control and Prevention (CDC) reports that people 50 years and older make up approximately 10% of the total number of AIDS cases nationwide. In addition, HIV infection in older adults is increasing at an alarming rate. AIDS awareness programs, which teach people about AIDS and how to lower their risk of becoming infected with HIV, have traditionally been aimed at younger people, rather than older people. Many older people are not aware of how HIV is transmitted or behaviors that put them at risk for getting HIV. As a result, sexually active older couples may engage in unprotected sex, which puts them at risk for HIV infection.

PROTECTING THE RIGHTS OF A PERSON WITH HIV/AIDS

In many cultures, being HIV-positive or having AIDS is considered shameful. As a result, a person who is HIV-positive or who has AIDS may experience discrimination and poor treatment by others. There are many factors that contribute to the negative attitude many people have toward those who are HIV-positive or have AIDS:

- Because HIV infection is associated with many behaviors that people can control (such as whether or not they practice safe sex), some people may feel that the person with HIV/AIDS "has only himself to blame."
- Many of the behaviors associated with HIV infection are behaviors that many people do not approve of for moral or religious reasons (such as abusing street drugs or being homosexual).
- Many people lack information about how HIV is transmitted, and as a result, fear becoming infected with HIV through casual contact with an infected person.

Because a person with HIV/AIDS is at risk for discrimination, many states have laws designed specifically to protect the rights of people with HIV/AIDS. These laws ensure the person's right to employment, education, privacy, and health care. It would be difficult to detail all of the laws here, because they vary from state to state and they change frequently as lawmakers write and introduce new laws. However, as an example, in most states, people with AIDS are protected under the Americans with Disabilities Act.

As with all of your residents, protecting the person's privacy and right to confidentiality is very important. This is especially true when a person has a condition, such as HIV/AIDS, that could cause her to experience problems as a result of negative attitudes others may have about her condition. As a nursing assistant, you are responsible for maintaining absolute confidentiality about a person's HIV status. You need to know the HIV status of a person to whom you are providing care. However, no one else needs to know.

Know your facility's policies related to keeping health information private, and follow these policies carefully at all times, with all residents.

CARING FOR A PERSON WITH AIDS

In the advanced stage of AIDS, pain and weakness cause the person to become almost completely dependent on others for assistance with activities of daily living (ADLs). As a result, the person may need to move to a long-term care facility. Advanced AIDS is one reason a younger person might be admitted to a long-term care facility. Remember what you learned in Chapter 8 about the special needs of younger residents.

MEETING THE PHYSICAL NEEDS OF A PERSON WITH AIDS

A person with AIDS becomes more dependent on others for basic physical care as the disease progresses. Fatigue and disability will make it difficult for the person to perform basic activities, such as those related to personal hygiene and grooming. As a result, you will need to help the person with any ADLs that he can no longer manage. As always, encourage the person to do as much for himself as possible, for as long as possible. Special considerations with regard to physical care for the person with AIDS include the following:

- People with AIDS often develop painful sores on the inside of the mouth. These sores can make eating difficult, putting the person at risk for poor nutrition. In addition, people with AIDS often suffer from chronic diarrhea, which puts them at risk for dehydration. As a result, you may be required to measure and record intake and output. You should also offer the person fluids, as ordered.
- As a result of sores on the inside of the mouth, oral hygiene can be painful for a person with AIDS. A special mouthwash or spray to numb the inside of the person's mouth may be used before providing oral care. Rashes and other skin disorders may require the use of special cleansing agents, special bathing techniques, or both.
- Because people with AIDS are at high risk for opportunistic infections, the person with AIDS needs to avoid potential sources of

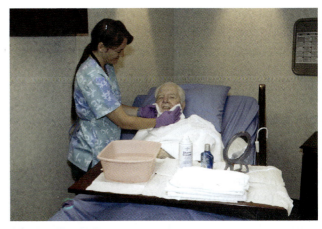

Figure 44-2
Practicing standard precautions is essential with all residents, not just those who are known to have an illness caused by a bloodborne pathogen (such as AIDS).

infection. You will need to ask visitors who have colds or other contagious illnesses to delay their visit until after they have recovered from their illness. Avoid coming to work if you have a contagious illness, and always practice proper infection control measures, especially good handwashing. This is important with all residents, but especially so when you are caring for people with weak immune systems.

You may find it frightening to provide physical care for a person who is known to have a communicable, potentially fatal illness. Know that with the proper and consistent use of standard precautions (see Chapter 16), your risk of exposure to HIV and other bloodborne pathogens in the workplace is actually quite low. Also, remember that you must use standard precautions with every resident, not just those who are known to be infected with HIV, because a person can be infected with HIV and not know it (Fig. 44-2).

TELL THE NURSE

When caring for a person with HIV/AIDS, it is very important for you to immediately report any of the following observations to the nurse:

- The person has a fever
- The person has sores or white patches in the mouth
- The person has diarrhea, nausea, or vomiting
- The person is coughing
- The person has a skin rash or bruises

● The person's mental status has changed (for example, he has become confused or disoriented)

● The person is bleeding from any body opening

MEETING THE EMOTIONAL NEEDS OF A PERSON WITH AIDS

People with HIV/AIDS can face a great deal of emotional stress. Because of increasing levels of stress, people with HIV/AIDS may lose their ability to cope. As a result, clinical depression and an increased risk for suicide are very common among people with HIV/AIDS. Sources of emotional stress include the following:

- Fear, shame, or disapproval can cause friends and even family members to abandon a person when they find out that she is HIV-positive. They may avoid the person, because they fear that they, too, could get the disease from casual contact or conversation. Or, they may just be ashamed to know a person with HIV/AIDS. Can you imagine how you would feel if your friends or family members could not give you emotional support when you needed it most?

- People with HIV/AIDS may lose their jobs as a result of their disease. Health care and the medications used to slow the progression of HIV are very expensive, and the loss of employment usually means the loss of health care benefits. For these reasons, the person with HIV/AIDS may have many worries about money.

- A person with HIV/AIDS may suffer from a lot of guilt, especially if the cause of infection was due to risky behavior. For example, a man who finds out that he is HIV-positive must face the fact that he may have transmitted a deadly disease to his sexual partner.

- A person with HIV/AIDS may have many fears related to his declining health and how this will affect his ability to care for himself. The person may also have fears about pain related to the disease, or about death itself.

Providing emotional care for the person with HIV/AIDS is an essential responsibility of the nursing assistant. When caring for a person with HIV/AIDS, you can use touch to comfort the person, spend time listening and talking, or share a simple hug (Fig. 44-3). None of these activities will transmit the virus to you. Many times, the only human touch a person with HIV or AIDS will experience will come from the person providing

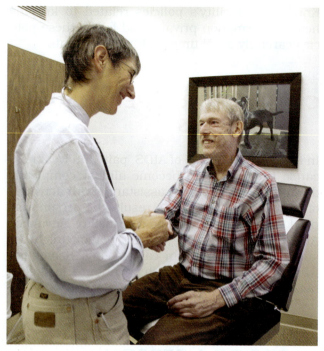

Figure 44-3
HIV cannot be transmitted from one person to another through touching or hugging. Lack of human touch can make a person feel unloved and alone. When caring for a person with HIV/AIDS, try not to let fear get in the way of your ability to provide compassionate care. (*AP Photo/ Paul Sakuma*)

care within the health care setting. How would you feel if people were afraid to touch you? Would you feel dirty, unloved, and alone? Instead of being afraid to care for people with HIV/AIDS, learn how to protect yourself from infection and practice what you have learned consistently.

Helping Hands and a Caring Heart

FOCUS ON HUMANISTIC HEALTH CARE

Remember that it does not really matter how a person became infected with HIV. Even if you do not approve of the person's lifestyle, you must not let your personal beliefs affect the care that you give the person. Instead of focusing on how the person got HIV, focus on who the person is. What does she enjoy about life? Whom does she admire? Try to remember that a person is defined by a lot more than just her HIV status. A resident with HIV/AIDS needs your care and support, perhaps more than anything else she has ever needed before. Your ability to provide supportive and compassionate care to your residents with HIV/AIDS will make a significant difference in their quality of life.

SUMMARY

- Acquired immunodeficiency syndrome (AIDS) is caused by infection with the human immunodeficiency virus (HIV). HIV invades the body's immune system, leaving it unable to do its job. As a result, the person eventually dies from infections or cancers that take over the body.
  - A person who has tested positive for having antibodies to HIV in his or her blood is said to be HIV-positive.
  - Most HIV-positive people eventually develop AIDS, an advanced stage of HIV infection. A person who is infected with HIV may live for many years before AIDS develops. AIDS is a terminal illness.
- Anyone can get HIV/AIDS, regardless of race, gender, sexual orientation, or age.
  - Behaviors that increase a person's risk of becoming infected with HIV include having unprotected sexual intercourse and using dirty needles to inject street drugs.
  - The virus can also be transmitted through tissue transplants or transfusions of blood or blood products, and from a mother to a child during birth or through breast milk.
  - Although HIV/AIDS is often thought of as a disease that affects young people, older people are at risk too.

- A person with HIV/AIDS may experience discrimination and poor treatment by others. It is important for the nursing assistant to keep information about a person's HIV status, or any other medical condition, private and confidential.
- In addition to providing physical care, the nursing assistant plays an important role in providing emotional care to the person with HIV/AIDS.
  - With the proper and consistent use of standard precautions, your risk of exposure to HIV and other bloodborne pathogens in the workplace is actually quite low.
  - Human touch is a very effective way of comforting a person and communicating care and concern. You cannot get HIV/AIDS from holding a person's hand or giving a person a hug.
  - Remember that it is not important how a person became infected with HIV. Try not to let your personal beliefs or fears get in the way of your ability to provide compassionate, competent care.

WHAT DID YOU LEARN?

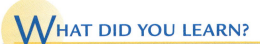

Multiple Choice

Select the single best answer for each of the following questions.

1. When are standard precautions used?
   a. When a person who is HIV-positive develops AIDS
   b. When a person is HIV-positive or has AIDS
   c. When caring for a resident who is homosexual
   d. When caring for any resident and contact with blood or body fluids is possible
2. Which one of the following statements about HIV infection and AIDS is true?
   a. Anyone can become infected with HIV, regardless of age, gender, sexual orientation, or race.

   b. The only people who become infected with HIV and get AIDS are drug abusers and homosexuals.
   c. HIV/AIDS is not a problem among the elderly.
   d. AIDS usually develops soon after a person is first exposed to HIV.
3. When caring for a person with HIV/AIDS, which one of the following observations should be reported to the nurse?
   a. The person has diarrhea
   b. The person seems depressed
   c. The person seems disoriented
   d. All of the above

4. Mr. Martin, one of the residents in your care, is HIV-positive. You should:
   a. Make sure that visitors are aware of Mr. Martin's HIV status
   b. Always put on gloves before touching Mr. Martin
   c. Respect Mr. Martin's right to have his medical information kept confidential
   d. Always put on a mask before going into Mr. Martin's room

5. Which one of the following physical problems is a person with AIDS at risk for?
   a. Alopecia (loss of hair), due to the medications used to slow the progression of HIV to AIDS
   b. Dehydration, due to chronic diarrhea
   c. Blindness, due to nerve damage as a result of HIV infection
   d. Heart failure, due to myocardial infarction

STOP and Think!

One of the residents you will be caring for today, Camilla, is a 34-year-old woman with advanced AIDS who has been admitted for end-stage care. You have never cared for a person with AIDS. Frankly, you are a little bit nervous about meeting Camilla and about providing hands-on physical care to a person who is known to have AIDS. In addition, you are not particularly used to caring for young people. Most of your residents are elderly. What will be your approach to Camilla?

Nursing Assistants Make a Difference!

"I am Clarence Wright and I live in the Sunny Shores Nursing facility. I came here about a year ago after my dear wife Callie passed away. We had been married for 53 years and I thought my heart was broken forever the day they lowered her into the grave. I didn't want to eat, get out of bed, or even take a bath; heck, I didn't want to go on living without her! A good friend visited me a week or so after the funeral and I guess I frightened him so much that he called the ambulance for me.

I went to the hospital and stayed a few days to be evaluated. There, a mental health specialist diagnosed me with severe depression. The doctor prescribed some medication to help me feel more "normal" and arranged for me to have counseling to help me come to terms with losing Callie. Shortly after I was released from the hospital, I decided to move to Sunny Shores.

After moving here, I was still pretty depressed. But, there was this really nice woman named Celia who helped care for me each day. She was my nursing assistant. At first she would help me get dressed and shaved and out for breakfast. Then she would ask me to go walk around the grounds with her. We didn't talk much at first. She didn't pry; instead, we just walked quietly. After I started feeling like talking, she let me talk about my life with Callie, and would sit and look at pictures of her with me. One day I broke down and just cried like a baby and Celia just sat quietly with me and held my hand. That day, I knew I would be able to make it.

Yes, I still get sad when I think of Callie's death. But I've learned to make use of what I have left of my life. I help Celia out with some of the residents who aren't as fortunate as I am. I read to one fellow who is blind and we have some of the most wonderful conversations. Also, a group of us meet every Thursday night to play cards. I have regained the feeling that my life has meaning and I know that Celia had a major part in that. Medicine is great for helping people with depression, but no medicine ever created can take the place of knowing that a person cares about you. And Celia shows that she cares about me and all the other residents down this hall. We love her and think that she's our angel in disguise."

You can listen to more stories about how nursing assistants make a difference on the CD in the front of your book.

Photo credit: Jupiterimages Corporation

ENTERING THE WORKFORCE

45 Job-Seeking Skills

As a nursing assistant trained to work in long-term care, you will find many opportunities to put your training to use. The population of the United States is rapidly aging, and future projections are already showing that there will always be a need for skilled and knowledgeable people prepared to provide care in the nation's long-term care facilities. Finding a job in which you will be happy and satisfied with your work is the focus of Unit 9.

Photo: A professional appearance and attitude are key during a job interview.

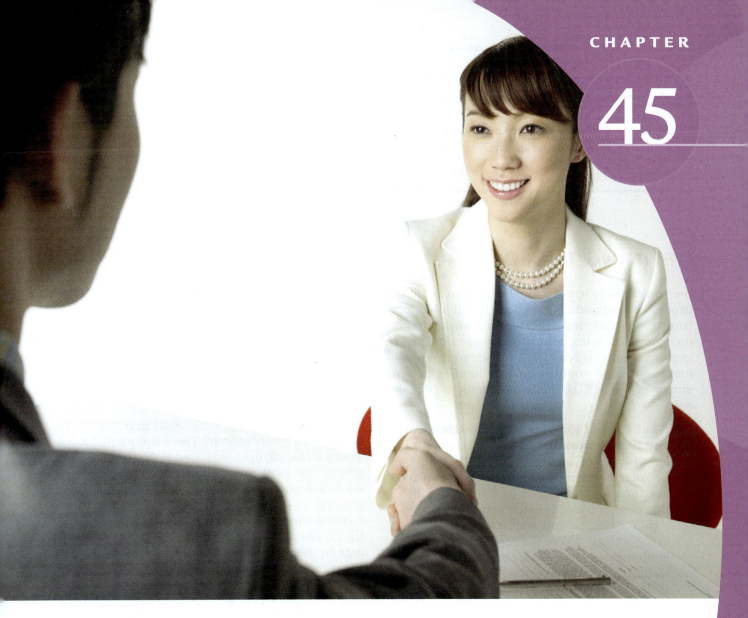

Job-Seeking Skills

⬤ WHAT WILL YOU LEARN?

As a nursing assistant trained to work in long-term care, there will be many job opportunities available to you. Perhaps you already know what type of long-term care facility you would like to work in, or perhaps you will have to try a few different things before you find your special place. In this chapter, we will discuss how to take a methodical approach to finding a job that you will enjoy. When you are finished with this chapter, you will be able to:

1. Describe questions a person should consider before beginning a job search.
2. List places to search for job openings.
3. Describe how to complete a job application.

Photo: A job interview is an opportunity for a potential employer to evaluate you, and for you to evaluate the potential employer.

4. Describe how to make a good impression during a job interview.

5. Describe the proper way to resign from a job.

Vocabulary Use the CD in the front of your book to hear these terms pronounced and defined:

Résumé   Reference list   Job application   Interview

DEFINING THE IDEAL JOB

So, you're ready to get a job. Before you begin the process of responding to notices about job opportunities, completing applications, and going on interviews, it is important that you take time to explore what you really want from your employment and what you will be able to offer to your employer (Fig. 45-1). Some questions to consider are:

- **What kind of long-term care setting would you like to work in?** You learned about different types of long-term care settings in Chapter 2. Perhaps you are most interested in caring for older, more frail residents. In this case, a nursing home setting might be right for you, as opposed to an assisted-living setting, where the residents need more limited assistance. Also, consider your special interests. For example, if you would really like to work with residents who have dementia, you could look for a job in a facility that has a specialty unit for dementia care. Focusing on your interests, likes, and dislikes will help you to narrow the search, increasing the chance that you will find a job you will enjoy.
- **Are there limitations on the hours or shifts you are available to work?** If you are a parent with small children, you may be limited to working certain shifts depending on your childcare arrangements. Do not lead an employer to believe that you are available for any shift if you can realistically work only evenings.
- **Do you have reliable transportation to get to work?** Your employer will rely on you to come to work as scheduled and on time. If you rely on public transportation, apply for work at facilities serviced by that particular transportation method.
- **What are some of your personality strengths?** Are you self-motivated and independent, or do you like more supervision and guidance? A nursing assistant who works well with minimal supervision would be an asset for an assisted-living facility, while one who prefers more supervision would probably be better suited for working in a nursing home or sub-acute care facility.

FINDING JOB OPENINGS

Once you have some specific goals in mind, where do you start your search? There are many places to search for job openings. Certainly, the classified ads in the local newspaper are a great place to start. Telephone directories list facilities that hire nursing assistants. You could try calling these facilities directly, or checking the Internet to see if the facilities you are interested in post job openings on their websites. In addition, you can use the Internet to check sites dedicated to helping people find jobs. The school that you are attending may offer a job placement service, where you can check job listings and obtain help with writing a résumé. You could also check for job postings on the bulletin board in the facility where you are receiving clinical training. Last but not least, friends and co-workers may know of openings. Start a list of positions that you hear of that interest you, so that you will have the information readily available.

PREPARING RÉSUMÉS, COVER LETTERS, AND REFERENCE LISTS

YOUR RÉSUMÉ

Before actually making application for a particular job, you must prepare a **résumé,** a brief document that gives a possible employer general information about your education and work experience. Résumés should be typed or printed using a computer on white or off-white paper.

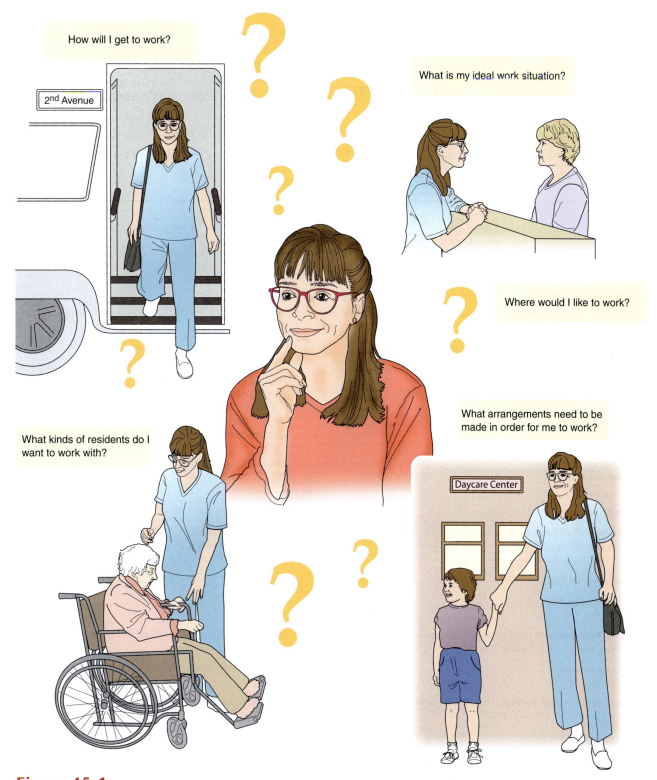

Figure 45-1
The first step to finding a job is thinking about what sort of situation best fits your personality, lifestyle, and interests.

With résumés, "plain" is best—no fancy lettering or designs are necessary! A résumé contains only facts and should be kept to one page, if at all possible (Fig. 45-2). Your résumé should include:

- Your full name, address, telephone number and, if you have one, your e-mail address
- A short objective, or career goal
- A history of your education (list the schools you attended most recently first, and for each school, include the dates you attended the school and the degree you graduated with)
- An employment history (list each of your previous employers, and for each employer, include the dates that you worked there, your job title, and your primary job duties)

Listing volunteer work on your résumé is appropriate, but only if it relates to the job you are applying for. There is some information that

---

SUZIE SMITH
123 NORTH AVENUE
ANYWHERE, US 12345
(123) 456-7890

Career Objectives:

To obtain a position as a Certified Nursing Assistant in a rehabilitation-centered health care facility that will allow me to use my skills to assist those in need.

Education:

Anywhere Vocational Center Anywhere, US	May–July 2009 Nursing Assisting Course CNA Certification: August 2009
State Jr. College Anywhere, US	August–December 2008 General Studies
Anywhere High School Anywhere, US	Graduated: June 2008 High School Diploma

Certifications:

Certified Nursing Assistant CPR Certification	August 2009 (Current) July 2009 (Current)

Employment History:

Sunshine Assisted Living Anywhere, US	August 2009–Present

CNA, Rehabilitation Unit. Provided assistance with activities of daily living for residents, with an emphasis on rehabilitation. Worked closely with physical therapists to carry out therapy plan with meals and ambulation.

Quality Printing Anywhere, US	July 2008–July 2009

Cashier/Customer Service: Worked part-time while attending college. Responsible for assisting customers with print orders and making end-of-day bank deposits.

Volunteer History:

Hospice Anywhere, US	June 2007–July 2009

Respite Volunteer. Provided respite for families receiving hospice care. Sat with patients and read to them.

Figure 45-2

A résumé is a short, precise document with information about you, your work experience, and your education.

should never be included on a résumé, including your age, marital status, weight, religion, sexual preference, and whether or not you have children (or are planning to have them). This information should not matter to an employer who is considering you as an employee. It is against the law for an employer to ask a candidate questions related to these subjects at any time during the hiring process.

YOUR COVER LETTER

You may also want to prepare a cover letter to send out with your résumé. A cover letter is written as a way of introducing yourself to a potential employer. Your résumé contains information about your education, training, and experience, but a cover letter goes beyond the straight facts. In the cover letter, you can explain why you are interested in the job you are applying for, and why you feel you are a well-qualified candidate for the job (Fig. 45-3). Your cover letter should be fairly short and typed or printed using a computer on white or off-white paper. Pay special attention to your grammar and spelling.

YOUR REFERENCE LIST

The last document you should prepare before applying for a job is a reference list. A **reference list** is a list of three or four people who would be willing to talk to a potential employer about your abilities. When considering people to include on your reference list, think about people who know you well and have worked with you in a professional capacity, such as your teachers, co-workers, or previous supervisors. Before listing a person as a reference, make sure you have his or her permission to do so. Some people may hesitate to act as a reference. For example, they may not want their contact information given out, they may be too busy, or they may not think you did as good a job for them as you thought you did. After a person has agreed to be your reference, make sure you have accurate contact information for that person, including his or her full name and title (if any), a current and complete address, and a telephone number. Type your reference list on a sheet of paper that matches your résumé. Some employers will ask for a list of references at the time you turn in an application; others will want you to write your references on the actual application

Suzie Smith
123 North Avenue
Anywhere, US 12345
February 1, 2010

Sandra Jones, Director of Human Resources
Sunny Hills Rehabilitation Center
1234 South Avenue
Anywhere, US 12345

Dear Ms. Jones,

I would like to express my interest in the certified nursing assistant position at Sunny Hills Rehabilitation Center that was listed in the local want ads. In July 2009, I completed my nursing assitant training at Anywhere Vocational Center. Since that time, I have been employed at Sunshine Assisted Living as a CNA in their rehabilitation unit.

I am a hard worker and I learn new skills easily. I love working with the elderly and have heard that your facility is a very enjoyable place to work.

Thank you for taking the time to review and consider my application. I am available for an interview at your convenience and look forward to meeting with you soon.

Sincerely,

Suzie Smith

Suzie Smith, CNA

Figure 45-3
A cover letter is a letter that you write to go along with your résumé. Your cover letter allows you to explain more fully why you want to work for a particular organization, and what qualities you have that make you the ideal person for the job opening in question.

form. Either way, you will be prepared with correct and current information. How efficient and organized you will appear at that first meeting!

PLACING APPLICATIONS

Now that you have thought about your ideal work situation, prepared a list of job opportunities to pursue, written your résumé and cover letter, and gathered your references, you are ready to place applications. A **job application** is a standardized form used by employers to obtain basic information about a potential employee, such as which position the person is applying for, how the person can be reached, and what shifts the person can work (Fig. 45-4). Although it is acceptable and common practice to just stop by facilities where you are interested in working and ask to complete an application, you may want to call ahead to ask if there are any positions open for nursing assistants. Even if there are not any immediate openings, most facilities will keep applications on file for approximately 6 months, so ask if you may place an application to be kept on file.

In some facilities, the director of nursing (DON) handles the hiring of nursing assistants. In others, hiring is handled through the human resources (HR) department (personnel). Usually, when you go to a facility to complete a job application, the receptionist at the main desk will give you the application to complete (Fig. 45-5). When you go to complete your application, take your résumé and references with you and dress appropriately, even though you expect only to complete the application and leave. Some facilities may choose to interview you at that time, especially if there is an opening. Appropriate dress means "clean and neat" and appropriate for business. Make sure your clothes are pressed and clean and your shoes are polished. Hair should be neatly arranged and out of your face. Jewelry should be simple and minimal, and if you wear perfume or cologne, the fragrance should be light. Women should make sure that their make-up is tastefully applied. Even if you do not interview, this will be the first impression you make on a possible employer. You can be sure that the people who do the hiring for the organization will do some preliminary screening by asking the receptionist whether you appeared neat and well-organized, and what your attitude was like.

Some facilities will allow you to take the application home to be filled out and returned at a later date. Others will require you to complete the application while you are there, so go prepared to complete the application form in the facility. Have notes available with details that you will need to complete the application. Remember the time you spent earlier thinking about practical factors that needed to be taken into consideration, such as childcare arrangements and transportation? Now you will be able to easily answer the questions on the application about your availability for work. The application form will also require you to provide information about your education, your work history, and the reasons you left previous jobs. There are many legitimate reasons why a person would leave a job. For example:

- "I left to take a position that was closer to home."
- "I left for family reasons." (For example, to take care of an aging parent or to be home with young children)
- "I left to go to school."
- "I left because we moved to a new city or town."
- "I left because I was laid off."

The reason for leaving a job could be that you were fired. If so, be honest. Your chances of finding new employment are much better if a potential employer hears the truth from you, instead of finding it out by calling your references. When giving a reason for leaving a job, avoid speaking negatively about your previous employer, even if the situation was not ideal. Doing so reflects poorly on you as a potential employee.

Answer all of the questions on the application form. Use blue or black ink, and write clearly. You will be required to sign and date the application form at the bottom. The application form is a legal document, and your signature states that all the information is true and accurate. An employer who finds out that you lied about any information on the application form has grounds to fire you without notice.

Most facilities will also request a copy of your résumé and reference list along with the completed application. Ask for an appointment for an interview when you submit your cover letter, résumé, reference list, and completed application. Some facilities will make the appointment at this time. Others may want to review your résumé and application and call you for an appointment at a later date. If you have not heard from a potential employer in 1 week's time, it is appropriate to call and ask about the status of your application. A follow-up call shows a potential employer that you have initiative and are interested in the job.

HIGHLAND CARE CENTER
APPLICATION FOR EMPLOYMENT

Highland Care Center is an equal opportunity employer, dedicated to a policy of non-discrimination in employment on any basis, including race, color, age, sex, religion, national origin, or disability. Highland supports hiring people who have disabilities and meets all ADA requirements to provide reasonable accommodations for people with disabilities who are qualified to do the job. A mandatory drug test will be performed within 90 days of hire. Criminal background checks will be made on all new employees.

PERSONAL INFORMATION

Name:_____   Date:_____

  Please list any other names you have been known by or employed under:_____

Phone Number:_____   Social Security Number:_____

Position Desired:_____   Salary Desired:_____

Present Address:_____
         Street   City   State   Zip Code

Permanent Address (if different from above):_____
         Street   City   State   Zip Code

Have you ever applied for employment with Highland before? Yes _____ No_____ If yes, when?_____

Have you ever worked for Highland before? Yes _____ No_____ If yes, when?_____

Available for: Full Time _____ Part Time _____ On Call _____ Shifts available for: Morning _____ Afternoon _____ Night _____

If hired, when would you be available to begin work? _____

Are you eligible for employment in the United States? Yes _____ No _____

How did you learn about Highland Care Center? _____

Have you ever been convicted of a felony or misdeamor? Yes _____ No _____ Do you smoke? Yes _____ No _____

Upon hire a criminal background check will be conducted.

EDUCATION	Name and Location of School	Graduate?
High School		
College		
Business/Trade/Tech.		

List Other Job-Related Skills: _____

_____

Special Skills or Qualifications: _____

_____

Figure 45-4
A job application is a standardized form used to obtain basic information about each person who applies for a job with the organization. It is a legal document, and your signature at the bottom states that all of the information you have provided is true and accurate.

Please list your previous work experience below beginning with your present or most recent employer for the past 5 years or your last three employers, whichever you feel will provide us with the most helpful information about you.

Dates of Employment Must list month and year	Name, Address, Phone Number of Employer Name of Supervisor	Ending Wage	Ending Position	Reason for Leaving
Begin Date _____ End Date _____				
Begin Date _____ End Date _____				
Begin Date _____ End Date _____				

If a previous employer is not to be contacted, designate which

one: _____

Are there any comments you would like to share ? _____

The information provided in this Application for Employment is true, correct and complete. If employed, any misstatement or omission of fact on this application may result in my dismissal. I understand that acceptance of an offer of employment does not create a contractual obligation upon Highland Care Center to continue to employ me in the future. Daywest HealthCare Services, Inc. Is a drug & alcohol free workplace. As a condition of employment all employees must successfully pass a drug test, which will be administered some time during their orientation period. Criminal background checks will be made on all new employees.

Signature: _____   Date: _____

FOR HIGHLAND USE ONLY

Interviewed by: _____   Date: _____

References:

Person Contacted, Place and Date: _____

Person Contacted, Place and Date: _____

Person Contacted, Place and Date: _____

Remarks: _____

_____

_____

**HIGHLAND CARE CENTER
RELEASE OF INFORMATION**

Applicant Name: _____

Social Security #: _____   Date: _____

I authorize Highland Care Center to seek and obtain information from employers, supervisors, and colleagues regarding the following as well as any other job-related information, which will enable the facility to evaluate my suitability for employment.

____ work habits   ____ technical skills

____ performance record   ____ vaccination records

____ ability to form effective working relationships with co-workers

____ other: _____

I authorize those contacted to release this information to Highland Care Center.

By initialing below, I authorize Highland Care Center to obtain information from:

        ____ All former employers and current employer

        ____ Former employers only

Signature: _____   Date: _____

Figure 45-4 (*Continued*)

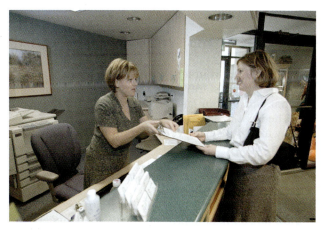

Figure 45-5
When you go to complete your application form, take your résumé, cover letter, and references with you, and dress neatly.

GOING ON INTERVIEWS

An **interview** is the chance for a potential employer to meet you personally and learn more about you in an effort to determine if you are the right person for the job. Equally as important, the interview is a chance for *you* to learn more about the employer and the position, in an effort to determine if they are right for you. Being properly prepared for the interview will allow you to ask targeted questions during the interview, so that you can obtain information you need to make an informed decision about the job, if it is offered to you. In addition, being properly prepared can make all the differ-

ence in how a potential employer views your potential! Your résumé and application contain all of the "hard" facts about your education and experience, but you are the one responsible for persuading the interviewer of your interest in the job, dedication to your profession, and abilities.

Before going to the interview, make a list of questions you would like answers to, and refer to this list during the interview. This shows that you are interested in the position and are taking the opportunity to interview seriously. Some questions you might want to ask include:

- "What are the major responsibilities or duties of the position? May I have a copy of the job description?"
- "May I see the unit where I will be working and meet the person who will be supervising me?"
- "What do you think nursing assistants like best about working here? Least?"
- "How many residents would I be assigned to care for?"
- "When would I be eligible for a performance evaluation, and what are the standards I will be evaluated against?"
- "What qualities are you looking for in a nursing assistant?"
- "What opportunities exist for career growth and furthering my education?"

You are interviewing for a job in the health care setting, so help the interviewer see you as a part of the staff. Present yourself as a well-groomed professional (see Guidelines Box 3-1 in Chapter 3, and Fig. 45-6). Make sure your clothing is pressed

Figure 45-6
Dress like the professional that you are when you go for your interview! Clean, neat hair and nails and polished shoes are appropriate for both men and women. **(A)** An appropriate outfit for a man would be slacks, a button-down shirt or a polo shirt, and a belt. A tie is optional. **(B)** For a woman, an appropriate outfit would be a skirt and a blouse. Make-up and jewelry should be kept to a minimum.

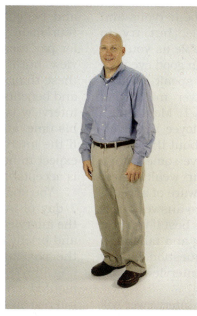

A

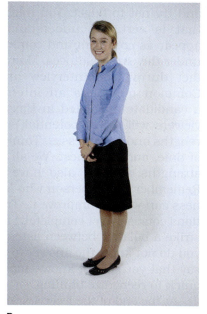

B

and all repairs, such as missing buttons or loose seams, have been taken care of before the interview. Your shoes should be clean and polished, and appropriately styled for a place of business. If you are a man, wear slacks (not jeans), a button-down shirt or a polo shirt, and a belt, and possibly a sport jacket if the weather is cool. A tie is optional. If you are a woman, wear a skirt (or dress slacks) and a blouse or a simple dress. Wear stockings, and make sure that the hem length of your skirt or dress is modest. Be aware that midriff tops and halter tops are not considered appropriate business attire.

You only have one chance to make a first impression, so make it a good one! If you have children, make arrangements for childcare so that you do not have to bring your children along with you to the interview. It is difficult to make a good impression during an interview if you are distracted by your childcare responsibilities. Give yourself adequate time to get to the interview. Ideally, you will arrive a few minutes early. Bring along a folder or briefcase containing certain key documents, such as a list of the questions you want to ask during the interview, an extra copy of your résumé and reference list, and your nursing assistant certification or registration. Before arriving at the facility, turn your cellular phone off and, if you were chewing gum, dispose of it.

After being introduced to the interviewer, shake his hand and take a seat when you are invited to do so. Do not address the interviewer by his first name, unless the interviewer specifically asks you to. Thank the person for the opportunity to interview at the beginning of the interview. During the interview, sit up straight and try not to fidget. You might be nervous and that is certainly understandable, but try to appear as confident and comfortable as you can under the circumstances. Maintain good eye contact during the interview and speak clearly. Common questions an interviewer might ask a candidate are listed in Box 45-1. Most interviewers will ask a potential employee about strengths and weaknesses. Think about this ahead of time, and be honest. We all have some terrific strengths and we also have our weaknesses. Remember that a person who is aware of a weakness can work to improve it. Try to answer questions concisely yet completely; it is best if you can strike a balance between listening and talking. If you do not know the answer to a question, simply say that you do not know—most interviewers are quick to recognize bluffing.

At the end of the interview, the interviewer will usually give you an opportunity to ask any ques-

---

BOX 45-1 Common Interview Questions

"Tell me about yourself. Why did you become a nursing assistant?"

"What part of your last job did you like the most? The least?"

"Why are you leaving your current job?" (or, "Why did you leave your last job?")

"What are you looking for in a manager?"

"How do you describe your work habits?"

"How do you set priorities?"

"How do you handle yourself under stress?"

"How do you handle problems with residents or co-workers?"

"Tell me about a specific situation that interfered with your ability to do your job, and how you handled it."

"What is the most satisfying workday you have had this year? Why?"

"Do you have a mentor? What have you learned from this person?"

"Who in your life would you consider to be 'successful'? Why?"

"What do you consider to be your greatest strength? Your greatest weakness?"

"Where do you want to go with your career? What steps have you taken to achieve your goal?"

"What is it about our organization that appeals to you?"

---

tions that you may have. Now is the time to refer to your list! Asking questions of your own indicates that you have an active interest in making sure that you are a good fit for the job and the organization. The interviewer may have discussed salary and benefits (medical benefits, dental benefits, retirement plans, holiday and sick time, schedule for pay increases) during the course of the interview, but if he did not, it is best not to ask about these things now. The proper time to discuss pay and benefits is when a job offer is made. When the interview is over, thank the interviewer again for his time, and for considering you for the position. If the interviewer did not mention when you can expect to hear from him regarding the position, it is acceptable to ask this question before leaving.

You should write a short thank-you note within 1 day of interviewing for the position, thanking the interviewer for considering you for the position and briefly explaining why you are excited about the possibility of working for his organization (Fig. 45-7). Everyone appreciates being complimented on his or her organization, and your interest in being a part of that organization is a compliment. You may hand-write your thank you

February 6, 2010

Dear Ms. Jones,

I would like to thank you for the opportunity to interview for the nursing assistant position at Sunny Hills Rehabilitation Center. I was impressed by the quality of your facility and the competence of your staff and would like very much to become a member of your health care team. I look forward to hearing from you in the near future.

Thank you,

Suzie Smith

Figure 45-7
After your interview, send a thank-you note to the person who interviewed you, thanking her for her time and restating your interest in the position and the organization.

note on a plain note card, or type it. As always, double-check your spelling and grammar!

As with dropping off the application, if you do not hear from the facility you interviewed with within the amount of time specified at the close of the interview, it is appropriate to follow up with a telephone call. When a representative of the organization calls to offer you a job, you can take this opportunity to ask any questions that may have occurred to you since the interview, or that were not appropriate to ask during the interview. If you need time to think about the offer, it is acceptable to ask the person who has offered you the job if

you can call him back with an answer within the next day or so.

Applying and interviewing for jobs can be a time-consuming process that requires a lot of effort. By taking the time to prepare, you increase your chances of finding a situation where you will be happy and satisfied with your work. Remember that getting the perfect job is just the beginning. Keeping the job and growing professionally are just as important. Remember the qualities that a person with a strong work ethic possesses? By demonstrating these qualities daily at work, you will quickly become a valuable member of the health care team. You will be open to learning new information and skills, which will help to keep your job fresh and challenging. When you are happy in your job, both you and your residents benefit.

LEAVING A JOB

Chances are, you will accept many different jobs over the course of your career. When leaving a job, give your employer at least 2 weeks' notice so that arrangements can be made to cover your shifts. Write a letter stating your desire to leave the job and the date of your last day on the job. Even if you were not happy at that particular place of employment, the professional thing to do is to thank your employer for the opportunity to work there. Leave on a positive note because you may need a reference from your present place of employment for a future job opportunity. You may even wish to work for your present employer again sometime in the future.

SUMMARY

- Advance planning about the type of employment you want helps to give your job search direction.
- The Internet, the telephone directory, and the newspaper are all tools you can use to find potential employers in your area. Friends, family members, and professional contacts (such as teachers or people you work with during your clinicals) may also know of job openings.
- Résumés, cover letters, and reference lists are key documents you prepare ahead of time.

- A résumé provides potential employers with information about your education and work history.
- A cover letter is your chance to introduce yourself to the employer and explain in more detail why you are interested in a particular job.
- A reference list contains names and contact information of people who would be willing to speak to the employer about your abilities.
- A job application is a standardized form that employers use to obtain basic information

about you. Job applications are legal documents.

- A job interview is an opportunity for the potential employer to evaluate you, and for you to evaluate the potential employer.

- A professional appearance and attitude are important.
- Being well-prepared for the interview and sending a thank-you note afterwards also help to make a good impression.

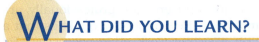

WHAT DID YOU LEARN?

Multiple Choice

Select the single best answer for each of the following questions.

1. A short, precise document with information about you, your work experience, and your education is called a:
   a. Minimum Data Set (MDS)
   b. Résumé
   c. Reference
   d. Cover letter

2. All of the following information should be included on your résumé, except for your:
   a. Name
   b. Address
   c. Employment history
   d. Religion

3. Which of the following should be included on a reference list?
   a. The reference's relationship to you
   b. Current contact information for the reference
   c. The hours you are available to work
   d. The questions you would like to ask during the interview

4. Which one of the following is a standardized form that is also a legal document used when applying for a job?
   a. Résumé
   b. Cover letter
   c. Reference list
   d. Job application

5. The chance for a potential employer to meet you personally occurs during the:
   a. Application process
   b. Interview process
   c. Job posting process
   d. Reference checking process

6. You are completing a job application. You should do all of the following except:
   a. Write neatly, in blue or black ink
   b. Provide information about your marital status when it is requested
   c. Sign the application when you are finished
   d. Provide information about your previous employment

STOP and Think!

- Raul is a nursing assistant student completing his clinical training in a long-term care facility. How could this experience benefit Raul in the future, when he begins to look for a paid position as a nursing assistant?

- Helene has worked at Sunny View Assisted Living for 6 months. Although she has

formed relationships with many of the residents there and generally enjoys her work, she is beginning to think that she might like to explore other long-term care environments. Do you have any advice for Helene as she looks to further define her career goals?

Nursing Assistants Make a Difference!

Wow, another busy day at the office! I am the Director of Nursing here at Sunrise Villa. I'm responsible for managing our nursing staff and making sure that the care they provide to our residents is of the highest quality. Yesterday, I interviewed six nursing assistants for an open position at our facility. I pride myself on making good hiring decisions whenever we have an open position, but especially when the position is for a nursing assistant. Nursing assistants are the staff members who spend the most time with the residents, so they really play an important role in ensuring our residents' happiness and well-being.

All of the candidates I interviewed yesterday seemed well-trained and eager to work here. It can be difficult to choose among so many good candidates! One thing I always tell a candidate during the interview is that I expect the care he or she gives to be good enough for my own mother. Then, I ask the candidate to explain how he or she would achieve that goal. One of yesterday's applicants, a young lady named Rachel, really impressed me with her answer. She didn't talk about how she would always go the extra mile to perform her daily duties with care, although that is important. No, what really impressed me was her comment that she would want to get to know my mother as a person—who she is and what she really likes. Then she talked about how she felt it was important for residents to feel that the person caring for them was doing her job because she loved it and cared about them, not just for a paycheck. The look on Rachel's face and the light in her eyes as she said this proved to me that she was speaking from her heart. Later, when I called the people on Rachel's reference list, they confirmed that Rachel was indeed one special nursing assistant and we would be very lucky to have her on our staff.

Well, needless to say, I offered Rachel the job today. After accepting it, she asked me why I had chosen her over the other qualified applicants. My answer was simple: "Because you really will be caring for my mother. She is a resident here."

You can listen to more stories about how nursing assistants make a difference on the CD in the front of your book.

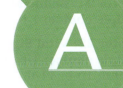

Answers to the
What Did You Learn? Exercises

Chapter 1: The Health Care System
Matching: 1-i, 2-f, 3-c, 4-h, 5-e, 6-d, 7-b, 8-a, 9-g, 10-j, 11-n, 12-m, 13-l, 14-k

Chapter 2: Overview of Long-Term Care
Multiple choice: 1-a, 2-a, 3-c, 4-b, 5-c
Matching: 1-i, 2-b, 3-a, 4-c, 5-h, 6-g, 7-j, 8-f, 9-e, 10-d

Chapter 3: The Nursing Assistant and The Nursing Team
Multiple choice: 1-c, 2-b, 3-c, 4-b, 5-b, 6-d, 7-b, 8-c, 9-c, 10-d, 11-a, 12-b, 13-c, 14-b

Chapter 4: Legal and Ethical Issues
Multiple choice: 1-b, 2-b, 3-b, 4-b, 5-d, 6-d, 7-c, 8-a, 9-b, 10-a, 11-d, 12-a
Matching: 1-e, 2-a, 3-d, 4-b, 5-c

Chapter 5: Communication Skills
Multiple choice: 1-b, 2-a, 3-d, 4-b, 5-c, 6-a, 7-c, 8-b, 9-b
Matching: 1-d, 2-a, 3-c, 4-b

Chapter 6: The Survey Process
Multiple choice: 1-b, 2-a, 3-a, 4-a, 5-a, 6-d, 7-b, 8-d
Matching: 1-c, 2-b, 3-d, 4-a, 5-g, 6-f, 7-e

Chapter 7: Understanding Human Needs
Multiple choice: 1-d, 2-a, 3-b, 4-c, 5-a, 6-d, 7-b, 8-c
Matching: 1-d, 2-c, 3-f, 4-g, 5-a, 6-b, 7-e

Chapter 8: The Long-Term Care Resident
Multiple choice: 1-d, 2-b, 3-d, 4-d, 5-a, 6-d, 7-a, 8-d, 9-d, 10-b
Matching: 1-g, 2-e, 3-b, 4-c, 5-f, 6-d, 7-a

Chapter 9: The Resident With Dementia
Multiple choice: 1-d, 2-a, 3-b, 4-c, 5-d, 6-b, 7-a, 8-b, 9-a, 10-d, 11-a, 12-a

Chapter 10: The Resident in Need of Rehabilitation and Restorative Care
Multiple choice: 1-d, 2-a, 3-c, 4-c, 5-b, 6-a, 7-c, 8-a, 9-b, 10-b

Chapter 11: Assisting With Admissions, Transfers, and Discharges
Multiple choice: 1-d, 2-b, 3-a, 4-d, 5-b, 6-c, 7-c, 8-c, 9-c

Chapter 12: Assisting With Assessments and Care Planning
Multiple choice: 1-c, 2-b, 3-a, 4-d, 5-c, 6-a, 7-d

Chapter 13: Providing Customer Service
Multiple choice: 1-c, 2-a, 3-b, 4-a, 5-a, 6-b, 7-a

Chapter 14: The Resident's Environment
Multiple choice: 1-c, 2-d, 3-c, 4-b, 5-a, 6-b, 7-d
Matching: 1-e, 2-d, 3-a, 4-b, 5-c

Chapter 15: Communicable Disease and Infection Control
Multiple choice: 1-d, 2-b, 3-b, 4-a, 5-d, 6-c, 7-d, 8-d, 9-a, 10-c, 11-b, 12-b, 13-c
Matching: 1-c, 2-d, 3-f, 4-g, 5-e, 6-a, 7-h, 8-I, 9-j, 10-b

Chapter 16: Bloodborne and Airborne Pathogens
Multiple choice: 1-d, 2-d, 3-d, 4-b

Chapter 17: Workplace Safety
Multiple choice: 1-a, 2-b, 3-d, 4-b, 5-c, 6-c, 7-c, 8-a, 9-a, 10-c, 11-b, 12-b, 13-b, 14-d, 15-b

Chapter 18: Resident Safety
Multiple choice: 1-a, 2-d, 3-b, 4-c, 5-d, 6-b, 7-b, 8-a, 9-c, 10-b, 11-c, 12-d

Chapter 19: Basic First Aid and Emergency Care
Multiple choice: 1-d, 2-b, 3-c, 4-c, 5-b, 6-d, 7-d, 8-d
Matching: 1-g, 2-f, 3-i, 4-b, 5-c, 6-e, 7-j, 8-h, 9-d, 10-a

Chapter 20: Positioning, Lifting, and Transferring Residents
Multiple choice: 1-a, 2-a, 3-d, 4-c, 5-d, 6-d, 7-d, 8-c, 9-b, 10-c, 11-d, 12-b, 13-d, 14-c, 15-d, 16-a

Chapter 21: Bedmaking
Multiple choice: 1-b, 2-d, 3-c, 4-c, 5-c, 6-a, 7-d

Chapter 22: Vital Signs, Height, and Weight
Multiple choice: 1-c, 2-a, 3-b, 4-c, 5-d, 6-d, 7-a, 8-d, 9-d, 10-b, 11-d, 12-b, 13-b

Chapter 23: Cleanliness and Hygiene
Multiple choice: 1-a, 2-c, 3-d, 4-d, 5-c, 6-d, 7-b, 8-a, 9-d, 10-d, 11-d, 12-c
Matching: 1-f, 2-e, 3-c, 4-b, 5-d, 6-a

Chapter 24: Grooming
Multiple choice: 1-c, 2-a, 3-a, 4-c, 5-b, 6-d, 7-d, 8-c, 9-d, 10-c, 11-a, 12-d
Matching: 1-d, 2-b, 3-e, 4-c, 5-a

Chapter 25: Basic Nutrition
Multiple choice: 1-c, 2-b, 3-c, 4-b, 5-b, 6-a, 7-c, 8-c, 9-b, 10-c, 11-b, 12-d
Matching: 1-c, 2-f, 3-a, 4-e, 5-d, 6-b

Chapter 26: Urinary and Bowel Elimination
Multiple choice: 1-b, 2-a, 3-a, 4-a, 5-c, 6-d, 7-b, 8-d, 9-a, 10-c, 11-a, 12-a
Matching: 1-i, 2-j, 3-e, 4-f, 5-b, 6-c, 7-g, 8-d, 9-h, 10-a

Chapter 27: Comfort, Rest, and Sleep
Multiple choice: 1-d, 2-c, 3-d, 4-c, 5-b, 6-a, 7-c, 8-b, 9-b, 10-c
Matching: 1-f, 2-h, 3-g, 4-a, 5-e, 6-b, 7-c, 8-d

Chapter 28: Caring for People During the End-of-Life Period
Multiple choice: 1-d, 2-d, 3-d, 4-a, 5-c, 6-d

Chapter 29: Caring for People Who Are Dying
Multiple choice: 1-c, 2-c, 3-b, 4-b, 5-a, 6-d, 7-b, 8-a
Matching: 1-d, 2-e, 3-b, 4-c, 5-a

Chapter 30: Basic Body Structure and Function
Multiple choice: 1-d, 2-c, 3-d, 4-a, 5-c
Matching: 1-c, 2-g, 3-a, 4-h, 5-b, 6-e, 7-d, 8-f

Chapter 31: The Integumentary System
Multiple choice: 1-d, 2-c, 3-a, 4-d, 5-b, 6-d, 7-b, 8-a, 9-b
Matching: 1-g, 2-j, 3-i, 4-f, 5-a, 6-h, 7-e, 8-d, 9-c, 10-b

Chapter 32: The Musculoskeletal System
Multiple choice: 1-b, 2-b, 3-d, 4-b, 5-d, 6-b, 7-d, 8-c, 9-b, 10-b, 11-a, 12-c
Matching: 1-f, 2-c, 3-d, 4-e, 5-b, 6-a

Chapter 33: The Respiratory System
Multiple choice: 1-c, 2-c, 3-d, 4-a, 5-c, 6-a, 7-b, 8-d

Matching: 1-f, 2-g, 3-e, 4-a, 5-d, 6-b, 7-I, 8-c, 9-j, 10-h

Chapter 34: The Cardiovascular System
Multiple choice: 1-a, 2-d, 3-b, 4-d, 5-b, 6-d, 7-a, 8-d, 9-b, 10-d
Matching:
   Set 1: 1-g, 2-d, 3-h, 4-j, 5-a, 6-b, 7-c, 8-i, 9-e, 10-f
   Set 2: 1-e, 2-a, 3-f, 4-g, 5-c, 6-d, 7-b

Chapter 35: The Nervous System
Multiple choice: 1-b, 2-a, 3-b, 4-d, 5-c, 6-b, 7-c, 8-c, 9-a, 10-a
Matching: 1-g, 2-i, 3-b, 4-h, 5-a, 6-c, 7-e, 8-d, 9-f

Chapter 36: The Sensory System
Multiple choice: 1-b, 2-b, 3-c, 4-d, 5-d, 6-a, 7-b, 8-a
Matching: 1-c, 2-b, 3-g, 4-a, 5-e, 6-h, 7-d, 8-f, 9-i, 10-j

Chapter 37: The Endocrine System
Multiple choice: 1-d, 2-a, 3-b, 4-b, 5-d, 6-a
Matching: 1-h, 2-b, 3-c, 4-i, 5-e, 6-f, 7-g, 8-j, 9-a, 10-d

Chapter 38: The Digestive System
Multiple choice: 1-c, 2-d, 3-c, 4-a, 5-a, 6-d, 7-c

Chapter 39: The Urinary System
Multiple choice: 1-b, 2-d, 3-c, 4-a, 5-a, 6-a, 7-b, 8-d, 9-b, 10-b
Matching: 1-e, 2-d, 3-a, 4-b, 5-c

Chapter 40: The Reproductive System
Multiple choice: 1-d, 2-b, 3-a, 4-d
Matching: 1-c, 2-e, 3-h, 4-g, 5-d, 6-f, 7-a, 8-b, 9-i

Chapter 41: Caring for People With Developmental Disabilities
Multiple choice: 1-b, 2-b, 3-a, 4-b, 5-c, 6-a, 7-c, 8-b, 9-b, 10-c

Chapter 42: Caring for People With Mental Illness
Multiple choice: 1-c, 2-b, 3-a, 4-b, 5-b, 6-a
Matching: 1-e, 2-b, 3-d, 4-c, 5-g, 6-f, 7-a

Chapter 43: Caring for People With Cancer
Multiple choice: 1-a, 2-d, 3-b
Matching: 1-c, 2-e, 3-a, 4-f, 5-b, 6-g, 7-d

Chapter 44: Caring for People With HIV/AIDS
Multiple choice: 1-d, 2-a, 3-d, 4-c, 5-b

Chapter 45: Job-Seeking Skills
Multiple choice: 1-b, 2-d, 3-b, 4-d, 5-b, 6-b

Introduction to the Language of Health Care

All professions have their own sets of words and abbreviations that are used to describe objects and situations that are specific to that particular profession. The health care profession is no different. In fact, the health care profession has so many unique words and abbreviations, you might think that health care professionals are speaking a different language from everyone else!

Understanding the words and abbreviations that are unique to the health care profession is essential if you expect to be able to communicate effectively with the other members of the health care team. Not knowing these words and abbreviations will make it difficult for you to read and follow orders for resident care. In addition, you will need to know these words and abbreviations to accurately record and report.

In this appendix, you will learn some tricks that will allow you to figure out the meaning of many unfamiliar words you may hear or read. We will also introduce you to some commonly used medical words and abbreviations. Finally, you should always make it a point to look up new words or abbreviations in a medical dictionary as soon as you hear or read them. Or, you can ask the nurse to explain the meaning of the word or abbreviation to you. Before long, you will become very comfortable using and understanding the language of the health care profession!

MEDICAL TERMINOLOGY

Although the strange-sounding language of the health care profession may seem overwhelming at first, it is really quite easy to pick up. Some medical words come from the names of people (for example, Down syndrome, Alzheimer's disease, Parkinson's disease). Other words come from Greek or Latin words, just as many everyday English, Spanish, French, and Italian words do. For example, you know what a rhinoceros looks like, right? A rhinoceros is a large animal with a huge horn growing out of its nose (Fig. B-1). *Rhin-* comes from the Greek word for "nose," and *-ceros* comes from the Greek word *keras*, or "horn." Now, where else might you find the Greek word *rhin-*? Well, if the mucous membranes on the inside of your nose are inflamed because you have a cold or allergies, the doctor might say that you have *rhinitis* (*rhin-*, nose + *itis*, inflammation). If a movie star has had a "nose job," then her publicist may tell the press that the celebrity has had *rhinoplasty*, the medical term for a nose job (*rhin-*, nose + *-plasty*, surgical repair).

Perhaps you have noticed a pattern here. Big words can be broken down into smaller parts, and if you know the meaning of the individual parts, you can figure out the meaning of the entire word. There are four types of word parts (Fig. B-2):

- **Roots** contain the essential, basic meaning of the word. For example, *cardi-* means "heart." Common roots are listed in Table B-1, at the end of this appendix.
- **Suffixes** are attached to the end of a root to make the root more specific. For example, *carditis* is "inflammation of the heart" (*cardi-*, heart + *-itis*, inflammation). Common suffixes are listed in Table B-2, at the end of this appendix.
- **Prefixes** are attached to the beginning of a root to make the root more specific. For example, *pericarditis* is "inflammation of the sac that surrounds the heart" (*peri-*, around + *cardi-*, heart + *-itis*, inflammation). Common prefixes are listed in Table B-3, at the end of this appendix.
- **Combining vowels** are often added in between the root and the suffix to make the new word easier to pronounce. When a word has more than one root, combining vowels may also be used between the roots. For example, *cardiomyopathy* is "disease of the heart muscle" (*cardi-*, heart + *o* + *my-*,

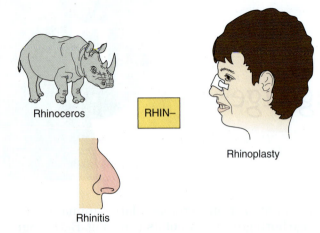

Figure B-1

Many of the words you use in everyday conversation have the same Greek or Latin origins as medical words that you may be less familiar with. For example, the Greek word *rhin-* means "nose." You see *rhin-* in words such as *rhinoceros, rhinitis,* and *rhinoplasty.* When you are trying to figure out the meaning of a new medical word, think about similar-sounding words that you may already know!

muscle + *o* + *-pathy,* disease). The combining vowel is usually "o," but "a" or "i" may also be used sometimes. The combining vowel that is used most often with each root is listed in Table B-1.

You will come across many medical words as you study each chapter in this textbook. When you come across a term in your reading that is new to you, try using what you have learned about the different word parts to guess at the

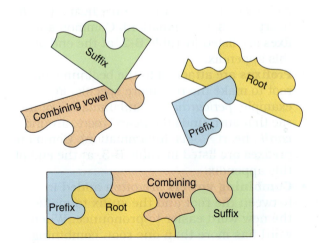

Figure B-2

Big words can be broken down into smaller parts, and if you know the meaning of the individual parts, then you can figure out the meaning of the entire word.

word's meaning. Then look up the word in the glossary and see how well you did!

ANATOMICAL TERMS

Anatomy is the study of the structure of the body. To describe the location of one body part in relation to another, health care professionals use specific terms. To ensure that these terms always have the same meaning to everyone, we always imagine the body to be in *normal anatomical position* when we describe it. A person who is in normal anatomical position is standing upright and facing forward, with his feet slightly spread apart, and with his arms to the sides and the palms facing forward (Fig. B-3). *Anatomical planes* are used as standard points of reference when describing the body. A *plane* is a flat surface, like a pane of glass. Health care professionals use three main imaginary planes to divide the body (Fig. B-4):

- The **sagittal plane** is a vertical plane that divides the body into right and left sides. A sagittal plane that divides the body into exact right and left halves is sometimes called the *mid-sagittal plane.*

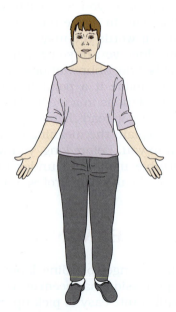

Figure B-3

When describing the location of one part of the body in relation to another, we imagine the body to be in normal anatomical position. In normal anatomical position, the person is standing upright, facing forward, with the legs slightly apart and the arms at the sides, with the palms facing forward.

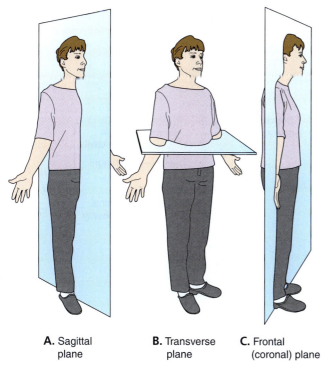

A. Sagittal plane   **B.** Transverse plane   **C.** Frontal (coronal) plane

Figure B-4

The body is divided into imaginary planes, which are used as points of reference when describing the location of one body part with relation to another. **(A)** The sagittal plane is a vertical plane that divides the body into right and left segments. Shown here is the mid-sagittal plane, which divides the body into equal right and left halves. **(B)** The transverse plane is a horizontal plane that divides the body into upper and lower segments. **(C)** The frontal (coronal) plane is a vertical plane that divides the body into front and back segments.

- The **transverse plane** is a horizontal plane that divides the body into upper and lower segments.
- The **frontal (coronal)** plane is a vertical plane that divides the body into front and back segments.

DIRECTIONAL TERMS

When describing the body, health care professionals often need to describe something that is above, under, to the side of, or further away from something else. To do this, they use standard directional terms. Directional terms are used to describe the location of one body part in relation to another. When we use directional terms, we need a point of reference that stays the same. If not, just changing a person's body position would change a directional reference. This is where normal anatomical position and the anatomical planes come in.

Using the anatomical planes as reference points gives us the following directional terms (Fig. B-5):

- **Medial:** closer to the mid-sagittal plane of the body (toward the inner side). For example, the nose is medial to the eyes.
- **Lateral:** further away from the mid-sagittal plane of the body (toward the outer side). For example, the ears are lateral to the nose.
- **Superior:** closer to the top of the body (closer to the head). For example, the chin is superior to the breast.

Figure B-5

Directional terms are used to describe the location of one body part in relation to another.

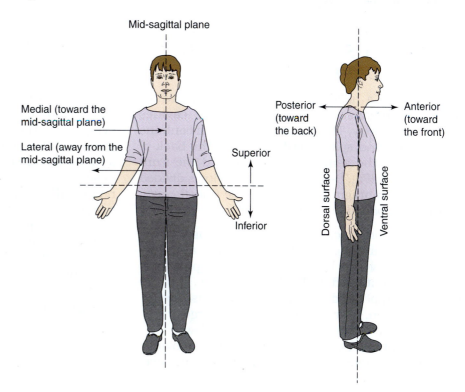

Mid-sagittal plane

Medial (toward the mid-sagittal plane)

Lateral (away from the mid-sagittal plane)

Superior

Inferior

Posterior (toward the back)

Anterior (toward the front)

Dorsal surface

Ventral surface

- **Inferior:** further away from the top of the body (closer to the feet). For example, the belly button is inferior to the breast.
- **Anterior:** toward the front, or *ventral surface*, of the body. For example, the abdomen is anterior to the buttocks.
- **Posterior:** toward the back, or *dorsal surface*, of the body. For example, the buttocks are posterior to the abdomen.

Two other directional terms are used to describe the location of one body part in relation to another. These terms describe the relationship between parts of the extremities (the arms and legs) and their points of attachment to the body (the shoulders and hips):

- **Proximal:** closer to the point of origin in relation to something else (for example, the elbow is proximal to the wrist)
- **Distal:** further away from the point of origin in relation to something else (for example, the wrist is distal to the elbow)

Like other words used in the health care profession, many of these directional terms have similar meanings to words you use every day. For example, *distal* sounds like *distant*, or "further away." Similarly, *proximal* sounds like *proximity*, which means "close by." If you find the terms *ventral* and *dorsal* hard to remember, just think of a shark swimming close to the surface of the water. The shark's dorsal fin, the fin located on the shark's back, is usually visible above the water.

TERMS USED TO DESCRIBE BODY CAVITIES

A *cavity* is a hollow space. In the body, cavities contain organs. There are two major cavities inside the body. The *dorsal cavity*, which contains the brain and spinal cord, is toward the back of the body. The *ventral cavity* is toward the front of the body (Fig. B-6). The ventral cavity is divided by the diaphragm into the *thoracic (chest) cavity* and the *abdominal (belly) cavity*.

- The thoracic cavity contains the lungs, the heart, and the large blood vessels that enter and leave the heart. Most of the esophagus is also contained in the thoracic cavity.
- The upper abdominal cavity contains the stomach, liver, pancreas, spleen, large intestine, and small intestine. The lower abdominal cavity contains the urinary bladder, the rectum, and the female reproductive

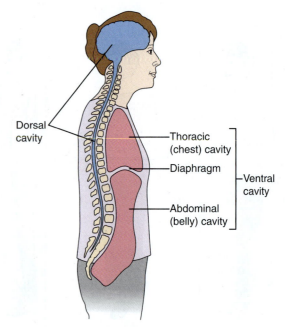

Figure B-6
The body has two major cavities, the dorsal cavity (*blue*) and the ventral cavity (*pink*). The diaphragm divides the ventral cavity into the thoracic (chest) cavity and the abdominal (belly) cavity.

organs. The kidneys lie behind the abdominal cavity. Sometimes the upper and lower abdominal cavity are referred to together as the *abdominopelvic cavity*.

TERMS USED TO DESCRIBE THE ABDOMINAL AREA

Many residents will experience pain or discomfort in the abdominal area. Often, knowing exactly where the pain or discomfort is occurring can provide clues to the source of the person's symptoms. Therefore, health care professionals use a number of different words to describe the abdominal area. The abdominal area can be described in terms of quadrants (fourths) or regions (Fig. B-7). Quadrants are typically used to describe general information, such as where a person is experiencing pain. Regions are used when it is necessary to be very specific (for example, when describing where an incision is located).

Quadrants

Quad means "four." The simplest way to describe the abdominal area is to divide it into fourths, or quadrants. The quadrants are named according

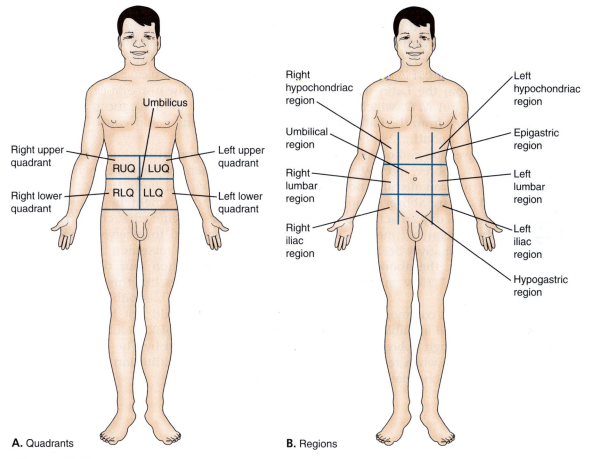

Figure B-7
The abdominal area can be described in terms of **(A)** quadrants or **(B)** regions. (Remember that when you are using the terms *right* and *left*, these terms are used in relation to the resident's right or left, not your right or left.)

to their location: right upper quadrant (RUQ), left upper quadrant (LUQ), right lower quadrant (RLQ), and left lower quadrant (LLQ). By using these quadrants as reference, you can describe where your resident is experiencing pain by saying, "Mrs. Jones is complaining of a sharp pain in her RUQ."

Regions

The abdomen can also be divided into smaller sections, called *regions*, for the purpose of description. There are nine regions (three rows of three):

- The upper row consists of the right and left hypochondriac regions and the epigastric region. The hypochondriac regions are named for their relationship to the ribs: *hypo-* means "below" and *chondr/o-* means "cartilage" (of the ribs). The epigastric region is named for its relation to the stomach: *epi-* means "above" and *gastric* means "stomach."

- The middle row consists of the right and left lumbar regions and the umbilical region. The right and left lumbar regions are named for the region of the spinal column in that area. The umbilical region is named for the umbilicus, or belly button.
- The lower row consists of the right and left iliac regions and the hypogastric region. The iliac regions are named after the iliac crest, the bone that forms the hip bones. The iliac regions are also sometimes called the inguinal (groin) regions. The hypogastric region is named for its relation to the stomach: *hypo-* means "below" and *gastric* means "stomach."

ABBREVIATIONS

Abbreviations are shortened versions of words or phrases. Health care professionals use abbreviations to make recording more efficient. Some abbreviations come from English words. For example, you just learned that *RUQ* means "right upper quadrant." Other abbreviations come from Latin or Greek words, and therefore may seem foreign at first. For example, *bid* is the abbreviation for "twice daily," from the Latin words **b**is (twice) **in** (a) **d**ie (day). And *NPO*, which means "nothing by mouth," comes from the Latin words **n**ils (nothing) **p**er (by) **o**s (mouth). As with other terms used in health care, you can often remember the meaning of a new abbreviation by relating it to an everyday word that you already know. For example, *bid, tid,* and *qid* are abbreviations that describe how many times a day an action is to be carried out. The abbreviation *bid* means "twice daily." Now think of how many wheels a *bi*cycle has: two, right? Similarly, the abbreviation *tid* means "three times daily." How many wheels does a *tri*cycle have?

Abbreviations that are commonly used in health care settings are listed in Table B-4, at the end of this appendix. Although abbreviations can help us save time and space when recording, it is very important to use only abbreviations that are

approved for use in your facility. Otherwise, other members of the health care team may be confused by your meaning. In addition, if you are unsure of the meaning of an abbreviation that you read in a resident's care plan, please either look the abbreviation up or ask the nurse to explain it to you. It is important not to just guess at the meaning, because guessing could cause harm to the resident.

Some abbreviations are easy to confuse, especially when they are handwritten. For example, *qd* (daily), *qid* (four times a day), and *qod* (every other day) might be easily mistaken for one another. Imagine what could happen if a resident is supposed to receive a medication daily (*qd*) but someone misreads the abbreviation and gives the medication four times a day (*qid*)! To help prevent errors like this from occurring, The Joint Commission has published a list of abbreviations that should not be used (Table B-5A; also see Table B-5B). Health care organizations that are accredited by The Joint Commission or are seeking accreditation will not use these abbreviations.

Table B-1   Common Roots and Their Combining Vowels

ROOT / COMBINING VOWEL	MEANING	ROOT / COMBINING VOWEL	MEANING
abdomin / o	abdomen	col / o	colon
aden / o	gland	cost / o	ribs
adip / o	fat	crani / o	cranium (skull)
adren / o	adrenal glands	cutane / o	skin
angi / o	vessel (usually blood or lymph)	cyan / o	blue
arteri / o	artery	cyst / o	bladder
arthr / o	joint	dent / o	teeth
blephar / o	eyelid	dermat / o	skin
bronchi / o	bronchus	dipl / o	double
calc / o	calcium	electr / o	electric
carcin / o	cancer	encephal / o	brain
cardi / o	heart	enter / o	intestine (usually the small intestine)
cephal / o	head	erythr / o	red
cerebr / o	cerebrum (brain)	esophag / o	esophagus
chol / e	bile, gall	femor / o	femur (thigh bone)
cholecyst / o	gallbladder	gastr / o	stomach
choledoch / o	bile duct	gingiv / o	gum
chondr / o	cartilage	gluc / o	sugar, glucose

(continued)

Table B-1 Common Roots and Their Combining Vowels (continued)

ROOT / COMBINING VOWEL	MEANING	ROOT / COMBINING VOWEL	MEANING
glyc / o	sugar, glucose	pancreat / o	pancreas
gynec / o	woman, female	pelv / i / o	pelvis
hemangi / o	blood vessel	pharyng / o	pharynx (throat)
hemat / o	blood	phleb / o	vein
hepat / o	liver	pleur / o	pleura
hydr / o	water	pneum / o	lung, air
hyster / o	uterus	proct / o	anus, rectum
irid / o	iris	pyel / o	renal pelvis
lapar / o	abdomen	radi / o	x-rays, radiation
laryng / o	larynx (voice box)	ren / o	kidney
leuk / o	white	retin / o	retina
lingu / o	tongue	rhin / o	nose
lip / o	fat	salping / o	fallopian tube
lith / o	stone, calculus	scler / o	hardening, sclera (white of the eye)
lumb / o	lower back	sigmoid / o	sigmoid colon
lymphangi / o	lymph vessel	spermat / o	sperm
lymph / o	lymph	spin / o	spine
mamm / o	breast	spondyl / o	vertebra (backbone)
mast / o	breast	stern / o	sternum (breastbone)
megal / o	enlargement	stomat / o	mouth
melan / o	black	tend / o	tendon
mening / o	meninges	therm / o	heat
men / o	menses, menstruation	thorac / o	chest
muc / o	mucus	thromb / o	blood clot
myel / o	spinal cord, bone marrow	thyr / o	thyroid gland
my / o	muscle	toxic, tox / o	poison
myring / o	tympanic membrane (eardrum)	trache / o	trachea (windpipe)
nas / o	nose	tympan / o	tympanic membrane (eardrum)
necr / o	death	ureter / o	ureter
nephr / o	kidney	urethr / o	urethra
neur / o	nerve	ur / o	urine
noct / o	night	uter / o	uterus
odont / o	teeth	vagin / o	vagina
oophor / o	ovary	vascul / o	blood vessel
ophthalm / o	eye	vas / o	vas deferens, vessel
orchi / o	testis	ven / o	vein
os / o	mouth	ventricul / o	ventricle (of brain or heart)
oste / o	bone	vesic / o	bladder
ot / o	ear	vertebr / o	vertebra (backbone)

Table B-2   Common Suffixes

SUFFIX	MEANING	SUFFIX	MEANING
-al	pertaining to	-oid	resembling
-algia	pain	-oma	tumor
-ar, -ary	pertaining to	-opia	vision
-cele	hernia, swelling	-osis	abnormal condition
-centesis	surgical puncture	-pathy	disease
-cyte	cell	-pause	cessation
-derma	skin	-penia	decrease
-dipsia	thirst	-pepsia	digestion
-ectomy	excision, removal of	-pexy	fixation
-edema	swelling	-phagia	swallow, eat
-emesis	vomiting	-phasia	speech
-emia	blood	-phobia	fear
-gram	record	-plasty	surgical repair
-graphy	process of recording	-plegia	paralysis
-ia	condition	-pnea	breathing
-ic	pertaining to	-rrhaphy	suture
-ism	condition	-rrhea	flow, discharge
-ist	specialist	-scope	instrument to view
-itis	inflammation	-scopy	visual examination
-lith	stone, calculus	-stenosis	structure, narrowing
-logist	specialist in the study of	-stomy	forming a new opening
-logy	study of	-therapy	treatment
-lysis	separation, destruction, loosening	-tome	instrument to cut
-malacia	softening	-tomy	incision, cut into
-megaly	enlargement	-tripsy	crushing
-meter	measure, instrument for measuring	-uria	urine, urination

Table B-3   Common Prefixes

PREFIX	MEANING	PREFIX	MEANING
a- , an-	without, not, absent	hypo-	under, below
ab	away from	inter-	between
amb-, ambi-	both, on two sides	intra-	within
auto-	self	macro-	large
bi-	two, double	micro-	small
brady-	slow	neo-	new
dys-	bad, painful, difficult	para-	near, beside, around
epi-	above, upon	peri-	around
hemi-	half, partly	poly-	many, much
hyper-	excessive	post-	after, behind

(continued)

Table B-3   Common Prefixes (continued)

PREFIX	MEANING	PREFIX	MEANING
pre-	before	supra-	above
quadri-	four	tachy-	rapid
sub-	under, below	tri-	three

Table B-4   Common Medical Abbreviations

ABBREVIATION	MEANING	ABBREVIATION	MEANING
Ab	antibody	cc	cubic centimeter
abd	abdomen	CCU	coronary care unit
ac	before a meal	CHD	coronary heart disease
ADL	activities of daily living	CHF	congestive heart failure
ad lib	as desired	cl liq	clear liquids
Adm (adm)	admitted or admission	CNA	certified nursing assistant
AFB	acid-fast bacillus (usually tuberculosis)	c/o	complains of
AIDS	acquired immunodeficiency syndrome	COPD	chronic obstructive pulmonary disease
AKA	above-the-knee amputation	CPR	cardiopulmonary resuscitation
AM (am)	morning	CVA	cerebral vascular accident (stroke)
amb	ambulate, ambulatory	dc (d/c)	discontinue
AMI	acute myocardial infarction (heart attack)	disch	discharge
amt	amount	DJD	degenerative joint disease
ap	apical	DNR	do not resuscitate
approx	approximately	DOA	dead on arrival
ASAP	as soon as possible	DOB	date of birth
as tol	as tolerated	DON	director of nursing
ax	axillary	drsg	dressing
bid	twice a day	Dx	diagnosis
BKA	below-the-knee amputation	ECG (EKG)	electrocardiogram
BM (bm)	bowel movement	EEG	electroencephalogram
BP, B/P	blood pressure	ER	emergency room
B.R.	bed rest	F	Fahrenheit
BRP	bathroom privileges	FBS	fasting blood sugar
BSC	bedside commode	FF	force fluids
C	centigrade, Celsius	fl (fld)	fluid
c̄	with	ft	foot or feet
CA	cancer	Fx	fracture
cath	catheter, catheterize	gal	gallon
CBC	complete blood count	GB	gallbladder
CBR	complete bed rest	GI	gastrointestinal
		GSW	gunshot wound
		GU	genitourinary

(continued)

Table B-4	Common Medical Abbreviations (continued)		
ABBREVIATION	**MEANING**	**ABBREVIATION**	**MEANING**
h (hr)	hour	O	oral
H_2O	water	OR	operating room
HBV	hepatitis B virus	OT	occupational therapy
HIV	human immunodeficiency virus	oz (Oz)	ounce
HOB	head of bed	PAR	post anesthesia recovery
HS (hs)	hour of sleep (bedtime)	pc	after a meal
ht	height	Peds	pediatrics
ICU	intensive care unit	per	by, through
IDDM	insulin-dependent diabetes mellitus	PM (pm)	afternoon or evening
in	inch	po (per os)	by mouth
I&O	intake and output	post op	postoperative
IV	intravenous	pre op	preoperative
L	left, liter	prep	preparation
lab	laboratory	prn	as necessary
lb	pound	Pt (pt)	patient
lg	large	PT	physical therapy
liq	liquid	q	every
LLQ	left lower quadrant	qd	every day
LMP	last menstrual period	qh	every hour
LPN	licensed practical nurse	q2h, q3h, q4h, etc.	every 2 hours, every 3 hours, every 4 hours, etc.
lt	left	qhs	every night at bedtime
LVN	licensed vocational nurse	qid	four times a day
LUQ	left upper quadrant	qod	every other day
meds	medications	qs	sufficient quantity
MI	myocardial infarction (heart attack)	qt	quiet
mid noc	midnight	R	rectal
min	minute	RBC	red blood cell, red blood cell count
ml	milliliter	rehab	rehabilitation
NA	nursing assistant	resp	respiration
NB	newborn	RLQ	right lower quadrant
neg	negative	RN	registered nurse
NIDDM	non-insulin–dependent diabetes mellitus	ROM	range of motion
nil	none	RR	recovery room
no	number	rt (R)	right
noc, noct	night	RT	respiratory therapy
NPO (npo)	nothing per mouth (nils per os)	RUQ	right upper quadrant
N&V	nausea and vomiting	Rx	treatment
O_2	oxygen	s̄	without
OB	obstetrics	s̄s̄	half
OJ	orange juice	SOB	shortness of breath
OOB	out of bed	Spec (spec)	specimen

(continued)

Table B-4   Common Medical Abbreviations (continued)

ABBREVIATION	MEANING	ABBREVIATION	MEANING
SSE	soapsuds enema	Tx	treatment
ST	speech therapy	ty	tympanic
STAT, stat	at once, immediately	UA (u/a)	urinalysis
STD	sexually transmitted disease	UK	unknown
Surg	surgery	URI	upper respiratory infection
Sx	symptoms	UTI	urinary tract infection
tbsp	tablespoon	VS (vs)	vital signs
tid	three times a day	WA	while awake
TIA	transient ischemic attack	WBC	white blood cell, white blood cell count
TLC	tender loving care		
TPN	total parenteral nutrition	w/c	wheelchair
TPR	temperature, pulse, and respirations	WNL	within normal limits
tsp	teaspoon	wt	weight

Table B-5A   The Joint Commission's Official "Do Not Use" List

DO NOT USE	POTENTIAL PROBLEM	USE INSTEAD
U (unit)	Mistaken for "0" (zero), the number "4" (four), or "cc"	Write "unit"
IU (International Unit)	Mistaken for IV (intravenous) or the number 10 (ten)	Write "International Unit"
Q.D., QD, q.d., qd (daily)	Mistaken for each other	Write "daily"
Q.O.D., QOD, q.o.d, qod (every other day)	Period after the Q mistaken for "I" and the "O" mistaken for "I"	Write "every other day"
Trailing zero (X.0 mg)*	Decimal point is missed	Write X mg
Lack of leading zero (.X mg)		Write 0.X mg
MS	Can mean morphine sulfate or magnesium sulfate	Write "morphine sulfate"
MSO_4 and $MgSO_4$	Confused for one another	Write "magnesium sulfate"

This list applies to all orders and all medication-related documentation that is handwritten (including free-text computer entry) or on pre-printed forms.
*Exception: A "trailing zero" may be used only where required to demonstrate the level of precision of the value being reported, such as for laboratory results, imaging studies of lesions, or catheter/tube sizes. It may not be used in medication orders or other mdication-related documentation.

Source: The Joint Commission (2006).

Table B-5B	Additional Abbreviations, Acronyms, and Symbols for Possible Future Inclusion in the Official "Do Not Use" List

DO NOT USE	POTENTIAL PROBLEM	USE INSTEAD
> (greater than) < (less than)	Misinterpreted as the number "7"(seven) or the letter "L" Confused for one another	Write "greater than" Write "less than"
Abbreviations for drug names	Misinterpreted due to similar abbreviations for multiple drugs	Write drug names in full
Apothecary units	Unfamiliar to many practitioners Confused with metric units	Use metric units
@	Mistaken for the number "2" (two)	Write "at"
cc	Mistaken for U (units) when poorly written	Write "ml" or "milliliters"
μg	Mistaken for mg (milligrams), resulting in one thousand-fold overdose	Write "mcg" or "micrograms"

Source: The Joint Commission (2006).

The Minimum Data Set

The current version of the Minimum Data Set (MDS) is MDS 2.0. An updated version of the MDS, MDS 3.0, is expected to be put into use by October 2010, as this book is going to press. MDS 3.0 is expected to increase accuracy in the assessment process, and to provide greater focus on the issues important to the resident. However, the overall purpose and use of the MDS will remain the same.

Numeric Identifier_____

MINIMUM DATA SET (MDS) — *VERSION 2.0*
FOR NURSING HOME RESIDENT ASSESSMENT AND CARE SCREENING

BASIC ASSESSMENT TRACKING FORM

SECTION AA. IDENTIFICATION INFORMATION

1.	RESIDENT NAME⊛				
		a. (First)	**b.** (Middle Initial)	**c.** (Last)	**d.** (Jr/Sr)
2.	GENDER⊛	1. Male		2. Female	
3.	BIRTHDATE⊛	Month — Day — Year			
4.	RACE/ ETHNICITY	1. American Indian/Alaskan Native 4. Hispanic 2. Asian/Pacific Islander 5. White, not of 3. Black, not of Hispanic origin Hispanic origin			
5.	SOCIAL SECURITY⊛ AND MEDICARE NUMBERS⊚ [C in 1ˢᵗ box if non med. no.]	**a.** Social Security Number **b.** Medicare number (or comparable railroad insurance number)			
6.	FACILITY PROVIDER NO.⊛	**a.** State No. **b.** Federal No.			
7.	MEDICAID NO. ["+" if pending, "N" if not a Medicaid recipient]⊛				

8.	REASONS FOR ASSESS-MENT	[Note—Other codes do not apply to this form]
		a. Primary reason for assessment
		  1. Admission assessment (required by day 14)
		  2. Annual assessment
		  3. Significant change in status assessment
		  4. Significant correction of prior full assessment
		  5. Quarterly review assessment
		  10. Significant correction of prior quarterly assessment
		  0. *NONE OF ABOVE*
		
		b. *Codes for assessments required for Medicare PPS or the State*
		  1. Medicare 5 day assessment
		  2. Medicare 30 day assessment
		  3. Medicare 60 day assessment
		  4. Medicare 90 day assessment
		  5. Medicare readmission/return assessment
		  6. Other state required assessment
		  7. Medicare 14 day assessment
		  8. Other Medicare required assessment			

9. **Signatures of Persons who Completed a Portion of the Accompanying Assessment or Tracking Form**

I certify that the accompanying information accurately reflects resident assessment or tracking information for this resident and that I collected or coordinated collection of this information on the dates specified. To the best of my knowledge, this information was collected in accordance with applicable Medicare and Medicaid requirements. I understand that this information is used as a basis for ensuring that residents receive appropriate and quality care, and as a basis for payment from federal funds. I further understand that payment of such federal funds and continued partici- pation in the government-funded health care programs is conditioned on the accuracy and truthful- ness of this information, and that I may be personally subject to or may subject my organization to substantial criminal, civil, and/or administrative penalties for submitting false information. I also certify that I am authorized to submit this information by this facility on its behalf.

Signature and Title	Sections	Date
a.		
b.		
c.		
d.		
e.		
f.		
g.		
h.		
i.		
j.		
k.		
l.		

GENERAL INSTRUCTIONS

Complete this information for submission with all full and quarterly assessments (Admission, Annual, Significant Change, State or Medicare required assessments, or Quarterly Reviews, etc.)

⊛ = Key items for computerized resident tracking

☐ = When box blank, must enter number or letter   [a.] = When letter in box, check if condition applies

MDS 2.0 September, 2000

Resident _____   Numeric Identifier_____

MINIMUM DATA SET (MDS) — *VERSION 2.0*
FOR NURSING HOME RESIDENT ASSESSMENT AND CARE SCREENING

BACKGROUND (FACE SHEET) INFORMATION AT ADMISSION

SECTION AB. DEMOGRAPHIC INFORMATION

1.	DATE OF ENTRY	*Date the stay began. Note — Does not include readmission if record was closed at time of temporary discharge to hospital, etc. In such cases, use prior admission date*

☐☐ — ☐☐ — ☐☐☐☐
Month — Day — Year

2.	ADMITTED FROM (AT ENTRY)	1. Private home/apt. with no home health services 2. Private home/apt. with home health services 3. Board and care/assisted living/group home 4. Nursing home 5. Acute care hospital 6. Psychiatric hospital, MR/DD facility 7. Rehabilitation hospital 8. Other
3.	LIVED ALONE (PRIOR TO ENTRY)	0. No 1. Yes 2. In other facility
4.	ZIP CODE OF PRIOR PRIMARY RESIDENCE	☐☐☐☐☐
5.	RESIDEN-TIAL HISTORY 5 YEARS PRIOR TO ENTRY	(*Check all settings* resident **lived in** during 5 years prior to date of entry given in item AB1 above) Prior stay at this nursing home — a. Stay in other nursing home — b. Other residential facility—board and care home, assisted living, group home — c. MH/psychiatric setting — d. MR/DD setting — e. *NONE OF ABOVE* — f.
6.	LIFETIME OCCUPA-TION(S) [Put "/" between two occupations]	☐☐☐☐☐☐☐☐☐☐☐☐☐☐☐☐☐
7.	EDUCATION (*Highest Level Completed*)	1. No schooling 5. Technical or trade school 2. 8th grade/less 6. Some college 3. 9-11 grades 7. Bachelor's degree 4. High school 8. Graduate degree
8.	LANGUAGE	(*Code for correct response*) **a.** Primary Language 0. English 1. Spanish 2. French 3. Other **b.** If other, specify ☐☐☐☐☐☐☐☐
9.	MENTAL HEALTH HISTORY	Does resident's RECORD indicate any history of mental retardation, mental illness, or developmental disability problem? 0. No 1. Yes

10.	CONDITIONS RELATED TO MR/DD STATUS	(*Check all conditions* that are related to MR/DD status that were manifested before age 22, and are likely to continue indefinitely)
		Not applicable—no MR/DD (Skip to AB11) — a.
		MR/DD with organic condition
		  Down's syndrome — b.
		  Autism — c.
		  Epilepsy — d.
		  Other organic condition related to MR/DD — e.
		MR/DD with no organic condition — f.

11.	DATE BACK-GROUND INFORMA-TION COMPLETED	☐☐ — ☐☐ — ☐☐☐☐ Month — Day — Year

SECTION AC. CUSTOMARY ROUTINE

1.	CUSTOMARY ROUTINE (*In year prior to DATE OF ENTRY to this nursing home, or year last in community if now being admitted from another nursing home*)	(***Check all that apply.*** *If all information UNKNOWN, check last box only.*)

CYCLE OF DAILY EVENTS

Stays up late at night (e.g., after 9 pm)	a.
Naps regularly during day (at least 1 hour)	b.
Goes out 1+ days a week	c.
Stays busy with hobbies, reading, or fixed daily routine	d.
Spends most of time alone or watching TV	e.
Moves independently indoors (with appliances, if used)	f.
Use of tobacco products at least daily	g.
NONE OF ABOVE	h.

EATING PATTERNS

Distinct food preferences	i.
Eats between meals all or most days	j.
Use of alcoholic beverage(s) at least weekly	k.
NONE OF ABOVE	l.

ADL PATTERNS

In bedclothes much of day	m.
Wakens to toilet all or most nights	n.
Has irregular bowel movement pattern	o.
Showers for bathing	p.
Bathing in PM	q.
NONE OF ABOVE	r.

INVOLVEMENT PATTERNS

Daily contact with relatives/close friends	s.
Usually attends church, temple, synagogue (etc.)	t.
Finds strength in faith	u.
Daily animal companion/presence	v.
Involved in group activities	w.
NONE OF ABOVE	x.
UNKNOWN—Resident/family unable to provide information	y.

SECTION AD. FACE SHEET SIGNATURES

SIGNATURES OF PERSONS COMPLETING FACE SHEET:

a. Signature of RN Assessment Coordinator   Date

I certify that the accompanying information accurately reflects resident assessment or tracking information for this resident and that I collected or coordinated collection of this information on the dates specified. To the best of my knowledge, this information was collected in accordance with applicable Medicare and Medicaid requirements. I understand that this information is used as a basis for ensuring that residents receive appropriate and quality care, and as a basis for payment from federal funds. I further understand that payment of such federal funds and continued partici-pation in the government-funded health care programs is conditioned on the accuracy and truthful-ness of this information, and that I may be personally subject to or may subject my organization to substantial criminal, civil, and/or administrative penalties for submitting false information. I also certify that I am authorized to submit this information by this facility on its behalf.

Signature and Title	Sections	Date
b.		
c.		
d.		
e.		
f.		
g.		

☐ = When box blank, must enter number or letter   ☐a. = When letter in box, check if condition applies

MDS 2.0 September, 2000

Resident_____ Numeric Identifier_____

MINIMUM DATA SET (MDS) — *VERSION 2.0*
FOR NURSING HOME RESIDENT ASSESSMENT AND CARE SCREENING
FULL ASSESSMENT FORM
(Status in last 7 days, unless other time frame indicated)

SECTION A. IDENTIFICATION AND BACKGROUND INFORMATION

1.	RESIDENT NAME	
		a. (First)　　b. (Middle Initial)　　c. (Last)　　d. (Jr/Sr)

2.	ROOM NUMBER

3. ASSESSMENT REFERENCE DATE
a. Last day of MDS observation period
☐☐ — ☐☐ — ☐☐☐☐
Month　　Day　　Year
b. Original (0) or corrected copy of form (enter number of correction)

4a. DATE OF REENTRY — Date of reentry from most recent temporary discharge to a hospital in last 90 days (or since last assessment or admission if less than 90 days)
☐☐ — ☐☐ — ☐☐☐☐
Month　　Day　　Year

5. MARITAL STATUS
1. Never married　　3. Widowed　　5. Divorced
2. Married　　4. Separated

6. MEDICAL RECORD NO.

7. CURRENT PAYMENT SOURCES FOR N.H. STAY (Billing Office to indicate; **check all that apply in last 30 days**)
Medicaid per diem	a.	VA per diem	f.
Medicare per diem	b.	Self or family pays for full per diem	g.
Medicare ancillary part A	c.	Medicaid resident liability or Medicare co-payment	h.
Medicare ancillary part B	d.	Private insurance per diem (including co-payment)	i.
CHAMPUS per diem	e.	Other per diem	j.

8. REASONS FOR ASSESSMENT
[Note—If this is a discharge or reentry assessment, only a limited subset of MDS items need be completed]

a. Primary reason for assessment
1. Admission assessment (required by day 14)
2. Annual assessment
3. Significant change in status assessment
4. Significant correction of prior full assessment
5. Quarterly review assessment
6. Discharged—return not anticipated
7. Discharged—return anticipated
8. Discharged prior to completing initial assessment
9. Reentry
10. Significant correction of prior quarterly assessment
0. NONE OF ABOVE

b. Codes for assessments required for Medicare PPS or the State
1. Medicare 5 day assessment
2. Medicare 30 day assessment
3. Medicare 60 day assessment
4. Medicare 90 day assessment
5. Medicare readmission/return assessment
6. Other state required assessment
7. Medicare 14 day assessment
8. Other Medicare required assessment

9. RESPONSIBILITY/ LEGAL GUARDIAN (Check all that apply)
Legal guardian	a.	Durable power attorney/financial	d.
Other legal oversight	b.	Family member responsible	e.
Durable power of attorney/health care	c.	Patient responsible for self	f.
		NONE OF ABOVE	g.

10. ADVANCED DIRECTIVES (For those items with supporting **documentation** in the medical record, **check all that apply**)
Living will	a.	Feeding restrictions	f.
Do not resuscitate	b.	Medication restrictions	g.
Do not hospitalize	c.	Other treatment restrictions	h.
Organ donation	d.		
Autopsy request	e.	NONE OF ABOVE	i.

SECTION B. COGNITIVE PATTERNS

1. COMATOSE (Persistent vegetative state/no discernible consciousness)
0. No　　1. Yes　　(If yes, skip to Section G)

2. MEMORY (Recall of what was learned or known)
a. Short-term memory OK—seems/appears to recall after 5 minutes
0. Memory OK　　1. Memory problem
b. Long-term memory OK—seems/appears to recall long past
0. Memory OK　　1. Memory problem

3. MEMORY/ RECALL ABILITY (**Check all** that resident was **normally able to recall during last 7 days**)
Current season	a.		
Location of own room	b.	That he/she is in a nursing home	d.
Staff names/faces	c.	NONE OF ABOVE are recalled	e.

4. COGNITIVE SKILLS FOR DAILY DECISION-MAKING (Made decisions regarding tasks of daily life)
0. INDEPENDENT—decisions consistent/reasonable
1. MODIFIED INDEPENDENCE—some difficulty in new situations only
2. MODERATELY IMPAIRED—decisions poor; cues/supervision required
3. SEVERELY IMPAIRED—never/rarely made decisions

5. INDICATORS OF DELIRIUM— PERIODIC DISORDERED THINKING/ AWARENESS (Code for behavior in the last 7 days.) [Note: Accurate assessment requires conversations with staff and family who have direct knowledge of resident's behavior over this time].
0. Behavior not present
1. Behavior present, not of recent onset
2. Behavior present, over last 7 days appears different from resident's usual functioning (e.g., new onset or worsening)

a. EASILY DISTRACTED—(e.g., difficulty paying attention; gets sidetracked)
b. PERIODS OF ALTERED PERCEPTION OR AWARENESS OF SURROUNDINGS—(e.g., moves lips or talks to someone not present; believes he/she is somewhere else; confuses night and day)
c. EPISODES OF DISORGANIZED SPEECH—(e.g., speech is incoherent, nonsensical, irrelevant, or rambling from subject to subject; loses train of thought)
d. PERIODS OF RESTLESSNESS—(e.g., fidgeting or picking at skin, clothing, napkins, etc; frequent position changes; repetitive physical movements or calling out)
e. PERIODS OF LETHARGY—(e.g., sluggishness; staring into space; difficult to arouse; little body movement)
f. MENTAL FUNCTION VARIES OVER THE COURSE OF THE DAY—(e.g., sometimes better, sometimes worse; behaviors sometimes present, sometimes not)

6. CHANGE IN COGNITIVE STATUS Resident's cognitive status, skills, or abilities have changed as compared to status of **90 days ago** (or since last assessment if less than 90 days)
0. No change　　1. Improved　　2. Deteriorated

SECTION C. COMMUNICATION/HEARING PATTERNS

1. HEARING (With hearing appliance, if used)
0. HEARS ADEQUATELY—normal talk, TV, phone
1. MINIMAL DIFFICULTY when not in quiet setting
2. HEARS IN SPECIAL SITUATIONS ONLY—speaker has to adjust tonal quality and speak distinctly
3. HIGHLY IMPAIRED/absence of useful hearing

2. COMMUNICATION DEVICES/ TECHNIQUES (**Check all that apply** during last 7 days)
Hearing aid, present and used	a.
Hearing aid, present and not used regularly	b.
Other receptive comm. techniques used (e.g., lip reading)	c.
NONE OF ABOVE	d.

3. MODES OF EXPRESSION (**Check all used** by resident to make needs known)
Speech	a.	Signs/gestures/sounds	d.
Writing messages to express or clarify needs	b.	Communication board	e.
American sign language or Braille	c.	Other	f.
		NONE OF ABOVE	g.

4. MAKING SELF UNDERSTOOD (Expressing information content—however able)
0. UNDERSTOOD
1. USUALLY UNDERSTOOD—difficulty finding words or finishing thoughts
2. SOMETIMES UNDERSTOOD—ability is limited to making concrete requests
3. RARELY/NEVER UNDERSTOOD

5. SPEECH CLARITY (Code for speech in the last 7 days)
0. CLEAR SPEECH—distinct, intelligible words
1. UNCLEAR SPEECH—slurred, mumbled words
2. NO SPEECH—absence of spoken words

6. ABILITY TO UNDERSTAND OTHERS (Understanding verbal information content—however able)
0. UNDERSTANDS
1. USUALLY UNDERSTANDS—may miss some part/intent of message
2. SOMETIMES UNDERSTANDS—responds adequately to simple, direct communication
3. RARELY/NEVER UNDERSTANDS

7. CHANGE IN COMMUNICATION/ HEARING Resident's ability to express, understand, or hear information has changed as compared to status of **90 days ago** (or since last assessment if less than 90 days)
0. No change　　1. Improved　　2. Deteriorated

☐ = When box blank, must enter number or letter　|a.| = When letter in box, check if condition applies

MDS 2.0 September, 2000

Resident _____ Numeric Identifier _____

SECTION D. VISION PATTERNS

1.	VISION	(Ability to see in adequate light and with glasses if used) 0. ADEQUATE—sees fine detail, including regular print in newspapers/books 1. IMPAIRED—sees large print, but not regular print in newspapers/books 2. MODERATELY IMPAIRED—limited vision; not able to see newspaper headlines, but can identify objects 3. HIGHLY IMPAIRED—object identification in question, but eyes appear to follow objects 4. SEVERELY IMPAIRED—no vision or sees only light, colors, or shapes; eyes do not appear to follow objects	
2.	VISUAL LIMITATIONS/ DIFFICULTIES	Side vision problems—decreased peripheral vision (e.g., leaves food on one side of tray, difficulty traveling, bumps into people and objects, misjudges placement of chair when seating self)	a.
		Experiences any of following: sees halos or rings around lights; sees flashes of light; sees "curtains" over eyes	b.
		NONE OF ABOVE	c.
3.	VISUAL APPLIANCES	Glasses; contact lenses; magnifying glass 0. No 1. Yes	

SECTION E. MOOD AND BEHAVIOR PATTERNS

1.	INDICATORS OF DEPRES- SION, ANXIETY, SAD MOOD	(Code for indicators observed in last 30 days, irrespective of the assumed cause) 0. Indicator not exhibited in last 30 days 1. Indicator of this type exhibited up to five days a week 2. Indicator of this type exhibited daily or almost daily (6, 7 days a week)		

VERBAL EXPRESSIONS OF DISTRESS

a. Resident made negative statements—e.g., "Nothing matters; Would rather be dead; What's the use; Regrets having lived so long; Let me die"

b. Repetitive questions—e.g., "Where do I go; What do I do?"

c. Repetitive verbalizations—e.g., calling out for help, ("God help me")

d. Persistent anger with self or others—e.g., easily annoyed, anger at placement in nursing home; anger at care received

e. Self deprecation—e.g., "I am nothing; I am of no use to anyone"

f. Expressions of what appear to be unrealistic fears—e.g., fear of being abandoned, left alone, being with others

g. Recurrent statements that something terrible is about to happen—e.g., believes he or she is about to die, have a heart attack

h. Repetitive health complaints—e.g., persistently seeks medical attention, obsessive concern with body functions

i. Repetitive anxious complaints/concerns (non-health related) e.g., persistently seeks attention/reassurance regarding schedules, meals, laundry, clothing, relationship issues

SLEEP-CYCLE ISSUES

j. Unpleasant mood in morning

k. Insomnia/change in usual sleep pattern

SAD, APATHETIC, ANXIOUS APPEARANCE

l. Sad, pained, worried facial expressions—e.g., furrowed brows

m. Crying, tearfulness

n. Repetitive physical movements—e.g., pacing, hand wringing, restlessness, fidgeting, picking

LOSS OF INTEREST

o. Withdrawal from activities of interest—e.g., no interest in long standing activities or being with family/friends

p. Reduced social interaction

2.	MOOD PERSIS- TENCE	One or more indicators of depressed, sad or anxious mood were not easily altered by attempts to "cheer up", console, or reassure the resident over last 7 days 0. No mood 1. Indicators present, 2. Indicators present, indicators easily altered not easily altered	
3.	CHANGE IN MOOD	Resident's mood status has changed as compared to status of 90 days ago (or since last assessment if less than 90 days) 0. No change 1. Improved 2. Deteriorated	

4.	BEHAVIORAL SYMPTOMS	(A) Behavioral symptom frequency in last 7 days 0. Behavior not exhibited in last 7 days 1. Behavior of this type occurred 1 to 3 days in last 7 days 2. Behavior of this type occurred 4 to 6 days, but less than daily 3. Behavior of this type occurred daily (B) Behavioral symptom alterability in last 7 days 0. Behavior not present OR behavior was easily altered 1. Behavior was not easily altered	(A)	(B)
		a. WANDERING (moved with no rational purpose, seemingly oblivious to needs or safety)		
		b. VERBALLY ABUSIVE BEHAVIORAL SYMPTOMS (others were threatened, screamed at, cursed at)		
		c. PHYSICALLY ABUSIVE BEHAVIORAL SYMPTOMS (others were hit, shoved, scratched, sexually abused)		
		d. SOCIALLY INAPPROPRIATE/DISRUPTIVE BEHAVIORAL SYMPTOMS (made disruptive sounds, noisiness, screaming, self-abusive acts, sexual behavior or disrobing in public, smeared/threw food/feces, hoarding, rummaged through others' belongings)		
		e. RESISTS CARE (resisted taking medications/ injections, ADL assistance, or eating)		

5.	CHANGE IN BEHAVIORAL SYMPTOMS	Resident's behavior status has changed as compared to status of 90 days ago (or since last assessment if less than 90 days) 0. No change 1. Improved 2. Deteriorated	

SECTION F. PSYCHOSOCIAL WELL-BEING

1.	SENSE OF INITIATIVE/ INVOLVE- MENT	At ease interacting with others	a.
		At ease doing planned or structured activities	b.
		At ease doing self-initiated activities	c.
		Establishes own goals	d.
		Pursues involvement in life of facility (e.g., makes/keeps friends; involved in group activities; responds positively to new activities; assists at religious services)	e.
		Accepts invitations into most group activities	f.
		NONE OF ABOVE	g.
2.	UNSETTLED RELATION- SHIPS	Covert/open conflict with or repeated criticism of staff	a.
		Unhappy with roommate	b.
		Unhappy with residents other than roommate	c.
		Openly expresses conflict/anger with family/friends	d.
		Absence of personal contact with family/friends	e.
		Recent loss of close family member/friend	f.
		Does not adjust easily to change in routines	g.
		NONE OF ABOVE	h.
3.	PAST ROLES	Strong identification with past roles and life status	a.
		Expresses sadness/anger/empty feeling over lost roles/status	b.
		Resident perceives that daily routine (customary routine, activities) is very different from prior pattern in the community	c.
		NONE OF ABOVE	d.

SECTION G. PHYSICAL FUNCTIONING AND STRUCTURAL PROBLEMS

1.	(A) ADL SELF-PERFORMANCE—(Code for resident's PERFORMANCE OVER ALL SHIFTS during last 7 days—Not including setup) 0. INDEPENDENT—No help or oversight —OR— Help/oversight provided only 1 or 2 times during last 7 days 1. SUPERVISION—Oversight, encouragement or cueing provided 3 or more times during last 7 days —OR— Supervision (3 or more times) plus physical assistance provided only 1 or 2 times during last 7 days 2. LIMITED ASSISTANCE—Resident highly involved in activity; received physical help in guided maneuvering of limbs or other nonweight bearing assistance 3 or more times — OR—More help provided only 1 or 2 times during last 7 days 3. EXTENSIVE ASSISTANCE—While resident performed part of activity, over last 7-day period, help of following type(s) provided 3 or more times: —Weight-bearing support —Full staff performance during part (but not all) of last 7 days 4. TOTAL DEPENDENCE—Full staff performance of activity during entire 7 days 8. ACTIVITY DID NOT OCCUR during entire 7 days

		(B) ADL SUPPORT PROVIDED—(Code for MOST SUPPORT PROVIDED OVER ALL SHIFTS during last 7 days; code regardless of resident's self-performance classification) 0. No setup or physical help from staff 1. Setup help only 2. One person physical assist 8. ADL activity itself did not 3. Two+ persons physical assist occur during entire 7 days	(A) SELF-PERF	(B) SUPPORT
a.	BED MOBILITY	How resident moves to and from lying position, turns side to side, and positions body while in bed		
b.	TRANSFER	How resident moves between surfaces—to/from: bed, chair, wheelchair, standing position (EXCLUDE to/from bath/toilet)		
c.	WALK IN ROOM	How resident walks between locations in his/her room		
d.	WALK IN CORRIDOR	How resident walks in corridor on unit		
e.	LOCOMO- TION ON UNIT	How resident moves between locations in his/her room and adjacent corridor on same floor. If in wheelchair, self-sufficiency once in chair		
f.	LOCOMO- TION OFF UNIT	How resident moves to and returns from off unit locations (e.g., areas set aside for dining, activities, or treatments). If facility has only one floor, how resident moves to and from distant areas on the floor. If in wheelchair, self-sufficiency once in chair		
g.	DRESSING	How resident puts on, fastens, and takes off all items of street clothing, including donning/removing prosthesis		
h.	EATING	How resident eats and drinks (regardless of skill). Includes intake of nourishment by other means (e.g., tube feeding, total parenteral nutrition)		
i.	TOILET USE	How resident uses the toilet room (or commode, bedpan, urinal); transfer on/off toilet, cleanses, changes pad, manages ostomy or catheter, adjusts clothes		
j.	PERSONAL HYGIENE	How resident maintains personal hygiene, including combing hair, brushing teeth, shaving, applying makeup, washing/drying face, hands, and perineum (EXCLUDE baths and showers)		

Resident_____   Numeric Identifier_____

			(A)	(B)
2.	BATHING	How resident takes full-body bath/shower, sponge bath, and transfers in/out of tub/shower (EXCLUDE washing of back and hair.) **Code for most dependent** in self-performance and support. **(A)** BATHING SELF-PERFORMANCE codes appear below		

0. Independent—No help provided
1. Supervision—Oversight help only
2. Physical help limited to transfer only
3. Physical help in part of bathing activity
4. Total dependence
8. Activity itself did not occur during entire 7 days
(*Bathing support codes are as defined in Item 1, code B above*)

3.	TEST FOR BALANCE (see training manual)	(*Code for ability during test in the last 7 days*) 0. Maintained position as required in test 1. Unsteady, but able to rebalance self without physical support 2. Partial physical support during test; or stands (sits) but does not follow directions for test 3. Not able to attempt test without physical help	
		a. Balance while standing	
		b. Balance while sitting—position, trunk control	

4.	FUNCTIONAL LIMITATION IN RANGE OF MOTION (see training manual)	(*Code for limitations during last 7 days that interfered with daily functions or placed resident at risk of injury*) **(A)** RANGE OF MOTION **(B)** VOLUNTARY MOVEMENT 0. No limitation 0. No loss 1. Limitation on one side 1. Partial loss 2. Limitation on both sides 2. Full loss	(A)	(B)
		a. Neck		
		b. Arm—Including shoulder or elbow		
		c. Hand—Including wrist or fingers		
		d. Leg—Including hip or knee		
		e. Foot—Including ankle or toes		
		f. Other limitation or loss		

5.	MODES OF LOCOMO-TION	(***Check all that apply** during last 7 days*)	
		Cane/walker/crutch	a.	Wheelchair primary mode of locomotion	d.
		Wheeled self	b.		
		Other person wheeled	c.	NONE OF ABOVE	e.

6.	MODES OF TRANSFER	(***Check all that apply** during last 7 days*)	
		Bedfast all or most of time	a.	Lifted mechanically	d.
		Bed rails used for bed mobility or transfer	b.	Transfer aid (e.g., slide board, trapeze, cane, walker, brace)	e.
		Lifted manually	c.	NONE OF ABOVE	f.

7.	TASK SEGMENTA-TION	Some or all of ADL activities were broken into subtasks during **last 7 days** so that resident could perform them 0. No 1. Yes	

8.	ADL FUNCTIONAL REHABILITA-TION POTENTIAL	Resident believes he/she is capable of increased independence in at least some ADLs	a.
		Direct care staff believe resident is capable of increased independence in at least some ADLs	b.
		Resident able to perform tasks/activity but is very slow	c.
		Difference in ADL Self-Performance or ADL Support, comparing mornings to evenings	d.
		NONE OF ABOVE	e.

9.	CHANGE IN ADL FUNCTION	Resident's ADL self-performance status has changed as compared to status of **90 days ago** (or since last assessment if less than 90 days) 0. No change 1. Improved 2. Deteriorated	

SECTION H. CONTINENCE IN LAST 14 DAYS

1.	CONTINENCE SELF-CONTROL CATEGORIES (*Code for resident's PERFORMANCE OVER ALL SHIFTS*)

0. CONTINENT—Complete control [*includes use of indwelling urinary catheter or ostomy device that does not leak urine or stool*]

1. USUALLY CONTINENT—BLADDER, incontinent episodes once a week or less; BOWEL, less than weekly

2. OCCASIONALLY INCONTINENT—BLADDER, 2 or more times a week but not daily; BOWEL, once a week

3. FREQUENTLY INCONTINENT—BLADDER, tended to be incontinent daily, but some control present (e.g., on day shift); BOWEL, 2-3 times a week

4. INCONTINENT—Had inadequate control BLADDER, multiple daily episodes; BOWEL, all (or almost all) of the time

a.	BOWEL CONTI-NENCE	Control of bowel movement, with appliance or bowel continence programs, if employed	
b.	BLADDER CONTI-NENCE	Control of urinary bladder function (if dribbles, volume insufficient to soak through underpants), with appliances (e.g., foley) or continence programs, if employed	

2.	BOWEL ELIMINATION PATTERN	Bowel elimination pattern regular—at least one movement every three days	a.	Diarrhea	c.
				Fecal impaction	d.
		Constipation	b.	NONE OF ABOVE	e.

MDS 2.0 September, 2000

3.	APPLIANCES AND PROGRAMS	Any scheduled toileting plan	a.	Did not use toilet room/commode/urinal	f.
		Bladder retraining program	b.	Pads/briefs used	g.
		External (condom) catheter	c.	Enemas/irrigation	h.
		Indwelling catheter	d.	Ostomy present	i.
		Intermittent catheter	e.	NONE OF ABOVE	j.

4.	CHANGE IN URINARY CONTI-NENCE	Resident's urinary continence has changed as compared to status of **90 days ago** (or since last assessment if less than 90 days) 0. No change 1. Improved 2. Deteriorated	

SECTION I. DISEASE DIAGNOSES

Check only those diseases that have a relationship to current ADL status, cognitive status, mood and behavior status, medical treatments, nursing monitoring, or risk of death. (Do not list inactive diagnoses)

1.	DISEASES	(*If none apply, CHECK the NONE OF ABOVE box*)			
		ENDOCRINE/METABOLIC/NUTRITIONAL		Hemiplegia/Hemiparesis	v.
				Multiple sclerosis	w.
		Diabetes mellitus	a.	Paraplegia	x.
		Hyperthyroidism	b.	Parkinson's disease	y.
		Hypothyroidism	c.	Quadriplegia	z.
		HEART/CIRCULATION		Seizure disorder	aa.
		Arteriosclerotic heart disease (ASHD)	d.	Transient ischemic attack (TIA)	bb.
				Traumatic brain injury	cc.
		Cardiac dysrhythmias	e.	**PSYCHIATRIC/MOOD**	
		Congestive heart failure	f.	Anxiety disorder	dd.
		Deep vein thrombosis	g.	Depression	ee.
		Hypertension	h.	Manic depression (bipolar disease)	ff.
		Hypotension	i.	Schizophrenia	gg.
		Peripheral vascular disease	j.	**PULMONARY**	
		Other cardiovascular disease	k.	Asthma	hh.
		MUSCULOSKELETAL		Emphysema/COPD	ii.
		Arthritis	l.	**SENSORY**	
		Hip fracture	m.	Cataracts	jj.
		Missing limb (e.g., amputation)	n.	Diabetic retinopathy	kk.
		Osteoporosis	o.	Glaucoma	ll.
		Pathological bone fracture	p.	Macular degeneration	mm.
		NEUROLOGICAL		**OTHER**	
		Alzheimer's disease	q.	Allergies	nn.
		Aphasia	r.	Anemia	oo.
		Cerebral palsy	s.	Cancer	pp.
		Cerebrovascular accident (stroke)	t.	Renal failure	qq.
		Dementia other than Alzheimer's disease	u.	NONE OF ABOVE	rr.

2.	INFECTIONS	(*If none apply, CHECK the NONE OF ABOVE box*)			
		Antibiotic resistant infection (e.g., Methicillin resistant staph)	a.	Septicemia	g.
				Sexually transmitted diseases	h.
		Clostridium difficile (c. diff.)	b.	Tuberculosis	i.
		Conjunctivitis	c.	Urinary tract infection **in last 30 days**	j.
		HIV infection	d.	Viral hepatitis	k.
		Pneumonia	e.	Wound infection	l.
		Respiratory infection	f.	NONE OF ABOVE	m.

3.	OTHER CURRENT OR MORE DETAILED DIAGNOSES AND ICD-9 CODES	a. _____	·
		b. _____	·
		c. _____	·
		d. _____	·
		e. _____	·

SECTION J. HEALTH CONDITIONS

1.	PROBLEM CONDITIONS	(***Check all problems** present in last 7 days unless other time frame is indicated*)			
		INDICATORS OF FLUID STATUS		Dizziness/Vertigo	f.
				Edema	g.
		Weight gain or loss of 3 or more pounds within a 7 day period	a.	Fever	h.
				Hallucinations	i.
		Inability to lie flat due to shortness of breath	b.	Internal bleeding	j.
				Recurrent lung aspirations in **last 90 days**	k.
		Dehydrated; output exceeds input	c.	Shortness of breath	l.
		Insufficient fluid; did **NOT** consume all/almost all liquids provided during **last 3 days**	d.	Syncope (fainting)	m.
				Unsteady gait	n.
				Vomiting	o.
		OTHER		NONE OF ABOVE	p.
		Delusions	e.		

Resident _____   Numeric Identifier _____

2.	PAIN SYMPTOMS	(Code the **highest level of pain** present in the **last 7 days**)	
		a. FREQUENCY with which resident complains or shows evidence of pain 0. No pain (**skip to J4**) 1. Pain less than daily 2. Pain daily	**b. INTENSITY** of pain 1. Mild pain 2. Moderate pain 3. Times when pain is horrible or excruciating	

3.	PAIN SITE	(If pain present, **check all sites** that apply in **last 7 days**)			
		Back pain		Incisional pain	f.
		Bone pain	a.	Joint pain (other than hip)	g.
		Chest pain while doing usual activities	b. c.	Soft tissue pain (e.g., lesion, muscle)	h.
		Headache	d.	Stomach pain	i.
		Hip pain	e.	Other	j.

4.	ACCIDENTS	(Check all that apply)			
		Fell in **past 30 days**	a.	Hip fracture in **last 180 days**	c.
		Fell in **past 31-180 days**	b.	Other fracture in **last 180 days**	d.
				NONE OF ABOVE	e.

5.	STABILITY OF CONDITIONS	Conditions/diseases make resident's cognitive, ADL, mood or behavior patterns unstable—(fluctuating, precarious, or deteriorating)	a.
		Resident experiencing an acute episode or a flare-up of a recurrent or chronic problem	b.
		End-stage disease, 6 or fewer months to live	c.
		NONE OF ABOVE	d.

SECTION K. ORAL/NUTRITIONAL STATUS

1.	ORAL PROBLEMS	Chewing problem	a.
		Swallowing problem	b.
		Mouth pain	c.
		NONE OF ABOVE	d.

2.	HEIGHT AND WEIGHT	Record (**a.**) **height in inches** and (**b.**) **weight in pounds**. Base weight on most recent measure in **last 30 days**; measure weight consistently in accord with standard facility practice—e.g., in a.m. after voiding, before meal, with shoes off, and in nightclothes
		a. HT (in.) **b.** WT (lb.)

3.	WEIGHT CHANGE	**a.** Weight loss—5 % or more in **last 30 days**; or 10 % or more in **last 180 days** 0. No 1. Yes	
		b. Weight gain—5 % or more in **last 30 days**; or 10 % or more in **last 180 days** 0. No 1. Yes	

4.	NUTRITIONAL PROBLEMS	Complains about the taste of many foods	a.	Leaves 25% or more of food uneaten at most meals	c.
		Regular or repetitive complaints of hunger	b.	NONE OF ABOVE	d.

5.	NUTRITIONAL APPROACHES	(**Check all that apply in last 7 days**)			
		Parenteral/IV	a.	Dietary supplement between meals	f.
		Feeding tube	b.		
		Mechanically altered diet	c.	Plate guard, stabilized built-up utensil, etc.	g.
		Syringe (oral feeding)	d.	On a planned weight change program	h.
		Therapeutic diet	e.	NONE OF ABOVE	i.

6.	PARENTERAL OR ENTERAL INTAKE	(**Skip to Section L if neither 5a nor 5b is checked**)
		a. Code the proportion of **total calories** the resident received through parenteral or tube feedings in the **last 7 days** 0. None 3. 51% to 75% 1. 1% to 25% 4. 76% to 100% 2. 26% to 50%
		b. Code the average **fluid intake** per day by IV or tube in **last 7 days** 0. None 3. 1001 to 1500 cc/day 1. 1 to 500 cc/day 4. 1501 to 2000 cc/day 2. 501 to 1000 cc/day 5. 2001 or more cc/day

SECTION L. ORAL/DENTAL STATUS

1.	ORAL STATUS AND DISEASE PREVENTION	Debris (soft, easily movable substances) present in mouth prior to going to bed at night	a.
		Has dentures or removable bridge	b.
		Some/all natural teeth lost—does not have or does not use dentures (or partial plates)	c.
		Broken, loose, or carious teeth	d.
		Inflamed gums (gingiva); swollen or bleeding gums; oral abcesses; ulcers or rashes	e.
		Daily cleaning of teeth/dentures or daily mouth care—by resident or staff	f.
		NONE OF ABOVE	g.

SECTION M. SKIN CONDITION

			Number at Stage
1.	ULCERS (Due to any cause)	(Record the number of ulcers at each ulcer stage—regardless of cause. If none present at a stage, record "0" (zero). Code all that apply during **last 7 days**. Code 9 = 9 or more.) **[Requires full body exam.]**	
		a. Stage 1. A persistent area of skin redness (without a break in the skin) that does not disappear when pressure is relieved.	
		b. Stage 2. A partial thickness loss of skin layers that presents clinically as an abrasion, blister, or shallow crater.	
		c. Stage 3. A full thickness of skin is lost, exposing the subcutaneous tissues - presents as a deep crater with or without undermining adjacent tissue.	
		d. Stage 4. A full thickness of skin and subcutaneous tissue is lost, exposing muscle or bone.	

2.	TYPE OF ULCER	(For each type of ulcer, **code for the highest stage in the last 7 days** using scale in item M1—i.e., 0=none; stages 1, 2, 3, 4)	
		a. Pressure ulcer—any lesion caused by pressure resulting in damage of underlying tissue	
		b. Stasis ulcer—open lesion caused by poor circulation in the lower extremities	

3.	HISTORY OF RESOLVED ULCERS	Resident had an ulcer that was resolved or cured in **LAST 90 DAYS** 0. No 1. Yes	

4.	OTHER SKIN PROBLEMS OR LESIONS PRESENT	(**Check all that apply** during **last 7 days**)	
		Abrasions, bruises	a.
		Burns (second or third degree)	b.
		Open lesions other than ulcers, rashes, cuts (e.g., cancer lesions)	c.
		Rashes—e.g., intertrigo, eczema, drug rash, heat rash, herpes zoster	d.
		Skin desensitized to pain or pressure	e.
		Skin tears or cuts (other than surgery)	f.
		Surgical wounds	g.
		NONE OF ABOVE	h.

5.	SKIN TREATMENTS	(**Check all that apply** during **last 7 days**)	
		Pressure relieving device(s) for chair	a.
		Pressure relieving device(s) for bed	b.
		Turning/repositioning program	c.
		Nutrition or hydration intervention to manage skin problems	d.
		Ulcer care	e.
		Surgical wound care	f.
		Application of dressings (with or without topical medications) other than to feet	g.
		Application of ointments/medications (other than to feet)	h.
		Other preventative or protective skin care (other than to feet)	i.
		NONE OF ABOVE	j.

6.	FOOT PROBLEMS AND CARE	(**Check all that apply** during **last 7 days**)	
		Resident has one or more foot problems—e.g., corns, callouses, bunions, hammer toes, overlapping toes, pain, structural problems	a.
		Infection of the foot—e.g., cellulitis, purulent drainage	b.
		Open lesions on the foot	c.
		Nails/calluses trimmed during **last 90 days**	d.
		Received preventative or protective foot care (e.g., used special shoes, inserts, pads, toe separators)	e.
		Application of dressings (with or without topical medications)	f.
		NONE OF ABOVE	g.

SECTION N. ACTIVITY PURSUIT PATTERNS

1.	TIME AWAKE	(**Check appropriate time periods over last 7 days**) Resident awake all or most of time (i.e., naps no more than one hour per time period) in the:			
		Morning	a.	Evening	c.
		Afternoon	b.	NONE OF ABOVE	d.

(If resident is comatose, skip to Section O)

2.	AVERAGE TIME INVOLVED IN ACTIVITIES	(**When awake and not receiving treatments or ADL care**) 0. Most—more than 2/3 of time 2. Little—less than 1/3 of time 1. Some—from 1/3 to 2/3 of time 3. None	

3.	PREFERRED ACTIVITY SETTINGS	(**Check all settings** in which activities are **preferred**)			
		Own room	a.		
		Day/activity room	b.	Outside facility	d.
		Inside NH/off unit	c.	NONE OF ABOVE	e.

4.	GENERAL ACTIVITY PREFERENCES (adapted to resident's current abilities)	(**Check all PREFERENCES** whether or not activity is currently available to resident)			
		Cards/other games	a.	Trips/shopping	g.
		Crafts/arts	b.	Walking/wheeling outdoors	h.
		Exercise/sports	c.	Watching TV	i.
		Music	d.	Gardening or plants	j.
		Reading/writing	e.	Talking or conversing	k.
		Spiritual/religious activities	f.	Helping others	l.
				NONE OF ABOVE	m.

MDS 2.0 September, 2000

Resident _____   Numeric Identifier _____

5.	PREFERS CHANGE IN DAILY ROUTINE	Code for resident preferences in daily routines 0. No change 1. Slight change 2. Major change **a.** Type of activities in which resident is currently involved **b.** Extent of resident involvement in activities	

SECTION O. MEDICATIONS

1.	NUMBER OF MEDICA-TIONS	(*Record the number of different medications used in the last 7 days;* enter "0" if none used)	
2.	NEW MEDICA-TIONS	(*Resident currently receiving medications that were initiated during the **last 90 days**)* 0. No 1. Yes	
3.	INJECTIONS	(*Record the number of DAYS injections of any type received during the **last 7 days**; enter "0" if none used)	
4.	DAYS RECEIVED THE FOLLOWING MEDICATION	(*Record the number of DAYS during **last 7 days**; enter "0" if not used. Note—enter "1" for long-acting meds used less than weekly)* **a.** Antipsychotic **d.** Hypnotic **b.** Antianxiety **c.** Antidepressant **e.** Diuretic	

SECTION P. SPECIAL TREATMENTS AND PROCEDURES

1.	SPECIAL TREAT-MENTS, PROCE-DURES, AND PROGRAMS	**a. SPECIAL CARE**—*Check treatments or programs received during the **last 14 days***

TREATMENTS				
Chemotherapy	a.		Ventilator or respirator	l.
Dialysis	b.		**PROGRAMS**	
IV medication	c.		Alcohol/drug treatment program	m.
Intake/output	d.		Alzheimer's/dementia special care unit	n.
Monitoring acute medical condition	e.		Hospice care	o.
Ostomy care	f.		Pediatric unit	p.
Oxygen therapy	g.		Respite care	q.
Radiation	h.		Training in skills required to return to the community (e.g., taking medications, house work, shopping, transportation, ADLs)	r.
Suctioning	i.			
Tracheostomy care	j.			
Transfusions	k.		*NONE OF ABOVE*	s.

b. THERAPIES - *Record the number of days and total minutes each of the following therapies was administered (for at least 15 minutes a day) in the **last 7 calendar days** (Enter 0 if none or less than 15 min. daily)*
[Note—count only post admission therapies]

	DAYS	MIN
(A) = # of days administered for **15 minutes or more** (B) = total # of minutes provided in last 7 days	(A)	(B)
a. Speech - language pathology and audiology services		
b. Occupational therapy		
c. Physical therapy		
d. Respiratory therapy		
e. Psychological therapy (by any licensed mental health professional)		

2.	INTERVEN-TION PROGRAMS FOR MOOD, BEHAVIOR, COGNITIVE LOSS	**(Check all interventions or strategies used in last 7 days**—no matter where received)	
		Special behavior symptom evaluation program	a.
		Evaluation by a licensed mental health specialist in **last 90 days**	b.
		Group therapy	c.
		Resident-specific deliberate changes in the environment to address mood/behavior patterns—e.g., providing bureau in which to rummage	d.
		Reorientation—e.g., cueing	e.
		NONE OF ABOVE	f.

3.	NURSING REHABILITA-TION/ RESTOR-ATIVE CARE	*Record the NUMBER OF DAYS each of the following rehabilitation or restorative techniques or practices was **provided to the resident** for more than or equal to 15 minutes per day in the last 7 days (Enter 0 if none or less than 15 min. daily.)*

a. Range of motion (passive)		**f.** Walking	
b. Range of motion (active)		**g.** Dressing or grooming	
c. Splint or brace assistance		**h.** Eating or swallowing	
TRAINING AND SKILL PRACTICE IN:		**i.** Amputation/prosthesis care	
d. Bed mobility		**j.** Communication	
e. Transfer		**k.** Other	

4.	DEVICES AND RESTRAINTS	(*Use the following codes for **last 7 days**:*) 0. Not used 1. Used less than daily 2. Used daily

Bed rails		
a. — Full bed rails on all open sides of bed		
b. — Other types of side rails used (e.g., half rail, one side)		
c. Trunk restraint		
d. Limb restraint		
e. Chair prevents rising		

5.	HOSPITAL STAY(S)	Record number of times resident was admitted to hospital with an overnight stay **in last 90 days** (or since last assessment if less than 90 days). (Enter 0 if no hospital admissions)	
6.	EMERGENCY ROOM (ER) VISIT(S)	Record number of times resident visited ER without an overnight stay **in last 90 days** (or since last assessment if less than 90 days). (Enter 0 if no ER visits)	
7.	PHYSICIAN VISITS	In the **LAST 14 DAYS** (or since admission if less than 14 days in facility) how many days has the physician (or authorized assistant or practitioner) examined the resident? (Enter 0 if none)	
8.	PHYSICIAN ORDERS	In the **LAST 14 DAYS** (or since admission if less than 14 days in facility) how many days has the physician (or authorized assistant or practitioner) changed the resident's orders? Do not include order renewals without change. (Enter 0 if none)	
9.	ABNORMAL LAB VALUES	Has the resident had any abnormal lab values during the **last 90 days** (or since admission)? 0. No 1. Yes	

SECTION Q. DISCHARGE POTENTIAL AND OVERALL STATUS

1.	DISCHARGE POTENTIAL	**a.** Resident expresses/indicates preference to return to the community 0. No 1. Yes	
		b. Resident has a support person who is positive towards discharge 0. No 1. Yes	
		c. Stay projected to be of a short duration— discharge projected **within 90 days** (do not include expected discharge due to death) 0. No 2. Within 31-90 days 1. Within 30 days 3. Discharge status uncertain	

2.	OVERALL CHANGE IN CARE NEEDS	Resident's overall self sufficiency has changed significantly as compared to status of **90 days ago** (or since last assessment if less than 90 days)
		0. No change 1. Improved—receives fewer 2. Deteriorated—receives
		            supports, needs less more support
		            restrictive level of care	

SECTION R. ASSESSMENT INFORMATION

1.	PARTICIPA-TION IN ASSESS-MENT	**a.** Resident: 0. No 1. Yes **b.** Family: 0. No 1. Yes 2. No family **c.** Significant other: 0. No 1. Yes 2. None	
2.	**SIGNATURE OF PERSON COORDINATING THE ASSESSMENT:**		

a. Signature of RN Assessment Coordinator (sign on above line)

b. Date RN Assessment Coordinator signed as complete				
	Month	Day		Year

Resident _____   Numeric Identifier _____

SECTION T. THERAPY SUPPLEMENT FOR MEDICARE PPS

1.	SPECIAL TREAT-MENTS AND PROCE-DURES	**a. RECREATION THERAPY**—*Enter number of days and total minutes of recreation therapy administered (**for at least 15 minutes a day**) in the **last 7 days** (Enter 0 if none)*

DAYS (A) **MIN** (B)

(A) = # of days administered for 15 minutes or more
(B) = total # of minutes provided in last 7 days

Skip unless this is a Medicare 5 day or Medicare readmission/ return assessment.

b. ORDERED THERAPIES—*Has physician ordered any of following therapies to begin in FIRST 14 days of stay—physical therapy, occupational therapy, or speech pathology service?*
0. No   1. Yes

If not ordered, skip to item 2

c. Through day 15, provide an estimate of the number of days when at least 1 therapy service can be expected to have been delivered.

d. Through day 15, provide an estimate of the number of therapy minutes (across the therapies) that can be expected to be delivered?

2.	WALKING WHEN MOST SELF SUFFICIENT	*Complete item 2 if ADL self-performance score for TRANSFER (G.1.b.A) is 0,1,2, or 3 AND at least one of the following are present:*

• Resident received physical therapy involving gait training (P.1.b.c)
• Physical therapy was ordered for the resident involving gait training (T.1.b)
• Resident received nursing rehabilitation for walking (P.3.f)
• Physical therapy involving walking has been discontinued within the past 180 days

Skip to item 3 if resident did not walk in last 7 days

(FOR FOLLOWING FIVE ITEMS, BASE CODING ON THE EPISODE WHEN THE RESIDENT WALKED THE FARTHEST WITHOUT SITTING DOWN. INCLUDE WALKING DURING REHABILITATION SESSIONS.)

a. Furthest distance walked without sitting down during this episode.

0. 150+ feet   3. 10-25 feet
1. 51-149 feet   4. Less than 10 feet
2. 26-50 feet

b. Time walked without sitting down during this episode.

0. 1-2 minutes   3. 11-15 minutes
1. 3-4 minutes   4. 16-30 minutes
2. 5-10 minutes   5. 31+ minutes

c. Self-Performance in walking during this episode.

0. *INDEPENDENT*—No help or oversight
1. *SUPERVISION*—Oversight, encouragement or cueing provided
2. *LIMITED ASSISTANCE*—Resident highly involved in walking; received physical help in guided maneuvering of limbs or other nonweight bearing assistance
3. *EXTENSIVE ASSISTANCE*—Resident received weight bearing assistance while walking

d. Walking support provided associated with this episode (code regardless of resident's self-performance classification).

0. No setup or physical help from staff
1. Setup help only
2. One person physical assist
3. Two+ persons physical assist

e. Parallel bars used by resident in association with this episode.

0. No   1. Yes

3.	CASE MIX GROUP	Medicare [ ][ ][ ][ ][ ] State [ ][ ][ ][ ][ ]

MDS 2.0 September, 2000

Resident _____   Numeric Identifier_____

MINIMUM DATA SET (MDS) - *VERSION 2.0*
FOR NURSING HOME RESIDENT ASSESSMENT AND CARE SCREENING

SECTION W. SUPPLEMENTAL MDS ITEMS

1.	**National Provider ID**	Enter for all assessments and tracking forms, if available.	

		If the ARD of this assessment or the discharge date of this discharge tracking form is between July 1 and September 30, skip to W3.	

2.	**Influenza Vaccine**	a. Did the resident receive the Influenza vaccine in this facility for this year's Influenza season (October 1 through March 31)?
		
		    0. No (If No, go to item W2b)
		    1. Yes (If Yes, go to item W3)
		
		b. If Influenza vaccine not received, state reason:
		    1. Not in facility during this year's flu season
		    2. Received outside of this facility
		    3. Not eligible
		    4. Offered and declined
		    5. Not offered
		    6. Inability to obtain vaccine	

3.	**Pneumo-coccal Vaccine**	a. Is the resident's PPV status up to date?
		    0. No (If No, go to item W3b)
		    1. Yes (If Yes, skip item W3b)
		
		b. If PPV not received, state reason:
		    1. Not eligible
		    2. Offered and declined
		    3. Not offered	

MDS 2.0 May, 2005

Numeric Identifier _____

SECTION V. RESIDENT ASSESSMENT PROTOCOL SUMMARY

Resident's Name:	Medical Record No.:

1. Check if RAP is triggered.

2. For each triggered RAP, use the RAP guidelines to identify areas needing further assessment. Document relevant assessment information regarding the resident's status.

   - Describe:
     — Nature of the condition (may include presence or lack of objective data and subjective complaints).
     — Complications and risk factors that affect your decision to proceed to care planning.
     — Factors that must be considered in developing individualized care plan interventions.
     — Need for referrals/further evaluation by appropriate health professionals.

   - Documentation should support your decision-making regarding whether to proceed with a care plan for a triggered RAP and the type(s) of care plan interventions that are appropriate for a particular resident.

   - Documentation may appear anywhere in the clinical record (e.g., progress notes, consults, flowsheets, etc.).

3. Indicate under the <u>Location of RAP Assessment Documentation</u> column where information related to the RAP assessment can be found.

4. For each triggered RAP, indicate whether a new care plan, care plan revision, or continuation of current care plan is necessary to address the problem(s) identified in your assessment. The Care Planning Decision column must be completed within 7 days of completing the RAI (MDS and RAPs).

A. RAP PROBLEM AREA	(a) Check if triggered	Location and Date of RAP Assessment Documentation	(b) Care Planning Decision—check if addressed in care plan
1. DELIRIUM	☐		☐
2. COGNITIVE LOSS	☐		☐
3. VISUAL FUNCTION	☐		☐
4. COMMUNICATION	☐		☐
5. ADL FUNCTIONAL/ REHABILITATION POTENTIAL	☐		☐
6. URINARY INCONTINENCE AND INDWELLING CATHETER	☐		☐
7. PSYCHOSOCIAL WELL-BEING	☐		☐
8. MOOD STATE	☐		☐
9. BEHAVIORAL SYMPTOMS	☐		☐
10. ACTIVITIES	☐		☐
11. FALLS	☐		☐
12. NUTRITIONAL STATUS	☐		☐
13. FEEDING TUBES	☐		☐
14. DEHYDRATION/FLUID MAINTENANCE	☐		☐
15. DENTAL CARE	☐		☐
16. PRESSURE ULCERS	☐		☐
17. PSYCHOTROPIC DRUG USE	☐		☐
18. PHYSICAL RESTRAINTS	☐		☐

B.

1. Signature of RN Coordinator for RAP Assessment Process

2. Month __ Day __ Year __

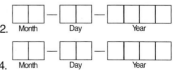

3. Signature of Person Completing Care Planning Decision

4. Month __ Day __ Year __

MDS 2.0 September, 2000

Glossary

Use the CD in the front of your book to hear these terms pronounced and defined. (The number following the entry refers to the chapter in which the entry is found.)

A

Abandonment: the act of withdrawing support or help from another person, despite duty or responsibility (4)

Absorption: transfer of nutrients from the digestive tract into the bloodstream (25)

Abuse: intentional act that causes harm to another person (4)

Acceptance: one of the stages of grief; the person comes to terms with the reality of his or her own impending death, and is finally at peace with this knowledge (28)

Accident: an unexpected, unintended event that has the potential to cause bodily injury (18)

Accreditation: official recognition that an organization meets certain standards of quality (1)

Acquired immunodeficiency syndrome (AIDS): a disease caused by human immunodeficiency virus (HIV), a bloodborne virus that attacks the body's immune system; death usually results when the body becomes unable to recognize and fight off infections (16)

Activities of daily living (ADLs): routine tasks of daily life, such as bathing, eating and grooming (compare with *instrumental activities of daily living*) (8)

Activity: a hobby or pursuit (pastime) that engages the mind, the body, or both, and may provide the opportunity for socializing with others (7)

Acute care setting: a place where health care is provided for people who require a high level of care; patients usually have severe illnesses, or are medically unstable, and length of stay in the facility is typically short (compare with *post-acute care setting* and *long-term care setting*) (1)

Acute illness: an illness with a rapid onset and a relatively short recovery time, usually unexpected (8)

Acute pain: sharp, sudden pain (27)

Addiction: a physical need for a substance that results in withdrawal signs and symptoms if the substance is withheld (42)

ADLs: see *activities of daily living*

Admission: official entry of a person into a health care setting (11)

Admissions assessment: an evaluation of the resident done by the nurse at the time of the resident's admission to obtain baseline information about the resident's condition (11)

Admission sheet: a form that is completed when a person is admitted to a health care setting; gathers standard information about the person, such as the person's name, address, date of birth, age, social security number, gender, insurance and employment information, emergency notification information, and advance directive information (11)

Advance directive: a document that allows a person to make his wishes regarding health care known to family members and health care workers, in case the time comes when he is no longer able to make those wishes known himself; examples include living wills and durable powers of attorney for health care (4)

Advocacy: the process of making a plea or providing support on another's behalf (4)

Aerobic: an adjective used to describe bacterium that need oxygen in order to live (compare with *anaerobic*) (15)

Afterlife: a state of being where the dead meet again with loved ones who have passed on before them (29)

Afternoon care: care that is provided before and after lunch and dinner (23)

Against medical advice (AMA): term used to describe a person's actions when a person leaves a health care facility without a doctor's order (11)

AIDS: see *acquired immunodeficiency syndrome*

Airborne pathogen: pathogens that can be transmitted through the air (16)

Airborne precautions: used when caring for people infected with pathogens that can be transmitted through the air; include placing the person in a private room with the door closed, wearing a mask when caring for the person, and minimizing the amount of time the person spends out of his or her private room (15)

Agnosia: difficulty recognizing information obtained using the five senses (9)

Alignment: good posture; the "A" in the ABCs of good body mechanics (17)

Alopecia: baldness, loss of hair (24)

Alzheimer's disease: a disorder characterized by the presence of abnormal protein deposits in the brain called plaques and tangles, which cause nerve cell death and gradual loss of brain function (9)

Alveoli (singular, alveolus): grape-like clusters of tiny air sacs in the lungs, where gas exchange takes place (33)

Ambulate: to walk (20)

Amino acids: molecules that are the building blocks of the body's cells; found in proteins (25)

Amnesia: difficulty remembering (9)

Amputation: the surgical removal of all or part of an arm or a leg (32)

Anaerobic: an adjective used to describe bacterium that can survive without oxygen (compare with *aerobic*) (15)

Anaphylactic shock: shock caused by a serious allergic reaction to a medication, bee sting, or certain foods (19)

Anatomy: the study of what body parts look like, where they are located, how big they are, and how they connect to other body parts (30)

Anemia: a condition that exists when the ability of the red blood cells to carry oxygen to the tissues is decreased (34)

Anger: one of the stages of grief; the person realizes that she is actually going to die as a result of her illness and has feelings of rage, which may be directed toward herself or others (28)

Angina pectoris: the classic chest pain that is felt as a result of the heart muscle being deprived of oxygen (34)

Anorexia: loss of appetite (25)

Antibodies: specialized proteins produced by the immune system that help our bodies to fight off specific microbes, preventing infection (15)

Anticoagulants: medications that are given to prevent the blood from clotting (34)

Antiperspirant: a grooming product that contains ingredients to stop or slow the production of sweat (23)

Antisepsis: practices that kill microbes or stop them from growing; one of the techniques of medical asepsis (compare with *sanitation, disinfection,* and *sterilization*) (15)

Anuria: the state of voiding less than 100 mL of urine over the course of 24 hours (26)

Anxiety: feeling of uneasiness, dread, apprehension, or worry (42)

Aphasia: difficulty using language; may be expressive (difficulty using words) or receptive (difficulty understanding words) (9)

Appetite: the desire for food (compare with *anorexia*) (25)

Apraxia: difficulty coordinating the steps needed to complete a task (9)

Arteries: vessels that carry blood away from the heart (34)

Arterioles: the smallest arteries (34)

Arteriosclerosis: "hardening of the arteries"; occurs when atherosclerotic plaques interfere with the elasticity of the arterial walls, making them brittle and prone to breaking (34)

Arthritis: inflammation of joints, usually associated with pain and stiffness (32)

Aspiration: the accidental inhalation of foreign material (such as food, liquids, vomitus) into the airway (19)

Assault: threatening or attempting to touch a person without the person's consent (4)

Assessment: the act of gathering information about a resident's condition and then interpreting what that information means (12)

Assisted-living facility: type of long-term care facility that provides residents with limited assistance with tasks such as medication administration, transportation, meals, and housekeeping (1)

Asthma: a condition that affects the bronchi and bronchioles of the lungs; triggers (such as cold weather, allergies, respiratory infections, stress, smoke, and exercise) cause the bronchi and bronchioles to become narrower, making breathing difficult (33)

Astigmatism: an inability to focus images properly because the cornea of the eye is not perfectly curved (36)

Atherosclerosis: blocking of the arteries, caused by the build-up of fatty deposits called plaque on the inside of the vessel wall (34)

Atria (singular, *atrium*): the upper chambers of the heart (34)

Atrophy: the loss of muscle size and strength (32)

Attitude: the side of ourselves that we display to the world, communicating outwardly how we feel about things (3)

Autism: a developmental disability characterized by extreme difficulty communicating and relating to other people and surroundings (41)

Automated external defibrillator (AED): a small, portable device that automatically detects a person's heart rhythm and delivers an electrical shock to the heart to stop fast, abnormal heart beats and restore the heart's normal rhythm (19)

Autonomy: an ethical principle that requires health care workers to respect a person's rights and personal preferences (4)

Autopsy: examination of a person's organs and tissues after the person has died, done to confirm or identify the cause of the person's death (29)

Axon: a long extension from the body of a neuron that *sends* information to other neurons (compare with *dendrites*) (35)

B

Balance: stability produced by the even distribution of weight; the "B" in the ABCs of good body mechanics (17)

Balanced Budget Act: an act, signed into law by President Bill Clinton in 1997, that created significant changes in the Medicare and Medicaid programs, including a major decrease in funding for Medicare, and the establishment of the prospective payment system (PPS) (2)

Bargaining: one of the stages of grief; the person wants to "make a deal" with someone he or she feels has control over his or her fate, such as God or a health care provider (28)

Barium: a radiopaque substance that coats the mucosa of the digestive tract, making the organs appear sharper and brighter on radiologic studies (x-rays) (38)

Barrier cream or ointment: a skin care product that is applied to the perineum to help protect the skin from contact with urine or feces (23)

Basic life support (BLS): basic emergency care techniques, such as rescue breathing and cardiopulmonary resuscitation (CPR) (19)

Bath blanket: a lightweight cotton blanket used to cover a person during a bed bath or linen change to help provide modesty and warmth (21)

Battery: touching a person without his or her consent (4)

Bed cradle: a metal frame that is placed between the bottom and top sheets to keep the top sheet, the blanket, and the bedspread away from the person's feet; used when pressure on the person's feet could result in pain or skin breakdown (21)

Bed hold: payments that secure a resident's place in the long-term care facility when the resident must be temporarily discharged from the facility for a period of time (for example, to receive care in a hospital or other health care facility) (11)

Bedpan: a device used for elimination when a person is unable to get out of bed; women use a bedpan for both urination and bowel movements; men use a bedpan for bowel movements only (26)

Bed protector: a square of quilted absorbent fabric backed with waterproof material that measures approximately 3 feet by 3 feet; used to prevent soiling of the bottom linens; sometimes called an *incontinence pad, soaker pad,* or *"chux"* (21)

Bedside commode: a device used for elimination when a person is able to get out of bed, but unable to walk to the bathroom; it consists of a chair-like frame with a toilet seat and a removable collection bucket (26)

Bell: the small, rounded surface on a stethoscope that is used to pick up faint sounds (22)

Beneficence: an ethical principle that requires health care workers to do good for those in their care by preventing harm and promoting the health and welfare of the person above all else (4)

Benefit period: a unit of time used by the Medicare program to track how many days of skilled health care services a person uses, and how many are still available; begins with hospitalization and ends when a person has not received any skilled health care services, either in the hospital or nursing home, for 60 days (2)

Benign: adjective used to describe a non-cancerous tumor (that is, a tumor that does not progress or invade other tissues) (compare with *malignant*) (43)

Bile: a substance produced by the liver that helps with the digestion of fats (38)

Biological death: occurs when the tissues of the brain and heart die from lack of oxygen; biological death is not reversible (compare with *clinical death*) (19)

Biopsy: a diagnostic procedure that involves obtaining a tissue sample and examining it under a microscope for cancerous cells (43)

Bipolar disorder (manic depression): a mental health disorder characterized by mood swings;

people with this disorder experience excessively "high" or happy periods, followed by excessively "low" or depressed periods (42)

Bisexual: a person who is sexually attracted to members of both sexes (7)

Bloodborne pathogen: a disease-producing microbe that is transmitted to another person through blood or other body fluids (16)

Blood pressure: the force that the blood exerts against the arterial walls; one of the vital signs (22)

Body alignment: positioning of the body so that the spine is not twisted or crooked (20)

Body fluids: liquid or semi-liquid substances produced by the body, such as blood, urine, feces, vomitus, saliva, drainage from wounds, sweat, semen, vaginal secretions, tears, cerebrospinal fluid, amniotic fluid, and breast milk (16)

Body mechanics: the efficient and safe use of the body (17)

Bony prominences: parts of the body where there is very little fat between the bone and the skin, such as the ankles, heels, hips, and elbows (31)

Body temperature: how hot the body is; one of the vital signs (22)

Bradycardia: a heart rate that is slower than normal (less than 60 beats/min in an adult) (22)

Bradypnea: a respiratory rate that is lower than normal (less than 10 breaths/min in an adult) (22)

Braille: a system that uses letters made from combinations of raised dots that allows a blind person to read (36)

Breakthrough pain: pain that occurs before a person's next regularly scheduled dose of pain medication (27)

Bronchi (singular, *bronchus*): passageways that carry air from the trachea ("windpipe") to the lungs, one bronchus goes to the right lung and the other goes to the left (33)

Bronchioles: the smallest branches of the bronchi (33)

Bronchitis: inflammation of the bronchi (33)

Bruise: discoloration of the skin caused by rupture of the blood vessels beneath the skin's surface (18)

C

Call light system: a system that allows a resident to call for help; usually consists of a call light control, a light in the hall, and a panel of lights at the nurses' station or some other central location (14)

Calorie count: an evaluation of the total number of calories and the amount of specific nutrients the resident has consumed over a specified amount of time (usually 3 days), done to determine if the resident's nutritional intake is adequate to meet assessed needs (25)

Calories: the unit of measure used to describe the energy content of food (25)

Capillary bed: the network of tiny vessels in the tissues where the oxygen and nutrients in the blood pass into the tissues, and carbon dioxide and other waste materials from the tissues pass into the blood (34)

Cardiac arrest: the condition that is said to occur when the heart stops beating (19)

Cardiac cycle: the pumping action of the heart in an organized pattern (all of the events associated with one heartbeat) (34)

Cardiac rehabilitation: therapy that helps a person regain strength and adopt habits that will help the cardiovascular system become healthier (34)

Cardiogenic shock: shock that occurs when the heart is unable to pump enough blood throughout the body to meet the tissues' need for oxygen (19)

Cardiopulmonary resuscitation (CPR): a technique used to sustain breathing and circulation for a person who has gone into respiratory or cardiac arrest (19)

Care plan: a specific plan of nursing care for each resident developed by the nursing team (3)

Carrier: a person who is infected with a virus but never develops symptoms of the disease; the virus lives in the person's body and can be transmitted to another person (16)

Cartilage: a tough, fibrous substance found in joints and other parts of the body; in slightly movable joints, the cartilage acts as a "shock absorber"; in freely movable joints, the cartilage provides a smooth surface for the bones of the joint to move against (32)

Cataract: the gradual yellowing and hardening of the lens of the eye (36)

Catastrophic reaction: an extreme reaction to a situation that would normally cause minimal or no stress; often seen in people with dementia (9)

Catheter: a tube that is inserted into the body for the purpose of administering or removing fluids (26)

Catheter care: thorough cleaning of the perineal area (especially around the urethra) and the catheter tubing that extends outside of the body, to prevent infection (26)

CDC: see *Centers for Disease Control and Prevention*

Cell: the basic unit of life (30)

Cell membrane: a membrane that surrounds the cytoplasm and gives the cell its shape (30)

Centers for Disease Control and Prevention (CDC): the government agency that provides statistics about health conditions and diseases, monitors for disease outbreaks, and implements prevention strategies; under the umbrella of the United States Department of Health and Human Services (DHHS) (16)

Centers for Medicare and Medicaid Services (CMS): the government agency that provides oversight of government-funded insurance programs and is responsible for monitoring nursing homes to ensure compliance with Omnibus Budget Reconciliation Act (OBRA) regulations; under the umbrella of the United States Department of Health and Human Services (DHHS) (2)

Central nervous system (CNS): the brain and spinal cord; responsible for receiving information, processing it, and issuing instructions (compare with *peripheral nervous system*) (35)

Cerebral palsy: a developmental disability caused by damage to the cerebrum, the part of the brain involved with motor control (41)

Cerebrospinal fluid (CSF): a clear fluid that circulates around the brain and spinal cord and acts as a "shock absorber" to protect these structures (35)

Certified nurse practitioner (CRNP): a registered nurse (RN) who has completed additional training for licensure in advanced practice, enabling him or her to do some tasks that usually only doctors are allowed to do (3)

Cerumen: a waxy substance that helps to protect the external auditory canal by trapping dirt and other particles; commonly referred to as "earwax" (36)

Cerumen impaction: a condition that occurs when earwax builds up and becomes packed in the external auditory canal (36)

Chain facility: a facility that is owned and operated by a corporation that owns multiple, similar facilities (compare with *free-standing facility*) (2)

Chain of infection: the six key conditions that must be met for a person to get a communicable infection (pathogen, reservoir, portal of exit, method of transmission, portal of entry, and susceptible host) (15)

Chain of survival: the series of events that must take place in an emergency situation to increase the person's ability to survive the emergency without any permanent damage (19)

Charge nurse: a registered nurse (RN) or licensed practical nurse/licensed vocational nurse (LPN/LVN) who supervises the other nurses for a particular shift (3)

Chemical digestion: the process of breaking down food through the use of chemical substances, such as enzymes (compare with *mechanical digestion*) (38)

Chemical restraint: any medication that alters a person's mood or behavior, such as a sedative or tranquilizer (compare with *physical restraint*) (18)

Chemotherapy: the use of medications to destroy malignant cancer cells (43)

Cheyne-Stokes respiration: very irregular, shallow breaths, in an alternating fast–slow pattern; often seen in people who are dying (29)

Chronic bronchitis: a disorder caused by long-term irritation of the bronchi and bronchioles, such as that caused by inhaling tobacco smoke; one of two forms of chronic obstructive pulmonary disease (COPD) (33)

Chronic condition: a condition that is ongoing and often needs to be controlled through continuous medication or treatment (8)

Chronic obstructive pulmonary disease (COPD): a general term used to describe two related lung disorders, emphysema and chronic bronchitis; the leading cause of COPD is smoking (33)

Chronic pain: pain that lasts beyond the usual time that it would take for the tissues to heal (27)

Chyme: the liquid substance produced by the digestion of food in the stomach (26)

Circulation: the continuous movement of the blood through the blood vessels; powered by the pumping action of the heart (34)

Circumcision: a procedure involving the removal of the foreskin, the fold of loose skin that covers the head of the penis; often performed on male infants for religious or cultural reasons (23)

Civil laws: laws concerned with relationships between individuals (4)

Clean utility room: a storage room for clean or sterile supplies (14)

Clinical death: the state of not having a pulse or breathing; can sometimes be reversed with prompt emergency treatment that restarts the heart and breathing (compare with *biological death*) (19)

Closed bed: an empty, made bed (21)

CNS: see *central nervous system*

Coagulation: clotting of the blood (34)

Co-existent medical conditions: more than one medical condition at the same time in the same person (8)

Cognitive impairment: problems processing, learning, or remembering information (8)

Coitus: sexual intercourse (7)

Collagen: a protein that supports connective tissue, such as that found in the dermis; loss of collagen contributes to the formation of wrinkles (31)

Colonies: groups of bacteria (15)

Colostomy: an alternate way of eliminating feces from the body; done when only part of the large intestine must be removed due to disease; after removing the diseased part of a person's large intestine, an artificial opening, called a stoma, is made in the abdominal wall and the remaining portion of the large intestine is connected to it (compare with *ileostomy*) (26)

Coma: a state of unconsciousness from which a person cannot be aroused (35)

Comatose: an adjective used to describe a person who is in a coma (35)

Communicable disease: a disease that can be given from one person to another (15)

Communication: the exchange of information (5)

Competency evaluation: an exam consisting of a written portion and a skills portion that must be passed at the end of the nursing assistant training course to obtain certification (3)

Compliance: the state of meeting established regulations, standards, or requirements (6)

Conception (fertilization): occurs when the male and female sex cells join, forming a cell that contains the complete number of chromosomes (40)

Condom catheter: a device used to manage urinary incontinence in men; it consists of a soft plastic or rubber sheath, tubing, and a collection bag for the urine (26)

Conductive hearing loss: hearing loss that results when something prevents sound waves from reaching the receptors in the cochlea of the ear; see also sensorineural hearing loss (36)

Confidentiality: keeping personal information that someone shares with you to yourself (4)

Conflict: discord resulting from differences between people; can occur when one person is unable to understand or accept another's ideas or beliefs (5)

Conjunctivitis ("pink eye"): infection and inflammation of the conjunctiva, a clear membrane that lines the inside of the eyelids and covers most of the surface of the eye; characterized by redness, swelling, itching, burning, and excessive tearing (36)

Constipation: a condition that occurs when the feces remain in the intestines for too long, resulting in hard, dry feces that are difficult to pass (26)

Contact precautions: used when caring for people infected with pathogens that can be transmitted directly (by touching the person), or indirectly (by touching fomites); include using barrier methods whenever contact with the infected person or items contaminated with wound drainage or body substances is necessary (15)

Contaminated: adjective used to describe an object that is soiled by pathogens (15)

Continuing Care Accreditation Commission (CCAC): an independent, non-profit organization that sets national standards for continuing care retirement communities (CCRCs), as well as for some other types of organizations that provide long-term care services (such as adult day care centers), and officially recognizes (accredits) organizations that meet these standards (2)

Continuing care retirement community (CCRC): a type of long-term care setting that provides many different levels of care (that is, independent living, assisted living, and nursing home care) and multiple services on the same campus (2)

Continuous positive airway pressure (CPAP) therapy: a treatment that involves forcing air into the airway to keep it open; used in the treatment of sleep apnea (27)

Continuum of care: the delivery of health care over time as a person moves from being independent to needing assistance with personal care, medical care, or both (2)

Contracture: a condition that occurs when a joint is held in the same position for too long a time; the tendons shorten and become stiff, possibly causing permanent loss of motion in the joint (10)

Coordinated body movement: using the weight of the body to help with movement; the "C" in the ABCs of good body mechanics (17)

COPD: see *chronic obstructive pulmonary disease*

Coping mechanisms: conscious and deliberate ways of dealing with stress (compare with *defense mechanisms*) (42)

Coronary artery disease: a disorder that occurs when the arteries that supply the heart (the coronary arteries) narrow as a result of atherosclerosis, preventing adequate blood flow to the heart muscle (34)

CPR: see *cardiopulmonary resuscitation*

Criminal laws: laws concerned with the relationship between the individual and society (4)

Cross-contamination: occurs when microbes are transferred from one person to another on the hands of a health care worker or through contact with a fomite (15)

Culture: the beliefs (including religious or spiritual beliefs), values, and traditions that are customary to a group of people; a view of the world that is handed down from generation to generation (7)

Culture change: an ongoing process that focuses on changing attitudes, goals, and practices in order to improve the long-term care environment and the way care is delivered (2)

Customer: a person who buys or uses a product or service (13)

Customer expectation: an assumption the customer makes about the qualities or characteristics of the service or product that is being provided (13)

Customer need: a service or product that the customer requires (13)

Customer service: the attention and assistance that is provided to a customer (13)

Cuticle: the skin along the edges of the nail (24)

Cyanotic: adjective used to describe skin, lips, or nail beds that have a blue or gray tinge (29)

Cyanosis: blue or gray discoloration of the skin, lips, and nail beds; develops when the skin does not receive enough oxygen and is a sign of a respiratory or circulatory disorder (31)

Cystitis: infection of the bladder (39)

Cystocele: a condition that occurs when the bladder shifts downward, pressing into the front (anterior) vaginal wall (40)

Cytoplasm: the jelly-like substance within a cell, within which the organelles float (30)

D

Dandruff: excessive itching and flaking of the scalp (24)

Decision-making capacity: the ability to make a thoughtful decision based on an understanding of the potential risks and benefits of taking a certain course of action (4)

Deep venous thrombosis (DVT): formation of a blood clot (thrombus) in one of the deep veins of the lower leg (34)

Defamation: the act of making untrue statements that hurt another person's reputation (4)

Defecate: to have a bowel movement (26)

Defense mechanisms: unconscious ways of dealing with stress (compare with *coping mechanisms*) (42)

Deficiency citations: statements included in the report produced by the survey team at the end of the survey that identify standards that the facility did not meet, as well as the findings that indicate how the facility failed to meet the standards (6)

Degenerative condition: a condition that gets progressively worse over time (8)

Dehydration: too little fluid in the tissues of the body (compare with *edema*) (25)

Delegate: to authorize another person to perform a task on your behalf (3)

Delirium: a temporary state of confusion (19)

Delusion: a false idea or belief that the person holds to be true and that cannot be changed (9)

Dementia: the permanent and progressive loss of mental functions (such as thinking, reasoning, and remembering), caused by damage to the brain tissue (9)

Dendrites: short extensions from the body of a neuron that *receive* information from other neurons (compare with *axon*) (35)

Denial: one of the stages of grief; the person refuses to accept the diagnosis or feels that a mistake has been made (28)

Dental caries: dental cavities or tooth decay, caused by poor oral hygiene (23)

Dentition: the type of teeth a person has, how many teeth, and the arrangement of those teeth in the mouth (25)

Deodorant: a grooming product that covers or masks odor (23)

Depression: 1) a disorder characterized by a persistent "low" mood and decreased pleasure (42); 2) one of the stages of grief; the person fully realizes that death will be the end result of the illness and experiences sadness and regret (28)

Depth of respiration: the quality of each breath (22)

Dermatitis: a general term for inflammation of the skin (31)

Dermis: the deepest layer of skin, where sensory receptors, blood vessels, nerves, glands, and hair follicles are found (31)

Development: changes that occur psychologically or socially as a person passes through life (7)

Developmental disability: a permanent disability that affects a person before he or she reaches adulthood (that is, before 19 to 22 years of age) and interferes with the person's ability to achieve developmental milestones (41)

Diabetes mellitus: an endocrine disorder that results when the pancreas is unable to produce enough insulin, the body's cells are unable to properly use the insulin that is produced, or both (37)

Diabetic retinopathy: a complication of diabetes that can lead to blindness (36)

Diagnosis-related groups (DRGs): a system for controlling health care costs in which the length of a person's hospital stay, as well as payment for hospitalization, surgery, or other treatment, is specified according to the person's diagnosis; used as a basis for Medicare payments in advanced (acute) care settings (compare with *resource utilization groups [RUGs]*)(1)

Dialysis: a procedure that is done to remove waste products and fluids from the body when a person's kidneys fail and can no longer perform this task (39)

Diaphoretic: adjective used to describe a person who has a medical condition that causes him to sweat a great deal (23)

Diaphragm: 1) the large flat surface of the stethoscope that is used to hear loud, harsh sounds (22); 2) the strong, dome-shaped muscle that separates the chest cavity from the abdominal cavity and assists in breathing (33)

Diarrhea: the passage of liquid, unformed stool (26)

Diastole: the resting phase of the cardiac cycle; during which the myocardium relaxes, allowing the chambers to fill with blood (compare with *systole*) (34)

Diastolic pressure: the pressure that the blood exerts against the arterial walls when the heart muscle relaxes; the second blood pressure measurement that is recorded (compare with *systolic pressure*) (22)

Dietitian: a person who has a degree in nutrition (6)

Digestion: the process of breaking food down into simple elements (nutrients) (25)

Digital examination: examination that is done when a person is thought to have a fecal impaction; a finger is inserted into the person's rectum to feel for the impacted mass (26)

Director of Nursing (DON): the registered nurse who directs all of the nursing care within a facility (3)

Disability: impaired physical, mental, or emotional function (10)

Disaster: a sudden, unexpected event that causes injury to many people, major damage to property, or both (17)

Discharge: the official release of a person from a health care facility (11)

Discharge planning: the process used by the members of the health care team to help prepare a resident to leave the facility; helps to make sure that the person continues to receive quality care, either from a home health care agency or from family members, after the discharge (11)

Disease: a condition that occurs when the structure or function of an organ or an organ system is abnormal (30)

Disinfection: the use of strong chemicals to kill pathogens on non-living objects that come in contact with body fluids or substances, such as bedpans, urinals, and over-bed tables; one of the techniques of medical asepsis (compare with *antisepsis, sanitization,* and *sterilization*) (15)

Disoriented: the state of being unable to answer basic questions about person, place, or time; a state of confusion (compare with *oriented to person, place, and time*) (19)

Diuretics: medications that help the kidneys remove extra water from the body (26)

Diuresis: excessive output of urine; also called *polyuria* (26)

Do not resuscitate (DNR) order: an order written on a person's chart specifying the person's wishes that the usual efforts to save his life will not be made; also called a *no-code order* (28)

Down syndrome: a developmental disability that is the result of having 47 chromosomes instead of 46; people with this disorder have mental retardation and certain key physical features, such as almond-shaped eyes and square hands with short, stubby fingers (41)

Draw sheet: a small, flat sheet that is placed over the middle of the bottom sheet, covering the area of the bed from above the person's shoulders to below his or her buttocks; see also *lift sheet* (21)

Droplet precautions: used when caring for people infected with pathogens that can be transmitted by direct exposure to droplets released from the mouth or nose (for example, when the person coughs, sneezes, or talks) (15)

Durable power of attorney for health care: a type of advance directive that transfers the responsibility for making medical decisions on a person's behalf to a family member, friend, or other trusted individual, in the event that the person is no longer able to make these decisions on his or her own behalf (4)

Dysphagia: difficulty swallowing (10)

Dyspnea: labored or difficult breathing (22)

Dysrhythmia: an irregular pulse rhythm (22)

Dysuria: painful or difficult urination (26)

E

Early morning care: care provided after a person wakes up to prepare him or her for breakfast or other early morning activities (23)

Eczema: a type of chronic dermatitis that is usually accompanied by severe itching, scaling, and crusting of the surface of the skin (31)

Edema: too much fluid in the tissues of the body (compare with *dehydration*) (25)

Edentulous: without teeth (23)

Egg (ovum, ova): female sex cell (40)

Ejaculation: the forceful release of semen from the body; method by which sperm cells leave the man's body through the penis (40)

Elopement: an incident that occurs when a resident leaves the facility without the knowledge of facility staff (18)

Embolus (plural, *emboli*): a blood clot (thrombus) that breaks loose and moves through the bloodstream (34)

Emergency: a condition that requires immediate medical or surgical evaluation or treatment to prevent the person from dying or having a permanent disability (19)

Emergency medical services (EMS) system: a network of resources (including people, equipment, and facilities) that is organized to respond to an emergency (19)

Empathy: the ability to imagine what it would feel like to be in another person's situation (3)

Emphysema: a disorder caused by long-term exposure of the alveoli to toxins, such as tobacco smoke; one of two forms of chronic obstructive pulmonary disease (COPD) (33)

Enabler: a device that helps to support a higher level of functioning for the resident (18)

Endocardium: the smooth inner lining of the heart wall (34)

Endospore: a protective shell that forms around some types of bacteria; the shell allows the bacterium to remain alive but enter a state of inactivity; when the bacterium's best growing conditions become available, the bacterium becomes active again (15)

Endotracheal tube: a device that is inserted into a person's nose or mouth and extends to the trachea; used when a person must receive mechanical ventilation for a short time (33)

End-stage disease: a medical condition that becomes progressively worse over time, causing irreversible changes that no longer respond to treatment (28)

Enema: the introduction of fluid into the large intestine by way of the anus for the purpose of removing stool from the rectum (26)

Enteral nutrition: placing food directly into a person's stomach or intestines, using a nasogastric tube, nasointestinal tube, gastrostomy tube, jejunostomy tube, or percutaneous endoscopic gastrostomy (PEG) tube (25)

Entrapment: an accident that occurs when a person becomes trapped in the side rail, or between the side rail and the mattress (18)

Enzymes: substances that have the ability to break chemical bonds (38)

Epicardium: the smooth outermost layer of the heart wall (34)

Epidermis: the outer layer of the skin (31)

Epilepsy: a disorder characterized by chronic seizure activity (35)

Erythema: redness of the skin (31)

Erythrocytes: red blood cells; responsible for carrying oxygen to all of the tissues of the body (34)

Esophageal (cardiac) sphincter: a circle of muscular tissue that surrounds the place where the esophagus enters the stomach and keeps food from going back up the esophagus after it has entered the stomach (38)

Esophagus: a long narrow tube that serves mainly as a passageway for food to get from the pharynx to the stomach (38)

Ethics: moral principles or standards that govern conduct (4)

Ethics committee: a group of people, each with different areas of expertise, brought together to help health care facilities resolve difficult ethical dilemmas (4)

Eupnea: a normal respiratory rate (22)

Evaluation statement: a statement in the interdisciplinary care plan that reviews the effectiveness of the interventions in helping the resident to meet the goal (12)

Evening (hour of sleep, hs) care: care provided in preparation for sleep (23)

Excoriation: an abrasion, or a scraping away of the surface of the skin; can be caused by trauma, chemicals, or burns (31)

Exhalation (expiration): the phase of ventilation during which carbon dioxide is transported out of the lungs (compare with *inhalation [inspiration]*) (22)

Exposure control plan: a plan that states what actions must be taken if an employee is exposed to blood or other body fluids while on the job (16)

External customer: a person from outside of your organization who relies on you to provide a product or service (compare with *internal customer*) (13)

F

Facemask: a device used for delivering oxygen that is made of soft, molded plastic material that fits over the nose and mouth (33)

False imprisonment: confining another person against his or her will (4)

Fanfolded: adjective used to describe the top sheet, blanket, and bedspread of a closed bed when they have been turned back (toward the foot of the bed) (21)

Fat-soluble: adjective used to describe a substance that dissolves in fat (for example, certain vitamins) (25)

Febrile: adjective used to describe the state of having a fever, or increased body temperature (22)

Fecal impaction: a condition that occurs when constipation is not relieved (26)

Fecal (bowel) incontinence: the inability to hold one's feces, or the involuntary loss of feces from the bowel (26)

Feces: the semi-solid waste product of digestion; stool (26)

Fetal alcohol syndrome: a combination of physical and mental problems that affect children whose mothers consumed alcohol during pregnancy (41)

Fiber supplement: a tablet or drink additive that is used to add bulk to the feces, causing them to hold fluid, and preventing constipation (26)

Fidelity: an ethical principle that requires health care workers to act with integrity to earn others' trust (4)

Filtrate: the liquid that forms the basis for urine (39)

Financial abuse: the misuse or theft of another person's money or property (4)

First aid: the care given to an injured or sick person while waiting for more advanced help to arrive (19)

Fissure: a crack in the skin (31)

Five rights of delegation: a set of guidelines that help nurses to make good decisions about which tasks to delegate and to whom (3)

Fixation: the process of holding a broken bone in one position until the fracture heals; may be *external* (accomplished through the use of a cast) or *internal* (accomplished through the use of metal plates, screws, rods, pins, or wires attached to the bone) (32)

Flatulence: the presence of excessive amounts of flatus (gas) in the intestines, causing abdominal distension (swelling) and discomfort (26)

Flatus: gas that is formed as part of the digestion process (26)

Flow meter: a device used to set the rate at which oxygen is delivered to a person who is receiving oxygen therapy (33)

Fluid balance: a state where the amount of fluid taken into the body equals the amount of fluid that leaves the body (25)

Flushing: redness of the skin (31)

Fomite: a non-living object that has been contaminated (soiled) by pathogens (15)

Footboard: a padded board that is placed upright at the foot of the bed; used to keep the person's feet in proper alignment (21)

Foreskin: the fold of loose skin that covers the head of the penis (23)

For-profit facility: a facility that is owned and operated by a company or organization with the intention of making money (compare with *non-profit [not-for-profit] facility*) (2)

Fowler's position: one of the basic positions in which the head of the bed is elevated to between 45 and 60 degrees; variations include *semi-Fowler's (low Fowler's) position* and *high Fowler's position* (20)

Fracture: a broken bone (32)

Fracture pan: a wedge-shaped bedpan that is used when a person has an injury or disability that makes it too uncomfortable or dangerous to use a regular bedpan (26)

Fragile X syndrome: an inherited type of mental retardation caused by a defect in the X chromosome (41)

Fraud: deception that could cause harm to another person (4)

Free-standing facility: a facility that is independently owned and operated (compare with *chain facility*) (2)

Frequency: the term used to describe voiding that occurs more often than usual (26)

Friction: a term used to describe the force created when two surfaces (such as a sheet and a person's skin) rub against each other; can lead to skin breakdown (20)

Frontotemporal dementia: a disorder characterized by damage to the areas of the brain that are responsible for personality, behavior, and language; in addition to a progressive decline in mental abilities, people with frontotemporal dementia have extreme changes in behavior and personality, difficulties with language, or both (9)

F-Tags: numerical headings used by the government to categorize the standards included in the long-term care regulations (6)

G

Gallbladder: a small pouch-like organ that is attached to the liver; it stores bile produced by the liver that is not secreted directly into the duodenum (38)

Gas exchange: the transfer of oxygen into the blood, and carbon dioxide out of it (33)

Gastrostomy tube: a tube used for enteral nutrition that is inserted into the stomach through a surgical incision in the abdomen (25)

Gatches: the joints at the hips and knees of the mattresses of most adjustable beds that allow the mattress to "break" so that the person's head can be elevated or his knees bent (14)

General lighting: lighting that supplies overall illumination (light), allowing a person to see and move about safely (compare with *task lighting*) (14)

Gingivitis: inflammation of the gums (23)

Glaucoma: a disorder of the eye that occurs when the pressure within the eye is increased to dangerous levels (36)

Glomerulus: part of the nephron, the functional unit of the kidney where blood is filtered to form urine (39)

Glucometer: a device used to monitor blood glucose levels (37)

Glucose: the body's most basic type of fuel; supplied by carbohydrates and sometimes referred to as "blood sugar" (25)

Goal statement (expected outcome): a statement in the interdisciplinary care plan of what the health care team expects the resident to be able to achieve within a specific time frame (12)

Goiter: enlargement of the thyroid gland (37)

Graduate: a measuring device used to measure fluids (25)

Grand mal seizure: a seizure characterized by generalized and violent contraction and relaxation of the body's muscles (compare with *petit mal [absence] seizure*) (19)

Grief: mental anguish, specifically associated with loss (28)

Grooming: activities related to maintaining a neat and attractive appearance, such as shampooing and styling the hair, shaving, and applying make-up (24)

Grounded: an adjective used to describe electrical equipment that has a way of returning stray electrical current to the outlet so that the risk of electrical shock is reduced (17)

Group insurance: insurance that is purchased at group rates by an employer or corporation (1)

Growth: changes that occur physically as a person passes through life (7)

Gynecologist: a doctor who specializes in diagnosing and treating disorders of the female reproductive system (40)

H

Halitosis: bad breath that does not go away (23)

Hallucination: an episode when a person sees, feels, hears, or tastes something that does not really exist (9)

Hangnails: broken pieces of cuticle (24)

HAV: see *hepatitis A virus*

HBV: see *hepatitis B virus*

HCV: see *hepatitis C virus*

HDV: see *hepatitis D virus*

Health care agent: the person named in a durable power of attorney for health care who is responsible for making decisions on a person's behalf, in the event that the person is no longer able to make decisions on his own behalf; may also be called the person's *durable power of attorney for health care* (4)

Health care–associated infections (HAIs): infections that patients or residents get while receiving treatment in a hospital or other health care facility, or that health care workers get while preforming their duties within a health care setting (15)

Health care team: group of people with different types of knowledge and skill levels who work together to provide holistic care to the resident (1)

Health Insurance Portability and Accountability Act (HIPAA): a federal privacy regulation that helps to keep personal information about patients and residents private (4)

Health maintenance organization (HMO): a managed care system that contracts with health care providers to provide health care services for a prepaid fee, and people seeking care agree to see only health care providers who are part of the HMO network (1)

Heart failure: a condition that occurs when the heart is unable to pump enough blood to meet the body's needs (34)

Hematuria: blood in the urine (26)

Hemiplegia: paralysis on one side of the body (compare with *paraplegia* and *quadriplegia*) (35)

Hemoglobin: a protein found in red blood cells that combines with oxygen to carry it to the tissues of the body (34)

Hemoptysis: the coughing up of blood or blood-stained sputum (33)

Hemorrhage: severe bleeding (19)

Hemorrhagic shock: shock that results from massive blood loss (19)

Hemostasis: the process of stopping blood loss from the circulatory system (34)

Hemothorax: a condition that occurs when blood builds up in the space between the lungs and the chest wall (33)

Hepatitis: inflammation of the liver (16)

Hepatitis A virus (HAV): a virus that is transmitted through the oral–fecal route and causes a form of acute hepatitis (16)

Hepatitis B virus (HBV): a bloodborne virus that causes a form of hepatitis that is acute in most people but may become chronic; a serious health threat for the health care worker (16)

Hepatitis C virus (HCV): a bloodborne virus that causes a form of chronic hepatitis that can eventually lead to end-stage cirrhosis (a fatal liver disease), liver failure, or liver cancer (16)

Hepatitis D virus (HDV): a bloodborne virus that is found only in people who are already infected with hepatitis B virus (HBV) (16)

Hepatitis E virus (HEV): a virus that is transmitted through the oral–fecal route and causes a form of hepatitis (16)

Hernia: a disorder that occurs when an internal organ bulges through a weakness in the muscular wall of the abdominal cavity (38)

Heterosexual: a person who is sexually attracted to members of the opposite sex (7)

HEV: see *hepatitis E virus*

High Fowler's position: one of the basic positions in which the head of the bed is elevated to between 60 and 90 degrees (20)

HIPAA: see *Health Insurance Portability and Accountability Act*

Hip fracture: a fracture that occurs at the top of the femur (thigh bone) (32)

HIV: see *human immunodeficiency virus*

HIV-positive: the state of being infected with human immunodeficiency virus (HIV) (44)

Holistic: an adjective used to describe care of the whole person, physically and emotionally (1)

Home health care agency: an agency that provides professional health care in a person's home (1)

Homeostasis: a state of balance (30)

Homosexual: a person who is attracted to members of the same sex (7)

Hopper: a sink-like fixture that empties into a sewer line and is used for tasks such as cleaning bedpans or rinsing soiled linens or clothing (14)

Hormones: chemicals that act on cells to produce a response (37)

Hospice organization: a health care organization that provides care for people who are dying and their families (1)

Hospital: a health care facility that provides treatment for people with acute medical or surgical conditions (1)

Human immunodeficiency virus (HIV): a virus transmitted in blood and other body fluids (such as semen) that targets the T cells of the immune system; most people infected with HIV go on to develop acquired immunodeficiency syndrome (AIDS), a fatal illness (16)

Hygiene: personal cleanliness (3)

Hyperglycemia: a blood glucose level that is too high (37)

Hyperopia: farsightedness; trouble seeing objects that are close (compare with *myopia*) (36)

Hypertension: high blood pressure; a blood pressure that is consistently greater than 140 mm Hg (systolic) and/or 90 mm Hg (diastolic) (22)

Hyperthyroidism: a condition caused by the excessive secretion of thyroxine, one of the thyroid hormones; characterized by increased hunger accompanied by weight loss, an irregular heartbeat, an inability to sleep, irritability, confusion, increased perspiration, and intolerance to heat (37)

Hyperventilation: increased rate and depth of breathing (22)

Hypoglycemia: a blood glucose level that is too low (37)

Hypotension: low blood pressure; a blood pressure that is consistently lower than 90 mm Hg (systolic) and/or 60 mm Hg (diastolic) (22)

Hypothyroidism: a condition caused by the low secretion of thyroxine, one of the thyroid hormones; characterized by fatigue, weakness, depression, anorexia, weight gain, constipation, and intolerance to cold (37)

Hypoventilation: decreased rate and depth of breathing (22)

Hypoxic: the state of being deficient of oxygen (33)

I

Ileostomy: an alternate way of eliminating feces from the body; done when the entire large intestine must be removed due to disease; after removing the person's diseased large intestine, an artificial opening, called a stoma, is made in the abdominal wall and the end of the small intestine is connected to it (compare with *colostomy*) (26)

Impotence (erectile dysfunction): the inability to achieve or maintain an erection long enough to engage in sexual activity (40)

Incident: an occurrence that is considered unusual, undesired, or out of the ordinary, and that disrupts the normal routine for the resident, the facility, or both (18)

Incident (occurrence) report: a preprinted document that is completed following an accident involving a resident (18)

Indwelling catheter: a urinary catheter that is left inside the bladder to provide continuous urine drainage; also known as a *retention catheter* or a *Foley catheter* (26)

Infection: disease caused by pathogenic microbes (15)

Infection control: basic practices designed to decrease the chance that an infection will spread from one person to another in a health care facility (15)

Influenza: an acute respiratory infection caused by the influenza virus; characterized by a sore throat, dry cough, stuffy nose, headache, body aches, weakness, and fever; commonly known as "the flu"(33)

Informed consent: written permission granted by a person to begin treatment or perform a procedure after receiving a full explanation of the treatment or procedure from the health care provider (4)

Ingestion: the intake of food or fluids (25)

Inhalation (inspiration): the phase of ventilation during which oxygen is taken into the lungs (compare with *exhalation [expiration]*) (22)

Insomnia: a disorder characterized by an inability to fall asleep, or to stay asleep (27)

Instrumental activities of daily living (IADLs): more complex tasks that a person must be able to do in order to continue to live independently, such as using the telephone or handling money (compare with *activities of daily living*) (8)

Intake and output (I&O) flow sheet: a document used for recording measurements of all the fluids that enter and leave the body (25)

Intentional tort: a violation of civil law committed by a person with the intent to do harm (4)

Intentional wound: a wound that is the result of a planned surgical or medical intervention (compare with *unintentional wound*) (31)

Interdisciplinary care plan: a specific plan of care for each resident developed with input from all members of the health care team (12)

Internal customer: a person from inside your organization who relies on you to provide a product or service (compare with *external customer*) (13)

Interventions: specific actions that members of the health care team take to help the resident (12)

Interview: a meeting between an employer and a potential employee, during which information is exchanged regarding the organization, the job, and the potential employee's qualifications for the job (45)

Intimacy: a feeling of emotional closeness to another human being (7)

Intravenous (IV) therapy: an alternate method of providing fluids and nutrition; fluids are given through a small catheter (tube) that is inserted into a vein (usually in the back of the hand) (25)

Invasion of privacy: the act of violating another person's right to keep certain information and aspects of himself away from the examination of others (4)

Ischemia: the state that occurs when the flow of oxygen-rich blood to the tissues is interrupted, leading to an oxygen deficiency in the tissues (34)

Isolation (transmission-based) precautions: guidelines, based on a pathogen's method of transmission, that health care workers follow to contain the pathogen and limit others' exposure to it as much as possible (15)

J

Jaundice: a yellow discoloration of the skin and the whites of the eyes; usually associated with liver disorders (31)

Jejunostomy tube: a tube used for enteral nutrition that is inserted into the jejunum (part of the small intestine) through a surgical incision in the abdomen (25)

Job application: a standardized form used to obtain basic information about a job candidate, such as which position the candidate is applying for, how the candidate can be reached, and what shifts the candidate can work (45)

Joint: the area where two bones join together (32)

Justice: an ethical principle that requires health care workers to be fair and treat people equally regardless of race, religion, culture, disability, or ability to pay (4)

K

Kardex: a card file that contains condensed versions of each resident's medical record (5)

Keratin: a substance that causes mature skin cells to thicken and become resistant to water (31)

Kidney stones (renal calculi): a painful disorder characterized by the formation of clumps of minerals ("stones") in the kidney and bladder (39)

Korotkoff sounds: sounds that are heard while taking a person's blood pressure (22)

Kyphosis: an abnormal forward curvature of the upper spine (32)

L

Larceny: the act of stealing another person's property (4)

Laryngitis: inflammation of the larynx (the "voice box") (33)

Larynx: part of the respiratory airway; also known as "the voice box" (33)

Lateral position: one of the basic positions in which the person lies on his or her side (20)

Laws: rules that are made by a controlling authority, such as the state or federal government, with the intent of preserving basic human rights (4)

Laxative: a medication that chemically stimulates the bowels to move; a treatment for constipation (26)

Lesion: a general term used to describe any break in the skin (31)

Leukemia: a general term for a group of disorders characterized by the excessive production of white blood cells that are abnormal in structure (34)

Leukocyte: white blood cell (34)

Lewy body dementia: a disorder characterized by the build-up of abnormal protein deposits (called Lewy bodies) in areas of the brain that are responsible for thinking and movement; in addition to a progressive decline in mental abilities, people with Lewy body dementia have problems controlling body movement similar to those seen in people with Parkinson's disease, visual hallucinations, and distinct changes in mental alertness (9)

Liability: the responsibility of an individual to act within the confines of the law (4)

Libel: written statements that injure someone's reputation; a form of defamation (4)

Licensed practical nurse (LPN): a specially trained person who is licensed by a state to provide routine care for the sick under the supervision of a registered nurse (RN); completes a 1- to 2-year program in a vocational school, community college, or hospital (3)

Licensed vocational nurse (LVN): another term for *licensed practical nurse*; used in the states of Texas and California (3)

Life-sustaining treatment: treatments that will prolong life, such as mechanical ventilation, cardiopulmonary resuscitation (CPR), and the placement of a feeding tube or intravenous (IV) line for the provision of nutrition (28)

Lift sheet: a draw sheet that is used to help lift or reposition a person who needs assistance with moving in bed (21)

Ligaments: very strong bands of fibrous tissue that cross over the joint capsule, attaching one bone to another and stabilizing the joint (32)

Litigation: the lawsuit, or legal action, taken against a person who is accused of breaking a law (4)

Liver: an organ that performs several important functions in the body, including the secretion of bile (a substance needed for digestion of fats), the production of clotting factors (chemicals that help our blood to clot), and the clearance of toxins (such as alcohol and drugs) from the body (38)

Living will: a type of advance directive that states a person's wish that death not be artificially postponed (4)

Logrolling: a technique for turning a person in which the person's body is moved in one fluid motion to keep the spine in alignment (20)

Long-term care facility: a health care facility that provides ongoing nursing care and personal assistance for people who can no longer live independently as a result of illness or disability; examples of long-term care facilities include nursing homes and assisted-living facilities (1)

Long-term care insurance: a private insurance policy that can be purchased by an individual to help pay for long-term care in the future, should it be needed (2)

Long-term care setting: a place where health care is provided for people who require ongoing nursing care, personal assistance, or both as a result of illness or disability; length of stay in the facility is usually longer than 30 days (compare with *advanced (acute) care setting* and *post-acute care setting*) (1)

Lungs: the primary organs for respiration, the process the body uses to obtain oxygen from the environment and remove carbon dioxide (a waste gas) from the body (33)

Lymph: fluid in the lymph vessels (vessels that return the fluid that leaks into the tissues to the bloodstream) (34)

Lymph nodes: masses of lymphatic tissue that "clean" the lymph by removing bacteria and other large particles before returning the fluid to the bloodstream (34)

M

Macular degeneration: a vision disorder that results from the build-up of deposits in the macula (part of the retina) and eventually leads to blindness (36)

Macule: a small, flat, reddened skin lesion (31)

Malignant: adjective used to describe a cancerous tumor (that is, a tumor that has the ability to progress or invade other tissues) (compare with *benign*) (43)

Malpractice: negligence committed by people who hold licenses to practice their profession, such as doctors, nurses, lawyers, dentists, and pharmacists (4)

Managed care system: a system designed to control health care costs by delivering health care to people who need it by arranging contracts with various health care providers; examples include preferred provider organizations (PPOs) and health maintenance organizations (HMOs) (1)

Mastication: chewing (38)

Masturbation: stimulation of the genitals for sexual pleasure or release, by a means other than sexual intercourse (7)

Materials Safety Data Sheet (MSDS): a document that summarizes key information about a chemical, such as its composition, which exposures may be dangerous, what to do if an exposure should occur, and how to clean up spills (17)

Mechanical digestion: the process of breaking down food through the use of physical means, such as chewing (compare with *chemical digestion*) (38)

Mechanical ventilation: a life-sustaining treatment in which a machine breathes for a person who cannot breathe on his or her own (33)

Medicaid: a federally funded and state-regulated plan designed to help people with low incomes to pay for health care (1)

Medical asepsis: techniques that are used to physically remove or kill pathogens (see also *sanitization, antisepsis, disinfection,* and *sterilization*) (15)

Medical record: a legal document where information about a resident's current condition, the measures that have been taken by the medical and nursing staff to diagnose and treat the condition, and the resident's response to the treatment and care provided is recorded; also called a "medical chart" (5)

Medicare: a type of insurance plan that is federally funded by Social Security and which all people 65 years and older, and some younger disabled people, are eligible to participate in (1)

Medication room: a storage room for medications and the supplies for administering medications (14)

Melanin: a dark pigment that gives our skin, hair, and eyes color (31)

Menarche: the onset of the first menstrual period (7)

Meninges: the three layers of connective tissue that cover and protect the brain and spinal cord (35)

Menopause: the cessation of menstruation and fertility that women typically experience in their early 50s (7)

Menstrual period: the monthly loss of blood through the vagina that occurs in the absence of pregnancy (40)

Mental illness: a disorder that affects a person's mind, causing the person to experience emotional difficulties, to act in unusual ways, or both (42)

Mental retardation: the state of having below-average intellectual functioning (that is, a decreased ability to reason, think, and understand) and problems with adaptive skills (that is, skills needed to live and work, such as communication skills, social skills, and self-care skills) (41)

Metabolism: the word used to describe the physical and chemical changes that occur when the cells of the body change the food that we eat into energy (22)

Metastasis: the process by which cancer cells spread from their original location in the body to a new location, which may be quite distant from the first (43)

Methicillin-resistant *Staphylococcus aureus* (MRSA): a type of bacteria that has become resistant to methicillin, a powerful antibiotic (15)

Microbe (microorganism): a living thing that cannot be seen with the naked eye; examples include bacteria and viruses (15)

Micturition: the process of passing urine from the body; also known as *urination* and *voiding* (26)

Midstream ("clean catch") urine specimen: a method of collecting urine that prevents contamination of the urine by the bacteria that normally exist in and around the urethra (26)

Minimum Data Set (MDS): a screening tool that is used to identify and document each resident's problem areas and the degree of assistance or skilled care that the resident needs; the first part of the Resident Assessment Instrument (RAI) (12)

Mission: the officially stated purpose of a health care facility or organization (1)

Mitered corner: a corner that is made by folding and tucking the sheet so that it lies flat and neat against the mattress (21)

Morning (A.M.) care: care provided in the morning, to ready the person for the day, such as completion of personal hygiene and grooming activities, and bedmaking (23)

Motor nerves: nerves that carry commands from the brain down the spinal cord and out to the muscles and organs of the body (35)

Mucous membrane: a special type of epithelial tissue that lines many of the organ systems in the body and is coated with mucus (33)

Mucus: a slippery, sticky substance that is secreted by special cells and serves to keep the surfaces of mucous membranes moist (33)

Multiple sclerosis (MS): a disorder of the nervous system in which the myelin sheaths that cover the nerves are damaged, resulting in faulty transmission of nerve impulses (35)

Muscle tone: the steady contraction of the skeletal muscles that helps us to maintain an upright posture, such as sitting or standing (32)

Muscular dystrophy: a general term for a group of disorders that cause the skeletal muscles to become more and more weak over time (32)

Myelin: a fatty, white substance that protects the axon and helps to speed the conduction of nerve impulses along the axon (35)

Myocardial infarction: a "heart attack"; occurs when one or more of the coronary arteries becomes completely blocked, preventing blood from reaching the parts of the heart that are fed by the affected arteries (34)

Myocardium: the thick, muscular middle layer of the heart wall; responsible for the pumping action of the heart (34)

Myopia: nearsightedness; trouble seeing objects that are far away (compare with *hyperopia*) (36)

N

Nasal cannula: a device used to deliver oxygen to a resident; consists of two prongs of soft plastic tubing that are inserted into the nostrils (33)

Nasal cavity: the inside of the nose (33)

Nasogastric tube: a tube used for enteral nutrition that is inserted through the nose, down the throat, and into the stomach (25)

Nasointestinal tube: a tube used for enteral nutrition that is inserted through the nose, down the throat, and into the small intestine (25)

Nasopharyngeal airway: a soft rubber tube that is inserted into a person's nose and extends back toward the throat to create an opening that air can flow through (33)

Necrosis: tissue death as a result of a lack of oxygen (31)

Need: something that is essential for a person's physical and mental health (7)

Neglect: the failure to provide for a dependent person's basic physical needs; a form of physical abuse (4)

Negligent: adjective used to describe a person who fails to do what a "careful and reasonable" person would do in any given situation (4)

Nephron: the basic functional unit of the kidney; consists of a glomerulus and a series of tubules (39)

Neurogenic bladder: a condition caused by problems with the nerves that control the bladder; the bladder may be overactive or underactive (39)

Neuron: a cell that can send and receive information (35)

Nits: the eggs of head lice, seen on the hair, near the scalp, in people with pediculosis capitis (head lice infestation) (24)

No-code order: an order written on a person's chart specifying the person's wishes that the usual efforts to save his life will not be made; see also *do not resuscitate (DNR) order* (28)

Nocturnal emission: the harmless involuntary discharge of semen during sleep; commonly called a "wet dream" (7)

Nocturia: the need to get up more than once or twice during the night to urinate, to the point where sleep is disrupted (26)

Non-maleficence: an ethical principle that requires health care workers to avoid harming those in their care (4)

Non-profit (not-for-profit) facility: a facility that is owned and operated by a service organization (such as a church or charitable group) with the intention of fulfilling a need in the community (compare with *for-profit facility*) (2)

Non-verbal communication: a way of communicating that uses facial expressions, gestures, and body language, instead of written or spoken language (5)

Normal (resident) flora: the harmless microbes that live in and on the body and help it to function properly (compare with *transient flora*) (15)

Nosocomial infections: infections that patients or residents get while receiving treatment in a hospital or other health care facility; a type of health care–associated infection (HAI) (15)

Nourishment room: a room on the unit of a nursing home that is used for storing and preparing snacks and beverages for residents (14)

NPO status: a doctor's order specifying that a resident is to have "*nils per os*" (nothing by mouth) (25)

Nucleus: the cell's "brain"; it contains all of the information the cell needs in order to do its job, grow, and reproduce (30)

Nurse practice acts: state laws that govern nursing practice and education (3)

Nurses' station: the area that serves as the central base of operations for the nursing staff (14)

Nursing home: type of long-term care facility that provides residents with around-the-clock nursing care and supervision (1)

Nursing process: a process that allows members of the nursing team to communicate with each other regarding a resident's specific needs (in regard to nursing care), what steps will be taken to meet those needs, and whether or not the steps were effective in meeting the resident's needs; consists of five steps: assessment, diagnosis, planning, implementation, and evaluation (3)

Nutrients: substances in foods and fluids that the body uses to grow, to repair itself, and to carry out processes essential for living (25)

Nutrition: the process of taking in and using food (25)

Nutritional supplement: a flavored shake or drink that is used to supply extra calories or protein; often served with meals or as a snack in between meals (25)

O

Obese: the state of being extremely overweight (25)

Objective data: information that is obtained directly, through measurements or by using one of the five senses (sight, smell, taste, vision, touch) (5)

Observation: something that you notice about the resident, typically related to a change in the resident's physical or mental condition (5)

Obsessive–compulsive disorder: an anxiety disorder that causes a person to suffer intensely from recurrent unwanted thoughts (obsessions) that are usually associated with rituals the person feels obligated to complete constantly (compulsions) (42)

Occult: an adjective used to describe something that is hidden or cannot be seen with the naked eye; often used in reference to blood in a urine or stool sample (26)

Occupational Safety and Health Administration (OSHA): an agency within the Department of Labor that establishes safety and health standards for the workplace, to protect the safety and health of employees (1)

Occupational therapy: a health care specialty that focuses on helping the person regain or maintain the skills needed for everyday life, such as those related to self care (10)

Occupied bed: a bed with a person in it (21)

Off-site preparation: the work the survey team does in advance to prepare for the survey, before arriving at the facility (6)

Oliguria: the state of voiding a very small amount of urine over a given period of time (26)

Ombudsman: a person from a state or local Office on Aging who regularly visits residents of long-term care facilities to check on their welfare and overall satisfaction with their care, and who advocates for the residents to ensure that their concerns are addressed (4)

Omnibus Budget Reconciliation Act (OBRA): an act passed in 1987 to improve the quality of life for people who live in nursing homes by making sure that residents receive a certain standard of care (2)

Open bed: a bed ready to receive a resident (21)

Opportunistic microbes: microbes that are considered normal (resident) flora when they are in or on one part of the body, but can cause infection if they move out of that area and into or onto another part of the body (15)

Oral–fecal route: a method of transmitting an infection; occurs when feces containing a pathogen contaminate food or water, which is then consumed by another person (16)

Organ: a group of tissues functioning together for a similar purpose (30)

Organelles: structures inside of the cell that help the cell to make the energy it needs to stay alive and to rid itself of waste products (30)

Organism: a living thing, such as an animal or a plant (30)

Organ system: a group of organs that work together to perform a specific function for the body (30)

Oriented to person, place, and time: the state of being able to answer basic questions about person, place, or time; alert (compare with *disoriented*) (19)

Oropharyngeal airway: a hard plastic device that is inserted into a person's mouth to stop the tongue from falling back into the throat; used to keep the airway open (33)

Orthostatic hypotension: a sudden decrease in blood pressure that occurs when a person stands up from a sitting or lying position (22)

Orthostatic blood pressures: a series of blood pressure measurements, usually taken first with the person lying down, then sitting, and then standing (22)

OSHA: see *Occupational Safety and Health Administration*

OSHA Bloodborne Pathogens Standard: standards created by the Occupational Safety and Health Administration that all employers must follow to help protect employees from exposure to bloodborne pathogens (16)

Osteomyelitis: infection of the bone tissue that can result in death of the bone (32)

Osteoporosis: a disorder characterized by the excessive loss of bone tissue (32)

Ostomy appliance: a specially designed plastic pouch worn on the outside of the body, fitted around a stoma, that is used for the collection of feces or urine (26)

Otitis externa: an infection of the lining of the external auditory canal; commonly referred to as "swimmer's ear" (36)

Otitis media: an infection of the middle ear (36)

Otosclerosis: an inherited form of hearing loss (36)

Over-bed table: a table that fits over a bed or a chair and can be raised or lowered as needed (14)

Ovulation: the release of a ripe, mature egg from the female ovaries each month (40)

P

Pain: an unpleasant sensation that can range from mild discomfort to intense suffering (27)

Pain scale: a tool or guide that helps to translate a person's subjective rating of his or her pain into an objective measurement (27)

Pain threshold: the point at which a person becomes aware of pain (27)

Pain tolerance: the level of pain that a person can endure before taking action to seek relief (27)

Palliative care: care that focuses on relieving uncomfortable symptoms, not on curing the problem that is causing the symptoms (28)

Pallor: paleness of the skin (31)

Pancreas: an organ that produces substances that aid in digestion, as well as the hormones insulin and glucagon (38)

Panic disorder: a mental health disorder in which a person experiences episodes of sudden, overpowering fright (panic) and anxiety, usually accompanied by chest or abdominal pain, a rapid heart rate, shortness of breath, and/or dizziness (42)

Papule: a small, raised, firm, skin lesion that can be easily felt by passing your fingers lightly over the affected area (31)

Paraplegia: paralysis from the waist down (compare with *quadriplegia* and *hemiplegia*) (35)

Parkinson's disease: a progressive neurologic disorder that is characterized by tremor and weakness in the muscles and a shuffling gait (35)

Pathogen: a microbe that can cause illness (15)

Pathologic fracture: a break in a bone that has been weakened by disease (32)

Patient: a person who is receiving health care in a hospital, clinic, or extended-care facility (1)

Pediculosis capitis: head lice (24)

Pelvic inflammatory disease (PID): infection of the fallopian tubes and abdominal cavity that can lead to infertility (40)

Pelvic organ prolapse: a condition that occurs when a pelvic organ shifts downward from its normal position (40)

Pension: regular cash payments paid to a person, usually after retirement (2)

Percutaneous endoscopic gastrostomy (PEG) tube: a special type of gastrostomy tube that is inserted into the stomach with the aid of an endoscope (25)

Pericardium: a double-layered protective sac that surrounds the heart (34)

Perineal care (peri-care): cleaning the perineum and anus, as well as the vulva (in women) and the penis (in men) (23)

Perineum: the area from the bottom of the vagina to the anus (in women) or the area from the root of the penis to the anus (in men) (23)

Periodontitis: infection and inflammation of the soft tissue and bones that support the teeth; can lead to tooth loss (23)

Peripheral nervous system (PNS): the nerves outside of the brain and spinal cord; receives information from the environment, and carries commands from the brain and spinal cord to the other organs of the body, such as the muscles (compare with *central nervous system*) (35)

Peripheral vascular disease: a disorder characterized by pain and cramping in the legs, caused by atherosclerosis of the arteries that supply the legs (34)

Peristalsis: involuntary wave-like muscular movements, such as those that occur in the digestive system to move chyme (partially digested food) through the intestines (26)

Perseveration: the inappropriate and constant repetition of a phrase or act; often seen in people with dementia (9)

Persistent vegetative state: a state of altered consciousness in which the person appears to be awake, but cannot respond in a deliberate or meaningful way to the environment (35)

Personal protective equipment (PPE): barriers that are worn to physically prevent microbes from reaching a health care provider's skin or mucous membranes such as gloves, gowns, masks, and protective eyewear (15)

Pessary: a device that is inserted into the vagina to support a prolapsed organ in the proper position (40)

Petit mal (absence) seizure: a seizure characterized by a sudden, brief break in consciousness or activity (compare with *grand mal seizure*) (19)

Phantom pain: the feeling that a body part is still present, after it has been surgically removed (amputated) (32)

Pharyngitis: inflammation of the throat (pharynx) (33)

Pharynx: throat region (33)

Phlebitis: inflammation of a vein (34)

Phobia: an excessive, abnormal fear of an object or situation (42)

Physical abuse: the use of force to cause pain or injury to the abused person's body, such as that caused by striking, biting, slapping, shaking, or failing to meet a dependent person's physical needs (for example, for food, water, and cleanliness) (4)

Physical restraint: a device that is attached to or near a person's body to limit a person's freedom of movement or access to his or her body (compare with *chemical restraint*) (18)

Physical therapy: a health care specialty that focuses on helping the person regain or maintain strength, endurance, coordination, balance, posture, and flexibility (10)

Physiology: the study of how the body parts work (30)

Pioneer Models for Culture Change: models for improving the delivery of long-term care, developed by the Pioneer Network, that emphasize providing individualized care to the maximum extent possible in a home-like environment (2)

Pioneer Network: a small group of professionals working in long-term care that began meeting in 1997 to share ideas and create a new vision for the future of long-term care (2)

Plan of correction: a report prepared by the facility following a survey that outlines specific actions the facility will take to address any deficiency citations and achieve compliance; also includes a description of how the facility will identify other residents at risk, and the actions the facility will take to prevent similar problems from happening in the future (6)

Plaque: a fatty deposit that builds up on the inside of the artery wall, blocking blood flow to the tissues and making the artery wall brittle and prone to breaking (34)

Plasma: the liquid part of the blood (34)

Platelets (thrombocytes): pinched-off pieces of larger cells that are found in the red bone marrow and are responsible for clotting of the blood (34)

Pleura: the membrane that lines the chest cavity and covers the outside of the lungs (33)

Pleurisy: inflammation of the pleura, the membrane that lines the chest cavity and covers the lungs (33)

Pneumonia: inflammation of the lung tissue, caused by infection with a virus or a bacterium, and resulting in impaired gas exchange (33)

Pneumothorax: the build-up of air in the space between the lungs and the chest wall (33)

Podiatrist: a doctor who specializes in the care of the feet (24)

Polyuria: excessive urine output; see also *diuresis* (26)

Poorhouses: community-supported facilities that provided shelter for those without the means of supporting themselves from the mid-1800s until the 1930s in the United States, also known as *almshouses* or *poor farms* (2)

Post-acute care setting: a place where health care is provided for people who have recovered enough from an acute illness to be out of immediate danger, but are still in need of some type of professional health care (compare with *advanced [acute] care setting* and *long-term care setting*) (1)

Postmenopausal bleeding: uterine bleeding after menopause (40)

Postmortem care: the care of a person's body after the person's death (29)

Post-procedure actions: steps that are routinely performed at the end of each resident care procedure, called "Finishing Up" actions in this book (compare with *pre-procedure actions*) (17)

Pre-certification (pre-approval) process: a system for controlling health care costs, in which the health care provider must prove that a person's medical condition meets certain criteria and obtain the insurance company's go-ahead for the proposed treatment before starting treatment (1)

Preferred provider organization (PPO): a managed care system that contracts with an insurance company to accept a standard payment as total payment for services rendered; in return for seeking care only from health care providers who are part of the PPO network, the insured person usually receives that care at a reduced cost to herself (1)

Pre-procedure actions: steps that are routinely performed before each resident care procedure; called "Getting Ready" actions in this book (compare with *post-procedure actions*) (17)

Presbycusis: age-related hearing loss (36)

Presbyopia: age-related loss of the eye's ability to focus on objects that are close (36)

Pressure points: bony areas where pressure ulcers are most likely to form; include the heels, ankles, knees, hips, toes, elbows, shoulder blades, ears, the back of the head, and along the spine (31)

Pressure-relieving mattress: a mattress that is placed on top of the regular mattress to help prevent skin breakdown in a resident who must stay in bed for long periods of time (21)

Pressure ulcer: a difficult-to-heal (and possibly even fatal) sore that forms when part of the body presses against a surface (such as a mattress or chair) for a long period of time; also known as *pressure sores* and *decubitus ulcers* (20)

Private pay: adjective used to describe an expense that is paid "out-of-pocket," using one's own money (2)

PRN (as-needed) care: personal hygiene care that is provided whenever a resident needs it, throughout the day or night (23)

Problem statement: a statement in the interdisciplinary care plan of exactly what problem (or potential problem) is being addressed (12)

Procedure: a series of steps followed in a particular order when providing care to a resident that helps to ensure that the care provided is safe and correct (17)

Professional: a person who has credentials, obtained through education and training, that enable him or her to become licensed or certified to practice a certain profession; also, a person who demonstrates a professional attitude (3)

Professionalism: the attitude of being a professional, characterized by a positive outlook and a commitment to doing one's best at all times (3)

Prognosis: a doctor's prediction of the course of a person's disease, and his or her estimation of the person's chances for recovery (43)

Prone position: one of the basic positions in which the person lies on his abdomen with his head turned to one side (20)

Prospective payment system (PPS): the method by which Medicare pays health care facilities for services provided; payment is a set fee based on anticipated or expected care (1)

Psychiatrist: a doctor who specializes in the diagnosis and treatment of mental illness (42)

Psychological (emotional) abuse: the use of words or actions to cause emotional pain or injury, such as that caused by threatening a person with physical harm or abandonment, teasing a person in a cruel way, or preventing a person from interacting with others (4)

Psychologist: a health care professional who is trained to provide counseling services for people with mental illness (42)

Puberty: the period during which the secondary sex characteristics appear and the reproductive organs begin to function (7)

Pulmonary circulation: the pattern of circulation that takes blood from the heart to the lungs to pick up oxygen and release carbon dioxide (compare with *systemic circulation*) (34)

Pulmonary embolism: a life-threatening condition that occurs when an embolus becomes stuck in the pulmonary artery, the artery that carries unoxygenated blood from the heart to the lungs (34)

Pulse: the wave of blood sent through the arteries each time the heart beats (22)

Pulse amplitude: the force or quality of the pulse (22)

Pulse deficit: the difference between the apical pulse rate (the pulse that is measured by listening over the apex of the heart with a stethoscope) and the radial pulse rate (the pulse that is measured by placing the middle two or three fingers over the radial artery, located on the inside of the wrist) (22)

Pulse points: the points where the large arteries run close enough to the surface of the skin to be felt as a pulse (19)

Pulse pressure: the difference between the systolic and diastolic pressures (22)

Pulse rate: the number of pulsations that can be felt over an artery in 1 minute; an indication of the heart rate (one of the vital signs) (22)

Pulse rhythm: the pattern of the pulsations and the pauses between them (22)

Pustule: a small, blister-like skin lesion that contains pus, a thick, yellowish fluid that is a sign of infection (31)

Pyelonephritis: a kidney infection (39)

Pyloric sphincter: a circle of muscular tissue that surrounds the place where the stomach empties into the small intestine and helps to prevent food from returning to the stomach once it enters the small intestine (38)

Q

Quadriplegia: paralysis from the neck down (compare with *paraplegia* and *hemiplegia*) (35)

Quality: the excellence, worth, or value of something, as perceived by the customer (13)

Quality Indicator Profile report: a report that identifies markers of quality in specific care areas; compares the facility's performance in these areas to that of other facilities in the state; and provides information about the care concerns of specific residents, based on assessment data pulled from the Minimum Data Set (MDS) (6)

Quality Measures: indicators of quality that are based on the outcomes of the care and services provided by the facility (13)

Quality of life: a way of expressing the amount of satisfaction and comfort we are getting from the way we are living (7)

R

Race: a general characterization that describes skin color, body stature, facial features, and hair texture (7)

RACE fire response plan: the general actions that are taken in the event of a fire emergency (remove to safety, activate the alarm, contain the fire, extinguish or evacuate) (17)

Radiation therapy: a type of therapy that uses energy transmitted by waves to destroy cancer cells (43)

Radiating pain: pain that travels from one area to another (27)

Range of motion: the complete extent of movement that a joint is normally capable of without causing pain (32)

Rash: a group of skin lesions (31)

Reciprocity: the principle by which one state recognizes the validity of a license or certification granted by another state (3)

Recording: communicating information about a resident to other health care team members in written form; sometimes called *charting* (5)

Rectocele: a condition that occurs when the front wall of the rectum shifts downward, pushing into the back (posterior) vaginal wall (40)

Reduction: the word used to describe the process of bringing the ends of a broken bone into alignment (32)

Reference list: a list of three or four people who would be willing to talk to a potential employer about a job candidate's abilities (45)

Referred (radiating) pain: pain that is felt somewhere other than where it originated (36)

Registered nurse (RN): a specially trained person who is licensed by a state to develop care plans and coordinate all aspects of patient or resident care, as well as to provide that care; holds a baccalaureate degree from a liberal arts college or university (4 years) or an associate degree from a junior or community college (2 years) (3)

Registry: an official record maintained by the state of the people who have successfully completed the nursing assistant training program (3)

Rehabilitation: the process of helping a person with a disability to return to his highest level of physical, mental, or emotional function (10)

Reincarnation: the idea that a person's spirit or soul will live again on Earth in the form of an animal or human being yet to be born (29)

Religion: a person's spiritual beliefs (7)

Reminiscence therapy: a technique used for interacting with people who have dementia, in which the person with dementia is encouraged to remember and share experiences from his or her past with others (9)

Renal: related to, involving, or located in the region of the kidneys (39)

Reporting: the spoken exchange of information between health care team members (5)

Reproduction: the process by which a living thing makes more living things like itself (40)

Rescue breathing: a basic life support (BLS) technique in which the rescuer blows air into the person's mouth to perform the function of breathing for the person until the person begins breathing again on her own (19)

Resident: a person who is receiving care in a long-term care facility, such as a nursing home or an assisted-living facility (1)

Resident Assessment Instrument (RAI): an assessment tool that all nursing homes in the United States are required by the Omnibus Budget Reconciliation Act (OBRA) to use; consists of two parts, the Minimum Data Set (MDS) and the Resident Assessment Protocols (RAPs) (12)

Resident Assessment Protocols (RAPs): a series of questions to answer or points to consider for each problem identified on the Minimum Data Set (MDS) that is used to gain additional insight into the cause of the problem; the second part of the Resident Assessment Instrument (RAI) (12)

Resident inventory sheet: a document that lists and briefly describes all of the resident's personal belongings; completed when a resident is admitted to a long-term care facility (11)

Resource utilization groups (RUGs): a system for controlling health care costs in which payment for services provided is based on the estimated amount of resources that a person is expected to use; used as a basis for Medicare payments in long-term care settings (compare with *diagnosis-related groups [DRGs]*) (1)

Respiration: the process the body uses to obtain oxygen from the environment and remove carbon dioxide (a waste gas) from the body (33)

Respiratory arrest: the condition where breathing has stopped (19)

Respiratory rate: the number of times a person breathes in 1 minute (one breath is both an inhalation and an exhalation); one of the vital signs (22)

Respiratory rhythm: the regularity with which a person breathes (22)

Respiratory therapy: any treatment that is used to help a person achieve satisfactory respiration (33)

Restraint alternatives: measures taken to avoid the use of chemical or physical restraints (18)

Résumé: a brief document that gives a possible employer general information about a job candidate's education and work experience (45)

Restorative care: care provided by the health care team to help a resident reach or maintain his highest level of function (10)

Reverse Trendelenburg's position: one of the basic positions in which the head of the mattress is raised so the person's head is higher than her feet (compare with *Trendelenburg's position*) (14)

Rigor mortis: the stiffening of the muscles that usually develops within 2 to 4 hours of death (29)

Rounds: the process of checking on each assigned resident every 2 hours throughout all shifts to provide for any needs the person may have (23)

Rugae: folds in the lining of the stomach (38)

S

Salivary glands: glands located near the mouth that produce and secrete saliva, a substance that helps with chewing and swallowing by moistening the food (38)

Sanitarian: a person who evaluates the safety and cleanliness of a building (6)

Sanitization: practices associated with basic cleanliness, such as handwashing, cleansing of eating utensils and other surfaces with soap and water, and providing clean linens and clothing; one of the techniques of medical asepsis (compare with *antisepsis, disinfection,* and *sterilization*) (15)

Schizophrenia: a mental health disorder that affects how a person thinks, feels and acts; the person has difficulty determining what is real from what is imaginary (42)

Scope of practice: the range of tasks that a nursing assistant is legally permitted to do (3)

Seborrheic dermatitis (cradle cap): severe scaling of the scalp with thick, yellow, crusty patches (24)

Sebum: an oily substance secreted by glands in the skin that lubricates the skin and helps to prevent it from drying out (31)

Semi-Fowler's (low Fowler's) position: one of the basic positions in which the head of the bed is elevated approximately 30 to 45 degrees (20)

Sense organs: a general term used to describe the eyes, the ears, the nose, and the taste buds (36)

Sensorineural hearing loss: hearing loss that occurs when the receptors in the ear are unable to receive stimuli or transmit nerve impulses (see also *conductive hearing loss*) (36)

Sensory nerves: nerves that carry information from the internal organs and the outside world to the spinal cord and up into the brain so that the brain can analyze the information (35)

Sensory receptors: specialized cells or groups of cells associated with a sensory nerve (36)

Sentinel events: problems that should rarely, if ever, be seen in a resident of a nursing home (6)

Septic shock: shock caused by a severe bacterial infection that involves the entire body (19)

Sex: the physical activity one engages in to obtain sexual pleasure and reproduce (7)

Sex cell (gamete): special cells contributed by each parent that contain half of the normal number of chromosomes (40)

Sexual abuse: subjecting a person to unwanted attention of a sexual nature, forcing a person to engage in unwanted sexual activity, or sexually exploiting a person (for example, by taking nude photographs of the person) (4)

Sexuality: how a person perceives his or her maleness or femaleness (7)

Sexually transmitted infection (STI): an infection that is most commonly transmitted by sexual contact; also known as a *sexually transmitted disease (STD)* or *venereal disease* (40)

Shingles (herpes zoster): a disorder, caused by the same virus that causes chickenpox, that is most frequently seen in people older than 65 years and is characterized by a blistering, painful rash that typically follows the pathway of a nerve (31)

Social Security Act: an act, signed into law by President Franklin D. Roosevelt in 1935, that established a program designed to provide regular cash payments for retired people age 65 years and older (2)

Shearing: a term used to describe the force created when something or someone is pulled across a surface that offers resistance; can lead to skin breakdown (20)

Shelter in place: the ability of a facility to be self-sufficient for several days during a disaster, in the event that help from emergency or support services is delayed (17)

Shift supervisor: a licensed nurse who is in charge of a particular floor or section of the facility for the duration of the shift (3)

Shock: the condition that results when the organs and tissues of the body do not receive enough oxygen-rich blood; see also *cardiogenic shock*, *hemorrhagic shock*, *anaphylactic shock*, and *septic shock* (19)

Shroud: a covering used to wrap the body of a person who has died (29)

Signs: objective observations (that is, observations based on information that is obtained directly, through measurements or by using one of the five senses) (compare with *symptoms*) (5)

Sims' position: one of the basic positions in which the person lies on his side with his head turned to one side and his knee sharply bent and supported by a pillow; the corresponding arm is bent at the elbow with the hand in front of the face, palm down, resting on a pillow; the lower leg is straight and the lower arm extends out from the side with the hand down near the hips and the palm turned upward (20)

Skeleton: the framework for the body formed by the bones (32)

Skin tear: an injury that occurs when the top layer of the skin is separated from the bottom layers (18)

Slander: spoken statements that injure someone's reputation; a form of defamation (4)

Sleep apnea: a disorder that causes the person to stop breathing for varying periods of time during sleep (27)

Soiled utility room: a holding place for dirty items, such as linens that need to be laundered, trash that needs to be disposed of, and used equipment that needs to be cleaned and disinfected (14)

Speech–language pathology: a health care specialty that focuses on helping the person regain or maintain the ability to communicate with others, chew, and swallow (10)

Sperm cell: male sex cell (40)

Sphygmomanometer: a device used to measure blood pressure (22)

Spina bifida: a congenital defect of the spinal column that occurs when the vertebrae do not close properly during development, leaving the spinal cord exposed (41)

Sputum: mucus and other respiratory secretions that are coughed up from the lungs, bronchi, and trachea; also known as *phlegm* (33)

Standard precautions: precautions that a health care worker takes with each resident to prevent contact with bloodborne pathogens; include the use of barrier methods (such as gloves) as well as certain environmental control methods (15)

Sterilization: the process of completely eliminating microbes from the surface of an object using an autoclave or chemicals; one of the techniques of medical asepsis (compare with *antisepsis*, *disinfection*, and *sanitation*) (15)

Stethoscope: a device that amplifies sound and transfers it to the listener's ears (22)

STI: see *sexually transmitted infection*

Stoma: an opening that is surgically made on the abdominal wall, often used for drainage of feces or urine from the body (26)

Stomach: a hollow, muscular pouch for holding food (38)

Stomatitis: inflammation of the mouth, often seen in people who are receiving chemotherapy (43)

Stool: a term used to refer to fecal material after it has left the body (26)

Stool softener: a medication that helps to prevent constipation by keeping fluid in the feces (26)

Straight catheter: a urinary catheter that is inserted and then removed immediately, after the urine in the bladder has drained out (26)

Stress: a physical or emotional factor that changes the body's normal balance or equilibrium (42)

Stroke: a disorder that occurs when blood flow to a part of the brain is completely blocked, causing the tissue to die; also known as a cerebrovascular accident (CVA) (35)

Stump: the end of an amputated limb that is left after surgery (32)

Sub-acute care setting: a place where health care is provided for people who require a high level of skilled care and monitoring that is less than what is provided in a hospital, but more than is provided in other health care settings; length of stay in the facility is usually 30 days or less; a type of post-acute care setting (1)

Subcutaneous tissue: the layer of fat that supports the dermis (the deepest layer of the skin) (31)

Subjective data: information that cannot be objectively measured or assessed (5)

Substance abuse disorders: disorders that involve the excessive or inappropriate use of drugs (legal or illegal), alcohol, or inhalants (42)

Suctioning: the process of removing fluid and mucus from a person's airway (33)

Suicide: the act of taking one's own life intentionally and voluntarily (42)

Sundowning: the worsening of behavioral symptoms in the late afternoon and evening (as the sun goes down) in a person with dementia (9)

Supine (dorsal recumbent) position: one of the basic positions in which the person lies on his back, with the bed flat and the head supported by a pillow (20)

Supportive care: treatments that will not prolong life, but will make a person more comfortable, such as oxygen therapy, nutritional supplementation, pain medication, range-of-motion exercises, grooming and hygiene, and positioning assistance (28)

Supportive devices: *1)* devices used when positioning a person to help the person maintain proper body alignment, such as pillows or rolled sheets, towels, or blankets (20); *2)* devices that help to stabilize a weak joint or limb; used in physical therapy to help a person with a disability regain function (10)

Suprapubic catheter: a urinary catheter that is inserted into the bladder through a surgical incision made in the abdominal wall, right above the pubic bone (26)

Surgical bed: a closed bed that has been opened to receive a person who will be arriving by stretcher; the top sheet, blanket, and bedspread are folded toward the side of the bed, leaving one side open and ready to receive the person (21)

Survey: an inspection of a nursing home carried out by the government to ensure that care is being provided according to standards and regulations (6)

Surveyor: an individual member of the survey team (6)

Survey team: the group of government officials who perform the survey (6)

Symptoms: subjective observations (that is, observations that are based on information that cannot be measured or observed firsthand, such as a resident's complaint of pain) (compare with *signs*) (5)

Synapse: the gap between the axon of one neuron and the dendrites of the next (35)

Syncope: fainting (19)

Systemic circulation: the pattern of circulation that takes blood from the lungs to the rest of the body to release oxygen and pick up carbon dioxide (compare with *pulmonary circulation*) (34)

Systole: the active phase of the cardiac cycle, during which the myocardium contracts, sending blood out of the heart (compare with *diastole*) (34)

Systolic pressure: the pressure that the blood exerts against the arterial walls when the heart muscle contracts; the first blood pressure measurement that is recorded (compare with *diastolic pressure*) (22)

T

Tachycardia: a heart rate that is faster than normal (more than 100 beats/min in an adult) (22)

Tachypnea: a respiratory rate that is higher than normal (more than 24 breaths/min in an adult) (22)

Tactile receptors: receptors found in the skin that are stimulated when something comes in contact with the surface of the body and presses on them, causing them to change shape (36)

Task lighting: bright light directed toward a specific area, used for activities that require good lighting to prevent eyestrain (compare with *general lighting*) (14)

Tasks: growth and development milestones that must be completed before a person can move on to the next stage of growth and development (7)

TB: see *tuberculosis*

T cells: special white blood cells (leukocytes) that play a role in the immune response to invading pathogens; the main target of the human immunodeficiency virus (HIV) (16)

Tendons: bands of connective tissue that attach the skeletal muscles to the bones (32)

Terminal illness: an illness or condition that has no cure and that will ultimately result in the person's death (28)

Tetany: a condition that occurs when the body's calcium level drops too low; characterized by cramping of the skeletal muscles and an irregular heart beat (37)

The Joint Commission: an independent, non-profit organization that sets national standards for all types of health care organizations and officially recognizes (accredits) organizations that meet these standards (1)

Thrombi (singular, *thrombus*): blood clots that form in the blood vessels (34)

Thrombophlebitis: inflammation of a vein caused by the presence of a blood clot (thrombus) (34)

Tinea capitis: a fungal infection of the scalp (24)

Tinea pedis: a fungal infection of the skin and nails, commonly known as "athlete's foot" (24)

Tinnitus: ringing in the ear (36)

Tissue: a group of cells similar in structure and specialized to perform a specific function (30)

Toe pleat: loosening of the top linens over a person's feet to relieve pressure and promote comfort (21)

Tort: a violation of civil law (4)

Total parenteral nutrition (TPN, hyperalimentation): an alternate method of providing fluid and nutrition; nourishment is delivered directly into the bloodstream through a large catheter (tube) inserted into a large vein near the heart (25)

Trachea: the passage that carries air from the larynx down into the chest toward the lungs; commonly known as the "windpipe" (33)

Tracheostomy: a surgically created opening in the neck that opens into the trachea; often used with a tracheostomy tube (instead of an endotracheal tube) when a person must be on a mechanical ventilator for more than a week or so (33)

Traction: a treatment for fracture in which the ends of the broken bone are placed in the proper alignment and then weight is applied to exert a constant pull and keep the bone in alignment (32)

Transfer: *1)* to move a person from one place to another, for example, from the bed to a wheelchair (20); *2)* to move a person within or between health care settings (11)

Transfer belt (gait belt): a webbed or woven belt with a buckle that is used to assist a weak or unsteady person with standing, walking, or transferring; called a *gait belt* when used to help a person walk (20)

Transient flora: microbes that are picked up by touching contaminated objects or people who have an infectious disease (compare with *normal [resident] flora*) (15)

Transient ischemic attack (TIA): a temporary (transient) episode of dysfunction caused by decreased blood flow to the brain (35)

Transmission-based precautions: precautions that a health care worker takes when a person is known to have a disease that is transmitted in a certain way; include airborne precautions, droplet precautions, and contact precautions (15)

Transsexual: a person who believes that he or she should be a member of the opposite sex (7)

Transvestite: a person who becomes sexually excited by dressing as a member of the opposite sex (7)

Trapeze bar: a device used to assist with movement that is attached to a frame over the person's bed (10)

Trendelenburg's position: one of the basic positions in which the foot of the mattress is raised so that the person's head is lower than her feet (compare with *reverse Trendelenburg's position*) (14)

Tuberculosis (TB): an airborne infection caused by a bacterium that usually infects the lungs (16)

Tumor: an abnormal growth of tissue; the cells that form the tumor may be benign or malignant (43)

Type 1 diabetes mellitus: a type of diabetes caused by destruction of the insulin-producing cells of the pancreas (37)

Type 2 diabetes mellitus: a type of diabetes caused by the inability of the cells of the body to respond to insulin; the pancreas still produces some insulin (37)

U

Ulcer: a shallow crater on the surface of the skin that is formed when the tissue dies and is shed (31)

Unintentional tort: a violation of civil law that occurs when someone causes harm or injury to another person or that person's property without the intent to cause harm (4)

Unintentional wound: an unexpected injury that usually results from some type of trauma (compare with *intentional wound*) (31)

United States Department of Health and Human Services (DHHS): the primary government agency responsible for protecting this nation's health; includes organizations such as the Food and Drug Administration (FDA), the Centers for Disease Control and Prevention (CDC), the National Institutes of Health (NIH), and the Centers for Medicare and Medicaid Services (CMS) (1)

Unit: a resident's living space (14)

Unit manager: a licensed nurse (usually a registered nurse [RN]) who has 24-hour-a-day responsibility for the operation of a particular floor or section of a facility; may also be called a *nurse* manager or *head nurse* (3)

Unresponsive: an adjective used to describe a person who is unconscious and cannot be aroused, or conscious but not responsive when spoken to or touched (19)

Urethritis: infection of the urethra, the passageway that carries urine from the bladder to the outside of the body (39)

Urgency: a need to urinate immediately (26)

Urinal: a device used for urination when a man is unable to get out of bed (26)

Urinalysis: examination of the urine under a microscope and by chemical means (26)

Urinary incontinence: the inability to hold one's urine, or the involuntary loss of urine from the bladder (26)

Urinary retention: the inability of the bladder to empty either completely during urination, or at all (26)

Urination: the process of passing urine from the body; also known as *micturition* and *voiding* (26)

Urine: formed by the kidneys; consists of waste products that have been filtered from the bloodstream, along with excess fluid (39)

Uterine prolapse (prolapsed uterus): a condition that occurs when the uterus shifts downward, into the vaginal canal (40)

V

Vaginitis: inflammation of the vaginal tissues (40)

Validation therapy: a technique used for interacting with people who have dementia, in which the caregiver acknowledges the person's reality, even if it is not correct (9)

Value: a cherished belief or principle (4)

Vancomycin-resistant enterococcus (VRE): a type of bacteria that has become resistant to vancomycin, a powerful antibiotic (15)

Varicose veins: a condition that results from pooling of blood in the veins just underneath the skin, causing them to become swollen and "knotty" in appearance (34)

Vascular dementia: a disorder characterized by the loss of function in areas of the brain due to tissue death caused by a lack of adequate oxygen and nutrients (9)

Vector: a living creature, such as an insect, that can transmit disease (15)

Veins: vessels that return blood to the heart (34)

Venous (stasis) ulcers: open sores that occur on the lower legs, usually in the ankle area, as a result of pooling of blood in the veins (34)

Venous thrombosis: the formation of blood clots (thrombi) in the veins as a result of pooling of the blood (34)

Ventilation system: a system that provides fresh air and keeps air circulating throughout a building (14)

Ventricles: the lower chambers of the heart (34)

Venules: the smallest veins (34)

Verbal communication: a way of communicating that uses written or spoken language (5)

Vertigo: dizziness (36)

Vesicle: a small, blister-like skin lesion that contains fluid (31)

Villi (singular, *villus*): tiny, finger-like structures on the lining of the small intestine that increase the small intestine's ability to absorb nutrients (38)

Virulence: the strength or disease-producing potential of a pathogen (15)

Vital signs: certain key measurements that provide essential information about a person's health (22)

Voiding: the process of passing urine from the body; also known as *urination* and *micturition* (26)

W

Water-soluble: adjective used to describe a substance that dissolves in water (for example, certain vitamins) (25)

Weight bearing: a term used to refer to a person's ability to stand on one or both legs (20)

Will: a legal statement that expresses a person's wishes for the management of his or her affairs after death (28)

Withdrawal: an emotional and physical reaction that occurs when use of an addictive substance is discontinued (42)

Work ethic: a person's attitude toward his or her work (3)

Wound: an injury that results in a break in the skin (and often the underlying tissues as well) (31)

Index

Note: A t following a page number indicates tabular material, an f indicates a figure, a p indicates procedure material, and a b indicates a boxed feature.

Quality health care, ensuring, 9–10, 10f, 11f
Quality Improvement (QI) Nurse, 41–42
Quality Indicator Profile report, 89, 90f, 91f
Quality Indicator Survey (QIS), 96. *See also* Surveys
Quality Measures, 197
Quality of life, 114–116
    activities in, 115–116, 115f, 116b
    definition of, 114
    OBRA on, 114
    personal choice in, 115
Quick-release knot, 299, 299f

R
Race, 113, 113f
RACE fire response plan, 272–273, 273f
Radial pulse, 387f, 388, 389, 406p
Radiating pain, 547, 717, 717f
Radiation therapy, for cancer, 817–818
Radiography, chest, 694
Range of motion, 625–626
    active, 159
    passive, 158–159
Range-of-motion exercises, 643–646
    guidelines for, 644b
    for multiple sclerosis, 709
    procedure for, 643, 646p–651p
    scope of practice and, 646
    types of, 643
Rapid eye movement (REM) sleep, 553, 553f
RAPs, *See* Resident Assessment Protocols
Rash, 617, 617f
Rationalization, 802
Receiver, 66, 67f, 68
Receptive aphasia, 139, 140, 707
Receptors
    sensory, 716
    tactile, 716, 717f
Reciprocity, 34
Recognizing people, difficulty with, 140
Recording, 76–82
    definition of, 76
    guidelines for, 80–82, 81b
    Kardex in, 82, 82f
    medical record (chart) in, 76–82
        computerized, 80–82, 80f
        flow sheet in, 79–80, 79f
        forms and documents in, 77, 78t
        organization of, 77, 77f
        progress notes in, 77–79, 77f, 78t
        time in, 80, 80f
Recreational drug use. *See also specific drugs*
    by nursing assistant, 40, 40f
    by resident, 803, 803f, 808–809
Rectal suppositories, 526
Rectal temperature, 386, 402p–403p
Rectocele, 777, 777f
Rectum, 752, 752f
Red blood cells, 678–679, 679f
    impaired production of, 687
    increased destruction of, 687
Reduction, fracture, 638
Reference list, 837–838
Referred pain, 717, 717f
Reflex incontinence, 519
Regenerative community, 21
Regions, abdominal, 853, 853f

Registered Nurse Assessment Coordinator (RNAC), 42–43, 42f, 182
Registered nurses (RNs), 41, 42t
Registry, 34
Regression, 802
Regular diet, 485b
Rehabilitation, 152–158, 155t
    cardiac, 694–695
    criteria for, 153–154
    definition of, 153, 154
    with developmental disabilities, 796
    devices in, 155, 157f
    disability in, 152
    discharge assistance in, 176f, 177
    humanistic health care in, 161
    nursing assistant's role in, 160–163, 161f, 162b
    OBRA on, 153, 154b
    occupational therapy in, 156, 158f
    for pain, 155t, 156
    physical therapy in, 154–157, 156f, 157f
    rehabilitation services in, 154–158, 155t (*See also* Rehabilitation services)
    speech–language pathology in, 156–158, 158f
    stroke, 707, 708f
    in sub-acute care setting, 8, 8f
    types of, 155t
Reincarnation, 580
Relaxation, for pain relief, 551
Reliability, 36
Religion
    culture and, 114, 114f
    on diet, 479–481
Reminiscence therapy, 148, 148f
Renal, 760
Renal calculi, 765–766, 765f
Renal failure, 766, 767f, 768b
Renal pelvis, 761
Repetition, 142
Rephrasing, 70
Report
    incident (occurrence), 294, 295f
    Quality Indicator Profile, 89, 90f, 91f
Reporting
    of accidents/incidents, 293–294, 295f
    general, 76, 76f
Repositioning, 334–337
    frequency of, 334
    friction in, 335
    guidelines for, 336b–337b
    lifting and turning in, 334–335
    logrolling in, 334–336, 348p–349p
    moving to side of bed in
        one assistant, 334, 343p
        two assistants, 334, 344p
    moving up in bed in
        one assistant, 334, 334f, 345p
        two assistants, 334, 334f, 346p
    for pressure ulcer prevention, 609–610, 609f
    raising head and shoulders in, 334, 347p
    shearing in, 334
    turning onto side in, 334, 347p–348p
Repression, 802
Reproduction, 772
Reproductive system, 595f, 596
Reproductive system disorders, female, 776–779
    cancer, 778–779, 778f
    cysts and non-cancerous growths, 776